AF615541

## Accessing the E-book edition

# ACUTE CARE SURGERY AND TRAUMA: EVIDENCE-BASED PRACTICE, SECOND EDITION

**Using the VitalSource® ebook**

Access to the VitalBook™ ebook accompanying this book is via VitalSource® Bookshelf – an ebook reader which allows you to make and share notes and highlights on your ebooks and search across all of the ebooks that you hold on your VitalSource Bookshelf. You can access the ebook online or offline on your smartphone, tablet or PC/Mac and your notes and highlights will automatically stay in sync no matter where you make them.

1. **Create a VitalSource Bookshelf account at** ***https://online.vitalsource.com/user/new*** or log into your existing account if you already have one.

2. **Redeem the code provided in the panel below to get online access to the ebook.** Log in to Bookshelf and select **Redeem** at the top right of the screen. Enter the redemption code shown on the scratch-off panel below in the **Redeem Code** pop-up and press **Redeem**. Once the code has been redeemed your ebook will download and appear in your library.

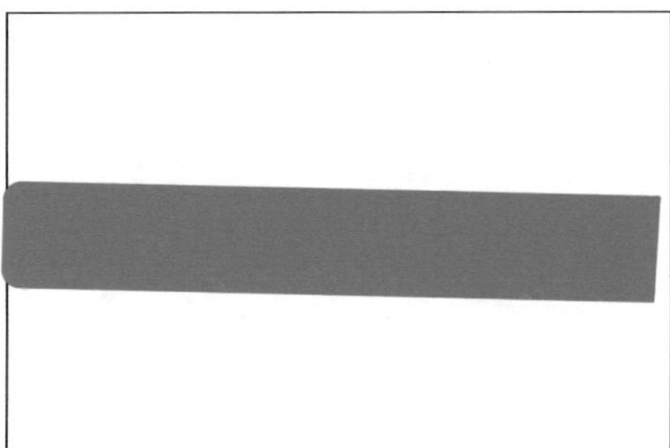

No returns if this code has been revealed.

**DOWNLOAD AND READ OFFLINE**

To use your ebook offline, download BookShelf to your PC, Mac, iOS device, Android device or Kindle Fire, and log in to your Bookshelf account to access your ebook:

***On your PC/Mac***

Go to ***https://support.vitalsource.com/hc/en-us*** and follow the instructions to download the free **VitalSource Bookshelf** app to your PC or Mac and log into your Bookshelf account.

***On your iPhone/iPod Touch/iPad***

Download the free **VitalSource Bookshelf** App available via the iTunes App Store and log into your Bookshelf account. You can find more information at ***https://support.vitalsource.com/hc/en-us/categories/200134217-Bookshelf-for-iOS***

***On your Android™ smartphone or tablet***

Download the free **VitalSource Bookshelf** App available via Google Play and log into your Bookshelf account. You can find more information at ***https://support.vitalsource.com/hc/en-us/categories/200139976-Bookshelf-for-Android-and-Kindle-Fire***

***On your Kindle Fire***

Download the free **VitalSource Bookshelf** App available from Amazon and log into your Bookshelf account. You can find more information at ***https://support.vitalsource.com/hc/en-us/categories/200139976-Bookshelf-for-Android-and-Kindle-Fire***

*N.B. The code in the scratch-off panel can only be used once. When you have created a Bookshelf account and redeemed the code you will be able to access the ebook online or offline on your smartphone, tablet or PC/Mac.*

**SUPPORT**

If you have any questions about downloading Bookshelf, creating your account, or accessing and using your ebook edition, please visit ***http://support.vitalsource.com/***

SECOND EDITION

# ACUTE CARE SURGERY AND TRAUMA

## EVIDENCE-BASED PRACTICE

SECOND EDITION

# ACUTE CARE SURGERY AND TRAUMA

## EVIDENCE-BASED PRACTICE

Edited by

**STEPHEN M. COHN, MD, FACS**
Professor of Surgery, University of Texas Health Science Center
San Antonio, TX, USA

**MATTHEW O. DOLICH, MD, FACS**
Professor of Surgery, University of California, Irvine Medical Center
Orange, CA, USA

**KENJI INABA, MD, FRCSC, FACS**
Professor of Surgery and Emergency Medicine, University of Southern California
Los Angeles, CA, USA

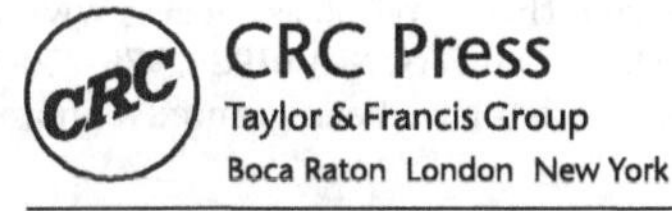

CRC Press
Taylor & Francis Group
Boca Raton London New York

CRC Press is an imprint of the
Taylor & Francis Group, an **informa** business

CRC Press
Taylor & Francis Group
6000 Broken Sound Parkway NW, Suite 300
Boca Raton, FL 33487-2742



Printed on acid-free paper
Version Date: 20151104

International Standard Book Number-13: 978-1-4822-9929-8 (Pack - Book and Ebook)



**Visit the Taylor & Francis Web site at**
**http://www.taylorandfrancis.com**

**and the CRC Press Web site at**
**http://www.crcpress.com**

# Contents

## Section III Surgical Critical Care

# *Foreword*

**Basil A. Pruitt, Jr.**

This new edition of one of the first textbooks promoting evidence-based surgical practice has been revised and expanded as testimony to the fact that evidence-based surgery (EBS) is a perpetual work-in-progress. The new material and organization of the contents of this second edition place an emphasis on trauma care, which was virtually ignored in the first edition, and feature surgical emergencies and surgical critical care in recognition of the curriculum of acute care surgery, which is emerging as a new career pathway for surgeons.

Evidence-based medicine (EBM), as defined by Sackett and colleagues, is "the conscientious, explicit, and judicious use of current best evidence in making decisions about the care of individual patients."[1] In the assessment of medical evidence, a systematic review (SR) of randomized controlled trials (RCTs) and RTCs per se are considered to provide the highest levels of medical evidence, i.e., 1a and 1b, respectively.[2] Randomized controlled trials are widely and relatively readily conducted in the evaluation of various drugs and medical treatments but are more difficult to apply in comparative evaluations of surgical procedures. The relative rarity of Class I citations in the tables presented with the various chapters in this book, particularly those related to operative procedures, attests to that difficulty.

Specific limitations affecting the usefulness and validity of a randomized controlled trial comparing surgical procedures include ethical concerns about sham operations and, conversely, the variable influence of the placebo effect in the absence of a sham operation. Other limitations include variations in the operating surgeons' technical skills and experience (minimized by specific training before starting the trial), evolution of surgical procedures across time, and differences in postoperative care among surgeons and among institutions. Difficulty in blinding both patients and surgeons is also of concern if effect on symptoms or quality of life is the outcome of interest. That potential for bias can be reduced by the use of independent investigators for outcome evaluation. Other limitations in the application of RCTs to address surgical questions include excessive limitation of eligibility criteria that can compromise external validity and generalizability of the results. Conversely, in less restricted nonrandom studies, the selection of treatment on the basis of surgical preference can bias the results. Finally, there are few if any readily accessible funding sources for surgical clinical studies or the evaluation of an operative innovation.[2–4]

In recognition of those limitations, it was reported in the late 1990s that although roughly comparable percentages of medical treatments and surgical practice were evidence based, i.e., 82% and 95%, respectively, 53% of medical treatments were based on Level I data but only 25% of surgical practice was supported by RCTs.[2] Despite the difficulties in applying RCTs to address surgical questions, more and more surgical studies have generated higher levels of evidence that have been utilized to develop treatment guidelines. In 2011, it was claimed that surgical practice had been revolutionized by the application of the results of randomized controlled trials (RCTs).[5] Changes in the treatment of breast cancer are cited as particular examples of the benefits of evidence-based surgery but more than half of the published surgical RCTs have compared medical therapies in surgical patients and less than half have compared surgical procedures per se.[2,5] The relative scarcity of PTCs for surgical procedures is considered by some to represent an imbalance, if not a waste of research effort, which should be addressed by the conduct of more RCTs comparing operations, the results of which can be used to define evidence-based surgery.[6,7]

Groups of research methodologists and clinicians have formed to advance the use of evidence-based surgery and promote the conduct of RCTs to compare operative interventions. Members of the Surgical Outcomes Research Centre (SOURCE) at McMaster University, representing "various subspecialties," have produced articles focused on clinically relevant surgical issues to transfer to the surgical community the skills needed "to critically appraise evidence."[8] Similar organizations, the BALLIOL Collaboration and its successor, the IDEAL Collaboration, have proposed a five-stage process by which innovative surgical procedures can be developed and evaluated, i.e., innovation (Stage 1), development (Stage 2a), exploration (Stage 2b), assessment (Stage 3), and long-term study (Stage 4).[9]

At each stage of the development of a surgical procedure, reports regarding that procedure become progressively more demanding and scientifically rigorous. At Stage 1, innovation, in which proof of concept is the goal, reports are commonly structured case reports. In Stage

2a, development, the studies of patients from whom ethical approval is required should be reported as consecutive cases in prospective development studies. At Stage 2b, exploration, studies should be prospective with data collected systematically and reported as prospective uncontrolled studies or if controlled as feasibility or exploratory RCTs. At Stage 3, assessment, in which the innovation is compared with the current standard to determine which is best, reporting takes the form of an RCT. At Stage 4, long-term studies, the procedure is monitored for rare outcomes and long-term effects with the results used to form a registry.[10,11] When assessing the strength of evidence in evaluating an innovative procedure or comparing two established procedures one should, as the authors of this text have done, grade the strength of the supporting evidence with regard to the location of the procedure of interest in the IDEAL framework for developing surgical procedures. The successful transit of an operative procedure or surgical innovation through the early stages of this process delivers a relatively mature product to the doorstep of an RTC. Such a preparation decreases the high risk of RTC failure of operative procedures without such staging.[12]

Fortunately, EBS is not captive to the RTC and evidence-based surgery can be predicated on well-designed prospective observational research. Observational studies may also have limitations that include systematic overestimation of treatment effect, confounding, and bias that can be reduced or eliminated by patient matching, cohort selection, use of sophisticated statistical techniques, and standardized data collection.[5] Those limitations should influence the grading and acceptance of evidence generated by observational studies.

The ultimate goal of EBS is the development of practical guidelines for decision support and patient education. To that end, the American College of Surgeons has produced "clinical guideline summaries" to formulate "evidence-based decisions in surgery," which offer recommendations for the diagnosis and treatment of, at present, 35 surgical conditions.[13] The grading of the evidence supporting the recommendations by the American College of Surgeon members considered to be "experts" is generic and ranges from "weak" to "strong" without the granularity of evidence level grading provided in this text by the authors, who have used the levels of evidence defined by the National Health Services Research and Development, Centre for Evidence-Based Medicine.[2]

The increased use of EBS in the development of clinical guidelines has led to many improvements in care, but flaws and misuse of the process have become apparent to such an extent that EBM has been questioned as "a movement in crisis."[14] Specific concerns include misattribution of clinical significance to statistically significant benefits; shift from patient-centered care to system-driven care by imposition of inflexible rules; difficulty in managing an excessive number of clinical guidelines; uncertain application of guidelines to patients, particularly the elderly, with multiple comorbid conditions; and abuse of the process by commercial and other special interests. The identification of those problems, which both authors and readers should have in mind when grading evidence, has prompted a call for "a return to real evidence-based medicine" in which care of individual patients based on studies focused on clinical usefulness and free of commercial interference and bias is enlightened by clinical expertise. The editors and authors of this book have provided rigorous grading of the papers supporting their recommendations for diagnosis and treatment, which have been tempered by invited comments of recognized clinical experts to realize the goal of scientifically based resource conserving patient-oriented EBS.

This second edition of *Acute Care Surgery and Trauma: Evidence-Based Practice* confirms the fact that EBS is not, to paraphrase Sackett, "cookbook surgery"[1] but is a perpetually evolving process. The differences between EBM and EBS suggest that clinical reality and the intrinsic characteristics of surgery that limit the application of RCTs support affixing the word "best" to the term "evidence-based surgery." The inclusion of EBM in the medical education process and EBS in surgical education has been justified by the increasing emphasis on EBM in clinical practice.[15] This book, which promotes that trend, should be in the library of every medical school, every department of surgery, and with all surgeons.

## References


1. Sackett DL, Rosenberg WMC, Gray JAM, Haynes RB, Richardson WS. Evidence based medicine: What it is and what it isn't. *BMJ* 1996; 312:71–72.
2. Wente MN, Seiler CM, UHL W, Büchler MV. Perspectives of evidence-based surgery. *Digestive Surgery* 2003; 20:263–269.
3. Johnson J, Rogers W, Lotz M, Townley C, Meyerson D, Tomassy G. Ethical challenges of innovative surgery: A response to the IDEAL recommendations. *The Lancet*, 2010; 376:1113–1115.
4. Cook JA. The challenges faced in the design, conduct and analysis of surgical randomised controlled trials. *Trials*, 2009;10:9.
5. Merkow RP, Ko CY. Evidence-based medicine in surgery. The importance of both experimental and observational study designs. *JAMA* 2011; 306(4):436–437.
6. Students 4 Best Evidence, Evidence-based surgery: What sets it apart? Available at http://www.students4bestevidence.net/evidence-based-surgery/. Accessed January 14, 2015.
7. Ioannidis J. Editorial. Clinical trials: What a waste. *BMJ* 2014; 349;g7089.

8. McMaster University, Surgical Outcomes Research Centre (SOURCE), EBS. Evidence based surgery. Available at http://www.fhs.mcmaster.ca/source/ebs.html. Accessed January 14, 2015.
9. McCulloch P, Altman DG, Campbell WB, Flum DR, Glasziou P, Marshall JC, Nicholl J, for the Balliol Collaboration. Surgical Innovation and Evaluation 3. No surgical innovation without evaluation: The IDEAL recommendations. *The Lancet* 2009;374:1105–1112.
10. The IDEAL Collaboration. Stages of innovation in surgery. Available at http://www.ideal-collaboration.net/the-collaboration/. Accessed January 22, 2015.
11. Köckerling F. The need for registries in the early scientific evaluation of surgical innovations. *Frontiers in Surgery* 2014;1:12.
12. McColloch PG. Editorial. Re: Clinical trials: What a waste. Available at http://www.bmj.com/content/349/bmj.g7089. Accessed March 3, 2015.
13. American College of Surgeons. *Evidence-Based Decisions in Surgery (Based on Practice Guidelines)*, Chicago, IL. Available at https://www.facs.org/education/resources/ebds-guidelines. Accessed February 17, 2015.
14. Greenhalgh T, Howick J, Maskrey N, for the Evidence Based Medicine Renaissance Group. Evidence based medicine: A movement in crisis? *BMJ* 2014;348:g3725.
15. Kwaan MR, Melton GB. Evidence-based medicine in surgical education. *Clinics in Colon and Rectal Surgery* 2012;25:151–155.

# Contributors

**Gregory A. Abrahamian**
The University of Texas Health Science Center at San Antonio
San Antonio, Texas

**Mitu Agarwal**

**Suresh K. Agarwal**
School of Medicine and Public Health
University of Wisconsin–Madison
Madison, Wisconsin

**Hasan B. Alam**
University of Michigan
Ann Arbor, Michigan

**Abdul Alarhayem**
The University of Texas Health Science Center at San Antonio
San Antonio, Texas

**Hirra Ali**
Albert Einstein College of Medicine
Bronx, New York

**Casey J. Allen**
University of Miami
Miami, Florida

**Antonio Aponte-Feliciano**
University of Massachusetts Medical School
Worcester, Massachusetts

**Jayson D. Aydelotte**
Dell Medical School
The University of Texas at Austin
Austin, Texas

**Hany Bahouth**
Rambam Health Care Campus
Haifa, Israel

**Chad G. Ball**
University of Calgary
Calgary, Alberta, Canada

**Jonathan Barasch**
Columbia University Medical Center
New York, New York

**Philip S. Barie**
Weill Cornell Medicine
and
NewYork-Presbyterian Hospital
Weill Cornell Medical Center
New York, New York

**Erik Barquist**
University of South Florida
Orlando, Florida

**Zachary M. Bauman**
University of Arizona Medical Center
Tucson, Arizona

**Rachel E. Beard**
Beth Israel Deaconess Medical Center
Boston, Massachusetts

**Heidi I. Becker**
South Texas Veterans Health Care System
San Antonio, Texas

**Stephen W. Behrman**
The University of Tennessee Health Science Center
Memphis, Tennessee

**Greg J. Beilman**
University of Minnesota
Minneapolis, Minnesota

**Peleg Ben-Galim**
Kaplan Medical Center
Rehovot, Israel

**Elizabeth Benjamin**
University of Southern California
Los Angeles, California

**David Bennett**
Columbia University Medical Center
New York, New York

**Eileen Bernal**
University of Texas Southwestern Medical Center
Dallas, Texas

**Shanel B. Bhagwandin**
Icahn School of Medicine at Mount Sinai
New York, New York

**John K. Bini**
Wright State University
The Uniformed Services University of the Health Sciences
Dayton, Ohio

**Lorne H. Blackbourne**
San Antonio Military Medical Center
San Antonio, Texas

**Juan J. Blondet**
University of Minnesota
Minneapolis, Minnesota

**Daniel J. Bonville**
Albany Medical College
Albany, New York

**Mina L. Boutrous**
The University of Texas Health Science Center at Houston
Houston, Texas

**Steven B. Brandes**
Department of Urology
Columbia University
New York, New York

**Susan Brien**
Royal College of Physicians and Surgeons of Canada
Ottawa, Ontario, Canada

**Steven Brower**
Icahn School of Medicine at Mount Sinai
New York, New York

**Carlos V.R. Brown**
Dell Medical School
The University of Texas at Austin
and
University Medical Center Brackenridge
Austin, Texas

**Timothy G. Buchman**
School Of Medicine
Emory University
Atlanta, Georgia

**Eileen M. Bulger**
Harborview Medical Center
University of Washington
Seattle, Washington

**Peter A. Burke**
Division of Acute Care/Trauma Surgery
Boston Medical Center
Boston, Massachusetts

**Christopher J. Busken**
The University of Texas Health Science Center at San Antonio
San Antonio, Texas

**Rafael M. Bustamante**
Lehigh Valley Health Network
Allentown, Pennsylvania

**Leopoldo C. Cancio**
U.S. Army Institute of Surgical Research
JBSA Fort Sam Houston, Texas

**Ramon F. Cestero**
The University of Texas Health Science Center at San Antonio
San Antonio, Texas

**Howard Champion**
Department of Surgery
Uniformed Services University of the Health Sciences
Bethesda, Maryland

**Clarence E. Clark III**
Morehouse School of Medicine
Atlanta, Georgia

**Michael S. Clemens**
San Antonio Military Medical Center
San Antonio, Texas

**Mark Cockburn**
Aventura Hospital and Medical Center
Miami, Florida

**Panna A. Codner**
Medical College of Wisconsin
Milwaukee, Wisconsin

**Mitchell Jay Cohen**
Department of Surgery
University of California, San Francisco
San Francisco, California

**Stephen M. Cohn**
Staten Island University Hospital
Staten Island, New York

**Raul Coimbra**
Department of Surgery
and
Division of Trauma, Surgical Critical Care, Burns, and Acute Care Surgery
University of California San Diego Health Sciences
La Jolla, California

**Kristin P. Colling**
University of Minnesota
Minneapolis, Minnesota

**Ben Coopwood**
Dell Medical School
The University of Texas at Austin
Austin, Texas

**Marshall A. Corson**
University of Washington
Seattle, Washington

**Todd W. Costantini**
Department of Surgery
University of California, San Diego
San Diego, California

**Martin A. Croce**
University of Tennessee Health Science Center
Memphis, Tennessee

**Bruce A. Crookes**
Medical University of South Carolina
Charleston, South Carolina

**James W. Davis**
University of California, San Francisco
Fresno, California

**Lori A. DeFreest**
Albany Medical Center
Albany New York

**E. Patchen Dellinger**
University of Washington
Seattle, Washington

**Demetrios Demetriades**
University of Southern California
and
Los Angeles County and
University of Southern California Medical Center
Los Angeles, California

**Marc A. de Moya**
Harvard Medical School
Boston, Massachusetts

**Daniel L. Dent**
The University of Texas Health Science Center at San Antonio
San Antonio, Texas

**Andrew DeRoo**
Albany Medical College
Albany, New York

**James C. Doherty**
Advocate Christ Medical Center
Oak Lawn, Illinois
and
The University of Illinois at Chicago
Chicago, Illinois

**Matthew O. Dolich**
University of California, Irvine
Orange, California

**Margaret Dorlon**
Medical University of South Carolina
Charleston, South Carolina

**Joseph J. DuBose**
Wilford Hall Medical Center
Lackland AFB, Texas

**Brian J. Eastridge**
The University of Texas Health Science Center at San Antonio
San Antonio, Texas

**Sara B. Edwards**
Icahn School of Medicine at Mount Sinai
New York, New York

**Akpofure Peter Ekeh**
Wright State University
Dayton, Ohio

**Marvin H. Eng**
Center for Structural Heart Disease
Henry Ford Hospital
Detroit, Michigan

**Robert M. Esterl, Jr.**
The University of Texas Health Science Center at San Antonio
San Antonio, Texas

**Timothy C. Fabian**
Department of Surgery
The University of Tennessee Health Science Center
Memphis, Tennessee

**Samir M. Fakhry**
Department of Surgery
Medical University of South Carolina
Charleston, South Carolina

**Ara J. Feinstein**
The University of Arizona College of Medicine, Phoenix
Phoenix, Arizona

**David V. Feliciano**
IU Division of General Surgery
and
Indiana University Hospital
Indiana University Medical Center
Indianapolis, Indiana

**Aaron M. Fields**
San Antonio Military Medical Center
Fort Sam Houston, Texas

**Lewis Flint**
Division of Education
American College of Surgeons
Chicago, Illinois

**Catherine S. Forster**
Cincinnati Children's Hospital Medical Center
Cincinnati, Ohio

**Antonio Jorge V. Forte**
Mayo Clinic
Jacksonville, Florida

**Spyridon Fortis**
The University of Iowa
Iowa City, Iowa

**Shannon M. Foster**
Reading Hospital
and
University of Pennsylvania
Reading, Pennsylvania

**Charles J. Fox**
Denver Health Medical Center
and
University of Colorado
Denver, Colorado

**Heidi L. Frankel**
Los Angeles, California

**Lane L. Frasier**
University of Wisconsin School of Medicine and Public Health
Madison, Wisconsin

**Stephen L. Freiberg**
The Johns Hopkins Hospital
Baltimore, Maryland

**Donald E. Fry**
Feinberg School of Medicine
Northwestern University
Chicago, Illinois

**Roy M. Fujitani**
Department of Surgery
University of California, Irvine
Irvine, California

**Enrique Ginzburg**
University of Miami
Miami, Florida

**Joseph E. Glaser**
Radiologic Associates, PC
and
Touro College of Osteopathic Medicine
Middletown, New York

**Adam Lee Goldstein**
Tel Aviv Sourasky Medical Center
Tel Aviv, Israel

**Gerald Gollin**
Rady Children's Hospital
San Diego, California

**Steven Granger**
School of Medicine
University of Utah
Salt Lake City, Utah

**Jonathan Green**
Department of General Surgery
University of Massachusetts Medical School
Worcester, Massachusetts

**Mark Kelly Green**
Marble Falls, Texas

**Wendie Grunberg**
The University of Texas Health Science Center
at San Antonio
San Antonio, Texas

**Fahim Habib**
Allegheny Health Network
Pittsburgh, Pennsylvania

**Ryan Hagino**
The University of Texas Health Science Center
at San Antonio
San Antonio, Texas

**Georges Haidar**
The University of Texas Health Science Center
at San Antonio
San Antonio, Texas

**S. Morad Hameed**
University of British Columbia
Vancouver, British Columbia, Canada

**Stephen O. Heard**
University of Massachusetts Medical School
UMass Memorial Medical Center
Worcester, Massachusetts

**Antonio Hernandez**
Vanderbilt University Medical Center
Nashville, Tennessee

**Michael P. Hirsh**
Department of General Surgery
University of Massachusetts Medical School
Worcester, Massachusetts

**John B. Holcomb**
Department of Surgery
The University of Texas Health
Houston, Texas

**John J. Hong**
Lehigh Valley Health Network
Allentown, Pennsylvania

**David B. Hoyt**
American College of Surgeons
Chicago, Illinois

**David K. Imagawa**
Irvine Medical Center
University of California
Orange, California

**Kenji Inaba**
University of Southern California
Los Angeles, California

**Rao R. Ivatury**
Virginia Commonwealth University
Richmond, Virginia

**Ronald Iverson**
Division Obstetrics & Gynecology
Boston Medical Center
Boston, Massachusetts

**Lenworth M. Jacobs**
Trauma Institute Hartford Hospital
Hartford, Connecticut

and

School of Medicine
University of Connecticut
Farmington, Connecticut

**Donald H. Jenkins**
Mayo Clinic
Rochester, Minnesota

**Igor Jeroukhimov**
Assaf Harofeh Medical Center
Zerefin, Israel

**Brent Jewett**
Medical University of South Carolina
Charleston, South Carolina

**Victor C. Joe**
Department of Surgery
University of California, Irvine
Orange, California

**Scott B. Johnson**
Department of Cardiothoracic Surgery
The University of Texas Health Science Center
at San Antonio
San Antonio, Texas

**Bellal Joseph**
College of Medicine
The University of Arizona, Tucson
Tucson, Arizona

**Gregory J. Jurkovich**
Denver, Colorado

**Krista L. Kaups**
University of California, San Francisco
Fresno, California

**Natasha Keric**
The University of Arizona College of Medicine, Phoenix
Phoenix, Arizona

**David R. King**
Harvard Medical School
Boston, Massachusetts

**Yoram Klein**
Sheba Medical Center
Tel Hashomer, Israel

**Yoram Kluger**
General Surgery and Pancreas Surgery Center
Haifa, Israel

**M. Margaret Knudson**
Department of Surgery
University of California, San Francisco
San Francisco, California

**Kenneth A. Kudsk**
Department of Surgery
University of Wisconsin–Madison
Madison, Wisconsin

**Marcelo J. Lacayo Baez**
Cleveland Clinic Florida
Weston, Florida

**Jeffrey H. Lawson**
Department of Surgery
Duke University
Durham, North Carolina

**Shari Lawson**
The University of Texas Health Science Center at San Antonio
San Antonio, Texas

**Elizabeth A. Lax**
Michigan State University
Southfield, Michigan

**J. Kayle Lee**
Advocate Christ Medical Center
Oak Lawn, Illinois
and
University of Illinois College of Medicine at Chicago
Chicago, Illinois

**Michael E. Lekawa**
School of Medicine
University of California, Irvine
Orange, California

**David M. Levi**
Carolinas Medical Center
Charlotte, North Carolina

**Aaron Lewis**
The University of Texas Health Science Center at San Antonio
San Antonio, Texas

**Edward B. Lineen**
University of Miami
Miami, Florida

**Alan Lisbon**
Harvard Medical School
Boston, Massachusetts

**David H. Livingston**
Department of Surgery
Rutgers-New Jersey Medical School
Newark, New Jersey

**Peter P. Lopez**
Michigan State University
Clinton Township, Michigan

and

Wayne State University
Southfield, Michigan

**Robert C. MacKersie**
Department of Surgery
University of California, San Francisco
San Francisco, California

**Alexandra A. MacLean**
Plasma Surgical, Inc.
Atlanta, Georgia

**Firas G. Madbak**
Reading Hospital
and
University of Pennsylvania
Reading, Pennsylvania

**Robert D. Madoff**
Department of Surgery
University of Minnesota
Minneapolis, Minnesota

**Mark A. Malangoni**
School of Medicine
University of Pennsylvania
Philadelphia, Pennsylvania

**Juan Marcano**
The University of Texas Health Science Center at San Antonio
San Antonio, Texas

**Matthew J. Marini**
Banner-University Medical Center Phoenix
Phoenix, Arizona

**Jennifer L. Marti**
Icahn School of Medicine at Mount Sinai
New York, New York

**Pedro Mascaro**
University of Miami
Miami, Florida

**Kenneth L. Mattox**
Michael E. DeBakey Department of Surgery
Baylor College of Medicine
Houston, Texas

**Kimball I. Maull**
University of Pittsburgh Medical Center
Pittsburgh, Pennsylvania

**Addison K. May**
Department of Surgery
Vanderbilt University Medical Center
Nashville, Tennessee

**J. Wayne Meredith**
Wake Forest Baptist Health
Winston-Salem, North Carolina

**Joseph L. Mills**
The University of Arizona Health Sciences Center
Tucson, Arizona

**Joesph P. Minei**
University of Texas Southwestern Medical Center
Dallas, Texas

**Thomas A. Mitchell**
San Antonio Military Medical Center
San Antonio, Texas

**Jorge A. Montes**
The University of Texas Health Science Center at San Antonio
San Antonio, Texas

**Ernest E. Moore**
University of Colorado, Denver
Denver, Colorado

**Frederick A. Moore**
University of Florida
Gainesville Florida

**Jay A. Motola**
Department of Urology
Mount Sinai Roosevelt
New York, New York

**Deborah L. Mueller**
The University of Texas Health Science Center at San Antonio
San Antonio, Texas

**Mark Muir**
The University of Texas Health Science Center at San Antonio
San Antonio, Texas

**Nicholas Namias**
Miller School of Medicine
University of Miami
Miami, Florida

**Avery B. Nathens**
Sunnybrook Health Sciences Centre
and
University of Toronto
and
Trauma Research
and
American College of Surgeons Trauma Quality Improvement Program
Toronto, Ontario, Canada

**Heather Norman**
Lehigh Valley Health Network
Allentown, Pennsylvania

**Brian O'Gara**
Harvard Medical School
Boston, Massachusetts

**Terence O'Keeffe**
University of Arizona Medical Center
Tucson, Arizona

**Adrian W. Ong**
Reading Hospital
and
University of Pennsylvania
Reading, Pennsylvania

**Matthew O'Rourke**
Cincinnati Children's Hospital and Medical Center
Cincinnati, Ohio

**Damaris Ortiz**
University of Illinois College of Medicine at Chicago
Chicago, Illinois

**David S. Owens**
University of Washington Medical Center
Seattle, Washington

**H. Leon Pachter**
Department of Surgery
New York University School of Medicine
New York, New York

**Andrew B. Peitzman**
Department of Surgery
and
School of Medicine
University of Pittsburgh
Pittsburgh, Pennsylvania

**Erin E. Perrone**
University of Michigan
Ann Arbor, Michigan

**W. Brian Perry**
South Texas Veterans Health Care System
San Antonio, Texas

**Edgar J. Pierre**
University of Miami
Miami, Florida

**Michelle A. Price**
The University of Texas Health Science Center
at San Antonio
San Antonio, Texas

**Basil A. Pruitt, Jr.**
Department of Surgery
University of Texas Health Science Center
at San Antonio
San Antonio, Texas

**Hemn Qader**

**Elie P. Ramly**
Massachusetts General Hospital
Boston, Massachusetts

**Megan Rashid**
University of Miami
Miami, Florida

**Todd E. Rasmussen**
Wilford Hall USAF Medical Center
Lackland Air Force, Texas
and
The Uniformed Services University of the Health Sciences
Bethesda, Maryland

**Bipin K. Ravindran**
Michigan Heart and Vascular Institute
Ypsilanti, Michigan

**Juliet J. Ray**
University of Miami
Miami, Florida

**Amirhossein Razavi**

**Peter M. Rhee**
The University of Arizona, Tucson
Tucson, Arizona

**J. David Richardson**
University of Louisville
Louisville, Kentucky

**Oscar Rios**
The University of Texas at Austin
Austin, Texas

**Raul J. Rosenthal**
Florida International University
University Park, Florida

**Michael F. Rotondo**
University of Rochester Medical Center
Rochester, New York

**Noelle N. Saillant**
Perelman School of Medicine
Hospital of the University of Pennsylvania
Philadelphia, Pennsylvania

**Edward Y. Sako**
The University of Texas Health Science Center
at San Antonio
San Antonio, Texas

**Ali Salim**
Brigham and Women's Hospital
Boston, Massachusetts

**Patrick C. Samson**
North Shore-Long Island Jewish Health Care System
New Hyde Park, New York

**Shevonne S. Satahoo**
University of Miami
Miami, Florida

**Stephanie A. Savage**
Indiana University School of Medicine
Indianapolis, Indiana

**Mark D. Sawyer**
Mayo Clinic
Rochester, Minnesota

**Tom Scalea**
R Adams Cowley Shock Trauma Center
Baltimore, Maryland

**William Schecter**
University of California, San Francisco
San Francisco, California

**Martin A. Schreiber**
Department of Surgery
Oregon Health & Science University
Portland, Oregon

**Carl I. Schulman**
University of Miami
Miami, Florida

**C. William Schwab**
Perelman School of Medicine
Hospital of the University of Pennsylvania
Philadelphia, Pennsylvania

**Steven D. Schwaitzberg**
Cambridge Health Alliance
and
Harvard Medical School
Cambridge, Massachusetts

**Wayne H. Schwesinger**
The University of Texas Health Science Center at San Antonio
San Antonio, Texas

**Joseph H. Shin**
Dartmouth Hitchock Medical Center
Lebanon, New Hampshire

**Richard K. Simons**
University of British Columbia
Vancouver, British Columbia, Canada

**Conrad H. Simpfendorfer**
Cleveland Clinic Florida
Weston, Florida

**Meghan E. Sise**
Massachusetts General Hospital
Boston, Massachusetts

**Michael J. Sise**

**Pieter J.S. Smit**
Division of Acute Care/Trauma Surgery
Boston Medical Center
Boston, Massachusetts

**Dror Soffer**
The Yitzhak Rabin Trauma Division
and
Tel Aviv Sourasky Medical Center
Tel Aviv, Israel

**David A. Spain**
Department of Surgery
Stanford University
Stanford, California

**K. Vincent Speeg**
The University of Texas Health Science Center at San Antonio
San Antonio, Texas

**Kenneth Stahl**
University of Miami
Miami, Florida

**Michael J. Stamos**
School of Medicine
University of California, Irvine
Irvine, California

**Chad N. Stasik**
The University of Texas Health Science Center at San Antonio
San Antonio, Texas

**Ronald Stewart**
The University of Texas Health Science Center at San Antonio
San Antonio, Texas

**Mary Stuever**
Wright State University
Dayton, Ohio

**Balachundhar Subramaniam**
Harvard Medical School
and
Beth Israel Deaconess Medical Center
Boston, Massachusetts

**Mark Y. Sun**
Department of Surgery
University of Minnesota
Minneapolis, Minnesota

**Marcel Tafen**
Albany Medical College
Albany, New York

**Pedro G.R. Teixeira**
University of Southern California
Los Angeles, California

**Burke Thompson**
Moses Cone Memorial Hospital
Greensboro, North Carolina

**Eric A. Toschlog**
Division of Trauma and Acute Care Surgery
The Brody School of Medicine
East Carolina University
and
Trauma Vidant Medical Center
Greenville North Carolina

**Boulos Toursarkissian**
The University of Texas Health Science Center at San Antonio
and
Peripheral Vascular Associates
San Antonio, Texas

**Donald Trunkey**

**Olga N. Tucker**
The Queen Elizabeth Hospital
Birmingham, United Kingdom

**Jacquelyn Turner**
Morehouse School of Medicine
Atlanta, Georgia

**Andreas G. Tzakis**
Cleveland Clinic Florida
Weston, Florida

**Evan J. Valle**
University of Miami
Miami, Florida

**Kent Van Sickle**
The University of Texas Health Science Center at San Antonio
San Antonio, Texas

**George C. Velmahos**
Harvard Medical School
and
Massachusetts General Hospital
Boston, Massachusetts

**Cynthia L. Villarreal**
The University of Texas Health Science Center at San Antonio
San Antonio, Texas

**Mohan N. Viswanathan**
School of Medicine
Stanford University
Stanford, California

**Kelly Vogt**

**Howard T. Wang**
The University of Texas Health Science Center at San Antonio
San Antonio, Texas

**Elizabeth Windell**
University of Arizona Medical Center
Tucson, Arizona

**David H. Wisner**
University of California, Davis
Davis, California

**Steven E. Wolf**
The University of Texas at Dallas
Dallas, Texas

**Katherine Xu**
Columbia University Medical Center
New York, New York

# Introduction

**Brad H. Pollock**

This textbook focuses on important surgical management issues where one or more problems are addressed using scientific evidence from the published literature. This introduction describes the rationale, process, and criteria used for obtaining and weighing the evidence provided by published research studies. Why evidence-based medicine? The primary use of evidence-based medicine (EBM) is to help make informed decisions by combining individual clinical expertise with the best available external clinical evidence. This approach optimizes decision-making for the care of individual patients.[1]

Surgical management issues presented in this textbook are oriented toward interventions. While gathering evidence from intervention studies is the most common use of EBM, the objectives of patient-oriented research studies can alternatively include determining the etiology of a health problem, determining the accuracy and utility of new tests, and identifying prognostic factors, including biomarkers. In this textbook, EBM is used to assess the safety and efficacy of new treatments and rehabilitative or preventive interventions. The evidence from multiple studies is often combined to make more precise clinical inferences in order to select the most appropriate treatment plan for individual patients. The goal of this introduction is to describe the ways in which evidence is evaluated and integrated.

## Assessing the Validity of Intervention Studies

Four attributes define the strength of evidence provided by a published intervention study. The first is the level of the evidence—dictated by the type of study design that was used. The second is the quality of evidence—directly related to lack of bias. The third is statistical precision—the degree to which true effects can be distinguished from spurious effects due to random chance alone. The fourth is the choice of a study endpoint to measure an effect—an endpoint's appropriateness to truly represent a clinically meaningful outcome—and the magnitude of the observed effect. For practical reasons, the selection of study subjects is almost always a compromise. The degree to which a chosen study population represents an intended target population must also be considered; selection bias can compromise a study's weight of evidence.

### Clinical Study Design

There are several different types of studies that are used in clinical research. Each study type (or design) has relative advantages but also limitations, including a unique profile of potential study biases. Case reports and case series can document the effects of an intervention or clinical course. However, these are subject to selection bias, often use subjective outcome assessment, and are imprecise due to the small samples. Case reports and case series have no control groups for comparisons. Case-control studies include subjects who have already developed the outcome of interest (cases) and a group of unaffected subjects (controls). Case-control studies can be performed in a more timely manner and are often much less expensive than other study designs. However, a temporal relationship between cause and effect can only be inferred and not directly observed because of the retrospective nature of case-control studies. Also, case-control studies are subject to biased recall of antecedent events and exposures. Selection bias is an important concern, especially the selection of controls. Case-control studies are most often used for very rare outcomes or when there is a long latency between exposure and the subsequent effect, i.e., development of an outcome.

Prospective cohort studies recruit subjects who are free of the outcome of interest. Subjects are then actively followed over time for the occurrence of the outcome. Recruitment may be selective and based on accruing an equal number of subjects into preselected exposure categories; matching on other factors is possible to reduce confounding and improve the precision of comparisons across exposure groups. Alternatively, recruitment to prospective cohort studies need not be based on predetermined categories of exposure; nonselective recruitment is common when there are multiple exposures of interest. An alternative design is the historical cohort study. These studies utilize preexisting information, often in a comprehensive database, to historically classify exposure status. The database is then gleamed for information about subsequent outcome events. Except for randomized controlled trials, prospective cohort studies are more expensive than alternative designs. An exposure of interest, such as a new surgical procedure vs. a conventional procedure, may be linked to unknown or unmeasurable potential confounders. Because cohort studies are not randomized, the distribution of these unknown or unmeasurable confounders may not be balanced between treatment groups, thus leading to confounding. Prospective studies are typically more resource intensive and time consuming than case-control studies. A major advantage of cohort designs is that they provide a clear picture of the temporal relationship between a cause and an effect. Matching can efficiently reduce confounding. Cohort designs are generally simpler and less expensive to conduct than a randomized controlled trial.

Randomized controlled trials (RCTs) provide the greatest weight of evidence compared to other designs. These are studies in which the allocation of subjects to an exposure of interest is done solely for the purpose of obtaining an unbiased estimate of the treatment effect. The key advantage of RCTs is the lower likelihood of confounding bias. While controlling for *known* confounders can be performed using techniques such as restriction, stratified block design, or statistical adjustment, randomization controls for confounding bias by balancing the distribution of *unknown* or *unmeasurable* confounding factors between treatment groups. RCTs can also be blinded more easily. Some of their disadvantages include higher costs and recruitment barriers, particularly for subjects who prefer not to be experimented on. Because of their prospective nature, RCTs are generally much costlier than nonprospective designs such as case-control studies. Even with those limitations, RCTs represent the gold standard; they provide the strongest weight of evidence for causal inference.

Other study designs are used less frequently in medical research. Cross-sectional studies collect both exposure and outcome information simultaneously and may be more applicable for prevalent rather than for acute or episodic conditions, but cannot directly address cause and effect temporal relationships. Crossover designs are studies in which all subjects serve as their own controls. For a typical simple crossover study, half the study population receives the primary treatment first and then crosses over to receive the second treatment; the other half receives the treatments in reverse order. A major assumption in crossover studies is that the residual effects of a treatment disappear by the time the groups are crossed over. This is clearly not applicable for many surgical interventions where a subject's condition is permanently altered by the therapy (e.g., limb amputation) or for certain pharmaceutical trials where the washout period for the new drug is too long or of unknown duration.

### Bias and Internal Validity

The strength of scientific evidence provided by an individual study is dependent on a number of key factors. All of these factors must be properly considered before attempting to make clinical inferences from a published study. Ideally, results are published for studies that are both internally and externally valid. Compromised validity lowers a study's weight of evidence.

The design of all patient-oriented research studies is strongly associated with the degree to which bias can potentially impact the study results and conclusions. The internal validity for a particular study is affected by selection bias, measurement bias, observer bias, confounding, and statistical precision. These potential problems can manifest themselves in different ways and degrees for different types of study designs.

Internal validity refers to a study's lack of bias; bias is a systematic error that affects inferences derived from the results of a study. Internally valid studies are free of bias. External validity refers to the generalizability of a study and addresses the issue of whether results derived from the assessment of a study-specific population can be extrapolated to another population of interest. Internal validity should be the primary consideration when reviewing a publication. If a study is not internally valid, one need not consider whether it is externally valid; i.e., biased study results should never be extrapolated to another population. For intervention studies, internal validity addresses whether observed changes (study results) can be attributed to the treatment effect or whether they are attributed to other, alternate explanations such as bias or lack of statistical precision.

There are a number of internal validity considerations. Selection bias results when an unrepresentative sample of subjects is included in a study. For retrospective designs such as case-control studies, selection bias can alter a study's measures of effect; for prospective studies such as randomized clinical trials, selection bias can compromise the study's generalizability. Measurement bias is inaccuracy related to the method of measuring values for a study. Examples include miscalibrated blood pressure readings, inaccurate height measurements, flawed laboratory methods that give erroneous values, and study variable coding that fails to accurately reflect clinically meaningful categories. Observer bias is inaccuracy related to measuring a study outcome typically when an observer knows the intervention group assignment. Observer bias is more likely to occur when the chosen outcome measure is subjective. Examples of more subjective measures include the occurrence of symptoms or toxicities, patient self-report measures, and interpretations of physical examination findings. If observers know which treatment a patient is receiving, their outcome assessments may be biased. Blinding is used to reduce observer bias for trials. Most common is the use of double blinding, where neither the observer nor the patient knows the treatment assignment. However, for many surgical interventions such as total limb vs. partial limb amputation, or for regimens with very idiosyncratic symptom or toxicity profiles, blinding may be impractical. Confounding bias is the mixing up of effects so that the primary effect under study cannot be separated from the influence of extraneous factors. For example, failing to account for preoperative disease severity in a randomized trial evaluating two surgical approaches might lead to confounding if the severity distribution differed between treatment groups.

### Statistical Precision

In the context of a clinical research study, statistical precision refers to the ability to distinguish real effects from those due to random chance, i.e., chance associations. For example, with just 10 subjects (5 in each group) in a randomized clinical trial comparing a new postsurgical antibiotic regimen to a conventional regimen for sepsis prophylaxis, an extreme finding could likely be attributed to random chance alone, not to a true biological drug effect. Chance errors are less likely to occur with larger sample sizes. Trials are always planned to limit the likelihood of chance errors; acceptable levels of error (for Type 1 and Type 2 statistical errors) are selected and the target minimum detectable effect size is chosen. Formal sample size/power calculations are performed during the study's design to ensure adequate statistical precision.

## External Validity

External validity refers to the ability to appropriately generalize a study's results to the population of interest such as the U.S. general population. The question is, "Does the study population possess unique characteristics that might modify the effect of an intervention in a way that would render it ineffective in some other group?" Subjects that are accrued to a trial may not be representative of the population to which the intervention is intended to be applied. There is a tendency for published surgical and nonsurgical intervention studies to enroll subjects at larger academic institutions. The characteristics for these referred patients may not be representative of patients seen at smaller nonacademic centers. Even within a center, subjects that volunteer to participate in a study may not be representative of the institution's entire clinical population.

Selection bias can occur with the self-selection of individuals who volunteer to participate in a research study. Both researchers and participants bring a multitude of characteristics associated with outcome measures to a clinical study, some inherent and some acquired. These can include factors such as gender; race/ethnicity; hair, eye, and skin color; personality; mental capability; physical status; and psychological attitudes like motivation or willingness to participate. Differences in the distribution of these factors between a source population and a protocol-enrolled study population may introduce selection bias. For example, some investigators may preferentially select more athletic-looking subjects for an elective orthopedic surgery clinical trial. Larger multicenter trials from geographically disparate locations may improve the generalizability of a study, but such studies may still suffer from selection bias.

## Weight of Evidence

Study design, lack of bias, statistical precision, and external validity are elements that affect a study's weight of evidence for causal inference. Each of these factors must be considered when evaluating a published study. For practical reasons, the investigator who is designing a new study is always confronted with trade-offs between these factors and cost. For example, having highly restrictive eligibility criteria reduces confounding but lowers the generalizability of a study. The choice of a more objective end point for an antibiotic trial (e.g., death versus confirmed sepsis) decreases observer bias at the cost of decreased statistical precision—fewer deaths compared to the number of incident sepsis cases. Investigators are faced with many challenges when designing intervention studies. Because resources are almost always limited, design compromises are made that ultimately impact the overall weight of evidence provided by a study.

### Literature Reviews

Reviews of the results of published studies can take multiple forms. Reviews can be done of single studies. Single studies may be used as the basis for making treatment decisions. There may be a very large randomized clinical trial that appropriately evaluated a single clinical end point with high validity. This may be sufficient for medical decision-making. Alternatively, narrative reviews or systematic reviews evaluate multiple publications.

### Narrative Reviews

Narrative reviews often address a broad set of clinical questions and are thus less focused on a specific question; they appear more often in the literature and are more qualitative and less quantitative. In contrast, systematic reviews are usually focused on a specific clinical issue, incorporate objective criteria for the selection of published studies, include an evaluation of quality and worthiness, and often use a quantitative summary to synthesize combined results.

Narrative reviews are often one of the first academic endeavors that young physicians complete during their training. The subjective nature of narrative reviews increases the likelihood that inferences are affected by imprecision and bias. For example, a count of included studies supporting or refuting a particular issue is determined and a winner is declared. For narrative reviews, little consideration may be given to issues of study design, sample size/statistical power, or study validity, or in the case of study counts, the possibility that there was a bias against publication of studies with null results.

### Systematic Reviews

Systematic reviews are a staple of EBM.[2] They provide the best means to combine evidence from multiple studies. They follow a defined protocol to identify, summarize, and combine information. Systematic reviews may restrict the inclusion of studies to specific study designs, such as randomized controlled trials, or they may include a broader set of designs. Systematic reviews can be very labor intensive and costly. They may attempt to use information from unpublished studies. There are significant challenges in combining evidence from studies that use different designs or different end points or that vary by other methodological characteristics.

A protocol for a systematic review uses a strict set of guidelines for selecting and amalgamating information from the literature. Cochrane Collaboration (http://www.cochrane.org/) guidelines for developing a systematic review protocol requires the following: a background section explaining the context and rationale for the review, a statement of the objectives, a clear definition of the inclusion and exclusion criteria for studies (including study designs, study populations, types of interventions, and outcome measures), the search strategy for identification of studies, and the methodological approach to the review process including the selection of trials, assignment of methodological quality, data handling procedures, and data synthesis. Data synthesis includes statistical considerations such as choice of summary effect measures, assessment of heterogeneity of effect across studies, subgroup analyses, use of random or fixed effects statistical models, and assessment of publication bias.

The existence of many clinical studies is often not reflected by resultant publications in the medical literature. The U.S. Food and Drug Administration initiated a public registry and results database called *ClinicalTrials.gov*. The Food and Drug Administration Amendments Act of 2007 mandated that certain clinical trials be registered at trial initiation and that summary results after the trial was completed be made available in *ClinicalTrials.gov*. This has been one source to identify trials that may not have been reported in the medical literature. Beyond *ClinicalTrails.gov*, work has been completed to develop a more complete clinical research ontology, the Ontology of Clinical Research (OCRe).[3] The OCRe was developed to accommodate a more diverse set of human study types (beyond clinical trials) with a much richer set of study characteristics descriptors, including attributes such as study design type, treatments, study population, outcome metrics and statistical analyses. Using such an ontological approach to classify human studies would aid in the review and interpretation of results of previous studies to address scientific questions, particularly to aid in systematic reviews.

### Meta-Analysis

Systematic reviews often, but not always, include a meta-analysis. The goals of meta-analysis are to provide a precise estimate of the effect, and to determine if the effect is robust across a range of populations.[4] Often a component of systematic reviews, meta-analyses calculate the results of each study identified by the reviewer and then calculate the average of those results—if appropriate. Data are first extracted from each individual study and then used to calculate a point estimate of effect along with a measure of uncertainly, e.g., the 95% confidence interval. This is repeated for each of the studies included in the meta-analysis. Then a decision is made about whether the results can be pooled to calculate an average result across all of the studies. The decision to combine or not combine studies is made by an assessment of the heterogeneity of effect across studies. Observed statistical heterogeneity suggests the true underlying treatment effects in the trials are not identical; i.e., the observed treatment effects have a greater difference than one should expect due to random error alone. Importantly, uncovering heterogeneity may be the primary goal of a meta-analysis. Analysis of heterogeneity may elucidate previously unrecognized differences between studies. Only in the absence of significant heterogeneity can study results be numerically combined and a summary measure of effect calculated. The calculation of summary measures relies on a mathematical process that gives more weight to the results from studies that provide more information (usually those with larger study populations) or with higher quality. Often, data for all included studies are plotted on a graph known as a "forest plot," which includes a graphical representation of the magnitude of effect for each study and its degree of uncertainty (plotted as confidence intervals). Meta-analysis can reveal the impact of potential confounders on the treatment effect.

### Publication Bias

All studies are subject to Type I errors, where evidence is found to reject a null hypothesis of no effect, or Type II errors, where evidence is found to not reject the null hypothesis when a true effect exists. Studies with statistically significant results ("positive" studies) are more likely to be accepted for publication than studies without statistically significant results ("negative" studies). Even adequately powered studies with very low Type II error rates are less likely to be accepted for publication than are smaller positive studies. With this gap, publication bias can adversely impact causal inferences about the efficacy of an intervention.

## Levels of Evidence and Grades of Recommendations

All reviews evaluate historical information and are therefore subject to systematic bias and random error. For different study objectives (e.g., determining the impact of a therapeutic or preventive intervention), the Oxford Centre for Evidence-Based Medicine Levels of Evidence displays the level of evidence based on a review of the literature, study design, and quality. The highest level of evidence for a therapeutic intervention is provided by systematic reviews of large RCTs that show homogeneity of effect across trials (Level 1a). The next highest is for an individual RCT with a narrow confidence interval (Level 1b); this is followed by an all or none effect related to the introduction of a treatment (Level 1c). The level of evidence decreases with weaker study designs such as cohort studies (Level 2) followed by case-control studies (Level 3), case series (Level 4), and, at the lowest level, expert opinion (Level 5). Grades of recommendations are based on the consistency of higher-level studies: an "A" grade shows consistency across Level 1 studies; a "B" grade shows consistency across Level 2 or 3 studies or extrapolations from Level 1 studies; a "C" grade shows consistency across Level 4 studies or extrapolations from Level 2 or 3 studies; a "D" grade shows Level 5 evidence or inconsistency across studies of any level.

## Development of Expanded Clinical Research Infrastructure

As the major driver of evidence-based medicine, clinical research has been in transition from work performed by isolated researchers in individual clinics toward larger team science-initiated multi-institutional investigations. This transition began many years ago such as with the initiation of the National Cancer Institute–sponsored clinical trials cooperative groups some 58 years ago, through to the formation of the Clinical Translational Research Award Consortium of the NIH and, most recently, the Patient-Centered Outcomes Research Institute (PCORI)-sponsored PCORnet.[5] These large transdisciplinary, multi-institution consortia have at their core the goal of addressing important clinical and translational hypotheses that contribute to the improved practice of medicine. In common, these groups have developed clinical research infrastructure emphasizing study population inclusiveness, quality control, harmonized research information technology infrastructure, adherence to best statistical practices for planning, monitoring and analysis, and dissemination of knowledge for new discoveries. Clinical research and evaluation of interventions in particular will increasingly rely on the use of the electronic health record for cohort discovery, subject recruitment, and collection of primary study data. For example, PCORnet is developing infrastructure to conduct national intervention and observational studies by trying EHR information together across the United States and potentially representing tens of millions of individuals. These developments are likely to accelerate the pace at which we gather scientific evidence, leading to improved care.

## Summary

Evidence-based medicine is not limited to the evaluation of RCTs and meta-analysis. A broader range of external evidence can be brought to bear on addressing clinical questions.[1] Practice guidelines developed using evidence-based medicine can have a positive impact on patient outcomes. Evidence-based medicine guidelines have reduced mortality from myocardial infarctions, and also improved care for persons with diabetes and other common medical problems. Evidence-based medicine supplements physicians' judgments that might otherwise be based solely on anecdotal clinical experience. Ultimately, developing systems to incorporate previous evidence and incorporating accessible information and prediction models at the bedside for decision support are tenets of the Learning Health System.[6] Surgical practice can benefit from EBM and should be incorporated into the standard of care.

## References

1. Sackett DL, Rosenberg WM, Gray JA, Haynes RB, Richardson WS. Evidence based medicine: what it is and what it isn't. 1996. *Clin Orthop Rel Res.* 2007;455:3–5.
2. Egger M, Smith GD, Altman DG. London, U.K.: BMJ Publishing Group; 2001.
3. Sim I, Tu SW, Carini S et al. The ontology of clinical research (OCRe): An informatics foundation for the science of clinical research. *J Biomed Inform.* 2013.
4. Borenstein M, Hedges LV, Higgins JPT, Rothstein HR. *Introduction to Meta-Analysis.* Wiley; 2008.
5. Collins FS, Hudson KL, Briggs JP, Lauer MS. PCORnet: Turning a dream into reality. *JAMIA.* 2014;21:576–577.
6. Friedman CP, Wong AK, Blumenthal D. Achieving a nationwide learning health system. *Sci Transl Med.* 2010;2:57cm29.

# Section I

# Trauma

# 1

# *Patient Safety in the Care of Trauma Patients*

**Kenneth Stahl and Susan Brien**

**CONTENTS**



## 1.1 Introduction

The aim of trauma care is to save the lives of injured patients and prevent further organ damage from the metabolic and physiologic derangements caused by their injuries. In order to achieve this goal, a critical judgment affecting a trauma patient's survival is required every 72 s during the first hours of their care [1]. Despite best efforts from the trauma team, the urgency and accuracy required for this decision-making process are conducive to producing errors. The circumstances likely to result in errors are unstable patients, fatigued operators, incomplete clinical information, delayed decisions, multiple concurrent tasks involving complex teams, transportation of unstable patients, and multiple hand-offs of patients' care. Due to these factors, the management of trauma patients poses significant challenges and creates a "perfect storm for medical errors" [2].

## 1.2 Incidence

Adverse outcome and error reporting in healthcare is sporadic at best [3]. For this reason, the actual number of errors that occur in the care of trauma victims is difficult to accurately assess. However, adverse outcomes as a result of errors in patient care do occur and some patients are seriously and sometimes fatally harmed [4]. Preventable deaths secondary to human and system errors account for up to 10% of fatalities in patients with otherwise survivable injuries treated at Level I trauma centers [5–7]. This number of unintended deaths equates to as many as 15,000 lost lives per year in the United States or almost two lives lost every hour [8]. This is two to four times higher than deaths due to errors reported in the general hospital patient population [9].

## 1.3 Mechanisms of Errors

In-hospital errors in the management of trauma patients that ultimately lead to adverse outcomes can occur at any time during their management and start right on admission. The primary survey is a rapid assessment and concurrent stabilization of the patient and is usually complete within the first 30 min of the resuscitative phase of trauma care. During this time period, 2.5 errors per patient (760 errors in 300 patients) have been observed [1]. Patients with low Glasgow Coma Score, psychiatric history, or drug and alcohol use provide trauma teams with additional challenges. Older patients, who already pose diagnostic challenges due to concurrent diseases, have an increased risk of adverse events [10].

Life-threatening errors include inadequate airway management, missed tension pneumothorax, underestimates of the severity of bleeding, and failure to manage acute shock states [11]. Delay in the diagnosis or mishandling of any of these conditions during the initial resuscitation will lead to the failure of the trauma team to rescue the patient. Studies indicate that 16% of preventable trauma deaths are due to failure of airway management, 28% failure to identify or control hemorrhage, 14.5% errors in diagnosis, and 11.8% missed diagnosis during the primary survey [12]. Errors in triage of hemodynamically precarious patients in need of prompt operative intervention can lead to hemodynamic collapse and avoidable cardiac arrest in the radiology suite or observation area. A diagnostic peritoneal lavage may be required to make the correct decision for disposition of the patient to the operating room for immediate surgery or radiology for further evaluation [13].

The secondary survey begins when the primary survey is completed, resuscitation efforts are well established, and vital signs are stabilized. The secondary survey is a head-to-toe evaluation of the trauma patient, including as complete a history and physical examination as the clinical circumstances allow. In addition, a careful reassessment of the patient's response to the initial resuscitation and search for more subtle injuries are carried out. Injuries can be missed during the secondary survey and lead to significant morbidity or mortality that occurs in up to 8.1% of trauma patients. Seventeen percent of these missed injuries are abdominal, 16.3% intra-thoracic, and 40.8% extremity injuries [14]. This same study demonstrated that 65.1% of injuries were missed due to inadequate or incorrect primary or secondary surveys, with 34.9% due to radiographic misinterpretations and 34.1% delayed surgeries.

## 1.4 Errors in the Operative Phase of Trauma Care

The surgical procedure itself has been the subject of numerous safety analyses, and avoiding technical mishaps in the surgical management of individual injuries and organ systems is detailed elsewhere in this text. As a general principle, it is important for the trauma surgeon to understand that, regardless of the patient's injuries, excellent surgical outcomes depend upon expeditious and skilled surgical procedures and meticulous attention to the cognitive and physiological aspects of the operation. Failure of the surgeon to maintain constant awareness of the physiological condition of the patient, including fluid and transfusion requirements, coagulation state, acid/base balance, and core temperature, leads to prolonged operations and increases mortality of patients with otherwise survivable injuries [15]. This is the concept of damage-control surgery that has been well established by recent meta-analysis [16]. The trauma surgeon needs the cognitive discipline and judgment to abort complex and timely organ repairs and defer to damage control surgery when the patient's condition demands this for survival. Persistence in an operation that is compromised by the bigger picture of the patient's deteriorating physiology is known as "cognitive anchoring bias" [17] and must be avoided by knowing and staying within the boundaries of the trauma safety box (see Section 1.7).

Additionally, the environment in the operating room needs to be managed by the trauma surgeon. This is necessary to ensure accurate communication of critical patient information and minimize distractions in order to avoid adverse outcomes [18]. The maintenance of situational awareness (the "big picture") and crew resource management skills are equally important [19]. This promotes good teamwork function and is another essential element of optimizing surgical outcomes and patient safety efforts [20].

## 1.5 Errors in the Intensive Care Unit and Postoperative Phase of Trauma Care

The risk of error during the ICU management of trauma patients is in the range of 1.7 adverse events per patient per day of which 13% are life threatening or fatal [21]. Forty-five percent of these errors were judged to have been preventable. Level II evidence-based studies indicate that the presence of at least one adverse event increased the odds ratio of mortality as much as 17-fold over matched controls with no adverse events [22]. Errors such as failure to recognize the development of abdominal or limb compartment syndrome [23], failure to recognize occult bleeding, and delayed onset of shock and respiratory failure are potentially avoidable events that contribute to adverse outcomes [7].

## 1.6 Result of Errors in Trauma Care

The actual rate of adverse events leading to death in trauma patients may be higher than reported if autopsy statistics are included. Studies that included autopsy findings document mortality due to errors ranges between 15% and 28% [24]. In a retrospective observational analysis of admissions to a Level I center, 1032 avoidable errors were found in the care of 893 (4%) patients. These errors contributed to 76 preventable or potentially preventable deaths. This same study found that 5.6% of fatalities over the study period could have been prevented. This study also indicated that errors occur in all three phases of management of trauma victims. Thirty-six percent of errors led to fatality in the resuscitative phase, 14% in the operative phase, and 50% in the intensive care unit phase [25].

## 1.7 Methods to Reduce Errors in Trauma Care

The nature of human and system errors that lead to adverse outcomes has been investigated in complex systems such as the commercial aviation industry and the nuclear power industry, environments that closely mimic trauma care. Organizations such as these are collectively known as "high-reliability organizations" (HROs); detailed descriptions can be found in safety literature [2]. HROs are defined as high-risk, error-intolerant systems that repeatedly carry out potentially dangerous procedures with minimal actual error. HROs understand circumstances that are likely to lead to adverse events known as "error-producing conditions" (EPCs). Sets of these conditions have been arrived at after careful analysis of accidents and near-miss incidents with the use of mathematical modeling of contributing factors [26,27]. The most important EPCs that affect trauma patient care are fatigue; high-risk, low-frequency events; time pressure; normalization of deviancy; poor supervision; faulty risk (injury severity) perception; and task overload.

High-reliability safety theories have generated strategies to avoid both individual and organizational errors. Application of these error-management strategies can reduce adverse outcomes in trauma care [2]. Safety in trauma care can be achieved by understanding and anticipating chances for errors and thus effectively trapping these small missteps before major adverse events take place [28]. Several safety methods of HROs have led to this kind of consistent error trapping and reductions in adverse outcomes and can be emulated by trauma systems. These include a preoccupation with studying and recognizing error patterns with root cause analysis, a reluctance to simplify interpretations of critical situations, attention to system operations, developing resiliency to recover from unexpected events, and deference to expertise. The HRO safety literature has described successful adoption of these principles as culminating in a state of "collective HRO mindfulness" that enhance team function [29].

In addition to this safety mindfulness, there are important sets of specific and teachable team skills that can be added to bring an overarching system for patient safety in trauma care. These HRO safety skills are divided into six broad categories: crew resource management (CRM), situational awareness (SA), time-critical decision-making (DM), team leadership and supervision, communication skills, and human factors (HF). These skills are closely interrelated and combine the central principles of teamwork and communication capabilities with individual performance. Level II evidence-based studies indicate that these methods can be utilized to enhance and improve surgical outcomes [30,31].

Combining these concepts of mental preparedness and error avoidance with team competencies can enhance safety outcomes in the management of trauma victims. This will result in an overarching "high-reliability mindset" [32] incorporating error awareness theories of HROs with error avoidance strategies of personal and team behaviors. This is an effective error mitigation strategy given that trauma centers operate in an environment demanding perfection without an HRO-like system safety net [33].

The concept of a "high-reliability mindset" has already transitioned into HRO and aviation safety with "scenario-based training" (SBT) that stresses advanced risk awareness and management and decision-making skills. Threat and error management is not new, and using this knowledge to create "mindset training" has received broad HRO industry acceptance [34]. This mindset, as it applies to trauma training and practice, includes the understanding of the specific conditions that define times when error is more likely to occur and thus predict unsafe circumstances to which patients may be exposed [35].

Derived from this understanding of inherently risk-producing conditions is the final component of the "high-reliability mindset," which is the concept of operating within the confines of a theoretical "box" that has specific safety boundaries and provides a safety net. James Reason's reference to this as the "safety space" offers a useful mental model of a three-dimensional area within which safe operations are assured [36]. The trauma safety box has sides defined by patient physiology, individual skills and currency of the primary surgeon, surgical team training, and human and environmental factors. To assure safe outcomes, trauma surgeons must mentally define this box and all team members must understand the safety boundaries, as they exist in any clinical situation. Operating "outside the box" is sometimes required due to variances in the condition of trauma patients, but it is essential to understand when such events occur. During these times, additional error-producing conditions may exist and dominate the environment. Therefore, a heightened level of individual vigilance and team performance is needed to prevent complications as the greatest risk to the patient is when the surgeon and the team are outside this safety box but are not aware they are there. See Figure 1.1.

The "high-reliability mindset" ingrains in the adopter a sense of enhanced vigilance during such times when increased risk of error exists. The importance of the individual surgeon adopting this mindset in trauma care is emphasized by Helmreich who showed that, although individual error occurs infrequently, it leads to a high

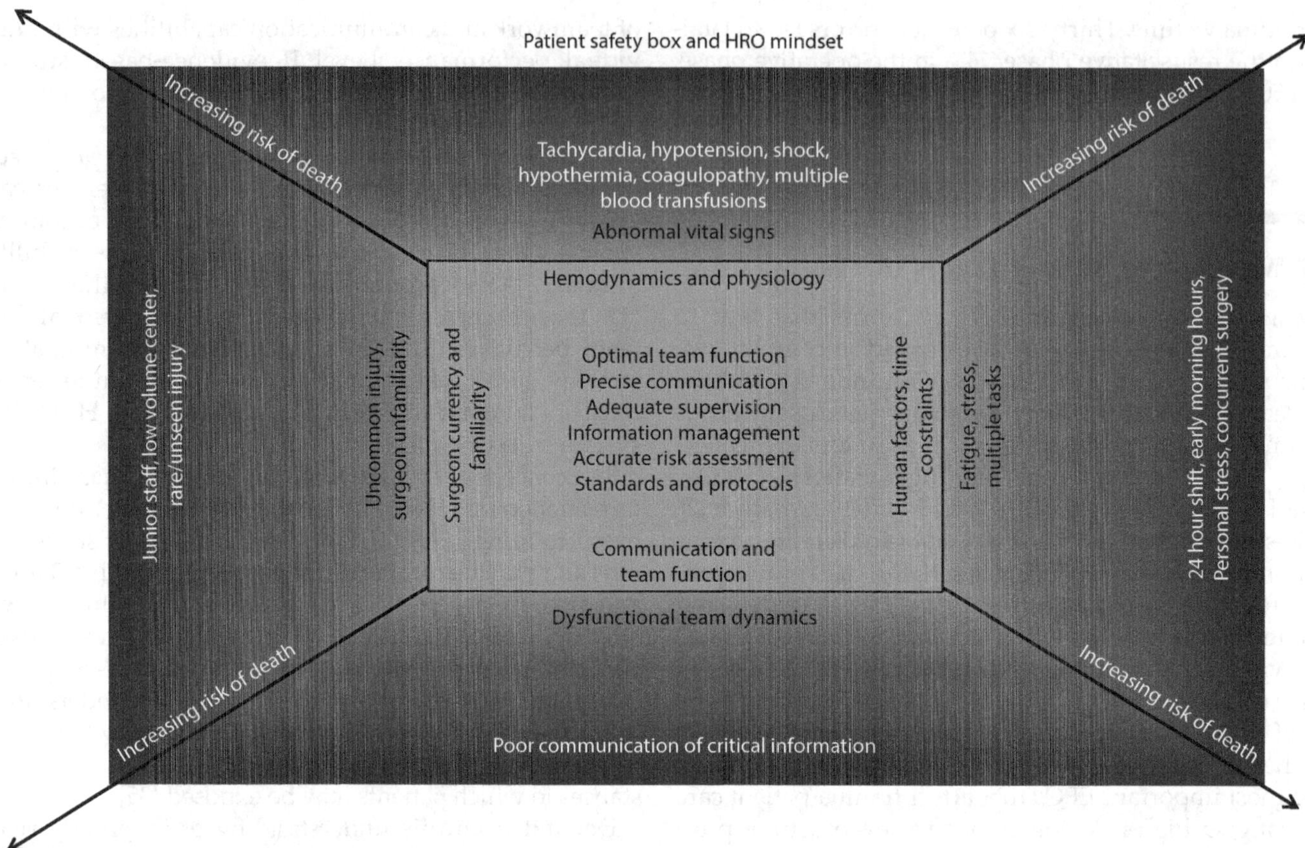


**FIGURE 1.1**
Conceptual model of the "high-reliability mindset" combines concepts of error avoidance by understanding circumstances when error is more likely to occur and strategies to manage these risks. The HRO mindset encompasses a global awareness of the "safety space" including a central "safety box" that defines the boundaries of safe operations with minimal risks of adverse outcome. The areas outside the box are also part of the overall safety mindset and predict increasing risk of error and conditions that make these errors more likely to occur. Best outcomes in the management of trauma victims come with the knowledge of the boundaries of the safety box, understanding risks of operating outside these boundaries, awareness of when the trauma surgeon and patient are outside the safety box, and a treatment strategy for returning inside the safety envelope.

risk of fatal or near-fatal outcomes [37]. This has critical implications in trauma care because of the role of human factors such as fatigue on individual performance.

### 1.7.1 Teamwork

Another integral part of the high-reliability mindset is teamwork. In every aspect of healthcare, teamwork has been shown to be more effective than non-team care [38]. Studies of high-performance, trained healthcare teams show a reduction in relative risk for major complication, reduction in relative risk of postoperative death, and reduction of postoperative length of stay [39]. Observational studies in the operating room have consistently demonstrated that training clinicians in teamwork skills provides important safety benefits [40–42].

Advanced teamwork skills include precise communication with "read-backs" and acknowledgments of understanding with "hear-backs" by team members to avoid errors while exchanging critical patient information. This also reduces the risk of adverse events occurring during the transfer of care and handoffs to other trauma teams [43]. Failure to carry out precise communications led to serious adverse patient consequences in over one-third of cases evaluated in a study of surgical information transfer within surgical teams [44]. A communication adjunct for high-reliability team skills is the use of aviation-style checklists to prevent team members from losing critical information. Published data document that checklists designed in a style that has been perfected in the cockpit can be adopted for team care of critically ill surgical patients with excellent results [45].

Another important team function is to define the roles and duties of each member of the trauma team. Key components of this training model have been taught as a curriculum known as "crew resource management" and emphasize organizing workloads and task assignments, clinical task planning, and review and critique strategies with preprocedure briefs and postprocedure debriefs.

Level II evidence-based data support the conclusion that these skills enhance the performance of the operating team leading to improved patient outcomes [16].

### 1.7.2 Simulation

HRO- and aviation-style simulation, both high and low fidelity, can be used to train and practice these key elements of the high-reliability mindset. Simulation training can be used for teaching safe trauma care because specific team actions as well as surgical tasks can be taught, practiced, and perfected in a simulated environment. A prospective observational study of trauma resuscitations demonstrated significant improvements in outcomes after aviation-style simulation practice sessions in study teams caring for multiple injured patients [46].

An innovative approach to teach safety in laparoscopic cholecystectomy designed to reduce the risk of common bile duct injury has been proposed, which is based on the aviation training principles of situational awareness and spatial disorientation [47]. This is an excellent demonstration of the cross-applicability of the two training methods and shows that simulated presentations of uncommon but critical scenarios that require immediate recognition and attention can be programmed and practiced for both pattern recognition and technical management skills [48].

## 1.8 Conclusions and Algorithm

Errors that lead to serious adverse outcomes in trauma management occur at a significant rate and can cause death in patients who might otherwise have survived their injuries. An understanding of the circumstances that make the occurrence of errors more likely is necessary to avoid adverse outcomes. Aviation and HRO safety theory can be used to teach individual skills and team behaviors that lead to enhanced trauma patient safety. These safety skills can be coalesced into a useful "high-reliability safety mindset" that forms overarching principles for the safe management of trauma patients. Successful adaption of these skills for use in our trauma practice and current curriculum training has been demonstrated [49]. Incorporation of this error understanding and avoidance strategy will help reduce the risks or unintended outcomes that trauma patients are exposed to during their hospital care (Table 1.1).

**TABLE 1.1**

Common Errors in Trauma and Error-Producing Conditions

| Common Errors in Trauma Care | Error-producing Conditions | Solutions |
|---|---|---|
| Resuscitation | | |
| Airway management | High-risk/low-frequency event<br>Information overload<br>One-way decision gate | Simulation training, procedural checklists, algorithms |
| Missed injuries on surveys | Poor information transfer<br>Time pressure<br>Information overload<br>Low signal to noise ratio<br>Volume overload and task saturation | Checklist use, adherence to established standard procedures, mass casualty simulation, drills |
| Inappropriate triage | Time pressure<br>Task overload<br>Faulty risk assessment<br>Normalization of deviance | Diminish reliance on "normal vitals and x-rays," high-level supervision |
| Operative | | |
| Delayed surgery | Time pressure<br>High-risk/low-frequency event<br>Task overload<br>Poor information transfer<br>Faulty risk assessment | Adherence to standards of care, teamwork decision-making, communication skills training |
| Prolonged surgery | Fatigue<br>Faulty risk assessment<br>Time pressure | Situational awareness strategies, team training and empowerment, HRO mindset adoption |
| Critical care | | |
| Missed diagnosis | Poor information transfer<br>High-risk/low-frequency event | Cognitive bias prevention strategies, simulation training |
| Prophylaxis | Lack of standardization<br>Faulty risk assessment<br>Inaccurate communication | Standardized orders, team training, communication skills training |

## References


1. Fitzgerald M, Cameron P, Mackenzie C et.al. Trauma resuscitation errors and computer-assisted decision support. *Arch Surg.* 2011;146(2):218–225.
2. Stahl KD, Brien SB. Reducing patient errors in trauma care. In: Cohn S, ed. *Acute Care Surgery: Evidenced-Based Practice.* Informa Healthcare USA Inc.: New York, pp. 276–287, 2009.
3. Pietro DA, Shyavitz LJ, Smith RA et al. Detecting and reporting medical errors; why the dilemma? *Br Med J.* 2000;320:794–798.
4. Weingart SN, Wison RM, Gibberd RW et al. Epidemiology of medical error. *Br Med J.* 2000;320:774–777.
5. Ivatury RR, Guilford K, Malhotra AK et al. Patient safety in trauma: Maximal impact management errors at a Level I trauma center. *J Trauma.* 2008;64:265–272.
6. Gruen RL, Jurkovich GJ, McIntyre LK et al. Patterns of errors contributing to trauma mortality: Lessons learned from 2594 deaths. *Ann Surg.* 2006;244:371–380.
7. Teixeira PG, Inaba K, Hadjizacharia P et al. Preventable or potentially preventable mortality at a mature trauma center. *J Trauma.* 2007;63:1338–1346.
8. Miniño AM, Anderson RN, Fingerhut LA et al. Deaths: Injuries, 2002. *National Vital Statistics Reports.* Vol. 54, No. 10. National Center for Health Statistics: Hyattsville, MD, pp. 32–37, 2006.
9. Institute of Medicine. *To Err Is Human: Building a Safer Health System.* National Academy Press: Washington, DC, 2000.
10. Ackroyd-Stolarz S, Read Guerney J, MacKinnon NJ et al. The association between a prolonged stay in the emergency department and adverse events in older patients admitted to hospital: A retrospective cohort study. *BMJ Qual Saf.* 2011;20:564–569.
11. Mackersie MC. Pitfalls in the evaluation and resuscitation of the trauma patient. *Emerg Med Clin N Am.* 2010;(28):1–27.
12. Houshian S, Larsen MS, Holm C. Missed injuries in a Level I trauma center. *J Trauma.* 2002;52:715–719.
13. Gonzalez RP, Ickler J, Gachassin P. Complementary roles of diagnostic peritoneal lavage and computed tomography in the evaluation of blunt abdominal trauma. *J Trauma.* December 2001;51(6):1128–1134.
14. Buduhan G, McRitchie D. Missed injuries in patients with multiple trauma. *J Trauma.* 2000;49:600–605.
15. Johnson J, Gracias V, Schwab C et al. Evolution in damage control for exsanguinating penetrating abdominal injury. *J Trauma.* 2001;51:261–271.
16. Cirocchi R, Montedori A. Damage control surgery for abdominal trauma. *Cochrane Database Syst Rev.* March 28, 2013;(3):1–14.
17. Epley N, Gilovich T. Putting adjustment back in the anchoring and adjustment heuristic: Differential processing of self-generated and experimenter-provided anchors. *Psychol Sci.* 2001;12(5):391–396.
18. McCarthy D, Blumenthal D. Committed to safety: Ten case studies on reducing harm to patients. The Commonwealth Fund, New York, April 2006.
19. Hurlbert S, Garrett J. Improving operating room safety. *Patient Saf Surg.* 2009;3:25.
20. Pronovost P, Freischlag JA. Improving teamwork to reduce surgical mortality. *JAMA* 2010;304(15):1721–1722.
21. Rothschild JM, Landrigan CP, Cronin JW et al. The critical care safety study: The incidence and nature of adverse events and serious medical errors in intensive care. *Crit Care Med.* 2005;33(8):1694–1700.
22. Orgeas MG, Timsit JF, Soufir L et al. Impact of adverse events on outcomes in intensive care unit patients. *Crit Care Med.* 2008;36(7):2041–2047.
23. Maxwell RA, Fabian TC. Croce M. Secondary abdominal compartment syndrome: An underappreciated manifestation of severe hemorrhagic shock. *J Trauma.* December 1999;47(6):995.
24. Lau G. Perioperative deaths: A further comparative review of coroner's autopsies with particular reference to the occurrence of fatal iatrogenic injury. *Ann Acad Med Singapore* July 2000;29(4):486–487.
25. Davis JW, Hoyt DB, McArdle MS et al. An analysis of errors causing morbidity and mortality in a trauma system: A guide for quality improvement. *J Trauma.* 1992;32:660–666.
26. Williams JC. A data-based method for assessing and reducing human error to improve operational performance. In: *Fourth IEEE Conference on Human Factors in Nuclear Power Plants*, Monterey, CA, pp. 436–450, June 6–9, 1988.
27. Hendy K. Defense R&D Canada—Toronto technical report DRDC Toronto TR 2002-057, March 2003.
28. Sundt TM, Brown JP, Uhlig PN, STS Workforce on Patient Advocacy, Communications, and Safety. Focus on patient safety: Good news for the practicing surgeon. *Ann Thorac Surg.* 2005;79:11–15.
29. Weick KE, Sutcliffe KM, Obstfeld D. Organizing for high reliability: Processes of collective mindfulness. *Crisis Manage.* 2008;3:31–67.
30. Shojania KG, Duncan BW, McDonald KM et al. eds. *Making Health Care Safer: A Critical Analysis of Patient Safety Practices.* Evidence Report/Technology Assessment No. 43 (Prepared by the University of California at San Francisco–Stanford Evidence-based Practice Center under Contract No. 290-97-0013), AHRQ Publication No. 01-E058. Agency for Healthcare Research and Quality: Rockville, MD, July 2001.
31. Risser DT, Rice MM, Salisbury ML et al. The potential for improved teamwork to reduce medical errors in the emergency department. The MedTeams Research Consortium. *Ann Emerg Med.* 1999;34:373–383.
32. Stahl K. Doctors don't die, pilots do (sometimes), and parachutes work. The Patient Safety Initiative Blog, http://www.thepatientsafetyinitiative.com/2011/04. Accessed November 23, 2014.
33. Stahl K, Brien S. Patient safety in surgical care. In: Stephen C, ed. *Surgery Evidenced-Based Practice.* People's Medical Publishing House: Shelton, Connecticut, pp. 14–22, 2012.
34. Wright R. Training's future. *Aviat Saf.* 2011;31(1):8–11.
35. Hollnagel E. *Barriers and Accident Prevention.* Ashgate Publishing Limited: Hampshire, U.K., 2004.
36. Reason J. *The Human Contribution.* Ashgate Publishing Ltd.: Farnham, England, 2008, pp. 265–279.

37. Helmreich R. On error management: Lessons from aviation. *BMJ*. 2000;320:781–785.
38. Jeffcott SA, MacKenzie CF. Measuring team performance in healthcare: Review of research and implications for patient safety. *J Crit Care*. 2008;23:188–196.
39. Bellomo R, Goldsmith S, Uchino J et al. Prospective controlled trial of effect of medical emergency team on post-operative morbidity and mortality rates. *Crit Care Med*. 2004;32(4);916–921.
40. Healey AN, Undre S, Vincent CA. Defining the technical skills of teamwork in surgery. *Qual Saf HealthCare*. 2004;15:231–234.
41. Awad SS, Fagan SP, Bellows C et al. Bridging the communication gap in the operating room with medical team training. *Am J Surg*. November 2005;190(5):770–774.
42. Lingard L, Epsin S, Whyte S et al. Communication failures in the operating room: An observational classification of recurrent types and effects. *Qual Saf Health*. 2004;13:330–334.
43. Arora V, Johnson J, Lovinger D et al. Communication failures in patient sign-out and suggestions for improvement: A critical incident analysis. *Qual Saf Health Care*. 2005;14:401–407.
44. Williams RG, Silverman R, Schwind C et al. Surgeon information transfer and communication: Factors affecting quality and efficiency of inpatient care. *Ann Surg*. 2007;245:159–169.
45. Stahl K, Palileo A, Schulman C et al. Enhancing patient safety in the trauma/surgical intensive care unit. *J Trauma*. 2009;67:430–435.
46. Holcomb JB, Dumire RD, Cormmett JW et al. Evaluation of trauma team performance using an advanced human patient simulator for resuscitation training. *J Trauma*. 2002;52:1078–1086.
47. Hugh TB. New strategies to prevent laparoscopic bile duct injury—Surgeons can learn from pilots. *Surgery* 2002;132(5):826–835.
48. Gaba DM. Anesthesiology as a model for patient safety in healthcare. *BMJ*. 2000;320:785–788.
49. Stahl K, Augenstein J, Schulman C. et al. Assessing the impact of teaching patient safety principles to medical students during surgical clerkship. *J Surg Res*. 2011:e1–e12.

# 2

# *Evidence-Based Injury Prevention Strategies*

**Michelle A. Price and Cynthia L. Villarreal**

**CONTENTS**



## 2.1 Introduction

Traumatic injury is a preventable disease. In the United States, unintentional and intentional injuries are the leading cause of death among persons aged <35 years and the fourth leading cause of death among persons of all ages [1]. In 2010, 180,811 persons in the United States suffered fatal injury, 2,529,169 were hospitalized and 28,550,424 were treated in emergency departments for nonfatal injuries. Medical treatment and work loss costs for civilian fatal and nonfatal injuries in the United States totaled more than $586 billion in 2005 [2]. These estimates, however, do not represent the true economic burden on society because they do not include the lives lost due to premature mortality, loss of patient and caregiver time, insurance costs, property damage, litigation, and diminished quality of life.

The development of trauma systems from the prehospital arena to rehabilitation services has been effective in reducing morbidity and mortality from injury. Nevertheless, 50% of deaths still occur at the scene or within minutes of the event. Thus, the mission of trauma care must also include injury prevention in addition to advances in resuscitation, definitive care, and rehabilitation. The American College of Surgeons (ACS) has recognized the importance of injury prevention initiatives in reducing the injury death and disability rate [3]. For this reason, an organized injury prevention program is required for trauma center verification. Similarly, the ACS Committee on Trauma has added a requirement for trauma centers to provide alcohol screening followed by a brief intervention for those testing positive for alcohol or those identified with an alcohol problem.

Injury prevention strategies in the health-care system are provided on a continuum ranging from hospital-funded community-based educational programs to anticipatory guidance in a primary care setting (prior to injury) and targeted interventions with injured patients with the goal of reducing the likelihood of future reinjury. Community education programs are usually conducted by trauma center outreach staff and include unintentional injury prevention (e.g., infant car seat installation training and home safety) and violence prevention programs (e.g., domestic violence and suicide prevention). The most effective programs are empirically based, conducted for a sufficient duration, and delivered in a culturally appropriate format to a cohesive target community [4].

In this chapter, we systematically review the available literature concerning the prevention of unintentional and violent injury and the effectiveness of physician-provided prevention counseling. We focus on the most prevalent mechanism of unintentional injury (motor vehicle collisions and falls) and violent injuries (e.g., domestic violence and handguns). Finally, we review the effectiveness of physician or health-care provider injury prevention counseling in primary care settings.

## 2.2 What Is the Estimated Number of Lives Saved by the Implementation of Primary Safety Belt Laws in the United States?

Motor vehicle traffic collisions are the leading cause of death among people aged 5–24 years in the United States [2]. Studies indicate that motor vehicle collisions are the leading cause of traumatic brain injuries, where the brain is injured in 70% of all collisions and the spinal cord in 5% of all collisions [5,6]. Unrestrained motor vehicle occupants account for 52% of the vehicle occupants killed on roadways in the United States [7]. Research has shown that safety belts are the single most effective means of reducing collision-related injury and mortality. Due to the fact that safety belts are very effective, laws have been established to encourage safety belt use. Safety belt laws are divided into two categories: primary and secondary. A primary safety belt law allows a law enforcement officer to stop a vehicle and issue a citation when the officer observes an unbelted driver or passenger in a motor vehicle, whereas secondary laws allow law enforcement officers to issue a ticket for not wearing a seat belt only when there is another citable traffic violation [8]. In the United States, only 34 states have primary safety belt use laws [9]. Over time, with the expansion of safety belt use laws to additional states, seat belt use rates have steadily increased, especially in the past decade in response to a national push to increase safety belt use.

Studies suggest that passing a primary law can increase safety belt use rates among nonusers by 40% [10]. In 1994, the overall observed shoulder belt use rate was 58%, a decade later, that number had risen to 80%, and in 2005, the national average was 82% [10]. Among states with primary versus secondary safety belt use laws, the average safety belt use rate was about 8% points higher in those states who had primary enforcement laws; 83 versus 75% [8]. In a study done by the Insurance Institute for Highway Safety [11], it was found that states that strengthened their laws from secondary enforcement to primary saw an estimated 7% decline in driver death rate. If the 28 states that still have secondary safety belt laws would have changed their safety belt law, more than 5000 lives could have been saved since 1996 [11]. The National Highway Traffic Safety Administration [10] suggests that lap/shoulder belts, when used properly, reduce the risk of fatal injury to front seat passenger car occupants by 45% and the risk of moderate to critical injury by 50%. Furthermore, for light truck occupants, safety belts reduce the risk of total injury by 60% and moderate to critical injury by 65%.

*Recommendation*: Educating patients and supporting community-based initiatives to increase safety belt use has great potential in the continuum of saving lives, preventing injuries, and reducing the economic costs associated with motor vehicle collisions. Physicians and other health-care providers should encourage patients to use safety belts, as well as participate in the policy-making process in those states without primary safety belt laws. Trauma surgeons can play a particularly poignant role in advocating for the passage of these laws, as they can speak to state legislators and the media regarding their experiences with motor vehicle collision patients who were unrestrained.

*Grade of recommendation*: A

## 2.3 What Evidence Exists on the Effectiveness of Screening and Brief Intervention for Alcohol Problems for Reducing Subsequent Injury among Emergency Room Patients?

In trauma systems today, estimates show that between 50% and 70% of patients have positive blood alcohol concentrations at the time of admission [12]. According to the Center for Disease Control and Prevention, alcohol is the leading contributor to both intentional and unintentional injuries [13]. Research has also shown that alcohol use contributes to patients having multiple traumatic injuries over time, supporting the need to provide screening and brief intervention (SBI) to reduce the likelihood of subsequent trauma among patients [14]. Yet, until recently, relatively few trauma patients who were under the influence of alcohol were screened for alcohol abuse, referred for treatment, or even acknowledged as having alcohol in their system. One of the greatest challenges to addressing alcohol problems is identifying patients who are in need of treatment. A promising technique is SBI. Hospital emergency rooms in many states are using this strategy to identify patients with problem drinking and addiction. In 2007, the ACS instituted the requirement that all ACS-verified Level I trauma centers screen all trauma patients for high-risk alcohol use and provide intervention to patients with elevated blood alcohol levels [14].

The purpose of SBI in trauma settings is to prevent substance abuse-related disabilities in persons at risk or to prevent further harm among those in the early stage of substance abuse [15]. SBI can be accomplished using a variety of tools that assist clinicians in asking about alcohol use, assessing the problem severity, advising the patient to decrease alcohol use, and monitoring progress. Two widely used brief instruments are Alcohol Use Disorders Identification Test (AUDIT) and CAGE. The AUDIT helps identify excessive drinking as the cause of the presenting illness and provides a framework for intervention to help risky drinkers reduce alcohol use (thus avoiding dangerous consequences) [16]. The CAGE instrument has been shown to be both sensitive and specific to identifying persons who meet criteria for alcohol abuse and dependence [17]. The CAGE is a very short and simple screening instrument that asks about attempting to *C*ut down on alcohol, being *A*nnoyed by other criticizing you about your drinking, feeling *G*uilty about drinking, and having an *E*ye-opener (an alcoholic beverage) in the morning.

SBI is not only effective in reducing subsequent injuries, but reduces alcohol-related costs to health-care facilities. Brief alcohol counseling sessions have reduced recidivism by 50% and have significantly reduced both binge drinking episodes and drinks consumed per week [18,19]. Studies have shown that SBI among trauma patients significantly reduces self-reported drinking, injuries, and other alcohol dependence symptoms [20–23]. Monti et al. [21] found that a single intervention session in the emergency department, versus standard treatment, reduced alcohol-related injuries 50 versus 21%. Gentilello found that a single 40 min session reduced weekly drinking by 22 drinks compared to 7 drinks among the control group, with a 47% reduction in hospital readmission among study participants [20].

Further, cost–benefit analysis research conducted by Gentilello et al. showed that SBI conducted in trauma centers could save hospitals $1.82 billion a year, and that for every dollar spent on screening and intervention, $3.81 in health-care costs was saved [19]. The Substance Abuse and Mental Health Services Administration indicates that trauma centers are in an ideal position to take advantage of the teachable moment generated from an injury by implementing SBI for at-risk and dependent drinkers [24]. Although data show that screening injured patients for the presence of an alcohol problem has been shown to reduce subsequent alcohol use, hospital readmissions, and related consequences, many trauma centers do not provide the service [19].

A review conducted by Field et al. (2010) suggests that the general efficacy of brief alcohol interventions is recognized as having mixed reviews [25]. The implementation of SBI varies from provider to provider, therefore; Eisenberg and Woodruff, recommend using provider training and development protocols that lead to high skill mastery [26]. With successful implementation of injury prevention strategies such as SBI, the overall public health approach available in trauma hospital settings will make great strides in improving prevention services among this vulnerable population (Table 2.1).

*Recommendation*: Trauma surgeons, emergency department physicians, and other health-care providers can detect alcohol problems using screening tools that are easy to administer, reliable, and effective in reducing repeat traumas. Screening tools and physician guides are available on the ACS website (https://www.facs.org/~/media/files/quality%20programs/trauma/publications/sbirtguide.ashx) and the National Institute of Alcohol Abuse and Alcoholism website (http://pubs.niaaa.nih.gov/publications/aa65/AA65.htm).

*Grade of recommendation*: A

## 2.4 What Are the Applications of Preventive Medicine to the Control of Domestic Violence?

Violence prevention encompasses a wide spectrum of interpersonal violence (i.e., child maltreatment, intimate partner violence [IPV], sexual violence, and elder abuse) and self-directed violence (i.e., self-harm and suicide). Much of the research on evidence-based prevention practices in health-care settings has focused on domestic or IPV. Annually, in the United States, women experience approximately 4.8 million IPV assaults or rapes and men experience about 2.9 million IPV assaults [27]. In a study of the prevalence of domestic violence victimization among women attending general practice, Richardson et al. found that 41% of female patients had experienced IPV and 17% had experienced it within the past year [28].

Health-care services play a central role in the care of IPV victims; however, the effectiveness of health-care professionals' responses has been a focus of concern since the 1970s [29]. Nelson et al. [30] systematically reviewed the evidence for screening women and the elderly for IPV and found that despite the extensive literature on IPV, few studies provide data on detection and management to guide clinicians. Ramsay et al. [31] conducted a systematic review of the effectiveness of health professional screening and intervention for IPV among women presenting in emergency departments, primary care

**TABLE 2.1**

Summary of Evidence-Based Injury Prevention Studies

| Author | References | Year | Evidence Level | Groups | Design | Median Follow-up | End Point |
|---|---|---|---|---|---|---|---|
| Dunn et al. | [18] | 2003 | II | Trauma patients (no control group) | CS | 6 and 12 months | Hazardous drinking patterns |
| Gentilello et al. | [19] | 2005 | II | Injured patients, 18 years or older, positive BAC | PCS | None | None |
| Monti et al. | [21] | 1999 | I | Motivation interview versus standard care | RCT | 3 and 6 months | Alcohol interventions, harm reduction |
| Longabaugh et al. | [22] | 2001 | I | Brief intervention versus brief intervention with booster session versus standard care | RCT | 12-months follow-up | Ongoing intervention, decrease alcohol recidivism |
| Hungerford et al. | [23] | 2003 | II | Convenience sample of alcohol positive patients | PCS | 4 months | Increased feasibility of alcohol screening and counseling |
| Nelson et al. | [30] | 2004 | II | Varied | SR | Varied | Varied |
| Ramsay et al. | [31] | 2002 | II | Varied | SR | Varied | Varied |
| Carbone et al. | [42] | 2005 | II | Gun safety counseling session, STOP 2 brochure plus a gun lock versus anticipatory guidance | PCS | 1 month | Gun ownership, gun storage practices |
| Albright and Burge | [48] | 2003 | I | Verbal counseling alone versus counseling plus a gun safety brochure versus no counseling | RCT | 60–90 days | Gun ownership, gun storage practices |
| Oatis et al. | [44] | 1999 | IV | STOP gun safety counseling plus brochure (no control group) | CS | ≥1 year | Gun ownership, gun storage practices |
| Grossman et al. | [45] | 2000 | I | Gun safety counseling with STOP brochure plus gun lock coupon versus standard care | RCT | 3 months | Gun ownership, gun storage practices |
| DiGuiseppi and Roberts | [51] | 2000 | I | Varied | SR | Varied | Varied |
| DiGuiseppi and Higgins | [52] | 2001 | I | Varied | SR | Varied | Varied |
| Bass et al. | [53] | 1993 | II | Varied | SR | Varied | Varied |

*Note:* CS, case study; RCT, randomized controlled trial; PCS, prospective cohort study; BAC, blood alcohol content; SR, systematic review.

facilities, or antenatal clinics. Eight of the nine screening studies found higher rates of IPV identification at the sites utilizing various screening tools. However, the one randomized controlled trial did not find evidence of increased identification rates related to the introduction of screening procedures [32]. The authors also reviewed six studies evaluating the effectiveness of IPV interventions in health-care settings and found no relation between type of intervention or health-care setting and the effect of the intervention [31]. In 2012, Klevens et al. conducted a randomized clinical trial at 10 primary health-care centers and found that providing a partner violence resource list with or without screening did not result in improved health [33]. In 2013, Taft et al. reviewed 11 trials that recruited 13,027 women and found that while screening was not harmful, there is insufficient evidence to justify universal screening in health-care settings [34].

*Recommendation*: IPV screening programs moderately increase rates of victim identification in health-care settings; however, there is limited evidence of effectiveness of associated interventions. Therefore, it would be premature to recommend implementation of a universal screening program. Further research utilizing randomized clinical trials is required to better quantify the effectiveness of IPV prevention strategies in health-care settings. Health-care professionals should, however, receive training on selectively screening for IPV for patients who meet specific criteria with well-validated, brief screening tools such as the Hurt, Insulted, Threatened, or Screamed at instrument [35] or the Partner Violence Screen instrument [36].

*Grade of recommendation*: B

## 2.5 What Is the Evidence for the Effectiveness of Clinician Counseling Regarding Firearm Safety?

In 2012, there were 33,563 firearm deaths in the United States (or 10.5 deaths per 100,000 population) [37]. Since the mid-1980s, organized medicine has crafted policies and programs to reduce firearm morbidity and mortality [38]. Longjohn and Christoffel found 5 consensus areas among 14 national medical societies: access prevention, gun commerce, research, public education, and clinical counseling [39]. The American Academy of Pediatrics recommends violence prevention anticipatory guidance at every health maintenance visit, including urging gun removal from homes [40]. However, the evidence on the effectiveness of patient counseling regarding gun removal or safer storage behaviors has been equivocal [41]. In an investigation of gun safety counseling coupled with a gun lock giveaway in a pediatric outpatient setting, Carbone et al. [42] found significant improvements in safe gun storage behaviors among families in the intervention group (62%) versus the control group (27%). In a similar study conducted in a family practice clinic, Albright and Burge [43] found improved gun storage behaviors among gun-owning patients who received either verbal counseling alone (64%) or verbal counseling plus a gun safety brochure (58%) compared to controls (33%). Conversely, two earlier studies that used Steps to Prevent Firearm Injury (STOP) did not find significant effects. Oatis et al. [44] did not find statistically significant declines in gun ownership or improvement in gun storage practices among participants who received gun safety counseling and written materials during a well-child visit at a pediatric practice. Similarly, Grossman et al. found that the gun safety counseling intervention did not lead to changes in gun ownership or significant changes in storage practices [45].

In the aftermath of the school shooting that killed 20 children and 6 educators in Newtown, Connecticut, President Obama issued 23 executive orders directing federal agencies to improve knowledge of the causes of firearm violence, prevention efforts, and strategies to reduce the public health burden of firearm violence. The Centers for Disease Control and Prevention (CDC) commissioned the Institute of Medicine to develop a research agenda based on gaps in the evidence [46]. The Institute of Medicine (IOM) research agenda focuses on the characteristics of firearm violence, risk and protective factors, interventions and strategies, gun safety technology and the influence of video games and other media [47]. Among the priorities for research on prevention and other intervention, the IOM report called for research to determine the degree to which various childhood education or prevention programs (including routine primary care counseling) reduce firearm violence.

*Recommendation*: Research on the effectiveness of physician counseling regarding gun removal and safe storage has been limited with mixed results. Further study is warranted cost–benefit ratio of these brief interventions is warranted [48].

*Grade of recommendation*: B

## 2.6 What Is the Effectiveness of Injury Prevention Counseling Delivered by a Health-Care Provider in Improving Safety Practices among Pediatric Patients?

Unintentional injuries are a leading cause of death for all Americans, regardless of age, race, gender, or economic status [13]. In particular, injury is the leading cause of death and a substantial cause of disability for children and adolescents [49]. Given the pervasive and preventable nature of these injuries, injury prevention counseling or anticipatory guidance should be integrated into physician visits and other health-care settings to educate parents, caretakers, and children about age-appropriate behavioral risks and safety strategies. However, the proportion of children receiving injury prevention counseling was relatively unchanged from 40% in 1994 to 42.4% in 2003 [50].

Injury prevention topics for office-based counseling include motor vehicle restraints, smoke detectors, pool fencing, hazards of infant walkers, and the safe storage of poisons and medications. There is sufficient evidence that clinical counseling can influence child safety seat use and use of a functioning smoke alarm in the home [51–53]. Due to the fact that children and adolescents are at greatest risk for concussions, it is important that injury prevention counseling encompass topics such as helmet use, seat belt or restraint system use, and the use of protective equipment while participating in athletic activities [54]. A review of the literature on childhood injury prevention counseling in primary care settings illustrated that the majority of studies, 18 of 20, demonstrated positive outcomes in increasing overall knowledge and safety practices along with decreasing childhood injury rates [53]. Furthermore, a systematic review of over 22 randomized controlled trials of a variety of injury prevention interventions in clinical settings suggested a strong improvement in safety practices, which included child safety seat and safety belt restraint use [51].

Research shows that parents and children are often receptive to injury prevention counseling during a sick visit, especially if it is related to an injury, a recent emergency department visit, or injury to a sibling [55]. Due to the fact that pediatricians come into contact with parents a great deal in the first 5 years of a child's life for routine care, the American Academy of Pediatrics and Bright Futures recommends that clinicians use this opportunity to provide injury prevention counseling [56,57]. The Injury Prevention Program, developed in 1983 by the American Academy of Pediatrics, includes a safety counseling schedule, age-appropriate safety sheets for families, and interventions that have been proven to effectively improve safety practices among parents and caregivers [53,58,59].

*Recommendation*: Physicians and health-care providers should use routine doctor visits, emergency department visits, and other health-care visits as teachable moments to educate the patient and their parent on age-appropriate injury prevention.

*Grade of recommendation*: A

## 2.7 What Is the Effectiveness of Injury Prevention and Medication Safety Counseling Delivered by a Health-Care Provider in Improving Safety Practices among Geriatric Patients?

As our population continues to grow, the number of older adults is on the rise. Older adults are at an increased risk for various types of unintentional injuries [60,61]. Unintentional injures rank among the top 10 leading causes of death and disability among adults aged 65 years and older with falls and motor vehicle crashes as leading causes [60]. According to Rosen et al., falls are the most common cause of injury death, hospitalization, and emergency department visits in this population with various injuries such as hip fractures and traumatic brain injuries [61]. The study suggests that injury prevention counseling be conducted by emergency physical and primary care physicians regarding fall prevention strategies such as asking about environmental circumstances surrounding an incident and suggesting potential modifications [61]. In 2010, the CDC published a compendium of effective fall interventions for older adults recommending exercise interventions to maintain or improve balance and mobility and home environment modifications [62].

Furthermore, injury prevention counseling to older adults on medication safety can be used as a strategy to reduce unintentional poisoning exposures to this population. Health-care providers are in a position to educate patients on medication safeguards such as how to read and follow prescriptions, importance of taking medications on time, and discarding old unused medications. Health-care providers should also use medication reviews to assess potential issues that may lead to falls [61]. A combination of strategies such as medication discharge summaries coupled with medication safety counseling, and reminder cards can lead to improved patient outcomes [63]. A study conducted by Shields et al. provides evidence that the majority of older adults are not aware of vital safety information needed to protect themselves adequately [64]. As trusted providers, health-care providers must maximize encounters with this population to increase awareness and reduce injury risks (Table 2.2).

**TABLE 2.2**
Evidence-Based Injury Prevention Summary

| No. | Question | Answer | Grade | References |
|---|---|---|---|---|
| 1 | Do state-based primary enforcement safety belt laws save lives in the United States? | Evidence supports the benefit of primary belt laws in reducing injuries and fatalities. | A | [8,10,11] |
| 2 | What evidence exists on the effectiveness of SBI for alcohol problems for reducing subsequent injury among emergency room patients? | Evidence supports SBI to reduce short-term recidivism, but additional research on long-term effects is needed. | A | [16,18–26] |
| 3 | What are the applications of preventive medicine to the control of domestic violence? | Screening programs increase victim identification however evidence on intervention effectiveness is limited. | B | [30–36] |
| 4 | What is the evidence for the effectiveness of clinician counseling regarding firearm safety? | Evaluation of gun safety programs in primary care settings have resulted in inconsistent outcomes. | B | [41–45] |
| 5 | What is the effectiveness of injury prevention counseling delivered by a health-care provider in improving safety practices among pediatric patients? | There is sufficient evidence to suggest that injury prevention counseling improves safety practices among the pediatric population. | A | [51–55] |
| 6 | What is the effectiveness of injury prevention and medication safety counseling delivered by a health-care provider in improving safety practices among geriatric patients? | There is sufficient evidence to support educating aging patients on injury prevention and medication safety. | A | [60–64] |

*Recommendation*: Physicians and health-care providers should use routine doctor visits, emergency department visits, and other health-care visits as teachable moments to educate aging patients on injury prevention and medication safety.

*Grade of recommendation*: A

## 2.8 Conclusions

Physicians in office-based practices, hospital outpatient/follow-up clinics, and emergency departments all have a unique opportunity to educate patients on injury prevention. Major influences in physicians' decisions to incorporate injury prevention counseling into routine care include physicians' confidence in their ability to counsel, perceptions regarding counseling effectiveness, training, practice setting, and office time constraints. Injury prevention counseling does not have to be very time-consuming and extensive, but rather substantive enough to increase knowledge. Effective prevention programs can include physician or nurse counseling, the use of computerized education materials, public service announcements, and educational videos in waiting areas. Due to the fact that physicians and health-care providers have time constraints, the most efficient strategy is to educate patients or caregivers on specific topics that are appropriate for the patient's age, time of year, and other common injuries seen in that population.

## Source of Funding and Disclaimer

This work was partially funded (M.A.P.) by NTI Subaward # NTI-TRA-10-101 from the National Trauma Institute and sponsored by the Department of the Army, Prime award #W81XWH-11-1-0841. The U.S. Army Medical Research Acquisition Activity, 820 Chandler Street, Fort Detrick MD 21702-5014 is the awarding and administering acquisition office. The opinions or assertions contained herein are the private views of the authors and are not to be construed as official or as reflecting the view of the Department of the Army or the Department of Defense.

## References

1. Centers for Disease Control and Prevention. 2002. Web-based Injury Statistics Query and Reporting System (WISQARS). US Department of Health and Human Services, National Center for Injury Prevention and Control. Atlanta, GA.
2. Centers for Disease Control and Prevention and National Center for Injury Prevention and Control. 2014. Web-based Injury Statistics Query and Reporting System (WISQARS). Atlanta, GA. Available from: http://www.cdc.gov/injury/wisqars (cited November 24, 2014).
3. American College of Surgeons Committee on Trauma. 2006. Resources for optimal care of the injured patient. Chicago, IL.
4. Nilsen, P. What makes community based injury prevention work? In search of evidence of effectiveness. *Inj Prev.* 2004;10(5):268–274.
5. Ruff RM, Marshall LF, Klauber MR et al. Alcohol abuse and neurological outcome of the severely head injured. *J Head Trauma Rehabil.* 1990;5:21–31.
6. Kreutzer JS, Doherty K, Harris J et al. Alcohol abuse among persons with traumatic brain injury. *J Head Trauma Rehabil.* 1990;5:9–20.
7. U.S. Department of Transportation and National Highway Traffic Safety Administration. 2014. Quick Facts 2012, pp. 1–6.
8. National Highway Traffic Safety Administration. 2004. Traffic Safety Facts: Strengthening safety belt use laws—Increase belt use, decrease crash fatalities and injuries. U.S. Department of Transportation: Washington, DC.
9. Governors Highway Safety Association. State Seat Belt Laws. 2015 (cited 2015 08/04/2015); Available from: http://www.ghsa.org/html.stateinfo/laws/seatbelt_laws.html.
10. National Highway Traffic Safety Administration. 2007. Traffic Safety Facts: Estimated minimum savings to a state's Medicaid budget by implementing a primary seat belt law. U.S. Department of Transportation: Washington, DC.
11. Insurance Institute for Highway Safety. 2005. Effectiveness of primary belt laws. Arlington, VA.
12. Cowperthwaite MC, Burnett MG. Treatment course and outcomes following drug and alcohol-related traumatic injuries. *J Trauma Manage Outcomes* 2011;5:3.
13. Centers for Disease Control and Prevention. 2007. Web-based Injury Statistics Query and Reporting System (WISQARS). US Department of Health and Human Services, National Center for Injury Prevention and Control. Atlanta, GA.
14. American College of Surgeons Committee on Trauma. 2007. Alcohol screening and brief intervention for trauma patients. Chicago, IL.
15. Babor TF, Kadden RM. Screening and interventions for alcohol and drug problems in medical settings: What works? *J Trauma Injury Infect Crit Care* 2005;59(3):S80–S87.
16. Saunders JB, Aasland OG, Babor TF et al. Development of the Alcohol Use Disorders Identification test (AUDIT): WHO collaborative project on early detection of persons with harmful alcohol consumption-II. *Addiction* 1993;88:791–804.
17. Ewing JA. Detecting alcohol: The CAGE questionnaire. *JAMA.* 1984;252(14):1905–1907.
18. Dunn CW, Zatzick DF, Russo J. Hazardous drinking by trauma patients during the year after injury. *J Trauma Injury Infect Crit Care* 2003;54(4):707–712.

19. Gentilello LM, Ebel BE, Wickizer TM et al. Alcohol interventions for trauma patients treated in emergency departments and hospitals: A cost benefit analysis. *Ann Surg.* 2005;241(4):541–550
20. Gentilello LM, Rivara FP, Donovan DM. Alcohol interventions in a trauma center as means of reducing the risk of injury recurrence. *Ann Surg.* 1999;230:473–483.
21. Monti PM, Colby SM, Barnett NP. Brief intervention for harm reduction with alcohol positive older adolescents in a hospital emergency department. *J Consult Clin Psychol.* 1999;67:989–994.
22. Longabaugh R, Woolard RF, Nirenbert TD. Evaluating the effects of a brief motivational intervention for injured drinkers in the emergency department. *J Stud Alcohol* 2001;62:806–816.
23. Hungerford DW, Williams JM, Furbee PM. Feasibility of screening and intervention for alcohol problems among young adults. *Am J Emerg Med.* 2003;21:14–22.
24. Substance Abuse and Mental Health Services Administration. 2006. Results from the 2005 National Survey on Drug Use and Health: National Findings, in Series H-30. Washington, DC.
25. Field CA, Baird J, Saitz R et al. The mixed evidence for brief intervention in emergency departments, trauma care centers, and inpatient hospital settings: What should we do? *Alcohol Clin Exp Res.* 2010;34(12):2004–2010.
26. Eisenberg K, Woodruff SI. Randomized controlled trial to evaluate screening and brief intervention for drug-using multiethnic emergency and trauma department patients. *Addict Sci Clin Practice* 2013;8(1):8.
27. Tjaden P, Thoennes N. 2000. Extent, nature, and consequences of intimate partner violence: Findings from the National Violence Against Women Survey. Department of Justice: Washington, DC.
28. Richardson J, Coid J, Petruckevitch A et al. Identifying domestic violence: Cross sectional study in primary care. *BMJ* 2002;324(7332):274.
29. Stark E, Flitcraft A. 1996. *Women at Risk: Domestic Violence and Women's Health.* Sage: London, U.K.
30. Nelson HD, Nygren P, McInerney Y et al. Screening women and elderly adults for family and intimate partner violence: A review of the evidence for the U.S. Preventive Services Task Force. *Ann Intern Med.* 2004;140(5):387–404.
31. Ramsay J, Richardson J, Carter YH et al. Should health professionals screen women for domestic violence? Systematic review. *BMJ* 2002;325(7359):314.
32. Thompson RS, Rivara FP, Thompson DC et al. Identification and management of domestic violence: A randomized clinical trial. *Am J Prevent Med.* 2000;19:253–263.
33. Klevens J, Kee R, Trick W et al. Effect of screening for partner violence on women's quality of life: A randomized controlled trial. *JAMA* 2012;308(7):681–689.
34. Taft A, O'Doherty L, Hegarty K et al. Screening women for intimate partner violence in healthcare settings. *Cochrane Database Systemat Rev.* 2013;4:1–72.
35. Sherin KM, Sinacore JM, Li XQ et al. HITS: A short domestic violence screening tool for use in a family practice setting. *Family Med.* 1998;30:508–512.
36. Feldhaus KM, Koziol-McLain J, Amsbury HL et al. Accuracy of 3 brief screening questions for detecting partner violence in the emergency department. *JAMA.* 1997;277:1357 1361.
37. National Vital Statistics System. 2012. Age-adjusted death rates = # of deaths per 100,000 total population. Atlanta, GA.
38. United States Department of Health and Human Services, Bureau of Maternal and Child Health and Resources Development, and Office of Maternal and Child Health. 1986. Surgeon general's workshop on violence and public health. US Department of Health and Human Services: Rockville, MD.
39. Longjohn MM, Christoffel KK. Are medical societies developing a standard for gun injury prevention? *Injury Prevent.* 2004;10:169–173.
40. American Academy of Pediatrics; Committee of Practice and Ambulatory Medicine. Recommendations for preventive pediatric health care. *Pediatrics* 2000;105: 645–646.
41. Dowd MD. Firearm injury prevention: Reasons for optimism. *Arch Pediatr Adolesc Med.* 2005;159(11):1081–1082.
42. Carbone PS, Clemens CJ, Ball TM. Effectiveness of gun-safety counseling and a gun lock giveaway in a Hispanic community. *Arch Pediatr Adolesc Med.* 2005;159(11):1049–1054.
43. Albert WG, Simpson RI. Evaluating an educational program for the prevention of impaired driving among grade 11 students. *J Drug Educ.* 1985;15(1):57–71.
44. Oatis PJ, Fenn Buderer NM, Cummings P et al. Pediatric practice based evaluation of the Steps to Prevent Firearm Injury program. *Injury Prevent.* 1999;5(1):48–52.
45. Grossman DC, Cummings P, Koepsell TD et al. Firearm safety counseling in primary care pediatrics: A randomized, controlled trial. *Pediatrics* 2000;106(1):22–26.
46. Kuehn BM. IOM details an ambitious agenda for US gun violence research. *JAMA* 2013;310(1):21.
47. Institute of Medicine and National Research Council of the National Academies; Committee on Priorities for a Public Health Research Agenda to Reduce the Threat of Firearm-Related Violence; Leshner, A. et al., eds. 2013. *Priorities for Research to Reduce the Threat of Firearm-Related Violence.* The National Academy of the Sciences: Washington, DC.
48. Albright TL, Burge SK. Improving firearm storage habits: Impact of brief office counseling by family physicians. *J Am Board Fam Pract* 2003;16(1):40–46.
49. Pressley JC, Barlow BA. Preventing injury and injury-related disability in children and adolescents. *Sem Pediatr Surg.* 2004;13:133–140.
50. Chen J, Kresnow MJ, Simon TR et al. Injury-prevention counseling and behavior among US children: Results from the second Injury Control and Risk Survey. *Pediatrics* 2007;119(4):958–965.
51. DiGuiseppi C, Roberts IG. Individual-level injury prevention strategies in the clinical setting. *Future Child* 2000;10:53–82.
52. DiGuiseppi C, Higgins JP. Intervention for promoting smoke alarm ownership and function. *Cochrane Database Systemat Rev.*, 2001;2001(2):CD002246.

53. Bass JL, Christoffel KK, Widome M et al. Childhood injury prevention counseling in primary care settings: A critical review of the literature. *Pediatrics* 1993;92:544–550.
54. U.S. Department of Health and Human Services and Centers for Disease Control and Prevention. 2009. Heads up: Facts for physicians about mild traumatic brain injury (MTBI), in Facts for Physicians. Atlanta, GA.
55. Gielen AC, Wilson MEH, McDonald EM et al. Randomized trial of enhanced anticipatory guidance for injury prevention. *Arch Pediatr Adolesc Med.* 2001;155:42–49.
56. Green M, ed. 1994. *Bight Futures: Guidelines for Health Supervision of Infants, Children, and Adolescents.* National Center for Education in Maternal and Child Health: Arlington, VA.
57. Committee on Practice and Ambulatory Management. Recommendation for preventive health care. *Pediatrics* 1995;96:373.
58. Gardner HG. Office-based counseling for unintentional injury prevention. *Pediatrics* 2007;119(1):202–206.
59. Barkin S, Fink A, Gelber L. Predicting clinician injury prevention counseling for young children. *Arch Pediatr Adolesc Med.* 1999;153:1226–1231.
60. Scheetz LJ. Life-threatening injuries in older adults. *AACN Adv Crit Care* 2011;22(2):128–139; quiz 140–141.
61. Rosen T, Mack KA, Noonan RK. Slipping and tripping: Fall injuries in adults associated with rugs and carpets. *J Injury Violence Res.* 2013;5(1):61–69.
62. Centers for Disease Control and Prevention. 2010. *Compendium of Effective Fall Interventions: What Works for Community-Dwelling Older Adults.* United States Department of Health and Human Services: Atlanta, GA.
63. Al-Rashed SA, Wright DJ, Roebuck N et al. The value of inpatient pharmaceutical counselling to elderly patients prior to discharge. *Br J Clin Pharmacol.* 2002;54(6):657–664.
64. Shields WC, Perry EC, Szanton SL et al. Knowledge and injury prevention practices in homes of older adults. *Geriatric Nurs.* 2013;34(1):19–24.

## Commentary on Evidence-Based Injury Prevention Strategies

*Avery B. Nathens*

In 1966, the National Academy of Sciences published *Accidental Death and Disability: the Neglected Disease of Modern Society,* which revolutionized how injuries were managed in North America. The publication of this report led to a number of developments in acute care for trauma victims including regional trauma systems to ensure access and designated trauma centers to ensure high-quality care. These efforts have led to tremendous reductions in injury-related mortality. Today, most deaths occur very early after the injury incident, with approximately half occurring at the scene and the vast majority of the remainder occurring within the first 24–48 h after arrival to hospital—often due to exsanguinating hemorrhage or severe traumatic brain injury. Clearly, the implementation of injury prevention initiatives with a strong evidence base will reduce injury-related mortality. Effective injury prevention initiatives have the potential for tremendous societal benefit.

It is this potential for benefit that underlies the American College of Surgeons' requirement for trauma centers to implement their own injury prevention programs. With the exception of alcohol screening and brief intervention, which is specified separately, the nature and scope of these programs are determined locally. Many of these programs might have limited effectiveness and are rarely scrutinized to the extent of other trauma center verification criteria. The implementation of injury prevention programs without an evidence base leads to trauma center stakeholders "feeling good" about their potential contributions to their local community but might have opportunity costs where budgets and human resources are limited.

Implementation of evidence-based injury prevention strategies is very different from other medical interventions. Specifically, only in this particular area is there a need to balance what might be good for the individual and/or society at large with potential infringements on civil liberties. This theme will become apparent in my commentary on some the questions addressed in this chapter.

### What Is the Estimated Number of Lives Saved by the Implementation of Primary Safety Belt Laws in the United States?

There is no question that relevant legislation and enforcement of restraint use saves lives with primary restraint laws more effective than secondary restraint laws. New York State was the first state to put in place restraint legislation in 1984. Over 30 years later, only 33 states have primary restraint laws and one state has no seat belt legislation relevant to adults (New Hampshire)*. The variability in the scope of legislation—e.g., some laws cover front seat use and/or back seat use, and/or children—suggests that evidence-based legislation is a more practical challenge with barriers related to a need to balance civil liberties and injury prevention. For example, the American Civil Liberties Union's opposition is that primary restraint laws give "law enforcement one more reason to unfairly target and selectively enforce laws against motorists who legitimately fear being stopped based solely on their appearances" (i.e., racial profiling)†. As well, such a law would give law enforcement further power to harass law-abiding citizens and erode the privacy and personal freedom of law-abiding citizens. In theory, because it is difficult to see through tinted windows or to tell if backseat passengers are wearing seat belts, almost any vehicle on the road could come under suspicion‡.

### What Evidence Exists on the Effectiveness of Screening and Brief Intervention for Alcohol Problems for Reducing Subsequent Injury among Emergency Room Patients?

The strong foundation of evidence underlying alcohol screening and brief intervention in trauma centers has led to this becoming a requirement for verification by the American College of Surgeons. In controlled clinical studies where the intervention is offered by well-trained, engaged providers, this intervention appears to be very effective. What isn't clear, however, is how effective this program might be with broad implementation where the intervention is being provided outside of a clinical study. Acknowledging the potential for diminished effectiveness in this context, there is work underway to understand how best to educate providers. The Disseminating Organizational Screening and Brief Intervention Services (DO-SBIS) for Alcohol at Trauma

* Governor's Highway Association. Seatbelt Laws (February 2015). Accessed February 3, 2015 at http://www.ghsa.org/html/stateinfo/laws/seatbelt_laws.html.

† American Civil Liberties Union of Ohio (April 1999). ACLU of Ohio opposes primary seat belt legislation. Accessed February 3, 2015 at http://www.acluohio.org/archives/press-releases/aclu-of-ohio-opposes-primary-seat-belt-legislation.

‡ American Civil Liberties Union of Nevada (February 2009). Opposition to S.B. 116, making the failure to wear a safety belt a primary offense. Accessed February 3, 2015 at http://aclunv.org/files/SB116_Primary-Seatbelt.pdf.

Centers Study is a randomized controlled trial designed to evaluate how workshop training in evidence-based motivational interviewing interventions might impact provider interviewing skills and patient alcohol consumption*. While there is no doubt that incorporating ASBI into the ACS trauma center verification requirements was a coup for injury prevention advocates, implementation as it was designed is critical to ensure patients and society reap the benefits.

### What Are the Applications of Preventive Medicine to the Control of Domestic Violence?

The authors cover this relatively broad topic markedly well and conclude that there is only limited evidence for effective prevention strategies in health care settings for intimate partner violence (IPV). The authors indicate that healthcare professionals should receive training on selectively screening for IPV and indicate that the limited effectiveness is likely related to the availability of effective intervention programs.

There is no doubt that screening for IPV is high yield. In an international assessment of the prevalence of IPV in orthopedic fracture clinics, 1 in 6 women had a history of physical abuse and one in 50 injured women presented to clinic as a direct result of IPV†. In spite of the benefits of screening, it is evident that we have a long way to go before broad use of screening tools in surgical practice. In a qualitative analysis of orthopedic surgery trainees, residents did not see their faculty mentors screen patients or advocate for screening‡. Further, they did not view IPV screening or intervention as part of their role as a surgeon. Their focus was primarily "getting through clinic" and "dealing with the surgical problem."

In the absence of strong evidence for effectiveness and many other competing priorities, IPV screening by surgeons in the acute care environment is simply not practicable. Perhaps screening done by other providers might be possible, but the benefits would be contingent on having suitable intervention strategies.

### What Is the Evidence for the Effectiveness of Clinician Counseling regarding Firearm Safety?

The authors conclude that research on the effectiveness of physician counseling regarding gun removal and safe storage has been limited and the results somewhat mixed. They call for further study on the cost–benefits of these brief interventions related to firearm safety. It would appear that very brief interventions and even the provision of reading materials would have very limited cost. Given the potential benefit and low cost, it would seem that the right thing to do would be clear. That it is not might speak to other barriers.

One such barrier might be the sensitivities related to these discussions in the broader context of the gun control debate in the United States. For example, the "Docs vs. Glocks law" in Florida prohibits physicians from asking patients about their ownership of guns or recording that information in medical records unless it is medically necessary§. The primary intent of this law is to protect the privacy of firearms owners. Like the controversy surrounding the benefits of any firearm legislation and the challenges in using federal research monies to study gun control, this is an area where the politics of prevention will likely stymy further research for years to come.

### What Is the Effectiveness of Injury Prevention Counseling Delivered by a Health Care Provider in Improving Safety Practices among (1) Pediatric and (2) Elderly Patients?

The evidence behind counseling relevant to injury prevention in children and the geriatric population in the outpatient setting appears to be strong and incontrovertible. However, when it comes to the elderly, the challenges, particularly related to the preservation of autonomy, become considerable. This is one of the reasons why "mature driver" laws are relatively controversial. Should re-evaluation of skills, more frequent license renewal, or vision testing be required on the basis of age alone? The single published nationwide study suggests

* Zatzick DF, Donovan DM, Dunn C et al. Disseminating Organizational Screening and Brief Intervention Services (DO-SBIS) for alcohol at trauma centers study design. *Gen Hosp Psychiatry*. 2013 March–April;35(2):174–180.

† PRAISE Investigators, Sprague S, Bhandari M, Della Rocca GJ, Goslings JC, Poolman RW, Madden K, Simunovic N, Dosanjh S, Schemitsch EH. Prevalence of abuse and intimate partner violence surgical evaluation (PRAISE) in orthopaedic fracture clinics: A multinational prevalence study. *Lancet*. 2013 September 7;382(9895):866–876.

‡ Gotlib Conn L, Young A, Rotstein OD, Schemitsch E. "I've never asked one question." Understanding the barriers among orthopedic surgery residents to screening female patients for intimate partner violence. *Can J Surg*. 2014 December;57(6):371–378.

§ Associated Press (July 2014). Federal Court Upholds Fla.'s Docs vs. Glocks Law. *New York Times*. Accessed February 4, 2015 at http://www.nytimes.com/aponline/2014/07/25/us/ap-us-docs-vs-glocks.html?_r=0.

there is no benefit to this form of legislation*. Perhaps the only prevention strategy to address safety in older drivers is the requirement for "in-person" license renewal†. It is likely that in-person renewal selects out unsafe or severely debilitated elderly drivers from re-licensure.

There might be a more appropriate approach than screening based on age. Many jurisdictions require the reporting of patients to motor-vehicle licensing authorities if there is a belief that they have a condition that might make it dangerous to operate a motor vehicle. Typically, physician compliance with reporting is poor. However, there is evidence to suggest that this is a very effective injury prevention strategy with a 45% reduction in the rate of motor-vehicle crashes following a reporting event‡. The impact on autonomy cannot be overstated. In this same study, patients who were reported had higher rates of depression and were less likely to return to the reporting physician. These data suggest that reporting has value but should be used when only appropriate.

* Bell TM, Qiao N, Zarzaur BL. Mature Driver Laws and State Predictors of Motor Vehicle Crash Fatality Rates among the Elderly: A Cross-sectional Ecological Study. *Traffic Inj Prev.* 2015 January 8;16(7):669–676.

† Grabowski DC, Campbell CM, Morrisey MA. Elderly licensure laws and motor vehicle fatalities. *J Am Med Assoc.* 2004 June 16;291(23):2840–2846.

‡ Redelmeier DA, Yarnell CJ, Thiruchelvam D, Tibshirani RJ. Physicians' warnings for unfit drivers and the risk of trauma from road crashes. *N Engl J Med.* 2012 September 27;367(13):1228–1236.

# 3

# *Trauma Systems*

**S. Morad Hameed and Richard K. Simons**

**CONTENTS**



## 3.1 Introduction: Trauma Systems at Work

**Case 1**: *Two 27-year-olds are shot as they emerge from a popular restaurant on a busy downtown street in a large metropolitan area. Police immediately secure the area. A basic life support ambulance crew arrives on the scene within 2 min, and is followed within 4 min by an advanced life support crew. The first responders take immediate action at the scene and make a quick decision about whether to transport the patients to a Level 3 trauma center 4 min away or to a Level 1 trauma center 10 min away. Meanwhile, trauma teams at both sites are mobilized. As the first patient arrives at the emergency department of the Level 1 trauma center, his pulse becomes undetectable. An emergency department thoracotomy tray has been opened by the waiting trauma team, and an operating room is standing by.*

**Case 2**: *A 19-year-old road worker is pinned against a wall by a crane during a highway construction project. Initial responders note that she is pale, cool, tachycardic, and hypotensive and is complaining of severe abdominal and pelvic pain. The work site is 90 min away from a Level 3 trauma center and 100 min away from a Level 1 trauma center by road. The on-scene paramedics, concerned about the severity of the patient's shock, activate the regional helicopter emergency medical service. Trauma surgeons at both centers are connected by phone to the transport crews.*

Cases like these create defining moments in the careers of trauma surgeons. Successful outcomes depend on knowledge, judgment, technical skills, and leadership. But, equally importantly, they depend on the reach and preparedness of entire *systems* of trauma care. Modern trauma systems are dynamic networks that span cities and remote environments, collecting data to prevent injury, and, when injuries do occur, facilitating quick and seamless transfers of patients to optimal, state-of-the-art trauma care. Trauma systems have evolved both as a strategy to deliver coordinated, acute care when it is most urgently needed, and as a comprehensive response to one of the greatest public health challenges of our time (Figure 3.1).

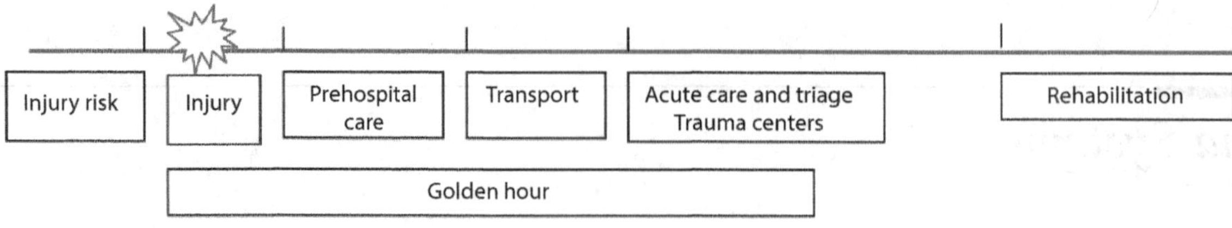


**FIGURE 3.1**
Structure of trauma systems. Trauma systems represent society's most complete and multimodal response to injury, from prevention to prompt and effective acute care and to rehabilitation and reintegration into society.

## 3.2 A Defining Challenge in Public Health

There are few problems in surgery, or in health care in general, that are more pressing than trauma. Each year, more than 100 million people are injured, and another 5.8 million people die as a result of injury [1]. The epidemic is global, with low- and middle-income countries shouldering 90% of the burden of injury [2]. In the United States, trauma is the fifth leading cause of death, but because of its heavy impact among the young, it results in the loss of more years of life than the three other leading causes of death (heart disease, stroke, and cancer) combined. When nonfatal injuries are accounted for, injury results in the loss of 5.1 million years of productive life annually. Americans spend over $150 billion in direct costs each year on the consequences of trauma [3]. The emotional and social costs to patients and families, though difficult to quantify, are also staggering.

In 1966, while considering the impact of injury on society, the U.S. National Academy of Sciences and the National Research Council observed that "public apathy to the mounting toll from accidents must be transformed into an action program under strong leadership" [4]. Its recommendations for a national strategy for injury control, which included mobilization of public awareness, and wide and formal collaboration on injury prevention, emergency medical care, and trauma research, transformed fatalistic attitudes about trauma into the perception of trauma as a public health problem with achievable solutions, and ushered trauma care into the modern era. But trauma is a complex epidemic to confront. Risk is highly influenced by the interplay of social, economic, environmental, and even geographic factors, and outcome is highly influenced by our ability to rapidly interrupt shock and its downstream consequences, and restore cognitive and musculoskeletal integrity and function. To be effective, injury control must, therefore, begin even before the moment of impact, be prepared to efficiently integrate and apply multidisciplinary knowledge to acute, lifesaving care, and end only when risk is eliminated and patients return to their places in society.

## 3.3 Trauma Systems: The Evolution of a Public Health Response

> From time to time [surgeons] must leave the sterile environment of the operating room and attempt to influence public health policy on behalf of their future patients [5].
>
> **HR Champion FRCS FACS (1988)**

In the decades since 1966, surgeons have taken critical roles in the development of a comprehensive approach to injury control. The American College of Surgeons (ACS) was decades ahead of the National Academy of Sciences/National Research Council in recognizing injury as a priority for advocacy and action. In 1922, it established the Committee on Trauma (ACS-COT) to provide surgical leadership in trauma care. Later, as surgeons returned home from wars in Korea and Vietnam "with their organizational and technical skills honed in combat," the ACS began to play an increasingly important role in the care of trauma patients [6]. Since its publication in 1976, the ACS-COT *Resources for Optimal Care of the Injured Patient* has set the standards for trauma care, and each new edition has been broader in scope and more influential than the last. Increasingly, governments are using the criteria described in this document to guide designation of trauma centers and regionalization of injury control efforts.

The ACS-COT considers injury control to be most effectively accomplished in a public health framework that includes approaches to prevention, optimization of access to acute care, acute care itself, rehabilitation, and research. In each of these areas, the ACS-COT promotes a public health approach that includes ongoing *assessment* of injury data and the epidemiology of injury, evidence-based *policy development*, and ongoing *assurance* of efficacy of processes [7]. These core functions are driven by the systematic collection and analysis of injury data in ACS-COT-mandated trauma registries.

A *trauma system* is defined as an organized and comprehensive public health response to injury within a specified geographic area that includes injury prevention, prehospital care, triage and transport, acute medical and surgical care, rehabilitation, education, and research. In just five decades since their conception, rapid access to trauma systems has become a reality for 80% of the populations of the United States and Canada [8,9], and trauma systems have been referred to as "an astounding achievement of modern health care" [10].

Trauma systems have been built out of necessity, often without the luxury of high-level evidence, but their rapid evolution has been guided by the careful analysis of available data. This chapter summarizes some of the best recent evidence on the impact of trauma systems on injury prevention and trauma care, outlines areas where more data are required, and briefly describes the exciting threshold to which trauma system development has brought us.

## 3.4 Injury Prevention: Can Trauma Systems Prevent Injury?

Traumatic deaths occur in a trimodal distribution, with 45% of deaths occurring within 1 h of injury, 34% occurring within 1–4 h, and 20% occurring after a week [11]. Although streamlined trauma systems and improvements in acute trauma care reduce the risk of delayed deaths [12], even the fastest and best acute care cannot address the high proportion of immediate deaths at the scene, which are often due to devastating central nervous system and cardiovascular injuries. This first mortality peak is thought to be more amenable to injury prevention efforts than to advances in acute care. The magnitude of this peak is so great that some investigators believe that the most significant advances in injury control in the future will come mainly from prevention initiatives [13].

When considered carefully, most injuries can be found to result from a combination of potentially modifiable personal, mechanical, and environmental risk factors. An understanding of the elements of this combination of risks is fundamental to the development of effective countermeasures that reduce risk and prevent injury. In 1970, William Haddon developed an elegant framework to deconstruct the complex determinants of injury. The Haddon Matrix considers three phases of injury: *pre-event* (which is a focus for primary prevention efforts), *event* (a focus for secondary prevention efforts), and *post-event* (a focus for tertiary prevention efforts). Within each phase, the risk or impact of injury is determined by the interplay of four types of factors: *host factors* (individual characteristics or behaviors that increase susceptibility to injury), *agent factors* (characteristics of the objects or vectors that inflict energy transfer and injury), *physical environment factors* (characteristics of the built environment that may predispose populations to injury), and *social environment factors* (the social, economic, and political milieu that influence the risk of injury) [14]. Haddon's phase-factor matrix has become the basis for thought and action in modern injury prevention.

The biggest gains in injury control will likely result from the identification of populations that remain vulnerable to injury, followed by thoughtful and comprehensive approaches to the modification of risk factors within each phase of injury in these groups. Evidence of the success of this approach is beginning to accumulate. Primary prevention efforts, which take place before an injury occurs (pre-event) in the effort to prevent it completely, have addressed host factors (graduated licensing has reduced motor vehicle crashes among inexperienced drivers by 28%), agent factors (restrictions of motorcycle engine size for young riders has decreased casualties in this group by 25%), physical environment factors (bicycle lanes have reduced casualties among cyclists by 35%), and social environment factors (legislation on motor vehicle speeding law enforcement and driver alcohol consumption have reduced injury mortality substantially) [15]. Perhaps the best evidence of the promise of trauma center-based injury prevention is provided by a prospective randomized controlled trial of a brief intervention for alcohol abuse, which demonstrated substantial reductions in alcohol consumption (22 versus 7 drinks per week) and re-injury risk (47%) [16]. As with primary prevention, secondary prevention efforts, which diminish the risk of injury once an event has occurred (seatbelts, airbags) [17], and tertiary prevention efforts, which seek to minimize the consequences of established injury (prehospital care, acute trauma care, rehabilitation), have also been shown to substantially reduce the burden and impact of injury.

Trauma systems are uniquely positioned to document the burden of injury, identify modifiable risks, and inform health policy at the highest levels. Recognizing this potential, the ACS-COT has placed significant value on the role of injury prevention coordinators at Level 1 and Level 2 trauma centers. However, a comprehensive survey of American trauma centers revealed that, despite a strong interest in injury prevention, less than 20% of them have dedicated coordinators, and greater than two-thirds have no specific funding for injury prevention programs [18]. Even where evidence exists for the cost-effectiveness of hospital-based injury prevention strategies, as is the case with the alcohol screening and brief intervention initiative [19], resource limitations and competing priorities resulted in its adoption by only half of surveyed trauma centers.

Despite these challenges, public health measures directed at injury control have already achieved some great successes and should be pursued further in mature trauma systems. In the United States, as a result of consistent efforts to change legislation, engineering, and behavior, the annual mortality rate from motor vehicle crashes has fallen from 18 to 1.7 deaths per million miles traveled since 1925 [20]. Similarly, deaths from occupational injuries fell from 37 to 4 per 100,000 workers between 1933 and 1997 [21]. But more work is needed. Injuries from all causes are still extremely common, and some segments of the population remain particularly vulnerable to the devastating consequences of injury morbidity and mortality [22–26].

*Recommendation*: Trauma systems have a key role in primary, secondary, and tertiary injury prevention.

*Grade of recommendation*: A

## 3.5 Clinical Trauma Care

Over the years, the focus of trauma systems has widened from trauma center-based injury care to multidimensional approaches to injury control that include public policy, prevention, prehospital care, acute medical care, and rehabilitation. All of these areas have grown up together and it is difficult to examine their progress and effects in isolation. Still, some insights into their value and potential can result from this approach.

### 3.5.1 Prehospital Care: Scoop and Run or Stay and Play?

Prompt control of injuries, including achievement of hemostasis and reversal of shock, has strong physiologic justification [27,28] and, as the basis of the golden hour concept of trauma care [29], has become a first principle of trauma systems. The exact logistics of the delivery of life-saving care in the critical first hours after injury, including in the prehospital setting, are a central focus of injury research with practical policy implications. For example, early advanced life support of trauma patients by well-trained paramedics in the field (including thorough assessment, invasive airway control, and prompt resuscitation with intravenous fluids), although intuitively appealing as a means to correct hypoxia and hypotension, has not consistently been shown to improve outcomes. In fact, several observational studies have suggested that prehospital intubation for airway protection and ventilatory support is associated with hypotension [30] and similar or worse outcomes in trauma patients with head injuries [31,32]. A prospective, alternate day trial of prehospital bag valve mask ventilation versus intubation in children requiring ventilatory support also did not reveal benefit from the more invasive approach [33]. There is also some evidence that a less invasive approach to initial fluid resuscitation may be beneficial: another prospective, alternate day trial of penetrating trauma in an urban environment suggested that survival increases if paramedics defer intravenous fluid resuscitation in patients sustaining penetrating torso trauma until a time when surgical hemostasis has been achieved [34]. The conclusions from these early studies have favored the notion that a "scoop and run" prehospital strategy, minimizing potentially harmful on-site interventions and prolonged scene times, may improve outcomes after severe injury.

Prehospital care issues were reexamined in one of the largest and most comprehensive studies of prehospital care to date. Stiell et al. investigated the effect of system-wide introduction of advanced life support skills for paramedics on survival after severe injury in 2867 patients. This before–after, controlled clinical trial suggested that augmentation of paramedic skills was not associated with improved survival (81.8% basic and 81.1% advanced) and was associated with *worse* survival in the subset of patients ($n$ = 598) with Glasgow Coma Scale score of less than 9 (60.0% basic and 50.9% advanced). Intubation in the field was associated with increased mortality (odds ratio [OR] 2.8). Interestingly, administration of prehospital intravenous fluids did not appear to be associated with improved outcome [35].

The reasons for failure of advanced paramedic training to make a significant impact on trauma outcomes are not well understood. Recent studies of jurisdictions that place a strong emphasis on prehospital care were not able to show a difference between field resuscitation versus rapid transport approaches [36]. It is possible that a combination of technical factors leading to inadvertent hypoxia or hyperoxia, aspiration, hypocapnea, hypotension, or intracranial hypertension during intubation can compound or exacerbate the primary injury and compromise recovery [37]. Until these factors are better characterized individually, it is reasonable to apply advanced life support measures in the prehospital setting selectively and cautiously, and to continue to expedite patients' transfer to definitive care.

This brings us to the issue of mode of transport. As trauma systems have been designed to minimize time to definitive care, considerable attention has been focused on the role and value of helicopters in modern trauma systems. Despite the ubiquity of air transport, its use is not supported by high-level evidence. In general, ground ambulance transport (GAT) is widely available and can be readily dispatched. Air medical transport (AMT) by helicopter may, in some jurisdictions, take longer to dispatch, but often has more sophisticated medical capability (advanced paramedics or physicians) and is faster once launched. Geographic analyses have suggested that distance thresholds from trauma centers to injury locations exist: beyond certain distances AMT is consistently faster than GAT [38]. For trauma patients living at considerable distance from trauma centers, AMT is generally considered to be potentially life saving [39]. However, the consistency of this association appears highly dependent on trauma system-specific factors such as numbers of helicopters, locations of landing pads, and weather conditions [40]. More studies are needed to characterize the value and optimum algorithms for helicopter transport in trauma.

*Recommendation*: Prehospital care should attempt to minimize scene time and prioritize immediately life-saving measures only, with rapid and efficient transfer to the most appropriate trauma center for resuscitation and definitive care.

*Grade of recommendation*: B

### 3.5.2 Trauma Centers: Are They Accessible?

Assuming patients in the early golden hour receive prompt and judicious prehospital care, where do they go next?

At the heart of trauma systems, trauma centers focus expertise and resources to bring high-quality care to patients with severe and complex injuries and take the lead in their communities on prevention and quality improvement initiatives, and scientific research. Between 1991 and 2002, the number of trauma centers in the United States more than doubled from 471 to 1154 (190 Level 1, 263 Level 2, and 701 Levels 3–5 hospitals) [41]. Access to Level 1 and Level 2 centers has grown to provide coverage to 69.2% Americans within 45 min and 84.1% within 60 min of injury [8]. This level of access is a phenomenal achievement, but more work is still needed for access to become universal. Approximately, 46.7 million Americans, mostly in rural areas, still cannot get to Level 1 or Level 2 care within 1 h of injury. The observation that injuries sustained in rural environments have higher injury severity-adjusted mortality than those in urban environments [42,43] may, in part, be attributable to the poor reach of trauma systems into these areas. Promotion of policies, such as the Emergency Medical Treatment and Active Labor Act, which requires trauma centers to receive severely injured patients if capacity exists, may help to establish access as an entrenched and fundamental property of trauma systems [44].

*Recommendation*: Rural and remote communities shoulder a heavy burden of injury and do not have ready access to urban trauma systems. Reappraisal of access to systems of trauma care in these environments and new ideas to reduce early mortality in these populations are urgently needed.

*Grade of recommendation*: B

### 3.5.3 Do Trauma Systems Save Lives?

Access to trauma centers is important because trauma centers are widely considered to improve outcomes. But do we know this for sure? Numerous investigators have explored this question from three different angles. The *structure* of trauma centers might include the presence of in-house trauma-attending and multidisciplinary trauma teams, well-equipped trauma bays, ready access to operating theaters, the presence of clinical protocols and educational curricula, research capacity and injury prevention activity, and participation in external review and designation. A few studies have suggested that the presence of trauma-attending in-house and other structural interventions reduces time to definitive treatment, cost, and even mortality [45–47], prompting organizations such as the ACS-COT and the Trauma Association of Canada to provide trauma surgeon response time guidelines. *Process* in trauma systems is assessed using measures of function: how fast does the team respond, how long do patients spend in the emergency department, how long to get to the operating room? Implementation of trauma systems has been shown to improve processes of care [48]. Finally, and most importantly, *outcome* of trauma patients, including mortality, length of stay, and functional measures, may all provide insights into how well a trauma center is fulfilling its mandate.

The trauma systems literature is dominated by this outcome bottom line, and particularly by mortality, as it has been most consistently measured. Because randomized trials of trauma center versus non-trauma center performance are not feasible (and probably no longer ethical), assessments of trauma centers have mostly used three types of observational designs. *Analyses of preventable deaths* by expert panels provided the earliest justification for the regionalization of trauma care in dedicated centers. In a striking example, West et al. compared the proportion of preventable in-hospital trauma deaths in San Francisco County, where trauma care was regionalized to a single trauma center, to that in Orange County, where over 40 centers participated in trauma care. They found only 1% of deaths in San Francisco to be preventable, while a staggering 73% of deaths would have been preventable in Orange County with access to high-quality trauma care [49]. Four years later, after the implementation of regionalized trauma care in Orange County, the proportion of preventable deaths fell to an eighth of its previous level [50]. Other analyses of preventable death such as the one by Gruen et al. [51] are also interesting because they demonstrate the scope and intensity of the clinical work carried out by trauma centers everyday and the impact of process on outcome. These investigators noted that some preventable deaths might have been, in part, due to problems with airway control, delayed control of acute thoracic/abdominal/

pelvic hemorrhage, inadequate venous thromboembolism or gastrointestinal prophylaxis, lengthy initial operative procedures rather than damage control surgery in unstable patients, over-resuscitation with fluids, and complications of feeding tubes. Other early trauma center studies have involved *comparisons of trauma center patient outcomes to national norms* (using Trauma and Injury Severity Score methodology and comparisons with reference data from the Major Trauma Outcomes Study) [52], and use of *population-based methods* to examine populations with and without access to trauma systems. Each of these strategies provided early evidence in favor of trauma centers and systems [53].

In one of the most widely cited population-based studies of trauma system effectiveness, investigators from the University of Washington led by Nathens examined the effect of trauma systems on motor vehicle crash mortality in 22 states using the national Fatality Analysis Reporting System database. After adjusting for differences in injury prevention legislation, and general injury mortality trends, the study found that an 8% mortality reduction attributable to trauma systems was evident by 15 years following trauma system implementation [54]. Celso et al. recently published another landmark study [55] of the effectiveness of trauma systems. Their review of the literature and meta-analysis examined 14 population-based studies, published between 1992 and 2004, comparing mortality rates before and after implementation of trauma systems or comparing mortality in jurisdictions with and without trauma systems. Like the Nathens study noted earlier, these were all *ecological studies;* retrospective observational studies examining the health of populations or communities using time trends (mortality before and after trauma system implementation) and geographical comparisons (mortality in jurisdictions with and without trauma systems) [56]. Improved odds of survival were noted in 8 of the 14 studies, and a meta-analysis including 6 of the studies demonstrated a 15% reduction in mortality where trauma systems were present. Since the publication of this meta-analysis, more rigorous evidence for trauma system effectiveness has accumulated. In another landmark trial, Mackenzie et al. used data from the National Study on the Costs and Outcomes of Trauma (NSCOT) to compare mortality between Level 1 trauma centers and large non-trauma centers in metropolitan areas of 14 states. After carefully adjusting for differences between the patient populations, the authors found that in-hospital and 1-year mortality were significantly lower for trauma centers (RR 0.80 and 0.75, respectively), and that this effect was more pronounced in younger patients with more severe injuries [57].

Trauma centers have also shown promise in the management of pediatric injuries [58]. Based on observed improved traumatic brain injury outcomes in high-level pediatric trauma centers, the ACS has recommended that children with such injuries be managed at these facilities. However, a recent study of six U.S. states suggests that almost one-third of children do not get to high-level care. Access for children is an important research priority.

*Recommendation*: Trauma systems improve injury survival and should be widely implemented based on this evidence alone.

*Grade of recommendation*: B

### 3.5.4 What Features of Trauma Systems Make a Difference?

The mounting evidence for trauma system effectiveness suggests that benefits of trauma systems have been established: New research efforts should focus on the further refinement of the structure and processes of trauma care. In the absence of high-quality evidence, early trauma systems were built on a foundation of expert opinion. But their rapid evolution has depended on (and will continue to depend on) close and ongoing evaluation of their structure and processes. In Quebec, such evaluation and evidence-based and context-specific evolution has resulted in a decline in mortality from severe injury from 51.8% in 1992 to 8.6% in 2002 [59]. In a study of over 72,000 patients, trauma investigators in Quebec probed the specific strengths of trauma systems and demonstrated that mortality following severe injury is strongly affected by structural and process issues such as advance notification of trauma centers by prehospital crews (OR 6.1), the presence of hospital-based performance improvement programs (OR 0.44), and by trauma center experience (OR 0.98) and tertiary designation (OR 0.68) [60]. More recent studies have confirmed the vital importance of nursing care and leadership on trauma center performance [61,62], and the significant impact of comprehensive performance and patient safety on trauma patient mortality rates [63].

The effects of experience and trauma center designation have also received attention from other trauma research groups. To define the experience effect, Nathens et al. compared outcomes in trauma patients treated at 31 university-affiliated Level 1 and Level 2 trauma centers. They observed that as trauma center volumes increase, hospital lengths of stay decrease, reflecting, perhaps, more rapid recovery in more experienced centers. This relationship descends to a plateau once injury admissions exceeded 600 (Injury Severity Score >15) per year. Also, odds of death from severe injuries relative to the smallest centers were shown to start decreasing above the 600 admissions threshold, again suggesting that about 600–650 major trauma admissions per year might be the boundary between low- and high-volume trauma centers. After adjustment for confounders, Nathens' group found significantly lower mortality among patients presenting to high-volume trauma centers with penetrating abdominal trauma and hypotension (OR 0.02!) and with multisystem injuries with low Glasgow Coma Scale (GCS) (OR 0.49) [64]. However, an analysis of 12,254 patients from the National Trauma Data Bank, focusing on a slightly different population of severely injured patients and using different volume thresholds, found ACS-COT trauma center *designation* level (i.e., degree of preparedness and resources for trauma care) to be more predictive of outcome than patient volume [65]. Disability at discharge (20.3 versus 33.8%) and mortality (25.3 versus 29.3) were significantly lower in Level 1 than in Level 2 centers, but trauma volumes were not associated with outcome differences. These studies are not directly comparable, but both suggest that care provided in dedicated trauma centers, either because of experience or preparedness, has the potential to reduce morbidity and save lives.

*Recommendation*: Specific structure and process features of trauma systems, including integrated prehospital care, trauma center volumes, verification/accreditation by external expert agencies such as the ACS-COT, and ongoing dedication to leadership and quality, influence trauma system performance. These features of trauma systems should be ongoing areas of focus and optimization.

*Grade of recommendation*: B

### 3.5.5 Beyond Saving Lives: What Are the Long-Term Outcomes of Trauma Systems?

Virtually all of the studies cited earlier use in-hospital survival as the metric for trauma system success. However, as mortality from multisystem trauma has fallen, both in military and civilian settings, many survivors are returning home to their communities and to productive life. Unfortunately, data on the long-term functional outcomes after traumatic conditions such as shock, multiorgan failure, traumatic brain injury, and pelvic and long bone fractures are expensive and not routinely collected. When these data are collected, the results are often very interesting. Recently, Moore et al. validated trauma center re-admission rates as a key indicator of trauma system performance. This is a welcome measure that will assist trauma systems in the optimization of intermediate term outcomes [66]. In the longer term, Gabbe et al. found that 6 months after major trauma, only 42% of patients had returned to work and only 32% characterized their recovery as good [67]. Outcome measures at the time of hospital discharge such as the modified Functional Independence Measure and the Glasgow Outcome Score, which are often used as indicators of functional recovery, were not found to be reliably predictive of long-term outcomes, emphasizing how little insight we get from hospital data on ultimate outcomes. Holbrook et al. at the University of California San Diego found that adolescents sustaining major trauma have significant and sustained deficits in quality of life compared with national norms [68]. These findings, and others by this group, highlight the urgency of data collection, continued research, and action in this area (Table 3.1).

*Recommendation*: Long-term outcomes after severe injury are poor and poorly understood. Consensus on specific indicators of long-term outcomes and systematic measurement of these outcomes are essential to inform the ongoing evolution of trauma systems.

*Grade of recommendation*: B

## 3.6 Future Directions

### 3.6.1 Integrated Systems of Trauma Care

In recent years, the concept of trauma systems has transitioned from regionalization of trauma care in (often single) specialized high-volume trauma centers, to a more holistic and multidisciplinary or *systems* approach, to injury control that starts with injury prevention and emphasizes a wider response to trauma including pre and posthospital care. Nathens' studies of the effect of trauma systems on motor vehicle crash survival have suggested that successful injury control may depend on a broad-based, systematic, and coordinated approach that includes seatbelt legislation, helmet use, and established speed limits, in addition to presence of trauma centers [54,69]. It is becoming increasingly evident that the observed successes of trauma systems cannot be attributed to any one component or measure, but rather to a systematic approach to injury control.

More effective and universal acute care of injury continues to be an area of intense interest for trauma systems. Trauma investigators have speculated that a more participatory or *inclusive* approach to trauma care, which involves all of a region's acute hospitals (to the extent that their resources permit), could streamline the triage and early care of injured patients and extend the reach of trauma systems beyond the catchments of large, urban trauma centers to more rural and remote regions. A recent comparison of American states with the traditional single trauma center-based exclusive trauma systems with states with inclusive trauma systems used administrative discharge data from 24 states

**TABLE 3.1**

Evidence and Recommendations

| Statement | Evidence | Recommendation |
|---|---|---|
| *Injury prevention* | | |
| Trauma systems prevent injury recidivism associated with alcohol abuse. | 1b | A |
| Trauma system implementation has been associated with reductions in mortality from motor vehicle crashes. | 2c | B |
| Trauma systems should play a more active role in injury prevention. | 2c | B |
| *Prehospital care* | | |
| Prehospital intubation in traumatic brain injury should be selective and attempted with caution. | 2b | B |
| Prehospital fluid resuscitation should be limited in patients with penetrating mechanisms in urban environments. | 1b | B |
| Scene time and interventions in trauma should be minimized until more is known about the effects of specific interventions. | 2a | B |
| Local analyses should be done to determine trauma center catchments that may be more rapidly served by AMT. | 2b | B |
| *Accessibility* | | |
| Systems of trauma care in rural, low-resource environments require a thorough reappraisal and new ideas on how to address the disproportionate burden of early mortality in these settings. | 2c | B |
| *Survival* | | |
| Trauma systems increase survival. | 2c | B |
| *Features of trauma systems* | | |
| Specific structural and process factors influence trauma system performance. | 2b | — |
| Trauma center volume influences outcome. | 2c | B |
| Trauma center verification influences outcome. | 2c | B |
| *Long-term outcomes* | | |
| Long-term outcomes in severe trauma are poor. | 2b | — |
| Trauma systems should collect and account for long-term outcome data. Broad consensus on specific indicators or benchmarks of long-term trauma outcomes is required. | — | — |
| *Integrated systems of trauma care* | | |
| A systematic approach to trauma care improves survival. | 2a | B |
| Inclusive trauma systems improve survival. | 2c | B |
| Inclusive trauma systems may improve survival in mass casualty and multicasualty situations. | Needed | |
| Trauma systems are cost-effective. | 2b | B |
| *Global health* | | |
| Trauma systems reduce morbidity and mortality in low-income settings. | Needed | — |

to demonstrate that states with the highest levels of inclusiveness (38%–100% of hospitals designated as Levels 1–5 trauma centers) had the lowest odds of mortality (OR 0.77) after adjustment for factors such as injury mechanism and trauma system maturity. The authors of this study speculated that early care of patients in inclusive systems at local trauma centers, and more efficient transfers to higher levels of trauma care when needed, may have been responsible for the observed advantage of inclusive systems [70]. These conclusions about sharing the work in inclusive trauma systems may seem to be at odds with other studies documenting the importance of the volume–outcome relationship in severe trauma [64]. It is true that increasing the profile of Level 1 and Level 2 trauma centers decreases trauma volumes at nearby Level 1 trauma centers, but it may do so without decreasing injury severity at the Level 1 centers, and while reducing mortality [71]. Although the ACS-COT is moving toward a more inclusive approach to trauma system design [72], the designation of new Levels 2, 3, and 4 centers within a given health-care ecosystem must be thoughtful, must carefully account for a population's needs, and must preserve the critical clinical, education, and research activities of regional Level 1 centers [73]. The process of trauma center designation must follow uniformly high standards and be governed by external agencies with experience and expertise to ensure that trauma system development remains focused on best practices, inter facility collaboration, and regional needs [74,75].

Inclusive trauma systems depend on great attention to triage, or the sorting and movement of patients, both from the scene and between hospitals, and the networks that include emergency medical systems and all levels of trauma systems must be evidence-driven, responsive, and dynamic. The need for rapid and accurate assessment of patient needs and accurate triage to appropriate facilities is underscored in a report by Sampalis et al. [76] in Montreal, who found that severely injured patients initially taken to less specialized hospitals and then transferred to trauma centers had almost twice the mortality of those transferred directly to trauma centers. The importance of this undertriage phenomenon was also observed by Haas et al., who estimated that transportation of injured patients directly to Level 1 or Level 2 trauma centers was associated with 30% lower mortality [77].

The increasing threats of multiple and mass casualty situations will also shape the role of trauma systems in building safer societies. Natural disasters and acts of war and terrorism have already tested both military and civilian trauma systems in North America and around the world. It is believed that more inclusiveness in the delivery of trauma care, with a high proportion of hospitals being able to respond promptly and according to their established capabilities, will increase the capacity of our response to these situations. Disaster preparedness has become an essential mandate of trauma systems, and research in this area using simulation or extrapolation from previous experiences is a priority if trauma systems are to remain effective and relevant [78–80].

The interesting challenge of modern trauma systems will be to reconcile observations about volume–outcome relationships, benefits of inclusive systems, and challenges of triage and transport. Trauma systems will be increasingly customized to match local needs. What seems clear is that this effort is not confined to a single agency, center, or discipline, but requires an integrated approach. Germany initiated a process to build a nationwide trauma program in 2006. By 2014, a system of 44 regional trauma networks, with an average of 14.5 trauma centers each, covering 90% of the country, and supported by an integrated national trauma registry, was in place. This was a large-scale effort that has laid the foundation for the optimization of trauma care and injury prevention on a national scale and could serve as a template for other countries [81,82].

### 3.6.2 Vulnerability and Access

Ensuring universal access to excellent trauma care is a core principle of trauma systems development and has been discussed on a broad level in this chapter. However, the architects of modern trauma systems must also remain aware of vulnerable populations at high risk of injury or with poor access to care to achieve meaningful advances in injury control. Socioeconomic status [23], race [22], insurance status [83], and residence in rural areas [43] have been associated with vulnerability to injury or poor access to care. Despite great advances in trauma systems development in Canada and the United States, millions of people still do not have prompt access to injury care [9,41]. One great area of concern is trauma among the elderly, which is an impending epidemic. Trauma systems must remain sensitive to the risk and implications of injury among the elderly and focus their care on the preservation of functional independence [84,85]. The ongoing optimization of trauma systems will require new strategies to understand vulnerability and risk, including geographic information science [86,87], and new ways to extend the reach of systems, including inclusive systems, education and outreach, and telehealth, and applications of web-based technologies.

### 3.6.3 Economic Considerations

Such considerations would seem to justify the high cost of maintaining trauma system preparedness. A survey of the additional capabilities and costs associated with 24 h trauma system preparedness in 10 trauma centers in Florida suggested that the annual costs of such preparedness is $2.7 million per center. Most of these costs were attributed to physician on-call coverage. The authors note that these costs of preparedness may not translate to billable patient care and are, therefore, not recouped [88]. The financial benefits of preparedness in terms of reductions in morbidity and mortality, however, are difficult to accurately quantify and are probably undervalued. A more global economic evaluation of trauma care examined the cost per quality-adjusted life year (cost/QALY) gained by treatment at a tertiary trauma center in Ottawa, Canada. The investigators found that the increase in cost/QALY for treatment at a tertiary trauma center compared with a non-trauma center ($4,303) compared favorably with other established health-care interventions [89]. Another analysis of the Florida trauma system confirmed that although care at trauma centers was more expensive, it was associated with a reduction in mortality of 18%, resulting in a cost of $35,000 per life saved at trauma centers. Again, when restored productivity was considered, the authors concluded that trauma center care compared very favorably with other established medical interventions. However, Fishman et al. raised an important issue regarding the unintended consequences of trauma systems: does trauma care adversely affect outcomes of non-trauma patients? They found that patients presenting to the emergency department with acute coronary syndromes during a concurrent trauma activation had nearly twice the number of adverse cardiac events at 30 days. Although this was a small study, it does suggest that future evaluations of trauma system costs should take into account possible collateral consequences [90].

*Recommendation*: The creation of more integrated systems of trauma care that balance inclusivity with trauma center performance, that continue to address issues of vulnerability and poor access, and that remain focused on the economic value of injury prevention and effective trauma care are key future directions in the ongoing evolution of trauma systems.

*Grade of recommendation*: B

### 3.6.4 Global Health: Can Trauma Systems Save Lives in Low-Resource Settings?

Perhaps the greatest frontier in the development of trauma systems is to extend their reach into remote and underserviced areas, and to implement them more widely in low-resource settings. Low- and middle-income countries, with stretched health-care and public health budgets, shoulder an immense burden of injury. But a lack of resources should not be a deterrent to the pursuit of advances in trauma care; millions of lives stand to be improved or even saved if trauma systems can find more universal applications [2,91]. Trauma systems prevent injury and improve outcomes in part because they are successful in reorganizing scarce resources and focusing them on achieving high standards of injury control.

Recognizing the promise of a public health/trauma systems approach to injury control in low-resource settings, the International Association for Trauma and Surgical Intensive Care and the World Health Organization, along with a number of prominent trauma organizations from around the world, set out to identify fundamental priorities for trauma care that must be achieved regardless of the level of individual or societal wealth. The results of their deliberations were published in 2004 in the document *Guidelines for Essential Trauma Care* [92]. These guidelines are the low-resource counterpart to the ACS-COT *Resources for Optimal Care of the Injured Patients.* They are geared to economies that spend as little as $3–4 per capita per year on health, are rallying points for advocacy, create tangible goals, and can be modified to fit local circumstances [2]. They represent the starting point for action on injury control at the global level.

A key first step in the development of trauma systems is the collection and analysis of high-quality injury data or injury surveillance [92]. Data collection is a necessary prerequisite for the improvement of clinical care, for the allocation of finite resources to acute care and rehabilitation, and for evidence-based injury prevention. While North American trauma systems have been built on a foundation of injury surveillance in the form of hospital-based trauma registries, in lower-resource settings, the costs of data collection and analysis have often proven to be prohibitive [93]. However, early initiatives in this area have suggested that trauma registries may be feasible and would play an important role [94]. Now, for the first time, the widespread availability and computational power of mobile informational technology tools are poised to create transformational change in injury surveillance, and the way data are applied to guide global trauma systems development. For example, an inexpensive iPad-based app designed by trauma surgeons as a mobile point of care electronic health record for trauma care [95] helped frontline physicians document 10,000 consecutive trauma admissions (including resuscitation, operative, and discharge notes) in its first 10 months of implementation at a busy South African trauma center. Data from these records wirelessly populated an electronic trauma registry in real time with an estimated 3.5 million data points, providing unprecedented insights in an environment with no previous formal data collection.

*Recommendation*: The ongoing development of trauma systems is a global public health priority. Injury surveillance and the application of data to addressing issues in injury control are feasible in low- and middle-income countries (LMICs) and should be major areas of thought and action in an ambitious global trauma systems agenda.

*Grade of recommendation*: E

## 3.7 Summary

> Every critically ill or injured person had the 'right to the best medical care, according to the state of the art and not according to location, severity of injury or ability to pay'.
>
> **R. Adams Cowley, MD**

In recent years, the value of trauma systems has been confirmed by a wealth of Level 2 data (population-based cohort and ecological studies) and trauma systems have become an important feature of the public health landscape. They provide data for injury prevention and stand ready for injury and mass casualty. They also illustrate that comprehensive public health approaches can make a difference in diseases with complex determinants and rapid and severe consequences. Perhaps, because of these factors, the principles of trauma systems have been applied widely. But gaps in the trauma systems literature and the persistence of injury as a major public health issue in North America and around the world mean that the work is still far from accomplished. New insights into the specific factors that make trauma systems effective are beginning to emerge and will continue to guide trauma system development. More studies are needed, including economic evaluations so that long-term benefits can be accounted for, and so that trauma systems remain efficient. More analyses involving outcomes other than hospital death are also needed [3], so that the heavy impact of prehospital deaths, including suicide [96] and nonfatal mortality on society, can be measured, and so that trauma systems may adjust accordingly. Also, innovative analyses of access to trauma systems are needed so that their reach might be extended further into rural and remote communities [97,98]. Trauma systems, which provide the framework for emergency response, must also clarify their roles in mass casualty and disaster situations. Ongoing insights from military experiences may be essential to this effort [99]. From the start, trauma systems have emphasized accountability and improvement and have worked to ensure that evidence is collected and acted on. Initiatives such as the NSCOT, collecting high-quality data, will provide important insights for the future development of trauma systems on many fronts. Finally, local successes have global implications. In the era of mobile information technology, surgeons working in trauma systems around the world will have unprecedented power to collect, analyze, and share data, implement best practices, and more fully realize the public health ideals of Drs. Champion and Cowley and the other architects of trauma systems.

## References


1. Krug EG, Sharma GK, Lozano R. The global burden of injuries. *Am J Public Health*. April 2000;90(4):523–526.
2. Mock C, Joshipura M, Goosen J, Lormand JD, Maier R. Strengthening trauma systems globally: The essential trauma care project. *J Trauma*. November 2005;59(5): 1243–1246.
3. Mann NC, Mullins RJ, MacKenzie EJ, Jurkovich GJ, Mock CN. Systematic review of published evidence regarding trauma system effectiveness. *J Trauma Acute Care Surg*. September 1999;1;47(3): S25.
4. National Academy of Sciences (US) and National Research Council (US) Committee on Trauma, National Academy of Sciences (US) and National Research Council (US) Committee on Shock. 1966. *Accidental Death and Disability: The Neglected Disease of Modern Society*. National Academies Press: Washington, DC.
5. Champion HR, Teter H. Trauma care systems: The federal role. *J Trauma*. June 1988;28(6):877–879.
6. Nathens AB, Brunet FP, Maier RV. Development of trauma systems and effect on outcomes after injury. *Lancet*. May 2004;363(9423):1794–1801.
7. American College of Surgeons Committee on Trauma. 2014. Resources for the optimal care of trauma patients. Chicago, IL; https://www.facs.org/, accessed September 22, 2015.
8. Branas CC, MacKenzie EJ, Williams JC et al. Access to trauma centers in the United States. *JAMA*. June 1, 2005; 293(21):2626–2633.
9. Hameed SM, Shuurman N, Razek T et al. Access to trauma systems in Canada. *J Trauma*. 2010 Dec;69(6):1350–1361; discussion 1361.
10. Ciesla DJ. Trauma systems and access to emergency medical care. *J Trauma*. June 2007;62(Supplement):S51.
11. Trunkey DD. Trauma. Accidental and intentional injuries account for more years of life lost in the U.S. than cancer and heart disease. Among the prescribed remedies are improved preventive efforts, speedier surgery and further research. *Sci Am*. August 1983; 249(2):28–35.
12. Demetriades D, Kimbrell B, Salim A et al. Trauma deaths in a mature urban trauma system: Is "trimodal" distribution a valid concept? *J Am Coll Surg*. September 2005; 201(3):343–348.
13. Stewart RM, Myers JG, Dent DL et al. Seven hundred fifty-three consecutive deaths in a Level I trauma center: The argument for injury prevention. *J Trauma*. January 2003;54(1):66–70; discussion 70–71.
14. Runyan CW. Introduction: Back to the future—Revisiting Haddon's conceptualization of injury epidemiology and prevention. *Epidemiol Rev*. 2003;25:60–64.
15. Ameratunga S, Hijar M, Norton R. Road-traffic injuries: Confronting disparities to address a global-health problem. *Lancet*. May 2006;367(9521):1533–1540.
16. Gentilello LM, Rivara FP, Donovan DM et al. Alcohol interventions in a trauma center as a means of reducing the risk of injury recurrence. *Ann Surg*. October 1999;230(4):473–480; discussion 480–483.
17. McGwin G, Jr., Metzger J, Alonso JE, Rue LW III. The association between occupant restraint systems and risk of injury in frontal motor vehicle collisions. *J Trauma*. June 2003;54(6):1182–1187.
18. McDonald EM, MacKenzie EJ, Teitelbaum SD, Carlini AR, Teter H, Jr, Valenziano CP. Injury prevention activities in U.S. trauma centres: Are we doing enough? *Injury*. May 2007;38(5):538–547.
19. Gentilello LM, Ebel BE, Wickizer TM, Salkever DS, Rivara FP. Alcohol interventions for trauma patients treated in emergency departments and hospitals. *Ann Surg*. April 2005;241(4):541–550.
20. Centers for Disease Control and Prevention (CDC). Ten great public health achievements—United States, 1900–1999. *MMWR*. April 2, 1999;48(12):241–243.
21. Centers for Disease Control and Prevention (CDC). Improvements in workplace safety—United States, 1900–1999. *MMWR*. June 11, 1999;48(22):461–469.
22. Karmali S, Laupland K, Robert Harrop A et al. Epidemiology of severe trauma among status Aboriginal Canadians: A population-based study. *CMAJ*. April 12, 2005;172(8):1007–1011.
23. Cubbin C, LeClere FB, Smith GS. Socioeconomic status and the occurrence of fatal and nonfatal injury in the United States. *Am J Public Health*. January 2000;90(1):70–77.
24. Centerwall BS. Race, socioeconomic status, and domestic homicide. *JAMA*. June 14, 1995;273(22):1755–1758.
25. Birken CS, Parkin PC, To T, Macarthur C. Trends in rates of death from unintentional injury among Canadian children in urban areas: Influence of socioeconomic status. *CMAJ*. October 10, 2006;175(8):867.

26. Bell N, Schuurman N, Hameed SM. A multilevel analysis of the socio-spatial pattern of assault injuries in greater Vancouver, British Columbia. *Can J Public Health*. January 2009;100(1):73–77.
27. Hameed SM, Aird WC, Cohn SM. Oxygen delivery. *Crit Care Med*. December 2003;31(Supplement):S658–S667.
28. Durham RM, Moran JJ, Mazuski JE, Shapiro MJ, Baue AE, Flint LM. Multiple organ failure in trauma patients. *J Trauma*. October 2003;55(4):608–616.
29. Cowley RA, Hudson F, Scanlan E et al. An economical and proved helicopter program for transporting the emergency critically ill and injured patient in Maryland. *J Trauma Acute Care Surg*. December 1, 1973;13(12):1029.
30. Shafi S, Gentilello L. Pre-hospital endotracheal intubation and positive pressure ventilation is associated with hypotension and decreased survival in hypovolemic trauma patients: An analysis of the national trauma data bank. *J Trauma*. November 2005;59(5):1140–1147.
31. Eckstein M, Chan L, Schneir A, Palmer R. Effect of prehospital advanced life support on outcomes of major trauma patients. *J Trauma*. April 2000;48(4):643–648.
32. Davis DP, Peay J, Sise MJ et al. The impact of prehospital endotracheal intubation on outcome in moderate to severe traumatic brain injury. *J Trauma*. May 2005;58(5): 933–939.
33. Gausche M, Lewis RJ, Stratton SJ et al. Effect of out-of-hospital pediatric endotracheal intubation on survival and neurological outcome: A controlled clinical trial. *JAMA*. February 9, 2000;283(6):783–790.
34. Bickell WH, Wall MJ, Jr., Pepe PE et al. Immediate versus delayed fluid resuscitation for hypotensive patients with penetrating torso injuries. *N Engl J Med*. October 27, 1994;331(17):1105–1109.
35. Stiell IG, Nesbitt LP, Pickett W et al. The OPALS major trauma study: Impact of advanced life-support on survival and morbidity. *CMAJ*. April 22, 2008;178(9):1141–1152.
36. Liberman M, Mulder D, Lavoie A, Denis R, Sampalis JS. Multicenter Canadian study of prehospital trauma care. *Ann Surg*. February 2003;237(2):153–160.
37. Davis DP. Should invasive airway management be done in the field? *CMAJ*. April 22, 2008;178(9):1171–1173.
38. Mitchell AD, Tallon JM, Sealy B. Air versus ground transport of major trauma patients to a tertiary trauma centre: A province-wide comparison using TRISS analysis. *Can J Surg*. April 2007;50(2):129–133.
39. Rhinehart ZJ, Guyette FX, Sperry JL et al. The association between air ambulance distribution and trauma mortality. *Ann Surg*. June 2013;257(6):1147–1153.
40. Karanicolas PJ, Bhatia P, Williamson J et al. The fastest route between two points is not always a straight line: An analysis of air and land transfer of nonpenetrating trauma patients. *J Trauma*. August 2006;61(2):396–403.
41. MacKenzie EJ, Hoyt DB, Sacra JC et al. National inventory of hospital trauma centers. *JAMA*. March 26, 2003; 289(12):1515–1522.
42. Muelleman RL, Wadman MC, Tran TP, Ullrich F, Anderson JR. Rural motor vehicle crash risk of death is higher after controlling for injury severity. *J Trauma*. January 2007;62(1):221–226.
43. Simons R, Brasher P, Taulu T et al. A population-based analysis of injury-related deaths and access to trauma care in rural-remote Northwest British Columbia. *J Trauma*. July 2010;69(1):11–19.
44. Spain DA, Bellino M, Kopelman A et al. Requests for 692 transfers to an academic Level I trauma center: Implications of the emergency medical treatment and active labor act. *J Trauma*. January 2007;62(1):63–68.
45. Rogers FB, Simons R, Hoyt DB, Shackford SR, Holbrook T, Fortlage D. In-house board-certified surgeons improve outcome for severely injured patients: A comparison of two university centers. *J Trauma*. June 1993;34(6):871–875; discussion 875–877.
46. Luchette F, Kelly B, Davis K et al. Impact of the in-house trauma surgeon on initial patient care, outcome, and cost. *J Trauma*. March 1997;42(3):490–495; discussion 495–497.
47. Cornwell EE, Chang DC, Phillips J, Campbell KA. Enhanced trauma program commitment at a Level I trauma center: Effect on the process and outcome of care. *Arch Surg*. August 2003;138(8):838–843.
48. Olson CJ, Arthur M, Mullins RJ, Rowland D, Hedges JR, Mann NC. Influence of trauma system implementation on process of care delivered to seriously injured patients in rural trauma centers. *Surgery*. August 2001;130(2):273–279.
49. West JG, Trunkey DD, Lim RC. Systems of trauma care. A study of two counties. *Arch Surg*. April 1979;114(4):455–460.
50. West JG, Cales RH, Gazzaniga AB. Impact of regionalization. The Orange County experience. *Arch Surg*. June 1983;118(6):740–744.
51. Gruen RL, Jurkovich GJ, McIntyre LK, Foy HM, Maier RV. Patterns of errors contributing to trauma mortality. *Ann Surg*. September 2006;244(3):371–380.
52. Champion HR, Copes WS, Sacco WJ et al. The Major Trauma Outcome Study: Establishing national norms for trauma care. *J Trauma*. November 1990;30(11):1356–1365.
53. Mullins RJ, Mann NC. Population-based research assessing the effectiveness of trauma systems. *J Trauma*. September 1999;47(3 Suppl):S59–S66.
54. Nathens AB, Jurkovich GJ, Cummings P, Rivara FP, Maier RV. The effect of organized systems of trauma care on motor vehicle crash mortality. *JAMA*. April 19, 2000;283(15):1990–1994.
55. Celso B, Tepas J, Langland-Orban B et al. A systematic review and meta-analysis comparing outcome of severely injured patients treated in trauma centers following the establishment of trauma systems. *J Trauma*. February 2006;60(2):371–378.
56. Coggon D, Rose G, Barker D. 1997. *Epidemiology for the Uninitiated*. BMJ Publishing Group: London, U.K.
57. MacKenzie EJ, Rivara FP, Jurkovich GJ et al. A national evaluation of the effect of trauma-center care on mortality. *N Engl J Med*. January 26, 2006;354(4):366–378.
58. Wang NE, Saynina O, Vogel LD, Newgard CD, Bhattacharya J, Phibbs CS. The effect of trauma center care on pediatric injury mortality in California, 1999 to 2011. *J Trauma Acute Care Surg*. October 2013;75(4): 704–716.

59. Liberman M, Mulder DS, Lavoie A, Sampalis JS. Implementation of a trauma care system: Evolution through evaluation. *J Trauma*. June 2004;56(6):1330–1335.
60. Liberman M, Mulder DS, Jurkovich GJ, Sampalis JS. The association between trauma system and trauma center components and outcome in a mature regionalized trauma system. *Surgery*. June 2005;137(6):647–658.
61. Evans T, Rittenhouse K, Horst M et al. Magnet hospitals are a magnet for higher survival rates at adult trauma centers. *J Trauma Acute Care Surg*. July 2014;77(1):89–94.
62. Collins N, Miller R, Kapu A et al. Outcomes of adding acute care nurse practitioners to a Level I trauma service with the goal of decreased length of stay and improved physician and nursing satisfaction. *J Trauma Acute Care Surg*. February 2014;76(2):353–357.
63. Sarkar B, Brunsvold ME, Cherry-Bukoweic JR et al. American College of Surgeons' Committee on Trauma Performance Improvement and Patient Safety program: Maximal impact in a mature trauma center. *J Trauma*. November 2011;71(5):1447–1454.
64. Nathens AB. Relationship between trauma center volume and outcomes. *JAMA*. March 7, 2001;285(9):1164–1171.
65. Demetriades D, Martin M, Salim A, Rhee P, Brown C, Chan L. The effect of trauma center designation and trauma volume on outcome in specific severe injuries. *Ann Surg*. October 2005;242(4):512–517; discussion 517–519.
66. Moore L, Stelfox HT, Turgeon AF et al. Derivation and validation of a quality indicator for 30-day unplanned hospital readmission to evaluate trauma care. *J Trauma Acute Care Surg*. May 2014;76(5):1310–1316.
67. Gabbe BJ. Functional measures at discharge. *Ann Surg*. May 2008;247(5):854–859.
68. Holbrook TL, Hoyt DB, Coimbra R et al. Trauma in adolescents causes long-term marked deficits in quality of life: Adolescent children do not recover preinjury quality of life or function up to two years postinjury compared to national norms. *J Trauma*. March 2007;62(3): 577–583.
69. Shafi S, Nathens AB, Elliott AC, Gentilello L. Effect of trauma systems on motor vehicle occupant mortality: A comparison between states with and without a formal system. *J Trauma*. December 2006;61(6):1374–1379.
70. Utter GH, Maier RV, Rivara FP, Mock CN, Jurkovich GJ, Nathens AB. Inclusive trauma systems: Do they improve triage or outcomes of the severely injured? *J Trauma*. March 2006;60(3):529–537.
71. Carr BG, Geiger J, McWilliams N, Reilly PM, Wiebe DJ. Impact of adding Level II and III trauma centers on volume and disease severity at a nearby Level I trauma center. *J Trauma Acute Care Surg*. November 2014;77(5):764–768.
72. ACS. Resources for the optimal care of the injured patient 2014; https://www.facs.org/~/media/files/quality programs/trauma/vrc resources/resources for optimal care 2014 v11.ashx, accessed September 23, 2015.
73. Tepas JJ III, Kerwin AJ, Ra JH. Unregulated proliferation of trauma centers undermines cost efficiency of population-based injury control. *J Trauma Acute Care Surg*. March 2014;76(3):576–581.
74. Simons R, Kirkpatrick A. Assuring optimal trauma care: The role of trauma centre accreditation. *Can J Surg*. August 2002;45(4):288–295.
75. Simons R, Kasic S, Kirkpatrick A, Vertesi L, Phang T, Appleton L. Relative importance of designation and accreditation of trauma centers during evolution of a regional trauma system. *J Trauma*. May 2002;52(5):827–833; discussion 833–834.
76. Sampalis JS, Denis R, Fréchette P, Brown R, Fleiszer D, Mulder D. Direct transport to tertiary trauma centers versus transfer from lower level facilities: Impact on mortality and morbidity among patients with major trauma. *J Trauma*. August 1997;43(2):288–295; discussion 295–296.
77. Haas B, Stukel TA, Gomez D et al. The mortality benefit of direct trauma center transport in a regional trauma system. *J Trauma Acute Care Surg*. June 2012;72(6):1510–1517.
78. Hoyt DB, Coimbra R. Trauma systems. *Surg Clin North Am*. February 2007;87(1):21–35.
79. Champion HR, Mabee MS, Meredith JW. The state of US trauma systems: Public perceptions versus reality—Implications for US response to terrorism and mass casualty events. *J Am Coll Surg*. December 2006; 203(6):951–961.
80. Currier M, King DS, Wofford MR, Daniel BJ, de Shazo R. A Katrina experience: Lessons learned. *Am J Med*. November 2006;119(11):986–992.
81. Ruchholtz S, Lefering R, Lewan U et al. Implementation of a nationwide trauma network for the care of severely injured patients. *J Trauma Acute Care Surg*. June 2014; 76(6):1456–1461.
82. Ruchholtz S, Lewan U, Debus F, Mand C, Siebert H, Kühne CA. TraumaNetzwerk DGU(®): Optimizing patient flow and management. *Injury*. October 2014;45(Suppl 3):S89–S92.
83. Delgado MK, Yokell MA, Staudenmayer KL, Spain DA, Hernandez-Boussard T, Wang NE. Factors associated with the disposition of severely injured patients initially seen at non-trauma center emergency departments. *JAMA Surg*. May 1, 2014;149(5):422.
84. Goodmanson NW, Rosengart MR, Barnato AE, Sperry JL, Peitzman AB, Marshall GT. Defining geriatric trauma: When does age make a difference? *Surgery*. October 1, 2012;152(4):668–675.
85. Ang D, Norwood S, Barquist E et al. Geriatric outcomes for trauma patients in the state of Florida after the advent of a large trauma network. *J Trauma Acute Care Surg*. July 2014;77(1):155–160.
86. Schuurman N, Hameed SM, Fiedler R, Bell N, Simons RK. The spatial epidemiology of trauma: The potential of geographic information science to organize data and reveal patterns of injury and services. *Can J Surg*. October 2008;51(5):389–395.
87. Ciesla DJ, Pracht EE, Cha JY, Langland-Orban B. Geographic distribution of severely injured patients. *J Trauma Acute Care Surg*. September 2012;73(3):618–624.
88. Taheri PA, Butz DA, Lottenberg L, Clawson A, Flint LM. The cost of trauma center readiness. *AJS*. January 2004;187(1):7–13.

89. Séguin J, Garber BG, Coyle D, Hébert PC. An economic evaluation of trauma care in a Canadian lead trauma hospital. *J Trauma*. September 1999;47(3 Suppl):S99–S103.
90. Fishman PE, Shofer FS, Robey JL et al. The impact of trauma activations on the care of emergency department patients with potential acute coronary syndromes. *Ann Emerg Med*. October 2006;48(4):347–353.
91. Mock C, Joshipura M, Arreola-Risa C, Quansah R. An estimate of the number of lives that could be saved through improvements in trauma care globally. *World J Surg*. March 15, 2012;36(5):959–963.
92. Mock C, Lormand JD, Goosen J et al. 2004. WHO 2004 guidelines for essential trauma care [Internet]. World Health Organization: Geneva, Switzerland, pp. 1–106.
93. O'Reilly GM, Joshipura M, Cameron PA, Gruen R. Trauma registries in developing countries: A review of the published experience. *Injury*. June 2013;44(6):713–721.
94. Schultz CR, Ford HR, Cassidy LD et al. Development of a hospital-based trauma registry in Haiti: An approach for improving injury surveillance in developing and resource-poor settings. *J Trauma*. November 2007;63(5): 1143–1154.
95. Zargaran E, Schuurman N, Nicol AJ et al. The electronic Trauma Health Record: Design and usability of a novel tablet-based tool for trauma care and injury surveillance in low resource settings. *J Am Coll Surg*. January 2014;218(1):41–50.
96. Schecter WP, Klassen C, O'Connor P, Potts M, Ochitill H. Suicide: The unmet challenge of the trauma system. *Arch Surg*. September 2005;140(9):902–904.
97. Schuurman N, Bell N, Hameed MS, Simons R. A model for identifying and ranking need for trauma service in nonmetropolitan regions based on injury risk and access to services. *J Trauma*. July 2008;65(1):54–62.
98. Osterwalder JJ. Could a regional trauma system in eastern Switzerland decrease the mortality of blunt polytrauma patients? A prospective cohort study. *J Trauma*. June 2002;52(6):1030–1036.
99. Eastridge BJ, Jenkins D, Flaherty S, Schiller H, Holcomb JB. Trauma system development in a theater of war: Experiences from operation Iraqi freedom and operation enduring freedom. *J Trauma*. December 2006; 61(6):1366–1373.

## Commentary on Trauma Systems

*Howard Champion*

As identified in this excellent dissertation on trauma systems, the early post-Vietnam civilian development of trauma centers and systems was often sporadic and powered by the force and commitment of individual personalities. These included F. William Blaisdell in San Francisco, who not only exemplified the commitment and competence needed to advance trauma care at that time, but created a dynasty that was effective throughout the country, thanks to Drs. Donald Trunkey, Frank Lewis, George Sheldon, and others. Robert Freeark had similar influence in Illinois, albeit aided by David Boyd who was the government custodian of the US civilian Trauma and Emergency Medical Services Systems (EMSS). The EMSS Act was passed by Congress in 1973 (and amended in 1976 and 1979) with the help of Senator Alan Cranston (D-CA) and Congressman Henry Waxman (D-CA).

I was privileged to be involved in the development of the Shock Trauma Center at the University of Maryland and what is regarded at the first statewide trauma system linked by state police helicopters. When I arrived in the United States from the University of Edinburgh in 1972, I brought lessons learned from the Birmingham Accident Hospital, specifically the three-team system of care delivery that is now commonplace, and was able to participate in the helicopter transport of patients from all over the state on my first day on the job. The helicopter crews were straight out of Vietnam, not averse to taking a patient out of the back of an ambulance at gunpoint, and landing in locations that would not be permitted today. Dr. R. Adams Cowley, "the father of trauma medicine," embodied the tenacity needed to develop trauma systems in the face of significant pushback from the medical and surgical communities. To do so, he leveraged the political environment, which is essential in developing trauma systems, politics was instrumental in creating a mandate for trauma care systems both in the United States and at the federal level in Australia. Dr. Cowley also ordered me to document the beneficial effects of what we were doing, creating a challenge that this chapter reviews in some detail, i.e., to provide evidence of the beneficial effects of trauma systems.

### Prehospital Care

Marshalling evidence of effectiveness of prehospital care is phenomenally challenging because of the emergency nature of the interactions among healthcare providers, the stranger who is their patient, and the knowledge that the patient's death could be imminent. Controlled trials are extraordinarily difficult to implement and even data collection is fraught with hazard. Nonetheless, since the early 1970s, the prehospital emphasis in the United States has been on prompt access to definitive care capabilities so that difficult-to-access torsal and head injuries can be given optimal chance of mitigation and treatment in the controlled clinical environment.

Warfare always results in significant advances in trauma care as a result of the exigencies and nature of combat trauma care in a tactical environment. The decade of war commencing in 2002 was no exception, and is characterized by additions to the prehospital care armamentarium. These include a resurgence in the use of tourniquets and clamps to address hemorrhage, new fluid resuscitation tactics and techniques, and an increasing emphasis on cricothyroidotomy as a first-line airway maneuver. Thanks to military medical leadership from such luminaries as COL John Holcomb, USA (Ret.); COL Brian Eastridge, USA (Ret.); LTC Robert Mabry, USA; Col. Russ Kotwal, USA (Ret.); Col. Donald Jenkins, USAF (Ret.); COL Lorne Blackbourne, USA (Ret.); and others, the needs of combat casualties have been rigorously documented and the standard of practice made uniform and appropriate under the operational guidance of those deployed and the leadership of the Committee on Tactical Combat Casualty Care (CoTCCC) under Capt. Frank Butler, USN (Ret.). Military-funded combat casualty care research continues to illuminate and increase the ability of care providers. All of these initiatives are slowly trickling into the civilian EMS environment and have spawned initiatives such as the Committee on Tactical Emergency Casualty Care (CTECC) with medical protocols for active shooter and tactical EMS settings.

With respect to helicopter transport, a paper soon to be published documents the benefits of former Secretary of Defense Robert Gates' order to bring helicopter evacuation times to within the "golden hour" in Afghanistan. Although it is clear that of the 285 helicopter services in the United States that fly 1515 helicopters from 846 U.S. bases and that the fact that abuses occur for a variety of economic and nonhealthcare reasons, helicopters remain a valuable tool in EMS and trauma systems.

### Do Trauma Centers Save Lives?

The body of evidence in the affirmative comports with the intuition of every trauma surgeon who has opened a chest or abdomen with expediency and put a stop to exsanguinating hemorrhage in a patient in extremis. However, teasing these data from various denominators is challenging. Furthermore the knock-on effect of trauma centers in the system that provides care of a lesser at risk patients in both trauma and acute care surgery must be considerable. Again, the data to support these prejudices are difficult to marshal. This contemporary review, in its reference to the many studies that quantify the connection between the existence of trauma centers/systems and reductions in morbidity and mortality, presents as strong a case as is possible.

### What Features Make a Difference in Trauma Centers?

The discipline, focused care, and constant review that have been part of the standard operating procedure in trauma centers since the early 1970s make a significant difference in the rigor, scrutiny, transparency, and accountability of patient care. Another significant element, as noted in the chapter, is patient volume. The fact that increases in trauma center volumes are associated with better outcomes (as reflected in shorter hospital lengths of stay, risk of death, and other indicators) raises the conundrum of urban versus rural disparities. Access, minimum patient volumes, time, distance, and cost are significant drivers of patient outcome that are easily used in goal-setting and performance evaluation in urban centers, but are often unattainable in rural and remote ones.

Perhaps no entity has dealt with this issue more successfully than the most effective trauma system ever created: the Joint Trauma System (JTS) that was developed over the past 15 years by the US Department of Defense (DoD) to service the needs of the combat injured in Afghanistan and Iraq. Using the tenets of Tactical Combat Casualty Care (i.e., point of wounding care including care under fire, tactical field care, and care during tactical evacuation to a Role 2 or Role 3 facility in theatre), the JTS has continually reduced the time to definitive care in adverse environments, and casualty morbidity and mortality have continued to decrease despite increasing injury severity. In the JTS, theater evacuation occurs from Afghanistan and Iraq to the Role 4 facility at Landstuhl in Germany where care can be continued before prompt evacuation to Role 5 facilities in the United States, predominantly Walter Reed National Military Medical Center in the Washington, DC area, and the Brooke Army Medical Center (BAMC) in San Antonio, CA (which also houses the Army Burn Center). Rehabilitation through the DoD-Veterans Administration collaboration and the BAMC Center for the Intrepid (a rehabilitation facility for Iraq/Afghanistan casualties who with burns, loss of limb function, or amputation) is cutting edge.

The DoD system of care is subject to weekly video teleconference mortality morbidity rounds and case discussions and is backed by a comprehensive system of data collection and assembly into a number of trauma registries. The analytic product continues to drive patient care and research. There is no doubt that lessons learned from this formidable array of capability will feed into civilian trauma systems worldwide for several years, just as lessons learned from Vietnam spurred the civilian trauma systems that are making such a difference in many parts of the world today.

### Future Directions

This chapter rightly lays out the continuing challenges in trauma systems. Not only do more than half of all trauma deaths occur prior to hospital care, this immediate mortality rate increases when special populations such as the elderly and when rural settings, where low–frequency, high-risk injuries are of particular concern, are factored in. Regionalization of trauma care has

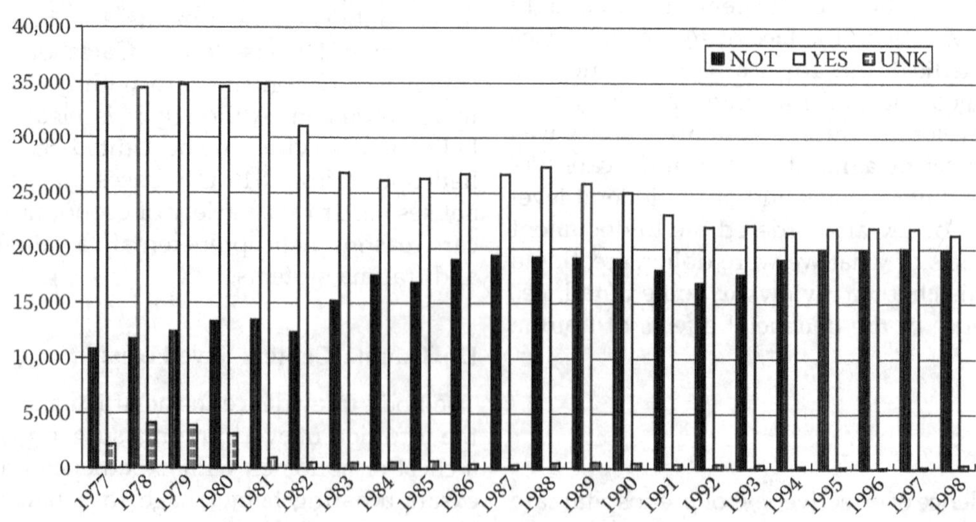


**FIGURE C3.1**
Automobile crash deaths of people not transported/transported (or transport status unknown) to an injury treatment facility.

paved the way not only for wider access to acute care surgery and critical care, but to the prehospital arena as well. Mentioned in the chapter is the German system that provides trauma system coverage to most of the country. A particular strength of the German trauma system is its integration of rehabilitation, a component that is still needed in most U.S. systems.

Having been involved in the development of a trauma system in the complex environment surrounding Washington, DC, I also must mention the jurisdictional boundaries that present challenges to regional integration and effectiveness, and take years to resolve.

As enumerated in this chapter, tremendous work has been done to build trauma systems in the 40 years since the Vietnam War ended. Inhospital crash deaths fell as trauma systems grew over 21 years from 1977 to 1998. (Figure C3.1) Further challenges remain and an enormous amount of talent is being applied to impose a public health approach to injury control so that prevention, mitigation, acute care systems, and rehabilitation processes and outcomes are documented in a manner that ensures continued improvement. The lesson I learned from R. Adams Cowley in the early 1970s is not only the importance of tenacity in pursuit of these goals, but that "when you are right, you have a moral obligation to impose your will on others." Let's all rise to that challenge, guided by this excellent chapter.

As experienced in the military over the past 14 years, the emphasis must now be on prehospital care and inclusive, seamless trauma systems.

# 4

# *Evidence-Based Surgery: Military Injury Outcomes*

**Brian J. Eastridge**

**CONTENTS**



## 4.1 Introduction

The development of trauma care has been a synergistic relationship between the military and civilian medical environments and has paralleled the history of war for the past several centuries [1,2]. "He who would become a surgeon should join an army and follow it for war is the only proper school for a surgeon." In the sixteenth century, Ambrose Pare conceptualized novel methods for the management of gunshot wounds as well as the ligation of large vessels, particularly during amputation. Jean Dominique Larrey, as surgeon-in-chief of the Napoleonic armies, introduced the concepts of triage and battlefield evacuation with his "ambulance volante" or flying ambulance during the French conflicts of the late eighteenth and early nineteenth centuries. During the Civil War, military physicians realized the utility of prompt attention to the wounded, early debridement and amputation to mitigate the effects of tissue injury and infection, and evacuation of the casualty from the battlefield. World War I saw further advances in the concept of evacuation, topical antisepsis, and the development of echelons of medical care. With World War II, antibiotics, blood transfusion, and resuscitative fluids, including plasma, were widely introduced into the combat environment, and surgical practice was improved to care for wounded soldiers. From his World War II experiences, Dr Michael Debakey, the surgical consultant to the Army Surgeon General, noted that wars have always promoted advances in trauma care due to the concentrated exposure of military hospitals to large numbers. Wartime medical experience fostered a fundamental drive to improve outcomes by improving practice [3]. Technological advances in aviation and medicine at the beginning of the Korean conflict led to the increase in deployed surgical capability, helicopters for patient evacuation from the locations where injury occur, and primary repair and grafting for vascular injury. In Vietnam, more highly trained medics at the location of the wounded and more prompt aeromedical evacuation decreased the battlefield mortality rate even further [4]. In addition, concerted efforts to gather combat injury data led to increased insights into the management of injury and improvements in trauma care in the United States [5–7]. The following chapter will review the current evidence substantiating the medical knowledge yield of the current conflicts of the twenty-first century.

## 4.2 What Is the Role of a Trauma System in Combat Injury Outcomes?

Trauma centers and trauma systems in the United States have had a remarkable impact on improving outcomes of injured patients [1,4,8–20], reducing mortality by up to 15% in evolved systems. With the onset of the conflicts in Iraq and Afghanistan, a military trauma system was developed and modeled after the successes of civilian systems, but modified to address the realities of combat.

The stated vision of the joint theater trauma system was to ensure that every soldier, marine, sailor, or airman injured on the battlefield had the optimal chance for survival and maximal potential for functional recovery. The system implementation mandated emplacement of infrastructure elements, including a trauma registry, performance improvement capability, and research. Data derived from the trauma registry were responsible for several hundred scientific manuscripts and more than 40 evidence-based clinical practice guidelines utilized to optimize combat casualty care. The joint trauma system improved information dissemination and performance enhancement along the continuum of care from battlefield wounding through the entire evacuation process, resulting in the lowest fatality rate (10.4%) in the history of warfare [21]. In the past several years, this military trauma system has published several manuscripts validating the value of performance improvement activities from the combat trauma registry to provide evidence-based benchmarks for battlefield trauma care [22]. Notable among these works were demonstrations of the system's capability to minimize post-injury complications such as hypothermia and compartment syndrome [23].

Telecommunication and technology advances since the Vietnam War have enabled us with access to robust and improved battlefield combat casualty care data. Based upon the military conflicts of antiquity, the epidemiology of combat injury has largely been documented by individuals, collated from medical administrative data, or by post hoc evaluation of data sources such as the Wound and Munitions Effectiveness Team data from Vietnam [24]. One central tenet evaluated by these previous data sets was the notion of combat survivability and it noted that in the past century, 90% of battlefield casualties happen on the battlefield before ever reaching medical care. Data derived from these sources were consistently based upon Levels 4 and 5 evidence. However, this evidence alluded to the fact that pre-hospital injury care was a critical and perhaps underappreciated aspect of the trauma system [25–27]. Following the recent conflicts in Southeast Asia, collaborative investigations linking combat casualty care outcomes to post-mortem evaluations have resulted in a large amount of detailed data. From an analysis of 558 combat casualties in a military medical treatment facility, 51.4% were considered to have potentially survivable injury, whereas 48.6% had non-survivable injury. The majority of the non-survivable injury was related to traumatic brain injury. In those casualties with potentially survivable injury, the primary pathology resulting in death was hemorrhage (80%) [28]. In a successive review, 87% of combat casualty mortality occurred before reaching a medical treatment facility. Of this pre-hospital casualty mortality number, 24% was potentially survivable, the majority of which (90%) died due to secondary hemorrhage [29]. The value of such analyses is based on their potential to justify allocation of resources and training with a specific focus.

Evidence to support battlefield evacuation was also augmented by the current conflicts in Southeast Asia. Mabry and his colleagues demonstrated that mortality outcomes for patients transported by trained flight paramedics (4.9%) were dramatically improved over flight medics with only Emergency Medical Technician-Basic training (15.8%) [30]. Subsequent work demonstrated that specialized medical evacuation teams with physicians and advanced resuscitative resources even further improved casualty survival of high-acuity injuries over that of paramedics [31–32].

*Recommendations*:

1. Trauma systems are responsible for improvements in outcomes following combat injury and should be a key element of the battlefield medical system.
2. Most combat casualty death occurs pre-hospital. Hemorrhage is the most substantial etiology of potentially survivable battlefield injury death that validates pre-hospital care as a key entity in combat casualty care continuum.
3. Mortality of combat casualties' improvement is associated with improved capabilities and training of flight medical providers. Flight medical personnel should be trained to at least the paramedic level to optimize combat casualty outcomes.

*Grade of recommendations*: 1. B 2. B 3. C

## 4.3 What Are the Impacts of Damage Control Measures on the Morbidity and Mortality of Combat Injury?

The concept of damage control resuscitation that was developed on the premise of concurrent hemostatic and hypotensive resuscitation strategies in order to manage hemorrhage and coagulopathy after combat injury was born out of the current war in Southeast Asia. This resuscitative principle was predicated upon the equally balanced ratio of packed red blood cells (PRBC) to plasma, and later platelets. Utilization of this strategy was optimized by the ability to predict patients at risk for massive transfusion [33]. In those requiring massive transfusion, Borgman demonstrated a decrease in mortality from 60% to approximately 20% after combat injury [34]. Subsequent studies from the military injury population, including a more recent performance improvement analysis of the outcomes of damage control resuscitation techniques, have established that the evolution of the balanced ratio resuscitation principle has further reduced the battlefield mortality of casualties, requiring massive transfusion to approximately 15% [35–37]. With the shift in resuscitation strategy, there has been a significant shift in the causation of in-hospital combat casualty mortality. Since the inception of this paradigm, casualties reaching a medical treatment facility were relatively more likely to succumb to severe brain injury secondary to the fact that this strategy decreased the number of hemorrhage deaths.

Damage control surgery techniques have dramatically altered the outcomes of troops injured on the battlefield. In the Vietnam War, in several case series it was observed that temporizing surgical procedures demonstrated a survival advantage when compared to definitive surgical therapy [5]. Although apparently temporarily misplaced as a technical relic after the Vietnam War, the technique regained popularity in the treatment of civilian trauma after a hallmark publication by Stone in 1983, which advocated abbreviated celiotomy in patients with abdominal injury with associated coagulopathy and hypothermia [38]. Within the past decade, a number of authors have also described the expansion of this life-saving surgical practice to include thoracic, vascular, orthopedic, and neurosurgical procedures [39–43]. In one of the largest studies of damage-control surgery in combat, prospective data was collected between April 2003 and January 2009 on 170 patients, who underwent an exploratory laparotomy for injury sustained on battlefield. Damage-control laparotomy, defined as an abbreviated exploratory laparotomy resulting in an open abdomen, was performed on 86 (51%) patients. Analyses revealed blood transfusion as the most significant risk factor for damage control. Patients after damage-control surgery had increased complications when compared to non-damage-control cohort but, despite this fact, survival between the groups was the same [44]. In a related study by Edens, 12,536 trauma admissions yielded 101 resuscitative thoracotomies (0.01%). In patients undergoing thoracotomy, penetrating trauma accounted for the majority of injuries (93%). There were no survivors after emergency department thoracotomy for blunt trauma ($N$ = 7). Expanding the indication for resuscitative thoracotomy to abdomen (30%) and extremities (22%), 12% (12/101) of all patients requiring thoracotomy survived [45].

*Recommendations*:

1. Damage control resuscitation has proven effective in minimizing mortality in high-acuity combat casualties and should be the resuscitative strategy of choice in casualties at risk for massive transfusion.
2. Damage control surgery techniques, including extra-abdominal procedures, should be followed for severe battlefield injury with unstable physiology.
3. The indication for resuscitative thoracotomy should be considered in all patients in extremis, excluding isolated brain injury.

*Grade of recommendations*: 1. B 2. C 3. C

## 4.4 What Are the Contemporary Techniques and Outcomes of Colon Surgery Performed on the Battlefield?

The practice of colon repair after injury has been intimately related to the lessons learned on the battlefield. In World War II, the propensity for complications and attributable mortality from failed primary colon repair led to a mandate from the British Surgeon General to exteriorize all colon injury [46]. This paradigm was pervasive for the subsequent 50 years of surgical history. Civilian trauma surgeons in the 1990s challenged the veracity of this dogmatic approach and found that primary repair of colon injury was both safe and effective [47–50]. However, there remains a controversy as to whether the ballistic energy of the combat injury makes this type of enteric injury a different entity from that of the civilian environment. Duncan demonstrated an overall complication rate of 48% and a leak rate of 30% in a small population of combat injured marines with colon injury managed by primary repair [51]. In a separate analysis of casualties from contemporary contingency operations, diversion was compared to primary repair/primary anastomosis. Primary repair was associated with a leak rate of only 10%, but once again, there was an attendant bias to divert colon injuries distal to the splenic flexure and repair those that occurred more proximally in the colon. Diversion was associated with a significantly lower incidence of complication. However, despite the differences in complication between the treatment modalities, there was no attributable increase in sepsis or mortality in the patient population with complications [52]. In a series of 65 patients with colon injury, Vertrees noted that primary repair was attempted in right-sided ($n$ = 18, 60%), transverse ($n$ = 11, 85%), and left-sided ($n$ = 9, 38%) colon injuries. Delayed definitive treatment of colon injuries occurred in 42% of patients after damage control celiotomy. Failure of colon repair occurred in 16% of patients and was more likely with concomitant pancreatic, stomach, or renal injury. The associated complication rate for diversion was 30% but increased dramatically to 75% in patients with primary repair or delayed definitive reconstruction failure [53]. A more contemporary analysis of military casualties with colorectal injuries was notable for a colostomy rate of 37%. The diversion rate for rectal injuries was 56%, whereas left-sided and right-sided injuries were diverted at rates of 41% and 20%, respectively. ISS ≥16 and the requirement for a damage control surgical intervention were likewise associated with higher diversion rates [54].

*Recommendation*:

1. In the combat environment, colon diversion should be strongly considered in patients with high-energy colon injury who would not tolerate complications such as anastomotic leak.

*Grade of recommendation*: 1. B

## 4.5 What Are the Contemporary Techniques and Outcomes of Vascular Surgery Performed on the Battlefield?

Advances in vascular surgery have been made in times of war. Although conceptualized for over two centuries, the first successful arterial repair for injury was done in 1896 by Murphy [55]. During World War I, German surgeons reported repair of more than 100 arterial injuries and pioneered autogenous reconstruction of injured vessels. However, the proclivity for mass casualty, significant soft tissue injury, and protracted transport times made routine reconstruction impractical, and subsequently ligation of vessels became the standard practice [55]. DeBakey reported 2471 arterial injuries treated by ligation in World War II with a 49% amputation rate [55]. Hughes in Korea reported arterial repair as a standard of practice with a 13% amputation rate [56]. Similar success was demonstrated by Rich from the conflict in Vietnam [6,7,55].

Improvements in the paradigm of casualty resuscitation during the current conflict have dramatically affected the capability of deployed surgeons to effectively perform vascular repair after injury on the battlefield. Damage control surgery techniques available to surgeons include temporary vascular shunts. Rasmussen et al. demonstrated that 57% of casualties had shunts placed at forward surgical facilities and 86% of proximal shunts were patent on admission to the combat support hospital. This patency of flow allowed for ongoing resuscitation in the context of a perfused extremity [57]. In two separate analyses, Fox showed that damage control resuscitation and damage control surgery techniques applied in the context of vascular injury were associated with the ability to perform prolonged complex limb revascularizations with limb salvage rates of 95% [58, 59]. Clouse, Sohn, and Fox independently demonstrated acute limb salvage rates for revascularization in theater of 92%–95% [60–62]. Late complications associated with revascularization included thrombosis, infection, and compartment syndrome [60]. The factor most significantly associated with post-revascularization morbidity was the use of prosthetic graft implants. In this population, the incidence of graft loss was 80% [60,63].

The management of venous injuries on the battlefield included ligation in 63% and repair in 37%. All patients developed post-operative edema. Thrombosis of the repair was demonstrated in 16% of the repaired veins. There was no acute limb loss associated within venous ligation or venous graft failure [64]. In a study of 111 U.S. military casualties with limb salvage for extremity vascular injuries, 25% were revascularized by a primary repair or end anastomosis, 72% were revascularized by saphenovenous reconstruction, and 3% revascularized with prosthetic conduit. With a mean follow-up of 347 days, 86% of the vascular reconstructions remained patent and the remaining 14% required a delayed amputation. Of this group, casualties with popliteal arterial injuries had the highest rate of amputation manifested by an amputation rate of 30% (7/23). The authors concluded that definitive vascular surgical intervention procedures performed at battlefield medical treatment facilities had excellent limb salvage results [65].

Proximity injury in the civilian penetrating extremity trauma population has been classically managed expectantly after studies by Thal and Frykberg demonstrated no increased incidence of vascular lesions requiring surgical therapy [66–68]. However, the high-energy nature of combat wounds has led investigators to reevaluate this diagnostic/management paradigm in the proximity combat penetrating extremity population. In a study of 99 patients who underwent angiography after evacuation for wound proximity, 47% had vascular abnormalities noted on angiography. Two-thirds of this group had a normal physical examination. Of this population with an abnormal angiogram, 52% required operative intervention [69]. In a similar analysis by Fox and Gillespie, a similar study of cervical vascular proximity by computerized tomographic angiography detected occult injury in 30% of studies, of which 50% required interventional or surgical management [70].

*Recommendations*:

1. Damage control techniques, including shunting, should be utilized to optimize survival and revascularization outcomes.
2. In the combat environment, arterial reconstruction can be performed with good long-term outcomes. Autogenous tissue optimizes outcome benefit potential.

3. In the context of battlefield venous injury, venous ligation is a safe and effective option for the management of venous vascular injury.
4. In the combat environment, proximity extremity injury should be evaluated by angiography to mitigate the risk of occult vascular injury.

*Grade of recommendations*: 1. B 2. B. 3. B 4. C

## 4.6 What Are the Contemporary Techniques and Outcomes of Burn Surgery Performed on the Battlefield?

The complexity of burn management in the combat environment is manifest across the spectrum of medical care from point of injury through resuscitation, intensive care through the continuum, and ultimately definitive surgical care. Contemporary data from the battlefield demonstrate that 52%–63% of burn injuries are battle injury [71,72]. The majority of these burns are associated with explosive etiology. Early surgical care for burn injury is limited to escharotomy and debridement of devitalized tissue. The most challenging phase of the battlefield burn casualty is the intensive care evacuation process performed by the U.S. Air Force Critical Care Air Transport Team and the U.S. Army Burn Flight Team. Classically, burn resuscitation has been practiced on a paradigm based upon weight and body surface area burned, according to the guidelines developed at the Parkland Memorial Hospital and the Brooke Army Burn Center. Ennis reported that a urine output-based resuscitation paradigm tracked by a flow sheet resulted in a decrease in the rate of resuscitation-associated abdominal compartment syndrome from 16% to 5% with an attendant decrease in mortality [73]. In a separate study of burn injuries from combat versus the civilian environment, Wolf and colleagues showed that the most important effectors of burn-related mortality were total body surface area (TBSA) burned, age ≥40 years, and the presence of inhalation injury [72]. The conflict in Southwest Asia presents an opportunity to develop contemporary resource requirements to manage combat-related burn injury. Military burn surgeons discovered a relationship of approximately one acute operative intervention required per 5% TBSA burn consisting of all operations performed during the acute and convalescent/reconstructive phases of care. Truncal burn involvement was demonstrated to be a significant determinant of acute surgical therapy, whereas upper extremity burns were a significant determinant of reconstruction surgical necessity [74].

*Recommendations*:

1. Burn casualties should be resuscitated based on urine output.
2. Combat burn mortality is related to TBSA burn, age >40 years, and the presence of inhalation injury.
3. Combat burn surgical requirements can be predicted based upon TBSA burn as well as burn location.

*Grade of recommendations*: 1. B 2. B 3. B

## 4.7 What Are the Contemporary Techniques and Outcomes of Severe Brain Injury Sustained on the Battlefield?

The management of severe traumatic brain injury on the battlefield demonstrates many unique complexities in addition to the inherent difficulty of managing this severely injured patient population. In cases where the primary brain injury has already occurred and the injured tissue is not amenable to repair, and thus unrecoverable, the focus of managing these patients is directed toward minimizing secondary brain injury. Multiple circumstances, including a medically austere environment, limited critical care resources, and prolonged aeromedical evacuation prompted a more aggressive surgical approach to limit secondary brain injury in severe traumatic brain injury incurred on the battlefield. DuBose evaluated a cohort of isolated severe traumatic brain injury garnered from the Joint Theater Trauma Registry and compared with a case-matched cohort of like patients from the National Trauma Data Bank [75]. From this analysis, the cohort of military patients had a greater propensity to have surgical intervention (27.0%), including operative cranial decompression, lobectomy, or debridement. Most prominently, the data demonstrated substantial differences in intracranial pressure monitoring (13.8% military vs. 1.7% civilian) and craniectomy (8.8% military vs. 0.6% civilian). Most importantly, the survival was also significantly better among military casualties overall (92.3% military vs. 79% civilian), particularly after penetrating mechanisms of injury (94.4% military vs. 52.1% civilian). The survival benefit was even more pronounced with increasing severity of traumatic brain injury from AIS 3 to AIS 5 (Table 4.1).

**TABLE 4.1**

Summary of Evidence and Recommendations

| Question | Answer | Level of Evidence | Grade of Recommendation | References |
|---|---|---|---|---|
| Do trauma systems improve outcome after combat injury? | Trauma systems are responsible for improvements in outcome after combat injury and should be a key element of the battlefield medical system. | 2b | B | [8–23] |
| Where do combat casualty deaths occur? | Most combat casualty death occurs pre-hospital. Hemorrhage is the most substantial etiology of potentially survivable battlefield injury death, which validates pre-hospital care as a key entity in combat casualty care continuum. | 2c | B | [24–29] |
| Does training of pre-hospital providers affect outcome? | Mortality of combat casualties improvement is associated with improved capabilities and training of flight medical providers. | 3b | C | [30–32] |
| Is damage control resuscitation effective in severely injured patients? | Damage control resuscitation has proven to be effective at minimizing mortality in high-acuity combat casualties and should be the resuscitative strategy of choice in casualties at risk for massive transfusion. | 2b | B | [33–44] |
| When is fecal diversion necessary for colon injury incurred on the battlefield? | Colon diversion should be performed in patients with high-energy colon injury that would not tolerate complications. | 2b | C | [47–54] |
| Is arterial reconstruction after combat vascular injury safe and effective? | In the combat environment, arterial reconstruction should be performed with good long-term outcomes. Autogenous tissue optimizes outcome benefit potential. | 2b | B | [55–65] |
| Should diagnostic studies be done for vascular proximity? | Proximity is an indication for vascular interrogation, secondary to the high-energy mechanism and associated increase in vascular injury. | 2b | C | [68–70] |
| How should burn casualties be resuscitated? | Urine output | 2b | B | [71–73] |
| Is surgical management of battlefield brain injury warranted? | Aggressive surgical management of severe traumatic brain injury in combat improves mortality and is indicated after severe traumatic brain injury. | 2b | C | [75] |

*Recommendations*:

1. Aggressive surgical management of severe traumatic brain injury in combat improves mortality.
2. Prompt and aggressive surgical management of traumatic brain injury is indicated.

*Grade of recommendations*: 1. C 2. C

## References


1. Trunkey DD. History and development of trauma care in the United States. *Clin Orthop Relat Res.* 2000;374:36–46.
2. Trunkey DD. In search of solutions. *J Trauma.* 2002;53(6):1189–1191.
3. DeBakey ME. History, the torch that illuminates: Lessons from military medicine. *Mil Med.* 1996;161(12): 711–716.
4. Hoff WS, Schwab CW. Trauma system development in North America. *Clin Orthop Relat Res.* 2004;422:17–22.
5. Rich NM. Vietnam missile wounds evaluated in 750 patients. *Mil Med.* 1968;133(1):9–22.
6. Rich NM, Baugh JH, Hughes CW. Acute arterial injuries in Vietnam: 1,000 cases. *J Trauma.* 1970;10(5):359–369.
7. Rich NM, Hughes CW. Vietnam vascular registry: A preliminary report. *Surgery.* 1969;65(1):218–226.
8. Demetriades D, Kimbrell B, Salim A et al. Trauma deaths in a mature urban trauma system: Is "trimodal" distribution a valid concept? *J Am Coll Surg.* 2005;201(3):343–348.
9. Jurkovich GJ, Mock C. Systematic review of trauma system effectiveness based on registry comparisons. *J Trauma.* 1999;47(3 Suppl):S46–S55.
10. Mann NC. Assessing the effectiveness and optimal structure of trauma systems: A consensus among experts. *J Trauma.* 1999;47(3 Suppl):S69–S74.
11. Mann NC, Mullins RJ. Research recommendations and proposed action items to facilitate trauma system implementation and evaluation. *J Trauma.* 1999;47(3 Suppl):S75–S78.
12. Mann NC, Mullins RJ, MacKenzie Ef et al. Systematic review of published evidence regarding trauma system effectiveness. *J Trauma.* 1999;47(3 Suppl):S25–S33.
13. Mullins RJ. A historical perspective of trauma system development in the United States. *J Trauma.* 1999;47(3 Suppl):S8–S14.
14. Mullins RJ, Mann NC. Population-based research assessing the effectiveness of trauma systems. *J Trauma.* 1999;47(3 Suppl):S59–S66.

15. Mullins RJ, Mann NC. Introduction to the academic symposium to evaluate evidence regarding the efficacy of trauma systems. *J Trauma*. 1999;47(3 Suppl):S3–S7.
16. Mullins RJ, Veum-Stone J, Hedges JR et al. Influence of a statewide trauma system on location of hospitalization and outcome of injured patients. *J Trauma*. 1996;40(4):536–545; discussion 545–546.
17. Nathens AB, Jurkovich GJ, Rivara FP et al. Effectiveness of state trauma systems in reducing injury-related mortality: A national evaluation. *J Trauma*. 2000;48(1):25–30; discussion 30–31.
18. O'Keefe GE, Jurkovich GJ, Copass M et al. Ten-year trend in survival and resource utilization at a level I trauma center. *Ann Surg*. 1999;229(3):409–415.
19. Trunkey DD. Trauma care systems. *Emerg Med Clin North Am*. 1984;2(4):913–922.
20. West JG, Williams MJ, Trunkey DD et al. Trauma systems: Current status—Future challenges. *JAMA*. 1988;259(24):3597–3600.
21. Eastridge BJ, Jenkins D, Flaherty S et al. Trauma system development in a theater of war: Experiences from Operation Iraqi Freedom and Operation Enduring Freedom. *J Trauma*. 2006;61(6):1366–1372; discussion 1372–1373.
22. Eastridge B, Wade CE, Spott MA et al. Utilizing a trauma systems approach to benchmark and improve combat casualty care. *J Trauma*. July 2010;69(Suppl 1):S5–S9.
23. Palm K, Apodaca A, Spencer D, Costanzo G, Bailey J, Fortuna G, Blackbourne LH, Spott MA, Eastridge BJ. Evaluation of military trauma system practices related to complications after injury. *J Trauma Acute Care Surg*. December 2012;73(6 Suppl 5):S465–S471.
24. Carey ME. Learning from traditional combat mortality and morbidity data used in the evaluation of combat medical care. *Mil Med*. 1987;152(1):6–13.
25. Bellamy RF, Maningas PA, Vayer JS. Epidemiology of trauma: Military experience. *Ann Emerg Med*. 1986;15(12):1384–1348.
26. Bellamy RF. The causes of death in conventional land warfare: Imply cations for combat casualty care research. *Mil Med*. 1984;149(2):55–62.
27. Champion HR, Holcomb JB, Lawnick MM et al. Improved characterization of combat injury. *J Trauma*. 2010;68(5):1139–1150.
28. Eastridge BJ, Hardin M, Cantrell J et al. Died of Wounds (DOW): Cause of death after battlefield injury. *J Trauma*. July 2011;71:S4–S8.
29. Eastridge BJ, Mabry RL, Seguin P et al. Death on the battlefield (2001–2011): Implications for the future of combat casualty care. *J Trauma Acute Care Surg*. December 2012;73(6 Suppl 5):S431–S437.
30. Holland SR, Apodaca A, Mabry RL. MEDEVAC: Survival and physiological parameters improved with higher level of flight medic training. *Mil Med*. May 2013;178(5):529–536.
31. Apodaca AN, Morrison JJ, Spott MA, Lira JJ, Bailey J, Eastridge BJ, Mabry RL. Improvements in the hemodynamic stability of combat casualties during en route care. *Shock*. 2013;40(1):5–10.
32. Apodaca A, Olson CM, Jr, Bailey J, Butler F, Eastridge BJ, Kuncir E. Performance improvement evaluation of forward aeromedical evacuation platforms in Operation Enduring Freedom. *J Trauma Acute Care Surg*. 2013;75:S157–S163.
33. Cancio LC, Wade CE, West SA et al. Prediction of mortality and of the need for massive transfusion in casualties arriving at combat support hospitals in Iraq. *J Trauma*. 2008;64(2 Suppl):S51–S55; discussion S55–S56.
34. Borgman MA, Spinella PC, Perkins JG, Grathwohl KW, Repine T, Beekley AC, Sebesta J, Jenkins D, Wade CE, Holcomb JB. The ratio of blood products transfused affects mortality in patients receiving massive transfusions at a combat support hospital. *J Trauma*. October 2007;63(4):805–813.
35. Spinella PC, Perkins JG, Grathwohl KW et al. Effect of plasma and red blood cell transfusions on survival in patients with combat related traumatic injuries. *J Trauma*. 2008;64(2 Suppl):S69–S77; discussion S77–S78.
36. Palm K, Apodaca A, Spencer D, Costanzo G, Bailey J, Blackbourne LH, Spott MA, Eastridge BJ. Evaluation of military trauma system practices related to damage-control resuscitation. *J Trauma Acute Care Surg*. December 2012;73(6 Suppl 5):S459–S464.
37. Langan NR, Eckert M, Martin MJ. Changing patterns of in-hospital deaths following implementation of damage control resuscitation practices in US forward military treatment facilities. *JAMA Surg*. September 2014;149(9):904–912.
38. Stone HH, Strom PR, Mullins RJ. Management of the major coagulopathy with onset during laparotomy. *Ann Surg*. 1983;197(5):532–535.
39. Johnson JW, Gracias VH, Reilly PM et al. Evolution in damage control for exsanguinating penetrating abdominal injury. *J Trauma*. 2001;51(2):261–269; discussion 269–271.
40. Rotondo MF, Bard MR. Damage control surgery for thoracic injuries. *Injury*. 2004;35(7):649–654.
41. Rotondo MF, Schwab CW, McGonigal MD et al. 'Damage control': An approach for improved survival in exsanguinating penetrating abdominal injury. *J Trauma*. 1993;35(3):375–382; discussion 382–383.
42. Rotondo MF, Zonies DH. The damage control sequence and underlying logic. *Surg Clin North Am*. 1997;77(4):761–777.
43. Shapiro MB, Jenkins DH, Schwab CW et al. Damage control: Collective review. *J Trauma*. 2000;49(5):969–978.
44. Bograd B, Rodriguez C, Amdur R et al. Use of damage control and the open abdomen in combat. *Am Surg*. August 2013;79(8):747–753.
45. Edens J, Beekley A, Chung KK, et al. Longterm outcomes after combat casualty emergency department thoracotomy. *J Am Coll Surg*. August 2009;209(2):188–197.
46. Imes PR. The emergency management of abdominal trauma. *Surg Clin North Am*. 1956:1289–1294.
47. George SM, Jr, Fabian TC, Mangiante EC. Colon trauma: Further support for primary repair. *Am J Surg*. 1988;156(1):16–20.
48. Fabian TC. Infection in penetrating abdominal trauma: Risk factors and preventive antibiotics. *Am Surg*. 2002;68(1):29–35.

49. Stone HH, Fabian TC. Management of perforating colon trauma: Randomization between primary closure and exteriorization. *Ann Surg.* 1979;190(4):430–436.
50. Croce MA, Fabian TC, Mangiante EC. Penetrating colon trauma. *J Tenn Med Assoc.* 1986;79(11):706–707.
51. Duncan JE, Corwin CH, Sweeney WB et al. Management of colorectal injuries during Operation Iraqi Freedom: Patterns of stoma usage. *J Trauma.* 2008;64(4):1043–1047.
52. Steele SR, Wolcott KE, Mullenix PS et al. Colon and rectal injuries during Operation Iraqi Freedom: Are there any changing trends in management or outcome? *Dis Colon Rectum.* 2007;50(6):870–877.
53. Vertrees A, Wakefield M, Pickett C et al. Outcomes of primary repair and primary anastomosis in war-related colon injuries. *J Trauma.* May 2009;66(5):1286–1291; discussion 1291–1293.
54. Watson JD, Aden JK, Engel JE, Rasmussen TE, Glasgow SC. Risk factors for colostomy in military colorectal trauma: A review of 867 patients. *Surgery.* June 2014;155(6):1052–1061.
55. Rich NM, Rhee P. An historical tour of vascular injury management: From its inception to the new millennium. *Surg Clin North Am.* 2001;81(6):1199–1215.
56. Hughes CW. The primary repair of wounds of major arteries; an analysis of experience in Korea in 1953. *Ann Surg.* 1955;141(3):297–303.
57. Rasmussen TE, Clouse WD, Jenkins DH et al. The use of temporary vascular shunts as a damage control adjunct in the management of wartime vascular injury. *J Trauma.* 2006;61(1):8–12; discussion 12–15.
58. Fox CJ, Gillespie DL, Cox ED et al. Damage control resuscitation for vascular surgery in a combat support hospital. *J Trauma.* 2008;65(1):1–9.
59. Fox CJ, Gillespie DL, Cox ED et al. The effectiveness of a damage control resuscitation strategy for vascular injury in a combat support hospital: Results of a case control study. *J Trauma.* 2008;64(2 Suppl):S99–S106; discussion S106–S107.
60. Fox CJ, Gillespie DL, O'Donnell SD et al. Contemporary management of wartime vascular trauma. *J Vasc Surg.* 2005;41(4):638–644.
61. Clouse WD, Rasmussen TE, Peck MA et al. In-theater management of vascular injury: 2 years of the Balad Vascular Registry. *J Am Coll Surg.* 2007;204(4):625–632.
62. Sohn VY, Arthurs ZM, Herbert GS et al. Demographics, treatment, and early outcomes in penetrating vascular combat trauma. *Arch Surg.* 2008;143(8):783–787.
63. Rasmussen TE, Clouse WD, Jenkins DH et al. Echelons of care and the management of wartime vascular injury: A report from the 332nd EMDG/Air Force Theater Hospital, Balad Air Base, Iraq. *Perspect Vasc Surg Endovasc Ther.* 2006;18(2):91–99.
64. Quan RW, Gillespie DL, Stuart RP et al. The effect of vein repair on the risk of venous thromboembolic events: A review of more than 100 traumatic military venous injuries. *J Vasc Surg.* 2008;47(3):571–577.
65. Dua A, Patel B, Kragh JF, Jr, Holcomb JB, Fox CJ. Long-term follow-up and amputation-free survival in 497 casualties with combat-related vascular injuries and damage-control resuscitation. *J Trauma. Acute Care Surg.* December 2012;73(6):1517–1524.
66. Dennis JW, Frykberg ER, Crump JM et al. New perspectives on the management of penetrating trauma in proximity to major limb arteries. *J Vasc Surg.* 1990;11(1):84–92; discussion 92–93.
67. Frykberg ER, Crump JM, Vines FS et al. A reassessment of the role of arteriography in penetrating proximity extremity trauma: A prospective study. *J Trauma.* 1989;29(8):1041–1050; discussion 1050–1052.
68. Francis H 3rd, Thal ER, Weigelt JA et al. Vascular proximity: Is it a valid indication for arteriography in asymptomatic patients? *J Trauma.* 1991;31(4):512–514.
69. Johnson ON 3rd, Fox CJ, White P et al. Physical exam and occult post-traumatic vascular lesions: Implications for the evaluation and management of arterial injuries in modern warfare in the endovascular era. *J Cardiovasc Surg (Torino).* 2007;48(5):581–586.
70. Fox CJ, Gillespie DL, Neber MA et al. Delayed evaluation of combat-related penetrating neck trauma. *J Vasc Surg.* 2006;44(1):86–93.
71. Kauvar DS, Wolf SE, Wade CE et al. Burns sustained in combat explosions in Operations Iraqi and Enduring Freedom (OIF/OEF explosion burns). *Burns* 2006;32(7):853–857.
72. Wolf SE, Wolf SE, Wade CE et al. Comparison between civilian burns and combat burns from Operation Iraqi Freedom and Operation Enduring Freedom. *Ann Surg.* 2006;243(6):786–792; discussion 792–795.
73. Ennis JL, Chung KK, Renz EM et al. Joint Theater Trauma System implementation of burn resuscitation guidelines improves outcomes in severely burned military casualties. *J Trauma.* 2008;64(2 Suppl):S146–S151; discussion S151–S152.
74. Chan RK, Aden J Wu, Hale RG, Renz EM, Wolf SE. Operative utilization following severe combat-related burns. *J Burn Care Res.* 2015 March–April;36(2): 287–296.
75. DuBose JJ, Barmparas G, Inaba K, Stein DM, Scalea T, Cancio LC, Cole J, Eastridge B, Blackbourne L. Isolated severe traumatic brain injuries sustained during combat operations: Demographics, mortality outcomes, and lessons to be learned from contrasts to civilian counterparts. *J Trauma.* January 2011;70(1):11–16; discussion 16–18.

## Commentary on Evidence-Based Surgery: Military Injury Outcomes

*Donald Trunkey*

Following WWII and the Korean conflict, surgical care focused on the treatment of shock, wounds, and the physiology of organ failure. During the conflict in Korea, a major problem was the high incidence of acute tubular necrosis due to shock. There was not much that could be done since dialysis was in the embryonic stages of doing support to the patient post injury. During the Vietnam War, patients were given excess amounts of fluid, which put them into ARDS. During the next conflict desert storm, multiple problems were identified. This led to meetings with the General Accounting Office. They documented some of the medical problems including full medical army capability was not achieved. Additionally, the General Accounting Office stated there was needed improvement required in the Navy's wartime medical care program. The other problems involved the air force, particularly medical readiness. They also stated the readiness system used to regulate movement of patients did not function adequately. They documented a poor system of forming teams which was problematic. Troop morale was a problem and there were numerous units, after action lessons learned, documented problems submitted had no action, or minimal action, taken.

As the war progressed in Afghanistan, excellence in wound care was the norm. DuBose did an excellent study on traumatic brain injuries sustained in combat operations. They compared the mortality outcomes and the lessons to be learned from contrast to civilian counterparts. The authors had access to the Joint Trauma Theater Registry (JTTR) and National Trauma Database (NTDB). There were 181 matched patients from the JTTR and an equal amount from the NTDB. They looked at any operative intervention, the number of patients that had ICP monitoring, craniotomy, craniectomy, brain lobectomy, other brain incision, skull debridement, and brain debridement. The number of patients in the JTTR was impressive and 39 patients had operative intervention, 25 patients had ICP monitoring, 12 had craniotomy, 16 had craniectomy, 4 had brain lobectomy, 2 had brain incisions, 14 had skull debridement, and 9 patients had brain debridement. The operative intervention in ICP monitoring received a p-value of less than 0.001. Craniectomy was done in 16 patients in the JTTR and only 1 in the NTDB.

Another table shows comparison of mortality in JTTR and NTDB matched patients. The JTTR patients had an overall mortality of 7.7% or 14 patients out of a 181. The NTDB had 21% mortality rate or 38 out of 181 patients. The p-value is 0.001. Mortality of penetrating trauma is 5.6% in the JTTR and 38.1% in the NTDB. P-value is 0.001. The most remarkable number is the mortality in the patients who had AIS Head 5 was 68.6% in the NTDB and only 5.7% in the JTTR registry. The p-value was 0.001.

There are other issues of civilian neurosurgery including manpower. There are approximately 3000 neurosurgeons in the United States. There are 130–140 new trainees each year; however, this has increased slightly. About 250 neurosurgeons retire each year. Approximately 8 years is required to start new programs. Neurosurgeons limit their practice. Among these 57% have eliminated pediatrics, 13% no longer do trauma, 11% no longer do craniotomies, and many neurosurgeons limit their practice to back surgery. During the 1996 match in neurosurgery, there were 140 residents and in 2006, there were 165 residents.

Another issue is on-call pay in trauma hospitals. Neurosurgeons require $4000–$7000 a night, orthopedists get $2000–$4000 a night, and general surgeons get $1000–$2000 a night. Specialty surgeons operative cases per Annum in level 1 hospital for neurosurgeon and orthopedics. In neurosurgery, there are 45 centers with an average of 33 patients during the year, with the range running from 0–105. Orthopedics has 33 centers. Their operative cases are 256 averaged. The range is 12–754.

# 5

# *Evidence-Based Surgery: Traumatized Airway*

**Edgar J. Pierre, Stephen L. Freiberg, Megan Rashid, and Pedro Mascaro**

CONTENTS



## 5.1 Introduction

Airway management is of paramount importance in caring for the trauma patient. The primary goals of airway intervention are to relieve or prevent airway obstruction, to secure the unprotected airway from aspiration, to provide adequate gas exchange, and to maintain cervical spine stabilization. Acute airway trauma is a rare yet potentially lethal injury that is often difficult to diagnose. Recent literature estimates the incidence of airway trauma is less than 0.1% of all trauma patients; however, the mortality of these injuries is high—up to 20% for blunt trauma and up to 40% for penetrating trauma [1,2]. Long-term outcomes are usually favorable if the patient is treated within 24 hours of presentation, but more than 60% of patients have other associated injuries, making diagnosis and management problematic [1,3,4].

Gaining control of the traumatized airway is the ultimate test of the provider's adeptness and clinical acumen. When the airway is secured, it is important to complete a diagnostic workup to determine the severity of the injury, as structures that can potentially be damaged after trauma to the face and neck include the upper airway, vascular structures, cervical spine, and aerodigestive tract [1]. Once the extent of the injury is determined, the choice remains whether to treat the injury conservatively or surgically.

First, some of the key questions are presented that a provider must understand to properly manage the airway for these patients. Next, a discussion directed at successfully navigating the challenge of airway management in the presence of acute airway trauma is addressed.

## 5.2 What Is the Optimal Pre-Hospital Airway?

Endotracheal intubation remains the gold standard for securing the airway in a trauma patient. However, endotracheal intubation is not without its risks and, therefore, should be performed in controlled settings by the most experienced personnel if at all possible [2]. However, pre-hospital intubation can rarely be performed under these conditions.

Pre-hospital intubation has failed to show mortality benefit in several studies [5–8]. This also holds true for additional advanced airway devices. Although not specific to trauma patients, a prospective trial of nearly 650,000 patients with out-of-hospital cardiac arrest had worse neurologic outcomes when advanced airway management was employed [9]. This, in combination with the heterogeneity of training in advanced airway management among pre-hospital providers, and the variation of usage of pre-hospital neuromuscular blockade, suggests that the optimal pre-hospital airway is, in fact, an effective ventilation with a bag-valve-mask. Only if ventilation with a bag-valve-mask is unsuccessful, should attempts be made for endotracheal intubation or placement of advanced airway devices.

*Recommendation*: The optimal pre-hospital airway is effective ventilation with a bag-valve-mask.

*Grade of recommendation*: B

## 5.3 What Is the Role of Pre-Hospital Intubation?

Data in the literature regarding the safety and efficacy of pre-hospital intubation are almost entirely derived from retrospective and descriptive studies, as randomization and standardization of such an intervention are nearly impossible to achieve. Studies from the United States suggest a success rate of pre-hospital endotracheal intubation of 86%–90%, but it can be as low as 50% when performed by rescuers that do not often perform the procedure [7]. Additionally, pre-hospital intubation routinely fails to show benefit in the literature: in a prospective observational study at a large Level I trauma center study by Cobas et al., there was a 31% incidence of failed pre-hospital intubation, and there was no difference in mortality between patients who were properly intubated and those who were not [7]. Furthermore, pre-hospital intubation has been associated with increased mortality both in patients with traumatic brain injury [6] and in patients with penetrating trauma [5]. Also, in another retrospective study by Stockinger et al., trauma patients who underwent pre-hospital intubation had increased mortality compared to those ventilated with a bag-valve-mask. Given the limitations of pre-hospital emergency medicine providers in the United States (who are generally paramedics and often are unable to administer neuromuscular blocking agents) and a lack of difference in mortality between patients who were properly intubated and those who were not, pre-hospital endotracheal intubation in the United States should be limited to experienced providers only if ventilation with a bag-valve-mask is unsuccessful.

*Recommendation*: Pre-hospital endotracheal intubation in the United States should be limited to experienced providers only if ventilation with a bag-valve-mask is unsuccessful.

*Grade of recommendation*: B

## 5.4 What Is the Optimal Size for an Endotracheal Tube?

In 1928, Magill recommended the placement of "the largest endotracheal tube which the larynx will comfortably accommodate" [10]. Even 30 years ago, it was common to place 9.0 or even 10.0 mm tubes for men and 8.0 mm tubes for women [11]. In recent years, there has been a trend to place increasingly smaller tubes, primarily because of data correlating larger tube sizes with increased incidence of sore throat [12]. As such, major anesthesiology textbooks now recommend the placement of an 8.0–9.0 mm tube for men and a 7.0–8.0 mm tube for women [13,14]. The fact remains, however, that evidence-based guidelines for endotracheal tube size selection do not exist. In a recent prospective cross-sectional study by Coordes et al., they evaluated tracheal morphometry of patients by computed tomography (CT) scan and, subsequently, made the recommendation of 8.0 mm tube for an average height man and a 7.0 mm tube for average height woman (even though they also assert the need for uniform tube labeling based on biometric data) [15].

In trauma patients, providers may be quick to select a smaller tube, as visualization of the larynx while using a smaller tube is often described as subjectively better [16]. However, important consideration should be given to the fact that trauma patients will often have prolonged intensive care unit (ICU) stays. In this regard, a larger tube size may be beneficial for two important reasons: first, it allows for decreased work of breathing and potential resultant ease with which to wean from a ventilator [17]. Second, a larger tube size allows for better pulmonary toilet and easier insertion of a fiberoptic bronchoscope, both critical aspects of the care of trauma and burn patients [11]. For this reason, it is the authors' recommendation that a minimum of a half size increase in tube size be considered for trauma patients for whom a prolonged ICU stay is anticipated.

In children, selection of endotracheal tube size is far more complex, but equally lacking in evidence-based guidelines. It is frequently taught that the internal diameter of the appropriately sized endotracheal tube will roughly approximate the size of the child's little finger, but this estimation is frequently difficult and unreliable. Age-based formulas are frequently utilized, but endotracheal tube size selection is more reliably based on a child's body length, and length-based resuscitation tapes are helpful for children up to 35 kg. Cuffed endotracheal tubes are equally safe for infants beyond the newborn period and in children [18,19].

*Recommendation*: The optimal sized endotracheal tube is 8.5 mm for men, 7.5 mm for women, and a length-based size selection for children.

*Grade of recommendation*: C

## 5.5 What Medications Should Be Used for Rapid Sequence Intubation?

Rapid sequence intubation (RSI) is the procedure of choice for securing the airway in trauma patients. In the Guidelines for Emergency Tracheal Intubation Immediately after Traumatic Injury by Dunham et al., it is recommended that if orotracheal intubation is required and the patient's jaws are not flaccid, a drug regimen should be administered to accomplish the following objectives: neuromuscular paralysis, sedation as needed, maintaining hemodynamic stability, preventing intracranial hypertension, preventing vomiting, and preventing intraocular content extrusion [20]. However, the specific drug regimen selected is highly dependent on the patient's particular injuries and clinical condition, and remains a topic of continued debate.

Commonly selected induction agents for trauma patients include etomidate and ketamine for their favorable hemodynamic effects. In a randomized controlled trial by Jabre et al., there was no difference in mortality found between the use of etomidate and ketamine for intubation of acutely ill patients [21]. The main concern with the usage of etomidate is that it can produce adrenal insufficiency; however, studies have failed to conclusively prove that this increases morbidity or mortality [21,22]. Ketamine has generally been avoided in patients with suspected traumatic brain injury due to concern that it increases intracranial pressure, but that fact remains controversial, and some newer data suggest that ketamine may even be neuroprotective [23].

Commonly selected paralytic agents include rocuronium and succinylcholine due to their rapid onset of action. In a systematic review by Perry et al., succinylcholine was found to be clinically superior, as it produced excellent intubating conditions with a slightly faster onset of action [24]. However, important contraindications to succinylcholine include severe burn or crush injuries beyond 48 h, ocular injury, and spinal cord injury.

*Recommendation*: For RSI, a drug regimen should be administered to accomplish the following objectives: neuromuscular paralysis, sedation as needed, maintaining hemodynamic stability, preventing intracranial hypertension, preventing vomiting, and preventing intraocular content extrusion.

*Grade of recommendation*: A

## 5.6 What Airway Adjuncts Should Be Considered if Unable to Intubate?

As per the American Society of Anesthesiologist Practice Guidelines for the Management of a Difficult Airway, if a patient cannot be intubated (and cannot be adequately ventilated by facemask), a supraglottic airway (SGA) is indicated [25]. The best studied and most often utilized is the laryngeal mask airway (LMA). If ventilation with the LMA is adequate, the provider has time and options to consider alternative methods of intubation, including but not limited to intubating stylets/exchange catheters, utilizing SGAs as a conduit to intubation, lightwands, or fiberoptic intubation. If ventilation with the LMA is inadequate, this places a provider on the emergency arm of the pathway. In a suggested modified algorithm for the trauma patient, additional adjuncts to be considered if ventilation with an LMA is inadequate, including the esophageal combitube, laryngeal tube, rigid bronchoscope, or transtracheal jet ventilation. Selection between these methods of emergency non-invasive ventilation is far more controversial, and if these methods fail, steps must be taken to obtain an emergency invasive airway.

*Recommendation*: If unable to intubate, an SGA should be placed.

*Grade of recommendation*: A

## 5.7 What Is the Role of Video Laryngoscopy?

Compared with direct laryngoscopy, video laryngoscopy has been associated with improved laryngeal views, higher frequency of successful intubations, and a higher frequency of first attempt intubations. There was no difference in time to intubation, airway trauma, lip/gum trauma, or dental trauma. As such, video laryngoscopy should be considered a useful initial approach to intubation in a predicted difficult airway, or as an adjunct if initial intubation attempt by direct laryngoscopy is unsuccessful [25,26].

*Recommendation*: Video laryngoscopy can be considered a useful approach to intubation in a predicted difficult airway or as an adjunct if initial intubation attempt by direct laryngoscopy fails.

*Grade of recommendation*: A

## 5.8 What Is the Role of Cricothyroidotomy?

When assessing difficult airway scenarios, it is essential to have a systematic approach to avoid significant morbidity and mortality. The American Society of Anesthesiologists has provided the framework in their algorithm to manage the unanticipated difficult airway [25]. As one progresses to the end of the algorithm, the "can't intubate, can't ventilate" scenario recommends the use of invasive airway access via cricothyroidotomy. The incidence of this scenario was estimated to be 0.01–2 per 10,000 cases in 1991 [27,28]. However, the emergence of LMAs as well as lighted stylets has decreased the need for invasive airway access [29].

To determine the best methodology to obtain airway access invasively, a number of studies have required the use of porcine trachea models to assess the efficacy, complications, overall ease, and procedural speed when comparing open versus percutaneous versus hybrid (incision first method) techniques. In a randomized controlled crossover design study by Kanji et al., physicians were compared on their time to successful cannulation, number of needle insertion(s), incision(s), and dilatation attempts. The hybrid approach was found to provide better anatomy localization and faster access times with fewer complications compared to the percutaneous technique [30]. In another study comparing the percutaneous versus open technique among emergency room attending and resident physicians, the results showed no significant differences other than the attending's ability to perform both procedures more quickly than the residents. The complication rates, ease of performance, and times were not significantly different [31].

Ultimately, an individual provider's level of experience in a given technique has shown to be the determining factor as to the speed and efficacy at which airway access is secured.

*Recommendation*: If a patient cannot be intubated or ventilated by other measures, surgical airway access is indicated via cricothyroidotomy.

*Grade of recommendation*: A

## 5.9 What Is the Best Strategy for Establishing an Emergency Airway in Children?

In the assessment of the emergency airway in children, it is vital to be aware of the unique challenges present in the pediatric patient. The presence of a prominent occiput, large tongue, tonsils, adenoids, and a large, floppy epiglottis relative to the size of the oral cavity impedes the visualization of the deeper airway during direct laryngoscopy [32]. The position of the larynx in children is also more cephalad when compared to that of adults, causing a more anterior view due to the acute angle between the epiglottis and the base of the tongue. Once the trachea and vocal cords have been visualized and the endotracheal tube has been placed, it is imperative to recognize that children's trachea is narrower and shorter compared to that of adults, leading to a greater risk of right mainstem bronchus intubations or inadvertent extubations [33–35].

From a physiologic standpoint, children have smaller functional residual capacity and increased oxygen consumption. This results in hypoxemic episodes and shorter safe apneic time during intubation. Hence, it is essential to provide adequate pre-oxygenation and then proceed to rapid sequence induction as the method of choice for the majority of pediatric emergency intubations, as it had a high success rate with a low rate of adverse events [36].

*Recommendation*: The best strategy for emergency airway management in children is RSI.

*Grade of recommendation*: B

## 5.10 How Should One Evaluate for Airway Injury?

The most sensitive way to diagnose airway injury is by history and physical exam. Signs and symptoms vary widely and often do not manifest for hours, particularly in blunt trauma [37]. In a study by Randall et al., the most common signs and symptoms found in laryngotracheal trauma include airway obstruction, subcutaneous emphysema, stridor, hoarseness, and odynophagia [1]. It is worth noting, however, that 14.6% of patients had no presenting indicator of airway injury, thus making diagnosis more difficult [38].

If the patient is stable and tracheal injury is suspected, the airway should be evaluated with a fiberoptic bronchoscope to identify the extent of the injury. In addition, computer tomography is a useful diagnostic tool in a patient with severe blunt force trauma to the anterior neck, unknown extent of injury, or physical exam findings obscuring examination (such as hematoma or edema) [1].

In a patient who presents with impending respiratory collapse, securing the airway is the first priority. Patients who have sustained airway injury often prefer to take the sitting position, as it is easier for the patients to maintain a patent airway seated as opposed to the supine position. Assuming that no absolute contraindications to this position exist, these patients should be allowed and encouraged to remain seated until the trauma team is ready to manage their airway definitively. After the airway is secured (generally defined as a tube present in the trachea with the cuff inflated distal to the injury [38]), further diagnostic workup can be initiated. Other than the aforementioned flexible fiberoptic bronchoscopy and CT, other diagnostic modalities include chest and lateral neck radiographs initially, then esophagogastroduodenoscopy and barium swallow to evaluate for aerodigestive injuries [39,40]. CT with angiography protocol (CTA) is becoming increasingly common, as it can provide information regarding the spine, airway, soft tissue of the neck, and, most importantly, the proximity of injury to vascular structures, identifying about a 99% sensitivity presence of dissection, pseudoaneurysm, occlusion, and transection.

*Recommendation*: History and physical exam are the first steps in the evaluation of a traumatic airway, but should be used in conjunction with imaging studies, as some patients can present with injury out of proportion to their symptoms.

*Grade of recommendation*: C

## 5.11 How Does One Secure the Airway in the Setting of Airway Trauma?

Securing the airway in the face of airway trauma poses an enormous challenge and may vary greatly, depending on the type of injury. Injuries that may compromise the airway include maxillofacial trauma, penetrating neck injuries, and blunt neck injuries, although there is often considerable overlap.

Facial trauma tends to be obvious, most often presenting with noticeable bleeding or facial distortion. However, sometimes, mild-appearing soft tissue injuries will mask more severe internal injuries [39]. In fact, even a patient able to speak requires regular reassessment, as his or her status can deteriorate quickly [41]. Facial injuries, generally characterized according to the Le Fort Classification, pose incredible risk for airway obstruction, and indications for early intubation in patients with facial injury include intraoral hemorrhage, pharyngeal edema, Glasgow Comma Score (GCS) less than 9, and voice change, as well as a patient unable to tolerate the supine position [42]. In these patients, it is recommended to maintain spontaneous ventilation for as long as possible, and keep them in the sitting or in prone position until one is ready to secure the airway [2].

In most trauma cases, endotracheal intubation is ideal; however, in maxillofacial trauma, it may not only be contraindicated but may also interfere with surgical repair. In these cases, nasotracheal intubation can be attempted, but a fiberoptic bronchoscope should be used to avoid worsening existing injuries. Le Fort II and III fractures are a contraindication to nasal intubation, and Le Fort III fractures require a tracheotomy almost half the time. When neither endotracheal nor nasotracheal intubation are feasible, a cricothyroidotomy or tracheotomy should be considered [42]. Cricothyroidotomy is more rapid than a tracheotomy and can be performed in the pre-hospital settings if needed.

Penetrating neck injuries provide their own challenges. In one study by Bhojani et al., the most common causes of penetrating trauma to the airway were gunshot wounds and stab wounds. About half of the patients in this study required emergency airways, about 0.1% of which were surgical airways [40]. Due to the extreme urgency of many penetrating neck injuries, assessment of the airway should be almost entirely clinical. Common findings include cervical ecchymoses or hematomas, stridor, wheezing, and hemoptysis. Rapid sequence induction with direct laryngoscopy and manual in-line stabilization remains the intubation method of choice, often utilized with the aid of a fiberoptic bronchoscope to evaluate the airway for signs of injury [2]. In addition, sometimes, it is easier and safer to intubate through an already existing neck wound, rather than creating another incision; however, due to the potential for creating or worsening a false lumen, confirmation of tracheal placement with fiberoptic bronchoscopy is mandatory after this maneuver. The caveat being a prolonged struggle to intubate may be a misuse of the golden hour, compromising the patient's respiratory status, and elevating intracranial pressure. Cricothyroidotomy is a useful alternative that Pierre et al. suggest would result in improved outcomes due to less hypoxia.

In contradistinction, motor vehicle collisions remain the most common cause of blunt airway injury. Blunt force trauma injuries to the trachea are less common, due in part to the flexibility of the tracheal cartilage and protection by the surrounding bony structures; however, many vital structures are associated with the cervical trachea, so injuries present in this area are often severe. Common symptoms of pending respiratory compromise from blunt trauma include pain when swallowing or rotating neck, subcutaneous emphysema, severe bruising of chest and neck, hemoptysis, dyspnea that is worse with neck extension, and hoarseness. Signs and symptoms indicative of a vascular injury include a bruit or thrill, an expanding or pulsatile hematoma or hemorrhage, and lack of a pulse, and

**TABLE 5.1**

Summary of Recommendations

| Question | Answer | Levels of Evidence | Strength of Recommendation | References |
|---|---|---|---|---|
| What is the optimal pre-hospital airway? | The optimal pre-hospital airway is effective ventilation with a bag-valve-mask. | IIb | B | [5–7] |
| What is the role of pre-hospital intubation? | Pre-hospital endotracheal intubation in the United States should be limited to experienced providers only if ventilation with a bag-valve-mask is unsuccessful. | IIc | B | [5–9] |
| What is the optimal sized endotracheal tube? | The optimal sized endotracheal tube is 8.5 mm for men, 7.5 mm for women, and a length-based selection for children. | IIIb, IV | C | [10–19] |
| What medications should be used for rapid sequence intubation? | For rapid sequence intubation, a drug regimen should be administered to accomplish the following objectives: neuromuscular paralysis, sedation as needed, maintaining hemodynamic stability, preventing intracranial hypertension, preventing vomiting, and preventing intraocular content extrusion. | Ib | A | [20] |
| What airway adjuncts should be considered if unable to intubate? | If unable to intubate, a supraglottic airway should be placed. | Ib | A | [25] |
| What is the role of video laryngoscopy? | Compared with direct laryngoscopy, video laryngoscopy has been associated with improved laryngeal views, higher frequency of successful intubations, and a higher frequency of first attempt intubations. | Ia | A | [25–26] |
| What is the role of cricothyroidotomy? | If a patient cannot be intubated or ventilated, surgical airway access via cricothyroidotomy is indicated. | Ib | A | [25] |
| What is the best strategy for establishing an emergency airway in children? | The best strategy for establishing emergency airway in children is rapid sequence intubation. | IIc | B | [36] |
| How should one evaluate for airway injury? | History and physical exam are the first step in evaluation of a traumatic airway, but should be used in conjunction with imaging studies. | 3b | C | [1,37–40] |
| How does one secure the airway in the setting of airway trauma? | Oral intubation or cricothyroidotomy should be performed early in patients with airway trauma. Unstable patients should be taken immediately to the operating room for exploration, but stable patients should be evaluated with imaging studies to determine the extent of the damage. | 5 | D | [37–42] |

these symptoms should prompt immediate definitive diagnostic testing. In addition, multiple injuries may obscure the presentation of airway injuries, as about 95% of patients with blunt vascular injuries of the neck had a concomitant major thoracic injury or a GCS less than 9 [43]. If there is any symptomatology of respiratory distress, the patient can deteriorate quickly as the injury progresses, so it is important to secure the airway early. Orotracheal intubation may be problematic in laryngeal fractures, as the endotracheal tube could extend the injury, create a false passage, or disrupt what little anatomy remains intact [39]. In addition, laryngoscopy can be hindered by the presence of a cervical collar in the setting of a suspected spine injury, but this difficulty can be attenuated with manual in-line stabilization. In one study, about 50% of patients who suffered blunt airway injury required a surgical airway, so a surgical airway may, in fact, be required in these patients [38]. Once the airway is secured, and if the patient is stable, the patient can undergo diagnostic tests to determine the extent of the injury, and decisions can be made regarding management. Unstable patients are taken directly to the operating room for surgical exploration of their injuries (Table 5.1).

*Recommendation*: Oral intubation or cricothyroidotomy should be performed early in patients with airway trauma. Unstable patients should be taken immediately to the operating room for exploration, but stable patients should be evaluated with imaging studies to determine the extent of the injury.

*Grade of recommendation*: D

## 5.12 Summary

In addition to mastery of basic airway management, the key to improving outcomes in traumatic airway injury is early recognition and intervention, which is complicated by the scarcity of these injuries at most centers. Unstable patients should have their airway secured by the most experienced airway personnel available, with surgical backup immediately available in case a surgical airway is needed. Stable patients should have their airway secured and undergo diagnostic evaluation, to determine the safest definitive treatment, which is surgical the majority of the time.

## References


1. Randall DR, Rudmik LR, Ball CG, Bosch JD. External laryngotracheal trauma: Incidence, airway control, and outcomes in a large Canadian center. *Laryngoscope.* 2014;124(4):E123–E133.
2. Pierre EJ, McNeer RR, Shamir MY. Early management of the traumatized airway. *Anesthesiol Clinics.* 2007;25(1):1–11, vii.
3. Farzanegan R, Alijanipour P, Akbarshahi H et al. Major airways trauma, management and long term results. *Ann Thorac Cardiovasc Surg.* 2011;17(6):544–551.
4. Mussi A, Ambrogi MC, Ribechini A, Lucchi M, Menoni F, Angeletti CA. Acute major airway injuries: Clinical features and management. *Eur J Cardio-Thorac Surg.* 2001;20(1):46–51, discussion 51–52.
5. Taghavi S, Vora HP, Jayarajan SN et al. Prehospital intubation does not decrease complications in the penetrating trauma patient. *Am J Surg.* 2014;80(1):9–14.
6. Davis DP, Peay J, Sise MJ et al. The impact of prehospital endotracheal intubation on outcome in moderate to severe traumatic brain injury. *J Trauma.* 2005;58(5):933–939.
7. Cobas MA, De la Pena MA, Manning R, Candiotti K, Varon AJ. Prehospital intubations and mortality: A level 1 trauma center perspective. *Anesth Analg.* 2009;109(2):489–493.
8. Lecky F, Bryden D, Little R, Tong N, Moulton C. Emergency intubation for acutely ill and injured patients. *Cochrane Database Systemat Rev.* 2008;(2):CD001429.
9. Hasegawa K, Hiraide A, Chang Y, Brown DF. Association of prehospital advanced airway management with neurologic outcome and survival in patients with out-of-hospital cardiac arrest. *JAMA* 2013;309(3):257–266.
10. Magill IW. Technique in endotracheal anaesthesia. *Br Med J.* 1930;2(3645):817–819.
11. Farrow S, Farrow C, Soni N. Size matters: Choosing the right tracheal tube. *Anaesthesia* 2012;67(8):815–819.
12. Stout DM, Bishop MJ, Dwersteg JF, Cullen BF. Correlation of endotracheal tube size with sore throat and hoarseness following general anesthesia. *Anesthesiology* 1987;67(3):419–421.
13. Barash PG, Cullen BF, Stoelting RK, Cahalan MK, Stock MC, Ortega R, eds. 2013. *Clinical Anesthesia,* 7th edn. Lippincott Williams & Williams: Philadelphia, PA.
14. Miller RD, Eriksson LI, Fleischer L, Wiener-Kronish JP, Young WL, eds. 2009. *Miller's Anesthesia,* 7th edn. Churchill Livingstone: New York.
15. Coordes A, Rademacher G, Knopke S et al. Selection and placement of oral ventilation tubes based on tracheal morphometry. *Laryngoscope* 2011;121(6):1225–1230.
16. Asai T and Shingu K. Difficulty in advancing a tracheal tube over a fiberoptic bronchoscope: Incidence, causes, and solutions. *Br J Anaesth.* 2004;92:870–871.
17. Bersten AD, Rutten AJ, Vedig AE, Skowronski GA. Additional work of breathing imposed by endotracheal tubes, breathing circuits, and intensive care ventilators. *Crit Care Med.* 1989;17(7):671–677.
18. King BR, Baker MD, Braitman LE, Seidl-Friedman J, Schreiner MS. Endotracheal tube selection in children: A comparison of four methods. *Ann Emerg Med.* 1993;22(3):530–534.
19. American Heart Association. 2005 American heart association (AHA) guidelines for cardiopulmonary resuscitation (CPR) and emergency cardiovascular care (ECC) of pediatric and neonatal patients: Pediatric basic life support. *Pediatrics* 2006;117(5):e989–e1004.
20. Dunham CM, Barraco RD, Clark DE et al. Guidelines for emergency tracheal intubation immediately after traumatic injury. *J Trauma.* 2003;55(1):162–179.
21. Jabre P, Combes X, Lapostolle F et al. Etomidate versus ketamine for rapid sequence intubation in acutely ill patients: A multicentre randomised controlled trial. *Lancet* 2009;374(9686):293–300.
22. de Jong FH, Mallios C, Jansen C, Scheck PA, Lamberts SW. Etomidate suppresses adrenocortical function by inhibition of 11 beta-hydroxylation. *J Clin Endocrinol Metab.* 1984;59(6):1143–1147.
23. Morris C, Perris A, Klein J, Mahoney P. Anaesthesia in haemodynamically compromised emergency patients: Does ketamine represent the best choice of induction agent? *Anaesthesia* 2009;64(5):532–539.
24. Perry JJ, Lee JS, Sillberg VA, Wells GA. Rocuronium versus succinylcholine for rapid sequence induction intubation. *Cochrane Database Systemat Rev.* 2008;(2):CD002788.
25. Apfelbaum JL, Hagberg CA, Caplan RA et al. Practice guidelines for management of the difficult airway: An updated report by the American Society of Anesthesiologists Task Force on Management of the Difficult Airway. *Anesthesiology* 2013;118(2):251–270.
26. Aziz M. Use of video-assisted intubation devices in the management of patients with trauma. *Anesthesiol Clinics* 2013;31(1):157–166.
27. Benumof JL. Management of the difficult adult airway. with special emphasis on awake tracheal intubation. *Anesthesiology* 1991;75(6):1087–1110.
28. Heard AM, Green RJ, Eakins P. The formulation and introduction of a 'can't intubate, can't ventilate' algorithm into clinical practice. *Anaesthesia* 2009;64(6):601–608.

29. Wong DT, Lai K, Chung FF, Ho RY. Cannot intubate-cannot ventilate and difficult intubation strategies: Results of a Canadian national survey. *Anesth Analg* 2005;100(5):1439–1446.
30. Kanji H, Thirsk W, Dong S et al. Emergency cricothyroidotomy: A randomized crossover trial comparing percutaneous techniques: Classic needle first versus "incision first". *Acad Emerg Med.* 2012;19(9):E1061–E1067.
31. Kocurek D, Seaberg D, McCabe J. Percutaneous versus open methods in cricothyroidotomy and thoracostomy. *Am J Emerg Med.* 1995;13(6):681.
32. Eastwood PR, Szollosi I, Platt PR, Hillman DR. Collapsibility of the upper airway during anesthesia with isoflurane. *Anesthesiology* 2002;97(4):786–793.
33. Griscom NT and Wohl ME. Dimensions of the growing trachea related to age and gender. *Am J Roentgenol.* 1986;146(2):233–237.
34. Weiss M, Balmer C, Dullenkopf A et al. Tracheal tube-tip displacement in children during head-neck movement—A radiological assessment. *Br J Anaesth.* 2006;96(4):486–491.
35. Litman RS, Weissend EE, Shibata D, Westesson PL. Developmental changes of laryngeal dimensions in unparalyzed, sedated children. *Anesthesiology* 2003;98(1):41–45.
36. Sagarin MJ, Barton ED, Chng YM et al. Rapid sequence intubation for pediatric emergency airway management. *Pediatr Emerg Care* 2002;18(6):417–423.
37. Schaefer SD. Management of acute blunt and penetrating external laryngeal trauma. *Laryngoscope* 2014;124(1):233–244.
38. Kummer C, Netto FS, Rizoli S, Yee D. A review of traumatic airway injuries: Potential implications for airway assessment and management. *Injury* 2007;38(1):27–33.
39. Rathlev NK, Medzon R, Bracken ME. Evaluation and management of neck trauma. *Emerg Med Clin North Am.* 2007;25(3):679–94, viii.
40. Bhojani RA, Rosenbaum DH, Dikmen E et al. Contemporary assessment of laryngotracheal trauma. *J Thorac Cardiovasc Surg* 2005;130(2):426–432.
41. Tuckett JW, Lynham A, Lee GA, Perry M, Harrington U. Maxillofacial trauma in the emergency department: A review. *Surgeon* 2014;12(2):106–114.
42. Mohan R, Iyer R, Thaller S. Airway management in patients with facial trauma. *J Craniofacial Surg.* 2009;20(1):21–23.
43. Ye D, Shen Z, Zhang Y, Qiu S, Kang, C. Clinical features and management of closed injury of the cervical trachea due to blunt trauma. *Scand J Trauma Resusc Emerg.* 2013;21:60.

## Commentary on Evidence-Based Surgery: Traumatized Airway

*Stephen O. Heard*

Over the past 25 years, vast improvements in airway management have occurred. The invention of supraglottic airways has decreased the incidence of "can't ventilate, can't intubate" situations. With the ability to ventilate through these devices, dire emergencies are turned into very manageable airway circumstances. Likewise, the development of rigid videolaryngoscopy has allowed clinicians to visualize better the glottis during difficult intubations. Despite these advances, the establishment of an airway in the trauma patient remains a challenge particularly for providers who do not routinely intubate patients. A full stomach, the presence of a rigid cervical collar, upper airway injuries, or head and neck injuries with bleeding and edema make tracheal intubation a very challenging proposition. Pierre et al. ask and answer a number of questions that are important in managing the airway of the trauma patient, particularly one who has suffered airway trauma. What is clear from perusing the chapter is the lack of high-quality studies that allow for definitive recommendations to be made regarding the management of the airway in these situations.

### What Is the Optimal Prehospital Airway and What Is the Role of Prehospital Intubation?

As pointed by out by Pierre et al., most prehospital emergency providers are paramedics. In many areas of the country, their training in emergency airway management is compromised, because they are competing with anesthesiology and emergency medicine residents, medical students, and student certified registered nurse anesthetists for the opportunity to manage the airway and intubate the trachea in controlled situations. Furthermore, an increasing number of patients in the operating room are being managed with supraglottic devices and with ultrasound-guided regional anesthesia, making it even more difficult to obtain the skills needed for advanced airway management. After becoming certified, if they are not exposed to adequate opportunities for airway management, their skills can atrophy. Too much time spent trying to establish an airway and intubate the patient can lead to hypoxia and hypotension, a deadly dyad in the trauma patient particular with traumatic brain injury.

### What Is the Optimal Size Endotracheal Tube?

I agree with the recommendations regarding the size of endotracheal tubes with the exception of women. Performing fiber-optic bronchoscopy through a tube with a 7.5 mm internal diameter can be challenging and may result in hypoventilation and damage to the bronchoscope. Use of a pediatric bronchoscope can be used, but the ability to provide pulmonary toilet with such a small scope and suction port is challenging. At my institution, we are frequently called to change the endotracheal tube to a larger one to allow for safer bronchoscopy. Changing endotracheal tubes can be associated with its own set of problems. Using a large tube (e.g., 8.0 mm ID) in woman at the time of intubation would preclude the need for a tube change.

### What Medications Should Be Used for Rapid Sequence Intubation?

The authors discuss the role of ketamine in rapid sequence intubation and its potential adverse effect on intracranial pressure. They also note that ketamine may be neuroprotective. I believe this issue should be put to rest. A recent systematic review* suggests that the intracranial pressure response (ICP) to ketamine is variable (decrease, no change, increase), but most importantly, there is no prolonged change in either ICP or cerebral perfusion pressure. In addition, there is no effect on long-term outcome.

Although this section is about medication use for rapid sequence intubation, I believe a few words regarding cricoid pressure for rapid sequence intubation are in order. Almost all trauma patients who require intubation have a full stomach. Cricoid pressure was originally described by Sellick† as a means to prevent passive regurgitation during laryngoscopy in patients with a full stomach. More recently,

* Cohen L, Athaide V, Wickham ME, Doyle-Waters MM, Rose NG, Hohl CM. The effect of ketamine on intracranial and cerebral perfusion pressure and health outcomes: A systematic review. *Ann Emerg Med.* 2015 January;65(1):43–51. e2.

† Sellick BA. Cricoid pressure to control regurgitation of stomach contents during induction of anesthesia. *Lancet.* 1961;2:404.

doubts have been cast on the utility of cricoid pressure to prevent aspiration. In an MRI study of normal volunteers, Smith et al.* found that cricoid pressure resulted in an unopposed esophagus over 70% of the time. However, Rice et al.†‡ point out the esophagus begins 1 cm distal to the cricoid ring, the cricoid ring and hypopharynx move together as a unit, and cricoid pressure will reliably compress the hypopharynx. Data reported by other investigators support the effectiveness of cricoid pressure§.

#### What Airway Adjuncts Should Be Considered If Unable to Intubate and What Is the Role of Video Laryngoscopy?

As mentioned previously, supraglottic airways can turn a "can't ventilate, can't intubate" emergency into a very manageable situation. Placement of these devices can be challenging at times and clinicians familiar with the American Society of Anesthesiologist's Guidelines for the Difficult Airway should be immediately available if there is difficulty in inserting these devices. At our institution (a Level I trauma center), we have a "code airway" team that is composed of an attending anesthesiologist, attending trauma surgeon, and respiratory therapist. This team will respond to all difficult airways in the emergency department if such a code is called by the attending emergency medicine physician. Providing extra assistance such as this has enabled the establishment of airways in very challenging situations.

Videolaryngoscopy provides better laryngeal views and higher frequency of successful intubations than with direct laryngoscopy; however, adequate training with these devices is required. Despite the better laryngeal views, it can be a challenge to insert the endotracheal tube into the trachea as the video laryngoscope is providing an indirect view of the glottis. Furthermore, significant mucosal damage has been reported during intubation with these devices.

#### What Is the Role of Cricothyroidotomy and What Is the Best Strategy for Establishing an Emergency Airway in Children?

Although I agree with the recommendations of the authors in these two sections, I urge a word of caution about cricothyroidotomy. In women (particularly obese women), it can be difficult to identify the cricothyroid membrane by palpation. Errors up to 3 cm can be realized¶. Use of the ultrasound will increase the accuracy of cricothyroid membrane identification.

#### How Should One Evaluate for Airway Injury and How Does One Secure the Airway in the Setting of Airway Trauma?

Establishing an airway in facial trauma can indeed be challenging. For those clinicians skilled with topical and regional anesthesia as well as the use of the bronchoscope, fiber-optic intubation is a reasonable choice in many situations. However, it does require a cooperative patient and significant bleeding in the oropharynx will make application of anesthesia difficult. Regardless of which method is used to secure the airway, a team approach is required and backup plans (Plans "B" and "C") should be in place. Simulation and crisis management training will improve the likelihood of the establishment of a successful airway.

---

* Smith KJMD, Dobranowski JMD, Yip GMD, Dauphin AMD, Choi PT-LMD. Cricoid pressure displaces the esophagus: An observational study using magnetic resonance imaging. *Anesthesiology.* 2003 July;99(1):60–64.

† Rice MJ, Mancuso AA, Gibbs C, Morey TE, Gravenstein N, Deitte LA. Cricoid pressure results in compression of the postcricoid hypopharynx: The esophageal position is irrelevant. *Anesth Analg.* 2009 November;109(5):1546–1552.

‡ Rice MJ, Mancuso A, Morey TE, Gravenstein N, Deitte L. The anatomy of the cricoid pressure unit. *Surg Radiol Anat.* 2010 April;32(4):419.

§ Zeidan AM, Salem MR, Mazoit JX, Abdullah MA, Ghattas T, Crystal GJ. The effectiveness of cricoid pressure for occluding the esophageal entrance in anesthetized and paralyzed patients: An experimental and observational glidescope study. *Anesth Analg.* 2014 March;118(3):580–586.

¶ Aslani A, Ng SC, Hurley M, McCarthy KF, McNicholas M, McCaul CL. Accuracy of identification of the cricothyroid membrane in female subjects using palpation: An observational study. *Anesth Analg.* 2012 May;114(5):987–992.

# 6

# Monitoring of the Trauma Patient

**Abdul Alarhayem and Natasha Keric**

**CONTENTS**



Traumatic injuries are the third leading cause of death among all age groups, and the leading cause of death among Americans aged 44 years and younger. To improve outcomes, life-threatening injuries must be diagnosed and treated expeditiously. The trauma surgeon must decide what type of monitoring will ensure an accurate diagnosis of shock, adequate and timely resuscitation, and early identification of potential problems.

## 6.1 Are Heart Rate and Blood Pressure Adequate Indicators of Shock?

Shock, originally described by Gross as "a manifestation of the rude unhinging of the mechanism of life" [1], is defined as a multisystem derangement caused by the body's inability to maintain organ perfusion necessary to sustain aerobic metabolism. In the setting of trauma, the old adage "All shock is hemorrhagic, until proven otherwise," still holds true.

Hemorrhage is still the most common cause of preventable death in both military and civilian settings. Recent data from combat operations such as Operation Enduring Freedom and Operation Iraqi Freedom found hemorrhage from major trauma to be the mechanism of death in more than 80% of potentially survivable cases [2].

Assessment of a trauma casualty in the prehospital and emergency department can be challenging. The use of traditional vital signs such as heart rate (HR) and systolic blood pressure (SBP) to identify patients at high risk of adverse outcomes has the advantage of simplicity, and trauma surgeons continue to place a high value on them during trauma alert activation and patient resuscitation.

However, numerous articles have displayed varying correlations between vital signs and major hemorrhage, patient survival, and the need for life-saving intervention.

Compensatory mechanisms allow for significant reductions in central circulating blood volume, stroke volume, and cardiac output well before changes in arterial blood pressure (BP) occur [3].

Clinicians routinely refer to hypotension as an SBP <90 mmHg; however, this often marks the beginning of circulatory decompensation rather than compromise, and mortality rates in these patients may approach 50% [4]. Trauma patients with an SBP <90 mmHg are twice as likely to die during hospitalization, and three times more likely to require emergency thoracic or abdominal surgery [5]. Unrecognized volume loss during the early compensatory phase of hemorrhage leads to poor perfusion and progressive acidosis and delays intervention, with the potential for sudden catastrophic decompensation [6]. A recent large review found an SBP of 110 mmHg to be a more clinically relevant definition of hypotension such that mortality was 4.8% greater for every 10 mmHg decrement in SBP [7]. Similar findings were reported in a large prospective European cohort study [8].

Although it may seem appropriate to expanding current trauma triage criteria to include patients with SBP between 90 and 110 mmHg, this may result in an unacceptably high degree of over triage [9].

Multiple studies have found that tachycardia does not reflect clinical reality accurately [11]. Animal and clinical studies have demonstrated that tachycardia is not always present even after major blood loss. In a study of more than 10,000 patients, it was found that HR was neither sensitive nor specific in determining the need for emergent intervention or packed red blood cell transfusion in the first 24 h of severe injury [12].

*Recommendation*: HR and BP are not adequate indicators of shock. Trauma patients with significant blood loss may present in compensated shock with normal vital signs. Other data in addition to HR and BP must be determined to detect occult hypoperfusion.

*Grade of recommendation*: B

## 6.2 Do Local Tissue Perfusion Measures Improve Our Ability to Diagnose Shock? Does Their Use Improve Outcomes?

Compensated shock may often be more accurately termed "unrecognized" shock [13]. Multiple measurements have been developed to identify occult hypoperfusion, i.e., before the onset of hemodynamic compromise. Oxygen delivery–consumption mismatch is the hallmark of shock; "upstream" or "downstream" markers are used to measure oxygen delivery and consumption, respectively.

Upstream measurements determine the amount of nutrients delivered to the tissue; they include both static and dynamic parameters. Static measures of preload, such as central venous pressure and pulmonary capillary wedge pressure are limited by significant inter- and intra-patient variability. In addition, these parameters do not correlate with intravascular volume status. The physiologic phenomenon of respiratory variability in preload can be used to assess fluid responsiveness. Large pulse pressure variation, systolic pressure variation, and stroke volume variation (SVV) are all dynamic measures and indicative of volume depletion. Although having consistently outperformed static measurements in predicting an increase in cardiac output in response to volume expansion, dynamic parameters have not been shown to improve outcomes, and thus their routine use is not recommended [14].

Downstream markers assess the adequacy of tissue nutrient delivery and extraction, given the level of metabolic demand. During normal metabolism, oxygen delivery ($DO_2$) far exceeds consumption. As systemic perfusion decreases, tissue beds compensate by increasing oxygen extraction from arterial blood, with a resultant decrease in oxygen saturation of venous hemoglobin.

Oxygen saturation of venous hemoglobin is measured readily in the pulmonary artery ($SvO_2$), or superior vena cava ($ScvO_2$) with acceptable correlation [15]. A low $SvO_2$ (<65%) is highly suggestive of tissue hypoperfusion. In patients with traumatic brain injury, $ScvO_2$ values <65% in the first 24 h have been associated with higher mortality [16].

Near-infrared spectroscopy (NIRS) is a novel monitoring strategy that enables direct measurement of oxygen saturation of hemoglobin found in peripheral muscle tissue or subcutaneous tissue ($StO_2$). Early studies suggest that $StO_2$ reflects global perfusion and may be as good as the base deficit (BD) for detecting shock [17,18]. Following a severe traumatic injury, patients with $StO_2$ >75% are highly unlikely to develop organ dysfunction and death [17]. Another study reported a threefold increase in mortality with every 10% decrease in $StO_2$ [19]. $StO_2$ has also been found to be an independent predictor for blood transfusions and life-saving interventions [20,21].

Once oxygen delivery falls below a critical level, blood flow to the most vulnerable organs (brain and heart) is maintained at the expense of other organs (skin, muscle, and intestines) [22]. Anaerobic metabolism ensues, and its metabolites accumulate in these tissue beds. Changes in hydrogen ion concentration may be measured at the cellular level through gastric intramucosal pH and sublingual $pCO_2$.

Gastric tonometry is an indirect measurement of gastric intramucosal pH (pHim), which is an indicator of splanchnic tissue ischemia [23]. A nasogastric tube is placed in the mid-gastric position with a silicone balloon, permeable to intraluminal $CO_2$, which is used to approximate intracellular $PCO_2$ and, thus, the degree of anaerobic metabolism.

Although it has the ability to predict outcomes based on early low pHim, only a single study demonstrated that therapeutic interventions guided by gastric tonometry were able to improve survival [24]. Follow-up randomized studies failed to show that pHim directed resuscitation improved individual patient outcomes [25–27]. Gastric tonometry is also logistically difficult, and this might be a significant factor inhibiting widespread use of this technology [28].

Measuring sublingual $PCO_2$ ($PslCO_2$) is technically more easily applied than gastric tonometry. Although the internal carotid artery provides lingual blood flow, blood flow to the tongue and splanchnic beds falls similarly in response to global hypoperfusion [29]. Initial studies show that $PslCO_2$ is equivalent to lactic acid levels and BD in predicting the severity of shock and, more importantly, survival in hypotensive trauma patients. $PslCO_2$ gap is also a useful prognosticator; patients with an initial $PslCO_2$ gap of >25 mmHg had higher mortality rates than those with a gap of <25 mmHg [30]. Further studies are required to determine the clinical utility of $PslCO_2$ as an end-point guiding resuscitation.

*Recommendations*: Routine use of dynamic measures of fluid responsiveness (e.g., pulse pressure variation [PPV], stroke volume variation [SVV]) is not recommended.

*Grade of recommendation*: B

Routine measurement of cardiac output for patients with shock is not recommended.

*Grade of recommendation*: B

Current local perfusion measures such as NIRS, gastric intramucosal pH, and sublingual capnography may help identify occult hypoperfusion; however, their lack of sensitivity limits their ability to guide resuscitation. Evidence suggesting they improve outcomes is lacking.

*Grade of recommendation*: B

## 6.3 Does Hemodynamic Monitoring with a Pulmonary Artery Catheter Improve Outcomes?

One may argue that no monitoring device, no matter how insightful, will improve outcome unless coupled with a treatment that itself improves outcome [31]. Although there is no debate about the measurements a pulmonary artery catheter (PAC) can offer, there is much controversy surrounding the benefits of this device [32].

A recent meta-analysis that included all randomized controlled trials evaluating the use of a PAC failed to show any associated benefit [33].

The Cochrane review shows that of the 12 studies included to evaluate the validity of the use of a PAC, there was no difference in mortality, complication rate, morbidity, cost, or length of stay with or without a PAC [34].

In severely injured trauma patients, Velmahos et al. found that there was no difference in mortality or organ failure even with a goal-directed resuscitation [35]. The ESCAPE trial, a randomized controlled trial in patients with severe symptomatic heart failure, found no mortality benefit in patients assigned to clinical assessment-guided therapy versus those receiving PAC and clinical assessment-driven therapy [36].

In addition, there are complications that may arise directly from the use of a PAC; a study of 70 critically ill patients demonstrated that 4% died from complications related to the PAC and 20%–30% had major complications [37].

As a result, the routine use of the PAC in the intensive care unit (ICU) has been clearly decreasing. Between 1993 and 2004, PAC use decreased by 65% from 5.66 to 1.99 per 1000 medical admissions, with a similar trend for surgical patients [38].

With the advent of none or minimally invasive devices that can provide accurate hemodynamic assessments, the use of PAC is all but extinct, except in very select circumstances (combined shock states, discordant ventricular heart failure, and pulmonary hypertension) [39].

*Recommendation*: The use of PACs has not been shown to improve outcomes; routine use should be discouraged.

*Grade of recommendation*: A

## 6.4 Is There a Biochemical Parameter That Best Identifies Shock and Guides Resuscitation?

Inadequate tissue $O_2$ delivery leads to anaerobic metabolism. Lactic acid and hydrogen ions, the two primary by-products of anaerobiasis, may serve as adjuncts in identifying "occult hypoperfusion" (i.e., normal hemodynamic parameters).

Lactate levels in the blood are a function of the balance between lactate production and clearance, with a normal value of less than 2.5 mg/dL.

Both the initial lactate level and time to normalization of lactate correlate with risk of multiple organ dysfunction syndrome and death [40–44]. Odom et al. demonstrated a dose–response relationship, with higher mortality seen in patients with higher lactate levels. Patients' mortality was found to be 5.4% when the lactate level was <2.5 mg/dL, but approached 20% in patients with a lactate level >4.0 mg/dL. Lactate clearance at 6 h also independently predicted mortality; the adjusted odds ratio for death was 1.0, 3.5, and 4.3 for patients with clearances of ≥60%, 30% to 59%, and <30%, respectively [45]. Abramson also found prolonged lactate clearance to be a predictor of increased mortality in severely injured trauma patients; those that did not normalize by 48 h had an 86% mortality rate, compared to a 100% survival rate in those who had normalized lactate levels at 24 h [42].

A recent multicenter randomized controlled trial found lactate-guided therapy (aiming to decrease lactate levels by 20% or more per 2 h for the initial 8 h of ICU stay) significantly reduced hospital mortality when adjusting for predefined risk factors (HR 0.61).

Lactate as an end point of resuscitation also allowed inotropes to be stopped earlier, and patients were weaned from mechanical ventilation and discharged from the ICU earlier [46].

Importantly, lactic acidosis may not correlate with tissue hypoperfusion in patients with malignancy, liver failure, and diabetic ketoacidosis and in those taking certain drugs and even following heavy exercise.

BD is calculated from arterial blood gas and is the amount of base required to return the pH of 1 L of blood back to a normal level. Thus, BD is a measure of uncompensated metabolic acidosis. Elevation of the BD beyond −3 correlates with the presence and severity of shock [47,48].

Trauma patients with an abnormal BD on admission or those who fail to normalize their BDs have a higher incidence of mortality and poor outcomes, such as acute lung injury, multiple organ failure, and a greater need for blood transfusion [49–51]. Also, a BD that increases (becomes more negative) with ongoing resuscitation may suggest the presence of uncontrolled hemorrhage [52].

Importantly, large-volume saline resuscitation results in a non-anion gap, hyperchloremic, metabolic acidosis, and, hence, a persistently elevated BD despite normalization of perfusion [53]. BD levels may also be confounded by alcohol intoxication, renal failure, chronic obstructive pulmonary disease, and other causes. Also, all measurements of BDs are rendered inaccurate in the setting of exogenous bicarbonate administration.

Measurement of the serum bicarbonate concentration may be used as surrogate for the BD with reasonable correlation and does not require an arterial sample [54,55]. Arterial pH is generally not useful because of the body's compensatory mechanisms.

*Recommendation*: In the absence of hypotension, abnormal serum lactate, arterial pH, bicarbonate, and BD suggest occult hypoperfusion. Failure to normalize these parameters correlates with poor outcome. Lactate may be the best biochemical parameter to follow over time; using it as an end point of resuscitation has been found to reduce hospital mortality.

*Grade of recommendation*: B

## 6.5 Should the Geriatric Trauma Patient Have More Invasive Monitoring?

Trauma in the elderly (≥65 years) is associated with higher mortality and complication rates compared with younger patients even after controlling for degree of injury [56,57]. Yet elderly patients are consistently under-triaged to major trauma centers, possibly due to

**TABLE 6.1**

Monitoring of the Trauma Patient: Evidence and Grades of Recommendation

| Question | Answer | Level of Evidence | Grade of Recommendation | References |
|---|---|---|---|---|
| Are HR and BP adequate indicators of shock? | HR and BP are not adequate indicators of shock. Trauma patients with significant blood loss may present in compensated shock with normal vital signs. Other data in addition to HR and BP must be determined to detect occult hypoperfusion. | IIB, IIC | B | [3–12] |
| Do local tissue perfusion measures improve our ability to diagnose shock? Does their use improve outcomes? | Routine use of dynamic measures of fluid responsiveness (e.g., PVV, SVV) and CO is not recommended. | IB | B | [14–30] |
| | Current local perfusion measures may help identify occult hypoperfusion; however, their lack of sensitivity limits their ability to guide resuscitation. Evidence suggesting they improve outcomes is lacking. | IB | B | |
| Does hemodynamic monitoring with a pulmonary artery catheter improve outcomes? | The use of pulmonary artery catheters (PAC) has not been shown to improve outcomes; routine use should be discouraged. | IA | A | [32–39] |
| Is there a biochemical parameter that best identifies shock and guides resuscitation? | In the absence of hypotension, abnormal serum lactate, arterial pH, bicarbonate, and base deficit suggest occult hypoperfusion. Failure to normalize these parameters correlates with poor outcome. Lactate may be the best biochemical parameter to follow over time; using it as an endpoint of resuscitation has been found to significantly reduce hospital mortality. | IB | B | [40–54] |
| Should the geriatric trauma patient have more invasive monitoring? | Transfer to a designated trauma center and ICU admission should be considered in elderly patients with one or more severe anatomic injuries (i.e., one or more body system AIS score ≥3) or an initial BD of −6 mEq/L or less. The indiscriminate use of pulmonary artery catheters in this population is not advocated. | IIB | B | [58–61] |

difficulty in accurately identifying the severity of injury due to comorbidities and age-related differences in physiology.

Following significant blood loss secondary to trauma, many elderly patients cannot appropriately augment their cardiac output, and therefore systemic vascular resistance is increased to maintain perfusion. As a result, elderly patients may demonstrate a normal BP, while having severely depressed and compromised cardiac function, leading to overall poor systemic perfusion.

The 2002 version of the Eastern Association for the Surgery of Trauma guidelines advocated the near-ubiquitous use of Swan-Ganz catheters in moderately to severely injured elderly patients, followed by optimization of cardiac output and oxygen delivery variables to supratherapeutic values. This was based on the work done by Scalea and colleagues, where it was found that elderly patients had high rates of occult hypoperfusion and that PAC-guided resuscitation to a cardiac index of at least 4 L/min/m$^2$ and an oxygen consumption of 170 mL/min/m$^2$ improved mortality [58].

We now know that noninvasive monitoring with bioelectrical impedance devices is comparable to PAC thermodilution techniques for estimating cardiac index in the geriatric trauma patient [59,60].

In addition, augmentation of post-injury oxygen delivery not only produces no survival benefit, but comes with an increased risk for intra-abdominal hypertension and death [61].

The use of PAC has not been shown to improve outcomes, irrespective of age or severity of injury; its use is thus not recommended (see Section 6.3).

Adequacy of resuscitation and the oxygen debt and tissue perfusion can be monitored by BD measurements [17]; a BD of −6 mmol/L indicates significant mortality, especially in patients older than 55 years. Normalizing lactate and BD levels can provide guidance as to the adequacy of hemodynamic resuscitation [62,63] (Table 6.1).

*Recommendation*: Transfer to a designated trauma center and ICU admission should be considered in elderly patients with one or more severe anatomic injuries (i.e., one or more body system Abbreviated Injury Scale [AIS] score of ≥3) or an initial BD of −6 mEq/L or less. The indiscriminate use of PACs in this population is not advocated.

*Grade of recommendation*: B

## References


1. Gross S. 1872. *A System of Surgery: Pathological.* Diagnostic, Therapeutique and Operative, Lea & Febiger: Philadelphia, PA.
2. Eastridge B, Mabry RL, Seguin P et al. Death on the battlefield (2001Y2011): Implications for the future of combat casualty care: Corrigendum. *J Trauma Acute Care Surg.* December 2012;73(6 Suppl 5):S431–S437.
3. Shires G, Carrico C, Canizaro P. 1973. *Response of the Extracellular Fluid.* WB Saunders Company: Philadelphia, PA, pp. 15–42.
4. Heckbert SR, Vedder NB, Hoffman W et al. Outcome after hemorrhagic shock in trauma patients. *J Trauma-Injury Infect Crit Care* 1998;45(3):545–549.
5. Lipsky AM, Gausche-Hill M, Henneman PL et al. Prehospital hypotension is a predictor of the need for an emergent, therapeutic operation in trauma patients with normal systolic blood pressure in the emergency department. *J Trauma* 2006;61(5):1228–1233.
6. Moulton SL, Mulligan J, Grudic GZ et al. Running on empty? The compensatory reserve index. *J Trauma Acute Care Surg.* 2013;75(6):1053–1059.
7. Eastridge BJ, Salinas J, McManus JG et al. Hypotension begins at 110 mmHg: Redefining "hypotension" with data. *J Trauma-Injury Infect Crit Care* 2007;63(2):291–299.
8. Hasler RM, Nüesch E, Jüni P et al. Systolic blood pressure below 110 mmHg is associated with increased mortality in penetrating major trauma patients: Multicentre cohort study. *Resuscitation* 2012;83(4):476–481.
9. Vandromme MJ, Griffin RL, Weinberg JA et al. Lactate is a better predictor than systolic blood pressure for determining blood requirement and mortality: Could prehospital measures improve trauma triage? *J Am Coll Surgeons* 2010;210(5):861–867.
10. Parks JK, Elliott AC, Gentilello LM et al. Systemic hypotension is a late marker of shock after trauma: A validation study of Advanced Trauma Life Support principles in a large national sample. *Am J Surg.* 2006;192(6):727–731.
11. Mutschler M, Nienaber U, Brockamp T et al. A critical reappraisal of the ATLS classification of hypovolaemic shock: Does it really reflect clinical reality? *Resuscitation* 2013;84(3):309–313.
12. Brasel KJ, Guse C, Gentilello LM et al. Heart rate: Is it truly a vital sign? *J Trauma* 2007;62(4):812–817.
13. Martin MJ and Beekley AC. 2010. *Front Line Surgery: A Practical Approach.* Springer: New York.
14. Antonelli M, Levy M, Andrews PJ et al. Hemodynamic monitoring in shock and implications for management. *Intens Care Med.* 2007;33(4):575–590.
15. Ladakis C, Myrianthefs P, Karabinis A et al. Central venous and mixed venous oxygen saturation in critically ill patients. *Respiration* 2001;68(3):279–285.
16. Di Filippo A, Gonnelli C, Perretta L et al. Low central venous saturation predicts poor outcome in patients with brain injury after major trauma: A prospective observational study. *Scand J Trauma Resusc Emerg Med.* 2009;17:23.
17. Cohn SM, Nathens AB, Moore FA et al. Tissue oxygen saturation predicts the development of organ dysfunction during traumatic shock resuscitation. *J Trauma-Injury Infect Crit Care* 2007;62(1):44–55.
18. Crookes BA, Cohn SM, Bloch S et al. Can near-infrared spectroscopy identify the severity of shock in trauma patients? *J Trauma-Injury Infect Crit Care* 2005;58(4):806–816.

19. Sagraves SG, Newell MA, Bard MR et al. Tissue oxygenation monitoring in the field: A new EMS vital sign. *J Trauma Acute Care Surg.* 2009;67(3):441–444.
20. Beekley AC, Martin MJ, Nelson T et al. Continuous noninvasive tissue oximetry in the early evaluation of the combat casualty: A prospective study. *J Trauma-Injury Infect Critical Care* 2010;69(1):S14–S25.
21. Moore FA, Nelson T, McKinley BA et al. Massive transfusion in trauma patients: Tissue hemoglobin oxygen saturation predicts poor outcome. *J Trauma Acute Care Surg.* 2008;64(4):1010–1023.
22. Tisherman SA, Barie P, Bokhari R et al. Clinical practice guideline: Endpoints of resuscitation. *J Trauma Acute Care Surg.* 2004;57(4):898–912.
23. Costello WT 2014. Gastric tonometry. In Ehrenfeld JM and Cannesson M (eds.), *Monitoring Technologies in Acute Care Environments*. Springer: New York, pp. 317–320.
24. Gutierrez G, Palizas F, Doglio G et al. Gastric intramucosal pH as a therapeutic index of tissue oxygenation in critically ill patients. *The Lancet* 1992;339(8787):195–199.
25. Gomersall CD, Joynt GM, Freebairn RC et al. Resuscitation of critically ill patients based on the results of gastric tonometry: A prospective, randomized, controlled trial. *Crit Care Med.* 2000;28(3):607–614.
26. Miami Trauma Clinical Trials Group. Splanchnic hypoperfusion-directed therapies in trauma: A prospective, randomized trial. *Am J Surg.* 2005;71(3):252–260.
27. Ivatury RR, Simon RJ, Islam S et al. A prospective randomized study of end points of resuscitation after major trauma: Global oxygen transport indices versus organ-specific gastric mucosal pH. *J Am Coll Surg.* 1996;183(2):145–154.
28. Marik PE. Regional carbon dioxide monitoring to assess the adequacy of tissue perfusion. *Curr Opin Crit Care* 2005;11(3):245–251.
29. Jin X, Weil MH, Sun S et al. Decreases in organ blood flows associated with increases in sublingual $PCO_2$ during hemorrhagic shock. *J Appl Physiol.* 1998;85(6):2360–2364.
30. Marik PE and Bankov A. Sublingual capnometry versus traditional markers of tissue oxygenation in critically ill patients. *Crit Care Med.* 2003;31(3):818–822.
31. Ehrenfeld JM and Cannesson M. 2014. *Monitoring Technologies in Acute Care Environments*. Springer: New York.
32. Barmparas G, Inaba K, Georgiou C et al. Swan-Ganz catheter use in trauma patients can be reduced without negatively affecting outcomes. *World J Surg.* 2011;35(8):1809–1817.
33. Shah MR, Hasselblad V, Stevenson LW et al. Impact of the pulmonary artery catheter in critically ill patients: Meta-analysis of randomized clinical trials. *JAMA* 2005;294(13):1664–1670.
34. Rajaram SS, Desai NK, Kalra A et al. Pulmonary artery catheters for adult patients in intensive care. *Cochrane Database Systemat Rev.* 2013;2:Cd003408.
35. Velmahos GC, Demetriades D, Shoemaker WC et al. Endpoints of resuscitation of critically injured patients: Normal or supranormal?: A prospective randomized trial. *Ann Surg.* 2000;232(3):409.
36. Binanay C, Califf RM, Hasselblad V et al. Evaluation study of congestive heart failure and pulmonary artery catheterization effectiveness: The ESCAPE trial. *JAMA* 2005;294(13):1625–1633.
37. Fein A, Goldberg SK, Walkenstein MD et al. Is pulmonary artery catheterization necessary for the diagnosis of pulmonary edema? *Am Rev Respirat Dis.* 1984;129(6):1006–1009.
38. Wiener RS, Welch HG. Trends in the use of the pulmonary artery catheter in the United States, 1993–2004. *JAMA* 2007;298(4):423–429.
39. Moore LJ, Turner KL, Todd SR. 2013. *Common Problems in Acute Care Surgery*. Springer: New York.
40. Moomey CB, Melton SM, Croce MA et al. Prognostic value of blood lactate, base deficit, and oxygen-derived variables in an LD50 model of penetrating trauma. *Crit Care Med.* 1999;27(1):154–161.
41. Suistomaa M, Ruokonen E, Kari A et al. Time-pattern of lactate and lactate to pyruvate ratio in the first 24 hours of intensive care emergency admissions. *Shock* 2000;14(1):8–12.
42. Abramson D, Scalea TM, Hitchcock R et al. Lactate clearance and survival following injury. *J Trauma-Injury Infect Crit Care* 1993;35(4):584–589.
43. Callaway DW, Shapiro NI, Donnino MW et al. Serum lactate and base deficit as predictors of mortality in normotensive elderly blunt trauma patients. *J Trauma-Injury Infect Crit Care* 2009;66(4):1040–1044.
44. Aslar AK, Kuzu MA, Elhan AH et al. Admission lactate level and the APACHE II score are the most useful predictors of prognosis following torso trauma. *Injury* 2004;35(8):746–752.
45. Odom SR, Howell MD, Silva GS et al. Lactate clearance as a predictor of mortality in trauma patients. *J Trauma Acute Care Surg.* 2013;74(4):999–1004.
46. Jansen TC, van Bommel J, Schoonderbeek FJ et al. Early lactate-guided therapy in intensive care unit patients. *Am J Respirat Crit Care Med.* 2010;182(6):752–761.
47. Davis JW, Shackford SR, Mackersie RC et al. Base deficit as a guide to volume resuscitation. *J Trauma-Injury Infect Crit Care* 1988;28(10):1464–1467.
48. Rutherford EJ, Morris JA, Reed GW et al. Base deficit stratifies mortality and determines therapy. *J Trauma Acute Care Surg.* 1992;33(3):417–423.
49. Davis JW, Parks SN, Kaups KL et al. Admission base deficit predicts transfusion requirements and risk of complications. *J Trauma-Injury Infect Crit Care* 1996;41(5):769–774.
50. Randolph LC, Takacs M, Davis KA. Resuscitation in the pediatric trauma population: Admission base deficit remains an important prognostic indicator. *J Trauma-Injury Infect Critical Care* 2002;53(5):838–842.
51. Eberhard LW, Morabito DJ, Matthay MA et al. Initial severity of metabolic acidosis predicts the development of acute lung injury in severely traumatized patients. *Crit Care Med.* 2000;28(1):125–131.
52. Davis JW, Kaups KL, Parks SN et al. Base deficit as a guide to volume resuscitation. *J Trauma* 1988;28(10):1464–1467.
53. Kellum JA, Bellomo R, Kramer DJ et al. Etiology of metabolic acidosis during saline resuscitation in endotoxemia. *Shock* 1998;9(5):364–368.

54. Eachempati SR, Reed RL, Barie PS. Serum bicarbonate concentration correlates with arterial base deficit in critically ill patients. *Surg Infect.* 2003;4(2):193–197.
55. Martin MJ, Fitzsullivan E, Salim A et al. Use of serum bicarbonate measurement in place of arterial base deficit in the surgical intensive care unit. *Arch Surg.* 2005;140(8):745–751.
56. Broos PL, Stappaerts KH, Rommens PM et al. Multiple trauma in elderly patients. Factors influencing outcome: Importance of aggressive care. *Injury* 1993;24(6):365–368.
57. Champion HR, Copes WS, Buyer D et al. Major trauma in geriatric patients. *Am J Public Health* 1989;79(9):1278–1282.
58. Scalea TM, Simon HM, Duncan AO et al. Geriatric blunt multiple trauma: Improved survival with early invasive monitoring. *J Trauma* 1990;30(2):129–134; discussion 134–136.
59. Brown CV, Shoemaker WC, Wo CC et al. Is noninvasive hemodynamic monitoring appropriate for the elderly critically injured patient? *J Trauma* 2005;58(1):102–107.
60. Callaway DW and Wolfe R. Geriatric trauma. *Emerg Med Clin North Am.* 2007;25(3):837–860.
61. Balogh Z, McKinley BA, Cocanour CS et al. Supranormal trauma resuscitation causes more cases of abdominal compartment syndrome. *Arch Surg.* 2003;138(6):637–643.
62. McNelis J, Marini CP, Jurkiewicz A et al. Prolonged lactate clearance is associated with increased mortality in the surgical intensive care unit. *Am J Surg.* 2001;182(5):481–485.
63. Husain FA, Martin MJ, Mullenix PS et al. Serum lactate and base deficit as predictors of mortality and morbidity. *Am J Surg.* 2003;185(5):485–491.

## Commentary on Monitoring of the Trauma Patient

*Stephen M. Cohn*

One of the fundamental problems in monitoring of the trauma patient is the lack of a gold standard for the diagnosis of *shock* in the clinical setting. In a recent study, we prospectively evaluated our ability to detect hypoperfusion using a variety of routine parameters such as systolic blood pressure (<90 mmHg), pulse (>100 beats/min), base deficit (>5 mEq/L), and added tissue oxygen saturation (NIRS STO2 < 75%)*. Investigators from seven major trauma centers agreed that it was critical to use the development of organ dysfunction as essential in our definition of "shock."

*A few years ago, a man was transported in extremis to our facility after sustaining a gunshot wound to the groin. Despite receiving four units of blood during his 90 min helicopter ride, he arrived with no detectable blood pressure and only a faint carotid pulse. We rushed him to the OR for repair of a severed iliac artery. Three days later, he was recovering nicely on the floor and was discharged soon after without complications. While everyone would agree that this individual experienced profound hypoperfusion or "shock" upon arrival, the fact that he developed no organ dysfunction suggests otherwise from a research perspective (as in our study above).*

Another difficulty encountered in making the diagnosis of hypoperfusion in the trauma patient are confounders that alter "normal" values. Pain, anxiety, illicit drugs, and alcohol can alter patient presentation. Pre-existing medical problems (COPD, CHF, renal dysfunction, cirrhosis) and medications (i.e., beta-blockers, antiplatelet drugs) may lead to baseline organ dysfunction and change the physiologic response of the trauma victim.

Drs. Alahayem and Keric have nicely summarized the limited evidence available on the topic of monitoring of the trauma patient. The paucity of Level I data presented underscores the difficulty in both conducting quality clinical trials in this field (where waiver of informed consent is required as severely injured subjects are unable to give approval to participation in studies), as well as problems deriving meaningful data from this highly heterogeneous population.

* Cohn SM, Nathens AB, Moore FA et al. Tissue oxygen saturation predicts the development of organ dysfunction during traumatic shock resuscitation. *J Trauma*. 2007;62(1):44–55.

### Are Heart Rate and Blood Pressure Adequate Indicators of Shock?

During "shock," heart rate elevation or diminished blood pressure is present only about 80% of the time, and therefore, 20% of the time are falsely normal in the setting of hypoperfusion, leading to organ dysfunction. Clearly, changing our threshold for concern to include those people, for example, with systolic pressures less than 110 mmHg, rather than 90 mmHg, will improve the test sensitivity while making the endpoint less specific. Unlike decades ago, we are better informed as to our ignorance in interpretation of vital signs and we utilize biochemical markers today and while continuing to investigate novel local tissue perfusion measures to assist us.

### Do Local Tissue Perfusion Measures Improve Our Ability to Diagnose Shock? Does Their Use Improve Outcomes?

There are a myriad of monitoring tools that have been employed in an attempt to help us identify and intervene earlier in the setting of hypoperfusion. Cardiac monitoring, blood and tissue oxygen saturation assessment, gastric tonometry, and sublingual capnometry are but a few examples. None of these technologies have been shown to produce data that consistently identifies patients with occult hypoperfusion, or lead to superior clinical outcomes. I have had the pleasure to have been involved in trials with all of the devices mentioned earlier.

Another issue is that most of our trauma patients do extremely well, with only a very small subset of patients developing organ dysfunction or death. These folks are not usually hard to identify as they are usually quite obviously severely injured and physiologically deranged. The challenge is to produce an inexpensive, safe, continuous, noninvasive monitor that can be used to diagnosis hypoperfusion in key organ beds, and inform us when to terminate resuscitation, ultimately leading to lower morbidity and mortality.

### Does Hemodynamic Monitoring with Pulmonary Artery Catheters Improve Outcome?

When I was a resident during the Jurassic Era, patients were admitted to the ICU prior to major elective cases or after major trauma for placement of a PA catheter. Aggressive fluid resuscitation was performed to facilitate the plotting of a Starling curve, and then the patients underwent crystalloid infusion, blood transfusion, and inotropic support to optimize oxygen delivery and consumption. Thankfully, this management scheme has been disproven, and tremendous resources are no longer consumed in this fashion. Use of PA catheters does not appear to convey benefit in clinical trials and may actually increase the risk of pulmonary embolism. Currently, PA catheter use is confined to a few scenarios where noninvasive technology is of limited value and the patient may benefit from monitoring of cardiac performance, such as hemodialysis patients or those individuals with severe cardiac dysfunction who are also septic.

## Is There a Biochemical Parameter That Best Identifies Shock and Guides Resuscitation?

Lactate and base deficit have been employed for a number of years, and provide another valuable method of estimating hypoperfusion. While a number of conditions can make interpretation of these two markers complicated (liver and renal dysfunction, for example), they appear essentially equally as accurate as heart rate and systolic blood pressure. Similar to these vital signs, base deficit identifies only about 80% of patients with hypoperfusion*. The magnitude of elevation in base deficit correlates with rising mortality. Normalization of lactate or base deficit is typically associated with improved outcomes. How well these markers can be used to guide or terminate resuscitation is uncertain particularly in the elderly and in patients with pre-existing medical problems.

In summary, we are not really much better at making the diagnosis of shock or guiding our management than we were 30 years ago. The major advances in resuscitation have been related to earlier infusion of blood products and avoiding massive volumes of crystalloids; the use of angioembolization to terminate bleeding in inaccessible regions; and the termination of operative procedures in patients who are clearly failing to respond to routine measures and have become hemodynamically unstable, hypothermic, or coagulopathic. Despite considerable efforts, we have made little progress in earlier or improved recognition of this potentially lethal entity. I find this shocking!

* Cohn SM, Nathens AB, Moore FA et al. Tissue oxygen saturation predicts the development of organ dysfunction during traumatic shock resuscitation. *J Trauma*. 2007;62(1):44–55.

# 7

# *Resuscitation of the Trauma Patient*

**David R. King and Elie P. Ramly**

**CONTENTS**



## 7.1 Introduction

The Edwin Smith Papyrus (1600 BC) described administering fluid by mouth following traumatic injury [1]. This may represent the earliest description of fluid resuscitation. Later, Cannon warned of the potential perils of aggressive fluid resuscitation, including exacerbating hemorrhage by (possibly) raising blood pressure and disrupting soft clots [2]. Indeed, it seems that the debates surrounding fluid resuscitation predate this evidence-based textbook by centuries.

This chapter will address several fundamental questions related to resuscitation of the trauma patient, within an evidence-based construct. The particular questions are important; however, they clearly do not represent all possible resuscitation-related dilemmas that may confront the surgeon/clinician. The goal, therefore, is to demonstrate and differentiate those maneuvers that are based on scientific evidence and discriminate them from those based solely in historical opinion. This is not to say that our surgical forefathers were wrong in their approaches and therapy (because in many cases, they were right on target), but to simply articulate those therapies that have a scientific basis from those whose basis should be questioned and improved upon if shown to be false.

## 7.2 Methods

An OVID Medline search was performed for all articles from 1950 to May 2014 using the terms "resuscitation" and "trauma." The search was limited to clinical trials and randomized controlled trials (RCTs) on human subjects. Multiple languages were accepted if there was an English language translation available. Manuscripts were screened for appropriateness to the topics listed below, and article references were examined for relevant similar articles using PubMed. A review was also performed of the Cochrane library using similar key terms. Manuscripts were discarded if there were significant methodological flaws or if the papers actually represented multiple case reports.

Several important questions were posed, and evidence was evaluated to address each question. Each question's level of evidence was classified using the classification system of the Oxford Center for Evidence-Based Medicine.

## 7.3 Question Results

### 7.3.1 What Type of Fluid Should Be Used for Acute Resuscitation of the Trauma Patient?

Despite the trauma surgeon's fascination with Lactated Ringer's solution, no evidence exists to suggest that this crystalloid solution has any survival benefit over others. Nearly every clinical trial demonstrates equivalence of a variety of resuscitation fluids, including Lactated Ringer's solution, normal saline, 3% or 7.5% hypertonic saline, hetastarch/pentastarch solutions, and gelatins [3–24]. A recent Cochrane systematic review of RCTs in critically ill patients with trauma, burns, or following surgery failed to show any difference in mortality between patients resuscitated with colloids (including albumin or plasma protein fraction, hydroxyethyl starch, modified gelatin or dextran) versus crystalloids. The results rather suggested a possible increase in mortality associated with the use of hydroxyethyl starch [25].

Newer-generation hetastarches with improved C2/C6 ratios, 1:20 branching, and 0.75° of substitution have no demonstrable effect on the coagulation system in small doses [14]. Although the use of hetastarches and gelatins has no proven morbidity or mortality advantage, less volume of these fluids is required to achieve similar resuscitation endpoints [4,10–14,16]. While this advantage may be of little significance in a resource-abundant civilian trauma center, there may be significant logistical advantages for the military, especially in far-forward units where supplies are limited by cubic weight. Colloids, however, are dramatically more expensive than crystalloid solutions, and this is important in all environments [9,24]. Colloids should be avoided if traumatic brain injury is suspected and limited to small volumes of infusion to avoid coagulation and renal insults [8–10,14,25].

The use of 7.5% hypertonic saline has some theoretical advantages (potential for sodium to act as an osmotic dehydrating agent in the injured brain and prevent edema formation) over isotonic fluid resuscitation in the multi-traumatized patient with a concurrent brain injury; however, results from multiple clinical trials are mixed with the majority of studies demonstrating equivalence with isotonic fluid resuscitation [4–6,12,13,18–20,26]. Resuscitation with normal saline may result in a hyperchloremic metabolic acidosis; however, the presence of said acidosis has never been convincingly demonstrated to worsen outcomes [8,9]. The use of hypotonic fluids for trauma resuscitation has never been studied; therefore, a specific analysis on this type of fluid cannot be generated.

The use of hemoglobin-based oxygen carriers for trauma resuscitation remains a research interest only. Despite convincing animal studies demonstrating survival advantages, all trauma-related clinical trials with these agents result in higher mortality rates [15,27–29]. There is currently not enough data to support their general use in trauma, although hemoglobin-based oxygen carriers remain the theoretical ideal resuscitation fluid.

*Recommendation*: Acute phase trauma resuscitation may be conducted safely with any isotonic crystalloid, as well as hypertonic saline, but not colloids. In general, crystalloid solutions remain preferred because of their low cost and similar outcomes compared to colloids.

*Level of evidence*: 1a

*Grade of recommendation*: A

### 7.3.2 How Does One Determine Whether a Traumatized Patient Requires Fluid Resuscitation?

Shock is generally defined as inadequate tissue perfusion. In trauma, this condition is often recognized on the basis of vital signs and mental status. Shock should generally be regarded as present if any trauma patient presents with a systolic blood pressure (SBP) less than 110 mmHg and a heart rate greater than 100 beats/min [12,30,31]. This is a significant departure from earlier classical teaching where blood pressure below 80 or 90 mmHg and heart rates above 120 beats/min was regarded as a reliable threshold for determination of shock. Altered mental status should also be regarded as a sign of shock until proven otherwise. If any of these parameters are present, fluid resuscitation and a hemostatic intervention (surgery, application of a tourniquet, angioembolization, etc.) should be immediately considered. One must understand that these parameters are meant to overtriage trauma patients such that few or no patients in hemorrhagic shock are inappropriately excluded from fluid resuscitation efforts.

*Recommendation*: Following trauma, any patient with a heart rate above 100 beats/min or systolic blood pressure less than 110 mmHg indicates shock and should trigger fluid resuscitation efforts combined with an aggressive hemorrhage control maneuver.

*Level of evidence*: 2c

*Grade of recommendation*: C

### 7.3.3 What Are the Endpoints for the Termination of Fluid Resuscitation?

Reliable and well-defined endpoints to resuscitation remain elusive. Multiple strategies have been proposed and tested, and none have proven to be better than clinical judgment based on vital signs, urine output, and simple laboratory tests such as arterial base deficit and lactate [30,32,33]. Oxygen delivery-based therapy and endpoints determined with a pulmonary artery catheter have excellent theoretical advantages; however, multiple clinical trials have shown no significant morbidity or mortality advantage [30,32]. Tissue-level near-infrared spectroscopy, as well as intramuscular polarographic Clark-type electrode tissue $pO_2$ monitoring, has been shown to be useful in animal studies; however, their role as resuscitation endpoints in humans remains no better than clinical judgment [34–36]. The available data suggest that resuscitation endpoints would be more usefully conceptualized as resuscitation spectrum, where fluid administration is not suddenly terminated once a specific criteria or point is reached, but rather slowly de-escalated as the patient's clinical condition improves. Certain exceptions to ongoing resuscitation endpoints exist in the setting of penetrating torso trauma; however, this will be addressed separately. One should also be aware that over-resuscitation may equally be as deleterious as under-resuscitation: recent evidence from retrospective cohorts suggests that aggressive early crystalloid resuscitation is associated with a substantial dose-dependent increase in morbidity, ICU, and hospital length of stay in blunt trauma patients [38]. Limiting the volume and rate of fluid administration while prioritizing hemorrhage control is advised. The surgeon should constantly re-evaluate the trauma patient to prevent overuse of resuscitation fluid and the consequences associated with this practice.

*Recommendation*: Clinical judgment combined with simple laboratory testing remains the best approach to deciding when to de-escalate fluid resuscitation. This should be approached as a continuum rather than a static point in care.

*Level of evidence*: 2b

*Grade of recommendation*: B

### 7.3.4 Does the Concept of Hypotensive (Delayed) Resuscitation Have a Role in Trauma Care?

Hypotensive resuscitation, or delayed fluid resuscitation, is a concept whereby fluid administration is intentionally withheld, slowed, or halted at some point before the standard endpoints of resuscitation are achieved. This technique has consistently been associated with a lower risk of death in RCTs of fluid resuscitation in animal models of severe hemorrhage [38]. There is evidence of survival benefit with the use of a delayed resuscitation paradigm following penetrating torso injury [40], although no conclusive data exist for blunt or extremity injuries [40]. Patients with a penetrating injury should have intravenous access established and fluid administered withheld until surgical intervention is available. A plethora of expert opinion has been generated from the battlefields of the War on Terror in Iraq and Afghanistan. Most experts generally suggest that hypotensive resuscitation is appropriate for patients in shock until definitive surgical intervention is available. This opinion, however, remains unstudied in a randomized controlled fashion. Special considerations, while caring for patients with traumatic brain injury or elderly trauma patients who may have coronary or carotid artery disease, include their relative intolerance to hypotensive resuscitation and concurrent susceptibility to fluid overload-related complications [41].

*Recommendation*: Hypotensive or delayed fluid resuscitation should be considered following penetrating torso injuries. Some evidence exists to support that this strategy may be considered on patients suffering from shock after blunt trauma as well as extremity injuries.

*Level of evidence*: 1b

*Grade of recommendation*: A

### 7.3.5 Should Blood or Blood Products Be Used as an Initial Resuscitation Fluid, When Available?

Some surgeons propose that in the setting of acute hemorrhage, one should replace lost intravascular volume with fresh whole blood or packed red blood cells (PRBC). Unfortunately, capillary refill across the interstitial space occurs rapidly, and this interstitial free water deficit must be restored to return the patient to fluid equilibrium. Additionally, although many patients present with acute blood loss, most will be successfully managed without blood transfusion. The use of blood and blood products also exposes the patient to risks associated with communicable diseases and transfusion reactions. No evidence exists demonstrating any clinical advantage to this practice, as pre-hospital randomization of patients to crystalloid or red blood cells is logistically difficult. Some evidence exists in the early hospital-based resuscitation environment, suggesting that patients who obviously have a large vascular injury and will require massive transfusion may benefit from early administration of blood and blood products [42–44]. Even in these series, however, the initial fluid of choice was crystalloid solution before switching to blood. Patients with penetrating torso injury have retrospectively been reported to have lower mortality rates when managed with damage control resuscitation—defined as an SBP of 90 mmHg maintained using early resuscitation with fresh frozen plasma and PRBC in a high ratio—combined with a restrictive rather than standard crystalloid resuscitation strategy [45].

*Recommendation*: Initial fluid resuscitation should begin with a crystalloid solution. There is no sufficient evidence to support initial resuscitation with blood products.

*Level of evidence*: 2c

*Grade of recommendation*: C

**TABLE 7.1**
Evidence Table

| Question | Answer | Grade of Recommendation | References |
|---|---|---|---|
| What type of fluid should be used for acute resuscitation of the trauma patient? | Isotonic crystalloid | A | [3–9,10–25,27,29] |
| How does one determine whether a traumatized patient requires fluid resuscitation? | Blood pressure less than 110 mmHg on presentation | C | [30,31] |
| What are the endpoints for termination of fluid resuscitation? | Clinical judgment | B | [30,32–36] |
| Does the concept of hypotensive (delayed) resuscitation have a role in trauma care? | Yes | A | [38–40] |
| Should blood or blood products be used as an initial resuscitation fluid, when available? | No | C | [42–44] |
| Do vasoactive drugs play a role in early resuscitation of the trauma patient? | No | C | [46–48] |

### 7.3.6 Do Vasoactive Drugs Play a Role in Early Resuscitation of the Trauma Patient?

The use of vasopressors in the acute resuscitation of trauma patients has regained substantial interest in recent years. Although multiple animal studies demonstrate dramatic survival advantage associated with early vasopressor use in trauma resuscitation, the clinical trial data squarely dispute these findings [46,47]. The available clinical data suggest no morbidity or mortality advantage [48], and one multicenter trial demonstrated a significantly greater mortality in the vasopressor group [46] (Table 7.1).

*Recommendation*: Although the early use of vasopressors after trauma remains an intense research interest, this practice is not currently supported by the existing body of clinical data. Hypotensive trauma patients should be managed with careful hypotensive fluid resuscitation with a focus on identification of the source of hemorrhage and a rapid hemostatic intervention.

*Level of evidence*: 2c

*Grade of recommendation*: C

## 7.4 Closing Comments

The practice of evidenced-based medicine allows the surgeon to make decisions based on the best science possible. By definition, evidence applies to populations of patients who share common characteristics. It would implore you, when your patient is failing to respond to conventional therapy, to re-evaluate how that patient is *different* from the evidence-based study population. Often, what is good therapy for the population may not be entirely appropriate for a specific individual or group of individuals who make up a subset of the population. Sometimes, these difficult patients provide insights and lead to the next great RCT that alters the way we practice surgery. Perhaps, such a study will be included in the next edition of this textbook.

## References

1. Rutkow IM. *Surgery: An Illustrated History*. Mosby: St. Louis, MO; *Medicine* 1991;84:554–557.
2. Cannon W, Fraser J, Cowell E. Preventive treatment of wound shock. *JAMA* 1918;70:618–621.
3. Vassar MJ, Perry CA, Gannaway WL, Holcroft JW. 7.5% sodium chloride/dextran for resuscitation of trauma patients undergoing helicopter transport. *Arch Surg.* September 1991;126(9):1065–1072.
4. Vassar MJ, Fischer RP, O'Brien PE, Bachulis BL, Chambers JA, Hoyt DB, Holcroft JW. A multicenter trial for resuscitation of injured patients with 7.5% sodium chloride. The effect of added dextran 70. The Multicenter Group for the Study of Hypertonic Saline in Trauma Patients. *Arch Surg.* September 1993;128(9):1003–1011; discussion 1011–1013.
5. Mattox KL, Maningas PA, Moore EE, Mateer JR, Marx JA, Aprahamian C, Burch JM, Pepe PE. Prehospital hypertonic saline/dextran infusion for post-traumatic hypotension. The U.S.A. Multicenter Trial. *Ann Surg.* May 1991;213(5):482–491.
6. Wade CE, Grady JJ, Kramer GC. Efficacy of hypertonic saline dextran fluid resuscitation for patients with hypotension from penetrating trauma. *J Trauma* May 2003;54(5 Suppl):S144–S148.
7. Tranbaugh RF and Lewis FR. Crystalloid versus colloid for fluid resuscitation of hypovolemic patients. *Adv Shock Res.* 1983;9:203–216.

8. SAFE Study Investigators; Australian and New Zealand Intensive Care Society Clinical Trials Group; Australian Red Cross Blood Service; George Institute for International Health, Myburgh J, Cooper DJ, Finfer S, Bellomo R, Norton R, Bishop N, Kai Lo S, Vallance S. Saline or albumin for fluid resuscitation in patients with traumatic brain injury. *N Engl J Med.* August 2007;357(9):874–884.
9. Finfer S, Bellomo R, Boyce N, French J, Myburgh J, Norton R; SAFE Study Investigators. A comparison of albumin and saline for fluid resuscitation in the intensive care unit. *N Engl J Med.* May 2004;27;350(22):2247–2256.
10. Shatney CH, Deepika K, Militello PR, Majerus TC, Dawson RB. Efficacy of hetastarch in the resuscitation of patients with multisystem trauma and shock. *Arch Surg.* July 1983;118(7):804–809.
11. Bulger EM, Jurkovich CJ, Nathens AB et al. Hypertonic resuscitation of hypovolemic shock after blunt trauma: A randomized controlled trial. *Arch Surg.* February 2008;143(2):139–148; discussion 149.
12. Rizoli SB, Rhind SG, Shek PN, Inaba K, Filips D, Tien H, Brenneman F, Rotstein O. The immunomodulatory effects of hypertonic saline resuscitation in patients sustaining traumatic hemorrhagic shock: A randomized, controlled, double-blinded trial. *Ann Surg.* January 2006;243(1):47–57.
13. Cooper DJ, Myles PS, McDermott FT, Murray LJ, Laidlaw J, Cooper G, Tremayne AB, Bernard SS, Ponsford J; HTS Study Investigators. Prehospital hypertonic saline resuscitation of patients with hypotension and severe traumatic brain injury: A randomized controlled trial. *JAMA* March 2004;291(11):1350–1357.
14. Allison KP, Gosling P, Jones S, Pallister I, Porter KM. Randomized trial of hydroxyethyl starch versus gelatine for trauma resuscitation. *J Trauma* December 1999;47(6):1114–1121.
15. Sloan EP, Koenigsberg M, Gens D, Cipolle M, Runge J, Mallory MN, Rodman G, Jr. Diaspirin cross-linked hemoglobin (DCLHb) in the treatment of severe traumatic hemorrhagic shock: A randomized controlled efficacy trial. *JAMA* November 1999;282(19):1857–1864.
16. Younes RN, Yin KC, Amino CJ, Itinoshe M, Rocha e Silva M, Birolini D. Use of pentastarch solution in the treatment of patients with hemorrhagic hypovolemia: Randomized phase II study in the emergency room. *World J Surg.* January 1998;22(1):2–5.
17. Nagy KK, Davis J, Duda J, Fildes J, Roberts R, Barrett J. A comparison of pentastarch and lactated Ringer's solution in the resuscitation of patients with hemorrhagic shock. *Circ Shock* August 1993;40(4):289–294.
18. Vassar MJ, Perry CA, Holcroft JW. Prehospital resuscitation of hypotensive trauma patients with 7.5% NaCl versus 7.5% NaCl with added dextran: A controlled trial. *J Trauma* May 1993;34(5):622–632; discussion 632–633.
19. Younes RN, Aun F, Accioly CQ, Casale LP, Szajnbok I, Birolini D. Hypertonic solutions in the treatment of hypovolemic shock: A prospective, randomized study in patients admitted to the emergency room. *Surgery* April 1992;111(4):380–385.
20. Holcroft JW, Vassar MJ, Turner JE, Derlet RW, Kramer GC. 3% NaCl and 7.5% NaCl/dextran 70 in the resuscitation of severely injured patients. *Ann Surg.* September 1987;206(3):279–288.
21. Modig J. Advantages of dextran 70 over Ringer acetate solution in shock treatment and in prevention of adult respiratory distress syndrome. A randomized study in man after traumatic-haemorrhagic shock. *Resuscitation* August 1983;10(4):219–226.
22. Moss GS, Lowe RJ, Jilek J, Levine HD. Colloid or crystalloid in the resuscitation of hemorrhagic shock: A controlled clinical trial. *Surgery* April 1981;89(4):434–438.
23. Lowe RJ, Moss GS, Jilek J, Levine HD. Crystalloid versus colloid in the etiology of pulmonary failure after trauma—A randomized trial in man. *Crit Care Med.* March 1979;7(3):107–112.
24. Wu JJ, Huang MS, Tang GJ, Kao WF, Shih HC, Su CH, Lee CH. Hemodynamic response of modified fluid gelatin compared with lactated ringer's solution for volume expansion in emergency resuscitation of hypovolemic shock patients: Preliminary report of a prospective, randomized trial. *World J Surg.* May 2001;25(5):598–602.
25. Perel P, Roberts I, Ker K. Colloids versus crystalloids for fluid resuscitation in critically ill patients. *Cochrane Database Systemat Rev.* February 2013;2:CD000567.
26. York J, Arrillaga A, Graham R, Miller R. Fluid resuscitation of patients with multiple injuries and severe closed head injury: Experience with an aggressive fluid resuscitation strategy. *J Trauma* March 2000;48(3):376–379; discussion 379–380.
27. Moore EE, Cheng AM, Moore HB, Masuno T, Johnson JL. Hemoglobin-based oxygen carriers in trauma care: Scientific rationale for the US multicenter prehosptial trial. *World J Surg.* July 2006;30(7):1247–1257.
28. Natanson C, Kern SJ, Lurie P, Banks SM, Wolfe SM. Cell-free hemoglobin-based blood substitutes and risk of myocardial infarction and death: A meta-analysis. *JAMA* May 2008;299(19):2304–2312.
29. Transcripts: Safety of hemoglobin-based oxygen carriers (Hbocs), April 29–30, 2008. Center for Biologics Evaluation and Research, FDA, The National Heart, Lung, and Blood Institute, NIH and Office of the Secretary and Office of Public Health and Science, DHHS, NIH Campus: Bethesda, Maryland. Updated April 9, 2013. http://www.fda.gov/BiologicsBloodVaccines/NewsEvents/WorkshopsMeetingsConferences/ucm092010.htm. Accessed August 7, 2015.
30. Velmahos GC, Demetriades D, Shoemaker WC et al. Endpoints of resuscitation of critically injured patients: Normal or supranormal? A prospective randomized trial. *Ann Surg.* September 2000;232(3):409–418.
31. Eastridge BJ, Salinas J, McManus JG, Blackburn L, Bugler EM, Cooke WH, Concertino VA, Wade CE, Holcomb JB. Hypotension begins at 110 mmHg: Redefining "hypotension" with data. *J Trauma* August 2007;63(2):291–297; discussion 297–299.

32. Miller PR, Meredith JW, Chang MC. Randomized, prospective comparison of increased preload versus inotropes in the resuscitation of trauma patients: Effects on cardiopulmonary function and visceral perfusion. *J Trauma* January 1998;44(1):107–113.
33. Durham RM, Neunaber K, Mazuski JE, Shapiro MJ, Baue AE. The use of oxygen consumption and delivery as endpoints for resuscitation in critically ill patients. *J Trauma* July 1996;41(1):32–39; discussion 39–40.
34. McKinley BA, Marvin RG, Cocanour CS, Moore FA. Tissue hemoglobin $O_2$ saturation during resuscitation of traumatic shock monitored using near infrared spectrometry. *J Trauma* April 2000;48(4):637–642.
35. Crookes BA, Cohn SM, Burton EA et al. Can near-infrared spectroscopy identify the severity of shock in trauma patients? *J Trauma* April 2005;58(4):806–813; discussion 813–816.
36. Ikossi DG, Knudson MM, Morabito DJ, Cohen MJ, Wan JJ, Khaw L, Stewart CJ, Hemphill C, Manley GT. Continuous muscle tissue oxygenation in critically injured patients: A prospective observational study. *J Trauma* October 2006;61(4):780–788; discussion 788–790.
37. Kasotakis G, Sideris A, Chang Y, De Moya M, Alam H, King DR, Tompkins R, Velmahos G. Aggressive early crystalloid resuscitation adversely affects outcomes in adult blunt trauma patients: An analysis of the glue grant database. *J Trauma Acute Care Surg.* May 2013;74(5):1215–1222.
38. Mapstone J, Roberts I, Evans P. Fluid resuscitation strategies: A systematic review of animal trials. *J Trauma* 2003;55:571–589.
39. Bickell WH, Wall MJ, Jr, Pepe PE, Martin RR, Ginger VF, Allen MK, Mattox KL. Immediate versus delayed fluid resuscitation for hypotensive patients with penetrating torso injuries. *N Engl J Med.* October 1994;331(17):1105–1109.
40. Dutton RP, Mackenzie CF, Scalea TM. Hypotensive resuscitation during active hemorrhage: Impact on in-hospital mortality. *J Trauma* June 2002;52(6):1141–1146.
41. Alam HB, Velmahos GC. New trends in resuscitation. *Curr Prob Surg.* August 2011;48(8):531–564.
42. Spinella PC, Perkins JG, Grathwohl KW, Beekley AC, Niles SE, McLaughlin DF, Wade CE, Holcomb JB. Effect of plasma and red blood cell transfusions on survival in patients with combat related traumatic injuries. *J Trauma* February 2008;64(2 Suppl):S69–S77; discussion S77–S78.
43. Stinger HK, Spinella PC, Perkins JG et al. The ratio of fibrinogen to red cells transfused affects survival in casualties receiving massive transfusions at an army combat support hospital. *J Trauma* February 2008;64(2 Suppl):S79–S85; discussion S85.
44. Borgman MA, Spinella PC, Perkins JG, Grathwohl KW, Repine T, Beekley AC, Sebesta J, Jenkins D, Wade CE, Holcomb JB. The ratio of blood products transfused affects mortality in patients receiving massive transfusions at a combat support hospital. *J Trauma* October 2007;63(4):805–813.
45. Duke MD, Guidry C, Guice J, Stuke L, Marr AB, Hunt JP, Meade P, McSwain NE, Jr, Duchesne JC. Restrictive fluid resuscitation in combination with damage control resuscitation: Time for adaptation. *J Trauma Acute Care Surg.* September 2012;73(3):674–678.
46. Sperry JL, Minei JP, Frankel HL, West MA, Harbrecht BG, Moore EE, Maier RV, Nirula R. Early use of vasopressors after injury: Caution before constriction. *J Trauma* January 2008;64(1):9–14.
47. Lienhart HG, Wenzel V, Braun J et al. Vasopressin for therapy of persistent traumatic hemorrhagic shock: The VITRIS at study. *Anaesthesist* February 2007;56(2):145–148, 150.
48. Cohn SM, McCarthy J, Stewart RM, Jonas RB, Dent DL, Michalek JE. Impact of low-dose vasopressin on trauma outcome: Prospective randomized study. *World J Surg.* February 2011;35(2):430–439.

## Commentary on Resuscitation of the Trauma Patient

*John B. Holcomb*

The review by King and Ramly attempts to place resuscitation practice for trauma patients into an evidenced-based context. Without explicitly saying so, it seems they were left wondering how we are supposed to know what to do (in an evidenced-based fashion), given the dearth of level 1 data to guide resuscitation products available today. One of the real conundrums in our supposedly evidenced-based world is that the clinical data supporting our recent resuscitation practice (serial using crystalloid, then RBCs, followed later by plasma and platelets) practiced for the last 30 years is very poor (level 5 data). After rereading their chapter, I am again reminded that it is unfortunate that the level 1 evidence base for trauma resuscitation is so poor.

This issue is really important. Death after injury in the United States has increased >20% in the last decade[*]. During the last decade, there have been >1.8 million civilians deaths from injury[†]. The toll that injury causes in the United States every year is staggering, and while well known to the readers of this textbook, it is not well understood by many outside our field. Worldwide, injury accounts for more deaths than malaria, TB, and HIV combined and has increased by >20% over the last decade[‡]. Because injury is still a disease of younger people (although the age of trauma patients are increasing), death after injury is far and away the leading cause of life years lost between the ages of 1 and 55 and costs the United States >400 billion dollars a year[§]. At the same time cancer, heart disease and HIV related deaths in the US have decreased[¶]. Why is this? There are likely multiple complex reasons. Primarily I believe it is because there are limited funds for clinical injury research. Importantly, there is not a NIH institute focused solely on injury and truly effective lobbying groups for injury research have not yet emerged[*].

In 1966, the National Academy of Science published the first report on the impact of injury in the United States[**]. Subsequently, the data describing the extraordinary impact of injury on the public health of the United States have been accurately documented in government websites. In 1983, Trunkey documented the disparity between the lives lost and funding available for trauma research[††]. In 2014, Rhee showed that this gap had actually widened[†]. These data have been well documented since the 1960s. Why is it that the federal government has yet to establish and appropriately fund an agency whose sole purpose is to decrease morbidity and mortality after injury?

The conclusions drawn from this chapter expose one of the fundamental problems in the field of trauma resuscitation. Namely, the lack of consistent funding to perform serial studies addressing the vast permutations of patient conditions we care for. Perhaps the best example of this approach is the work done by the National Cancer Institute[‡‡]. On their website, they report on the ongoing 12,000+ clinical trials accepting patients and the results of 25,000+ clinical trials that are no longer recruiting. They have and are addressing the important questions of the day and thus, cancer deaths are decreasing.

The most important theme of this chapter is the appalling lack of high-quality studies to guide our every day practice. This problem will not be solved by one large study addressing all permutations of which fluids, when to start, how much to give, and when to stop in all varieties of injury (age and mechanisms). Rather our patients need a series of studies that will answer the limited questions posed by the authors and many more. Importantly, phase 1 studies and so-called negative phase 3 studies are important to inform the field[§§¶¶***]. King and Ramly mention penetrating and blunt mechanism and cohorts that include hemorrhagic shock, head injury, and the elderly. They do not describe the commonly seen groups who present with mixed head injury and hemorrhagic shock, or the varying effects of extreme age, (high and low), confounded by various medications and co-morbidities. In fact many of their conclusions only reflect

* Rhee P, Joseph B, Pandit V et al. Increasing trauma deaths in the United States. *Ann Surg.* 2014;260:13–21.

† Injury Prevention & Control: Data & Statistics. CDC, 2011. Accessed November 30, 2014. http://www.cdc.gov/injury/wisqars/.

‡ Norton R, Kobusingye O. Injuries. *N Engl J Med.* 2013;368:1723–1730.

§ National Trauma Institute. Accessed November 30, 2014. http://www.nationaltraumainstitute.org/index.html.

¶ Rhee P, Joseph B, Pandit V et al. Increasing trauma deaths in the United States. *Ann Surg.* 2014;260:13–21.

** Division of Medical Sciences, Committee on Trauma and Committee on Shock. *Accidental Death and Disability: The Neglected Disease of Modern Society.* Washington, DC: National Academy of Sciences-National Research Council; September 1966.

†† Trunkey DD. Trauma. Accidental and intentional injuries account for more years of life lost in the U.S. than cancer and heart disease. Among the prescribed remedies are improved preventive efforts, speedier surgery and further research. *Sci Am.* 1983 August;249(2):28–35.

‡‡ National Cancer Institute. Accessed November 30, 2014. http://www.cancer.gov/clinicaltrials/search.

§§ Bulger EM, May S, Kerby JD et al. Out-of-hospital hypertonic resuscitation after traumatic hypovolemic shock: A randomized, placebo controlled trial. *Ann Surg.* 2011 March;253(3):431–441.

¶¶ Bulger EM, May S, Brasel KJ et al. Out-of-hospital hypertonic resuscitation following severe traumatic brain injury: A randomized controlled trial. *J Am Med Assoc.* 2010 October 6;304(13):1455–1464.

*** Cotton BA, Podbielski J, Camp E et al. A randomized controlled pilot trial of modified whole blood versus component therapy in severely injured patients requiring large volume transfusions. *Ann Surg.* 2013 October;258(4):527–532; discussion 532–533.

opinions. Unfortunately, with rare exceptions, the evidenced-based answer to all the questions is "I don't know." Until there are truly evidenced-based guidelines to account for the most common presenting conditions, we will continue to treat our patients as best we can.

Frankly, my practice has evolved over the last 13 years, based on experiences in the military and large civilian trauma centers*†‡§. We now extensively utilize damage control resuscitation practices, with a substantial focus on stopping bleeding§§. Tourniquets, hemostatic dressings, intra-aortic balloons, and rapid OR and IR use are employed. Resuscitation is always easier if the patient has stopped bleeding. If resuscitation is required, we start balanced blood product resuscitation prehospital and continue into the hospital with an approach using plasma, platelets, and RBCs as the primary resuscitation fluids¶**. Crystalloids are used sparingly, and we use the balanced electrolyte solution plasmalyte. In our experience, this approach minimizes the crystalloid-based iatrogenic resuscitation injury practiced for so many years and has improved our outcomes. Results from several randomized studies will soon be available, but they are only a starting point for truly evidenced-based decisions while caring for seriously injured patients.

The authors of this chapter have reviewed the literature and have commented on fewer than 25 level 1 studies. While many of us have contributed to the large number of lower grade studies, robust national funding and collaborative effort are required to generate the evidence that surely will decrease morbidity and mortality after injury and improve the quality of care. This is perhaps the dominant issue we face today.

* Holcomb JB, Jenkins D, Rhee P et al. Damage control resuscitation: Directly addressing the early coagulopathy of trauma. *J Trauma.* 2007 February;62(2):307–310.

† Holcomb JB, Wade CE, Michalek JE et al. Increased plasma and platelet to red blood cell ratios improves outcome in 466 massively transfused civilian trauma patients. *Ann Surg.* 2008 September;248(3):447–458.

‡ del Junco DJ, Holcomb JB, Fox EE et al. Resuscitate early with plasma and platelets or balance blood products gradually: Findings from the PROMMTT study. *J Trauma Acute Care Surg.* 2013 July;75(1 Suppl. 1):S24–S30.

§ Langan NR, Eckert M, Martin MJ. Changing patterns of in-hospital deaths following implementation of damage control resuscitation practices in US forward military treatment facilities. *J Am Med Assoc Surg.* 2014 September 1;149(9):904–912.

¶ Holcomb JB, Pati S. Optimal trauma resuscitation with plasma as the primary resuscitative fluid: The surgeon's perspective. *Hematology Am Soc Hematol Educ Program.* 2013;2013:656–659.

** Johansson PI, Stensballe J, Oliveri R, Wade CE, Ostrowski SR, Holcomb JB. How I treat patients with massive hemorrhage. *Blood.* 2014 November 13;124(20):3052–3058.

# 8

# *Diagnosis of Injury in the Trauma Patient*

**Elizabeth Benjamin, Pedro G.R. Teixeira, and Kenji Inaba**

**CONTENTS**



## 8.1 Introduction

Diagnostic imaging remains critical to the management of the acutely injured trauma patient, especially in the era of selective nonoperative management of many traumatic injuries. As diagnostic technology evolves, constant reassessment is required to ensure that the sensitivity and specificity parameters of any diagnostic test are well-understood and that the target population is well-defined so as to minimize cost, radiation burden, patient movement, and time. For the unstable trauma patient, operative exploration maintains a central role in diagnosis and management. These patients often have ongoing hemorrhage and shock, and although simple radiologic procedures can be used as adjuncts to operative decision-making, the core principles of trauma surgery that mandate operative management of the unstable patient remain unchanged. For the stable trauma patient, however, rapid assessment and cataloging of injury burden are essential for optimal outcomes and radiologic imaging plays a central role in data acquisition. Two main pathways result in the deterioration of the initially stable trauma patient. First, ongoing blood loss or underestimation of injury burden results in the conversion of the initially stable to the subsequently unstable patient. Hemorrhage remains a major cause of early death after trauma and the primary cause of preventable and potentially preventable death in both civilian and military populations [1,2]. Imaging is essential to identify areas of ongoing blood loss or potential hemorrhage in the otherwise stable patient. Second, missed injuries are a major component of potentially preventable morbidity and mortality. Delay in diagnosis can result in delayed treatment, increased infectious risk, or failure of early mobilization.

Ultrasonography and computerized tomography (CT) are widely available imaging modalities that have been fully incorporated into the armamentarium of the trauma surgeon and are essential components of trauma management algorithms. This chapter will review the evidence base to support the use of these modalities for the initial assessment of the injured patient.

## 8.2 Focused Abdominal Sonography for Trauma

Focused abdominal sonography for trauma (FAST) is a standardized ultrasound examination that aims to identify the presence of free fluid in the pericardium and peritoneal cavity. As an initial diagnostic adjunct, the ultrasound has several advantages: it is noninvasive, repeatable, accessible, portable, rapid, and cost-effective. Reliance on ultrasound has, however, been tempered by inter-operator variability and several patient-related factors such as subcutaneous emphysema, morbid obesity, and severe chest wall injury that can impair image acquisition. FAST was not designed to diagnose specific injuries but, instead, was designed as a screening assessment tool. In the unstable polytrauma patient, intra-abdominal fluid in the setting of a normal chest radiograph may influence operative planning. Alternatively, a positive abdominal FAST in a stable, asymptomatic blunt trauma patient may influence the decision to obtain further definitive imaging. FAST is not intended as an isolated study but, instead, most effective when utilized in combination with additional imaging modalities and clinical presentation.

## 8.3 What Is the Role of FAST in the Initial Assessment of the Hemodynamically Stable Blunt Trauma Patient?

Physical examination alone is unreliable for the diagnosis of intra-abdominal injuries in patients who have sustained blunt abdominal trauma [3]. Diagnostic imaging is, therefore, relied upon to diagnose or rule out intra-abdominal injuries. The ideal screening examination for intra-abdominal injuries has a high degree of sensitivity, which would allow for the safe exclusion of significant injuries while still maintaining an acceptable specificity, effectively decreasing the number of patients requiring definitive imaging.

Although early reports on abdominal FAST for the identification of intra-abdominal injury after blunt trauma were encouraging [4], more recent studies suggest that this modality may lack sufficient sensitivity to consistently be used as a reliable screening test. In the hemodynamically stable blunt trauma patient, FAST has several limitations. Current data suggest that a negative FAST is not sufficient to rule out intra-abdominal injury, and conversely, a positive scan in a stable patient does not mandate immediate operation [5,6]. In a well-designed prospective study with uniform application of CT scan as the standard reference, Miller and colleagues found that FAST had a 42% sensitivity for intra-peritoneal fluid in hemodynamically stable patients [7]. They concluded that the ultrasound should not be the sole screening method for the evaluation of blunt abdominal trauma. These results were supported by a 7-year single-center review of FAST in the stable blunt trauma patient, which defined the sensitivity and specificity of FAST at 41% and 99%, respectively, with the authors concluding that FAST did not add value in the initial assessment of the stable blunt trauma patient [8]. A Cochrane review analyzing the use of ultrasound-based treatment algorithms suggested that the utilization of ultrasound in the evaluation of trauma patients had minimal impact on management decisions [9]. It has been demonstrated that 18%–26% of patients with intra-abdominal injuries have no detectable free intra-peritoneal fluid, and that up to 29% of abdominal injuries may be missed if ultrasound is the only diagnostic adjunct utilized in blunt trauma patients [5,6]. Although there is some evidence suggesting that repeat imaging may improve sensitivity of FAST [10], there is insufficient evidence to support the use of a negative FAST as the sole modality to rule out intra-abdominal injury. In the era of selective nonoperative management of solid organ injuries, a positive FAST in the hemodynamically stable blunt trauma patient is similarly not sufficient to warrant operative intervention, and further definitive imaging is often indicated.

*Recommendation*: FAST should not be used as the only diagnostic modality to exclude significant intra-abdominal injury in the initial assessment of the blunt trauma patient (Grade B). Patients with suspected intra-abdominal injury should undergo clinical observation or further investigation, irrespective of the ultrasound findings (Grade B).

## 8.4 What Is the Role of FAST in the Initial Assessment of the Hemodynamically Unstable Blunt Trauma Patient?

In the hemodynamically unstable blunt trauma patient, FAST as a diagnostic adjunct is significantly more important. In this patient population, FAST has largely supplanted the diagnostic peritoneal lavage as the primary diagnostic adjunct for the identification of free intra-abdominal fluid. A positive FAST in the setting of hemodynamic instability mandates immediate surgical intervention to rule out intra-abdominal bleeding as a source of instability. A positive FAST in hemodynamically unstable blunt injured patients correlates to a therapeutic laparotomy in 83% of the cases [11]. Delay in operative intervention for additional imaging has been associated with increased mortality [12].

A negative FAST in the unstable blunt trauma patient, however, similar to a negative study in the hemodynamically stable patient, is of less value, with a significant number of false-negative results, especially in retroperitoneal injury and pelvic fracture [13]. Lee et al. demonstrated that 37% of the patients with a negative FAST on initial investigation required therapeutic laparotomy [11]. Holmes found that 32% of the unstable patients with a negative ultrasound had intra-abdominal injuries [14]. Even in the hands of a radiologist, a negative initial FAST is insufficient to rule out intra-abdominal injury with sensitivity, specificity, positive, and negative predictive values of 62%, 96%, 84%, and 89%, respectively [15].

*Recommendation*: A positive FAST warrants laparotomy in hemodynamically unstable patients (Grade B). Negative

FAST in a hemodynamically unstable patient is insufficient to rule out intra-abdominal injury (Grade B).

## 8.5 What Is the Role of Ultrasound in the Initial Assessment of Penetrating Trauma Patients?: Cardiac View and Abdominal View

Time is of essence in the management of cardiac injuries. Early diagnosis and treatment are critical factors for survival. Physical examination, however, is inaccurate for the diagnosis of cardiac injury.

The cardiac component of FAST, designed to assess the pericardial sac for the presence of fluid, is an immediately available, repeatable, and noninvasive diagnostic option. In a well-designed prospective study, Rozycki et al. investigated the role of ultrasound as the primary imaging modality used to determine the need for surgical intervention in patients with suspected cardiac injuries [16]. In this study, the ultrasound was 100% accurate in detecting hemopericardium, with no false-positive or false-negative results. This was followed with a prospective multicenter study including five Level I trauma centers confirming the reliability of ultrasound in identifying penetrating cardiac injuries with a 100% sensitivity and 97% specificity [17]. Similar results were described in a prospective observational analysis of 130 patients with penetrating torso injury in which cardiac FAST exam had a sensitivity and specificity of 100% for detection of cardiac injury [18]. A positive cardiac FAST, however, relies on the presence of fluid trapped in the pericardial space. The potential decompression of blood into the left chest with a concurrent cardiac and pericardial injury has been described as a potential source of false-negative exam. In a retrospective analysis of 228 patients, five false-negative pericardial FAST exams were identified, all of which were secondary to left chest penetrating injuries with associated hemothorax [19].

The pericardial FAST can be rapidly performed and has been shown to provide reliable information to influence clinical course. A negative exam in a hypotensive patient in the absence of hemothorax may direct attention to a noncardiac etiology, while a positive exam in a patient with multiple truncal and precordial wounds may reflect a cardiac injury, thus influencing operative incision order and choice.

As the role of nonoperative management in penetrating abdominal trauma expands, the utility of the abdominal windows of FAST in penetrating injuries is less clear. The decision for operative intervention is based less on peritoneal penetration or intra-abdominal fluid and more on clinical presentation, patient reliability, and wound trajectory [20]. In the stable patient with penetrating injury, a positive FAST may represent solid organ injury and may not require operative intervention. Conversely, an unstable patient with penetrating abdominal trauma and peritonitis will undergo laparotomy regardless of ultrasound results. Although some reports of high sensitivity and specificity of FAST exist [18], the majority of the literature supports that this modality is insufficient to diagnose or rule out intra-abdominal injury that will require operative intervention in the stable trauma patient after penetrating injury. In a Western Trauma Association multicenter trial of 134 stable patients with penetrating abdominal trauma, the sensitivity of FAST was 21% with a positive predictive value of 50% [21]. Similar results have been reported from the military experience with a reported FAST sensitivity of 56% in a largely penetrating injury population [22]. These results support previous prospective analyses that established the low sensitivity of abdominal FAST (46%–67%) to detect clinically significant penetrating abdominal injury [23–25]. In a study by Soffer et al. that included analysis of clinical indications for operative intervention, the abdominal FAST results changed management in only 1.7% of patients [23]. Although the reported specificity of the abdominal FAST after penetrating trauma is more compelling, reported at 94%–100%, the negative predictive value ranges from 60% to 90% [17,21–25]. The possibility of hollow viscus injury (HVI) causing a sonographically undetectable volume of abdominal fluid precludes the current FAST from acting as the sole indicator to rule out abdominal injury after penetrating trauma.

*Recommendation*: Ultrasound should be the initial diagnostic modality for patients with penetrating precordial wounds (Grade A), and a positive ultrasound for fluid in the pericardial sac warrants immediate surgical intervention (Grade A). FAST is not a reliable imaging modality in penetrating trauma for ruling out significant intra-abdominal injury (Grade B).

## 8.6 What Is the Current Evidence to Support the Use of Ultrasound for the Diagnosis of Pneumothorax in the Resuscitation Area?

Traditionally, the diagnosis of pneumothorax in acute trauma is established using plain radiography. CT is a highly sensitive and specific method for the detection of pneumothorax and is considered the gold standard imaging modality for this injury.

Plain radiography has several limitations for the detection of pneumothorax. Because air accumulates preferentially in the anteromedial and subpulmonic region in patients in the supine position, radiographic images obtained in supine trauma patients may miss pneumothoraces, although the clinical significance of these occult pneumothoraces is questionable [26].

The process of obtaining the plain radiographs is time consuming, involves radiation, and there is a delay in obtaining the images, all issues that may be obviated with the advantages of ultrasound.

EFAST, or Extended FAST, has been widely applied as a simple, rapid, and noninvasive adjunct in most civilian and military trauma patients. Rowan et al. demonstrated in a small prospective study that ultrasound was more sensitive and accurate than plain chest radiograph in the detection of pneumothorax and had sensitivity comparable to CT scan [27]. Further prospective studies using CT scan as a reference standard confirmed the higher sensitivity for ultrasound (92%–95%) compared to plain chest radiograph (52%–79%) [28,29]. Zhang et al. demonstrated in a prospective study that ultrasound outperformed plain radiograph for the detection of pneumothorax (86% vs. 28%, $p < 0.001$), allowed a significantly faster detection of pneumothorax ($2.3 \pm 2.9$ vs. $19.9 \pm 10.3$, $p < 0.001$), and had stronger agreement with CT scan findings [30]. Although thoracic ultrasound for trauma to identify pneumothorax has not been formally incorporated into national protocols, many centers rely heavily upon this information for patient procedures and triage [31]. The clinical significance of the often occult pneumothorax identified on ultrasound also remains unclear.

*Recommendation*: Ultrasound can be as sensitive as or more sensitive than plain chest radiography and can be utilized to diagnose pneumothorax in injured patients (Grade B).

## 8.7 What Is the Role of CT Scan in the Assessment of Hollow Viscus Injury after Blunt Abdominal Trauma?

Traditionally, abdominal CT is thought to be a poor predictor of blunt HVI with normal imaging identified in 13% of patients with known injury [32]. CT scan has been shown to be more sensitive and specific than clinical exam alone [33], but no single imaging modality has been shown to reliably rule in or out HVI [32]. With the advances of multidetector CT (MDCT) and reformatting software, however, the ability to detect HVI with CT imaging is again under investigation [34].

Intuitively, the presence of free air on CT scan should correlate with HVI; however, this is often not the case after blunt abdominal trauma. In a single-center retrospective study, the presence of intra-peritoneal free air on CT was benign in 60% of patients, often likely due to barotrauma [35]. The authors identified seatbelt sign, free fluid, and radiographic signs of bowel trauma to be predictors of clinically significant free air on CT scan. In a retrospective review, the presence of free intra-peritoneal air had a sensitivity of only 50% and a positive predictive value of 9.5% for HVI [36]. Extra-luminal free air in the presence of bowel wall discontinuity has also been shown to lack sensitivity but has high specificity and positive predictive value for bowel injury [37].

The significance of free fluid on CT scan, especially in the absence of solid organ injury, has also been the topic of much debate. In a review of 122 patients with free fluid on CT scan after blunt abdominal trauma in the absence of solid organ injury, small bowel injury was found in only 12 patients [38]. Conversely, in a review of 68 patients with blunt bowel and mesenteric injuries, all patients had free fluid present on CT imaging [39]. Gonser-Hafertepen et al. categorized the amount of free fluid to determine the predictive value for identifying HVI [40]. They found that no patient with trace free fluid required operation but that moderate to large amounts of fluid was an independent predictor of therapeutic laparotomy (OR 66, $p < 0.001$).

Aside from free fluid and pneumoperitoneum, several additional signs of potential injury have been described. Bowel wall thickening or increased contrast enhancement of the bowel wall can be a nonspecific findings after trauma when diffusely present, but focal enhancement or thickening has been described as a specific indicator or HVI [41,42]. The accuracy of HVI detection is also thought to be higher in the stomach and duodenum when compared to the colon and remaining small bowel [43].

While some signs have high sensitivity and low specificity, others have low sensitivity but high specificity. No one sign has emerged as the sole indicator of injury; however, especially with the advances in MDCT, the overall combination of radiologic findings, in conjunction with physical examination, remains an important adjunct in the diagnosis of blunt HVI. Finally, with current technology, patients with blunt HVI are unlikely to have a completely negative preoperative CT scan [39,44].

*Recommendation*: CT scan alone cannot be used to reliably rule in or rule out the presence of HVI after blunt abdominal trauma (Grade B). Using MDCT, pneumoperitoneum, free fluid, focal bowel wall thickening or enhancement, and bowel wall discontinuity are all signs suggestive of HVI, especially when present in combination (Grade B). In the presence of a completely negative CT scan, blunt HVI is unlikely (Grade B).

## 8.8 Can CT Scan Be Utilized to Diagnose or Rule Out Penetrating Diaphragmatic Injury?

The identification of diaphragmatic injury after penetrating trauma can be challenging. In the era of abdominal exploration for all penetrating abdominal injuries, the presence of diaphragmatic injury could be directly visualized. More recently, however, selective nonoperative management of penetrating torso trauma in the stable, evaluable patient has become widely accepted [20]. In this population, CT scan is often used as a diagnostic adjunct both to identify missile trajectory and injuries sustained. The utility of CT scan imaging to identify occult diaphragmatic injury, however, has been questioned. Diaphragmatic injuries occur in approximately 7%–24% of patients after left thoracoabdominal penetrating trauma [45,46]. Although small diaphragmatic injuries rarely cause immediate symptoms, they have the ability to expand over time and create a source of potential incarceration or strangulation of herniated abdominal contents. In contemporary practice, laparoscopy may be used as a diagnostic modality to identify occult diaphragmatic injury after penetrating left thoracoabdominal trauma prior to patient discharge [45].

Although traditionally thought to lack sensitivity, new MDCT technology, with thinner cuts and advanced reconstruction, has shown promising results in the identification of diaphragmatic injury after penetrating thoracoabdominal trauma [47]. In a retrospective review using intra-operative injury identification as the gold standard, 64-slice MDCT had a sensitivity ranging from 71% to 100% and specificity of 50%–92% for identification of diaphragmatic injury [48]. In addition, visualization of trans-diaphragmatic trajectory and contiguous injury improves sensitivity and specificity of CT scans [47,49]. In a retrospective analysis of 136 patients with penetrating trauma and injury trajectory in the vicinity of the diaphragm, radiologists, blinded to the operative findings, reviewed the images [50]. The authors reported the sensitivity and specificity of MDCT as 87.2% and 72.4%, respectively, increased to 88% and 82% when a contiguous injury was identified (Table 8.1).

**TABLE 8.1**

Summary Points with Recommendations Including Level of Evidence and Grade of Recommendations

| | Question | Answer | Levels of Evidence | Grade of Recommendation | References |
|---|---|---|---|---|---|
| 1 | What is the role of FAST in the initial assessment of the hemodynamically stable blunt trauma patient? | FAST should not be used as the only diagnostic modality to exclude significant intra-abdominal injury in the initial assessment of the blunt trauma patient. | IIb, IIIa | B | [6–9] |
| | | Patients with suspected intra-abdominal injury should undergo clinical observation or further investigation, irrespective of the ultrasound findings. | IIb, IIIa | B | [7–9] |
| 2 | What is the role of FAST in the initial assessment of the hemodynamically unstable blunt trauma patient? | A positive FAST warrants laparotomy in hemodynamically unstable patients. | Ib, IIb | B | [4,11] |
| | | Negative FAST in a hemodynamically unstable patient is insufficient to rule out intra-abdominal injury. | IIIb | B | [13–15] |
| 3 | What is the role of ultrasound in the initial assessment of penetrating trauma patients: cardiac view and abdominal view? | Ultrasound should be the initial diagnostic modality for patients with penetrating precordial wounds. | Ib, IIb | A | [4,16,17] |
| | | A positive ultrasound for fluid in the pericardial sac warrants immediate surgical intervention. | Ib, IIb | A | [4,16,17] |
| | | FAST is not a reliable imaging modality in penetrating trauma for ruling out significant intra-abdominal injury. | Ib, IIb | B | [21,22,24] |
| 4 | What is the current evidence to support the use of ultrasound for the diagnosis of pneumothorax in the resuscitation area? | Ultrasound can be as sensitive as or more sensitive than plain chest radiography and can be utilized to diagnose pneumothorax in injured patients (Grade A). | Ib | A | [29,31] |
| 5 | What is the role of CT scan in the assessment of hollow viscus injury after blunt abdominal trauma? | CT alone cannot be used to reliably rule in or rule out the presence of HVI after blunt abdominal trauma. | IIb | B | [32] |
| | | Using MDCT, pneumoperitoneum, free fluid, focal bowel wall thickening or enhancement, and bowel wall discontinuity are all signs suggestive of HVI, especially when present in combination. | IIb, IIIb | B | [33,35–37, 40,44] |
| | | In the presence of a completely negative CT scan, blunt HVI is unlikely. | IIb, IIIb | B | [39,40,44] |
| 6 | Can CT scan be utilized to diagnose or rule out penetrating diaphragmatic injury? | MDCT can be used as a diagnostic adjunct to identify occult diaphragmatic injury after penetrating trauma and has improved sensitivity and specificity with visualization of a trans-diaphragmatic trajectory or contiguous injury. | IIIb | B | [48–50] |
| | | Diagnostic laparoscopy can be used to identify or rule out occult diaphragmatic injury. | IIb | B | [45] |

*Recommendation:* MDCT can be used as a diagnostic adjunct to identify occult diaphragmatic injury after penetrating trauma and has improved sensitivity and specificity with the visualization of a trans-diaphragmatic trajectory or contiguous injury (Grade B).

## References


1. Teixeira PG, Inaba K, Hadjizacharia P et al. Preventable or potentially preventable mortality at a mature trauma center. *J Trauma* 2007;63(6):1338–1346; discussion 46–47.
2. Sauaia A, Moore FA, Moore EE et al. Epidemiology of trauma deaths: A reassessment. *The J Trauma* 1995;38(2):185–193.
3. Rodriguez A, DuPriest RW, Jr, Shatney CH. Recognition of intra-abdominal injury in blunt trauma victims. A prospective study comparing physical examination with peritoneal lavage. *Am Surgeon* 1982;48(9):457–459.
4. Rozycki GS, Ballard RB, Feliciano DV, Schmidt JA, Pennington SD. Surgeon-performed ultrasound for the assessment of truncal injuries: Lessons learned from 1540 patients. *Ann Surg.* 1998;228(4):557–567.
5. Yoshii H, Sato M, Yamamoto S et al. Usefulness and limitations of ultrasonography in the initial evaluation of blunt abdominal trauma. *J Trauma* 1998;45(1):45–50; discussion 1.
6. Chiu WC, Cushing BM, Rodriguez A et al. Abdominal injuries without hemoperitoneum: A potential limitation of focused abdominal sonography for trauma (FAST). *J Trauma* 1997;42(4):617–623; discussion 23–25.
7. Miller MT, Pasquale MD, Bromberg WJ, Wasser TE, Cox J. Not so FAST. *J Trauma* 2003;54(1):52–59; discussion 9–60.
8. Natarajan B, Gupta PK, Cemaj S, Sorensen M, Hatzoudis GI, Forse RA. FAST scan: Is it worth doing in hemodynamically stable blunt trauma patients? *Surgery* 2010;148(4):695–700; discussion 1.
9. Stengel D, Bauwens K, Rademacher G et al. Emergency ultrasound-based algorithms for diagnosing blunt abdominal trauma. *Cochrane Database Systemat Rev.* 2005;(2):CD004446.
10. Blackbourne LH, Soffer D, Mckenney MG et al. Secondary ultrasound examination increases the sensitivity of the FAST exam in blunt trauma. *J Trauma* 2004;57(5):934–938.
11. Lee BC, Ormsby EL, McGahan JP, Melendres GM, Richards JR. The utility of sonography for the triage of blunt abdominal trauma patients to exploratory laparotomy. *AJR* 2007;188(2):415–421.
12. Neal MD, Peitzman AB, Forsythe RM et al. Over reliance on computed tomography imaging in patients with severe abdominal injury: Is the delay worth the risk? *J Trauma* 2011;70(2):278–284.
13. Hoffman L, Pierce D, Puumala S. Clinical predictors of injuries not identified by focused abdominal sonogram for trauma (FAST) examinations. *J Emerg Med.* 2009;36(3):271–279.
14. Holmes JF, Harris D, Battistella FD. Performance of abdominal ultrasonography in blunt trauma patients with out-of-hospital or emergency department hypotension. *Ann Emerg Med.* 2004;43(3):354–361.
15. Gaarder C, Kroepelien CF, Loekke R, Hestnes M, Dormage JB, Naess PA. Ultrasound performed by radiologists-confirming the truth about FAST in trauma. *J Trauma* 2009;67(2):323–327; discussion 8–9.
16. Rozycki GS, Feliciano DV, Schmidt JA et al. The role of surgeon-performed ultrasound in patients with possible cardiac wounds. *Ann Surg.* 1996;223(6):737–744; discussion 44–46.
17. Rozycki GS, Feliciano DV, Ochsner MG et al. The role of ultrasound in patients with possible penetrating cardiac wounds: A prospective multicenter study. *J Trauma* 1999;46(4):543–551; discussion 51–52.
18. Tayal VS, Beatty MA, Marx JA, Tomaszewski CA, Thomason MH. FAST (focused assessment with sonography in trauma) accurate for cardiac and intraperitoneal injury in penetrating anterior chest trauma. *J Ultrasound Med.* 2004;23(4):467–472.
19. Ball CG, Williams BH, Wyrzykowski AD, Nicholas JM, Rozycki GS, Feliciano DV. A caveat to the performance of pericardial ultrasound in patients with penetrating cardiac wounds. *J Trauma* 2009;67(5):1123–1124.
20. Inaba K, Demetriades D. The nonoperative management of penetrating abdominal trauma. *Adv. Surg.* 2007;41:51–62.
21. Biffl WL, Kaups KL, Cothren CC et al. Management of patients with anterior abdominal stab wounds: A Western Trauma Association multicenter trial. *J Trauma* 2009;66(5):1294–1301.
22. Smith IM, Naumann DN, Marsden ME, Ballard M, Bowley DM. Scanning and war: Utility of FAST and CT in the assessment of battlefield abdominal trauma. *Ann Surg.* 2015;262(2):389–396.
23. Soffer D, McKenney MG, Cohn S et al. A prospective evaluation of ultrasonography for the diagnosis of penetrating torso injury. *J Trauma* 2004;56(5):953–957; discussion 7–9.
24. Udobi KF, Rodriguez A, Chiu WC, Scalea TM. Role of ultrasonography in penetrating abdominal trauma: A prospective clinical study. *J Trauma* 2001;50(3):475–479.
25. Boulanger BR, Kearney PA, Tsuei B, Ochoa JB. The routine use of sonography in penetrating torso injury is beneficial. *J Trauma* 2001;51(2):320–325.
26. Tocino IM, Miller MH, Fairfax WR. Distribution of pneumothorax in the supine and semirecumbent critically ill adult. *AJR* 1985;144(5):901–905.
27. Rowan KR, Kirkpatrick AW, Liu D, Forkheim KE, Mayo JR, Nicolaou S. Traumatic pneumothorax detection with thoracic US: Correlation with chest radiography and CT—Initial experience. *Radiology* 2002;225(1):210–214.
28. Nandipati KC, Allamaneni S, Kakarla R et al. Extended focused assessment with sonography for trauma (EFAST) in the diagnosis of pneumothorax: Experience at a community based level I trauma center. *Injury* 2011;42(5):511–514.

29. Soldati G, Testa A, Sher S, Pignataro G, La Sala M, Silveri NG. Occult traumatic pneumothorax: Diagnostic accuracy of lung ultrasonography in the emergency department. *Chest* 2008;133(1):204–211.
30. Zhang M, Liu ZH, Yang JX et al. Rapid detection of pneumothorax by ultrasonography in patients with multiple trauma. *Crit Care* 2006;10(4):R112.
31. Abdulrahman Y, Musthafa S, Hakim SY et al. Utility of extended FAST in blunt chest trauma: Is it the time to be used in the ATLS algorithm? *World J Surg.* 2015;39(1):172–178.
32. Fakhry SM, Watts DD, Luchette FA, Group EM-IHVIR. Current diagnostic approaches lack sensitivity in the diagnosis of perforated blunt small bowel injury: Analysis from 275,557 trauma admissions from the EAST multi-institutional HVI trial. *J Trauma* 2003;54(2):295–306.
33. Joseph DK, Kunac A, Kinler RL, Staff I, Butler KL. Diagnosing blunt hollow viscus injury: Is computed tomography the answer? *Am J Surg.* 2013;205(4):414–418.
34. Atri M, Hanson JM, Grinblat L, Brofman N, Chughtai T, Tomlinson G. Surgically important bowel and/or mesenteric injury in blunt trauma: Accuracy of multidetector CT for evaluation. *Radiology* 2008;249(2):524–533.
35. Marek AP, Deisler RF, Sutherland JB et al. CT scan-detected pneumoperitoneum: An unreliable predictor of intra-abdominal injury in blunt trauma. *Injury* 2014;45(1):116–121.
36. Hefny AF, Kunhivalappil FT, Matev N, Avila NA, Bashir MO, Abu-Zidan FM. Usefulness of free intraperitoneal air detected by CT scan in diagnosing bowel perforation in blunt trauma: Experience from a community-based hospital. *Injury* 2015;46(1):100–104.
37. Park MH, Shin BS, Namgung H. Diagnostic performance of 64-MDCT for blunt small bowel perforation. *Clin Imaging* 2013;37(5):884–888.
38. Mahmood I, Tawfek Z, Abdelrahman Y et al. Significance of computed tomography finding of intra-abdominal free fluid without solid organ injury after blunt abdominal trauma: Time for laparotomy on demand. *World J Surg.* 2014;38(6):1411–1415.
39. Petrosoniak A, Engels PT, Hamilton P, Tien HC. Detection of significant bowel and mesenteric injuries in blunt abdominal trauma with 64-slice computed tomography. *J Trauma Acute Care Surg.* 2013;74(4):1081–1086.
40. Gonser-Hafertepen LN, Davis JW, Bilello JF et al. Isolated free fluid on abdominal computed tomography in blunt trauma: Watch and wait or operate? *J Am Coll Surg.* 2014;219(4):599–605.
41. Khan I, Bew D, Elias DA, Lewis D, Meacock LM. Mechanisms of injury and CT findings in bowel and mesenteric trauma. *Clin. Radiol.* 2014;69(6):639–647.
42. Brofman N, Atri M, Hanson JM, Grinblat L, Chughtai T, Brenneman F. Evaluation of bowel and mesenteric blunt trauma with multidetector CT. *Radiographics* 2006;26(4):1119–1131.
43. Kim HC, Yang DM, Kim SW, Park SJ. Gastrointestinal tract perforation: Evaluation of MDCT according to perforation site and elapsed time. *Eur Radiol.* 2014;24(6):1386–1393.
44. Tan KK, Liu JZ, Go TS, Vijayan A, Chiu MT. Computed tomography has an important role in hollow viscus and mesenteric injuries after blunt abdominal trauma. *Injury* 2010;41(5):475–478.
45. Murray JA, Demetriades D, Cornwall EE et al. Occult injuries to the diaphragm: Prospective evaluation of laparoscopy in penetrating injuries to the left lower chest. *J Am Coll. Surg.* 1998;187(6):626–630.
46. Leppaniemi A and Haapiainen R. Occult diaphragmatic injuries caused by stab wounds. *J Trauma* 2003;55(4):646–650.
47. Dreizin D, Bergquist PJ, Taner AT, Bodanapally UK, Tirada N, Munera F. Evolving concepts in MDCT diagnosis of penetrating diaphragmatic injury. *Emerg Radiol.* 2015;22(2):149–156.
48. Dreizin D, Borja MJ, Danton GH et al. Penetrating diaphragmatic injury: Accuracy of 64-section multidetector CT with trajectography. *Radiology* 2013;268(3):729–737.
49. Hammer MM, Flagg E, Mellnick VM, Cummings KW, Bhalla S, Raptis CA. Computed tomography of blunt and penetrating diaphragmatic injury: Sensitivity and inter-observer agreement of CT Signs. *Emerg Radiol.* 2014;21(2):143–149.
50. Bodanapally UK, Shanmuganathan K, Mirvis SE et al. MDCT diagnosis of penetrating diaphragm injury. *Eur Radiol.* 2009;19(8):1875–1881.

## Commentary on Diagnosis of Injury in the Trauma Patient

*Kimball I. Maull*

As the technological revolution in medicine passes from the twentieth to the twenty-first century, my admonition to residents and students, "Don't let technology triumph over good judgment," appears to be less and less relevant. In a way, I welcome the change. I sleep while the radiologist works into the night interpreting imaging studies! By the same token, I regret the loss of reliance on one's clinical acumen to make a diagnosis and, thereby, take a patient to the operating theatre without further ado. Today, in all but the most technologically deprived environs, those days are gone. So, too, is the critical role of clinical assessment and the challenge that the injured patient presents to the surgeon and surgeon-in-training. If the clinician assesses the patient to be uninjured, and the imaging study shows otherwise, is there still an argument? Perhaps not. If the clinician assesses the patient to be injured and the imaging study is negative, is there still an argument? Perhaps so.

In this chapter, the authors have reviewed the role of sonography and computed tomography (CT) in the diagnosis of injuries and have provided conclusions for the role of each in both blunt and penetrating injury mechanisms. Instability is rightfully acknowledged as the bailiwick of the operating room and the discussion appropriately ends there. Imaging addresses the dual threats of unrecognized ongoing hemorrhage and injuries that may prove elusive at the time of presentation (missed injuries). The role of clinical examination is included but not emphasized. The authors dismiss the reliability of clinical assessment by reference to a study in the 1980s by Rodriguez et al. showing diagnostic peritoneal lavage to be superior to physical examination in detecting hemoperitoneum. I believe physical examination often holds the key to determining the significance of imaging findings and must be included in any algorithm, which attempts to define a diagnostic approach to the trauma patient. Notwithstanding this shortcoming, the chapter provides an up-to-date and reliable matrix to identify clinically significant injuries. The authors' recommendations provide timely recognition of the need for early operation, but also serve as reassurance for continued nonoperative management as the case may warrant.

The following comments refer to the specific questions addressed by the authors.

### What Is the Role of FAST in the Initial Assessment of the Hemodynamically Stable Blunt Trauma Patient?

There is little debate that FAST is helpful, when positive, and of limited value, when negative. The latter interpretation should not be a basis for dismissing further assessment if there is reason to believe that the patient is at risk. It is in this common situation that physical examination can play a pivotal role. Based on the experience of others and my own patient contact through the years, virtually all patients with blunt perforation of the intestine either complain of pain in the abdomen or have tenderness elicited by palpation of the abdomen, most commonly both. The very real and confounding variable relates to the trauma patient with CNS compromise, either by head injury, heavy alcohol ingestion, or therapeutic sedation or paralysis. In such situations, the role of physical examination becomes moot. Close clinical reassessment is vital in these situations. One has only to be consulted on a deteriorating severely head injured patient in the neurosurgical intensive care unit to bear witness to the lethality of missed bowel perforation. Often, the patient is "too sick to travel" for a CT and sonography is the sole diagnostic modality available short of peritoneal tap or operation. The portability and ability to repeat the examination is a true benefit of this modality.

The positive FAST is, indeed, helpful but can sonographic findings be quantitated? The authors do not address this specific aspect, but clearly, the answer to this is yes. It has long been recognized that the appearance of blood in all three zones (subdiaphragmatic, gutters, and pelvis) is more predictive of the need for operation than the actual anatomic organ disruption (grade of injury)*. The amount of fluid visible on sonography should heighten the clinician's awareness of impending instability.

### What Is the Role of FAST in the Initial Assessment of the Hemodynamically Unstable Blunt Trauma Patient?

Many of us have been in the position with the unstable patient where the FAST is positive—there is a thin crescent beneath the liver, no apparent perisplenic or pelvic fluid, and at operation, a nonbleeding liver laceration is

* Gould HR, Buntain WL, Maull KI. 1996. Imaging in blunt abdominal trauma. In: Maull KI, Cleveland HC, Strauch GO, Wolferth, CC, eds. *Advances in Trauma*. Year Book Medical Publishers: Chicago, IL, Vol. 3, pp. 53–100.

found and an intraperitoneal explanation for hypotension is lacking. The origins of the shock state lie elsewhere. Can this situation be avoided? My answer echoes the concise caveat of the authors: Delay in operative intervention for additional imaging more often leads to increased mortality. This remains a clinical conundrum.

### What Is the Role of Ultrasound in the Initial Assessment of Penetrating Trauma Patients: Cardiac View and Abdominal View?

In experienced hands, ultrasound via the cardiac window is highly accurate in detecting cardiac injury. Pericardial fluid is the tip-off, and the authors correctly define cardiac bleeding through a rent in the pericardium as a pitfall in making a conclusive diagnosis is some cases. Thus, their comment to be wary when injury results in an associated hemothorax is good advice. I also concur that FAST has little to offer in the diagnosis of clinically significant penetrating abdominal trauma. The patient's clinical status is the key to therapy.

### What Is the Current Evidence to Support the Use of US for the Diagnosis of Pneumothorax in the Resuscitation Area?

This is an evolving skill set, and again, in experienced hands, there appears to be solid evidence that the EFAST can aid in the diagnosis of pneumothorax. There is also ample evidence, beginning with the prospective study by this commentator, that the "occult pneumothorax" does not mandate decompression, but can be treated selectively*. I also concur that the supine chest film is often misleading. Data presented at the European Society for Trauma and Emergency Surgery in 2009 (Afifi et al.) showed that symptoms and signs at admission, related to the thorax, correlate more closely with significant thoracic CT findings than the admission chest film. The study confirmed tachypnea, chest wall tenderness, decreased air entry, and impaired oxygen saturation as particularly predictive. Again, the utility of physical diagnosis must be recognized.

### What Is the Role of CT Scan in the Assessment of Hollow Viscus Injury after Blunt Abdominal Trauma?

The jury is still out on whether multidetector computed tomography (MDCT) will enhance the reliability of CT scan to the point where it can reliably exclude the diagnosis of blunt intestinal injury. Be mindful that blunt intestinal trauma runs the gamut from simple bruising to bursting injury, from uncomplicated mesenteric hematoma to mesenteric laceration with continued hemorrhage. Further, injury, which may not appear to be significant initially, may lead to later complications. This is especially true for patients with mesenteric lacerations, which bleed, then cease bleeding, and are not explored. The mesenteric defect can lead to bowel herniation and strangulation obstruction. Intestinal stenosis from ischemia is also a recognized consequence of hollow viscus injury related to direct trauma or mesenteric vascular compromise. I do take issue with the author's final recommendation. When perforation exists, the value of physical examination cannot be overstated and, if the patient complains of pain and has evolving tenderness, a negative CT should not dissuade the surgeon from operating.

### Can CT Scan Be Utilized to Diagnose or Rule Out Penetrating Diaphragmatic Injury?

The discussion and recommendations for the use of CT to diagnose diaphragmatic injury are on target. CT may demonstrate findings that convince the clinician that there is a diaphragmatic injury, but—and this is a big but—in the patient at high risk, will the radiologist be willing to categorically exclude injury to the diaphragm? I think not. There are other modalities, which are superior to CT to confirm (and treat) this injury. Do not be misled by a negative CT, especially if the patient is at risk, and there are soft findings of trauma to the area. There is a certain irony when considering sonography and CT in the diagnosis of ruptured left hemidiaphragm. This injury was actually diagnosed *by ultrasound* in the pre-CT era, the first report of the use of ultrasound in diagnosing abdominal trauma in this country†.

* Enderson BL, Abdalla R, Frame SB, Maull KI. Tube thoracostomy for occult pneumothorax—A prospective randomized study. *J Trauma.* 1993;35:726–730.

† Jones TK, Walsh JW, Maull KI. Diagnostic imaging in blunt abdominal trauma. *Surg Gynecol Obstet.* 1983;157:389.

# 9

# *Evidence-Based Approach to Damage Control Laparotomy*

**Bruce A. Crookes and Brent Jewett**

**CONTENTS**



## 9.1 Introduction

Over the course of the past 20 years, the term "damage control" has become a part of the common vernacular among trauma surgeons, general surgeons, and orthopedists. Initially conceptualized as a temporizing measure to stabilize the victims of penetrating trauma, it is now a widely applied algorithm that has become a standard of care within the trauma community.

The term "damage control" has its origin within the U.S. Navy, where it was intended to describe a technique in which the damaged hull of a ship undergoes rapid assessment and stabilization, so that it may return to the controlled environment of port [1]. Although the original application of the term "damage control" to surgery is attributed to Rotondo et al. [2] in 1993, the origins of the surgical technique can be traced back to Pringle [3], who first applied hepatic packing to arrest hemorrhage. Most authors, however, attribute the formalization of the technique to Stone [4] who, in 1983, described the technique of laparotomy truncation in the setting of exsanguinating hepatic hemorrhage. Stone and his associates terminated the initial laparotomy of patients with hepatic injury once the patient became coagulopathic. Stone's work was replicated by several other authors, most typically, in the setting of hepatic injury [5–10].

With an increase in semiautomatic weapons use in the late 1980s, trauma surgeons began to see a marked increase in homicide rates [11]. Now faced with an average of 2.7 shots per body [11,12], traumatologists saw a concomitant increase in mortality as a result of these devastating injuries. From this crucible of interpersonal violence arose the sentinel report by Rotondo et al. [2], and the term "damage control" was applied to trauma surgery for the first time. Damage control is now readily practiced in trauma centers around the world [13] and, most recently, has been extensively applied to foreign conflicts [14].

The damage control sequence is commonly employed to avoid the "lethal triad" of hypothermia (defined as a core body temperature of <35°C), coagulopathy, and acidosis. Although there is no formal definition of the damage control technique, its steps are commonly acknowledged to include the following three-part sequence [15–18]:

1. Operating room (OR) (Part I)
   a. Rapid control of hemorrhage
   b. Control or containment of contamination
   c. Restoration of vascular flow when required
   d. Intra-abdominal packing
   e. Temporary abdominal closure
2. Intensive care unit (ICU) (Part II)
   a. Core rewarming
   b. Optimization of hemodynamics
   c. Correction of coagulopathy
   d. Ventilatory support
   e. Secondary survey and injury identification

3. OR (Part III)
    a. Pack removal
    b. Definitive repair of injuries

The purpose of this chapter is to provide an evidence-based review of the literature with respect to the indications for the implementation of damage control techniques, the morbidity and mortality associated with the use of damage control, as well as the optimal technique for temporary closure of the abdominal wall.

## 9.2 Does a "Damage Control" Approach Improve Mortality?

Reports of damage control procedures have denoted mortality rates ranging from 16% to 69% [2,19]. In a collective review of 961 damage control patients, published in 1994, Rotondo et al. [15] delineated a cumulative mortality rate from all of the known, published damage control series of 58%. More recent series, however, have shown a continued improvement in mortality rates. Johnson et al. [20] performed a retrospective cohort series comparing their damage control experience with that at their center from 10 years earlier. While the historical control group had a mortality rate of 58%, Johnson et al. had a mortality of 10% for their more recent series. The authors postulated that this was due to improved ICU care, increased experience with the open abdomen, and improved temperature control. Sutton et al. reported an initial mortality rate of 27% and, importantly, found no long-term deaths if the patient survived the initial hospitalization [21]. In a large case series of 344 patients, Miller et al.'s [22] series had a similar mortality rate of 25%. Arthurs et al. [23] examined the application of a damage control technique to soldiers who suffered multisystem penetrating pelvic injuries, with a resultant mortality of 28%. Wang et al. [19] reported a survival of 61.5% when damage control techniques were utilized to manage hemorrhagic shock in patients with blunt abdominal trauma. Most recently, the U.S. military has successfully employed the damage control paradigm, yielding a 16% mortality rate [24].

Asensio et al. [25] examined the mortality rate in damage control patients before and after the institution of intraoperative guidelines and found a consistent mortality rate of 24% pre- and post-implementation. Interestingly, the combination of a vascular injury and rectal injury resulted in a mortality of 36% and was found to be the most deadly injury complex. Nicholas et al. [26] used a retrospective cohort analysis to find that in penetrating abdominal trauma, an increasing application of damage control techniques resulted in a statistically significantly higher survival rate (73.3%). Unfortunately, it carried with it a significant morbidity load, including sepsis, intra-abdominal abscess, and gastrointestinal fistula rate.

Finally, Finlay et al. [27] used a damage control technique to control hemorrhage in general surgical patients. He then predicted their outcome by P-POSSUM and POSSUM scoring and found that the observed mortality rate (7.1%) was significantly reduced.

The combination of damage control resuscitation concepts with damage control laparotomy (DCL) has seemingly continued to decrease mortality rates even further. Cotton et al. [28] compared outcomes in 282 patients who underwent DCL prior to damage control resuscitation techniques with outcomes in 108 DCLs coupled with damage control resuscitation: the 24 h and 30-day survival was significantly higher with the addition of damage control resuscitation (88% vs. 97% and 76% vs. 86%).

Despite the enthusiasm for the technique, DCL may be over-utilized. Higa et al. [29] noted that the number of DCLs in their trauma population decreased from 36.3% (53 of 146) in 2006 to 8.8% (15 of 170) in 2008, which was paradoxically accompanied by a concomitant decrease in mortality from 21.9% to 12.9%.

*Recommendation*: The application of damage control techniques appears to have decreased mortality rates, although the absolute mortality reduction is difficult to quantify due to improvements in critical care and resuscitation. Practitioners of this resuscitation paradigm should consider combining the technique with a damage control resuscitation algorithm.

*Grade of recommendation*: C

## 9.3 How Do We Preoperatively Identify the Damage Control Patient?

The decision to employ a damage control technique initiates a sequence of events that require an intense utilization and commitment of resources: the patient must now undergo at least two operations, the ICU must assume the responsibility for a complex and time-consuming resuscitation, and the surgeon and the OR staff are obligated to return to the OR within the next several days after the injury. Thus, the decision to convert to a damage control approach is crucial.

Clearly, the majority of trauma patients will not require a damage control technique. Multiple authors have attempted to characterize patients who would benefit from a damage control approach, most employing objective markers, including mechanism of injury, injury severity score (ISS), temperature, pH, coagulopathy, lactate levels, and the number of units of blood transfused.

Wyrzykowski, in the definitive text *Trauma* [30], advocates that "In trauma patients, relative pre-operative indications for DCL include systolic blood pressure (SBP) <90 mmHg with penetrating torso, blunt abdominal, or severe pelvic trauma, and the need for resuscitative thoracotomy."

Ansensio et al. [31] retrospectively evaluated 548 patients for prehospital characteristics which predicted "exsanguination syndrome." Using a logistic regression model, they identified several independent risk factors for survival upon presentation to the ED: penetrating trauma, spontaneous ventilation, and the absence of an ED thoracotomy. As a result, the authors of this chapter recommend that patients arriving in the ED with a Revised Trauma Score (RTS) ≤5, patients requiring ≥2000 mL of crystalloids or ≥2 units of PRBCs for resuscitation, and those patients who have a pH of ≤7.2 are in the early stages of the "exsanguination syndrome" and were excellent candidates for a damage-control approach.

Preoperative indications for DCL in non-trauma patients have been published [32] and are similar to traumatic indications. In a review of 455 patients undergoing DCL for emergency abdominal surgery over the past 10 years, the indications for DCL have included uncontrolled bleeding during elective surgery, hemorrhage from complicated gastroduodenal ulcer disease, generalized peritonitis, acute mesenteric ischemia, and "other sources of intra-abdominal sepsis" [32]. Unfortunately, there is insufficient data to validate guidelines for emergency general surgery operations.

*Recommendation*: A "damage control approach" should be taken with any trauma patient who has any of the following characteristics:

- RTS ≤5
- Patients who require ≥2000 mL of crystalloids for their resuscitation in the ED
- Patients who require ≥2 units of PRBCs for their resuscitation in the ED
- Patients who have a pH ≤7.2
- SBP <90 mmHg with penetrating torso, blunt abdominal, or severe pelvic trauma, and the need for resuscitative thoracotomy

*Grade of recommendation*: C

## 9.4 How Do We Intraoperatively Identify the Damage Control Patient?

Once the patient is in the OR, how does one know when to convert to a "damage control" technique?

Rotondo et al. [2], in the original report on damage control, began to employ a damage control technique once a patient had received more than 10 units of PRBCs before the termination of the laparotomy, but did not evaluate the effectiveness of transfusion requirement as a trigger point for conversion to damage control. Cue et al. [33] noted that coagulopathy began to occur in patients who had received more than 15 units of PRBCs during their initial resuscitation and operation and recommended abdominal packing prior to reaching that transfusion threshold. Burch et al. [34] performed a retrospective review of 200 patients who were treated for over 7.5 years utilizing damage control techniques. This group used a logistic regression analysis to show that the two most powerful predictors of mortality were the rate of red cell transfusion (units per hour) and pH. When plotted as a scatter plot, these two variables correctly identified patient death within 48 h of injury 77% of the time. Asensio et al. [31] identified the following values as predictive of survival once a trauma patient was in the OR: ISS ≤20, spontaneous ventilation in the ED, OR blood product replacement of <4000 mL, no ED or OR thoracotomy, and the absence of abdominal vascular injury. His group recommended that damage control techniques be employed when transfusion volumes are >4000 mL of PRBCs (or >5000 mL if both PRBCs and whole blood are used), total OR volume of resuscitation is >12,000 mL (crystalloid and blood products), or when pH is ≤7.2 and a temperature of 1342 and a temperature of blood product of ≥5000 mL.

Sharp and Locicero [35], in a case series of 39 patients, identified several intraoperative risk factors for mortality, including a pH <7.18, a temperature of 9331°C, a prothrombin time of 16 s, a partial thromboplastin time of 50 s, and transfusion of 10 units or more, as being predictive of outcome. Patients with four to five risk factors had a 100% mortality rate, although this represents a small subset of the overall study (three patients). Those who had two to three risk factors had an 83% mortality rate, and those with zero to one risk factor had an 18% mortality rate.

Other non-traditional endpoints may be helpful in identifying the physiologically unstable patient, including end-tidal $CO_2$—arterial $CO_2$ difference and thenar eminence mixed tissue oxygen saturation ($StO_2$). In a database of 501 trauma patients, Tyburski et al. [36] found that patients with a difference >10 mmHg, which was persistent (i.e., initial OR, post-resuscitation, and final OR), predicted a 100% mortality. Minimum thenar eminence $StO_2$ may also be predictive of the need for massive transfusion and may ultimately provide a surrogate marker for the need for damage control [37].

Several reviews of damage control indicate that a damage control technique should be employed in the following circumstances [13,15,16,37]:

1. Inability to achieve hemostasis owing to a recalcitrant coagulopathy
2. Inaccessible major venous injury

3. Time-consuming procedure in the patient with suboptimal response to resuscitation
4. Management of extra-abdominal life-threatening injury
5. Reassessment of intra-abdominal contents
6. Inability to re-approximate abdominal fascia due to splanchnic reperfusion-induced visceral edema

Consensus statements, however, list the intraoperative indications for DCL in trauma patients to include "non-surgical" bleeding, pH ≤ 7.18, temperature ≤33°C, transfusion of ≥10 units of blood, total fluid replacement >12 L, and estimated blood losses of ≥5 L [4,35]. This also includes patients with evidence of visceral edema, peak inspiratory pressures >40 cm $H_2O$, or intra-abdominal pressure >21 mm Hg during attempted closure [38–42].

While these indications represent the application of sound surgical judgment, evidence-based guidelines to definitively support their implementation are lacking at present.

*Recommendation:* In the OR, a "damage control" technique should be considered when, and if, the following criteria apply:

- Patients who require transfusion of ≥10 units of blood or a total fluid replacement of >12 L
- Patients who have had an ED or OR thoracotomy
- Patients who have a pH ≤7.2
- Patients who have a temperature of ≤34°C
- If the patient has an inaccessible major venous injury
- If the surgeon cannot achieve hemostasis owing to a recalcitrant coagulopathy
- If the definitive operative repair is a time-consuming procedure in the patient with suboptimal response to resuscitation
- If the patient requires the management of an extra-abdominal life-threatening injury
- If the patient will require a reassessment of intra-abdominal contents
- If the surgeon cannot re-approximate the abdominal fascia due to splanchnic reperfusion-induced visceral edema
- Patients with peak inspiratory pressures >40 cm $H_2O$ or intra-abdominal pressure >21 mmHg during attempted closure

*Grade of recommendation*: D

## 9.5 When Should We Terminate the Initial "Damage Control" Operation?

In Rotondo et al.'s [2] initial description of the technique, the authors retrospectively included those patients who had penetrating injury resulting in exsanguination from an abdominal source who had received greater than 10 units of PRBCs prior to completion of the laparotomy.

It would seem obvious that the need to terminate an operation would be based upon the factors of coagulopathy, acidosis, or hypothermia. Ferrara et al. [43] examined a series of 45 trauma patients who required massive transfusions. They found that non-survivors were more likely to have had penetrating injuries (88% vs. 55%), received more transfusions (26.5 vs. 18.6), had lower pH (7.04 vs. 7.18), had lower core temperatures (31°C vs. 34°C), and had a higher incidence of clinical coagulopathy (73% vs. 23%). Severe hypothermia occurred in 80% of non-survivors vs. 6% of survivors.

Cosgrif et al. [44] used a logistic regression analysis to develop a predictive model for the development of coagulopathy. Factors that predicted the presence of coagulopathy included an ISS >25, a pH <7.10, a temperature <34°C, and an ISS >25. If all four of these variables were present, 98% of patients had a coagulopathy (defined as a prothrombin time and partial thromboplastin time greater than two times normal). Clearly, prolonging an operation in the setting of these factors would be unwise.

Garrison et al. [45] examined a series of 70 consecutive patients who underwent a damage control operation to control hemorrhage, comparing survivors and non-survivors. Significant differences included ISS (29 vs. 38), initial pH (7.3 vs. 7.1), platelet count (229,000 vs. 179,000), prothrombin time (14 s vs. 22 s), partial thromboplastin time (42 s vs. 69 s), and duration of hypotension (50 vs. 90 min).

*Recommendation*: Damage control operations should be rapidly terminated, and the patient should be transferred to the ICU when the patient meets any of the following criteria:

- Core temperature ≤34°C
- pH ≤7.2
- Prothrombin time ≥ twice normal
- Partial thromboplastin time ≥ twice normal

*Grade of recommendation*: B

## 9.6 What Is the Best Method to Temporarily Close the Abdomen in Order to Prevent Long-Term Morbidity?

Historically, multiple methods have been described to temporarily close the open abdomen, ranging from simple towel clips, to the "Bogota Bag," to polytetrafluoroethylene patches, to the Wittman Patch, to vacuum closures [46]. As damage control laparotomies have become more prevalent, there has also been an evolution in the methods used to close the abdomen. Offner et al. [47] retrospectively compared methods utilized to temporarily close the open abdomen, including primary fascial closure, towel clips, and the "Bogota Bag." The group found that primary fascial closure led to a statistically higher incidence of abdominal compartment syndrome, acute respiratory distress syndrome, and multisystem organ failure.

Barker et al. reported a case series of 717 general surgical and trauma patients who had a vacuum type closure of their abdominal wall, in which the overall complication rate was 15.5% (14.7% in trauma patients) [46]. In this series, 68.1% of the patients underwent a primary fascial closure of their abdomen. Garner et al. [48] achieved a 90% (13 out of the 14 patients) primary closure rate when the incision was managed with a vacuum closure dressing. Smith et al. [49] reported on a 4-year experience of treating open abdomens with a vacuum dressing and reported a 4.3% rate of intra-abdominal abscesses and a 4.3% rate of enterocutaneous fistulae.

Hougaard et al. [50] published a retrospective review of 115 patients who underwent temporary abdominal closure with a negative pressure wound dressing (either VAC or ABTHERA) for open abdomens secondary to abdominal compartment syndrome, damage control surgery, diffuse peritonitis, or wound dehiscence. This group achieved a 92% secondary fascial closure rate, a 17% mortality rate, and a 3.5% fistula rate.

Cothren et al. [51] used a modified closure technique, combining a vacuum dressing with persistent fascial tension (using #1 PDS suture) to accomplish a 100% fascial closure rate. Using a similar technique, Miller et al. [22] closed 88% of patients with an open abdomen, with a mean time to closure of 9.5 days. One patient who was successfully closed developed an incisional hernia. Fantus et al. [52] reported a 100% fascial closure rate in a small case series of patients who were treated with a Wittman patch with a vacuum dressing.

Miller et al. [53] have published the largest series in the literature (344 patients) that examined closure technique of the open abdomen. His group found that complications began to escalate after 8 days from the initial operative intervention to fascial closure. Patients undergoing primary closure had significantly fewer complications than those patients undergoing temporary abdominal closure (skin closure only, split thickness skin graft, and/or absorbable mesh), or prosthetic closures, despite equivalent mean ISS scores between the groups. Bee et al. prospectively followed 51 patients who underwent DCLs and noted that there was no statistical difference between fascial closure rates or development of enterocutaneous fistulas when comparing a mesh bridging closure vs. abdominal vacuum-assisted closure [54].

Pommerening et al. [55] analyzed 499 patients who underwent DCL and noted that only 327 (65.5%) achieved primary fascial closure; they found that each hour delay in return to the OR (24 h after initial laparotomy) was associated with a 1.1% decrease in the odds of primary fascial closure. In another analysis by Pommerening et al. [56], 301 of the 501 DCLs achieved primary fascial closure. Primary skin closure was associated with an increased risk of superficial abdominal site infection, but not fascial dehiscence. Of the patients who achieved skin closure, 85.6% did not develop abdominal surgical site infections and were spared the morbidity of managing an open wound at discharge.

Of note, the means of resuscitation of the damage control patient may ultimately justify the end: Harvin et al. [57] reviewed 77 patients undergoing DCL (23 received 3% hypertonic saline and 54 received isotonic maintenance fluid) and noted that early primary fascial closure (<7 days) was accomplished in 96% of patients who received hypertonic saline, as opposed to only 80% of the patients in the isotonic fluid arm.

*Recommendation*: Temporary closure of the open abdomen is best accomplished with a combination of a vacuum type device and a fascial tensioning system. Delays to the OR should be avoided in order to obtain primary fascial closure. Abdominal closure is best accomplished by hospital day number 8 in order to reduce morbidity.

*Grade of recommendation*: C

## 9.7 What Is the Morbidity Rate from a "Damage Control" Approach?

Carrillo et al. report a morbidity rate of 56% in their case series of 14 patients [58]. Sharp and Locicero [35] denoted a complication rate of 27% of survivors.

Nicholas et al. [26] denoted that an increase in the use of damage control techniques resulted in higher rates of sepsis, intra-abdominal abscesses, and gastrointestinal fistulas. Rotondo and Zonies [15] delineated a 40% morbidity rate when all damage control series were summated. Morris et al. [59] found an overall complication rate of 1.09 complications per patient, with eight positive blood cultures, six intra-abdominal abscesses, and abdominal compartment syndrome in 16 patients.

Abikhaled et al. [60] compared groups of damage control patients who were packed, noting that patients who were packed for more than 72 h had statistically significant lower rates of abscess rate and mortality. The duration of packing, however, may be more indicative of ongoing physiologic instability rather than serving as a conduit for higher mortality. In a cohort of 67 octogenarians undergoing DCL, Arhinful et al. [61] noted an overall complication rate of 62%, and an overall in-hospital mortality rate of 37%. Goussous et al. [62] examined 111 patients who underwent DCL (79 for sepsis and 32 for hemorrhage) and noted similar rates of overall morbidity (81% vs. 66), mortality (19% vs. 22%), intra-abdominal abscess (18% vs. 16%), deep wound infection (9% vs. 9%), enterocutaneous fistula (8% vs. 6%), and primary fascial closure (58% vs. 59%).

Brenner et al. [63] prospectively followed 88 trauma patients who underwent DCL and noted 44 intra-abdominal infections and 18 enterocutaneous fistulas. All 63 survivors were readmitted at least once, most commonly for ventral hernia repair followed by infection and fistula management. Despite these morbidities, 51 of the surviving 63 (81%) returned to normal daily activities. Sutton published a prospective series of 56 consecutive trauma patients who underwent a damage control approach and found that 76% of the patients were readmitted at least once, with the most common reasons for readmission being infection ($n = 19$), ventral hernia repair ($n = 17$), and fistula management ($n = 14$). Interestingly, if the patients survived their initial hospitalization to discharge, there was a 0% mortality rate [21]. Fox et al. [64] followed 34 patients following DCL and found that early closure patients (<7 days) had less daily pain (38% vs. 95%), had higher overall SF-36 scores (66 vs. 46), and were more likely to return to work (54% vs. 10%) than late closure patients (>7 days) with either primary fascial closure or vicryl bridging mesh. For patients who are discharged with a ventral incisional hernia, it appears that abdominal wall reconstruction is feasible within 6 months of discharge, with no increase in complications [65].

Finally, Cheatham and Safcsak [66] prospectively examined the effects of delayed abdominal closure post-hospital. Patients who were discharged with a chronic incisional hernia were compared with patients discharged with primary fascial closure and with the general population, utilizing SF-36 version 2 health survey at regular intervals for 2 years post-decompression. Cheatham's group looked at quality-adjusted life years and successful return to employment. At 6 months post-decompression, physical and social functioning were significantly decreased among patients with an open abdomen when compared with the general population, but not in patients whose abdomens were closed prior to discharge. At 18 months post-decompression and after formal abdominal closure, patients who had been discharged with an open abdomen demonstrated normal physical and mental health perception. When compared with the general population at the 18-month time point, both groups of patients exhibited decreased, but identical, quality-adjusted life years ($1.20 \pm 0.11$ vs. 1.23; $p = 0.39$) and similar ability to resume employment (41% vs. 55%; $p = 0.49$).

*Recommendation*: Expected complication rates from damage control laparotomies range from 25% to 40% of patients with the most common complications being intra-abdominal abscesses and enterocutaneous fistulae. Methods to avoid these complications are unclear from the literature. Patients who are discharged with an open abdomen should return to a quality of life that is similar to that of patients who are discharged with a closed abdomen by 18 months post-discharge.

*Grade of recommendation*: C

## Disclaimer

There were no sources of funding or conflicts of interest in the writing of this chapter.

## References

1. Department of Defense. *Surface Ship Survivability*. Naval War Publication 3-2031. US Government Printing Office: Washington, DC.
2. Rotondo MF, Schwab CW, McGonigal MD et al. Damage control: An approach for improved survival in exsanguinating penetrating abdominal injury. *J Trauma* 1993;35:375–382; discussion 82–83.
3. Pringle JHV. Notes on the arrest of hepatic hemorrhage due to trauma. *Ann Surg*. 1908;48:541–549.

4. Stone HH, Strom PR, Mullins RJ. Management of the major coagulopathy with onset during laparotomy. *Ann Surg.* 1983;197:532–535.
5. Lucas CE, Ledgerwood AM. Prospective evaluation of hemostatic techniques for liver injuries. *J Trauma* 1976;16:442–451.
6. Calne RY, McMaster P, Pentlow BD. The treatment of major liver trauma by primary packing with transfer of the patient for definitive treatment. *Br J Surg.* 1979;66:338–339.
7. Feliciano DV, Mattox KL, Jordan GL. Jr. Intra-abdominal packing for control of hepatic hemorrhage: A reappraisal. *J Trauma* 1981;21:285–290.
8. Svoboda JA, Peter ET, Dang CV, Parks SN, Ellyson JH. Severe liver trauma in the face of coagulopathy. A case for temporary packing and early reexploration. *Am J Surg.* 1982;144:717–721.
9. Carmona RH, Peck DZ, Lim RC Jr. The role of packing and planned reoperation in severe hepatic trauma. *J Trauma* 1984;24:779–784.
10. Ivatury RR, Nallathambi M, Gunduz Y, Constable R, Rohman M, Stahl WM. Liver packing for uncontrolled hemorrhage: A reappraisal. *J Trauma* 1986;26:744–753.
11. McGonigal MD, Cole J, Schwab CW, Kauder DR, Rotondo MF, Angood PB. Urban firearm deaths: A five-year perspective. *J Trauma* 1993;35:532–536; discussion 6–7.
12. Schwab CW. Violence: America's uncivil war—Presidential address, Sixth Scientific Assembly of the Eastern Association for the Surgery of Trauma. *J Trauma* 1993;35:657–665.
13. Shapiro MB, Jenkins DH, Schwab CW, Rotondo MF. Damage control: Collective review. *J Trauma* 2000;49:969–978.
14. Fox CJ, Gillespie DL, Cox ED et al. The effectiveness of a damage control resuscitation strategy for vascular injury in a combat support hospital: Results of a case control study. *J Trauma* 2008;64:S99–S106; discussion S7.
15. Rotondo MF, Zonies DH. The damage control sequence and underlying logic. *Surg Clin North Am.* 1997;77:761–777.
16. Moore EE, Burch JM, Franciose RJ, Offner PJ, Biffl WL. Staged physiologic restoration and damage control surgery. *World J Surg.* 1998;22:1184–1190; discussion 90–91.
17. Scalea T. What's new in trauma in the past 10 years. *Int Anesthesiol Clin* 2002;40:1–17.
18. Lee JC, Peitzman AB. Damage-control laparotomy. *Curr Opin Crit Care* 2006;12:346–350.
19. Wang SY, Liao CH, Fu CY et al. An outcome prediction model for exsanguinating patients with blunt abdominal trauma after damage control laparotomy: A retrospective study. *BMC Surg.* 2014;14:24.
20. Johnson JW, Gracias VH, Schwab CW et al. Evolution in damage control for exsanguinating penetrating abdominal injury. *J Trauma* 2001;51:261–269; discussion 9–71.
21. Sutton E, Bochicchio GV, Bochicchio K et al. Long term impact of damage control surgery: A preliminary prospective study. *J Trauma* 2006;61:831–834; discussion 5–6.
22. Miller PR, Meredith JW, Johnson JC, Chang MC. Prospective evaluation of vacuum-assisted fascial closure after open abdomen: Planned ventral hernia rate is substantially reduced. *Ann Surg.* 2004;239:608–614; discussion 14–16.
23. Arthurs Z, Kjorstad R, Mullenix P, Rush RM, Jr, Sebesta J, Beekley A. The use of damage-control principles for penetrating pelvic battlefield trauma. *Am J Surg.* 2006;191:604–609.
24. Smith IM, Beech ZK, Lundy JB, Bowley DM. A prospective observational study of abdominal injury management in contemporary military operations: Damage control laparotomy is associated with high survivability and low rates of fecal diversion. *Ann Surg.* 2014;261(4):765–773.
25. Asensio JA, Petrone P, Roldan G, Kuncir E, Ramicone E, Chan L. Has evolution in awareness of guidelines for institution of damage control improved outcome in the management of the posttraumatic open abdomen? *Arch Surg.* 2004;139:209–214; discussion 15.
26. Nicholas JM, Rix EP, Easley KA et al. Changing patterns in the management of penetrating abdominal trauma: The more things change, the more they stay the same. *J Trauma* 2003;55:1095–1108; discussion 108–110.
27. Finlay IG, Edwards TJ, Lambert AW. Damage control laparotomy. *Br J Surg.* 2004;91:83–85.
28. Cotton BA, Reddy N, Hatch QM et al. Damage control resuscitation is associated with a reduction in resuscitation volumes and improvement in survival in 390 damage control laparotomy patients. *Ann Surg.* 2011;254:598–605.
29. Higa G, Friese R, O'Keeffe T et al. Damage control laparotomy: A vital tool once overused. *J Trauma* 2010;69:53–59.
30. Feliciano DV, Mattox KL, Moore EE. 2008. *Trauma*, 6th edn. McGraw-Hill Medical: New York.
31. Asensio JA, McDuffie L, Petrone P et al. Reliable variables in the exsanguinated patient which indicate damage control and predict outcome. *Am J Surg.* 2001;182:743–751.
32. Weber DG, Bendinelli C, Balogh ZJ. Damage control surgery for abdominal emergencies. *Br J Surg.* 2014;101:e109–e118.
33. Cue JI, Cryer HG, Miller FB, Richardson JD, Polk HC. Jr. Packing and planned reexploration for hepatic and retroperitoneal hemorrhage: Critical refinements of a useful technique. *J Trauma* 1990;30:1007–1011; discussion 11–13.
34. Burch JM, Ortiz VB, Richardson RJ, Martin RR, Mattox KL, Jordan GL, Jr. Abbreviated laparotomy and planned reoperation for critically injured patients. *Ann Surg.* 1992;215:476–483; discussion 83–84.
35. Sharp KW, Locicero RJ. Abdominal packing for surgically uncontrollable hemorrhage. *Ann Surg.* 1992;215:467–474; discussion 74–75.
36. Tyburski JG, Carlin AM, Harvey EH, Steffes C, Wilson RF. End-tidal $CO_2$-arterial $CO_2$ differences: A useful intraoperative mortality marker in trauma surgery. *J Trauma* 2003;55:892–896; discussion 6–7.

37. Moore FA, Nelson T, McKinley BA et al. Massive transfusion in trauma patients: Tissue hemoglobin oxygen saturation predicts poor outcome. *J Trauma.* 2008;64:1010–1023.
38. Oelschlager BK, Boyle EM, Jr, Johansen K, Meissner MH. Delayed abdominal closure in the management of ruptured abdominal aortic aneurysms. *Am J Surg.* 1997;173:411–415.
39. Raeburn CD, Moore EE, Biffl WL et al. The abdominal compartment syndrome is a morbid complication of postinjury damage control surgery. *Am J Surg.* 2001;182:542–546.
40. Rasmussen TE, Hallett JW, Jr, Noel AA et al. Early abdominal closure with mesh reduces multiple organ failure after ruptured abdominal aortic aneurysm repair: Guidelines from a 10-year case-control study. *J Vasc Surg.* 2002;35:246–253.
41. Cheatham ML. It is time to pay attention--now more than ever! *Crit Care Med.* 2007;35:1629–1630.
42. Diaz JJ, Jr, Cullinane DC, Dutton WD et al. The management of the open abdomen in trauma and emergency general surgery: Part 1-damage control. *J Trauma* 2010;68:1425–1438.
43. Ferrara A, MacArthur JD, Wright HK, Modlin IM, McMillen MA. Hypothermia and acidosis worsen coagulopathy in the patient requiring massive transfusion. *Am J Surg.* 1990;160:515–518.
44. Cosgriff N, Moore EE, Sauaia A, Kenny-Moynihan M, Burch JM, Galloway B. Predicting life-threatening coagulopathy in the massively transfused trauma patient: Hypothermia and acidoses revisited. *J Trauma* 1997;42:857–861; discussion 61–62.
45. Garrison JR, Richardson JD, Hilakos AS et al. Predicting the need to pack early for severe intra-abdominal hemorrhage. *J Trauma* 1996;40:923–927; discussion 7–9.
46. Barker DE, Green JM, Maxwell RA et al. Experience with vacuum-pack temporary abdominal wound closure in 258 trauma and general and vascular surgical patients. *J Am Coll Surg.* 2007;204:784–792; discussion 92–93.
47. Offner PJ, de Souza AL, Moore EE et al. Avoidance of abdominal compartment syndrome in damage-control laparotomy after trauma. *Arch Surg.* 2001;136:676–681.
48. Garner GB, Ware DN, Cocanour CS et al. Vacuum-assisted wound closure provides early fascial reapproximation in trauma patients with open abdomens. *Am J Surg.* 2001;182:630–638.
49. Smith LA, Barker DE, Chase CW, Somberg LB, Brock WB, Burns RP. Vacuum pack technique of temporary abdominal closure: A four-year experience. *Am Surg.* 1997;63:1102–1107; discussion 7–8.
50. Hougaard HT, Ellebaek M, Holst UT, Qvist N. The open abdomen: Temporary closure with a modified negative pressure therapy technique. *Int Wound J.* 2014;11(Suppl 1):13–16.
51. Cothren CC, Moore EE, Johnson JL, Moore JB, Burch JM. One hundred percent fascial approximation with sequential abdominal closure of the open abdomen. *Am J Surg.* 2006;192:238–242.
52. Fantus RJ, Mellett MM, Kirby JP. Use of controlled fascial tension and an adhesion preventing barrier to achieve delayed primary fascial closure in patients managed with an open abdomen. *Am J Surg.* 2006;192:243–247.
53. Miller RS, Morris JA, Jr, Diaz JJ, Jr, Herring MB, May AK. Complications after 344 damage-control open celiotomies. *J Trauma* 2005;59:1365–13571; discussion 71–74.
54. Bee TK, Croce MA, Magnotti LJ et al. Temporary abdominal closure techniques: A prospective randomized trial comparing polyglactin 910 mesh and vacuum-assisted closure. *J Trauma* 2008;65:337–342; discussion 42–44.
55. Pommerening MJ, DuBose JJ, Zielinski MD et al. Time to first take-back operation predicts successful primary fascial closure in patients undergoing damage control laparotomy. *Surgery* 2014;156:431–438.
56. Pommerening MJ, Kao LS, Sowards KJ, Wade CE, Holcomb JB, Cotton BA. Primary skin closure after damage control laparotomy. *Br J Surg.*, 2014.
57. Harvin JA, Mims MM, Duchesne JC et al. Chasing 100%: The use of hypertonic saline to improve early, primary fascial closure after damage control laparotomy. *J Trauma Acute Care Surg.* 2013;74:426–430; discussion 31–32.
58. Carrillo C, Fogler RJ, Shaftan GW. Delayed gastrointestinal reconstruction following massive abdominal trauma. *J Trauma* 1993;34:233–235.
59. Morris JA, Jr, Eddy VA, Blinman TA, Rutherford EJ, Sharp KW. The staged celiotomy for trauma. Issues in unpacking and reconstruction. *Ann Surg.* 1993;217:576–584; discussion 84–86.
60. Abikhaled JA, Granchi TS, Wall MJ, Hirshberg A, Mattox KL. Prolonged abdominal packing for trauma is associated with increased morbidity and mortality. *Am Surg.* 1997;63: 1109–1112; discussion 12–13.
61. Arhinful E, Jenkins D, Schiller HJ, Cullinane DC, Smoot DL, Zielinski MD. Outcomes of damage control laparotomy with open abdomen management in the octogenarian population. *J Trauma* 2011;70:616–621.
62. Goussous N, Jenkins DH, Zielinski MD. Primary fascial closure after damage control laparotomy: Sepsis vs haemorrhage. *Injury* 2014;45:151–155.
63. Brenner M, Bochicchio G, Bocchicchio K et al. Long-term impact of damage control laparotomy: A prospective study. *Arch Surg.* 2011;146:395–399.
64. Fox N, Crutchfield M, LaChant M, Ross SE, Seamon MJ. Early abdominal closure improves long-term outcomes after damage-control laparotomy. *J Trauma Acute Care Surg.* 2013;75:854–858.
65. Ekeh AP, McCarthy MC, Woods RJ, Walusimbi M, Saxe JM, Patterson LA. Delayed closure of ventral abdominal hernias after severe trauma. *Am J Surg.* 2006;191:391–395.
66. Cheatham ML, Safcsak K. Long-term impact of abdominal decompression: A prospective comparative analysis. *J Am Coll Surg.* 2008;207:573–579.

## Commentary on Evidence-Based Approach to Damage Control Laparotomy

*C. William Schwab and Noelle N. Saillant*

Damage control surgery (DCS) emerged during the same time period as evidence-based medicine (EBM). EBM utilizes the available "evidence" (little, based on Level I science) to create clinical guidelines, thus providing a homogenized approach to simple clinical problems. Recall that use of a guideline carries the warning (usually in small print) that some patients should not be managed by prescription and that clinician judgment remains preeminently important. Complicated and dynamic conditions, where interactions of logistics, resources, individuals, and teams converge with a dynamic physiologic evolution, may not be amendable for a guideline. The damage control "situation," in our experience, is just that condition!

The semiautomatic pistol changed civilian gunshot injuries forever and demanded a highly cognitive, well-planned, but radically different surgical strategy. Rapid treatment confined to control of the damage alone was the answer. When we selected the term for the original paper, *Damage Control*, it described a specific application of surgical maneuvers to a distinct subset of "maximally injured" patients. Subsequently, the term "damage control" was applied to any form of abbreviated surgery with a resultant open abdomen. The term has also been applied in diverse patient populations (pediatrics, elders, septic, fecal peritonitis, etc.) and various delivery environments (low resource, mass causality, military, etc.). In addition, the past two decades have encompassed astounding advances in resuscitation, anesthesia, and surgical and critical care techniques. These incongruencies make any attempt to analyze, compare, and summarize the "damage control" literature very frustrating and leave us wanting for objective affirmations. At the same time, the collective experience concludes that DC works and patients with little chance of survival live!

*Wherein lays the truth?*

First let's define DCS for *Trauma*.

DCS for trauma is a deliberate and anticipated set of nontraditional resuscitative and surgical maneuvers to reverse the effects of exsanguination and massive tissue destruction from physical injury. It requires several coordinated phases or stages:

- DC 0: Decision, triage with DC resuscitation (DCR)
- DC I: OR, abbreviated laparotomy, arrest of hemorrhage, contamination control, packing, and open abdominal management
- DC II: ICU Physiologic restoration
- DC III: OR return, pack removal, definitive injury repair, possible closure
- DC IV: OR return(s), reevaluation and further repair, probable closure. In some cases, deliberate selection of long-term open abdomen and ventral hernia management
- DC V: OR, abdominal wall reconstruction (months later)

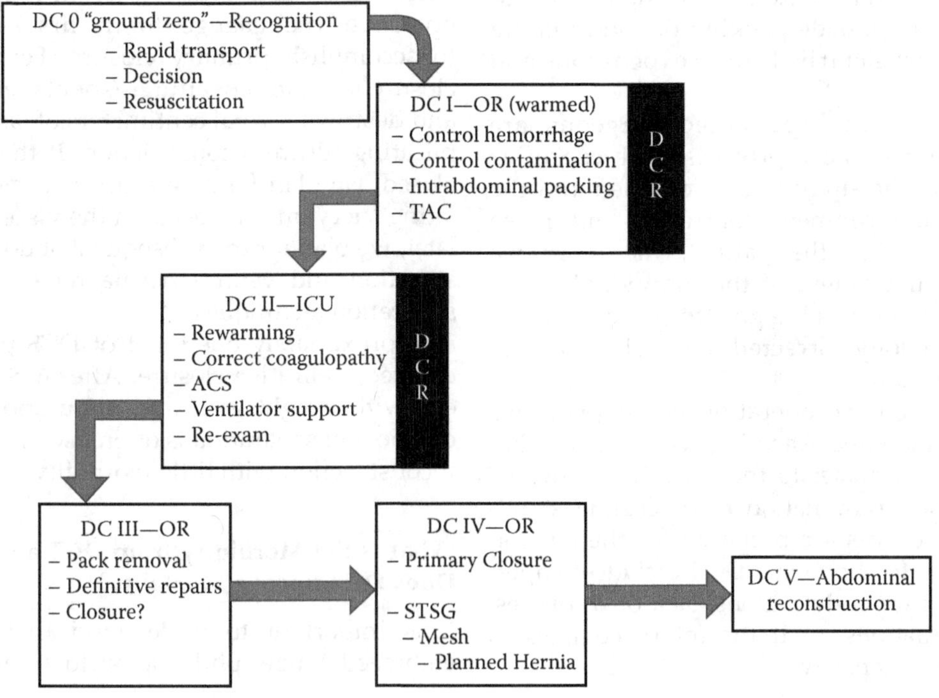

We have elected to combine some questions and save the most important discussion (survival and morbidity) for last.

## How Do We Identify the Need for DCS?

Simply put, it is the recognition of critical injury and exsanguination.

The *pattern recognition* of hypoperfusion (especially sustained low BP), low temperature (Temp < 36°C), and the need to transfuse blood in the face of significant mechanism (GSW, high energy blunt, etc.) demands DCS. Together, hypotension and bradycardia are harbingers of lethality unless expedient control of bleeding is accomplished. Acidosis is not usually determined within minutes of arrival, nor is coagulopathy.

The common reasons to initiate DCS during an operation are physiologic deterioration, changing clinical priorities, or the need for a complex operation that exceeds the capacities of the surgeon, team, or patient (see the following).

## When Should Initial OR End?

Termination of the resuscitative operation comes only when the compelling sources bleeding are controlled and contamination is limited. The principle of simplicity is *the discipline* of DCS. This guidon has necessitated creative solutions such as vascular shunting, limited intestinal resection, hybrid approaches with angio-embolizaiton and intra-luminal balloon occlusion. We find temporary vascular shunting for named vessels and *firm* tamponade packing of solid viscera or ragged musculoskeletal beds to be expeditious and efficacious.

We believe that two experienced surgeons are required for the technical prowess and cognitive demands of DC I. The surgery is disciplined and the operating room environment controlled and noise minimized. The sicker the patient, the more we abbreviate the management of the individual organ injuries. We set 120 min as the goal to complete DC I; rarely is the physiology corrected to the classical end points of resuscitation.

Occasionally, when the operation is complete, we continue resuscitation and warming with the anesthesia team and delay transfer to the ICU. This provides a period of further examination to determine stability and assure resources are prepared for the patient. Additional reasons to abbreviate DC I include competing priorities in other body regions, lack of resources, mass casualty situations, or if the injury complex is *beyond* the surgeons' capacity.

## What Is Best Closure Method?

The early days of DCS taught us to leave the abdomen open with a negative pressure/vacuum device at the conclusion of DC I. Regardless of device chosen, maintenance of negative pressure secures the egress, measurement, and control of fluid loss in order to ensure hygiene and ease of nursing care. This is our standard early management.

It was fortunate that we cared for the patients as the surgeon and as the surgical intensivist. This provided insight into the surgical morbidities associated with exposed viscera and the open abdomen. Each brought about adaptations of damage control I and III:

- Gentle handling of all tissues
- Avoiding closure under tension to preserve the fascia
- Supervision of senior surgeon at all vac changes
- Protecting intestinal anastomoses with omentum and viscera
- Relocating an ileocolic anastomosis laterally, away from fascial edges
- Placement of end ostomies far laterally between the anterior and mid axillary lines (to preserve the rectus fascia and limit stooling into the open abdomen)
- Delaying attempts at fascial closure if bowel protruded above the rectus fascia

The optimal definitive closure of the abdomen is with native tissue (primary fascial closure) without skin closure. We are comfortable performing bedside or intraoperative "vac" changes for the first 7–10 days post DC I to accomplish primary closure. Forcing early fascial closure leads to reopenings (spontaneous and planned) and destroys several centimeters of fascia, thereby complicating future reconstruction. If the fascia cannot be closed, we plan for skin graft placement over a granulating Vicryl mesh placed on the visceral block. Months later, we plan for the subsequent abdominal wall reconstruction and ventral hernia repair, with component separation techniques.

Approximately one-third of DCS patients will need delayed, definitive closure. After 6–8 months of recovery with weight gain and maturation of the STSG, a component separation is often used for the final elective reconstruction with little morbidity.

## What Is the Morbidity from DCT and Does DC Improve Mortality?

It is important to understand that damage control embraced a new philosophy: to accept *any* morbidity, to sustain the patient's life. At the present time, DCS combined with DCR appears to improve survival compared to historic controls. Overall morbidity remains significant and some complications require intensive (organ failure and sepsis) and prolonged care (enteroatmospheric fistula). However, recent longer-term observations have reported that the majority (>80%) of DC patients return to full activities of daily life.

*Wherein lays the truth?*

It is doubtful that any prospective randomized trial will ever be completed. Therefore, one must trust the collective experience for the evidence. DCS has been verified around the globe, in hospitals, military battle theaters, and mass disasters. In our view, DCS works and is the current and best paradigm for: (1) salvaging the exsanguinating trauma patient, or (2) surgical resourcing for mass casualty situations.[*†‡§]

* Brenner M, Bochicchio G, Bochicchio K, Ilahi O, Rodriguez E, Henry S, Joshi M, Scalea T. Long term impact of damage control laparotomy: A prospective study. *Arch Surg.* 2010;146:395–399.

† Cotton BA, Reddy N, Hatch QM et al. Damage control resuscitation is associated with a reduction in resuscitation volumes and improvement in survival in 390 damage control laparotomy patients. *Ann Surg.* 2011;254(4):1–15.

‡ Hoey BA, Schwab CW. Damage control surgery. *Scand J Surg.* 2002;91(1):92–103.

§ Smith IM, Beech ZKM, Lundy JB, Bowley DM. A prospective observational study of abdominal injury management in the contemporary military operations: Damage control laparotomy is associated with high survivability and low rates of fecal diversion. *Ann Surg.* 2014;00:1–9.

# 10

# *Evidence-Based Surgery: Coagulopathy in the Trauma Patient*

**Bellal Joseph and Peter M. Rhee**

**CONTENTS**



## 10.1 Introduction

Acute coagulopathy of trauma (COT) is a hypocoagulable state that can develop immediately after injury, and acute blood loss is a well-established factor associated with worse outcomes in trauma patients [1]. About 24%–36% of trauma patients are known to be hypocoagulable at the time of admission, which continues to remain one of the leading factors associated with mortality among trauma patients [2,3]. Tissue hypoperfusion associated with shock may be an important trigger for the development of COT, which initiates a complex interplay of mediators due to alteration in the protein C pathway and consumption of coagulation factors [1]. Dilution of blood with intravenous crystalloid fluid therapy in response to blood loss is another highly important variable.

Fresh frozen plasma (FFP) has been considered an effective substitute, as it provides volume support and coagulation factors to arrest the initial triggers for the development of COT. However, with the implementation of damage control resuscitation (DCR), there has been a paradigm shift in our resuscitation practices. DCR, which is also known as hemostatic resuscitation, is the adoption of permissive hypotension; early use of blood products, ratio-based blood product transfusion, minimization of crystalloid resuscitation, and factor replacement with drugs have been able to limit the development of hypothermia and acidosis, which are known factors that aggravate the COT [4]. In the military, fresh whole blood transfusion was found to be safe and efficacious without causing adult respiratory distress syndrome, multiple organ dysfunction syndrome, or COT. In the civilian trauma setting, COT remains a major problem, and to treat this, we first need to be able to recognize it. However, there continues to be a lack of consensus regarding the optimal method of measuring coagulopathy in trauma patients, treatment strategies of blood product use, type of factor replacement, role of permissive hypotension, and use of adjunct therapy preventing the COT. In this chapter, we aim to address and provide evidence to help manage coagulopathic trauma patient.

## 10.2 How Do We Measure Coagulopathy? INR versus TEG

The management of COT requires its detection early in the course of management of trauma patients. The conventional coagulation assays such as prothrombin time (PT), activated partial thromboplastin time (aPTT), and international normalized ratios (INR) have been used for the detection of COT, but these assays are limited in their ability to detect COT. One of the primary reasons is that COT is not a static but rather a dynamic state that goes through different stages of hypocoagulability, hypercoagulability, and fibrinolysis [5]. Moreover, PT, aPTT, and INR are performed under optimal conditions of coagulation in a laboratory, i.e., 37°C and normal physiologic pH. Because of this, the conventional coagulation assays fail to take into account the in vivo effects of hypothermia and acidosis on the coagulation cascade [1]. Conventional coagulation assays are conducted on plasma, and therefore they do not take into account the role of platelet function in clot formation. Moreover, most of these coagulation assays are not immediately available during the management of trauma patients. A more optimal coagulation test for trauma patients would be the one that provides urgent point-of-care testing, takes into account the in vivo state of clotting, and provides a dynamic measure of the coagulation [6].

In recent years, viscoelastic tests such as thromboelastography (TEG) and rotational thromboelastometry (ROTEM) have emerged as coagulation tests that detect thrombin formation and fibrinolysis, thus providing information about the global process of coagulation (Figure 10.1) [7]. They are performed on whole blood, instead of plasma and hence take into account the contribution of platelets to the final clot formation. TEG and ROTEM are based on the principle of detecting the clot strength, which is the ultimate endpoint of the coagulation cascade. Changes in clot strength from decreased fibrin synthesis, decreased platelet activity, or enhanced fibrinolysis can be detected by TEG and ROTEM and reflect abnormalities in coagulation [8].

TEG and ROTEM are performed in a cup filled with whole blood that has a pin suspended inside it connected to a transducer system. TEG and ROTEM are based on the same principle but slightly differ from each other in the mechanics involved. TEG involves the rotation of the cup, while ROTEM involves the pin oscillating inside a stationary cup. The movement of the cup mimics the sluggish venous flow inside a blood vessel, while the transducer system connected to the pin detects changes in clot strength [9].

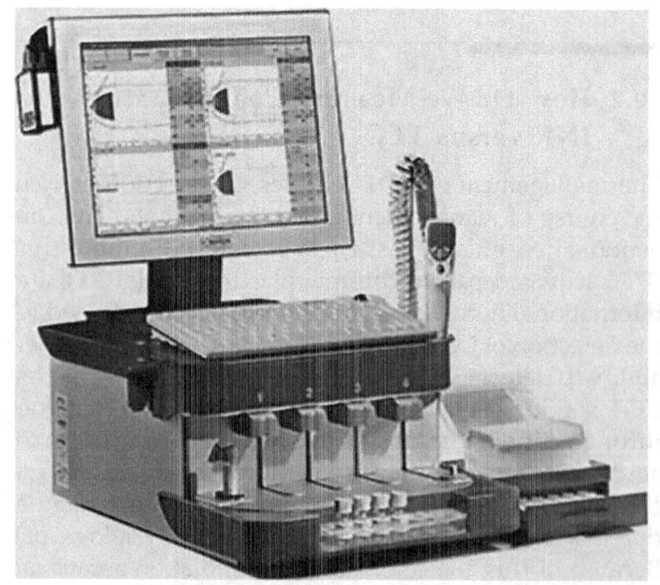

**FIGURE 10.1**
Thromboelastography.

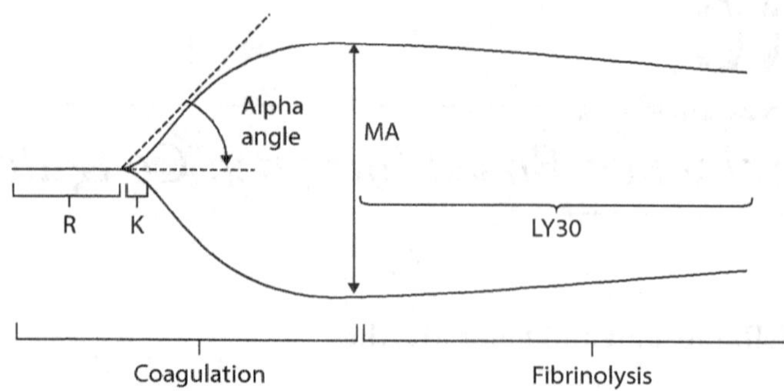


**FIGURE 10.2**
Thromboelastograph.

TEG parameters reflect clot formation time, clot strength, and clot breakdown. Reaction time or R time reflects the latent time until fibrin formation begins. A decrease in R time reflects hypocoagulability from factor deficiency or decreased factor activity, while shortened R time reflects hypercoagulability [10]. α angle reflects the rate of fibrin formation. Measures of clot strength are maximum amplitude (MA) and G, which measures clot elasticity. MA reflects the strength of platelet and fibrin interaction in the clot (Figure 10.2). Any defect in platelet count or function or decreased fibrin formation is reflected as a decrease in MA. High MA reflects hypercoagulability and is shown to be a risk factor for pulmonary embolism [11]. Fibrinolysis is measured by the parameters LY30 and LY60. LY30 and LY60 measure the rate of amplitude reduction at 30 and 60 min, respectively, after MA. A higher LY30 and LY60 reflect decreased clot stability and accelerated fibrinolysis (Figure 10.3) [1].

Viscoelastic tests have shown to be more sensitive than conventional coagulation assays in detecting the coagulation abnormalities that accompany COT [12]. They have shown to be useful in guiding resuscitation in these patients [13]. The ability to detect hyper fibrinolysis also provides the ability to initiate anti-fibrinolytic therapy in these patients that has shown to reduce mortality [14].

Despite these advantages, TEG and ROTEM have limitations. They are relatively newer tests with much higher costs than the conventional coagulation assays. The equipment requires daily calibration and greater expertise to use them and is still not widely available at most trauma centers.

*Recommendation*: There is a lack of Classes I, II, or III studies to determine the best tool to diagnose coagulopathy and determine resuscitation therapy in trauma patients. Although TEG has been gaining popularity, its implementation nationally is still very limited. PTT and PT/INR continue to remain the standard for measuring coagulopathy nationally.

*Grade of recommendation*: C

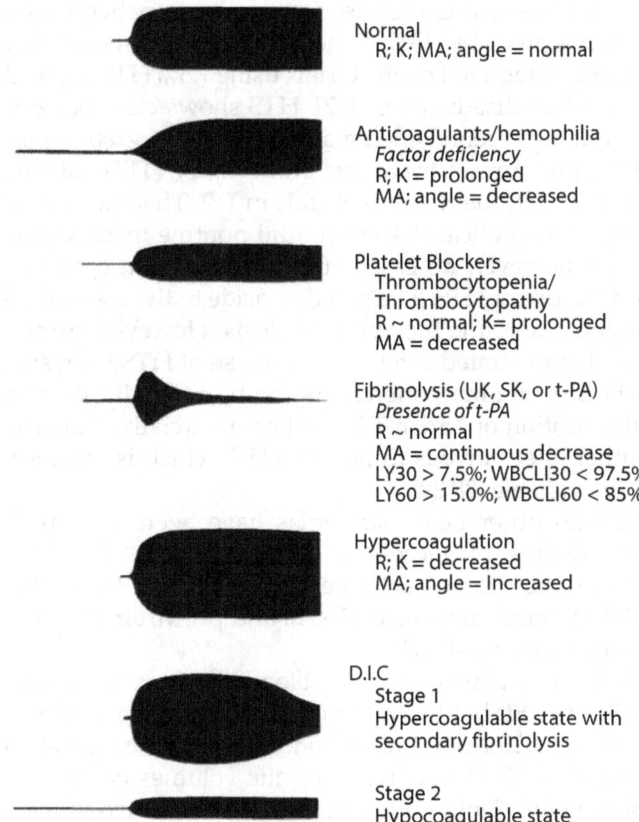


**FIGURE 10.3**
Interpretation of the thromboelastograph.

## 10.3 Blood Product Ratio: What Is the Optimum Ratio?

Severely injured trauma patients require large amounts of volume to resuscitate and restore the intravascular status. The ideal fluids for resuscitation have always been a matter of debate. Isotonic fluids have been, for long, considered the "ideal fluid" for resuscitation in trauma patients. This stems down from the work of Shires and Canizaro during the pre–Vietnam War era that proposed the use of isotonic fluids in a 3:1 ratio to replace intravascular fluid losses. Large-volume isotonic fluid replacement improves the blood pressure; however, it does not improve the oxygen-carrying capacity needed to correct the tissue hypoxia associated with shock. The use of isotonic fluids causes a temporary expansion in the intravascular compartment, but ultimately, most of this fluid redistributes into the interstitial and intracellular compartments. Current insights also show that crystalloids induce neutrophil activation and increased inflammatory responses in trauma patients [15,16]. Studies have shown that increased use of large amounts of crystalloids increases mortality, hospital and intensive care unit length of stay, acute respiratory distress syndrome, and abdominal compartment syndrome [17,18]. There are also concerns of metabolic acidosis associated with the supra-physiologic concentrations of chloride in normal saline. These findings have led to a paradigm shift away from an aggressive resuscitation to less aggressive and more hemostatic resuscitation. This approach, called damage control resuscitation, aims to minimize the use of crystalloids and decrease the incidence of lethal triad of acidosis, hypothermia, and coagulopathy.

The term "damage control resuscitation" is derived from the U.S. Navy, and the data are mostly based on military sources that showed improved survival with the use of fresh whole blood for resuscitation in trauma patients [19,20]. Although fresh whole blood is the ideal fluid for resuscitation, its availability and storage make it an unfeasible option in the civilian trauma setting. However, storage of whole blood even in the most optimum conditions at 4°C causes it to lose platelet and clotting factor activity and undergo morphological changes in red blood cells (RBCs). The advent of component therapy allowed for separation and storage of whole blood components in conditions that help maintain their functionality.

Up to 5% of trauma patients require massive transfusion (MT), i.e., the need for more than 10 units of packed red blood cells (PRBCs) in 24 h [21]. Despite the use of pRBC, many of these trauma patients continue to become coagulopathic due to the combined effects of COT and dilutional coagulopathy. Dilutional coagulopathy even occurs with the use of large amounts of PRBCs, which dilute the existing coagulation factors. Fresh whole blood was not available, and large amounts of PRBCs were still causing coagulopathy; this led to the idea of resuscitating early with all three blood components, i.e., PRBC, FFP, and platelets, in an attempt to reconstitute whole blood in a nearly physiologic ratio before any coagulopathy occurs. These observations called for the development of MT protocols and early use of fixed PRBC, FFP, and platelet ratios during resuscitation. In addition to providing RBCs for the delivery of oxygen, the coagulation factors that are lost through blood loss and consumed during blood loss can be replenished. In addition, it is an excellent way to restore blood volume with oncotic particles. The early use of blood products also has the desired effect of preventing coagulopathy rather than treating it. The development of these MT protocols has seemed to show improvement in outcomes in trauma patients [21,22]. The greatest advantage with the use of predefined ratios exists within the first 6 h when most deaths in trauma patients occur from exsanguinating hemorrhage. This requires the need to identify patients requiring MTs at the time of arrival. Some studies developed scoring systems to predict the need for MT. Trauma-Associated Severe Hemorrhage and Assessment of Blood Consumption scoring systems utilize vital signs, laboratory parameters, and Focused Assessment with Sonography for Trauma (FAST) exam to predict MT with a high degree of accuracy [23,24].

Numerous retrospective studies were performed using data from both civilian and military centers looking for the ideal ratio for transfusion. Despite the retrospective nature of the studies, they all consistently reported a lower mortality with the use of high PRBC and FFP ratios. In all of these studies, the use of PRBC:FFP in ratios close to 1:1 showed a decreased early mortality (24 h) [25–30]. The independent effect of high (≥1:2) versus low (≤1:2) platelet: PRBC ratios was also studied by Holcomb et al., and they found an improved 30-day survival with high ratios of plasma: PRBC [28]. However, some studies argued that the survivors lived longer to receive more transfusions and the mortality advantage was actually seen because of a survivor bias [31]. This debate was resolved after the large multi-institutional Pragmatic, Randomized Optimal Platelet and Plasma Ratios (PROPPR) trial that randomized patients to receive 1:1:1 versus 2:1:1 ratios of PRBC, FFP, and platelets found a lower 24 h mortality but no statistical difference in 30-day mortality with 1:1:1 ratio. The results of this study will be available soon. Despite these advantages, the increased FFP:PRBC is associated with heightened risk for transfusion-related acute lung injury and is the most common cause of transfusion-related deaths.

*Recommendation*: Evidence demonstrates whole blood transfusion to be a potential life-saving method of resuscitation in severely injured trauma patients. Additionally, Level I evidence from the PROPPR trail shows an early survival advantage but not a 28-day survival advantage with a PRBC:FFP:platelets ratio of 1:1:1.

*Grade of recommendation*: A

## 10.4 Adjuvant Measures

Resuscitation with hypertonic saline (HTS) has been extensively studied and has showed significant reduction in resuscitation volumes, with 250 mL of 7.5% HTS achieving similar results to 2–3 L of 0.9% normal saline [32]. It has shown improvement in the immunological response, leading to decreased lung and bowel injuries [33,34]. A meta-analysis of clinical studies showed improved survival rates with the use of HTS and dextran as compared to normal saline [35]. A multicenter, blinded, randomized clinical trial was performed to evaluate the combined role of HTS for a prehospital or emergency department resuscitation, which could not be completed because of concerns for futility of outcomes. This trial showed survival advantage with HTS in patients requiring MT; however, there was increased mortality in patients who did not require MT [36]. A meta-analysis has shown that the six randomized control trials using 7.5% HTS showed no survival disadvantage [37]. HTS shows clear benefits in reducing cerebral edema and improving cerebral perfusion pressure in traumatic brain injury (TBI) patients and still continues to enjoy its role in TBI. There were concerns of theoretical risks of central pontine myelinolysis (CPM); however, no cases of CPM have been observed with the use of HTS. The real downside to the use of HTS is hyperchloremic metabolic acidosis. However, studies have demonstrated safety with the use of HTS for resuscitation in trauma patients. As the traditionally studied concentration of 7.5% HTS is not commercially available, another alternative is to use 5% HTS, which is commercially available [38,39].

Several other novel strategies have been tried with some degree of success as adjuncts for DCR. These include the use of activated recombinant factor VII (rFVIIa), tranexamic acid (TXA), and prothrombin complex concentrate (PCC).

PCC is a plasma-derived blood product somewhat similar to FFP but has additional advantages. It contains as much as 25 times higher concentration of coagulation factors than FFP, thus reducing the volumes needed for resuscitation. Unlike FFP, PCC is present in lyophilized form, and therefore, it does not require thawing needed for FFP, thus expediting therapy [40]. PCC has two types—three-factor and four-factor PCC. Both these types contain factors C, S, II, IX, and X. Four-factor PCC additionally contains factor VII that is present in very small amounts in three-factor PCC [41]. Studies comparing the efficacy of three-factor with four-factor PCC are lacking. Clinical trial comparing PCC and FFP with FFP alone showed accelerated correction of INR with the addition of PCC [42]. Some retrospective studies have also shown improved outcomes with PCC as compared to FFP [43].

Hyperfibrinolysis is seen in up to 7% of trauma patients and is a known factor that aggravates the COT. The main inducers of hyperfibrinolysis in trauma patients are shock and injury severity. TXA is an antifibrinolytic agent that is used to inhibit this hyperfibrinolysis and reduce blood loss in trauma patients. The CRASH-2 trial was a double-blinded, prospective, randomized, placebo-controlled trial performed in 274 hospitals in 40 countries that decreased the risk of mortality if used within 3 h of injury [14]. Although the CRASH-2 trial provides Level I evidence that shows statistically significant survival advantage with the use of TXA, the main criticism is that this may lack clinical significance. The Military Application of Tranexamic Acid in Trauma Emergency Resuscitation trial was a retrospective study on patients receiving at least 1 unit of PRBC [44]. In this study when they did a subgroup analysis on patient receiving MT (greater than 10 units of PRBC), they found that there was improved measures of coagulopathy and survival with TXA use. Based on these findings, the military Tactical Combat Casualty Care Committee has recommended its use in the military setting.

rFVIIa has also been used as a possible adjunct for control of traumatic hemorrhage. rFVIIa is approved by FDA for use in hemophilia but has been extensively used for off-label purposes including trauma. Holcomb et al. proposed its use as a part of DCR early with plasma and PRBC. rFVIIa activates factor Xa at the site of tissue injury by complexing with tissue factor and also on the surface of platelets [45]. Two parallel randomized, placebo-controlled, double-blind trials were conducted to determine the use of rFVIIa use in blunt and penetrating trauma patients. rFVIIa effectively reduced the RBC transfusion requirement and the need for MT in patients with blunt trauma without any increased risk for thromboembolic complications [46]. Some studies have also reported improved 24 h survival with the use of rFVIIa in exsanguinating trauma patients [47]. Despite these benefits, the routine use of rFVIIa is limited by high costs. Moreover, the efficacy of rFVIIa decreases with co-existing hypothermia and acidosis. Therefore, rFVIIa should be used after the correction of these physiologic parameters [48].

*Recommendation*: In recent years, there has been Level II as well as Level III evidence supporting the use of rFVIIa in severely injured coagulopathic trauma patients; there is a lack of Level I data to demonstrate the mortality benefit of rFVIIa. Additionally, there has been increasing Levels II and III evidence highlighting the use of PCC in trauma patients and also the benefit of PCC over rFVIIa. The advantage of PCC is that it is approximately one eighth the cost of rFVIIa. Although survival advantage has not been shown with PCC, it has been shown to effectively and quickly treat coagulopathy. It is also notable that PCC is the recommended therapy for warfarin reversal. TXA has been also shown to be beneficial, and military too has recommended its use.

*Grade of recommendation*: A.

## 10.5 Permissive Hypotension: What Do We Know About It?

In recent years, there has been significant improvement in prehospital management of trauma patients. Many of these trauma patients are hypotensive at the time of arrival of prehospital personnel from hypovolemia. Reversal of this hypovolemic shock with aggressive fluid resuscitation to achieve normal or near-normal vital parameters seems to be the logical approach. However, recent data have shown that achieving near-normal blood pressure may actually disrupt normal hemostasis, "pop off" the clot, and worsen bleeding.

The most important study on this topic was by Bickell et al. that showed that prehospital fluid resuscitation in penetrating trauma patients was associated with lower mortality and fewer post-operative complications [49]. Although there were many critics of this study, it is notable that this trial was iconoclastic, and it definitively showed that it did not harm patients by not giving crystalloid fluids. Therefore, the previously proposed use of prehospital large-volume resuscitation began to lose traction. All animal models of hemorrhage have shown a reduction in mortality with the hypotensive resuscitation [50]. Similarly, a significant review of human studies has shown reduction in the incidence of coagulopathy with reduced volume of prehospital fluids [51]. Dutton et al. performed a randomized study in hemorrhagic shock patients where one group had a target systolic blood pressure (SBP) of >100 mmHg and the other 70 mmHg. They found no difference in the duration of hemorrhage and mortality rate in the two groups and concluded that titration of fluids to a lower than normal SBP did not affect mortality [52]. Following these studies, Advanced Trauma Life Support changed their aggressive resuscitation strategy to a more balanced resuscitative strategy and accepted the possible beneficial role of permissive hypotension in exsanguinating trauma patients.

The role of permissive hypotension stems from a logical argument that the goal of prehospital resuscitation in exsanguinating trauma patients is to maintain blood pressure just enough to maintain adequate tissue perfusion to the vital organs. The goal of prehospital resuscitation is not achieving the normal figures of blood pressure, as achieving those high pressures in trauma patients disrupts clot and potentially worsens bleeding. The most important question in this regard has been what pressure is adequate enough to maintain normal tissue perfusion without increasing the risk of mortality. Most studies have shown that achieving a mean arterial pressure (MAP) of 60 mmHg or an SBP of 90 mmHg maintains adequate tissue perfusion [53]. Pressures above this have shown to worsen the bleeding in uncontrolled hemorrhage models [54].

One of the major concerns about the role of permissive hypotension has been the risk of inducing a state of irreversible shock and end organ damage. However, maintaining a MAP of around 60 mmHg for 60–90 min is safe and does not increase the risk of irreversible shock and mortality [55]. The role of permissive hypotension needs to be understood in its context, and that permissive hypotension in uncontrolled hemorrhagic shock is not an alternative to definitive hemorrhage control. Hypotensive resuscitation with restricted use of fluids is most applicable in the scenario where rapid transport to a trauma center for definitive hemorrhage control can be carried out.

**TABLE 10.1**

Clinical Questions

| Question | Answer | Grade of Recommendation | References |
|---|---|---|---|
| How do we measure coagulopathy? INR versus TEG | TEG has higher sensitivity than conventional coagulation assays. However, no Level I evidence exists. | C | [17–19] |
| Blood product ratio: What is the optimum ratio? | Protocols improve blood product utilization and outcomes. Early empiric use of PRBC and FFP at ratios of 1:1 improves short-term mortality. | A | [35,36] |
| Adjuvant measures | Resuscitation with HTS may be beneficial in patients requiring MT, and rFVIIa reduces blood product requirement and need for MT in patients with blunt trauma. PCC, in combination with FFP, accelerates INR correction but does not improve clinical outcomes. | A | [23,53,54,68,61] |
| Permissive hypotension: What do we know about it? | Reduces mortality in the right scenario and for the right patient population. | C | [49–52] |

**TABLE 10.2**

Levels of Evidence

| Subject | Year | References | Level of Evidence | Strength of Recommendation | Findings |
|---|---|---|---|---|---|
| MT protocols | 2008, 2010 | [35,36] | III | B | MT protocols improve outcomes. |
| PRBC:FFP ratio | 2014 | | I | A | Early empiric use of PRBC and FFP at ratios of 1:1 improves 24 h mortality. |
| HTS | 2011 | [53,54] | II | B | Resuscitation with HTS may be beneficial in patients requiring MT. |
| Factor VIIa for trauma | 2005 | [68] | II | B | rFVIIa reduces blood product requirement and need for MT in patients with blunt trauma. |
| Antifibrinolytics | 2010 | [23] | I | B | TXA lowers mortality if used within 3 h of injury. |

The biggest risk with hypotensive resuscitation exists in patients with co-existing TBI. TBI patients require high blood pressure to maintain adequate cerebral perfusion pressure because of the raised intra-cranial pressures from ongoing cerebral edema. Hypotension in these patients has actually shown to cause secondary brain injury (Tables 10.1 and 10.2) [56].

*Recommendation*: Permissive hypotension is a double-edged sword. Evidence suggests that, if used appropriately in the right scenario and for the right population, permissive hypotension can significantly reduce mortality but can be detrimental if used otherwise.

*Grade of recommendation*: C

## Disclaimer

There are no identifiable conflicts of interests to report. The authors have no financial or proprietary interest in the subject matter or materials discussed in the chapter.

## References

1. Palmer L, Martin L. Traumatic coagulopathy—Part 1: Pathophysiology and diagnosis. *J Vet Emerg Crit Care.* 2014;24:63–74.
2. MacLeod JB, Lynn M, McKenney MG, Cohn SM, Murtha M. Early coagulopathy predicts mortality in trauma. *J Trauma.* 2003;55:39–44.
3. Maegele M, Lefering R, Yucel N et al. Early coagulopathy in multiple injury: An analysis from the German Trauma Registry on 8724 patients. *Injury.* 2007;38:298–304.
4. Santry HP, Alam HB. Fluid resuscitation: Past, present, and the future. *Shock.* 2010;33:229–241.
5. Brohi K, Cohen MJ, Ganter MT et al. Acute coagulopathy of trauma: Hypoperfusion induces systemic anticoagulation and hyperfibrinolysis. *J Trauma.* 2008;64:1211–1217; discussion 7.
6. Kashuk JL, Moore EE, Le T et al. Noncitrated whole blood is optimal for evaluation of postinjury coagulopathy with point-of-care rapid thrombelastography. *J Surg Res.* 2009;156:133–138.
7. Enriquez LJ, Shore-Lesserson L. Point-of-care coagulation testing and transfusion algorithms. *Br J Anaesth.* 2009;103(Suppl 1):i14–i22.

8. da Luz LT, Nascimento B, Rizoli S. Thrombelastography (TEG(R)): Practical considerations on its clinical use in trauma resuscitation. *Scand J Trauma Resusc Emerg Med.* 2013;21:29.
9. Espinosa A, Stenseth R, Videm V, Pleym H. Comparison of three point-of-care testing devices to detect hemostatic changes in adult elective cardiac surgery: A prospective observational study. *BMC Anesthesiol.* 2014;14:80.
10. Sankarankutty A, Nascimento B, Teodoro da Luz L, Rizoli S. TEG(R) and ROTEM(R) in trauma: Similar test but different results? *World J Emerg Surg.* 2012;7(Suppl 1):S3.
11. Dai Y, Lee A, Critchley LA, White PF. Does thromboelastography predict postoperative thromboembolic events? A systematic review of the literature. *Anesth Analg.* 2009;108:734–742.
12. Martini WZ, Cortez DS, Dubick MA, Park MS, Holcomb JB. Thromboelastography is better than PT, aPTT, and activated clotting time in detecting clinically relevant clotting abnormalities after hypothermia, hemorrhagic shock and resuscitation in pigs. *J Trauma.* 2008;65:535–543.
13. Cotton BA, Faz G, Hatch QM et al. Rapid thrombelastography delivers real-time results that predict transfusion within 1 hour of admission. *J Trauma.* 2011;71:407–414; discussion 14–17.
14. Shakur H, Roberts I, Bautista R et al. Effects of tranexamic acid on death, vascular occlusive events, and blood transfusion in trauma patients with significant haemorrhage (CRASH-2): A randomised, placebo-controlled trial. *Lancet.* 2010;376:23–32.
15. Rhee P, Burris D, Kaufmann C et al. Lactated Ringer's solution resuscitation causes neutrophil activation after hemorrhagic shock. *J Trauma Inj Infect Crit Care.* 1998;44:313–319.
16. Rhee P, Wang D, Ruff P et al. Human neutrophil activation and increased adhesion by various resuscitation fluids. *Crit Care Med.* 2000;28:74–78.
17. Joseph B, Zangbar B, Pandit V et al. The conjoint effect of reduced crystalloid administration and decreased damage-control laparotomy use in the development of abdominal compartment syndrome. *J Trauma Acute Care Surg.* 2014;76:457–461
18. Kasotakis G, Sideris A, Yang Y et al. Aggressive early crystalloid resuscitation adversely affects outcomes in adult blunt trauma patients: An analysis of the Glue Grant database. *J Trauma Acute Care Surg.* 2013;74:1215.
19. Spinella PC. Warm fresh whole blood transfusion for severe hemorrhage: U.S. military and potential civilian applications. *Crit Care Med.* 2008;36:S340–S345.
20. Spinella PC, Perkins JG, Grathwohl KW, Beekley AC, Holcomb JB. Warm fresh whole blood is independently associated with improved survival for patients with combat-related traumatic injuries. *J Trauma.* 2009;66:S69–S76.
21. Nunez TC, Young PP, Holcomb JB, Cotton BA. Creation, implementation, and maturation of a massive transfusion protocol for the exsanguinating trauma patient. *J Trauma.* 2010;68:1498–1505.
22. Cotton BA, Gunter OL, Isbell J et al. Damage control hematology: The impact of a trauma exsanguination protocol on survival and blood product utilization. *J Trauma.* 2008;64:1177–1182; discussion 82–83.
23. Yucel N, Lefering R, Maegele M et al. Trauma Associated Severe Hemorrhage (TASH)-Score: Probability of mass transfusion as surrogate for life threatening hemorrhage after multiple trauma. *J Trauma.* 2006;60:1228–1236; discussion 36–37.
24. Nunez TC, Voskresensky IV, Dossett LA, Shinall R, Dutton WD, Cotton BA. Early prediction of massive transfusion in trauma: Simple as ABC (assessment of blood consumption)? *J Trauma.* 2009;66:346–352.
25. Borgman MA, Spinella PC, Perkins JG et al. The ratio of blood products transfused affects mortality in patients receiving massive transfusions at a combat support hospital. *J Trauma.* 2007;63:805–813
26. Duchesne JC, Hunt JP, Wahl G et al. Review of current blood transfusions strategies in a mature level I trauma center: Were we wrong for the last 60 years? *J Trauma.* 2008;65:272–276; discussion 6–8.
27. Gunter OL, Jr., Au BK, Isbell JM, Mowery NT, Young PP, Cotton BA. Optimizing outcomes in damage control resuscitation: Identifying blood product ratios associated with improved survival. *J Trauma.* 2008;65:527–534.
28. Holcomb JB, Wade CE, Michalek JE et al. Increased plasma and platelet to red blood cell ratios improves outcome in 466 massively transfused civilian trauma patients. *Ann Surg.* 2008;248:447–458.
29. Sperry JL, Ochoa JB, Gunn SR et al. An FFP:PRBC transfusion ratio ≥1:1.5 is associated with a lower risk of mortality after massive transfusion. *J Trauma.* 2008;65:986–993.
30. Teixeira PG, Inaba K, Shulman I et al. Impact of plasma transfusion in massively transfused trauma patients. *J Trauma.* 2009;66:693–697.
31. Snyder CW, Weinberg JA, McGwin G, Jr. et al. The relationship of blood product ratio to mortality: Survival benefit or survival bias? *J Trauma.* 2009;66:358–362; discussion 62–64.
32. Alam HB. An update on fluid resuscitation. *SJS.* 2006;95:136–145.
33. Hypertonicity regulates the function of human neutrophils by modulating chemoattractant receptor signaling and activating mitogen-activated protein kinase p38. *J Clin Investig.* 1998;101:2768–2779.
34. Murao Y, Hata M, Ohnishi K et al. Hypertonic saline resuscitation reduces apoptosis and tissue damage of the small intestine in a mouse model of hemorrhagic shock. *Shock.* 2003;20:23–28.
35. Wade CE, Kramer GC, Grady JJ, Fabian TC, Younes RN. Efficacy of hypertonic 7.5% saline and 6% dextran-70 in treating trauma: A meta-analysis of controlled clinical studies. *Surgery.* 1997;122:609–616.
36. Bulger EM, May S, Kerby JD et al. Out-of-hospital hypertonic resuscitation after traumatic hypovolemic shock: A randomized, placebo controlled trial. *Ann Surg.* 2011;253:431–441.
37. Doyle JA, Davis DP, Hoyt DB. The use of hypertonic saline in the treatment of traumatic brain injury. *J Trauma.* 2001;50:367–383.
38. DuBose JJ, Kobayashi L, Lozornio A et al. Clinical experience using 5% hypertonic saline as a safe alternative fluid for use in trauma. *J Trauma.* 2010;68:1172–1177.

39. Joseph B, Aziz H, Snell M et al. The physiological effects of hyperosmolar resuscitation: 5% vs 3% hypertonic saline. *Am J Surg.* 2014;208:697–702.
40. Ferreira J, DeLosSantos M. The clinical use of prothrombin complex concentrate. *J Emerg Med.* 2013;44:1201–1210.
41. Bershad EM, Suarez JI. Prothrombin complex concentrates for oral anticoagulant therapy-related intracranial hemorrhage: A review of the literature. *Neurocrit Care.* 2010;12:403–413.
42. Boulis NM, Bobek MP, Schmaier A, Hoff JT. Use of factor IX complex in warfarin-related intracranial hemorrhage. *Neurosurgery.* 1999;45:1113–1118; discussion 8–9.
43. Joseph B, Aziz H, Pandit V et al. Prothrombin complex concentrate versus fresh-frozen plasma for reversal of coagulopathy of trauma: Is there a difference? *World J Surg.* 2014;38:1875–1881.
44. Morrison JJ, Dubose JJ, Rasmussen TE, Midwinter MJ. Military application of tranexamic acid in trauma emergency resuscitation (MATTERs) study. *Arch Surg.* 2012;147(2):113–119.
45. Franchini M, Lippi G, Guidi GC. The use of recombinant activated factor VII in platelet-associated bleeding. *Hematology.* 2008;13:41–45.
46. Boffard KD, Riou B, Warren B et al. Recombinant factor VIIa as adjunctive therapy for bleeding control in severely injured trauma patients: Two parallel randomized, placebo-controlled, double-blind clinical trials. *J Trauma.* 2005;59:8–15; discussion 8.
47. Rizoli SB, Nascimento B, Jr., Osman F et al. Recombinant activated coagulation factor VII and bleeding trauma patients. *J Trauma.* 2006;61:1419–1425.
48. Fries D. The early use of fibrinogen, prothrombin complex concentrate, and recombinant-activated factor VIIa in massive bleeding. *Transfusion.* 2013;53(Suppl 1):91s–95s.
49. Bickell WH, Wall MJ, Jr., Pepe PE et al. Immediate versus delayed fluid resuscitation for hypotensive patients with penetrating torso injuries. *New Engl J Med.* 1994;331:1105–1109.
50. Mapstone J, Roberts I, Evans P. Fluid resuscitation strategies: A systematic review of animal trials. *J Trauma.* 2003;55:571–589.
51. Kwan I, Bunn F, Chinnock P, Roberts I. Timing and volume of fluid administration for patients with bleeding. *Cochrane Database Syst Rev.* 2014;3:Cd002245.
52. Dutton RP, Mackenzie CF, Scalea TM. Hypotensive resuscitation during active hemorrhage: Impact on in-hospital mortality. *J Trauma Inj Infect Crit Care.* 2002;52(6):1141–1146.
53. Kentner R, Safar P, Prueckner S et al. Titrated hypertonic/hyperoncotic solution for hypotensive fluid resuscitation during uncontrolled hemorrhagic shock in rats. *Resuscitation.* 2005;65:87–95.
54. Sondeen JL, Coppes VG, Holcomb JB. Blood pressure at which rebleeding occurs after resuscitation in swine with aortic injury. *J Trauma.* 2003;54:S110–S117.
55. Palmer L, Martin L. Traumatic coagulopathy—Part 2: Resuscitative strategies. *J Vet Emerg Crit Care.* 2014;24:75–92.
56. Chesnut RM, Marshall LF, Klauber MR et al. The role of secondary brain injury in determining outcome from severe head injury. *J Trauma.* 1993;34:216–222.

## Commentary on Evidence-Based Surgery: Coagulopathy in the Trauma Patient

*Stephen M. Cohn*

There are no identifiable conflicts of interests to report.

The author has no financial or proprietary interest in the subject matter or materials discussed in the manuscript.

The resuscitation of the trauma patient has undergone a paradigm shift over the last decade. Many may remember with trepidation the era of large volume crystalloid–based resuscitation. The well-meaning care we provided made most of our students and residents believe that the archetypical trauma patient looked like the Michelin man (or woman); hugely swollen, edematous with resultant abdominal compartment syndrome, ARDS, kidney failure, and enteroatmospheric fistulae bubbling away in the corner of the ICU. Fortunately this conception of the post-trauma patient exists largely in the memory of those who cared for these patients. Gone are the days where the resident would announce proudly on morning ICU rounds that they gave a patient 20 units of packed red blood cells and 15 L of crystalloid in bolus after bolus for a bleeding trauma patient with a sagging blood pressure.

Two concurrent scientific and clinical discoveries have driven this paradigm shift. First was the initial description and subsequent characterization of acute traumatic coagulopathy. Initially described concurrently in 2003 in two separate papers, Brohi and Macleod suggested that there was an endogenous coagulopathy, which occurred nearly immediately after injury and was independent of the traditional iatrogenic causes of hypothermia, dilution, and acidosis. Subsequent work by multiple other groups has elucidated that this ATC occurs nearly immediately after severe injury and shock and is likely mediated by activation of the protein C system. This system has been extensively described in multiple clinical and basic science investigations. Interestingly the ATC that makes our patients bleed seems to be the unfortunate "too much of a good thing" sequalie of a cytoprotective activation of protein C as the body tries to keep itself alive through the acute phase after severe trauma. Later, if and when a patient has survived their initial injury they are left with "too little of a good thing" and a propensity for inflammatory-driven complications such as organ failure, ARDS, and infection. The continuum between early bleeding and later inflammatory and infectious complications represents an important biology essential to the understanding of the effects of injury and our resuscitative interventions on both bleeding and inflammation.

Along with the description and ultimate understanding of ATC, the other revolutionary finding that changed our resuscitative paradigm was the initial description and subsequent refinement of balanced component-based resuscitation. Initially discovered by Borgman, the ideal that we could recreate whole blood out of the components available in the blood bank all the while limiting our crystalloid resuscitation has become, as of 2015, the standard of care. While there remains considerable debate on the exact ratio and timing of blood products, mechanism of benefit and the dynamics of who will benefit especially in light of the mixed results of the PROPPR study, it is safe to say that the era of large volume crystalloid-based resuscitation is over and has been replaced by a standard of care that seeks a balanced blood product–based resuscitation.

In this nicely written chapter, Drs. Joseph and Rhee very nicely discuss the current state of coagulation science. Their topics include diagnosis, blood product ratio, adjuvant resuscitation, and permissive hypotension.

So what does the trauma surgeon need to know about coagulopathy in 2015?

### ATC Is a Real Issue and Needs To Be Addressed

As described earlier, acute traumatic coagulopathy is a real and important entity occurring in severely injured and shocked patients and results in increased bleeding, added resuscitation requirements, and incumbent increased morbidity and greater mortality. These patients need to be diagnosed and treated with an aggressive balanced resuscitation, which seeks to reverse ATC. Whether the balanced resuscitation provides benefit from correction of coagulopathy and improved hemostasis or from a balanced inflammatory milieu and prevention of endotheliopathy (or a likely combination of the two) remains an open experimental question. Either way understanding that ATC exists and must be addressed is paramount and has revolutionized the care of the injured patient.

### Diagnosis of Traumatic Coagulopathy Is an Evolving Field

While conventional coagulation tests have been appropriately questioned (and are nicely discussed in this chapter), they do have an important history and continued utility in 2015. Indeed the initial description and many of the characterizations of coagulopathy after trauma were done using prothrombin time and partial thromboplastin time. Subsequent work suggested that viscoelastic tests (TEG/ROTEM) could give more and potentially better data regarding when and how the coagulation system is perturbed after trauma. The literature remains mixed on this topic and new and better analyses are continuing. Indeed while TEG/ROTEM are being more widely adopted, their use is not yet widespread or completely validated and some of the literature claiming prediction suffers from circular logic from treatment bias. Of course not to be forgotten is the extremely important role of platelets after trauma where several studies have shown approximately 50% of patients suffering from platelet dysfunction despite normal platelet counts. As of 2015, both CCTs and functional testing both have a continued place in the treatment of the severely injured patient. CCTs appropriately diagnose the presence of ATC and functional testing can define which part of the cell-based model of coagulation is broken and needs repair. Ultimately, there is a huge amount of investigative effort, which should revolutionize and hopefully personalize diagnosis for ATC over the next several years.

### Diagnosis May Not Matter Initially? Resuscitation in 2015

While much has been made and considerable effort continues on the topic of diagnosis of ATC, whether the need is relevant remains an open question. The most severely injured and/or shocked trauma patient should be treated with a balanced blood product resuscitation beginning immediately without any delay for diagnosis. While it remains unclear whether balanced resuscitation saves lives because it fixes coagulation and helps achieve hemostasis or rather because it prevents inflammatory and endothelial dysfunction (or a likely dynamic mix of the two depending on the patient and injury), there is considerable evidence to suggest that all severely injured trauma patients who need resuscitation will benefit and hence, it should be rapidly initiated on all. As for PCC the data remains controversial. While PCC is effective at reversing warfarin-induced coagulopathy or correcting a specific factor deficit, it does not address the overwhelming anticoagulant milieu that exists post trauma and does not address platelet function issues, rendering its use in severe trauma resuscitation an open question. Additionally as much of the benefit from balanced resuscitation comes balancing the inflammatory milieu rather than just fixing the coagulation cascade, PCC should remain an adjunct to an aggressive balanced resuscitation, which seeks to recreate whole blood from the components available. While the mixed results of the PROPPR study provided more questions than answers about how/when and which specific patients should receive which resuscitation protocol, the overwhelming evidence suggests initial aggressive resuscitation benefits all patients. As the patient progresses and additional diagnostic data (lab tests, etc.) come back, the resuscitation should be tailored to a goal-directed, lab-based resuscitation what is needed (hemoglobin, fixing coagulation, etc.). Additional and better studies will no doubt be aimed at ferreting out which patients will benefit toward the ultimate goal of precision individual patient-targeted care.

# 11

# *Traumatic Brain Injury*

**Ara J. Feinstein and Matthew J. Marini**

**CONTENTS**



Traumatic brain injury (TBI) continues to be a major cause of death and disability. The Centers for Disease Control and Prevention reports a continued uptrend in the numbers of TBI-related emergency department visits, hospitalizations, and deaths between 2001 and 2010, peaking at 824 per 100,000. Most injuries are due to motor vehicle crashes, falls, and assaults, with falls more prevalent as age increases [1]. TBI is viewed as a dual cerebral insult composed of primary and secondary processes [2]. The primary injury occurs at the time of impact with immediate damage to brain cells. These subsequently become progressively vulnerable to further damage due to secondary cerebral changes such as intracranial hypertension (ICH), decreases in cerebral perfusion pressure, and cerebral hypoxia [3]. Treatment of these patients is often complicated by concomitant injuries that affect the ability of the clinician to effectively manage TBI. In an effort to improve outcomes, questions arise regarding monitoring, intervention, and pharmacologic management of these patients.

## 11.1 Does Repeat Head Computed Tomography after TBI Determine the Need for Clinical Intervention?

Head computed tomography (CT) is an invaluable tool in the evaluation of patients with suspected TBI. Any patient with blunt trauma and a Glasgow Coma Scale (GCS) score of less than 15 undergoes head CT at most institutions. Repeat head CT scans are routinely performed to evaluate progression of intracranial bleeding or to assess the need for neurosurgical intervention. Given the increased cost and risk of moving critically ill patients, several studies have called this practice into question.

Sifri et al. prospectively evaluated 130 consecutive patients with minor head injury (GCS ≥13 and loss of consciousness or amnesia) and intracranial bleeding on initial CT scan that did not require immediate intervention [4]. Ninety-nine of these patients (76%) had no deterioration of their exam prior to the second CT. Twelve patients had worsening of their bleeding on repeat CT (9%), but none of these required neurosurgical intervention. In contrast, of the 31 (24%) patients who had deterioration of their neurologic exam prior to the second CT, 14 (11%) had worse CT scans and two (1.5%) required surgical intervention. After the initial CT, a stable neurologic exam has a negative predictive value of 100% in predicting the lack of neurosurgical intervention.

Brown et al. prospectively studied 100 consecutive TBI patients with an abnormal initial head CT that did not require immediate neurosurgical intervention [5]. Sixty-eight of these patients underwent 90 repeat CT scans. Eighty-one (90%) of these scans were performed without neurological change, and none of these patients required medical or surgical intervention for TBI, despite the apparent worsening on 19 (23%) scans. Of the nine CT scans done in the setting of a deteriorating mental status, six (67%) were worse, requiring one medical and two surgical interventions.

In a subsequent study, Brown et al. prospectively examined 274 patients with an abnormal head CT not requiring immediate intervention [6]. Patients were stratified into mild (GCS 13–15), moderate (GCS 9–12), and severe (GCS ≤8) injury groups. Only two patients (0.7%) had changes on repeat CT that required intervention in the absence of clinical deterioration. Both were in the severe injury group.

Abdel Fattah et al. prospectively studied 145 consecutive patients with a GCS of 13–15 with intracranial hemorrhage [7]. These subjects were divided into two groups: 92 (63%) in the "routine" repeat CT group and 53 (37%) in the "selective" repeat CT group. Six subjects (11%) in the selective group received repeat scans due to physical exam changes, with one (1.9%) having a progression of hemorrhage not requiring intervention. Overall, the patients in the selective group had significantly fewer scans with shorter intensive care unit (ICU) and hospital length of stay.

Joseph et al. prospectively studied 1129 trauma patients with intracranial hemorrhage on initial CT [8]. These were divided into two groups: routine repeat CT within 6 h (1099) and repeat CT due to deteriorating neurologic exam (30). In the routine group, 216 (20%) had worsening on CT scan. Four of these patients required intervention. All four of these patients had a presentation GCS ≤8 and were intubated. In the selective group, 30 patients underwent repeat CT for a decline in neurologic exam. Sixteen (53%) of these scans showed progression and 12 (40%) required an intervention (Table 11.1).

*Recommendation*: Patients with intracranial hemorrhage and a deteriorating neurologic exam or the presence of moderate or severe injury (GCS ≤12) warrant a repeat

**TABLE 11.1**

Table of Evidence: Repeat Head CT

| Trial (Ref. No.) | Year | Level of Evidence | Randomized Groups (*n*) | Intervention/ Design | Median Follow-Up | Minor End Point | Major End Point | Interpretations/ Comments |
|---|---|---|---|---|---|---|---|---|
| [4] | 2006 | IIb | Prospective, observational study | 130 patients with minor TBI/ICH underwent serial CT scans to observe for progression of ICH. | | | Neurologic deterioration, neurosurgical intervention | In patients with minimal head injury and normal neurologic exam, repeat head CT should not be performed. |
| [5] | 2004 | IIb | Prospective, observational study | 100 TBI patients with abnormal CT scans were observed for use of repeat head CT and clinical outcomes. | | | Neurologic deterioration, number of head CTs performed, neurosurgical intervention | In patients with TBI and abnormal initial head CT, repeat head CT is not warranted unless there is acute change in neurologic status. |
| [6] | 2007 | IIb | Prospective, observational study | 274 TBI patients with abnormal initial CT scans were observed for use of repeat head CT and clinical outcomes. | | | Neurologic deterioration, medical and neurosurgical intervention | Repeat head CT is warranted in patients who sustain TBI and clinically decline, as it often results in need for intervention; routine repeat head CT is not warranted in patients with GCS >8 without change in neurologic status. |
| [7] | 2012 | IIb | Prospective, observational study | 145 patients with GCS 13–15 divided into routine repeat head CT and "selective" repeat head CT groups | | ICU days, hospital length of stay | Neurologic deterioration, progression of ICH, neurosurgical intervention | Use of selective repeat head CT results in decreased number of head CTs, ICU days, and hospital length of stay for TBI patients with GCS 13–15. |
| [8] | 2014 | IIb | Prospective, observational study | 1129 patients with ICH after TBI were divided into routine repeat head CT at 6 h and selective head CT groups. | | | Neurologic deterioration, progression of ICH | In the absence of deteriorating neurologic examination, repeat head CT is not warranted in TBI setting. |

head CT to guide therapy. Patients with a GCS of 13–15 and no change in neurologic exam do not require a routine repeat CT scan (Grade B recommendation).

## 11.2 Do Procoagulants Decrease Intracranial Hemorrhage Related to TBI?

The use of novel hemostatic agents in the setting of trauma to reverse coagulopathy has been a growing area of interest over the past decade. The frequency of intracranial hemorrhage in the setting of TBI has been reported to be as high as 75%. Furthermore, patients who sustain TBI while taking oral anticoagulation have a 30-day mortality approaching 60% [9]. Coagulopathy in the setting of secondary TBI due to ongoing hemorrhage, pretraumatic use of anticoagulants, and liberal administration of crystalloid results in worsening of the ICH and increased mortality [10]. Several agents have been investigated in trauma populations to reverse coagulopathy, including factor VII, prothrombin complex concentrate (PCC), and transexamic acid (TXA). PCC is a combination of FDA-approved vitamin K-associated clotting factors to reverse coagulopathy from warfarin use in patients with acute hemorrhage. There are two available versions of the drug: a four-factor formulation containing factor VII and a three-factor formulation without factor VII. Factor VII is available in recombinant form and has been studied in trauma populations. TXA is an anti-fibrinolytic agent that is often used in the setting of surgical bleeding, but recent studies have focused on its use in trauma.

Kluger et al. performed a post hoc analysis of study data from a prospective, randomized, placebo-controlled study, evaluating the safety and efficacy of intravenous recombinant activated factor VII (rFVIIa) versus placebo [11]. They identified 30 patients and showed no differences in outcomes or adverse events.

Narayan et al. performed a multicenter, randomized, double-blinded, placebo-controlled, dose-escalation trial to investigate the safety and preliminary effectiveness of rFVIIa in 97 patients with TBI [12]. There were no significant differences in outcomes or adverse events between the placebo ($n$ = 36) and factor VIIa ($n$ = 61) groups. There was, however, a nonsignificant trend toward smaller hemorrhage size and increased deep vein thrombosis (DVT) in the factor VIIa group. This study was a safety and dosing trial that likely lacked sufficient power to show clinical benefits.

Joseph et al. conducted a retrospective study of 85 coagulopathic TBI patients who received either PCC ($n$ = 64) or rFVIIa ($n$ = 21) [13]. The groups were not similar, with patients in the PCC group being significantly older, with a lower Injury Severity Score (ISS), more likely to be on warfarin pre-injury, and receiving fewer blood products prior to treatment. The authors found lower mortality and cost in the PCC group, but this is difficult to interpret, given the differences in the patient populations of the two groups.

Yanamadala et al. retrospectively compared PCC to FFP in 33 patients taking warfarin who sustained TBI with ICH, with five patients receiving PCC for their sole pharmacologic source of coagulopathy reversal [9]. Time to reversal was significantly shorter for the PCC group (65 min PCC vs. 265 min FFP). The time to anesthesia induction was also significantly shorter in the PCC group (159 min PCC vs. 307 min FFP).

The CRASH-2 trial studied the use of TXA in trauma patients and found that the use of TXA within 3 h of injury reduced the risk of death due to bleeding and reduced hospital costs [14]. Although this study did not use TBI specifically as its inclusion criteria, Perel et al. performed a nested study of the patients within the CRASH-2 study that sustained TBI. The study compared mortality, mean hemorrhage growth, and the presence of new ischemic lesions in the TXA and placebo groups. Although the TXA group appeared to have lower mortality, less progression of hemorrhage, and fewer new ischemic foci, none of the analyses reached statistical significance [15]. These data have prompted the creation of the CRASH-3 trial to specifically study the outcomes of TBI patients receiving TXA.

Yutthakasemsunt et al. performed a randomized, placebo-controlled trial in 238 patients with TBI and GCS 4–12. There were no statistically significant improvements in mortality, ICH progression, or Glasgow Outcome Scale in patients receiving TXA, stressing the need for larger studies (Table 11.2) [16].

*Recommendation*: PCC may be an adjunct to FFP to reverse coagulopathy due to warfarin in TBI (Grade B recommendation). There are insufficient data to recommend the use of TXA or factor VII in this population.

## 11.3 When Should DVT Prophylaxis Be Initiated in TBI?

Chemical DVT prophylaxis has been an intense area of research in the trauma literature. Grade B recommendations support low-molecular-weight heparin (LMWH) as the most effective method of prophylaxis to prevent DVT in trauma patients *without* TBI [17]. Prophylactic therapy for DVT and pulmonary embolism (PE) in patients with TBI must always be balanced against the risk of expansion of intracranial hematoma and re-bleeding [18]. This necessitates balancing evidence-based guidelines with

**TABLE 11.2**
Table of Evidence: Procoagulants

| Trial (Ref. No.) | Year | Level of Evidence | Randomized Groups (*n*) | Intervention/ Design | Median Follow-Up | Minor End Point | Major End Point | Interpretations/ Comments |
|---|---|---|---|---|---|---|---|---|
| [9] | 2014 | IIb | Prospective, observational study | Prospective analysis of 33 patients undergoing correction of coagulopathy with either PCC or FFP while treated for TBI | | | Time to INR correction, time delay until surgical intervention | Patients who were treated with PCC had faster correction of INR and shorter delay to surgical intervention; however, the study is very small and underpowered. |
| [11] | 2007 | Ib | Randomized, double-blinded trial | 30 hemodynamically unstable polytrauma patients with TBI, randomized to receiving rFVIIa vs. placebo | | | ICU-free days, mechanical ventilation-free days, thromboembolic events, serious adverse reactions | There were no differences in outcomes or adverse events; rFVIIa is safe to use. |
| [12] | 2008 | Ib | Randomized, double-blinded trial | 97 patients randomized to receive either placebo or rFVIIa | | | Death, DVT | There were no differences in outcomes; there was a trend toward increased DVT and smaller hemorrhage with large rFVIIa doses but was not statistically significant. |
| [13] | 2012 | IIb | Retrospective cohort observational study | Retrospective analysis of patient outcomes in patients receiving either PCC or rFVIIa | | | Amount of blood products transfused, cost of hospitalization and overall mortality | Patients receiving PCC required less blood product transfusion, had improved mortality, and less hospital cost than those treated with rFVIIa. |
| [15] | 2012 | Ib | Nested, randomized, controlled trial derived from CRASH-2 study | Nested data from CRASH-2 trial of TBI patients who were randomized to treatment with TXA or placebo | | Death, need for surgical intervention | Intracranial hemorrhage growth from admission to 24–48 h after admission | Patients receiving TXA had less progression of ICH and lower mortality; however, the findings failed to reach statistical significance. |
| [16] | 2013 | Ib | Randomized, double-blinded trial | 238 mild to severe TBI patients randomized to receive TXA or placebo | | Death | Progressive intracranial hemorrhage on CT scan 24 h after initial scan | No statistically significant difference in progression of intracranial hemorrhage or mortality between TXA and placebo groups. |

prophylactic regimens that are individualized based on injury patterns and risks of each patient.

Phelan et al. analyzed 62 patients randomized to enoxaparin ($n$ = 34) or placebo ($n$ = 28) after moderate TBI and a stable CT scan 24 h after admission [19]. Subclinical, radiographic TBI progression rates on the scans performed 48 h after injury and 24 h after the start of treatment were 5.9% for enoxaparin and 3.6% for placebo, a treatment effect difference of 2.3%, which was not significant. No clinical TBI progressions occurred, and one DVT occurred in the placebo arm. The study only randomized a small percentage of the total patients screened, with a large number excluded due to a TBI too severe. Although lacking in power, it does suggest that in patients with moderate TBI, initiation of enoxaparin 24 h after TBI with a stable repeat CT is safe.

In a prospective, nonrandomized study, Norwood et al. analyzed the use and safety of LMWH (enoxaparin) in patients with intracranial hemorrhage injuries (IHI) following blunt trauma [20]. The medication was started 24 h after injury or craniotomy except in patients with concomitant splenic injury being conservatively managed. Head CT scans were carried out on admission, 24 h after admission, and at various times during hospitalization. Although only 4% of patients managed nonoperatively had expansion of their hematoma while on enoxaparin, 9.1% of patients receiving surgical intervention suffered post-operative bleeding. This bleeding rate caused the study authors to change their protocol, so the drug was started later (24 h after surgical intervention). Venous color flow duplex studies were performed within 24 h of hospital discharge on 101 of the 150 patients that found a 2% DVT incidence in enoxaparin-treated patients (which they compare to historic controls), and no patient in the study group was documented to have suffered a PE.

In a follow-up study in 2008, Norwood et al. prospectively followed 525 patients with TBI who received enoxaparin within 48 h of admission [21]. Only 26% of eligible patients were enrolled in the study, with many being excluded for concomitant injuries or the surgeon's reluctance to initiate venous thromboembolism (VTE) prophylaxis. After starting enoxaparin, 18 (3.4%) patients had progression of their hemorrhage by serial CT. Six of these patients (1.1%) required craniotomy.

Salottolo et al. retrospectively analyzed 255 patients receiving enoxaparin or heparin for DVT prophylaxis after TBI with stable repeat head CT [22]. Therapy was initiated early (<72 h) in 108 patients and late (≥72 h) in 147 patients. Rates of hemorrhage progression or DVT did not differ significantly in patients who received VTE prophylaxis early or late. There were significant differences in the demographics of the two groups, and given the small sample size, it is difficult to draw conclusions from this study.

A retrospective evaluation of unfractionated heparin (UFH) use for DVT prophylaxis in patients sustaining severe closed head injuries (Abbreviated Injury Scale score of >3) was carried out by Kim et al [23]. They compared 47 patients who received UFH early after injury (<72 h) versus 17 patients treated late after injury (>72 h). They did not exclude patients with splenic and hepatic lacerations managed conservatively. They demonstrated no increase in the risk of increased intracranial bleeding in either group by CT and/or change in physical exam, but also no difference in the rate of DVT, PE, or death between the two groups. No conclusions as to the efficacy of UFH as a prophylactic agent for DVT can be drawn from this study, but it does suggest that prophylactic doses of heparin can be safely administered early to patients with TBI.

Dudley et al. retrospectively analyzed 287 patients with moderate to severe (GCS 3–12) TBI treated with dalteparin or enoxaparin initiated at 48–72 h post-injury after a minimum of two stable head CT scans [24]. They reported only one patient with a symptomatic expansion of ICH and no difference in DVT rates between groups.

In a retrospective cohort study, Koehler et al. reviewed 669 patients with TBI who received enoxaparin after TBI [25]. Two hundred and sixty-eight patients received prophylaxis early (<72 h), and 401 patients received prophylaxis late (>72 h). Following prophylaxis, no patients required craniotomy, and there was no difference in the rate of hemorrhage progression between the early and late groups. No deaths were attributable to DVT prophylaxis, but one patient in the late group died of PE (Table 11.3).

*Recommendation*: Early initiation (72 h after injury) of heparin or LMWH in patients with moderate TBI and without clinical or radiologic decline is supported by Levels II and III data (Grade B recommendation).

## 11.4 Is Standard Use of Anti-Epileptic Drugs for Seizure Prophylaxis Beneficial in Patients with TBI?

Post-traumatic seizure activity occurs both early and late after injury. Brain seizure activity is known to dramatically increase cerebral metabolic requirements, glucose metabolism [26], and intracranial pressure (ICP) [27].

If untreated, the overall risk of seizure activity following TBI in patients with no previous history of epilepsy is 2%–5%; however, this varies widely depending on the age, wounding mechanism, and severity of TBI [28]. The presence of early seizures (<7 days) after TBI has not been substantiated to correlate with an increased mortality in

**TABLE 11.3**
Table of Evidence: DVT Prophylaxis

| Trial (Ref. No.) | Year | Level of Evidence | Randomized Groups (*n*) | Intervention/ Design | Median Follow-Up | Minor End Point | Major End Point | Interpretations/ Comments |
|---|---|---|---|---|---|---|---|---|
| [19] | 2002 | IIb | Prospective, nonrandomized, observational study | LMWH given 24 h after admission or 24 h after surgery to patients with TBI | Variable—until hospital discharge or death | | Expansion of IHI or prevention of DVT/PE | Study group was small and nonrandomized. Variable study protocol changed during study due to bleeding complication. There was a trend toward safety of LMWH in TBI patients with CT scan follow-up. |
| [20] | 2012 | Ib | Randomized, double-blinded trial | 62 TBI patients randomized to LMWH or placebo 24 h after admission | | VTE occurrence, extracranial hemorrhagic complications | Radiologic worsening of TBI | TBI progression rates 24 h after injury in patients receiving LMWH were similar to placebo group; only small subset of patients were randomized, but the study suggests that VTE prophylaxis is safe to use in TBI patients. |
| [21] | 2008 | IIb | Prospective, nonrandomized, observational study | 525 patients received enoxaparin 48 h after sustaining TBI | Variable—until hospital discharge or death | | Intracranial bleeding complications, discharge GCS, death | Use of enoxaparin 48 h after sustaining TBI was deemed safe in the setting of stable head CT. |
| [22] | 2011 | IIb | Retrospective, observational study | 255 patients with TBI and stable head CTs were analyzed for use of chemical VTE prophylaxis before or after 72 h | | | VTE occurrence | There were no differences in outcomes between groups receiving chemical VTE prophylaxis before or after 72 h from injury; however, given the small sample size and variable demographics, it is difficult to derive a conclusion from this study. |
| [23] | 2002 | IIb | Retrospective, observational study | 64 patients with TBI and Abbreviated Injury Scale score of >3 divided into early (<72 h) vs. late (>72 h) administration of UFH | 12 months or until discharge or death | | | There was no significant difference between two groups of DVT prevention (4% early vs. 6% late) with no major increases in intracranial bleeding. Groups are too small to draw major conclusions. |

*(Continued)*

**TABLE 11.3 (*Continued*)**

Table of Evidence: DVT Prophylaxis

| Trial (Ref. No.) | Year | Level of Evidence | Randomized Groups (*n*) | Intervention/ Design | Median Follow-Up | Minor End Point | Major End Point | Interpretations/ Comments |
|---|---|---|---|---|---|---|---|---|
| [24] | 2010 | IIb | Retrospective, observational study | 287 TBI patients treated with enoxaparin or dalteparin prophylaxis 48–72 h after injury | | | Symptomatic expansion of ICH, occurrence of VTE | There was no difference between expansion of ICH or VTE occurrence in patients receiving either drug. |
| [25] | 2011 | IIb | Retrospective cohort study | 669 TBI patients received chemical VTE prophylaxis either before or after 72 h from injury | | | Progression of ICH, occurrence of VTE/PE | There was no difference in progression of ICH between early and late administration of chemical VTE prophylaxis; there were no deaths attributed to VTE prophylaxis; however, one patient died of PE in the late group. |

trauma patients but is predictive of the development of late seizure activity [29]. As such, patients who suffer post-TBI seizures have been shown to have significantly worse long-term functional outcomes as compared to patients who do not suffer seizure activity [30]. Therefore, pharmacologic suppression of post-TBI seizure activity is part of an overall brain protective strategy.

In a systematic review of Class I and Class II data, phenytoin was effective when used as prophylaxis against early post-TBI seizures given for 7 days following TBI [31]. Phenytoin demonstrated a significant benefit (3.4% early seizure rate vs. 13.3% in placebo group) in suppressing post-TBI seizures in patients with severe brain injuries. They further evaluated adverse events and drug complications and found that there were few serious side effects from anti-epileptic drug usage. From these data, the authors make practice recommendations for adult patients with severe TBI (defined as prolonged loss of consciousness, amnesia, intracranial hematoma or brain contusion on CT scan, and/or depressed skull fracture). These include prophylactic treatment with phenytoin, beginning with an intravenous loading dose as soon as possible after injury to decrease the risk of early (<7 days) post-TBI seizures.

The same study reviewed the use of anti-epileptic drugs in late (>7 days) post-TBI seizures. From their review, they concluded that data do not support the use of phenytoin for more than 7 days, as there was no difference in late post-TBI seizures in the anti-epileptic drug-treated group (10.0%) vs. placebo group (8.4%). From these data, the authors make additional practice guideline recommendations that prophylactic treatment with phenytoin, carbamazepine, or valproate should not routinely be used beyond the first 7 days after injury in an attempt to decrease the risk of post-TBI seizures.

Szaflarski et al. randomized 46 TBI and 6 stroke patients to receive either phenytoin or levetiracetam after severe TBI [32]. Patients were monitored in the ICU with electroencephalogram for 72 h and clinically thereafter. There was no difference in early seizures (levetiracetam 5/34 vs. phenytoin 3/18) or at 6 months (levetiracetam 1/20 vs. phenytoin 0/14). Surprisingly, patients in the levetiracetam group experienced significantly better 6-month outcomes than patients in the phenytoin arm by Glasgow Outcomes Scale-Extended and Disability Rating Scale.

Inaba et al. prospectively studied 813 consecutive blunt TBI patients admitted to two Level I trauma centers (mean admission GCS 12) [33]. Patients received either levetiracetam (407) or phenytoin (406). Although not randomized, the groups were similar in demographics. There were six seizures in each group (1.5%). This suggests that both drugs are effective in preventing seizures in the first 7 days after injury (Table 11.4).

*Recommendation*: There is a significantly lower risk of early (<7 days) post-injury seizures in patients with severe head injuries who are treated with either levetiracetam or phenytoin. There are insufficient data to recommend one drug over the other (Level II recommendations).

**TABLE 11.4**

Table of Evidence: Seizure Prophylaxis

| Trial (Ref. No.) | Year | Level of Evidence | Randomized Groups (*n*) | Intervention/ Design | Median Follow-Up | Minor End Point | Major End Point | Interpretations/ Comments |
|---|---|---|---|---|---|---|---|---|
| [31] | 2007 | Ia | Systematic review of the existing literature | Review of data Levels I–IV from the decade of 1996–2006 | | | | Summary of pooled data suggests benefits to anti-epileptic drugs in early (<7 days) post-injury seizure prophylaxis. |
| [32] | 2010 | Ib | Randomized, controlled, single-blinded trial | 52 patients randomized to receive either phenytoin or levetiracetam | 6 months | | Seizure occurrence, death | There were no differences between the two groups in preventing early seizures; the levetiracetam group had better functional outcomes on long-term follow-up. |
| [33] | 2013 | IIb | Prospective, observational study | 813 patients with TBI received either phenytoin or levetiracetam | | | Seizure occurrence with 7 days | Seizure occurrence was the same for both groups, suggesting that both medications are efficacious in preventing early post-TBI seizure. |

## 11.5 Do ICP Monitoring and Therapy Directed at Lowering ICP Improve Outcome?

In the management of patients with TBI, ICP monitoring has been one of the most important measures for goal-directed therapy. It is widely accepted that ICH (ICP >20 mmHg) is strongly associated with TBI-related mortality [34]. Thus, guidelines have been developed in an effort to minimize TBI-related mortality due to ICH. The Brain Trauma Foundation (BTF) 2007 guidelines recommend that all patients with head trauma, a GCS of 3–8, and abnormal CT imaging should have some form of ICP monitoring. It also recommends ICP monitoring in patients with severe TBI and a normal CT scan if two of the following conditions are met: the patient is more than 40 years old, the presence of posturing, or systolic blood pressure <90 mmHg. It also recommends that treatment for ICH should be initiated when ICP reaches the threshold of greater than 20 mmHg [35]. However, these guidelines are not based on any randomized, controlled data and are derived solely from Class II and Class III evidence. As the most recent guidelines were released, several studies have been published that question the efficacy of ICP-directed therapy in patients with TBI. These studies argue that improved outcomes associated with ICP monitoring may actually be coincidental to other improvements in TBI care.

A randomized controlled trial involving ICP monitoring was published by Chestnut et al [36]. The trial included 324 patients with severe TBI being treated in two different facilities that were randomized to a treatment protocol utilizing intra-parenchymal ICP monitoring to guide therapy or treatment based on imaging and clinical examination. The primary outcome of the study was based on a composite of survival time, functional status at 3 and 6 months, and neuropsychological status at 6 months. There were no significant differences between the two groups with regards to the primary outcome composite score, 6-month mortality, length of ICU stay, or adverse events. The imaging and clinical exam group did have a significantly greater time interval over which brain-specific therapy was provided (mannitol, hypertonic saline, etc.).

In a retrospective review of data from a prospective database, Farahvar et al. examined 223 patients managed without ICP monitors and 1084 patients managed with ICP monitors during the first 48 h after admission with TBI [37]. They demonstrated that patients in the ICP monitoring group had a significant decrease in mortality at 2 weeks, citing mortality of 19.6% in the monitored group versus 33.2% in the nonmonitored population. This is difficult to interpret, however, as the non-ICP monitor group had significantly higher proportions of patients over the age of 60 years and with pupillary changes compared to the ICP monitoring group.

Cremer et al. produced a retrospective cohort study comparing outcomes of TBI patients from two different trauma centers [38]. One of the centers did not use ICP monitoring and relied on treating patients by maintaining mean arterial pressures of 90 mmHg and providing therapeutic interventions based on clinical observations and CT imaging (122 patients). The other center used ICP monitoring with goals of therapy directed at maintaining an ICP <20 mmHg and cerebral perfusion pressure (CPP) >70 mmHg (142 patients). Outcomes for the two populations were similar for in-hospital mortality (34% without ICP monitoring vs. 33% with ICP monitoring) and functional outcomes. However, the ICP-directed group had prolonged mechanical ventilation time, as well as increased use of sedatives, vasopressors, mannitol, and barbiturates.

Shafi et al. also produced a retrospective review of 1646 patients with severe TBI from the National Trauma Data Bank comparing outcomes in patients with and without ICP monitoring [39]. This study found that only 43% of studied patients that met BTF criteria underwent placement of an ICP monitor and that among those patients there was a 45% reduction in survival when compared to the non-ICP monitored group (Tables 11.5 and 11.6).

*Recommendation*: Despite expert guidelines, there are insufficient data to support the use of ICP monitoring in TBI (Level B recommendations).

**TABLE 11.5**

Table of Evidence: ICP Monitoring

| Trial (Ref. No.) | Year | Level of Evidence | Randomized Groups (*n*) | Intervention/ Design | Median Follow-Up | Minor End Point | Major End Point | Interpretations/ Comments |
|---|---|---|---|---|---|---|---|---|
| [36] | 2012 | Ib | Randomized, double-blinded trial | TBI patients treated with or without ICP monitoring | 6 months | | Survival time, impaired consciousness, functional status at 3 and 6 months, neuropsychologic status at 6 months | Management of TBI using ICP monitoring to keep ICP <20 mmHg does not improve outcomes compared to treating patients based on imaging/ symptoms. |
| [37] | 2012 | IIb | Retrospective cohort of data from prospectively maintained database | Outcomes comparison of patients with TBI who underwent ICP monitoring vs. without ICP monitoring | | | Mortality at 2 weeks from injury | Patients undergoing ICP monitoring had lower mortality rates at 2 weeks than nonmonitored patients. |
| [38] | 2005 | IIb | Retrospective cohort study with prospective outcome assessment | Outcomes comparison of patients with TBI who underwent ICP monitoring vs. without ICP monitoring | | | Mortality, GCS at 12 months | For patients surviving for more than 24 h after injury, ICP monitoring provided no benefit to survival or functional outcomes. |
| [39] | 2008 | IIb | Retrospective cohort study, nonrandomized data | Outcomes comparison of patients with TBI who underwent ICP monitoring vs. without ICP monitoring | | | Survival to discharge | Patients who were treated with ICP monitoring per BTF guidelines were associated with worse survival outcomes when controlling for injury/TBI severity, comorbidities, and need for craniotomy. |

**TABLE 11.6**

Summary of Recommendations

| Question | Answer | Levels of Evidence | Grade of Recommendation | References |
|---|---|---|---|---|
| Does repeat head CT determine the need for intervention? | Only patients with ICH and deteriorating exam or moderate/severe injury (GCS ≤12) require repeat CT. | IIb | B | [4–8] |
| Do procoagulants decrease intracranial hemorrhage related to TBI? | PCC may be useful in conjunction with FFP in decreasing hemorrhage in coagulopathic TBI patients. TXA and factor VII have not been proven useful in this setting. | Ib–IIb | B | [9–16] |
| When and how should DVT prophylaxis be initiated? | Heparin and LMWH are safe after 72 h post-injury or surgery in the absence of clinical or radiologic progression. | Ia–IIb | B | [17–24] |
| Is seizure prophylaxis beneficial? | Yes, up to 7 days after TBI. It is not beneficial after 7 days. | Ia–IIb | B | [30–32] |
| Does the use of ICP monitoring improve outcomes? | No, there are insufficient data to suggest that ICP monitoring improves outcomes. | Ia–IIb | B | [35–38] |

## References


1. CDC. Traumatic brain inury in the United States: Fact sheet. http://www.cdc.gov/traumaticbraininjury/get_the_facts.html (accessed December 15, 2014).
2. Sarrafzadeh AS, Peltonen EE, Kaisers U et al. Secondary insults in severe head injury: Do multiply injured patients do worse? *Crit Care Med.* 2001;29:1116–1123.
3. Carlson A, Schermer C, Lu S. Retrospective evaluation of anemia and transfusion in traumatic brain injury. *J Trauma.* 2006;61: 567–571.
4. Sifri ZC, Homnick AT, Vaynman A, Lavery R, Liao W, Mohr A, Hauser CJ, Manniker A, Livingston D. A prospective evaluation of the value of repeat cranial computed tomography in patients with minimal head injury and an intracranial bleed. *J Trauma.* October 2006;61(4):862–867.
5. Brown CV, Weng J, Oh D, Salim A, Kasotakis G, Demetriades D, Velmahos GC, Rhee P. Does routine serial computed tomography of the head influence management of traumatic brain injury? A prospective evaluation. *J Trauma.* November 2004;57(5):939–943.
6. Brown CV, Zada G, Salim A, Inaba K, Kasotakis G, Hadjizacharia P, Demetriades D, Rhee P. Indications for routine repeat head computed tomography (CT) stratified by severity of traumatic brain injury. *J Trauma.* June 2007;62(6):1339–1344.
7. AbdelFattah KR, Eastman AL, Aldy KN. A prospective evaluation of the use of routine repeat cranial CT scans in patients with intracranial hemorrhage and GCS score of 13 to 15. *J Trauma Acute Care Surg.* September 2012;73(3):685–688.
8. Joseph B, Aziz H, Pandit V. A three-year prospective study of repeat head computed tomography in patients with traumatic brain injury. *J Am Coll Surg.* July 2014;219(1):45–51.
9. Yanamadala V, Walcott B, Fecci P et al. Reversal of warfarin associated coagulopathy with 4-factor prothrombin complex concentrate in traumatic brain injury and intracranial hemorrhage. *J Clin Neurosci.* 2014;21:1881–1884.
10. Perel P, Roberts I, Shakur H, Thinkhamrop B, Phuenpathom N, Yutthakasemsunt S. Haemostatic drugs for traumatic brain injury. *Cochrane Database Syst Rev.* 2010;(1):CD007877.
11. Kluger Y, Riou B, Rossaint R. Safety of rFVIIa in hemodynamically unstable polytrauma patients with traumatic brain injury: Post hoc analysis of 30 patients from a prospective, randomized, placebo-controlled, double-blind clinical trial. *Crit Care.* 2007;11(4):R85.
12. Narayan RK, Maas AI, Marshall LF. Recombinant factor VIIA in traumatic intracerebral hemorrhage: Results of a dose-escalation clinical trial. *Neurosurgery.* April 2008;62(4):776–786.
13. Joseph B, Pantelis H, Aziz H. Prothrombin complex concentrate: An effective therapy in reversing the coagulopathy of traumatic brain injury. *J Trauma Acute Care Surg.* 2012;74(1):248–253.
14. Roberts I, Shakur H, Coats T et al. The CRASH-2 trial: A randomized controlled trial and economic evaluation of tranexamic acid on death, vascular occlusive events and transfusion requirement in bleeding trauma patients. *Health Tech Assess.* 2013;17(10):1–79.
15. Perel P, Al-Shahi Salman R, Morris Z. CRASH-2 (Clinical Randomization of An Antifibrinolytic in Significant Hemorrhage) intracranial bleeding study: The effect of transexamic acid in traumatic brain injury—A nested randomized, placebo controlled trial. *Health Tech Assess.* 2012;17(10):1–11.
16. Yutthakasemsunt S, Kittiwatanagul W, Piyavechvirat P et al. Transexamic acid for patients with traumatic brain injury: A randomized, double-blinded, placebo controlled trial. *BMC Emerg Med.* 2013;22(13):20.

17. Rogers FB, Cipolle MD, Velmahos G, Rozychi G, Luchette FA. Practice management guidelines for the prevention of venous thromboembolism in trauma patients: The EAST practice management guidelines work group. *J Trauma*. 2002;53:142–164.
18. Hammond F, Meighben M. Venous thromboembolism in the patient with acute traumatic brain injury: Screening, diagnosis, prophylaxis and treatment issues. *J Head Trauma Rehabil*. 1998;13(1):36–50.
19. Phelan HA, Wolf SE, Norwood SH, Aldy K. A randomized, double-blinded, placebo-controlled pilot trial of anticoagulation in low-risk traumatic brain injury: The Delayed Versus Early Enoxaparin Prophylaxis I (DEEP I) study. *J Trauma Acute Care Surg*. December 2012;73(6):1434–1441.
20. Norwood SH, McAuley CE, Berne JD, Vallina VL, Kerns BD, Graham TW, Short K, McLarty JW. Prospective evaluation of the safety of enoxaparin prophylaxis for venous thromboembolism in patients with intracranial hemorrhagic injuries. *Arch Surg*. 2002;137:696–702.
21. Norwood SH, Berne JD, Rowe SA. Early venous thromboembolism prophylaxis with enoxaparin in patients with blunt traumatic brain injury. *J Trauma*. November 2008;65(5):1021–1026.
22. Salottolo K, Offner P, Levy AS. Interrupted pharmocologic thromboprophylaxis increases venous thromboembolism in traumatic brain injury. *J Trauma*. January 2011;70(1):19–24.
23. Kim J, Gearhart MM, Zurick A, Zuccarello M, James L, Luchette FA. Preliminary report on the safety of heparin for deep venous thrombosis after severe head injury. *J Trauma*. 2002;53:38–43.
24. Dudley RR, Aziz I, Bonnici A. Early venous thromboembolic event prophylaxis in traumatic brain injury with low-molecular-weight heparin: Risks and benefits. *J Neurotrauma*. December 2010;27(12):2165–2172.
25. Koehler DM, Shipman J, Davidson MA. Is early venous thromboembolism prophylaxis safe in trauma patients with intracranial hemorrhage. *J Trauma*. February 2011;70(2):324–329.
26. Darbina O, Rissob JJ, Carreb E. Metabolic changes in rat striatum following convulsive seizures. *Brain Res*. 2005;1050:124–129.
27. Shah AK, Fuerst D, Sood S. Seizures lead to elevation of intracranial pressure in children undergoing invasive EEG monitoring. *Epilepsia*. June 2007;48(6):1097–1103.
28. Wang HC, Chang WN, Chang HW. Factors predictive of outcome in posttraumatic seizures. *J Trauma*. 2008;64(4):883–888.
29. Jeremitsky E, Omert L, Dunham CM. Harbingers of poor outcome the day after severe brain injury: Hypothermia, hypoxia, and hypoperfusion. *J Trauma*. 2003;54:312–319.
30. Asikainen I, Kaste M, Sarna S. Early and late posttraumatic seizures in traumatic brain injury rehabilitation patients: Brain injury factors causing late seizures and influence of seizures on long-term outcome. *Epilepsia*. 1999:40(5)584–589.
31. Bratton SL, Chestnut RM, Ghajar J et al. Antiseizure prophylaxis. *J Neurotrauma*. 2007;24(S1):S83–S86.
32. Szaflarski JP, Sangha KS, Lindsell CJ. Prospective, randomized, single-blinded comparative trial of intravenous levetiracetam versus phenytoin for seizure prophylaxis. *Neurocrit Care*. April 2010;12(2):165–172.
33. Inaba K, Menaker J, Branco BC. A prospective multicenter comparison of levetiracetam versus phenytoin for early posttraumatic seizure prophylaxis. *J Trauma Acute Care Surg*. March 2013;74(3):766–771.
34. Marmarou A, Anderson R, Ward J et al. Impact of ICP instability and hypotension on outcome in patients with severe head trauma. *J Neurosurg*. 1991;75:S59–S66.
35. Brain Trauma Foundation; American Association of Neurological Surgeons; Congress of Neurological Surgeons. Guidelines for the management of severe traumatic brain injury. *J Neurotrauma*. 2007;24(Suppl 1):S1–S106.
36. Chestnut R, Temkin N, Carney N et al. A trial of intracranial-pressure monitoring in traumatic brain injury. *N Engl J Med*. December 2012;367(26):2471–2481.
37. Farahvar A, Gerber L, Chiu Y et al. Increased mortality in patients with severe traumatic brain injury treated without intracranial pressure monitoring. *J Neurosurg*. October 2012;117(4):729–734.
38. Cremer L, van Dijk G, Wensen E et al. Effect of intracranial pressure monitoring and targeted intensive care on functional outcome after severe head injury. *Crit Care Med*. 2005;33(10):2207–2213.
39. Shafi S, Diaz-Arrastia R, Madden C et al. Intracranial pressure monitoring in brain-injured patients is associated with worsening of survival. *J Trauma*. 2008;64:335–340.

## Commentary on Traumatic Brain Injury

*Eileen M. Bulger*

Management of patients with traumatic brain injury remains an ongoing challenge, and research in this area has been hampered by a number of retrospective and observational studies, which frequently suffer from significant selection bias. Randomized controlled trials are particularly challenging in this patient population as it is difficult to obtain informed consent for early interventions, and the heterogeneity of the population likely impacts the ability to see an effect. Randomized controlled trials focusing on specific therapeutic interventions have largely failed to demonstrate benefit, including studies of early hypertonic resuscitation, hypothermia, magnesium administration, steroid use, progesterone therapy, and so on. This has resulted in a lack of Level 1 evidence to guide the treatment of TBI. Treatment of patients with severe TBI has thus largely relied upon guidelines from the Brain Trauma Foundation, which are based on expert consensus with a moderate to low level of supporting evidence. A recent clinical trial discussed in this review has called into question the role of ICP monitoring, which is a fundamental principle of these guidelines. This trial, known as the BEST TRIP trial*, randomized patients with severe TBI (GCS ≤ 8) to two different, but aggressive, management protocols for intracranial hypertension. One arm relied on a traditional ICP-monitored treatment algorithm and the other arm utilized serial neurologic monitoring and imaging to guide therapy. Patients in the non-ICP-monitored arm actually received more interventions for suspected intracranial hypertension and there was no difference between the groups in functional outcome or mortality. This study is frequently misinterpreted as a call to abandon ICP monitoring as I will address in the following when I discuss each clinical question covered in this review.

### Does Repeat Head Computed Tomography (CT) after Traumatic Brain Injury Determine the Need for Clinical Intervention?

The authors have summarized the literature in this area well and I agree with their assessment that current evidence supports repeat CT imaging for any patient with neurologic deterioration and those with severe TBI (GCS ≤ 8). This is particularly important if one is using a non-ICP-monitored strategy as serial imaging was a key component of patient monitoring for the patients in the BEST TRIP trial who did not have an ICP monitor.

Another patient subgroup that is an increasing challenge are those patients who are injured while taking oral anticoagulants or antiplatelet agents for their medical comorbidities. This population has grown with the increase in elderly trauma and even a ground level fall may result in a significant injury. These patients appear to benefit from rapid correction of coagulopathy, when possible, but many of the newer oral anticoagulants do not have a specific reversal agent. While data is sparse, I would recommend given the high risk of progression of intracranial hemorrhage in these patients that this group also be considered for repeat imaging and close neurologic monitoring.

### Do Procoagulants Decrease Intracranial Hemorrhage Related to Traumatic Brain Injury?

The challenge in interpreting this literature is to distinguish between those studies that are assessing reversal of anticoagulant agents which the patient was taking preinjury versus those studies assessing the impact of procoagulant agents on a broader population of TBI patients. I agree with the authors' interpretation that for patients taking warfarin the evidence supports rapid reversal and PCC appears to be a good agent for this. As noted, we are in desperate need for reversal agents for some of the newer oral thrombin inhibitors.

The studies evaluating tranexamic acid have included a broader population of TBI patients and while they were able to demonstrate a decrease in the progression of intracranial hemorrhage for patients receiving TXA, they are clearly underpowered to demonstrate a difference in mortality or long-term neurologic function. There is a randomized controlled trial of early TXA administration that will begin enrolling patients this year with moderate to severe TBI based on prehospital GCS score (clinicaltrials.gov: NCT01990768). This study will add additional information to inform the potential role of TXA for early treatment of TBI patients.

### When Should Deep Vein Thrombosis Prophylaxis Be Initiated in TBI?

I agree with the author's assessment in that literature. This has been an area of contention between intensivists and neurosurgeons for many years. These data encourage the institutional development of protocols to standardize the timing of initiation of DVT prophylaxis for these patients.

* Chesnut RM, Temkin N, Carney N et al. A trial of intracranial-pressure monitoring in traumatic brain injury. *N Engl J Med.* 2012;367(26):2471–2481.

### Is Standard Use of Antiepileptic Drugs for Seizure Prophylaxis Beneficial in Patients with TBI?

Appropriate assessment and recommendation.

### Do Intracranial Pressure Monitoring and Therapy Directed at Lowering Intracranial Pressure Improve Outcome?

This is the most controversial of all the questions and while I agree with the fundamental conclusion that we have insufficient evidence to definitively guide therapy, I think it is important that we not abandon ICP monitoring all together. The BEST TRIP trial did not test ICP monitoring versus no monitoring. In fact, the "control" arm followed a very aggressive protocol of patient monitoring and intervention for suspected intracranial hypertension and actually received more interventions than the ICP arm. In several editorials written after publication of the BEST TRIP trial, the lead author, Dr. Chesnut, advocates continued use of ICP monitoring but suggests we should revisit our ICP thresholds for intervention and tailor our therapy based on individual patient's pathophysiology using a multimodal monitoring strategy[*†‡]. A recent systematic review of the literature on this topic using the GRADE methodology makes strong recommendations not to abandon the use of ICP monitors and ICP management pathways[§]. Clearly, we have a lot more to learn to optimize TBI management, but this is a circumstance where we should not misinterpret this single RCT as justification to abandon this treatment approach.

---

* Chesnut RM. A conceptual approach to managing severe traumatic brain injury in a time of uncertainty. *Ann N Y Acad Sci*. 2015 May;1345:99–107.

† Chesnut RM. Intracranial pressure monitoring: Headstone or a new head start. The BEST TRIP trial in perspective. *Intensive Care Med*. 2013;39(4):771–774.

‡ Chesnut RM. What is wrong with the tenets underpinning current management of severe traumatic brain injury? *Ann N Y Acad Sci*. 2015 May;1345:74–82.

§ Chesnut R, Videtta W, Vespa P, Le Roux P, The Participants in the International Multidisciplinary Consensus Conference on Multimodality Monitoring. Intracranial pressure monitoring: Fundamental considerations and rationale for monitoring. *Neurocrit Care*. 2014 December;21(Suppl. 2):S64–S84.

# 12

# *Spine and Spinal Cord Injuries*

**Yoram Klein and Peleg Ben-Galim**

**CONTENTS**



## 12.1 Introduction

Spine injuries are common in the modern urban trauma setting. Although rare, spinal cord injury (SCI) (1.3% of all trauma patients) carries an extremely high rate of morbidity and mortality. There are approximately 11,000 new traumatic SCIs annually in the United States with billions of dollars in treatment costs for the estimated 240,000 existing SCI patient population [1]. Although surgical techniques have dramatically improved and the ability to achieve reduction and maintain spinal alignment and stability enable earlier rehabilitation of the patients, the neurological recovery and the 10-year survival of this population have not changed significantly over the years.

The etiologies of SCI are as follows:

1. High-energy motor vehicle collisions (MVCs); most are thoracic and lumbar
2. Fall injuries; most are in the thoracolumbar zone
3. Sports injuries from diving or other head collisions; most are cervical
4. Violence/penetrating trauma
5. Other miscellaneous causes

Three other statistical points are worth mentioning:

1. Male to female ratio for these injuries is 4:1, without any racial predisposition.
2. In sports accidents related SCI, 92% resulted in quadriplegia as compared with 54% in MVC-related SCI.
3. The 10-year survival rate of SCI patients older than 30 years is about 50%.

## 12.2 Pathophysiology

Most SCIs are the result of contusion or traction forces rather than cord transection. Most of the damage to neural tissue is related to the primary injury, although some additional injury can be attributed to continuous cord compression or traction; therefore, early surgical decompression may be advocated and beneficial in selected cases. Secondary tissue damage (the "second hit") is thought to occur at a later stage because of continuous cord compression, which causes ischemia and hypoxia of the cord with an inflammatory tissue response.

## 12.3 Neurological Assessment

An initial neurological examination of the SCI patient is essential for the evaluation of the functional level and the prognosis. The examination should include sensory, motor, and proprioception evaluation together with perianal sensation, rectal sphincter tone, and bulbocavernous reflex. A simple and acceptable functional classification of SCI is the Frankel classification, as follows [2]:

1. Complete absence of motor and sensory function
2. Sensation present but no motor function
3. Sensation + motor function 2–3/5
4. Sensation present with motor function of 4/5
5. Normal sensory and motor function

Spinal cord syndromes classification:

1. Complete SCI: There is no motor or sensory function caudal to the level of injury and the bulbocavernous reflex is present.
2. Incomplete spinal cord injuries (ICSCIs): There are some motor or sensory functions below the level of injury. There are a few types of ICSCIs, as follows:
   a. Central cord syndrome is the most common ICSCI and is characterized by quadriparesis, in which the arms are weaker than the legs. About 75% of the patients will have partial recovery of the motor function.
   b. Brown-Sequard syndrome is a rare unilateral SCI (usually due to penetration injuries) characterized by motor deficit ipsilateral to the injury combined with contralateral sensory deficit. Most of these patients gain partial recovery with bowel and bladder continence and usually walking ability.
   c. Anterior cord syndrome is a relatively uncommon ICSCI characterized by complete motor and sensory loss with some remnant of trunk and lower extremity deep sensation and proprioception. The prognosis of this syndrome is poor and only 10% of them show some motor recovery.
   d. Posterior cord syndrome is a rare ICSCI and is characterized by loss of proprioception and deep sensation but intact motor functioning.
3. Spinal shock: Defined as a complete SCI with absent bulbocavernous reflex. It should not be confused with neurogenic shock, which is a hemodynamic condition characterized by hypotension and bradycardia. Only after the reappearance of the bulbocavernous reflex we can definitely classify the neurological status of the patient to one of the incomplete or complete SCI syndromes.

## 12.4 Initial Management

As with every other major trauma patient, the most urgent goal is to maintain and optimize oxygen delivery (airway, breathing, and circulation) followed by a quick neurological evaluation in order to promptly detect signs of severe brain injury.

### 12.4.1 Airway Management

Head injury with depressed level of consciousness is the most common indication for definitive airway control in trauma patients. Unfortunately, cervical spine injury (CSI) is more common among these patients. The overall incidence of CSI is found to be around 2% among blunt trauma patients, while in patients with a Glasgow coma score (GCS) of less than 8, the incidence SCI is rising to more than 10% [3]. Upper cervical spine ligamentous injuries with or without vertebral fractures are among the most common injuries in acceleration–deceleration MVA injuries and represent unstable injuries that mandate head–neck immobilization with airway control [4,5]. Although extremely rare, worsening of cervical spinal cord damage due to airway control maneuver is a dreaded complication [6].

#### *12.4.1.1 What Is the Impact of Airway Maneuvers on Cervical Spine Movement?*

Numerous studies have tried to define the spinal movement during airway management in patients with intact and injured cervical spine. Nevertheless, the evidence is limited owing to the heterogeneity of the measurement techniques and the controversy about the clinical importance of the biomechanical findings. Both basic and advanced airway maneuver were found to cause movement in different segments of the cervical spine. Even presumably safe maneuvers, such as chin lift and jaw thrust, were found to cause movements that theoretically might jeopardize the cord. Advanced airway interventions, such as blind nasotracheal intubation and direct laryngoscopy and orotracheal intubation (DLOI), were also found to cause relative segmental cervical spine movement (to a lesser extent than the preintubation maneuver) in patients with normal and injured cervical spine. The most accentuated movements were found to be at the atlanto-occipital and atlanto-axial joints, but other portions of the cervical spine were affected as well [7,8]. Occipito-cervical injuries warrant special attention, as these injuries are common and accentuated pathological motion at the atlanto-occipital and atlanto-axial joints has been documented during airway control, intubation, and cervical collar application. No significant difference in movement was found between curved or straight laryngoscope blades [9]. Although the measured movements can be considered within the physiological margins in the intact cervical spine, the injured spine might still be compromised by these maneuvers. This is the reason for the application of spine neck immobilization during airway intervention. The most common immobilization technique is the manual in-line stabilization that was found to be most effective in limiting segmental movement to 1–3 mm in various airway maneuvers [10,11]. Noteworthy is the tendency of paramedic teams to exert traction forces to the head in order to achieve in-line stabilization [12]. This is to be avoided and the head is to be held "in situ" and in-line with the longitudinal axis of the spine without exerting pulling or pushing forces. In particular, traction forces are to be avoided during in-line stabilization and airway management, especially with upper cervical spine injuries and the so-called "internal decapitation"-type injuries where "in situ" (no traction) in-line stabilization may be lifesaving [13]. Cervical collar application has also been shown to limit the ability to control airway and in itself exerts traction forces upon the neck and may cause abnormal pathological motion in the unstable injured cervical segment [14].

*Summary and recommendations*: There are no Level I clinical data. Cadaver experiments and the accumulated experimental data suggest that airway management in the trauma patient with suspected CSI might inflict relative spinal segmental movement. Manual in-line stabilization of the neck emphasizing in situ holding of the head over the shoulders without pulling during the airway intervention can safely be applied and significantly limit the allegedly dangerous spine motion.

*Grade of recommendation*: B

#### *12.4.1.2 What Is the Preferred Way to Achieve Tracheal Intubation in Patients with Suspected CSI?*

There are several options for achieving definitive airway control in a trauma patient with suspected CSI. Traditionally, DLOI was considered unsafe for patients with unstable CSI, and so blind nasotracheal intubation and surgical cricothyroidotomy were recommended as better options in that scenario. In the past decade, many series demonstrated the safety of DLOI. Although all series were retrospective, one fact aroused from them very clearly: Neurologic deterioration after orotracheal intubation is an extremely rare event even in patients with unstable CSI. In a review article from 2006, Crosby summarized the results of 12 retrospective series examining the outcome of tracheal intubations in patients with CSI; most of them were unstable. The accumulated number of DLOI was 395; only two experienced neurological deteriorations were not attributed to the airway intervention [15]. Regardless of the evident safety of DLOI, awake nasotracheal intubation is an option that many anesthesiologists choose as the preferred technique for definitive airway control in patients with suspected CSI [16]. This maneuver can be done blindly or, more commonly in recent years, with a fiber-optic endoscope. Minimal spine movement, the ability to continue the neurological examination after the intubation, and maintaining airway protective reflexes are some of the advantages of this procedure. The potential disadvantages are the slow learning curve that causes many caregivers to be uncomfortable with the procedure [17] and the potential for desaturation that might aggravate secondary cord injury [18]. No significant differences in success rate or safety were found between flexible and rigid endoscopes in establishing controlled airway in patients with a compromised cervical spine [19]. In recent years, video laryngoscopy has gained popularity in emergency airway management. Devices such as the GlideScope were shown to be effective in achieving tracheal intubation in patients with cervical collars [20]. To date, no data exist that can support its use as a safer technique to intubate patients with suspected CSI.

*Summary and recommendations*: Both DLOI and fiber-optic awake nasotracheal intubation are safe and effective options for securing the airway in a trauma patient with suspected CSI.

*Grade of recommendation*: B

No data exist to support one technique over the other. Because no special equipment or advanced expertise is needed for DLOI, it is probably preferred in emergency situations, whereas the fiber-optic option is preferred for more elective procedures.

*Grade of recommendation*: C

### 12.4.2 Breathing and Circulation

SCIs might inflict respiratory failure and hemodynamic compromise. On the other hand, hypoxemia and hypotension might increase the chance for secondary cord injury and worsening the neurological outcome. Cervical SCI might cause respiratory muscle paresis and paralysis, causing decreased ventilatory efficiency, hypoxemia, and hypoventilation. Patients with cervical SCI are at significant risk for ventilatory failure. This risk varies based on the level and completeness of injury. Ventilatory support is needed for the majority of patients with C5 and higher injuries and virtually all patients with C3 and higher injuries in the acute phase. Adequate fluid resuscitation and hemodynamic improvement was found to correlate with better neurological outcome [21]. High SCI (usually above the level of T6) can be associated with disruption of the sympathetic chain that will cause hypotension and bradycardia. This condition, called neurogenic shock, is caused by unopposed parasympathetic vasodilation and bradycardia. Its incidence in recent retrospective cohort study was found to be 19.3% [22]. In most patients, perfusion pressure can be maintained with fluid administration. Despite a lack of evidence-based literature on the subject, if systolic blood pressure of at least 90 mmHg, mean arterial pressure of 85 mmHg, and normal perfusion status are not achieved, early administration of vasoactive drug should be considered [23].

### 12.4.3 Diagnostic Options in Patients with Suspected Spine Injury

Imaging of the suspected injured spine has been the focus of many studies and analyses. Readily available computerized imaging has revolutionized the evaluation of the spine. On the other hand, large-scale studies demonstrated the safety of clearing the spine without any imaging in certain circumstances.

#### *12.4.3.1 What Criteria Should Be Used to Clear the Cervical Spine in a Trauma Patient?*

Two major research projects have been published in an attempt to establish a set of criteria by which a significant CSI can be safely ruled out based on clinical evaluation alone. Other smaller prospective studies basically reached the same conclusion. The NEXUS study enrolled 34,069 patients. There were five criteria for the definition of a low probability of CSI: no midline cervical tenderness, no focal neurological deficit, normal alertness, no intoxication, and no painful, distracting injury. The decision instrument missed 8 of the 818 patients who eventually were diagnosed with CSI (sensitivity, 99.0%; 95% confidence interval [CI], 98.0%–99.6%). The negative predictive value was 99.8% (95% CI, 99.6%–100%), the specificity was 12.9%, and the positive predictive value was 2.7% [24]. The Canadian study enrolled 8924 adults with blunt trauma to the head and neck, with normal vital signs and GCS of 15. Among the study population, there were 151 (1.7%) patients diagnosed with clinically important CSI. The decision to order C-spine radiography was based on three questions: (1) Is there any high-risk factor present that mandates radiography (i.e., age 65 years, dangerous mechanism, or extremities paresthesias)? (2) Is there any low-risk factor present that allows safe assessment of range of motion (i.e., simple rear-end MVC, sitting position in emergency department, ambulatory at any time since injury, delayed onset of neck pain, or absence of midline C-spine tenderness)? (3) Is the patient able to actively rotate neck 45° to the left and right? The results had 100% sensitivity (95% CI, 98%–100%) and 42.5% specificity (95% CI, 40%–44%) for identifying clinically important C-spine injuries [25]. In 2003, a prospective comparison of the two criteria sets was published. There were important CSIs among the 8283 study patients. The Canadian C-spine rule was more sensitive than the NEXUS rule (99.4% versus 90.7%; $p < 0.001$), more specific (45.1% versus 36.8%; $p < 0.001$), and resulted in lower radiography rates [26].

*Summary and recommendations*: Both the NEXUS and the Canadian C-spine set of criteria can be safely used to clinically clear the C-spine in adult, asymptomatic patients with blunt trauma. Patients that meet the low-risk criteria do not need any further radiographic investigation.

*Grade of recommendation*: A

#### *12.4.3.2 What Imaging Study Is Needed to Clear the C-Spine in the Obtunded Patient?*

Another controversial issue is the clearance of the C-spine in the comatose patient. Clearing the C-spine in these circumstances is important mainly to allow removal of the cervical collar and by that preventing side effects (neck and scalp pressure sores and elevated intra-cranial pressure) and improving the nursing and the physical therapy care. In the alert patient, C-spine is done by clinical examination combined with computerized tomography (CT). Clinical examination can detect ligamentous injury that might be missed by the CT. Coma or deep sedation in the intensive care unit prevents meaningful physical examination. Three options were traditionally suggested: passive flexion–extension fluoroscopy, magnetic resonance imaging (MRI), and clearing of the C-spine based on the CT alone. The limitations of the flexion–extension study were mentioned earlier. Passive flexion–extension study was also found to be unreliable in detecting C-spine instability in comatose patients [27]. The difficulties and risk of taking a ventilated multiple trauma patient to the MRI have led to attempts to show the safety of clearing the C-spine based on normal CT alone. Currently, the most comprehensive study was a meta-analysis, published by Raza et al. in 2013, that included 10 prospective studies. The authors found a cumulative negative predictive value and a specificity of cervical spine CT of 99.7% (95% CI, 99.4%–99.9%). The positive predictive value and sensitivity was 93.7% (95% CI, 84.0%–97.7%). They concluded that clearing the C-spine based on the CT was safe and recommended [28].

*Summary and recommendations*: In the obtunded trauma patient, the C-spine can be safely cleared based on a normal CT. MRI should be reserved for selected patients.

*Grade of recommendation*: B

#### 12.4.3.3 What Is the Imaging Modality of Choice to Evaluate the Spine?

Active flexion–extension cervical spine radiography has been suggested as adjacent to normal static radiographs in cases of continued neck tenderness or stiffness after a blunt trauma. However, despite its evident safety, it rarely is able to add important information in the alert patient where muscle guarding typically will not allow for more than a few degrees of motion due to pain. Moreover, it has been demonstrated that the threshold cervical range of motion needed to detect even significant instability is approximately 30° of flexion or extension, which is more than most painful patients can perform [29]. Finally, flexion–extension radiographs became a rare choice due to its high rate of technical inadequacy and the fact that it adds little information to CT or MRI, which became more available in recent years [30,31]. Traditionally, evaluation of the thoracic, lumbar, and sacral spine was done with plain radiographs augmented with CT in cases of evident fracture or technical inadequacy. In recent years, the availability of the high-resolution fast multisliced CT scanner makes it the screening modality of choice. With most victims of high-energy blunt trauma needing torso CT, regenerating the spine images has been found to be more effective than plain radiographs with proven cost reduction [32,33].

A known low sensitivity, together with the cumbersome task of obtaining at least three views (lateral, anteroposterior, and open-mouth odontoid), has led many trauma centers to choose cervical spine CT with coronal reconstruction as the primary screening modality for suspected CSI in the multiple trauma patients. The superiority of this approach was showed in a meta-analysis published in 2005. Despite some methodological flaws and the fact that no randomized controlled study was included, the authors presented a pooled sensitivity for plain radiography of 52% (95% CI, 47, 56), versus a pooled sensitivity for CT of 98% (95% CI, 96, 99) [34]. The American College of Orthopedic Surgeons now recommends routine cervical spine screening via CT scan instead of plain radiography [35]. The three-view radiographic study should be performed only when CT is not readily available and should not be considered a substitute for CT. Lateral cervical plain radiographs in the resuscitation area cannot rule out unstable CSI, so the information gained will not change the management of the patient. This is why we do not recommend this study.

The assumption that CSI increases the risk for other thoracolumbar spine injuries has been proven in a large retrospective study based on the nationwide trauma database. The occurrence of thoracolumbar spine fracture was doubled from 6.9% to 13.06% if a concomitant cervical spine fracture was found [36].

MRI is the most sensitive imaging method for evaluation of the neck structure, including soft tissue (ligaments, discs, etc.) and neural structures. This is why it is an appealing modality for diagnosis of a suspected injured spine. However, its relatively low availability and the technical problems of scanning trauma patients in the acute phase preclude its routine use in the initial evaluation. MRI is an important follow-up study in patients with CT signs that are suggestive of ligamentous or soft tissue and disc rupture injuries (noncongruent facet joins, chip avulsion fractures of end plates adjacent to disc space, and distended disc space). These may represent severely unstable cervical injuries that reduced via muscle spasm and guarding in the alert patient, and in this scenerio, MRI may add important additional information that no other modality can detect. MRI is also usually performed in patients with SCI to document the injury to the spinal cord itself and for reserved for cases of spinal-related signs and symptoms that are not explained by findings in the CT (i.e., continued neck pain or motion limitation or unexplained clinical neurological finding) [37].

*Summary and recommendations*: In patients where spine clearance cannot be achieved with clinical examination, CT of the cervical spine with reconstructions is the screening modality of choice. Views reconstructed from the thoracic and abdominal CT are adequate for the evaluation of the thoracic and lumbar spine. MRI should be reserved for selected cases of SCI patients and clinical/radiological discrepancy or inadequate CT.

*Grade of recommendation*: B

### 12.4.4 Medical Management of Spinal Cord Damage

Inflicting direct forces such as laceration, compression, and distraction on the spinal cord creates primary damage and cell death on impact. A secondary insult can occur within minutes as a result of hypoxia or hypoperfusion. The resulting inflammatory process, combined with other metabolic derangements, might further increase neural and glia cell apoptosis. These events will eventually lead to a worse neurological outcome. The relative contribution of the secondary insult to the final neurological outcome is not known but estimated to be no higher than 10% [38], and it is still the focus of numerous research projects. Several studies focus on the effort to promote neural tissue recovery and regeneration. Autologous incubated macrophages, oscillating field stimulation, autologous bone marrow cell transplantation with granulocyte–macrophage colony-stimulating factor, and autologous olfactory ensheathing cell transplantation are all in various stages of clinical studies after showing promising results in animal models. However, none have yet produced any evidence to support use in any human clinical condition [39–42]. Several compounds that may attenuate secondary cord injury are being clinically tested. The most prominent are minocycline and GTPase Ras homology protein inhibitor. Again, evidence for their routine use is yet to be found [43,44]. GM-1 ganglioside was thought to have neuroprotective properties via several mechanisms that participate in the secondary injury cascade. Despite promising initial results, a large multicenter study demonstrated no effectiveness for the drug, and, therefore, its use cannot be recommended [45]. Riluzole, a sodium channel–blocking benzothiazole anticonvulsant medication, has lately been advocated by Fehlings et al. for administration in the acute setting of SCI [46,47].

#### *12.4.4.1 Should High-Dose Corticosteroids Be Used in Trauma Patients with SCI?*

Few issues in medicine have stirred up as much controversy and dispute as the issue of corticosteroids administration in SCI. The complexity of interpretation of evidence-based data and its influence on medicolegal considerations are demonstrated in a survey of 60 Canadian neurosurgeons and orthopedic spine surgeons about their practice. Approximately 75% of the responders routinely prescribe steroids for acute SCI, but 70% of them do so due to fear from litigation or peer criticism. Only 17% of them believe that steroids actually improve their patient's neurological outcome [48]. The first study on administration of methylprednisolone (MP) was published in 1984 [49]. In 1992, the National Spinal Cord Injury Study was published with high-profile professional and popular media coverage. It was a prospective, randomized, double-blind, controlled, multicenter trial with 487 patients randomized to high-dose MP, naloxone, or placebo. A 1-year follow-up study summarized the results. No significant neurological improvement was achieved, and an insignificant trend toward increased complication rate (mainly infection) was demonstrated. A post hoc analysis found that patients who received high-dose MP within 8 h of their injury showed a statistically significant, although questionable, improvement in motor and sensory scores at 6 months [50]. The next pivotal study randomized 499 patients and compared 24 and 48 h MP administration with no significant outcome differences. Again, post hoc analyses showed that the 48 h MP group had a slightly better motor outcome if the drug was given 3–8 h after the trauma. The sensory scores were equal between the groups. As in all other similar studies, an increased infectious complications rate was evident [51]. In general, the same results were also obtained subsequently, including several prospective randomized studies.

*Summary and recommendations*: Current data do not support the routine use of high-dose MP in patients with SCI because accumulative results suggest questionable minimal functional recovery and a clear increase in complications.

*Grade of recommendation*: B

### 12.4.5 Surgical Management of Patients with SCI

#### *12.4.5.1 What Is the Optimal Timing for Surgical Intervention?*

The effect of early surgery on neurological outcomes remains a debatable topic. Vaccaro et al. designed a prospective randomized controlled study to determine whether functional outcome is improved in patients with traumatic cervical SCI who underwent early surgery (<72 h after injury) compared with those who underwent late surgery (>5 days after injury). They revealed no significant neurological benefit for the early surgical intervention [52]. Fehlings et al. conducted a meta-analysis study, which provide the following recommendations: (1) urgent decompression is recommended in case of bilateral locked facets and incomplete tetraplegia, or neurological deterioration; and (2) urgent decompression in any acute CSI is a reasonable practice option [53].

The dilemma of timing is much more complicated in multitrauma patients with an associated spinal injury. Though advocating urgent decompression, Fehling et al. found that in this setting, it is extremely difficult to obtain MRI of the cervical spine and to prepare the patients for urgent surgery if face of physiological insult that often mandates lifesaving efforts and intensive care unit stay [54]. Dai et al. retrospectively summarized their experience with 147 patients who sustained blunt high-energy

**TABLE 12.1**

Clinical Questions

| Question | Answer | Grade of Recommendation | References |
|---|---|---|---|
| What is the impact of airway maneuvers on cervical spine movement? | Relative segmental spine movement might happen, and can be minimized with in-line in situ immobilization. | B | [4–8] |
| What is the preferred way to achieve tracheal intubation in patients with suspected CSI? | Both direct oral and fiber-optic awake nasotracheal intubation are safe and effective. | B | [9–13] |
| | Oral intubation is preferred in emergency situations. | C | |
| What criteria should be used to clinically clear the cervical spine in a trauma patient? | The Nexus or the Canadian C-spine criteria can be used for clinical clearance of the spine. | B | [17–19] |
| What imaging study is needed to clear the C-spine in the obtunded patient? | Normal CT is sufficient to safely clear the C-spine in an obtunded patient. | B | |
| What is the imaging modality of choice for evaluation of the spine? | CT and MRI are indicated when CT findings suggest ligamentous injury. | B | [20–26] |
| Should high-dose corticosteroids be used in trauma patients with SCI? | No | B | [35–38] |
| What is the optimal timing to operate a patient with spinal injury? | Early reduction and operation for decompression within 6–12 h may be beneficial in incomplete SCI and in evolving neurological deterioration. | D | [39–41] |

*Abbreviations:* CSI, cervical spinal cord injury; CT, computed tomography; SCI, spinal cord injury.

multitrauma with thoracolumbar fractures. Although it is not the preferable study design in terms of evidence-based medicine, it is worthwhile to learn its results and conclusions. There was no statistically significant correlation between the timing of thoracolumbar surgery and the complications rate. Neither the severity of the injury nor the timing of surgery had any significant effect on the recovery rate [55]. One criticism of these earlier studies is that the threshold definition of early versus late surgery was randomly defined at 72 h. Animal models and clinical data have clearly demonstrated that if any recovery is to be expected in face of continuous cord compression and SCI, decompression and removal of cord pressure is to be achieved within 12–24 h and optimally even within 6 h. Therefore, this earlier trial that defined the threshold at 72 h compared two groups, both of which had surgery at a "late" stage. New trials that compare decompression surgery within 24 h and after 24 h have consistently shown a marked neurological improvement of two grades in SCI patients and represent a new trend toward very early surgery [56–58] (Table 12.1).

*Summary and recommendations*: To date, there are no defined standards regarding the timing of decompression and stabilization in acute SCI. The literature does infer urgent spinal cord decompression in the face of evolving neurological deficit. The question of surgery timing in multiple trauma patients with spinal injury remains open for debate because prospective studies are unlikely to be initiated.

*Grade of recommendation*: D

## References


1. Aashjian RZ, Majercik S, Biffl WL et al. Halo-vest immobilization increases early morbidity and mortality in elderly odontoid fractures. *J Trauma*. 2006;60:199–203.
2. Browner BD, Jupiter JB, Levine AM et al. 1998. *Skeletal Trauma: Fractures, Dislocations, Ligamentous Injuries*. WB Saunders: Philadelphia, PA.
3. Demetriades D, Charalambides K, Chahwan S et al. Non-skeletal cervical spine injuries: Epidemiology and diagnostic pitfalls. *J Trauma*. 2000;48:724–727.
4. Dreiangel N, Ben-Galim P, Lador R, Hipp JA. Occipito-cervical dissociative injuries: Common in blunt trauma fatalities and better detected with objective CT-based measurements. *Spine J*. August 2010;10(8):704–707.
5. Lador R, Ben-Galim P, Weiner BK, Hipp JA. The association of occipitocervical dissociation and death as a result of blunt trauma. *Spine J*. December 2010;10(12): 1128–1132.
6. Lador R, Ben-Galim P, Hipp JA, PhD. Motion within the unstable cervical spine during patient maneuvering: The Neck Pivot-Shift Phenomenon. *J Trauma*. January 2011;70(1):247–251.
7. Aprahamian C, Thompson BM, Finger WA et al. Experimental cervical spine injury model: Evaluation of airway management and splinting techniques. *Ann Emerg Med*. 1984;13:584–587.
8. Sawin PD, Todd MM, Traynelis VC et al. Cervical spine motion with direct laryngoscopy and orotracheal intubation: An in vivo cinefluoroscopic study of subjects without cervical abnormality. *Anesthesiology*. 1996;85: 26–36.

9. Gerling MC, Davis DP, Hamilton RS et al. Effects of cervical spine immobilization technique and laryngoscope blade selection on an unstable cervical spine in a cadaver model of intubation. *Ann Emerg Med.* 2000;36:293–300.
10. Lennarson PJ, Smith D, Todd MM et al. Segmental cervical spine motion during orotracheal intubation of the intact and injured spine with and without external stabilization. *J Neurosurg.* 2000;92:201–206.
11. Brimacombe J, Keller C, Kunzel KH et al. Cervical spine motion during airway management: A cinefluoroscopic study of the posteriorly destabilized third cervical vertebrae in human cadavers. *Anesth Analg.* 2000;91: 1274–1278.
12. Kalantar BS, Hipp JA, Reitman CA, Dreiangel N, Ben-Galim P. Diagnosis of unstable cervical spine injuries: Laboratory support for the use of axial traction to diagnose cervical spine instability. *J Trauma.* Oct 2010;69(4):889–895.
13. Ben-Galim P, Sibai TA, Hipp JA, Heggeness MH, Reitman CA. Internal decapitation: Survival following head to neck dissociation injuries. *Spine.* July 2008;33(16):1744–1749.
14. Ben-Galim P, Dreiangel N, Mattox KL, Reitman CA, Kalantar SB, Hipp JA. Extrication collars can result in abnormal separation between vertebrae in the presence of a dissociative injury. *J Trauma.* August 2010;69(2):447–450.
15. Crosby ET. Airway management in adults after cervical spine trauma. *Anesthesiology* 2006;104:1293–1318.
16. Rosenblatt WH, Wagner PJ, Ovassapian A et al. Practice patterns in managing the difficult airway by anesthesiologists in the United States. *Anesth Analg.* 1998;87:153–157.
17. Ezri T, Szmuk P, Warters RD et al. Difficult airway management practice patterns among anesthesiologists practicing in the United States: Have we made any progress? *J Clin Anesth.* 2003;15:418–422.
18. Fuchs G, Schwarz G, Baumgartner A et al. Fiberoptic intubation in 327 patients with lesions of the cervical spine. *J Neurosurg Anesth.* 1999;11:16–11.
19. Cohn AI, Zornow MH. Awake endotracheal intubation in 520 patients with cervical spine disease: A comparison of the Bullard laryngoscope and the fiberoptic bronchoscope. *Anesth Analg.* 1995;81:1283–1286.
20. Bathory I, Frascarolo P, Kern C, Schoettker P. Evaluation of the GlideScope for tracheal intubation in patients with cervical spine immobilisation by a semi-rigid collar. *Anaesthesia.* 2009;64:1337–1341.
21. Vale FL, Burns J, Jackson AB et al. Combined medical and surgical treatment after acute spinal cord injury: Results of a prospective pilot study to assess the merits of aggressive medical resuscitation and blood pressure management. *J Neurosurg.* 1997;87:239–246.
22. Guly HR, Bouamra O, Lecky FE. Trauma audit and research network. The incidence of neurogenic shock in patients with isolated spinal cord injury in the emergency department. *Resuscitation.* 2008;76:57–62.
23. Hadley MN, Walters BC, Grabb PA et al. Blood pressure management after acute spinal cord injury. *Neurosurgery.* 2002;50(Suppl):58–62.
24. Hoffman JR, Mower WR, Wolfson AB et al. Validity of a set of clinical criteria to rule out injury to the cervical spine in patients with blunt trauma. National Emergency X-Radiography Utilisation Study Group. *N Engl J Med.* 2000;343:94–99.
25. Stiell IG, Wells GA, Vandemheen KL et al. The Canadian C-spine rule for radiography in alert and stable trauma patients. *JAMA.* 2001;286:1841–1848.
26. Stiell IG, Clement CM, McKnight RD et al. The Canadian C-spine rule versus the NEXUS low-risk criteria in patients with trauma. *N Engl J Med.* 2003;349:2510–2518.
27. Freedman I, van Gelderen D, Cooper DJ, Fitzgerald M, Malham G, Rosenfeld JV, Varma D, Kossmann T. Cervical spine assessment in the unconscious trauma patient: A major trauma service's experience with passive flexion-extension radiography. *J Trauma.* June 2005;58(6):1183–1188.
28. Raza M1, Elkhodair S, Zaheer A, Yousaf S. Safe cervical spine clearance in adult obtunded blunt trauma patients on the basis of a normal multidetector CT scan—A meta-analysis and cohort study. *Injury.* November 2013;44(11):1589–1595.
29. Hwang H, Hipp JA, Ben-Galim P, Reitman CA. Threshold cervical range-of-motion necessary to detect abnormal intervertebral motion in cervical spine radiographs spine. *Spine.* April 2008;33(8):E261–E267.
30. Wang JC, Hatch JD, Sandhu HS et al. Cervical flexion and extension radiographs in acutely injured patients. *Clin Orthop Relat Res.* 1999;365:111–116.
31. Insko EK, Gracias VH, Gupta R et al. Utility of flexion and extension radiographs of the cervical spine in the acute evaluation of blunt trauma. *J Trauma.* 2002;53:426–429.
32. Sheridan R, Peralta R, Rhen J et al. Reformatted visceral protocol helical computed tomographic scanning allows conventional radiographs of the thoracic and lumbar spine to be eliminated in the evaluation of blunt trauma patients. *J Trauma.* 2003;55:655–669.
33. Brandt MM, Wahl WL, Yeom K et al. Computed tomographic scanning reduces cost and time of complete spine evaluation. *J Trauma.* 2004;56:1022–1026.
34. Holmes JF, Akkinepalli R. Computed tomography versus plain radiography to screen for cervical spine injury: A metaanalysis. *J Trauma.* 2005;58:902–905.
35. Mulkens TH, Marchal P, Daineffe S et al. Comparison of low-dose with standard-dose multidetector CT in cervical spine trauma. *Am J Neuroradiol.* 2007;28:1444–1450.
36. Winslow JE III, Hensberry R, Bozeman WP et al. Risk of thoracolumbar fractures doubled in victims of motor vehicle collisions with cervical spine fractures. *J Trauma.* 2006;61:686–687.
37. Karpova A, Arun R, Cadotte DW, Davis AM, Kulkarni AV, O'Higgins M, Fehlings MG. Assessment of spinal cord compression by magnetic resonance imaging—Can it predict surgical outcomes in degenerative compressive myelopathy? A systematic review. *Spine.* 2013;38(16): 1409–1421.

38. Young W, Yen V, Blight A. Extracellular calcium ion activity in experimental spinal cord contusion. *Brain Res.* 1982;235:105–113.
39. Knoller N, Auerbach G, Fulga V et al. Clinical experience using incubated autologous macrophages as a treatment for complete spinal cord injury: Phase I study results. *J Neurosurg Spine.* 2005;3:173–181.
40. Shapiro S, Borgens R, Pascuzzi R et al. Oscillating field stimulation for complete spinal cord injury in humans: A Phase I trial. *J Neurosurg Spine.* 2005;2:3–10.
41. Yoon SH, Shim YS, Park YH et al. Complete spinal cord injury treatment using autologous bone marrow cell transplantation and bone marrow stimulation with granulocyte macrophage-colony stimulating factor: Faze me/II clinical trial. *Stem Cells.* 2007;25:2066–2073.
42. Féron F, Perry C, Cochrane J et al. Autologous olfactory ensheathing cell transplantation in human spinal cord injury. *Brain.* 2005;128:2951–2960.
43. Yune TY, Lee JY, Jung GY et al. Minocycline alleviates death of oligodendrocytes by inhibiting pro-nerve growth factor production in microglia after spinal cord injury. *J Neurosci.* 2007;27:7751–7761.
44. Fournier AE, Takizawa BT, Strittmatter SM. Rho kinase inhibition enhances axonal regeneration in the injured. *J Neurosci.* 2003;23:1416–1423.
45. Geisler FH, Coleman WP, Griece G et al. The sygen multi-centre acute spinal cord injury study. *Spine.* 2001;26:87–98.
46. Wu Y, Satkunendrarajah K, Fehlings MG. Riluzole improves outcome following ischemia-reperfusion injury to the spinal cord by preventing delayed paraplegia. *Neuroscience.* 2014;18(265):302–312.
47. Grossman RG, Fehlings MG, Frankowski RF et al. A prospective, multicenter, phase I matched-comparison group trial of safety, pharmacokinetics, and preliminary efficacy of riluzole in patients with traumatic spinal cord injury. *J Neurotrauma.* February 2014;31(3): 239–255.
48. Hurlbert RJ, Moulton R. Why do you prescribe methylprednisolone for acute spinal cord injury? *Can J Neurol Sci.* 2002;29:236–239.
49. Bracken MB, Collins WF, Freeman DF et al. Efficacy of methylprednisolone in acute spinal cord injury. *JAMA.* 1984;251:45–52.
50. Bracken MB, Shepard MJ, Collins WF et al. Methylprednisolone or naloxone treatment after acute spinal cord 1-year follow-up data. *J Neurosurg.* 1992;76:23–31.
51. Bracken MB, Shepard MJ, Holford TR et al. Administration of methylprednisolone for 24 or 48 hours or tirilazad mesylate for 48 hours in the treatment of acute spinal cord injury. *JAMA.* 1997;277:1597–1604.
52. Vaccaro AR, Daugherty RJ, Sheehan TP et al. Neurologic outcome of early versus late surgery for cervical spinal cord injury. *Spine.* 1997;22:2609–2613.
53. Fehlings MG, Perrin RG. The role and timing of early decompression for cervical spinal cord injury: Update with a review of recent clinical evidence. *Injury.* 2005;36(Suppl 2):S13–S26.
54. Fehlings MG, Cuddy B, Dickman C, Fazl M, Green B, Hitchon P, Northrup B, Sonntag V, Wagner F, Tator CH. Surgical treatment for acute spinal cord injury study pilot study #2: Evaluation of protocol for decompressive surgery within 8 hours of injury. *Neurosurg Focus.* January 1999;6(1):e3.
55. Dai LY, Tao WF, Zhou O. Thoracolumbar fractures in patients with multiple injuries: Diagnosis and treatment—A review of147 cases. *J Trauma.* 2004;56:348–355.
56. Wilson JR, Singh A, Craven C, Verrier MC, Drew B, Ahn H, Ford M, Fehlings MG. Early versus late surgery for traumatic spinal cord injury: The results of a prospective Canadian cohort study. *Spinal Cord.* November 2012;50(11):840–843.
57. Umerani MS, Abbas A, Sharif S. Asian: Clinical outcome in patients with early versus delayed decompression in cervical spine trauma. *Spine J.* August 2014;8(4):427–434.
58. Fehlings MG, Vaccaro A, Wilson JR et al. Early versus delayed decompression for traumatic cervical spinal cord injury: Results of the Surgical Timing in Acute Spinal Cord Injury Study (STASCIS). *PLoS One.* 2012;7(2):e32037.

## Commentary on Spine and Spinal Cord Injuries

*Lenworth M. Jacobs*

Injuries to the spine and spinal cord continue to be a major diagnostic and management concern for practitioners. In spite of significant advances in surgical management of spinal column injuries relative to alignment and stabilization, neurological recovery with its attendant catastrophic disabilities has not changed significantly over the last number of years. The authors have focused on a number of vitally important issues that are of interest to the practitioner who is faced with a patient with spinal column and spinal cord injuries.

It is important to understand that the majority of spinal cord injuries are the result of severe contusions or traction forces applied either in a longitudinal or transverse vector to the cord itself. Virtually, no survivable injury results in physical cord transection. The consequences of these kinetic forces and physiologic changes result in physical and cellular damage, with resulting cord ischemia and local inflammation. The identification of the type of force and the physiologic changes along with the knowledge of how best to ameliorate these physiologically negative results will provide a better functional outcome for the patient.

An important issue for the practitioner is to solicit a detailed history of the cause of the event and how the forces were applied to the spinal column and the spinal cord. A detailed physical examination that identifies the anatomic and physiologic results of the injury must be elicited and recorded. This forms the first snapshot in a moving picture. The closer the examination is to the time of the injury provides insight into the severity of the injury and the likelihood of it progressing to ultimate catastrophic functional failure. The original exam coupled with frequent re-examinations at 15–30 min intervals will allow other practitioners to understand the evolution of the injury process and generate appropriate interventions.

A challenging management problem especially in those patients who have had blunt trauma to the cervical spine is the management of both the spinal column and the spinal cord. Preserving function to the diaphragm, the thoracic musculature, and the distal spinal cord is essential. Establishing, protecting, and maintaining an airway are critical. The practitioner must determine if the patient can protect their airway and ventilate themselves without external support. Another issue is whether this process can be maintained for the duration of the resuscitative process or if airway control is necessary to preserve adequate ventilation and oxygenation.

The authors discuss in an elegant and comprehensive manner the dilemmas that face the clinician relative to when and how to protect the spinal cord and when and how to maintain the airway with or without endotracheal intubation. A critical tenant in the immediate and early management of patients with cervical cord injury is to not to do any further harm to the patient.

The concept of cervical stabilization and inline traction are well discussed. The treating practitioner has to determine if manual traction and stabilization is sufficient or if stabilization of the entire spinal cord with long and short board devices along with a cervical collar is necessary for all patients. A critical decision is to identify if the patient is losing ventilatory function. Control of the airway should be performed early in the process to avoid rapid chaotic control of the airway in a patient who is becoming hypoxic. Not only is the hypoxia deleterious to the patient, but it will have significant negative effects relative to a second hypoxic injury to the spinal cord. The decision for early airway management has to be balanced with the potential to cause harm by the intubation process. The most experienced person should gain control of the airway. This is not a time for an inexperienced operator to practice their airway control skills. Awake nasotracheal intubation is an elegant way to control the airway in a person with an unstable spinal column and deteriorating ventilation. It is essential to engage the patient and establish rapport so that they do not inappropriately move or stress the upper cervical musculature. Careful explanation of the procedure enables excellent cooperation with an awake patient.

Correcting hypovolemia and maintaining sufficient intravascular volume to assure adequate central profusion is critical. Monitoring the cerebral status of the patient and their hemodynamic parameters including urinary output can give a functional guide to optimal volume resuscitation. If the hemodynamic parameters are stable and the patient is not showing signs of shock, it is reasonable to accept a systolic blood pressure of 90 mmHg and not employ vasoactive drugs to pursue normal or supernormal blood pressure.

### Clearing the Cervical Spine

The authors provide an excellent discussion of the dilemma of not missing a spinal column or spinal cord injury as opposed to spending many hours and multiple tests to clear a normal spinal column and a spinal cord that is uninjured and functions normally. It is very important to evaluate the patient to determine if there is a low possibility of cervical spine injury. The absence of tenderness, no focal neurologic deficits, and an alert patient with normal cerebral function who is not impaired by drugs, alcohol, or pain can be managed clinically with relatively minimal interventions. This is to be contrasted with the patient who has an altered sensorium secondary to alcohol or a cerebral injury especially if the patient is unresponsive or comatose. These patients require definitive objective evaluations.

The multislice CT scanner is an excellent tool for evaluating the spinal cord and the spinal column. In modern centers where CT scans are adjacent to the resuscitation suite and there is radiologic interpretation immediately available, the CT scanner is the investigatory agent of choice. An MRI is more effective in evaluating soft tissue, ligamentous and other injuries. Generally, the MRI suite is a more difficult environment to maintain and manage a patient who has airway and ventilation difficulties and may well be on a ventilator. The clinician has to be sensitive to the need for precision in diagnosis versus the risk of putting such a patient in an MRI suite, which may have suboptimal intensive care management personnel and equipment. The discussion and the evaluation of the appropriate literature in this chapter are extremely helpful to guide practitioners as they navigate through these difficult decisions.

## Management of Spinal Cord Injury

There has been a significant debate as to why spinal cord injuries, which initially are not devastating, progress to partial or complete loss of function. The sequelae of the initial injury whether it be edema, local hemorrhage, compression, or inflammation have been the subject of extensive investigation over the years. The concept of adequate oxygenation of the cord, decompression of hematomas pressing upon the cord, and amelioration of the inflammatory processes is important in obtaining the best functional outcomes. Each process requires a different therapeutic approach.

It is obvious that adequate tissue perfusion and oxygenation is essential to prevent ongoing injury. Similarly, an epidural hematoma of the cord, which is causing ischemia secondary to compression, must be decompressed. It is not quite so clear at the cellular level what processes will decrease the release of cytokines which exacerbate inflammation. This latter subject has been the focus of the use of steroids early in the injury process.

The authors have reviewed the literature and the evidence and conclude that the current data does not support the use of high-dose steroids and may, in fact, promote an increase in complications. This debate has been a fierce one since anything that will enhance functional outcomes has been the goal of practitioners who treat spinal cord patients. It is critical to evaluate the evidence to be sure that the natural progression of the disease would not have ended up with the same outcome as the introduction of high-dose steroids. Once the regimen of high-dose steroids has been introduced, it is not possible to reverse their effects. Therefore, with the increased incidence of complications, their use has been brought into sharp focus despite anecdotal stories of enhanced results with the application of high-dose steroids.

The authors also discuss surgical management of patients with spinal cord injury. They conclude that urgent decompression is recommended in bilateral locked facets and incomplete tetraplegia or neurologic deterioration. However, urgent decompression in all acute cervical spinal cord injuries is not a reasonable practice option. There are a number of new trials, which are focusing the issue of early versus late decompression and we eagerly await the results of these trials, which will provide more precise guidance for the timing of these interventions.

Spinal column and spinal cord injuries continue to be a serious challenge for all practitioners. It is essential to have a clear understanding of the etiologic processes and the appropriate therapeutic interventions, which maximize survival and increase neurologic function.

The authors have brought clarity to a number of the real dilemmas that practitioners face. There is also a continuing need to aggressively pursue research in this area in order to increase the ultimate function of patients who have spinal cord injuries.

# 13

# *Facial Injuries*

**Hirra Ali, Antonio Jorge V. Forte, and Joseph H. Shin**

**CONTENTS**



## 13.1 Introduction

Facial injuries are among the most common emergencies seen in an acute care setting. They range from simple soft tissue lacerations to complex facial fractures associated with significant craniomaxillofacial injuries with soft tissue loss. The management of these injuries generally follows standard surgical management priorities but is rendered more complex by the nature of the numerous areas of overlap in management areas such as airway, neurologic, ophthalmologic, and dental. In addition, the significant psychological nature of injuries affecting the face and the resultant aftermath of scarring can have devastating and long-lasting consequences. Despite the fact that these injuries are exceedingly common, they are cared for by a large group of different specialists and, as such, have a remarkably heterogeneous presentation and diverse treatment schema. Nonetheless, guiding principles in the care of these injuries will provide the basis for the best possible outcomes. The following questions will hopefully guide general management and provide a framework for understanding the principles in the acute care of patients with facial injuries and trauma.

## 13.2 What Is the Proper Timing and Method of Closure? What Is the Optimal Subsequent Care for Facial Lacerations and Wound after Closure?

There remains little standardization in the method of repair of traumatic lacerations and the subsequent care of these wounds, primarily because of the numerous different specialties involved in caring for the trauma patient. We reviewed the available literature in order to provide best practice guidelines to address the optimal timing of wound closure, the closure technique and material utilized, type of dressing, and adjunctive measures for facial laceration.

The timing of facial skin laceration closure is the same as that of any open wound. The presence of contaminating factors in the management of wounds would generally not allow closure after 6 h and would favor delayed closure [1]. However, clinical practice is slightly more variable with facial lacerations because of the uniquely sensitive nature of facial scarring. While we generally ascribe to experimental data regarding timing of closure, in practice, the 6 h rule is often overlooked with an attempt to be vigorous with cleaning of the wound.

The presence of exceptionally rich blood supply in the face is also deemed of benefit in extending the 6 h rule.

In 2013, Rui-feng et al. published a prospective, randomized controlled trial addressing whether primary closure of a dirty wound is possible. The authors randomly divided 600 facial lacerations inflicted by a dog bite into two groups, those closed primarily and those left open to allow for healing by secondary intention, and measured the infection rate and time to healing. The group found that primary closure of the dirty wound did not have an increased incidence of infection over the group left to heal by secondary intention and primary closure predictably shortens the time to healing. They concluded that immediate primary closure of dirty wounds after thorough irrigation and debridement was the preferred approach [2].

Regarding the suturing technique, Gandham and Menon published a prospective, randomized controlled trial in 2003 in which they compared the cosmetic appearance of skin lacerations closed by either traditional or dynamic sliding loop suture technique. Two independent observers blinded to the technique used a Visual Analogue Cosmetic Scale to assess the aesthetic result and found no statistical difference in cosmetic outcome between the two groups [3]. Then in 2005, Singer et al. conducted a prospective, randomized controlled trial that compared the short-term wound infection, dehiscence rates, and the cosmetic outcome after 3 months of traumatic facial lacerations closed with either a single or double layer of sutures. The study included 65 patients, all with simple, linear, nonbite, and nongaping (<10 mm in width) wounds. Wounds were evaluated at time of closure, 5 days later, and again 3 months later. Both the patient and a researcher who was blinded to the number of suture layers assessed cosmesis at the 3-month follow-up. The authors demonstrated that although skin closure with a single layer of suture was 7 min shorter, no statistical difference was found between groups regarding aesthetic result. Therefore, cosmetic outcome was not improved by the addition of a second layer of deep sutures to simple interrupted percutaneous sutures for treatment of short facial lacerations [4].

Traditional management of facial lacerations includes closure of the skin with nonabsorbable suture citing the low tissue reactivity that minimizes scar formation and the high tensile strength preventing dehiscence. However, several studies comparing absorbable and nonabsorbable suture in adults reported no statistically significant difference in infection rate or wound appearance [5–9]. In 2008, Luck et al. conducted a prospective, randomized controlled trial comparing absorbable catgut suture and nonabsorbable nylon suture for closure of pediatric facial lacerations. The authors showed that there was no statistically significant difference between the two groups in the rates of infection, wound dehiscence, keloid formation, parental satisfaction, and cosmetic outcome [10]. However in 2013, the same group published again a nearly identical prospective, randomized controlled trial comparing absorbable and nonabsorbable suture for skin closure of facial laceration in the pediatric population. The results largely echoed those of the previous study with no statistical difference in the rate of infection, wound dehiscence, and keloid formation. The aesthetic results were judged using the visual analogue scale (VAS) by caregivers and three blinded physicians. As in the prior study, there was no difference in caregiver VAS score; however, the 2013 results of the physician group found that nonabsorbable suture resulted in a better cosmetic outcome. One of the reasons for this disparity could be accounted by the difference between treatments of absorbable suture at the first physician visit; in 2008, any remaining suture was removed, and in 2013, it was not removed allowing it to completely resorb. Up to 50% of catgut repairs were still intact by day 9, while all nylon was removed by day 7; thus, the longer time to absorption possibly allowed for greater tissue reactivity and could account for the difference in cosmetic outcome, according to the authors [11].

Cyanoacrylates, commonly referred to as tissue adhesives, have revolutionized wound care because of the inexpensive, painless, and relatively easy means to repair low-tension facial lacerations. They provide good tensile strength and bactericidal or bacteriostatic properties and obviate the need for suture removal. A 2009 Cochrane review included 11 studies comparing tissue adhesive with standard wound closure with the aesthetic result being the primary outcome and secondary outcomes being patient pain, time of procedure, and any complications, including wound infection or dehiscence. There was no difference in the cosmetic outcomes between suture and tissue adhesive; pain and procedure time statistically significantly favored tissue adhesive, while only a small increased rate of wound dehiscence was found with tissue adhesives [12].

Two of the studies included in the Cochrane review compared different types of tissue adhesives, one of which published by Zempsky et al. compared Steri Strip® and Dermabond® for closure of pediatric facial laceration. They conducted a prospective, randomized trial that consisted of 100 children divided into two groups: one was treated with Steri Strips and the other was given Dermabond. Pain was measured using a 100 mm pain VAS and cosmetic outcome was measured by two blinded cosmetic surgeons using a 100 mm VAS. There was no statistical difference in pain, cosmetic score, or wound complication rates. The authors concluded that the use of Steri Strips for skin closure was less expensive and provided a clinically equivalent result when compared with Dermabond [13].

Botulinum toxin has also been studied as a therapeutic option to improve the quality of wound healing after facial laceration closure. In 2013, Ziade et al. addressed this issue by conducting a prospective, randomized controlled trial of 30 postoperative patients with facial wounds randomized into patients who received botulinum toxin within 72 h of repair and those who did not. The rationale behind this hypothesis is that botulinum toxin-induced immobilization of muscle activity around the healing wound reduces the muscle tension that acts on the wound edges, thereby decreasing the repeated microtrauma and the chance for hypertrophic and hyperpigmented scars. After 1-year follow-up, cosmetic outcome was judged by the patient, an independent evaluator, and six physicians using the VAS based on photographs. No statistically significant difference was found between the two groups based on patient and independent evaluator assessment; however, the physician group found a statistically significant improvement in scarring in the group that underwent postoperative botulinum injection [14].

The utility of ablative and nonablative lasers for treatment of scars has been well described, and recently, this approach has been applied to minimizing scarring from traumatic facial lacerations. A case series published in 2012 describes the use of ablative fractional resurfacing for traumatic facial scars using an Er:YAG laser after primary repair during the immediate postoperative period. All patients had treatment initiated 1 month after primary repair with laser treatment, occurring four times at monthly intervals. The results obtained 1 month after the last treatment revealed improvement as measured by the cosmetic scale used by patients, independent evaluators, and 10 physicians. The authors concluded that laser treatment is a safe and effective adjunct to postoperative care of facial lacerations; however, more studies including randomized controlled trials are required [15].

*Recommendation*: There is significant variation in the management of facial lacerations and wounds. In general, there appears to be little difference noted in terms of the ultimate outcome of the treatment of lacerations and injuries, depending on the method of repair. Early expeditious repair should be undertaken within 6 h if at all feasible or practical. Either absorbable or nonabsorbable sutures may be considered equal if performed with a small enough diameter and with good technique. The timing of removal is generally best done between 5 and 7 days. The advent of skin glues such as cyanoacrylates have obviated the need for this in some cases and are equally efficacious in providing satisfactory results. Postoperative care with the use of botulinum toxin may be effective in improving the appearance of scars in early studies. The use of ablative fractional resurfacing for traumatic facial scars using an Er:YAG laser shows early promise; however, it is still considered experimental and needs more study.

*Grade of recommendation*: B

## 13.3 What Is the Proper Timing of Repair of Facial Fractures, Especially in the Setting of Neurologic Trauma/Other Injuries?

Facial injuries, in particular facial fractures, have long been noted to be associated with concomitant head and cerebral injuries. A retrospective review of trauma in motorcycle riders found the odds of traumatic brain injury (TBI) were 3.5 times greater with a facial injury than without a facial injury and 6.5 times greater with a facial fracture than without a facial fracture. Additionally, while significantly increased odds of TBI were observed for fracture of all bones of the face, the highest odds of TBI were found in riders with fractures to bones of the upper face [16].

The timing of repair of facial fractures in the polytrauma patient, specifically patients with TBI, has been controversial. It is accepted that the outcome of facial fractures is improved by early repair, as demonstrated in orthopedic literature. Delay of fracture fixation clearly impedes the restoration of both function and aesthetic results by allowing fibroblast migration and potentially increasing scarring, leading to a poor result. The historical concern of deleterious impact on functional neurological outcome posed by the risks of anesthesia during operative intervention has been the basis of a delayed approach to operative repair. A study by Derdyn et al. retrospectively examined clinical and radiographic data in patients with displaced facial fracture and cerebral trauma. They found that a statistically significant worse neurological outcome was predicted by the presence of upper-level facial fracture, low presenting Glasgow Coma Scale (GCS), intracranial hemorrhage, displacement of midline cerebral structures, and multisystem trauma. More importantly, they found no significant difference in survival between individuals who underwent early, middle, or late operative intervention for facial fractures [17]. Furthermore, in 2007, another retrospective review of patients with TBI and facial fracture sought to determine if a difference in postoperative complications was changed by the timing of repair of facial fracture. Of the 99 patients studied, they found an 11% complication rate, and on multivariate logistic regression model analysis, it was found that the odds of a postoperative complication was increased not only by a prolonged surgical procedure but also by a delay in surgical repair [18].

Similarly, in 2008 Janus et al. retrospectively reviewed 34 charts of patients who underwent midface fracture repair at a level 1 trauma center. Early repair was defined as postinjury days 1–5; late repairs occurred after day 6. There was no statistically significant difference between the two groups with respect to operative time, median number of screws used for repair, complication rate, and estimated operative blood loss (although there was a trend toward increased blood loss in the early treatment group). The authors also suggest that midface fractures should be repaired before 14 days, as after this period bone begins to heal and manipulation becomes more difficult [19].

*Recommendation*: Despite the significant correlation between facial injuries as well as head injuries and other traumatic conditions, it appears at this time that there is support for performing early repair of facial fractures as soon as the patient's condition stabilizes. This support, though retrospective, demonstrates that there is little to gain from significant delay in fracture management and that there is no increase in complications from early (postinjury days 0–5) repair. The benefits of early repair in the neurologically stable patient appear to outweigh any possible issues related to delay.

*Grade of recommendation*: B

## 13.4 Are Antibiotics Indicated in the Management of Facial Lacerations or in Facial Fractures, and if So, When?

Antibiotics are used widely in surgery and the management of facial injuries. Growing awareness of the efficacy of antibiotic use in a perioperative setting must be balanced with the emerging threat of complications of prolonged use, the most serious of which is the development of antibiotic-resistant organisms. The profusion of opinion on the use of antibiotics is complicated again by the heterogeneous and varied presentations of the injuries as well as those presenting with dental and oral injuries with their exceedingly high risk of subsequent infection.

It has generally been accepted that patients with simple lacerations do not require either pretreatment or posttreatment antibiotic use [20]. The management of facial fractures and the use of antibiotics in these cases are more complicated. The presence of colonization and bacterial load in the paranasal sinuses and normal flora in the nasal and respiratory tract and then in the oral mucosa represent possible sources for bacterial contamination and the potential for a subsequent infection. Therefore, the use of perioperative antibiotic treatment in these cases has a justifiable basis. Chole and Yee, in 1987, studied 101 patients with facial fractures in a prospective, randomized controlled trial that investigated the role of the administration of cefazolin 1 g intravenously 1 h prior to surgery and 8 h later. They concluded that perioperative antibiotic use reduces the incidence of postoperative infection by demonstrating a reduction in facial and mandibular fracture infection rates from 42% to 9% and 44% to 13%, respectively [21].

In a prospective study that included 90 patients, Heit et al. compared the efficacy and cost of 1 g daily of ceftriaxone and 2 million units of penicillin G every 4 h in patients with compound mandible fractures undergoing surgery. Two patients in each group developed infections. They, therefore, conclude that ceftriaxone is equally effective and carries a lower cost than penicillin G without any increase in systemic toxicity. They also suggest that adding metronidazole to the regimen may extend anaerobic coverage [22].

Abubaker and Rollert conducted a prospective, randomized controlled study in 2001 evaluating the use of antibiotics postoperatively following mandibular fracture treatment. Thirty patients were randomly assigned into two groups, and each group received penicillin G, 2 million U intravenously, every 4 h through the preoperative period, intraoperative period, and for 12 h postoperatively. In addition, the study group received penicillin VK, 500 mg every 6 h for 5 days postoperatively, and the control group received oral placebo using the same schedule for the same duration. Patients were evaluated for signs of infection after 1, 2, 4, and 6 weeks. The study reports that in uncomplicated mandibular fractures, the use of postoperative antibiotic prophylaxis does not seem to reduce infection rate. However, one important limitation of this study was its relatively small sample size [23].

In 2006, Miles et al. sought to determine the benefit of postoperative antibiotic treatment of mandible fractures. They studied 291 patients who underwent open reduction and internal fixation (ORIF) of mandibular fractures in a prospective, randomized trial. The study group received 2.4 mIU of intramuscular penicillin G benzathine, or if allergic, a 5- to 7-day regimen of oral clindamycin. No antibiotics were given postoperatively to the control group. The follow-up period was 5–8 weeks. The authors did not find statistically significant effectiveness in the use of postoperative antibiotics when addressing open mandibular fractures with ORIF techniques. They conclude that there is no benefit to the use of postoperative antibiotics in the patient with the open mandible fracture [24].

Finally, Andreasen et al. published a systematic review in 2006 regarding the role of prophylactic administration of antibiotics in the treatment of maxillofacial fractures. They concluded that 1-day administration of antibiotics is as effective as a 7-day course. Additionally, the authors believe that because of the very low infection incidence in maxillary, zygoma, and condylar fractures, antibiotic treatment does not seem necessary [25].

*Recommendation*: In general, antibiotic use is best reserved for those indications in which there is an established infection. There is little to no role for antibiotics use in a prophylactic manner for facial injuries, such as simple lacerations or general uncomplicated nonbite injuries. There does appear to be a more compelling role for antibiotic use preoperatively/perioperatively in patients with fractures of the maxilla or mandible. This follows more traditional guidelines. As it is so in such cases, the postoperative use of antibiotics, even in mandibular fractures with oral contamination, does not generally seem warranted.

*Grade of recommendation*: B

## 13.5 Which Treatment Is Better for Mandible Fractures: Closed or Open Reductions?

Despite many years of experience with the management of mandible fractures with both a closed approach (maxillomandibular fixation [MMF]) and the use of ORIF, there remains significant controversy about management by proponents of each depending upon the situation as well as the type of fixation. The intervention is aimed at realignment of the fractured segments and prevention of movement by immobilization of the fractured bone, thereby allowing osseous union to occur. In closed reduction, the bone ends or fragments are realigned either manually or using traction devices, and in open reduction, the fracture site is exposed and then internal fixation carried out. The benefit of ORIF is clear as it has been shown that early mobilization and return to functionality is of vital importance to the patient. MMF still has a very important role in those patients who cannot tolerate a longer operation or potentially in complex fractures that require a combination of techniques or potentially in injuries affecting the condyle.

In 2010, Singh et al. conducted a prospective, randomized controlled study to compare these two options for treatment of displaced subcondylar fractures of the mandible angulated between 10° and 35° or the ascending ramus was shortened by more than 2 mm. Clinical and radiographic data were collected 6 months following intervention, and the authors concluded that while both treatment options for condylar fractures of the mandible yielded acceptable results, the open treatment was superior in all objective and subjective functional parameters except occlusion [26].

Eckelt et al. coordinated a prospective, randomized multicenter study in 2006, which included 66 patients with mandibular condylar process displaced fractures divided in two groups according to their modality of treatment: open or closed reductions. Patients had a follow-up at 6 weeks and at 6 months. There was no statistically significant difference in either clinical complications or accuracy of fracture reduction based on radiographs. However, patients who underwent open reduction presented statistically significant improvement of mandible mobility and subjective functional index, as well as statistically significant reduction in disturbance of function, disturbance of occlusion, subjective pain, and discomfort [27].

Collins et al. published in 2004 a prospective, randomized controlled trial that studied 90 patients with mandible fractures, comparing the outcomes of using 2 mm locking plates versus 2 mm nonlocking plates. The theoretical advantages of locking plates include less screw loosening, greater stability across fracture site, less precision required, and less alteration in osseous and occlusal relationship. The difference in overall complication rates according to the type of plate used was not statistically significant, and operative time was the same [28].

Kaplan et al. conducted a prospective, randomized single-blinded study to compare outcomes of patients who underwent ORIF of displaced mandible fractures followed by either immediate mobilization or 2 weeks of MMF. Twenty-nine patients were followed and examined at 6 weeks, 3 months, and 6 months after surgery. The rates of infection, wound breakdown, and inferior alveolar nerve paresthesia, as well as the dentition quality and the quality of occlusion, did not show any statistically significant difference between either patients after immediate mobilization or patients who underwent MMF [29].

All the aforementioned studies were included in a Cochrane review published in 2013, which included 14 studies totaling 830 mandibular fractures not affecting the condyle comparing open and closed management. The review included studies with different interventions including different plate materials, use of one or two lag screws, microplate versus miniplate, early and delayed mobilization, eyelet wires versus intraoperative intermaxillary fixation, and intramural versus transbuccal approach, which was composed of small trials with even smaller sample sizes for each comparison and outcome. As a result, the authors concluded that there was inadequate evidence to support open or closed reduction for the treatment of mandibular fractures without condylar involvement [30] (Table 13.1).

**TABLE 13.1**

Summary of Questions and Recommendations

| Question | Answer | Level of Evidence | Grade of Recommendation | References |
|---|---|---|---|---|
| What is the proper method and timing of closing and caring for facial lacerations and injuries after closure? | Repair should be performed within 6 h with either absorbable or nonabsorbable sutures. Postoperative care with botulinum toxin and Er:YAG laser may improve outcome. | IIB | B | [1–15] |
| What is the proper timing of repair of facial fractures, especially in the setting of neurologic trauma/other injuries? | Early repair in the neurologically stable patient appears to outweigh any possible issues related to delay. | IIIB | B | [16–19] |
| Are antibiotics indicated in the management of facial lacerations or in facial fractures, and if so, when? | Prophylactic antibiotics in nonbite wounds are not necessary. In fractures, perioperative antibiotic use reduces the incidence of infection. Postoperative antibiotic does not seem to reduce infection rate. | IIB | B | [20–25] |
| Which treatment is better for mandible fractures: closed or open reduction? | Performance of open reduction and internal fixation with appropriate size fixation is critical in the development of the best possible result and patient outcome. | IIB | B | [26–30] |

*Recommendation*: Technological advances in composition of rigid fixation with titanium alloys as well as the development of the self-drilling, self-tapping screws as well as the locking plate have greatly expanded the armamentarium of the surgeon caring for the patient with facial fractures. The use of MMF is well tolerated, especially in the medically compromised patient. However, when possible, the performance of ORIF with appropriate size fixation yields the best possible result and patient outcome. Early motion and rehabilitation will allow greater functional improvement and allow for maximal patient benefit, especially with regards to feeding and nutrition. Six weeks of rigid fixation and liquid diet have significant impact of the patient's overall weight and return to function. Therefore, optimal timing of surgery and use of optimal rigid fixation when possible is indicated.

*Grade of recommendation*: B

## 13.6 Conclusion

The management of facial injuries is often complex because of the different anatomic areas involved as well as the multiple specialties necessary to care for these separate issues. Ultimately, the outcome for these patients can be most rewarding, as the resultant outcome may be excellent depending upon proper management. These include appropriate timing as well as the optimal methods and materials used for management both in early and late care as well as in operative treatment. The aforementioned principles have been demonstrated to be effective guidelines in the care of patients with facial injuries.

## References


1. Edlich RF, Rogers W, Kaufman D, Kasper G, Tung MS, Wangeensteen OH. Studies in the management of the open contaminated wound: I Optimal timing for closure of the contaminated open wound; II Comparison of resistance to infection of open and closed wound during healing. *Am J Surg*. 1969;117:323–329.
2. Rui-feng C, Li-song H, Ji-bo Z et al. Emergency treatment on facial laceration of dog bite wounds with immediate primary closure: A prospective randomized trial study. *BMC Emerg Med*. 2013;13:1–5.
3. Gandham SG, Menon D. Prospective randomized trial comparing traditional suture technique with the dynamic sliding loop suture technique in the closure of skin lacerations. *Emerg Med J*. 2003;20:33–36.
4. Singer AJ, Gulla J, Hein M, Marchini S, Chale S, Arora BP. Single-layer versus double-layer closure of facial lacerations: A randomized controlled trial. *Plast Reconstr Surg*. 2005;116:363–368.
5. Fosko SW, Heap D. Surgical pearl: An economical means of skin closure with absorbable suture. *J Am Acad Dermatol*. 1998;39:248–250.
6. Gabel EA, Jimenez GP, Eaglstein WH et al. Performance comparison of nylon and an absorbable suture material (Polyglactin 910) in the closure of punch biopsy sites. *Dermatol Surg*. 2000;26:750–752.
7. Guyuron B, Vaughan C. A comparison of absorbable and nonabsorbable suture materials for skin repair. *Plast Reconstr Surg*. 1992;89(2):234–236.
8. Scaccia FJ, Hoffman JA, Stepnick DW. Upper eyelid blepharoplasty. A technical comparative analysis. *Arch Otolaryngol Head Neck Surg*. 1994;120:827–830.
9. Missori P, Polli FM, Fontana E et al. Closure of skin or scalp with absorbable sutures. *Plast Reconstr Surg*. 2003;112:924–925.

10. Luck RP, Flood R, Eyal D, Saludades J, Hayes C, Gaughan J. Cosmetic outcomes of absorbable versus nonabsorbable sutures in pediatric facial lacerations. *Pediatr Emerg Care*. 2008;24(3):137–142.
11. Luck R, Tredway T, Gerard J et al. Comparison of cosmetic outcomes of absorbable versus nonabsorbable sutures in pediatric facial lacerations. *Pediatr Emerg Care*. 2013;29(6):691–695.
12. Farion KJ, Russell KF, Osmond MH et al. Tissue adhesives for traumatic lacerations in children and adults. *Cochrane Database of Systematic Reviews* 2002; Issue 3. Art. Updated Issue 1, 2009; John Wiley & Sons, Ltd.
13. Zempsky WT, Parrotti D, Grem C, Nichols J. Randomized controlled comparison of cosmetic outcomes of simple facial lacerations closed with Steri Strip Skin Closures or Dermabond tissue adhesive. *Pediatr Emerg Care*. 2004;20(8):519–524.
14. Ziade M, Domergue S, Batifol D et al. Use of botulinum toxin type A to improve treatment of facial wounds: A prospective randomised study. *J Plast Reconstr Aesthet Surg*. 2013;66(2):209–214.
15. Kim SG, Kim EY, Kim YJ et al. The efficacy and safety of ablative fractional resurfacing using a 2,940-Nm Er: YAG laser for traumatic scars in the early posttraumatic period. *Arch Plast Surg*. 2012;39(3):232–237.
16. Kraus, JF, Rice TM, Peek-Asa C et al. Facial trauma and the risk of intracranial injury in motorcycle riders. *Ann Emerg Med*. 2003;41(1):18–26.
17. Derdyn C, Persing JA, Broaddus WC, Delashaw JB, Jane J, Levine PA, Torner J. Craniofacial trauma: An assessment of risk related to timing of surgery. *Plast Reconstr Surg*. 1990;86(2):238–245.
18. Shibuya TY, Karam AM, Doerr T et al. Facial fracture repair in the traumatic brain injury patient. *J Oral Maxillofac Surg*. 2007;65(9):1693–1699.
19. Janus SC, MacLeod SP, Odland R. Analysis of results in early versus late midface fracture repair. *Otolaryngol Head Neck Surg*. 2008;138(4):464–467.
20. Cummings P, Del Beccaro MA. Antibiotics to prevent infection of simple wounds: A meta-analysis of randomized studies. *Am J Emerg Med*. 1995;13(4):396–400.
21. Chole RA, Yee J. Antibiotic prophylaxis for facial fractures. A prospective, randomized clinical trial. *Arch Otolaryngol Head Neck Surg*. 1987;113(10):1055–1057.
22. Heit JM, Stevens MR, Jeffords K. Comparison of ceftriaxone with penicillin for antibiotic prophylaxis for compound mandible fractures. *Oral Surg Oral Med Oral Pathol Oral Radiol Endod*. 1997;83(4):423–426.
23. Abubaker AO, Rollert MK. Postoperative antibiotic prophylaxis in mandibular fractures: A preliminary randomized, double-blind, and placebo-controlled clinical study. *J Oral Maxillofac Surg*. 2001;59(12):1415–1419.
24. Miles BA, Potter JK, Ellis E III. The efficacy of postoperative antibiotic regimens in the open treatment of mandibular fractures: A prospective randomized trial. *J Oral Maxillofac Surg*. 2006;64(4):576–582.
25. Andreasen JO, Jensen SS, Schwartz O, Hillerup Y. A systematic review of prophylactic antibiotics in the surgical treatment of maxillofacial fractures. *J Oral Maxillofac Surg*. 2006;64(11):1664–1668.
26. Singh, V, Bhagol A, Goel M et al. Outcomes of open versus closed treatment of mandibular subcondylar fractures: A prospective randomized study. *J Oral Maxillofac Surg*. 2010;68(6):1304–1309.
27. Eckelt U, Schneider M, Erasmus F, Gerlach KL, Kuhlisch E, Loukota R, Rasse M, Schubert J, Terheyden H. Open versus closed treatment of fractures of the mandibular condylar process-a prospective randomized multi-centre study. *J Craniomaxillofac Surg*. 2006;34(5): 306–314.
28. Collins CP, Pirinjian-Leonard G, Tolas A, Alcalde R. A prospective randomized clinical trial comparing 2.0-mm locking plates to 2.0-mm standard plates in treatment of mandible fractures. *J Oral Maxillofac Surg*. 2004;62(11):1392–1395.
29. Kaplan BA, Hoard MA, Park SS. Immediate mobilization following fixation of mandible fractures: A prospective, randomized study. *Laryngoscope*. 2001;111(9): 1520–1524.
30. Nasser M, Pandis N, Fleming PS et al. Interventions for the management of mandibular fractures. *Cochrane Database Syst Rev*. 2013;7:CD006087.

## Commentary on Facial Injuries

*Krista L. Kaups*

Facial trauma encompasses a range of injuries from a simple laceration to a complex, contaminated fracture with associated airway and neurologic compromise. The significant heterogeneity of these injuries and the potential consequences of treatment choices, both from functional and cosmetic standpoints, contribute to the difficulty of defining optimal management for them. Several things are agreed upon in the care of patients with facial injuries, including the need to observe basic wound principles that have been taught for many decades, including the removal of debris and contaminants, wound cleansing and irrigation and meticulous closure technique, everting skin edges and matching wound edges both vertically and horizontally, as well as an awareness of anatomic forces.

Despite this, a general sense prevails among clinicians that facial injuries are somehow different from injuries to other parts of the body. While primary closure of injuries to other parts of the body after an interval of more than 6 h or so is strongly discouraged, we accept that facial lacerations can be closed even after a relatively prolonged delay. Likely because of the cosmetic implications (and a relative lack of data), debate continues over optimal closure materials and techniques. And, although fracture management for the axial skeleton is defined, the timing and methodology of surgical management for facial fractures has been somewhat more fluid.

### What Is the Proper Timing and Method of Closure? What Is the Optimal Subsequent Care for Facial Lacerations in Wounds after Closure?

As the authors observe, closure of skin lacerations on the face has been found to be acceptable even when longer than 6 h has elapsed from the time of injury. Interestingly, although 6 h is widely cited as a time when bacterial overgrowth becomes excessive, supporting evidence for this is minimal. A number of recent reviews, including a meta-analysis by Zehtabchi and colleagues, demonstrated that delayed closure even up to 24 h after injury was not associated with an increased infection rate*. Similarly, Eliya-Masamba and Banda, in a Cochrane database study, failed to turn up any randomized control trials that allowed comparison of primary closure with delayed closure†.

Closure methods are another area of discussion and dispute. In reviewing the literature, the authors support the idea that an absorbable suture can be used successfully, with less trauma to the patient and an appropriate cosmetic outcome. In a Cochrane review in 2007 without much standardized data, no statistically significant difference was found between suture types in relation to the incidence of wound infection or outcome of appearance. The use of nonsutured closure (either tissue adhesives or tape closure) offers a potentially quicker and less traumatic option to suturing with apparently good outcomes. Again, careful technique and judgment related to the size and specific location of the wound, on the part of the clinician, is essential.

With the limited available data, earlier removal of sutures (at 5–7 days) to minimize scarring appears appropriate. Despite the many adjunctive measures being described and marketed to minimize scarring (silicone sheets and gels, lasers, botulinum toxin, etc.), data to support routine use of any of them is not robust.

### What Is the Proper Timing of Repair of Facial Fractures, Especially in the Setting of Neurologic Trauma/Other Injuries?

From the standpoint of mechanism of injury, the occurrence of brain injury in the patient who sustains forces severe enough to cause facial fractures is to be expected. As our knowledge of traumatic brain injury has expanded, several principles have become clear. Among these are that any occurrence of hypoxia and hypotension in these patients are to be strenuously avoided as they contribute very significantly to worsened functional outcomes for the patient. Additionally, studies evaluating patients as they proceed through their hospital course demonstrate unrecognized and unheralded episodes of both hypotension and hypoxia, emphasizing the need for vigilance. The use of intracranial pressure monitoring and management of intracranial perfusion in patients, with major traumatic brain injuries, is also strongly supported. Close monitoring appears to be particularly important soon after injury. The timing of fracture fixation must be done in relation to the patient's overall status. If operative management of facial fractures can be accomplished with meticulous attention to patient monitoring and avoidance of hypotension and hypoxia, the presence of brain injury does not preclude this from taking place.

* Zehtabchi S, Tan A, Yadav K et al. The impact of wound age on the infection rate of simple lacerations repaired in the emergency department. *Injury*. 2012;43(11):1793–1798.

† Eliya-Masamba MC, Banda GW. Primary closure versus delayed closure for non-bite traumatic wounds within 24 hours post injury. *Cochrane Database Syst Rev*. 2013;10:CD008574.

Additionally, the presence of tissue edema may increase the operative difficulty or increase bleeding at the time of early fracture fixation. Thus, there may be some benefit for allowing edema to subside. Again, the principle of undertaking fixation when it can be most safely accomplished is paramount—while balanced with the need to act before bone healing is underway.

### Are Antibiotics Indicated in the Management of Facial Lacerations or in Facial Fractures and If So, When?

Essential guidelines for antibiotic use include proper drug selection, optimal dosing and route of administration considering the patient's size and metabolic status, and appropriate duration of use. Antibiotic use in the patient with facial injuries has been variable and often based on the preference of the individual practitioner rather than evidence. Certainly, the patient who has a clean laceration has no indication for antibiotic treatment. The management of the contaminated laceration may be more challenging. Copious irrigation of the wound, with normal saline, most likely allows for the best wound cleansing without deleterious effects on wound healing. Prophylaxis for the contaminated wound should be for the shortest period of time possible.

In the management of patients with facial fractures, antibiotic prophylaxis has frequently been continued for a more extended period of time because of concerns about injuries that traverse contaminated spaces including the mouth and sinuses. However as the authors note, reviews of antibiotic prophylaxis in patients with maxillofacial fractures showed equal or perhaps even better results with either a single dose or 24 h treatment. Other recent studies have supported this in comparison of 24 h or less regimens versus antibiotic administration for up to 10 days, showing no difference in infection rates[*†]. Simply stated, longer courses of antibiotic prophylaxis do not benefit the patient and put the patient at risk for the development of resistant organisms and antibiotic-associated complications.

### Which Treatment Is Better for Mandible Fractures: Closed or Open Reductions?

The essential endpoint and management goal for patients with mandible fractures is attaining stabilization of the fracture. As with other fractures, internal fixation, when appropriate, appears to provide the best results overall with the earliest mobilization and return to activity.

### Conclusion

In addressing facial injuries, it is essential that the practitioner evaluate the entire status of the patient, achieving airway and hemorrhage control is essential. Management of injuries should be done in a systematic fashion with wound irrigation, followed by wound approximation that, it appears, can be done even in delayed fashion. The importance of meticulous technique, following time-honored precepts regarding alignment of tissue edges, must be kept in mind. Suture approximation works well although other closure methods also have their place.

Fractures should be addressed when homeostasis is achieved and issues related to intracranial injuries are controlled. Straightforward, clean facial lacerations do not require antibiotic administration. The use of antibiotics for prophylaxis should be limited to the shortest possible time, likely a 24 h period.

* Lovato C, Wagner JD. Infection rates following perioperative prophylactic antibiotics versus postoperative extended regimen prophylactic antibiotics in surgical management of mandibular fractures. *J Oral Maxillofac Surg.* 2009;67(4):827–832.

† Kyzas PA. Use of antibiotics in the treatment of mandible fractures: A systematic review. *J Oral Maxillofac Surg.* 2011;69(4):1129–1145.

# 14

# *Ocular Trauma: An Evidence-Based Approach to Evaluation and Management*

**Jorge A. Montes, Heidi I. Becker, and Mark Kelly Green**

**CONTENTS**



## 14.1 Introduction

Eye injuries are varied and represent a small percentage of trauma cases. Trauma patients often have limited follow-up at the tertiary care centers where they are referred for acute care. Researchers have, therefore, found it challenging to address the paucity of high-quality randomized clinical trials guiding the treatment of ocular injuries because of difficulty with recruitment and follow-up. Ophthalmologists and their acute care colleagues have, in many cases, relied more on historical standard of care guidelines than evidence-based guidelines to treat the variety of ocular conditions that arise in the setting of trauma.

While the nature of ocular injuries has not changed dramatically in the past few decades, the medical and, particularly, the surgical tools available for treating such conditions have evolved significantly. In some cases, the literature has not kept pace with the technology. For example, the guidelines for surgical intervention rather than medical treatment for traumatic hyphema are largely based on the outcomes of studies performed prior to the introduction of refined micro-surgical techniques [1,2].

The goal of this review, therefore, is to clarify the current state of the literature addressing the evaluation and treatment of eye injury after trauma. The recommendations arising from this review are intended to guide clinicians and also identify potential areas of research.

## 14.2 Do Steroids or Orbital Decompression Surgery Improve Final Visual Acuity in Cases of Traumatic Optic Neuropathy?

Traumatic optic neuropathy (TON) occurs with blunt force frontal trauma and also in the setting of orbital hemorrhage or fractures. Patients present with decreased visual acuity, afferent pupillary defects, and decreased color vision in the affected eye. The optic nerve usually appears normal acutely.

Interest in treating patients with TON with high-dose corticosteroids arose in the wake of studies supporting steroid use in the setting of spinal cord trauma. A randomized controlled trial was begun in the 1990s to determine whether high-dose corticosteroid treatment or orbital decompression improved final visual acuity in cases of blunt force TON [3]. The trial, however, was converted to an observational case-control study after it became clear that insufficient numbers of patients would make the study difficult to complete even after years of recruitment. Selection bias thus arose in this retrospective study that relied on individual ophthalmologists, orbital surgeons, and neuro-ophthalmologists to report their management and outcomes in absence of a standardized protocol. Patients included in the study were diagnosed within 7 days of injury and had at least 1 month of follow-up.

The study found that neither optic canal decompression surgery nor corticosteroid treatment had a significant impact on final visual acuity and that improvement in visual acuity occurred in many patients whether they were simply observed, treated with surgery, corticosteroids, or both surgery and corticosteroids. The study was limited by its retrospective and observational nature.

More recently, a Cochrane review examined the literature on TON and found that the literature lacks randomized clinical trials and is limited to retrospective case series such as the study by Levin et al. The Cochrane review concludes that the current evidence does not support treating TON with either steroids or surgery [4,5].

*Recommendation*: TON cases should be observed rather than treated with corticosteroids or orbital decompression surgery.

## 14.3 Does Enucleation Have a Role in the Prevention or Treatment of Sympathetic Ophthalmia?

Sympathetic ophthalmia (SO) is a potentially devastating complication of ocular trauma first described during ancient times and further characterized during the Civil War era. There is the inciting eye, or eye that has been traumatized, and the sympathizing eye. The sympathizing eye is the untraumatized eye that is undergoing an autoimmune inflammatory response by the exposure of ocular antigens by the inciting eye. A bilateral granulomatous panuveitis arises after penetrating injury or surgery to one or both eyes. The majority of cases arise within 3 months of the initial insult with 90% manifesting within 1 year of injury [6]. Modern incidence varies in reports from 0.03/100,000 to 0.2%–0.5% after penetrating injury, a substantial drop from the 16% incidence reported during the Civil War [6]. The decrease in incidence is believed to reflect improved surgical techniques for primary closure of ruptured globes and also is thought to be due to better understanding and recognition of other etiologies of bilateral inflammatory ocular disease such as Vogt–Koyanagi–Harada disease.

Enucleation (complete removal of the eye and a portion of the optic nerve) of the injured eye within 2 weeks of the onset of SO has been advocated to improve final visual acuity. The recommended timing of enucleation is based on retrospective data from a clinicopathologic study conducted in the 1980s. The pathology specimens from patients with a diagnosis of SO at a single center from 1913 to 1978 were reviewed along with the patients' clinic charts. Penetrating injury accounted for just over half of the cases of SO, whereas intraocular surgery was associated with 40.4% of cases. The authors found that enucleation within 2 weeks of the onset of symptoms of SO correlated with visual acuity of 20/70 or better in 74% of patients, whereas acuity in patients who were enucleated later in the course of disease fared significantly worse [7].

Similarly, a second, smaller series examined the timing of enucleation and its effect on visual outcomes as well as the impact of steroid use on final visual acuity. Reynard et al. retrospectively reviewed the pathology specimens and clinical charts of 30 cases of SO. The authors compared the visual outcomes of patients treated with early (defined as less than 2 weeks after onset of SO) enucleation and later enucleation. Visual outcomes of patients treated with topical or systemic corticosteroids were also compared with those of patients who did not receive steroids. The visual outcomes as well as disease severity as graded histologically by the authors were significantly better in patients treated with early enucleation. Patients treated with steroids also had better outcomes than those who did not receive immunosuppressive therapy irrespective of enucleation status [8].

A prospective series published in 2000 examined the more recent incidence and clinical histories of newly diagnosed cases of SO in the United Kingdom and Ireland. This series relied on individual ophthalmologists to report cases to the authors over a 12-month period. The authors found a low incidence of SO of 0.03/100,000 and found that, of the 17 cases that met their inclusion criteria, over half arose after intraocular surgery rather than trauma. The mean age of 56 years and equal gender distribution also reflected the association with surgery rather than trauma. The authors found that enucleation was performed less frequently than in prior reports, and that in one case, a diagnosis of SO was made months after enucleation for recurrent choroidal melanoma. Patients who were enucleated required no less immunosuppression than those who retained both eyes. With immunosuppressive therapy such as corticosteroids, cyclosporine, and azathioprine, visual prognosis at 1 year from time of diagnosis was quite good with over 75% of patients reported to have vision of 20/40. The case series was limited by its small size and might not have similar findings if conducted in a different population where trauma is more prevalent [9].

With current surgical techniques and timely repair, in many cases, an injured eye retains reasonable visual function after penetrating injury. In the unlikely event that SO arises, prompt treatment is indicated. If the inciting eye is blind, painful, or unlikely to regain vision, enucleation may be considered. However, preserving vision in the sympathizing eye requires treatment with steroids or steroid-sparing agents [6]. With the current array of immunosuppressive agents, the inciting eye may also retain reasonable vision, and the literature does not support prophylactic or therapeutic enucleation for SO.

*Recommendation*: The literature regarding SO is limited to case series and clinicopathologic reports. As it stands, the literature does not support prophylactic or therapeutic enucleation for SO.

## 14.4 Does Patching Improve Outcomes of Corneal Abrasions?

Traumatic corneal abrasions are painful de-epithelializations caused by superficial trauma to the ocular surface. Corneal abrasions usually heal well in immunocompetent patients, but they are painful for the patient and have the potential to develop into infectious ulcers. Pain control and supportive measures such as patching the eye shut to speed healing are two areas of interest in the literature.

Turner and Rabiu provide a thorough review of the literature addressing patching. They reviewed 11 papers describing randomized clinical trials from 1960 to 2002. The authors comment that the papers reviewed were of varying quality in terms of randomization and blinding. A meta-analysis of the major outcome of time to heal of simple, traumatic corneal abrasions less than 10 $mm^2$ showed no improvement in healing time with patching [10]. In addition, patching did not reduce pain and also resulted in a loss of binocular vision [10].

*Recommendation*: Patching does not reduce pain or speed healing in simple corneal abrasions and does not have a role in the treatment of simple corneal abrasions.

## 14.5 Do Topical NSAIDs Provide Pain Control in Simple Corneal Abrasions?

Pain management for corneal abrasions has also received considerable attention in the literature. Topical non-steroidal anti-inflammatory drugs (NSAIDs) have been used successfully to treat post-operative pain from corneal de-epithelializations after refractive surgery. Several investigators have examined NSAID use for pain management in the setting of simple corneal abrasions. A meta-analysis in 2005 used stringent inclusion criteria to review the randomized trials in the literature. Eleven randomized clinical trials were identified by the authors, of which five met the authors' inclusion criteria for analysis. Three of the five used similar pain-rating scales, and the data from these studies were used for primary analysis. After meta-analysis of the three randomized controlled trial with similar pain-rating scales, the authors found a significant improvement in pain control in patients using topical non-steroidal anti-inflammatory agents [11]. Although the meta-analysis did not address whether the use of NSAIDs slowed healing of the corneal abrasions, one well-designed study that assessed the time to heal along with pain control showed no significant delay in healing time in NSAID-treated patients over placebo-treated controls [12].

*Recommendation*: Topical NSAIDs reduce pain without affecting time to heal of simple corneal abrasions.

## 14.6 What Medications (Systemic or Topical) Prevent Re-Bleeds of Traumatic Hyphemas?

Hyphema (bleeding in the anterior chamber) may arise spontaneously, after eye surgery, after penetrating trauma, and most classically, after blunt force trauma. Traumatic hyphemas are more common in young males and arise most commonly after assault and athletic accidents [13]. Sequelae of hyphema include corneal blood staining, increased intraocular pressure and resultant optic atrophy, and peripheral anterior synechiae, all of which can decrease final visual acuity. Although corneal blood staining may be transient, children can develop amblyopia and permanent loss of vision even as the blood clears. Final visual acuity may also be limited by other pathology such as macular holes or TON related to the original trauma rather than the hyphema.

Secondary hemorrhages (rebleeds) are associated with higher rates of ocular hypertension, corneal blood staining, and optic atrophy. Visual outcomes after hyphema are worse in cases of secondary hemorrhage, and preventing rebleeding remains a key goal. Those at higher risk for rebleeding include patients with bleeding diatheses or on blood thinners, patients with sickle cell disease or trait, and more darkly pigmented patients irrespective of sickle cell status. A substantial body of literature addresses the medical, environmental, and surgical treatment of hyphema with the goal of reducing the incidence of rebleeding.

Walton et al. provided an extensive review and meta-analysis of this literature in 2002. In several randomized controlled clinical trials, systemic medications such as corticosteroids and the antifibrinolytic agents α-aminocaproic acid (Amicar) and tranexamic acid (Cyklokapron) decreased the incidence of rebleeds over placebo-treated controlled. These studies, however, did not show improved final visual acuity over placebo-treated controls. These drugs, which have undesirable side effects, are, therefore, not uniformly used. The antifibrinolytics can cause undesirable side effects of nausea, vomiting, and orthostatic hypotension. They also must be renally dosed in cases of renal impairment, can precipitate renal failure in hemophiliacs, and are considered FDA pregnancy category C. Topical Amicar is not available in the United States [14].

A 2013 Cochrane review of medical interventions of traumatic hyphemas, which included 27 randomized studies, found that antifibrinolytic agents extended the number of days that the primary hyphema lasted, yet decreased the number of secondary hyphemas. The evidence was limited in supporting a decreased rate of secondary hyphemas by a small number of these events. They also reported no benefit from isolated use of corticosteroids, cycloplegics, or nondrug interventions (binocular patching, bed rest, or head rest) but could not comment on the additive effect of these interventions. No interventions showed an effect on final visual acuity at 2 weeks or less after trauma [15].

*Recommendation*: The literature supports the use of steroids to reduce rebleeds (both topical and systemic). Antifibrinolytics, topical or systemic, have a tendency to reduce rebleeds. The most recent Cochrane review reports lack of statistical significance in the use of antifibrinolytics due to the small occurrence of rebleeds. A larger study is needed to prove their usefulness statistically. If used, there should be caution in patients with a history of gastrointestinal bleeds, sickle cell, or low blood pressure. Antifibrinolytics should be avoided in pregnant patients.

## 14.7 Is Surgical Intervention Indicated to Reduce Complications from Traumatic Hyphemas?

If the intraocular pressure is uncontrolled or corneal blood staining is noted, the hyphema should be surgically removed from the anterior chamber. The studies that guide the timing and technique of surgical intervention were performed in the 1970s and found significantly worse visual outcomes in patients treated surgically versus medically [16]. Although the literature supports a conservative approach to surgical intervention (intraocular pressure above 60 mmHg for 2 days in non-sickle cell patients, for example), the tools and techniques available to the eye surgeon have evolved significantly since these studies. As suggested by other authors, earlier surgical intervention may be warranted, but the studies to support it are yet to be performed [13,14].

*Recommendation*: The literature does not advocate earlier surgical intervention to reduce complications from hyphemas, but the association of surgical intervention with worse visual outcomes arises from outdated data.

## 14.8 Do Intravitreal Antibiotics Prevent Post-Traumatic Bacterial Endophthalmitis? Does Their Use Affect Final Outcomes in Eyes That Are Already Infected?

Penetrating ocular trauma can not only destroy vital intraocular structures but can also, particularly in settings of contaminated wounds and intraocular foreign bodies, cause bacterial endophthalmitis. Treating bacterial endophthalmitis involves injection of intravitreal antibiotics and usually includes sampling the vitreous or anterior chamber fluid for cultures.

While the current standard of care for ruptured globes includes prompt surgical repair and systemic and topical antibiotics, some have questioned whether prophylactic injection with intraocular antibiotics could reduce the risk of developing endophthalmitis in eyes without signs of clinical infection.

A case control study in 2000 examined the effect of prophylactic intravitreal vancomycin and ceftazidime on the rate of endophthalmitis in patients treated for open-globe injuries. Exclusion criteria included full hyphema, endophthalmitis, history of eye surgery within 3 months of presentation, delayed presentation (greater than 72 h), delayed intra-ocular foreign body removal (greater than 1 week), and patients in whom visualization of the needle for intravitreal injection would have been difficult. Thirty-two patients were prospectively randomized to receive intravitreal injections at the time of primary repair, while 38 patients were repaired without intravitreal injections. The method of randomization was not described. All patients received systemic and topical antibiotics and topical steroids. Some patients received systemic steroids. In cases of intraocular foreign bodies diagnosed at presentation, the foreign bodies were removed within 1 week of presentation. Patients were followed-up for 3 months. Although the main outcome of clinically diagnosed endophthalmitis occurred more frequently in the control patients, the difference in the rate of endophthalmitis between controls and treated patients was not statistically significant. The *p* value became significant, however (0.03), if two patients in the treated group with initially undetected retained intra-ocular foreign bodies (eyelashes recovered at time of vitrectomy for endophthalmitis) were excluded from the statistical analysis [17].

A larger, multicenter double-blinded randomized controlled trial was undertaken by Sohelian et al. The authors randomized 346 eyes of 346 patients with open globes undergoing repair to receive either balanced salt solution or gentamicin and clindamycin by intraocular injection after open-globe repair. Exclusion criteria included vision of no light perception, "severe" hyphema, endophthalmitis at time of presentation, and opaque cornea. Monocular patients and children less than 3 years of age were also excluded. Patients received injections at the end of primary repair. Time to primary repair was reported, but time to removal of intraocular foreign body was not. Patients with trauma to the anterior segment were injected into the anterior chamber, and patients with posterior damage received intravitreal injections. Endophthalmitis was diagnosed based on either clinical impression or positive vitreous cultures taken at the time of primary repair. The study found a trend toward lower rates of endophthalmitis in patients treated with prophylactic intraocular antibiotics, and patients with intraocular foreign bodies had statistically significant lower rates of post-traumatic endophthalmitis when treated with prophylactic antibiotics ($p = 0.04$) [18].

*Recommendation*: Prophylactic intravitreal antibiotics reduce the risk of endophthalmitis in open globes with intraocular foreign bodies. Open globes without

**TABLE 14.1**

Summary of Evidence Regarding Evaluation and Management of Ocular Trauma

| Question | Answer | Levels of Evidence | Grade of Recommendation | References |
|---|---|---|---|---|
| Do steroids or orbital decompression surgery improve final visual acuity in cases of TON? | TON cases should be observed rather than treated with corticosteroids or orbital decompression surgery. | 3B, 1B, 3A | B | [3–5] |
| Does enucleation has a role in the prevention or treatment of SO? | The literature regarding SO is limited to case series and clinicopathologic reports. As it stands, the literature does not support prophylactic or therapeutic enucleation for SO. | 5, 4, 3B (Note no Level I or II evidence available) | C | [6–9] |
| Does patching improve outcomes of corneal abrasions? | Patching does not reduce pain or speed healing in simple corneal abrasions and does not have a role in the treatment of simple corneal abrasions. | 3A | B | [10] |
| Do topical NSAIDs provide pain control in simple corneal abrasions? | Topical NSAIDs reduce pain without affecting time to heal of simple corneal abrasions. | 1A, 1B | A | [11,12] |
| What medications (systemic or topical) prevent rebleeds of traumatic hyphemas? | The literature supports the use of steroids and antifibrinolytics to reduce rebleeds. Topical steroids and antifibrinolytics also reduce rebleeds. The decision to use systemic therapy versus or in addition to topical treatment should be influenced by the overall clinical picture and the patient's ability to tolerate the undesirable side effects of systemic therapy. | 3A, 2A | B | [13,14] |
| Is surgical intervention indicated to reduce complications from traumatic hyphemas? | The literature does not advocate earlier surgical intervention to reduce complications from hyphemas, but the association of surgical intervention with worse visual outcomes arises from outdated data. | 3A, 2A, 1A, 2B | B | [13–16] |
| Do intravitreal antibiotics prevent post-traumatic bacterial endophthalmitis? Does their use affect final outcomes in eyes that are already infected? | Prophylactic intravitreal antibiotics reduce the risk of endophthalmitis in open globes with intraocular foreign bodies. Open globes without intraocular foreign bodies may also benefit from prophylactic antibiotics. | 3B, 1B | B | [17,18] |
| Can CT scan accurately detect clinically occult ruptured globes? | CT scan is an important study to obtain in settings of ocular trauma to evaluate for intraocular foreign bodies and associated orbital and facial and head trauma. The findings on CT scan may heighten clinical suspicion for an occult ruptured globe, but CT cannot detect open globes accurately enough to preclude surgical exploration in unclear cases. | 3B | B | [19] |

intraocular foreign bodies may also benefit from prophylactic antibiotics.

## 14.9 Can CT Scan Accurately Detect Clinically Occult Ruptured Globes?

In cases of a full-thickness corneoscleral laceration or obvious uveal prolapse, little question exists as to the presence of a ruptured globe. However, in other cases, such as those with dense or diffuse subconjunctival hemorrhage and hyphema, it can be difficult to determine the integrity of the globe even with detailed slit lamp examination. An unconscious or uncooperative patient presents additional challenges. If the status of the globe cannot be determined clinically, surgical exploration to rule out the presence of an occult open globe is considered the gold standard.

As CT scans are commonly used in the evaluation of the trauma patient, some have questioned whether CT scans may be able to aid the clinician in determining the status of the globe in unclear cases. In a retrospective review of the CT scans of 48 eyes that underwent exploration for occult ruptured globe, Arey et al. found that certain CT findings increased the likelihood of ruptured globe. Three masked observers, two neuro-radiologists and one ophthalmologist, identified several findings on CT that increased the likelihood of the surgeon encountering a ruptured globe at surgery. The positive predictive value of the CT scan ranged from 86% to 100%, but the negative predictive value was much lower at 42%–50%. Although CT scan can be a useful adjunct in evaluating patients for open globes and may increase the pre-test probability of encountering a ruptured globe at surgery, it cannot replace surgical exploration [19] (Table 14.1).

*Recommendation*: CT scan is an important study to obtain in settings of ocular trauma to evaluate for intraocular foreign bodies and associated orbital and facial and head trauma. The findings on CT scan may heighten clinical suspicion for an occult ruptured globe, but CT cannot detect open globes accurately enough to preclude surgical exploration in unclear cases.

## References

1. Read J. Traumatic hyphema: Surgical vs medical management. *Ann Ophthalmol.* 1975;7(5):659–662, 664–666, 668–670.
2. Kunimoto DY, Kanitkar KD, Makar M et al. 2004. *The Wills Eye Manual: Office and Emergency Room Diagnosis and Treatment of Eye Disease*, 4th edn. Lippincott Williams & Wilkins: Philadelphia, PA, p. 22.
3. Levin LA, Beck RW, Joseph MP et al. The treatment of traumatic optic neuropathy: The international optic nerve trauma study. *Ophthalmology.* 1999;106(7):1268–1277.
4. Yu-Wai-Man P, Griffiths PG. Steroids for traumatic optic neuropathy. *Cochrane Database Syst Rev.* June 2013 17;(6):CD006032.
5. Yu-Wai-Man P, Griffiths PG. Surgery for traumatic optic neuropathy. *Cochrane Database Syst Rev.* 2005;(4):CD005024.
6. Chu DS, Foster CS. Sympathetic ophthalmia. *Int Ophthalmol Clin.* 2002;42(3):179–185.
7. Lubin JR, Albert DM, Weinstein, M. Sixty-five years of sympathetic ophthalmia: A clinicopathologic review of 105 cases (1913–1978). *Ophthalmology.* 1980;87(2):109–121.
8. Reynard M, Riffenburgh RS, Maes EF. Effect of corticosteroid treatment and enucleation on the visual prognosis of sympathetic ophthalmia. *Am J Ophthalmol.* 1983; 96:290–294.
9. Kilmartin DJ, Dick AD, Forrester JV. Prospective surveillance of sympathetic ophthalmia in the UK and the Republic of Ireland. *Br J Ophthalmol.* 2000;84(3):259–263.
10. Turner A, Rabiu M. Patching for corneal abrasion. *Cochrane Database Syst Rev.* 2006;(2):CD004764.
11. Calder L, Balasubramanian S, Fergusson D. Topical nonsteroidal anti-inflammatory drugs for corneal abrasions: Meta-analysis of randomized trials. *Acad Emerg Med.* 2005;12(5):467–473.
12. Goyal R, Shankar J, Fone DL et al. Randomised controlled trial of ketorolac in the management of corneal abrasions. *Acta Ophthalmol Scand.* 2001;79(2):177–179.
13. Campagna, J. December 2007. *Focal Points Clinical Module: Traumatic Hyphema: Current Strategies.* American Academy of Ophthalmology: San Francisco, CA, Vol. XXV, p. 10.
14. Walton W, Von Hagen S, Grigorian R et al. Management of traumatic hyphema. *Surv Ophthalmol.* 2002;47(4):297–334.
15. Gharaibeh A, Savage HI, Scherer RW, Goldberg MF, Lindsley K. Medical interventions for traumatic hyphema. *Cochrane Database Syst Rev.* Dec 2013;12:CD005431.
16. Rakusin W. Traumatic hyphema. *Am J Ophthalmol.* 1972;74(2):284–292.
17. Narang S, Gupta V, Gupta A et al. Role of prophylactic antibiotics in open globe injuries. *Indian J Ophthalmol.* 2003;51;39–44.
18. Soheilian M, Rafati N, Mohebbi MR et al. Prophylaxis of acute post-traumatic bacterial endophthalmitis. *Arch Ophthalmol.* 2007;125:460–465.
19. Arey ML, Mootha W, Whittemore AR et al. Computer tomography in the diagnosis of occult open-globe injuries. *Ophthalmology.* 2007;114(8):1448–1452.

# 15

# *Neck Trauma*

**Marc A. de Moya**

**CONTENTS**



## 15.1 Introduction

The neck has been an area that has spawned much debate and research in trauma over the past several decades. It is a region packed with vital structures vulnerable to both blunt and penetrating mechanisms. Penetrating neck injuries, defined as penetration of the platysma, account for approximately 5%–10% of all injuries [1]. Blunt neck injuries, including aerodigestive, vascular, and nerve injuries affect approximately 0.7%–4.2% of all significant blunt trauma patients. This excludes the most common neck structure injured, the cervical spine. This chapter will focus on a few of the most commonly asked questions regarding the evaluation and treatment of aerodigestive and vascular injuries in the neck.

In 1969, Cook County investigators divided the neck into three zones [2]. Roon and Christensen recapitulated this classification in 1979 [3] in an effort to standardize therapy and research efforts. Zone I refers to the area from the clavicles to the cricoid cartilage. Zone II refers to the area from the cricoid cartilage to the angle of the mandible, and Zone III refers to the area from the angle of the mandible to the base of the skull. However, since the first description of the three zones of the neck in 1969, much has changed in how we approach, image, and treat patients with neck trauma.

Mandatory exploration of the neck was the standard of care soon after World War II but led to a negative exploration rate of approximately 56% [4]. In the 1960s, routine operative explorations were challenged in the abdomen by Dr. Nance and Cohn [5] and in the neck by Dr. Shirkey et al. [6]. This initial push for nonoperative management eventually led to more careful selection of operative candidates. Clinicians began to use the hard signs of vascular injury—(1) active external hemorrhage, (2) expanding hematomas, (3) bruit or thrill over the wound, (4) pulse deficit, and (5) a central neurologic deficit—to select operative candidates. Hard signs of tracheobronchial injuries include (1) bubbling from the wound, (2) massive subcutaneous emphysema, or (3) hemoptysis. Some consider crepitance/dysphagia/hematemesis as soft signs of digestive tract injuries. Hard signs of digestive tract injuries usually do not manifest themselves immediately but are more insidious, leading to neck cellulitis/sepsis.

In an effort to decrease the number of negative neck explorations, more emphasis has been placed on the physical exam, new imaging technology, and close observation. As our technology has improved, so has the ability to see otherwise occult injuries, raising questions of treatment. In a series of 146 patients with penetrating neck trauma, 25% of the external wounds did not correlate with the zone of the internal injury, which questions the value of zone-specific treatment algorithms [7]. There are several questions that will be addressed later forming a foundation for the current assessment and treatment algorithms for neck trauma. The following recommendations are focused on the most recent literature.

## 15.2 Assessment of Neck Trauma

### 15.2.1 How Good Is the Physical Exam to Rule Out a Significant Aerodigestive or Vascular Injury?

The initial evaluation of a patient with a suspected neck trauma is the physical exam. Clinicians have been unsure of how reliable the physical exam is as a predictor of a significant aerodigestive or vascular injury. Atteberry et al., in 1994, studied 28 patients with penetrating zone II neck injuries [8]. They compared the physical exam with angiographic, operative, and ultrasonic findings. There were no missed injuries albeit a short follow-up period. The same group performed a follow-up study with a larger series in 2000 after having instituted strict physical exam–driven protocols for neck trauma [9]. This follow-up study with 145 patients over an 8-year period confirmed their earlier study. Again the false-negative rate was approximately 0.3%, which was quoted to be equivalent to false-negative rates of angiograms. The false-positive rate was 10%. In 1997, Demetriades et al. [10] reviewed their experience of 223 patients and claimed that the negative predictive value of physical exam was 100%. Of particular concern is the lack of significant signs following stab wounds to the cervical esophagus.

In penetrating neck trauma, cervical esophageal injuries occur in 0.5%–7%. Meyer et al. reported clinical exam findings indicative of an esophageal injury in approximately 68% of patients with penetrating neck injuries [11]. Weigelt et al. [12] discovered that up to 50% of esophageal injuries were missed in those stabbed, based on clinical exam. Conversely, they describe a 100% sensitivity in physical exam for gunshot wound victims. The early clinical findings described for an esophageal injury include crepitance [13], hematemesis, anterior tracheal deviation, or hoarseness. If the diagnosis is delayed, complications as a result of contamination arise including abscess, sepsis, mediastinitis, or neck cellulitis.

The role of physical exam in blunt neck trauma is not as clear. In those with angiographically confirmed carotid/vertebral injuries, some report that up to approximately 60% of patients lack any hard signs of injury. Therefore, the physical exam in blunt trauma is not consistently accurate in detecting vascular injuries. Injury secondary to blunt trauma has been reported but is exceedingly rare. Tracheobronchial injuries have similar findings as penetrating traumatic injuries with an equivalent sensitivity.

*Recommendation*: Physical exam is adequate to rule out significant airway and vascular injuries. Caution is required when ruling out a digestive tract injury based on physical exam and observation may be warranted.

*Grade of recommendation*: B

### 15.2.2 Are Both Esophagoscopy and Swallow Studies Necessary to Rule Out Esophageal Injuries?

Esophageal injuries can occur in both blunt and penetrating trauma; however, it is exceedingly rare to have a blunt cervical esophageal injury. The lack of more obvious signs, particularly in stab wounds, has led clinicians to use other diagnostic methods to rule out/in an esophageal injury. Clearly the early treatment of esophageal injuries significantly decreases complications and costs [14–16]. The delay in treatment may lead to stricture, dysfunction, and infectious complications.

The diagnostic modalities that one may choose from include an esophagogram, flexible esophagoscopy, or rigid esophagoscopy. Some have found that esophagograms were 90% accurate, while esophagoscopy was 86% accurate [17]. Weigelt et al. [18] reported a 100% sensitivity for the combination of esophagograms followed by rigid esophagoscopy if the esophagogram was equivocal in 118 patients with penetrating neck trauma. Srinivasan et al. [19] in a retrospective study of 55 patients discovered that flexible endoscopy yielded a sensitivity of 100% and specificity of 92.4%. However, this series had a small number of esophageal injuries and overall a small number of patients.

*Recommendation*: Contrast esophagography if completely negative may effectively rule out an esophageal injury; however, esophagoscopy should be added in those cases that the esophagography is equivocal.

*Grade of recommendation*: C

### 15.2.3 How Reliable Is CT Scan for Ruling Out a Vascular or Aerodigestive Tract Injury?

Since the advent of the modern-day CT scan, our diagnostic accuracy has significantly improved, not only achieving better patient selection but also detecting smaller injuries. Once the trauma community began to challenge the notion of mandatory explorations, the reliance on better imaging modalities has evolved. Gracias et al. [20] reported that if the trajectory of the injury was distant from vital structures, no further imaging was necessary. Mazolewski et al. examined the role of CT angiography and found that when compared with operative findings, the CT was 100% sensitive and 91% specific in a group of 14 patients [21]. Eastman et al. [22] compared 146 high-risk patients with both CT angiograms and digital subtraction angiograms. Of the 46 positive findings on digital subtraction, one false-negative CT angiogram was discovered. This injury was a Grade I vertebral artery injury. They concluded that the sensitivity, specificity, positive predictive value, negative predictive, and accuracy was 97.7%, 100%, 100%, 99.3%, and 99.3%, respectively. One other study similar to the parallel CTA versus DS-angio design was performed by Malhotra et al. in 2007. Malhotra et al. [23] did not agree with the Eastman trial and found the sensitivity, specificity, positive, and negative predictive values to be 74%, 86%, 65%, and 90%, respectively. However, if the initial values are eliminated from the study, the sensitivity and specificity values approach the Eastman values. In the discussion, Malhotra suggests that the early data may have been affected by the initial learning curve. Nevertheless, this study provided a warning that the initial optimism for CT angio needs to be tempered and critically analyzed further. In 2014, Paulus et al. [24] published a series of patients comparing 64-channel multidetector CTs to digital subtraction angiograms and found there was a 68% sensitivity versus the 51% sensitivity from their earlier study and the negative predictive value was 97.5%. In addition, 62% of the injuries missed were Grade I injuries with no significant sequelae. They concluded that 64-channel multidetector CTs were now reliable enough to use as a screening modality for blunt cerebrovascular injury (BCVI). Sliker et al. [25] compared the use of a whole body CT protocol with a dedicated CT angiogram for visualization of neck injuries and found them to be equivalent. Both modalities had high sensitivities and specificities for ruling out a cerebrovascular injury. Munera et al. [26] and Nunez et al. [27] demonstrated that the CT scan was also sensitive in detecting nonvascular injuries. Inaba et al. [28] report on 106 patients with penetrating neck trauma. No injuries requiring intervention were missed by CT scan, and it appeared that this potentially reduced the number of unnecessary explorations.

There has been ongoing debate regarding the use of CT scan to rule out esophageal injuries.

*Recommendations*:

1. A 16-slice CT scan can accurately identify vascular injuries and trajectory of bullets.

   *Grade of recommendation*: B
2. A 64-slice CT scan can have a high enough negative predictive value to be used to rule out significant cerebrovascular injury.

   *Grade of recommendation*: C
3. Reformatted images are helpful in detecting tracheobronchial injuries.

   *Grade of recommendation*: C
4. CT scan cannot be used to rule out an esophageal injury.

   *Grade of recommendation*: C

### 15.2.4 What Is the Role of Color Flow Doppler Imaging to Determine Vascular Injury?

Color flow Doppler imaging is noninvasive and readily available. In some series, the sensitivity when compared to digital subtraction angiography reaches 90%–95% [29]. Demetriades et al. [30] and Ginzburg et al. [31] have both published duplex sensitivities and specificities approaching 100%. However, the limitations of ultrasound include the inability to detect nonocclusive injuries with preserved flow, such as intimal flaps and pseudoaneurysms. The technique also fails to detect high internal carotid injuries, which is in fact the most common area injured in blunt trauma patients.

*Recommendation*: Duplex ultrasound may be used to rule out an arterial injury in zone II; however, it is limited in zone I or III.

*Grade of recommendation*: C

### 15.2.5 What Are the Risk Factors for Blunt Carotid/Vertebral Arterial Injuries (BCVI)?

Although the signs and symptoms of significant neck trauma secondary to penetrating mechanisms tend to be fairly straightforward, those for blunt trauma are more obsequious. In the study by Miller et al., only approximately 34% of carotid artery injuries were diagnosed by ischemic changes confirmed by either CT angiogram or digital subtraction angiogram. Thirty-eight percent of the carotid artery injuries were diagnosed based on the suspicion given injury patterns and mechanism. In Fabian's 1996 study [42] of 87 BCVIs, his group suggested in their discussion that the higher incidence of BCVI in their trial was as a result of "aggressive neurosurgical screening." Based on this and other suggestions, the "at risk" group was more actively sought after. The Denver group screened all those patients with mechanisms compatible with severe cervical hyperextension/rotation or hyperflexion, displaced midface or complex mandibular fractures, closed head injury consistent with diffuse axonal injury, near hanging, seat belt sign across the neck, basilar skull fractures particularly involving the carotid canal, and cervical body fractures. In addition to this list, some have advocated the presence of Horner's syndrome to suggest enough force to produce a BCVI, although in a recent study Malhotra et al. [32] discovered that the presence of Horner's syndrome was rarely associated (<10%) with BCVI, suggesting that it may not be necessary to add to the list of risk factors. These recent studies are based on studies almost 30 years ago that analyzed the associated injuries and found a high incidence associated with complex facial trauma, direct neck blows, cervical spine fractures, and near hanging [33–35].

In 2014, Bruns et al. [36] published a series of 256 patients with BCVI and found that 30% of the patients had no radiographic or physical findings, suggesting the need for additional imaging using the aforementioned screening criteria. Although this suggests that the screening criteria may be too strict, further study is required to identify other risk factors as our imaging modalities improve.

*Recommendations*:

1. Cervical spine fractures, carotid canal fractures, seat belt sign, unilateral neurologic deficits, near hanging, and Le Fort II or III.
   *Grade of recommendation*: C
2. A high mechanism of injury may also contribute a high risk for BCVI.
   *Grade of recommendation*: C

## 15.3 Treatment of Neck Trauma

### 15.3.1 Should Penetrating Neck Injuries Be Selectively Observed or Always Explored?

In 1956, Fogelman and Stewart demonstrated that mandatory exploration was associated with few complications and a diminished mortality [37]. Since that time, several authors have challenged the concept of mandatory explorations. This challenge comes around as a result of improved technologies and more careful critical analysis of physical exam. Mandatory exploration produced a negative exploratory rate of approximately 50%–60% [4,38,39]. Over the past decade, larger prospective observational trials have demonstrated success with a more selective approach. Biffl et al. [40] demonstrated in a series of 128 asymptomatic patients by physical exam that only one patient had a missed injury. This injury was from an ice pick. He went on to describe that only 15% of the patients required adjuvant tests. Sriussadaporn et al. [41] observed 17 asymptomatic patients. Only 2 of 40 patients who underwent exploration did not need the operation despite having a "deep" wound. Nason [42] found that 67% of those mandatorily explored had a negative exploration and all zone II injuries were symptomatic. Velmahos et al. [43] described in a large retrospective series that 3% of explorations were unnecessary, and in the monitored group, 9% had missed injuries; however, interpretation of the high missed injury rate was difficult. The only randomized clinical trial comparing mandatory exploration with selective observation was Golueke et al. [44], where there was no difference in hospital stay, morbidity, or mortality in 160 patients.

*Recommendation*: Mandatory exploration and selective explorations have equivalent outcomes.

*Grade of recommendation*: C

### 15.3.2 How Should BCVIs Be Treated?

Much has been written concerning carotid injuries but little is known about how to best treatment the spectrum of carotid and vertebral injuries. The overall incidence of BCVIs is between 0.33% and 1% of all traumas. In 1994, a Western Trauma Association multi-institutional trial described 60 carotid artery injuries [45]. The overall mortality was 43% and moderate to bad neurologic complications were present in over 22%. In 1996, Fabian et al. [46] described treatment and outcomes of 87 blunt carotid artery injuries over an 11-year period. The use of heparin with a goal partial thromboplastin time (PTT) of 40–50 s seemed to independently improve outcomes. In 1999, Biffl et al. [47] developed a grading system for studying and categorizing blunt carotid injuries: Grade I = <25% luminal stenosis, Grade II = >25% luminal stenosis or intimal flap, Grade III = pseudoaneurysm, Grade IV = complete occlusion, and Grade V = transection with active extravasation. They studied 76 patients with 109 blunt carotid injuries and determined that based on their protocol they had favorable outcomes with the use of systemic anticoagulation, however, lacked any controls. In 2001, Miller et al. [48] described 139 BCVIs in 96 patients. Of these, 75 were carotid artery injuries and 64 were vertebral artery injuries. Overall stroke rate for carotid injuries was 31% and the overall stroke rate for vertebral injuries was 14%. Those patients with carotid injuries who received systemic anticoagulation had a significant decrease in stroke rate (6.8% vs. 64%). Those with vertebral artery injuries who received systemic anticoagulation also benefited from systemic anticoagulation with a decreased stroke rate (2.6% vs. 54%).

*Recommendation*: Systemic anticoagulation with either IV heparin (PTT 40–50 s) or antiplatelet therapy decreases stroke rate in Grade II–IV injuries.

*Grade of recommendation*: C

### 15.3.3 Does Endovascular Repair Confer an Outcome Advantage over Medical Therapy for Grade II and III Traumatic BCVI?

There are no randomized controlled trials exploring this question. There are three trials that attempt to address the issue. In 2005, Cothren et al. [49] reviewed their institution's experience with stenting for BCVI. Of the 46 patients with Grade III (pseudoaneurysm) injuries, 50% underwent carotid stents. Of those who underwent carotid stents, 21% had a complication related to the stent and 45% occlusions, whereas 5% of those who were treated medically had a 5% occlusion rate.

In 2011, DiCocco et al. [50] described their series of selective endovascular stent repairs for Grade II and III BCVI. They reported an occlusion rate of 4% when stents were used with appropriate medical therapy, suggesting some patients with severe injuries may benefit from stenting.

**TABLE 15.1**
Summary of Clinical Recommendations

| Question No. | Question | Answer | Grade | References |
|---|---|---|---|---|
| 1 | Is physical exam adequate to r/o significant aerodigestive or vascular injury in penetrating trauma? | Physical exam is adequate to r/o significant airway and vascular injuries. Caution is required when ruling out a digestive tract injury based on physical exam and observation may be warranted. | B | [4,8–11,13,16] |
| 2 | Are both esophagoscopy and fluoroscopic studies required to rule out esophageal injuries? | Contrast esophagography if completely negative may effectively rule out an esophageal injury; however, esophagoscopy should be added in those cases where the esophagography is equivocal. | C | [15–18] |
| 3 | How reliable is CT scan for ruling out a vascular or aerodigestive tract injury? | A 16-slice CT scan can accurately identify vascular injuries and trajectory of bullets. | B | [20–23,25,28] |
| | | Reformatted images are helpful in detecting tracheobronchial injuries. | C | |
| | | CT scan cannot be used to rule out an esophageal injury. | C | |
| | | A 64-slice CT scan can have high enough negative predictive value to be used to rule out significant BCVI. | C | [2] |
| 4 | Can color flow Doppler rule out a vascular injury? | Duplex ultrasound may be used to rule out an arterial injury in zone II; however, it is limited in zone I or III. | C | [29–31] |
| 5 | What are the risk factors for BCVI? | Cervical spine fractures, carotid canal fractures, seat belt sign, unilateral neurologic deficits, near hanging, Le Fort II or III. | C | [46,47] |
| | | A high mechanism of injury may also contribute a high risk for BCVI. | C | [3] |
| 6 | Is selective exploration safe for penetrating neck trauma? | Mandatory exploration and selective explorations have equivalent outcomes. | C | [4,40,43,44] |
| 7 | How should BCVIs be treated? | Systemic anticoagulation with either IV heparin (PTT 40–50 s) or antiplatelet therapy decreases stroke rate in Grade II–IV injuries. | C | [46–48] |
| 8 | Does endovascular repair confer an outcome advantage over medical therapy for Grade II and III traumatic BCVI? | There is no appreciable difference in outcomes when comparing endovascular stents with medical therapy, including those with Grade II and III injuries. Stenting should be reserved for large pseudoaneurysms. | C | [4–6] |

This was followed up in 2014 by Burlew et al. [51] who reviewed 195 patients with Grade II or III injuries. After the aforementioned 2005 report they published, they only performed stents in 2% of patients and found that no patients (109) who were treated with medical therapy suffered a stroke. In addition, they found that none of those patients with Grade II had a rupture of the pseudoaneurysm. They concluded that stenting should only be reserved for those with large pseudoaneurysms (Table 15.1).

*Recommendation*: There is no appreciable difference in outcomes when comparing endovascular stents to medical therapy, including those with Grade II and III injuries. Stenting should be reserved for large pseudoaneurysms.

*Grade of recommendation*: C

## References


1. Demetriades D, Asensio JA, Velmahos G et al. Complex problems in penetrating neck trauma. *Surg Clin North Am*. 1996;6(4):661–683.
2. Monson DO, Saletta JD, Freeark RJ. Carotid vertebral trauma. *J Trauma*. 1969;9:987–999.
3. Roon AJ, Christensen N. Evaluation and treatment of penetrating cervical injuries. *J Trauma*. 1979;19(6): 391–397.
4. Elerding SC, Manart FD, Moore EE. A reappraisal of penetrating neck injury management. *J Trauma*. 1980;20: 695–697.
5. Nance FC, Cohn I, Jr. Surgical judgement in the management of stab wounds of the abdomen. A retrospective and prospective analysis based on a study of 600 stabbed patients. *Ann Surg*. 1969;170:569–645.
6. Shirkey AL, Beall AC, Jr., Debakey ME. Surgical management of penetrating wounds of the neck. *Arch Surg*. 1963;86:955–963.
7. Low GM, Inaba K, Chouliaras K et al. The use of the anatomic 'zones' of the neck in the assessment of penetrating neck injury. *Am Surg*. 2014;80(10):970–974.
8. Atteberry LR, Dennis JW, Menawat SS, Frykberg ER. Physical examination alone is safe and accurate for evaluation of vascular injuries in penetrating zone II neck trauma. *J Am Coll Surg*. 1994;179(6):57–62.
9. Sekharan J, Dennis JW, Veldenz HC et al. Continued experience with physical examination alone for evaluation and management of penetrating zone 2 neck injuries: Results of 145 cases. *J Vasc Surg*. 2000;32(3): 483–489.
10. Demetriades D, Theodorou D, Cornwell E III et al. Evaluation of penetrating injuries of the neck: Prospective study of 223 patients. *World J Surg*. 1997;21:41–48.

11. Meyer JP, Barrett JA, Schuler JJ et al. Mandatory vs selective exploration for penetrating neck trauma. A prospective assessment. *Arch Surg.* 1987;122:592.
12. Weigelt JA, Thal ER, Snyder WH III et al. Diagnosis of penetrating cervical esophageal injuries. *Am J Surg.* 1987;154:619.
13. Goudy SL, Miller FB, Bumpous JM. Neck crepitance: Evaluation and management of suspected upper aerodigestive tract injury. *Laryngosope.* 2002;112:791–795.
14. Symbas PN, Hatcher CR, Jr., Vlasis SE. Esophageal gunshot injuries. *Ann Surg.* 1980;191:703–707.
15. Shama DM, Odell J. Penetrating neck trauma with tracheal and esophageal injuries. *Br J Surg.* 1984;71: 534–536.
16. Asensio JA, Chahwan S, Fornao W et al. Penetrating esophageal injuries: Multicenter study of the American Association for the Surgery of Trauma. *J Trauma.* 2001;50:289.
17. Noyes LD, McSwain NE, Jr., Markowitz IP. Panendoscopy with arteriography versus mandatory exploration of penetrating wounds of the neck. *Ann Surg.* 1986;204:21–31.
18. Weigelt JA, Thal ER, Snyder WH III et al. Diagnosis of penetrating cervical esophageal injuries. *Am J Surg.* 1987;154:619–622.
19. Srinivasan R, Haywood T, Horwitz B et al. Role of flexible endoscopy in the evaluation of possible esophageal trauma after penetrating injuries. *Am J Gastroenterol.* 2000;95(7):1725–1729.
20. Gracias VH, Reilly PM, Philpott J et al. Computed tomography in the evaluation of penetrating neck trauma: A preliminary study. *Arch Surg.* 2001;136: 1231–1235.
21. Mazolewski PJ, Curry JD, Browder T et al. Computed tomographic scan can be used for surgical decision making in Zone II penetrating neck injuries. *J Trauma.* 2001;51:315–319.
22. Eastman AL, Chason DP, Perez CL et al. Computed tomographic angiography for the diagnosis of blunt cervical vascular injury: Is it ready for primetime? *J Trauma.* 2006;60(5):925–929.
23. Malhotra AK, Camacho M, Ivatury RR et al. Computed tomographic angiography for the diagnosis of blunt carotid/vertebral artery injury: A note of caution. *Ann Surg.* 2007;246(4):632–642.
24. Paulus EM, Fabian TC, Savage SA et al. Blunt cerebrovascular injury screening with 64-channel multidetector computed tomography: More slices finally cut it. *J Trauma Acute Care Surg.* 2014;76(2):279–283.
25. Sliker CW, Shanmuganathan K, Mirvis SE. Diagnosis of blunt cerebrovascular injuries with 16-MDCT: Accuracy of whole-body MDCT compared with neck MDCT angiography. *AJR.* 2008;190:790–799.
26. Munera F, Soto JA, Nuniz D. Penetrating injuries of the neck and the increasing role of CTA. *Emerg Radiol.* 2004;10:303–309.
27. Nunez DB, Jr., Torres-Leon M, Munera F. Vascular injuries of the neck and thoracic inlet: Helical CT-angiographic correlation. *Radiographics.* 2004;24(4):1087–1098.
28. Inaba K, Munera F, McKenney M et al. Prospective evaluation of screening multislice helical computed tomographic angiography in the initial evaluation of penetrating neck injuries. *J Trauma.* 2006;61(1):144–149.
29. Kuzniec S, Kauffman P, Molnar LJ et al. Diagnosis of limb and neck arterial trauma using duplex ultrasonography. *Cardiovasc Surg.* 1998;6:358–366.
30. Demetriades D, Theodorov D, Cornwell E III et al. Penetrating injuries to the neck in patients in stable condition: Physical examination, angiography or color flow imaging. *Arch Surg.* 1995;130:971–975.
31. Ginzburg E, Montavo B, Leblang S et al. The use of duplex ultrasound in penetrating neck trauma. *Arch Surg.* 1996;131:691–693.
32. Malhotra AK, Camacho M, Ivatury RR et al. Computed tomographic angiography for the diagnosis of blunt carotid/vertebral artery injury: A note of caution. *Ann Surg.* 2007;246(4):632–643.
33. Stringer WL, Kelly DL. Traumatic dissection of the extracranial internal carotid artery. *Neurosurgery.* 1980; 6:123.
34. Perry MO, Snyder WH, Tahl ER. Carotid artery injuries caused by blunt trauma. *Ann Surg.* 1980;192:74.
35. Davis JW, Holbrook TL, Hoyt DB et al. Blunt carotid artery dissection: Incidence, associated injuries, screening, and treatment. *J Trauma.* 1990;30:1514.
36. Bruns BR, Tesoriero R, Kufera J et al. Blunt cerebrovascular injury screening guidelines: What are we willing to miss? *J Trauma Acute Care Surg.* 2014;76(3):691–695.
37. Fogelman M, Stewart R. Penetrating wounds of the neck. *Am J Surg.* 1956;91:581–596.
38. Saletta JD, Lowe RJ, Lim LT et al. Penetrating trauma of the neck. *J Trauma.* 1976;16:579–587.
39. Bishara RA, Pasch AR, Douglas DD et al. The necessity of mandatory exploration of penetrating zone II neck injuries. *Surgery.* 1986;100:655–660.
40. Biffl WL, Moore EE, Rehse DH et al. Selective management of penetrating neck trauma based on cervical level of injury. *Am J Surg.* 1997;174:678–682.
41. Sriussadaporn S, Pak-Art R, Tharavej C et al. Selective management of penetrating neck injuries based on clinical presentations is safe and practical. *Int Surg.* 2001;86: 90–93.
42. Nason RW, Assuras GN, Gray PR et al. Penetrating neck injuries: Analysis of experience from a Canadian trauma centre. *Can J Surg.* 2001;44:122–126.
43. Velmahos GC, Souter I, Degiannis E et al. Selective surgical management in penetrating neck injuries. *Can J Surg.* 1994;37:487–491.
44. Golueke PF, Goldstein AS, Sclafani SJ et al. Routine versus selective exploration of penetrating neck injuries: A randomized prospective study. *J Trauma.* 1984;24:1010–1014.

45. Cogbil TH, Moore EE, Meissner M et al. The spectrum of blunt injury to the carotid artery: A multicenter perspective. *J Trauma*. 1994;37(3):473–479.
46. Fabian TC, Patton JH, Croce MA et al. Blunt carotid injury: Importance of early diagnosis and anticoagulant therapy. *Ann Surg*. 1996;223(5):513–525.
47. Biffl WL, Moore EE, Offner PJ et al. Blunt carotid arterial injuries: Implications of a new grading scale. *J Trauma*. 1999;47(5):845.
48. Miller PR, Fabian TC, Bee TK et al. Blunt cerebrovascular injuries: Diagnosis and treatment. *J Trauma*. 2001;51(2):279–286.
49. Cothren CC, Moore EE, Ray CE et al. Carotid artery stents for blunt cerebrovascular injury: Risks exceed benefits. *Arch Surg*. 2005;140(5):480–486.
50. DiCocco JM, Fabian TC, Emmett KP et al. Optimal outcomes for patients with blunt cerebrovascular injury (BCVI): Tailoring treatment to the lesion. *J Am Coll Surg*. 2011;212(4):549–557.
51. Burlew CC, Biffl WL, Moore EE et al. Endovascular stenting is rarely necessary for the management of blunt cerebrovascular injuries. *J Am Coll Surg*. 2014;218: 1012–1017.

## Commentary on Neck Trauma

*Kenji Inaba*

The management of penetrating injuries to the neck as outlined by the authors has undergone considerable change over the years. We have moved away from a zone-based approach and now look at the neck as an intact unit. This is due to our understanding that an external hole in one zone does not necessarily mean that the underlying damage will remain confined to that zone. In fact, even injuries that start outside of the neck itself can travel to and traverse the neck, injuring critical structures*. The other major advance driving this approach has been the advent of CT angiography as a screening examination. The contemporary approach to penetrating neck injuries now begins with a physical examination looking for the "hard signs," "soft signs," or "no signs" of vascular or aerodigestive tract injury. Those with hard signs can proceed directly to the operating room, those with soft signs to screening imaging with CT angiography, and those that have no signs can be discharged from the hospital.

In Question 1 (How Good is the Physical Exam to Rule Out a Significant Aerodigestive or Vascular Injury?), the authors address the sensitivity of the physical examination for deciding upon screening imaging, cautioning that digestive tract injuries in particular may be occult to the physical examination. While it is true that the literature reflects the relative rarity of this injury and the poor follow-up, the data cited does not take into account contemporary algorithms where soft signs of injury would trigger a screening CTA. In the Meyer study† for example, only hard signs were examined. Both this and the Weigelt study‡, due to the time period when they were conducted, actually did not have access to CTA. In the largest contemporary multicenter prospective examination of the utility of physical examination–directed CTA in 453 penetrating neck injuries§, the sensitivity of physical examination for clinically significant vascular and aerodigestive tract injuries was 100%. For Question 2 (Are Both Esophagoscopy and Fluoroscopic Studies Required to Rule Out Esophageal Injuries?), as pointed out by the authors, complementary use of the traditional workup modalities such as esophagoscopy and contrast swallow may still be required, even in the era of CTA. It is not uncommon to see a CTA with a trajectory close to the aerodigestive tract, with no discernible injury but significant air tracking suspicious for damage. In these equivocal studies, a conventional work-up should be performed utilizing contrast esophagography (if the patient is able to comply) and direct visualization with esophagoscopy. For Question 3 (How Reliable Is CT for Ruling Out a Vascular or Aerodigestive Tract Injury?), again, the sensitivity of CTA is near perfect across all of the available series using contemporary multislice CTA. Because of this, as well as the availability of CTA at all hours, and the nonradiologist friendly images produced, for Question 4 (Can Color Flow Doppler Rule Out a Vascular Injury?), we do not utilize color flow Doppler as part of our modern day practice. Finally for Question 6 (Is Selective Exploration Safe for Penetrating Neck Trauma?), because the study design, time frame, algorithms, and imaging technology utilized in these studies differ greatly, a head-to-head comparison of selective observation versus mandatory exploration is difficult to perform. In 2015, mandatory exploration should only be considered if there is no access to CTA as the morbidity, cost, and complication burden associated with the significant rate of negative explorations are very difficult to justify.

For blunt injuries, as pointed out by the authors, the data supporting the risk factors, indications for imaging and treatment algorithms is suboptimal. The screening criteria as outlined in Question 5 (What Are the Risk Factors for BCVI?) are the same ones that we follow practically; however, the standard practice across the country likely has significant variation. Once the diagnosis is made, for the treatment questions addressed in Questions 7 and 8 (How Should BCVI Be Treated and Does Endovascular Repair Confer an Outcome Advantage over Medical Therapy for Grade II and III Injuries?), what is clear is that there are no clear answers to what lesions deserve to be treated, the optimal medical therapy, or the indications for employing an endovascular solution. The data is well laid out by the authors; however, further large-scale validation studies are required prior to allowing for any definitive conclusions to be made.

* Low G, Inaba K, Chouliaras K et al. The use of the anatomic 'zones' of the neck in the assessment of penetrating neck injury. *Am Surg.* 2014;80(10):970–974.

† Meyer JP, Barrett JA, Schuler JJ et al. Mandatory versus selective exploration for penetrating neck trauma. *Arch Surg.* 1987;122:592.

‡ Weigelt JA, Thal ER, Snyder WH et al. Diagnosis of penetrating cervical esophageal injuries. *Am J Surg.* 1987;154:619.

§ Inaba K, Branco BC, Menaker J et al. Evaluation of multidetector computed tomography for penetrating neck injury: A prospective multicenter study. *J Trauma.* 2012;72(3):576–583.

# 16

# *Emergency Thoracotomy*

**Joseph J. DuBose and Mina L. Boutrous**

**CONTENTS**



## 16.1 Introduction

Emergency department thoracotomy (EDT) is used as a lifesaving maneuver in an attempt to facilitate resuscitation of patients in cardiovascular collapse following trauma. Despite the aggressive nature of this operation, it has been difficult to effectively evaluate the impact that EDT has on outcomes and resource utilization. Additionally, the definition of "signs of life" and specific indications and protocols for EDT are inconsistent across trauma centers and in the published literature. The conditions under which EDT is performed largely preclude validation in clinical trials. Research on this topic has, therefore, been limited to retrospective reviews and a number of small case series. In the era of evidence-based medicine, there is little evidence on which to establish concrete practice guidelines for this procedure [1–12].

In the absence of conclusive evidence to guide management, the burden for determining the appropriate use of EDT continues to rely on the clinical judgment of trauma providers. Although institutional protocols have been advocated [13], the utility of EDT continues to require a risk–benefit analysis on a case-by-case basis. The likelihood of a favorable outcome must be balanced against the misuse of limited resources, potential for occupational exposure to blood-borne pathogens, and the monetary cost of performing a potentially futile procedure. Appropriate patient selection, therefore, requires thorough knowledge of the available literature and appropriate application to each unique scenario.

## 16.2 Is There a Length of Prehospital CPR Time beyond Which the Performance of Emergency Thoracotomy for Penetrating Trauma Should Be Considered Futile?

Several large, retrospective reviews have suggested that the most favorable outcomes following EDT occur in patients with penetrating thoracic injuries and signs of life on arrival to the hospital [7,8,14,15]. Additionally, other reports have shown that EDT may benefit select patients who require prehospital CPR after penetrating injuries. In a 26-year review of 959 patients who underwent EDT, Powell and colleagues [7] found that among 26 survivors requiring prehospital CPR, 21 (81%) were neurologically functional at discharge. Patients with cardiac stab wounds and pericardial tamponade were the most likely to benefit from EDT, even if they arrived in asystole. Among these five survivors, four (80%) patients requiring CPR for less than 15 min experienced good functional outcomes. In contrast, of those patients with a penetrating injury who required more than 15 min of prehospital CPR, none survived.

In another review of EDT use, Rhee et al. [8] noted an overall survival following EDT after a penetrating injury of 8.8% (273 of 3173). These investigators found that survival following these mechanisms was associated with shorter intervals between the loss of signs of life and the performance of thoracotomy. As the authors pointed out, however, a lack of uniform definitions of "signs of life" across the literature confounded their review.

*Recommendation*: Based on available literature, the most favorable outcomes following EDT are achieved in patients with penetrating thoracic injuries and who have required CPR for less than 15 min. Patients with tamponade following cardiac stab wounds appear to be the most likely to benefit in this scenario. Conclusive evidence of an association between a specific duration of prehospital CPR and optimal outcome, however, has not been identified.

*Grade of recommendation*: C

## 16.3 Should Emergency Thoracotomy Be Performed on Blunt Trauma Patients Who Lose Vitals in the Prehospital Setting?

Favorable outcomes are relatively poor following EDT after blunt trauma. The largest retrospective reviews have documented that an average of 1.4% of these patients will survive; 2% of those presenting in shock and less than 1% if no vital signs are present on arrival [2,4,8]. Of 38 patients injured by blunt mechanisms who required CPR after a witnessed arrest, Fialka et al. reported 4 EDT survivors (10.5%) following CPR for a mean of 13 min [16]. Powell et al. [7], however, identified no survivors among those who had undergone EDT after more than 5 min of CPR. Of the survivors in this latter series, neurologic outcomes were universally poor.

*Recommendation*: Based on the retrospective data available, EDT after blunt trauma is associated with a very low survival and poor neurologic outcome. While rare survivors are reported, there is no evidence to effectively guide appropriate selection for EDT after blunt injury. Limiting EDT use to patients with penetrating injuries may result in a more appreciable survival rate and more efficient use of resources.

*Grade of recommendation*: C

## 16.4 Is Emergency Thoracotomy Effective at Reducing Mortality in Patients with Extrathoracic Injuries?

Some authors have suggested that EDT may improve survival of select patients with extrathoracic injuries [10,17,18]. Several small retrospective reports demonstrate that EDT with rapid cross-clamping of the thoracic aorta may allow temporary control of nonthoracic sources of exsanguinating arterial hemorrhage in agonal patients. In a review of 50 patients who underwent EDT for intra-abdominal hemorrhage, Seamon et al. [10] documented survival with good neurologic outcomes in 8 (16%) patients. All of these survivors presented with hemorrhagic shock secondary to major abdominal vascular (75%) or severe liver injuries (25%). The authors attributed the survival of these individuals to the ability of EDT to establish subdiaphragmatic aortic control and facilitate effective internal cardiac compressions until massive transfusion and definitive hemorrhage control could be accomplished at laparotomy.

Sheppard et al. [18] have specifically examined the utility of EDT in agonal patients with nontorso injuries. Among 959 patients who underwent EDT over a 26-year period, they found that 27 (3%) of them followed penetrating nontorso injuries. All of these patients who had sustained penetrating head injuries died. Of the remaining patients with penetrating injuries to the neck or extremities, three (11%) survived to leave the hospital with good neurologic function and one sustained a mild neurologic deficit.

*Recommendation*: The utility of emergency thoracotomy for patients with nonthoracic injuries has not been well examined. Very small retrospective reports have suggested that the use of this procedure may facilitate salvage in a very select group of agonal patients with exsanguinating vascular injuries to the abdomen, neck, extremity, or head injuries.

*Grade of recommendation*: C

## 16.5 Do Protocolized Approaches to the Performance of Emergency Thoracotomy Influence Outcomes?

Based on consideration of the reported survival rates, risks, and costs associated with EDT use, some authors have proposed the adoption of institutional protocols to guide the most effective utilization of this intervention [13]. The potential impact of such protocols, however, has not been well defined. Aihara et al. [13] described their experience before and after the implementation of an EDT protocol. Their protocol called for EDT only in the event of pericardial tamponade secondary to penetrating chest trauma on patients with obtainable vital signs and unaltered sensorium in the field or on arrival to the emergency room. Compared with the 6 years prior to implementation, protocol utilization resulted in an increase in survival rate from 4% to 20%. Furthermore, the total number of EDTs declined from 32.2 cases per year to 8.1 cases per year. The authors suggested that establishing an institutional protocol may improve survival and minimize potential exposure risk to staff.

*Recommendation*: There are no conclusive data that support institutional EDT protocols. One small, single-center retrospective report has suggested that a protocol confining EDT use to penetrating cardiac injuries with signs of life may improve patient survival and decrease the potential for staff exposure.

*Grade of recommendation*: C

## 16.6 Should the Pericardium Be Opened in All Cases of Emergency Thoracotomy?

Large retrospective reviews have suggested that the greatest survival benefit following EDT may occur in patients sustaining penetrating cardiac injuries, particularly stab wounds. Among these patients, the rapid release of pericardial tamponade and direct control of the source of hemorrhage is paramount to survival. Small retrospective series suggest that pericardial tamponade may be present in as many as 50% of penetrating injuries and approximately 20% of patients undergoing EDT after blunt mechanisms [19]. Among survivors of EDT, pericardial tamponade has been documented in as many as 87.5% [20]. Rapid pericardiotomy via EDT not only facilitates effective evacuation of these intrapericardial collections but also provides access to sources of cardiac hemorrhage and facilitates effective internal cardiac compressions.

*Recommendation*: Although limited to retrospective reports, EDT may have the greatest survival rate for those patients with pericardial tamponade resulting from a penetrating cardiac injury. Therefore, pericardiotomy should be performed as a routine component of EDT. Furthermore, this maneuver may allow direct control of cardiac hemorrhage and will facilitate optimal delivery of cardiac compressions.

*Grade of recommendation*: C

**TABLE 16.1**

Questions, Answers, and Evidence Regarding Emergency Thoracotomy

| Question | Answer | Grade of Recommendation | Level of Evidence | Findings | References |
|---|---|---|---|---|---|
| After which duration of prehospital CPR for penetrating thoracic injuries is EDT futile? | According to retrospective data, EDT after more than 15 min of prehospital CPR is futile. | C | III | According to retrospective reviews, EDT after more than 15 min of prehospital CPR is futile. | [7,8] |
| Should EDT be performed after blunt mechanism of injury in patients requiring prehospital CPR? | Limiting EDT use to patients with penetrating injuries results in better survival rates. | C | III | Retrospective reviews suggest that EDT survival after blunt trauma is <1%. | [2,4,7,8] |
| Is emergency thoracotomy effective at reducing mortality in patients with extrathoracic injuries? | EDT may facilitate salvage in a very select group of agonal patients with vascular injuries to the abdomen, neck, or extremities. | C | IV | Very small series have demonstrated EDT survivors following vascular injuries to abdomen, neck, and extremities. | [10,17,18] |
| Do protocolized approaches to the performance of EDT influence outcomes? | A protocol confining EDT use to penetrating injuries with signs of life may improve survival rates. | C | IV | Protocols dictating EDT use for only penetrating injuries will increase EDT survival and decrease overall number of EDT performed. | [13] |
| Should the pericardium be opened in all cases of emergency thoracotomy? | Pericardiotomy should be performed following penetrating thoracic injury for evacuation of tamponade, direct control of cardiac hemorrhage, and optimal delivery of cardiac compressions. | C | III | Expedient relief of tamponade is a common finding among EDT survivors. | [19,20] |
| Can REBOA serve as a potential replacement for conventional EDT? | REBOA has shown such promising results in the past few years, and there's reason to believe that REBOA could be replacing EDT in the near future. | D | IV | The largest case series to date shows that REBOA is an effective means of proactive aortic control for patients in end-stage shock from blunt and penetrating trauma. | [21,22] |

## 16.7 Can Resuscitative Endovascular Balloon Occlusion of the Aorta (REBOA) Serve as a Potential Replacement for Conventional EDT?

Previously utilized for the endovascular control or rupturing aortic aneurysms, Rasmussen et al. [21] were among the first to introduce the concept of proximal balloon occlusion for trauma in 2011. The technique, termed resuscitative balloon occlusion of the aorta, or REBOA, may serve as a useful adjunct in preserving blood flow to the brain and heart in the setting of hemorrhagic shock. The largest published series to date, consisting of preliminary experience with six patients with hemorrhagic shock after trauma, has demonstrated the potential of this approach [22]. A prospective multicenter observational study being conducted by the American Association for the Surgery of Trauma is designed to examine the results of this adjunct on a larger scale. Several groups have introduced curriculum designed to familiarize trauma providers with REBOA, including the Endovascular Skills for Trauma and Resuscitative Surgery course [22] (Table 16.1).

*Recommendation*: REBOA has shown such promising results in the past few years. However, future work should concentrate on formulating devises that can be feasibly used by trauma surgeons and emergency doctors alike. With larger prospective clinical trials underway, there's reason to believe that REBOA could be replacing EDT in the near future.

*Grade of recommendation*: D

## References


1. Arreola-Risa C, Rhee P, Boyle EM, Maier RV, Jurkovich GG, Foy HM. Factors influencing outcome in stab wounds of the heart. *Am J Surg.* 1995;169:553–556.
2. Cothren CC, Moore EE. Emergency department thoracotomy for the critically injured patient: Objectives, indications, and outcomes. *World J Emerg Surg.* 2006;1:4.
3. Hall BL, Buchman TG. A visual, timeline-based display of evidence for emergency thoracotomy. *J Trauma.* 2005;59:773–777.
4. Hunt PA, Greaves I, Owens WA. Emergency thoracotomy in thoracic trauma—A review. *Injury.* 2006;37:1–19.
5. Karmy-Jones R, Nathens A, Jurkovich GJ et al. Urgent and emergent thoracotomy for penetrating chest trauma. *J Trauma.* 2004;56:664–668; discussion 668–669.
6. Mejia JC, Stewart RM, Cohn SM. Emergency department thoracotomy. *Semin Thorac Cardiovasc Surg.* 2008;20:13–18.
7. Powell DW, Moore EE, Cothren CC et al. Is emergency department resuscitative thoracotomy futile care for the critically injured patient requiring prehospital cardiopulmonary resuscitation? *J Am Coll Surg.* 2004;199:211–215.
8. Rhee PM, Acosta J, Bridgeman A, Wang D, Jordan M, Rich N. Survival after emergency department thoracotomy: Review of published data from the past 25 years. *J Am Coll Surg.* 2000;190:288–298.
9. Seamon MJ, Fisher CA, Gaughan J et al. Prehospital procedures before emergency department thoracotomy: "Scoop and run" saves lives. *J Trauma.* 2007;63:113–120.
10. Seamon MJ, Fisher CA, Gaughan JP, Kulp H, Dempsey DT, Goldberg AJ. Emergency department thoracotomy: Survival of the least expected. *World J Surg.* 2008;32:604–612.
11. Soreide K, Petrone P, Asensio JA. Emergency thoracotomy in trauma: Rationale, risks, and realities. *Scand J Surg.* 2007;96:4–10.
12. Soreide K, Soiland H, Lossius HM, Vetrhus M, Soreide JA, Soreide E. Resuscitative emergency thoracotomy in a Scandinavian trauma hospital—Is it justified? *Injury.* 2007;38:34–42.
13. Aihara R, Millham FH, Blansfield J, Hirsch EF. Emergency room thoracotomy for penetrating chest injury: Effect of an institutional protocol. *J Trauma.* 2001;50:1027–1030.
14. Baxter BT, Moore EE, Moore JB, Cleveland HC, McCroskey BL, Moore FA. Emergency department thoracotomy following injury: Critical determinants for patient salvage. *World J Surg.* 1988;12:671–675.
15. Working Group, Ad Hoc Subcommittee on Outcomes, American College of Surgeons. Committee on Trauma. Practice management guidelines for emergency department thoracotomy. Working group, ad hoc subcommittee on outcomes, American college of surgeons-committee on trauma. *J Am Coll Surg.* 2001;193:303–309.
16. Fialka C, Sebok C, Kemetzhofer P, Kwasny O, Sterz F, Vecsei V. Open-chest cardiopulmonary resuscitation after cardiac arrest in cases of blunt chest or abdominal trauma: A consecutive series of 38 cases. *J Trauma.* 2004;57:809–814.
17. Asensio JA, Arroyo H, Jr., Veloz W et al. Penetrating thoracoabdominal injuries: Ongoing dilemma-which cavity and when? *World J Surg.* 2002;26:539–543.
18. Sheppard FR, Cothren CC, Moore EE et al. Emergency department resuscitative thoracotomy for nontorso injuries. *Surgery.* 2006;139:574–576.
19. Grove CA, Lemmon G, Anderson G, McCarthy M. Emergency thoracotomy: Appropriate use in the resuscitation of trauma patients. *Am Surg.* 2002;68:313–316; discussion 316–317.
20. Lewis G, Knottenbelt JD. Should emergency room thoracotomy be reserved for cases of cardiac tamponade? *Injury.* 1991;22:5–6.
21. Stannard A, Eliason JL, Rasmussen TE. Resuscitative endovascular balloon occlusion of the aorta (REBOA) as an adjunct for hemorrhagic shock. *J Trauma.* 2011;71(6):1869–1872.
22. Brenner ML, Moore LJ, DuBose JJ, Tyson GH, McNutt MK, Albarado RP, Holcomb JB, Scalea TM, Rasmussen TE. A clinical series of resuscitative endovascular balloon occlusion of the aorta for hemorrhage control and resuscitation. *J Trauma Acute Care Surg.* 2013;75(3):506–511.

## Commentary on Emergency Thoracotomy

*Ernest E. Moore*

Drs. DuBose and Boutrous have nicely addressed the prevailing controversies surrounding resuscitative emergency department thoracotomy (EDT), and emphasize the dearth of quality data to enable the development of evidence-based guidelines.

### Prehospital CPR Time Limit for Penetrating Trauma?

The fundamental issue is whether there is a definable time interval beyond which patients are unsalvageable or are revived but remain neurologic invalids. As acute care surgeons, we do not want to deny patients an opportunity for meaningful survival, but, on the other hand, we have a societal obligation to be financially responsible. A recent multicenter prospective study of the Western Trauma Association (WTA) has further validated the 15 min CPR threshold for penetrating wounds*. However, the topic is complicated by the prospect of organ donation for EDT survivors who are ultimately declared brain dead†.

### Role in Blunt Trauma?

While meaningful survival following EDT for blunt trauma is relatively low, there is undisputed documentation of success, even in those arriving in the ED without vital signs. The WTA study* reported survival with up to 10 min of prehospital CPR and, as the authors indicated, there is survival reported for even greater times of prehospital CPR for blunt trauma survivors.

### Role in Extrathoracic Trauma?

The rationale for EDT following extrathoracic trauma is to redistribute limited blood volume to the coronary and cerebral vascular beds and, arrest subdiaphragmatic arterial blood loss, and facilitate internal cardiac massage. There is clear evidence that this concept is life-saving in a select group of patients with near-exsanguination. However, REBOA achieves the first two objectives of EDT in this scenario, and may supplant EDT in those patients arriving in profound shock without cardiac arrest (see section "Pericardiotomy during EDT?").

### Protocols for EDT?

While there may be no randomized data to support protocols, most Level I trauma centers have guidelines for this relatively high cost/low yield procedure. The WTA has recently developed a consensus-driven algorithm for EDT‡.

### Pericardiotomy during EDT?

Pericardiotomy is an integral component of EDT for potential cardiac injuries to accomplish rapid control of cardiac bleeding. However, access for internal cardiac massage and direct observation of myocardial performance are also compelling arguments in the patient arriving with cardiac arrest.

### Will REBOA Replace EDT?

For patients with a detectable perfusion pressure, REBOA can replace EDT for Zone III injuries with the possible exception of a transected external iliac artery§. But application for Zone II injuries is controversial, and a viable role for Zone I injuries remains to be established when trained surgeons are available¶. Moreover, it is unlikely REBOA will replace EDT for patients arriving with CPR in progress.

---

* Moore EE, Knudson MM, Burlew CC et al. Defining the limits of resuscitative emergency department thoracotomy: A contemporary Western Trauma Association perspective. *J Trauma*. 2011;70(2):334–339.

† Schnuriger B, Inaba K, Bernardino BC, Salim A, Russell K, Lam L, Plurad D, Demetriades D. Organ donation: An important outcome after resuscitative thoracotomy. *J Am Coll Surg*. 2010;211:450–455.

‡ Burlew CC, Moore EE, Moore FA, Coimbra R, McIntyre RC Jr., Davis JW, Sperry J, Biffl WL. Western Trauma Association critical decisions in trauma: Resuscitative thoracotomy. *J Trauma Acute Care Surg*. 2012;73(6):1359–1363.

§ Morrison JJ, Percival TJ, Markov NP, Villamaria C, Scott DJ, Saches KA, Spencer JR, Rassmussen TE. Aortic balloon occlusion is effective in controlling pelvic hemorrhage. *J Surg Res*. 2012;177:341–347.

¶ Norii T, Grandall CS, Terasaka Y. Survival of severe blunt trauma patients with resuscitative endovascular balloon occlusion of the aorta compared to propensity score adjusted untreated patients. *J Trauma Acute Care Surg*. 2012;70:334–339.

# 17

# *Chest Wall Trauma*

**John K. Bini**

CONTENTS



Trauma to the chest wall is common and may account for up to one-quarter of all traumatic deaths. Because thoracic trauma accounts for a significant portion of traumatic morbidity and mortality, proper management of these injuries has the potential to significantly and positively impact trauma outcomes. Many clinical questions surround the management of chest wall trauma and significant clinical equipoise exists. Unfortunately, this is one area where robust data guiding management is often lacking. Questions exist regarding the optimal management of acute open pneumothorax, optimal treatment for tension pneumothorax, autotransfusion for hemothorax, optimal chest drainage tube size, and surgical stabilization of multiple rib fractures or flail chest. The lack of level 1, 2, and in some cases level 3 evidence makes answering all these questions in the setting of an evidence-based text impracticable. This chapter will answer and make recommendations in areas where sufficient evidence exists, specifically in the areas of surgical stabilization of the chest wall, autotransfusion, and selection of chest tube size.

## 17.1 Should Open Reduction and Internal Fixation Be Performed Routinely on Trauma Patients with Flail Chest?

### 17.1.1 What Patients Should Be Considered for Open Reduction Internal Fixation (ORIF) of Rib Fractures?

It has been reported that up to 25% of annual traumatic deaths result from chest trauma. Flail chest may be seen in as many as 6% of patients (82 of 1417) sustaining blunt chest trauma [1–3]. Mortality rates of up to 12% (84 of 711) for patients with multiple rib fractures and up to 33% (30 of 92) for patients with a flail chest have been reported [4–6]. A study of 181,331 adults in the National Trauma Data Bank showed that the odds ratio for death for younger patients and patients over 64 years of age. If two patients have similar nonrib trauma, the one with rib fractures will have a substantially higher expected risk of death than one without. This effect is more pronounced for older patients [6].

Studies have demonstrated a direct correlation between the number of rib fractures and intrathoracic injury, morbidity, and mortality [3]. In particular, patients who have had a flail chest often report long-term dyspnea and chest pain and have abnormal test results on spirometry [7]. Bulger et al. [8] found that elderly patients with rib fractures had twice the mortality and thoracic morbidity compared with younger patients with similar injuries. In their study, for each additional rib fracture in the elderly patient, mortality increased by 19% and the risk of pneumonia increased by 27%.

Rib fractures are frequently associated with pulmonary contusions [5] and multiple rib fractures predispose patients to pulmonary insufficiency and compromised ventilation. In patients with a flail chest, paradoxical chest wall motion and pain can result in low tidal volumes, alveolar collapse, arteriovenous shunting, and hypoxemia, resulting in prolonged mechanical ventilation [9]. This may cause complications such as pneumonia and sepsis [10,11].

Because the stability of the chest wall is intimately related to the ability to ventilate and subsequently oxygenate, it may seem almost intuitive that stabilization of the bony thorax would result in improved ventilation and ultimately improve outcomes in this patient population. Therefore, the structural integrity of the chest wall provides a theoretical advantage of improved lung functional reserve following surgical stabilization secondary to restoration of greater lung volumes.

Nonoperative management has been associated with substantial pain and discomfort [9]. Fractured ribs managed nonoperatively are cyclically displaced during breathing while they are healing. This may lead to malunion or nonunion, which may require future surgery [12,13]. The key to nonoperative management relies fully on various pain control methods (IV and oral narcotics, nonsteroidal anti-inflammatory medications, intercostal and paravertebral blocks, patient-controlled analgesia, pleural catheters, and epidural analgesia), pulmonary toilet, and, if necessary, positive pressure mechanical ventilation. Reported long-term problems are rare, and most broken ribs heal uneventfully.

Ultimately, significant clinical equipoise exists regarding the management of rib fractures surgically and operative intervention remains controversial [14]. Reported short-term benefits of ORIF of rib fractures and flail chest include earlier restoration of pulmonary function [9,11,15], fewer complications associated with mechanical ventilation [10,11,16,17], and more intensive care unit (ICU)- and hospital-free days [9,11]. Some of the potential long-term benefits of surgical fixation may be reduced long-term pain, pulmonary dysfunction, and skeletal deformity [20,34].

The Eastern Association for the Surgery of Trauma (EAST) Practice Management Guidelines for "Pulmonary Contusion—Flail Chest" [18] state that although improvement has not been definitively shown in any outcome parameter after surgical fixation of flail chest (FC), this modality may be considered in cases of severe FC failing to wean from the ventilator or when thoracotomy is required for other reasons. The patient subgroup that would benefit from early "prophylactic" fracture fixation has not been identified and there is insufficient clinical evidence to recommend any type of proprietary implant for surgical fixation of rib fractures. However, in vitro studies indicate that rib plating or wrapping devices are likely superior to intramedullary wires. EAST goes on to say that self-activating multidisciplinary protocols for the treatment of chest wall injuries may improve outcome and should be considered where feasible. All these recommendations, however, are level 3 because most studies are retrospective case series and the one prospective randomized trial by Tanaka et al. [11] had very few numbers (37 patients). They also noted that there are no prospective, randomized controlled studies comparing surgical fixation with modern conservative treatment with epidural analgesia and chest physiotherapy. Consequently, although surgical fixation clearly corrects the anatomic chest deformity, comparison of its efficacy with that of conservative treatment remains problematic.

Tanaka et al. [11] randomized 37 patients at 5 days after injury to be treated with surgical fixation or internal pneumatic stabilization. Ventilator management was the same for both groups and at 1 month following injury, patients who underwent surgery required less vent support ($p < 0.05$) and had lower rates of pneumonia ($p < 0.05$), more ICU-free days ($p < 0.05$), and lower medical costs ($p < 0.05$) than patients treated with intubation and mechanical ventilation. They also showed that patients who underwent surgical stabilization had improved early FEV1 and significantly more of them were able to return to their previous employment 6 months after injury.

Granetzny et al. [19] conducted a randomized trial of 40 patients with flail chest. The operatively treated group was compared with patients treated with external adhesive plaster. Eighty-five percent of the patients in the surgical group achieved chest wall stability, while only 50% of the nonoperative group achieved stability. The operatively managed patients required an average of 2 days on the ventilator, while the nonoperative patients spent an average of 12 days on the vent. Pulmonary function tests at 2 months indicated that the operatively treated group had a significantly less restrictive pattern ($p < 0.001$), as indicated by measurement of forced vital capacity and total lung capacity. The surgical group also had significantly fewer days in the ICU and as in-patients ($p < 0.001$) along with having a lower rate of pneumonia ($p = 0.014$).

Mayberry et al. [20] performed a retrospective review of long-term outcomes of 46 patients who had surgical repair of severe chest wall injuries. They reported the indications for surgery were: flail chest with an inability to be weaned from the ventilator, acute intractable pain, acute chest wall defects/deformity, acute pulmonary herniation, and thoracotomy for other traumatic indications. Fifteen patients with a mean age of 60.6 years (range, 30–91 years) were surveyed at a mean of 48.5 ± 22.3 months (range, 19–96 months) postinjury. RAND-36 indices [20] showed equivalent or better health status compared with reference populations, with the exception of role limitations due to physical problems when compared with the general population.

Ahmed and Mohyuddin [9] retrospectively reviewed 64 cases of flail chest over a 10-year period. Twenty-six patients were treated operatively and 38 were treated with intubation and mechanical ventilation. The surgical group had an average 3.9 ventilator days, and 80% of the patients were liberated from the ventilator in 1.3 days. The patients treated nonoperatively had an average of 15 ventilator days. The surgical group had a mortality rate of 8% compared with 29% in the nonoperative group. Thirty-seven percent of the nonoperative patients required tracheostomy compared with only 11% in the operative group. The surgical group in this study also had lower infectious complication rates and fewer days in the ICU. They concluded that surgical stabilization of chest wall injuries was superior to nonoperative management and resulted in lower complication rates, faster recovery, and better cosmetic results.

Nirula et al. [21] conducted a retrospective case–control study comparing 30 patients treated surgically with 30 controls and found a trend toward fewer vent days in the surgical group (2.9 days compared with 9.4 days in the control group). They concluded that surgical fixation of rib fractures may reduce ventilator days in trauma patients with multiple rid fractures with severe thoracic injuries.

Karev [16] reported on 133 consecutive patients with flail chest. Forty patients were treated surgically and 93 were treated nonoperatively. Surgical fixation was performed within 24 h of admission. Nonoperative treatment was done with mechanical ventilation and epidural and regional anesthesia. This group recommended that surgical fixation should be considered when extensive flail chest is present, particularly for patients with severe pulmonary and heart contusion.

Doben et al. [22] conducted a retrospective case–control study evaluating outcomes of patients undergoing surgical fixation of flail chest injuries ($n$ = 10) to those managed nonoperatively ($n$ = 11). Surgical fixation in this study was performed as a rescue therapy for those patients who failed to wean from mechanical ventilation. Failure to wean was defined as failing three consecutive spontaneous breathing trials. This small study showed a significant reduction in total ventilator days in patients who underwent surgery represents. Their results did not demonstrate significant decreases in ICU length of stay or hospital length of stay.

Voggenreiter et al. [15] attempted to address what may be the key question regarding surgical fixation of flail chest, patient selection. They retrospectively compared 20 patients treated operatively and 22 treated nonoperatively and divided them into four groups: group 1, operative chest wall stabilization in flail chest without pulmonary contusion ($n$ = 10); group 2, operative chest wall stabilization in flail chest with pulmonary contusion ($n$ = 10); group 3, flail chest without pulmonary contusion and without chest wall stabilization ($n$ = 18); and group 4, flail chest with pulmonary contusion and without chest wall stabilization ($n$ = 4). In patients with flail chest who did not have pulmonary contusions, surgical stabilization resulted in earlier ventilator liberation. Interestingly, those patients with significant pulmonary contusions did not benefit from surgery. The results of this study suggest that pulmonary contusion is a relative contraindication to operative fixation and is an independent risk factor for the failure of operative management to provide a clinical benefit.

*Recommendation*: Current literature shows no clear evidence that surgical stabilization of flail chest injuries should be performed on a routine basis. However, there is level 2 and 3 evidence that suggest surgical stabilization should be considered in patients with significant chest wall injury and no underlying pulmonary contusion. It should also be considered in patients with flail chest who fail to wean from mechanical ventilation or who are undergoing thoracotomy for another reason. Based on available trials and reviews, these are grade B recommendations.

## 17.2 In Trauma Patients with Traumatic Hemothorax Who Require Blood Transfusion, Should Blood Collected from the Hemothorax Routinely Be Autotransfused?

Historically, autotransfusion has been described in both the civilian and military literature [23,24]. In 1957, Ferrara published an article in the *Southern Medical Journal* describing the technique at his facility for performing autotransfusion in the setting of a traumatic hemothorax [24]. The technique of autotransfusion with blood drained from a hemothorax has been described clinically for nearly 80 years [25]. Concerns regarding the safety of transfused blood have prompted reconsideration of the use of allogeneic (from an unrelated donor) red blood cell (RBC) transfusion, and a range of techniques to minimize transfusion requirements [26].

Although the practice of autotransfusion is well described historically, it is not well studied in the trauma population. It has been most rigorously studied in the cardiac surgery population [27–30]. In the trauma literature, the majority of clinical reports are case series and case reports that are descriptive in nature [23,24,30,31]. There are prospective randomized studies in the trauma literature; however, they primarily look at variance in laboratory indicators of coagulation and not clinical outcomes or studies of efficacy [32,34,35].

Body et al. [27] conducted a multicenter prospective trial to determine the efficacy and safety of autotransfusion of mediastinal blood in 617 patients undergoing elective primary coronary artery bypass grafting. The independent effect of SMB (shed mediastinal blood) transfusion on postoperative RBC transfusion was examined by multivariable modeling. The investigators evaluated potential complications of SMB transfusion, such as bleeding and infection. Three hundred and twelve of the study patients (51%) received postoperative SMB transfusion (mean volume, 554 ± 359 mL).

Patients transfused with SMB had significantly lower volumes of RBC transfusion than those not receiving SMB (0.86 ± 1.50 vs. 1.08 ± 1.65 units; $p < 0.05$). However, multivariable analysis showed that SMB transfusion was not predictive of postoperative RBC transfusion. The volume of chest tube drainage on the operative day (707 ± 392 vs. 673 ± 460 mL; $p = 0.30$), reoperation for hemorrhage (3.1% vs. 2.5%; $p = 0.68$), and overall frequency of infection (5.8% vs. 6.6%; $p = 0.81$) were similar between patients receiving and not receiving SMB, respectively. However, in patients who did not receive allogenic RBC transfusion, there was a significantly greater frequency of wound infection in the SMB group (3.6% vs. 0%; $p = 0.02$). These findings led the authors to conclude that SMB is ineffective as a blood conservation method and may be associated with a greater frequency of wound infection [27].

Helm et al. [28] conducted a prospective randomized study of patients undergoing coronary artery bypass or cardiac valve surgery to determine the benefit of the acute removal and reinfusion of fresh autologous blood around the time of cardiopulmonary bypass—a technique known as intraoperative autologous donation (IAD). Ninety patients were prospectively randomized to either have (IAD group) or not have (control group) calculated maximum volume IAD performed. The investigators found that postoperative hematocrits were significantly greater at 12 and 24 h postoperatively in the IAD group versus the control group, despite a significant decrease in both the percentage of patients in whom allogeneic RBCs were transfused (17% vs. 52%; $p < 0.01$) and the number of RBC units transfused per patient per group (0.28 ± 0.66 and 1.14 ± 1.19 units; $p < 0.01$). However, they observed that chest tube output, incidence of excessive postoperative bleeding, postoperative prothrombin time, and platelet and coagulation factor transfusion requirement did not differ between groups. Based on their results, they concluded that intraoperative autologous donation serves to preserve RBC mass and its routine use in eligible patients was justified. However, they concluded that autotransfusion had no effect on postoperative bleeding or platelet and coagulation factor transfusion requirement [28].

Ward et al. [30] prospectively randomized 35 consecutive cardiac surgery patients into two groups. The experimental group ($n = 18$) received autotransfusion for 12 h after completion of the operative procedure. The control group ($n = 17$) was treated with standard chest drainage and fluid replacement. Both groups received homologous blood transfusion when the hemoglobin level fell to less than 8.0 g/dL. Packed RBCs were required postoperatively in 6 of the 17 control and 6 of the 18 autotransfusion patients ($p$ = not significant). Postoperative colloid fluid replacement was less in the autotransfused group (333 ± 78 mL; 95% confidence bounds, 168–498 mL) compared with the control group (615 ± 114 mL; 95% confidence bounds, 372–857 mL; $p = 0.048$). Homologous blood product exposure tended to be higher in autotransfusion patients (83%) than in control patients (47%) ($p = 0.057$). Fibrin split products were elevated only in the autotransfusion patients ($p < 0.002$). Neither group demonstrated transfusion-related complications, and autotransfusion of shed mediastinal blood did not decrease the need for homologous blood transfusion [30].

Eng et al. [29] conducted a prospective, randomized, controlled study in two matched groups of 20 patients undergoing elective coronary artery bypass surgery. The treatment group had shed mediastinal blood autotransfused. Use of homologous blood was reduced from 760.5 ± 108.37 mL in the control patients to 466.25 ± 87.44 mL in the autotransfusion (AT) patients, a reduction of 38.7% ($p < 0.05$). There was no statistically significant difference in the clinical outcome, overall blood loss, use of platelets, fresh frozen plasma and colloids, hematological indices, renal and hepatic functions, or clotting mechanism. There was a reduction in the fibrinogen level in the patients who received AT ($p < 0.05$). Mediastinal blood contained significant levels of hemoglobin (8.175 ± 0.506 g/dL), platelets (96.55 ± 10.39/mm$^3$ 10(3)), protein (42.5 ± 1.13 g/L), and calcium (2.385 ± 0.054 mmol/L) and was well oxygenated ($PO_2$ = 20.46 +/- 0.81 kPa). No patients developed bacteremia or had any AT-related infections [29].

Broadie et al. [32] collected from the body cavities of 31 trauma victims with indications for intraoperative transfusion. Blood was collected at thoracotomy or laparotomy prior to the institution of any anticoagulant measures and was assessed for clotting competence, the presence of fibrinogen, the presence of soluble fibrin monomere, and the appearance of fibrin degradation products. The prothrombin time, partial thromboplastin time, and thrombin time of this blood were markedly elevated; fibrinogen was absent; soluble fibrin monomer was absent; and fibrin degradation products were markedly elevated. They concluded that the blood collected from body cavities is incoagulable [32].

Lassié et al. [25] conducted a prospective study assessed an autotransfusion system in 30 patients suffering from hemothorax. The retransfusion took place in less than 4 h and patients with an isolated hemothorax did not receive any homologous blood. The shed blood was analyzed and found to have decreased platelets, fibrinogen, and is incoagulable. Its hematocrit was lower than the patient's, but the concentration of 2,3 DPG remained normal [25].

Barriot et al. [31] reviewed 18 patients with life-threatening traumatic hemothorax who received prehospital autotransfusion. Hemorrhagic blood was not coagulable and had a hematocrit of 20% ± 4%, few platelets, and low fibrinogen levels. Five patients died from irreversible hemorrhagic shock. Thirteen patients were alive on admission to the hospital, underwent emergency surgery, and were discharged alive. During autotransfusion, hematocrit decreased from 24% ± 3% to 19% ± 3%, and systolic arterial pressure increased from 78 ± 11 to 88 ± 12 mmHg. On admission to the hospital, platelet count was 90,800 ± 21,400/mm$^3$, prothrombin time 48% ± 3%, partial thromboplastin time 197% ± 18%, plasma-free hemoglobin levels 21 ± 7 mg/100 mL, and serum potassium levels 3.6 ± 0.5 mmol/L. No serious complications were attributed to autotransfusion [31].

Ahmed et al. [33] reported on a large series of patients undergoing autotransfusion during the Somali Civil War between 1992 and 2001. This was a retrospective study that looked at 45,900 war-wounded patients, 13,770 of whom had chest injuries. There was no blood bank and a lack of donors; therefore, it was necessary to set up a system for immediate autotransfusion in patients with massive hemothorax from penetrating chest war wounds. A total of 137 patients had autotransfusion. There were five deaths (3.6% mortality rate), and no major complications were detected in the autotransfused patients that survived [33].

A group of investigators at the University of Texas Health Science Center in San Antonio, Texas, conducted two prospective studies looking at blood from trauma patients who received thoracostomy tubes [34,35]. The first study was a prospective descriptive study of adult patients from whom ≥50 mL of blood was drained within the first 4 h after chest tube placement. Pleural and venous blood samples were analyzed for coagulation, hematology, and electrolytes. The group enrolled 22 subjects. The measured coagulation factors of hemothorax were significantly depleted compared with venous blood: international normalized ratio (>9 in contrast to 1.1, $p < 0.001$), activated partial thromboplastin time (>180 in contrast to 28.5 s, $p < 0.001$), and fibrinogen (<50 in contrast to 288 mg/dL, $p < 0.001$). The mean hematocrit (26.4 in contrast to 33.9, $p = 0.003$), hemoglobin (9.3 in contrast to 11.8 g/dL, $p = 0.004$), and platelet count (53 in contrast to 174 K/μL, $p < 0.001$) of hemothorax were significantly lower than venous blood. Hemothorax blood contains significantly decreased coagulation factors and has lower hemoglobin when compared with venous blood [34].

The second study was a prospective descriptive study of 34 adult patients with traumatic chest injury necessitating tube thoracostomy. Pleural and venous samples were analyzed for coagulation, hematology, and electrolytes at 1–4 h after drainage. Pleural samples were also analyzed for their effect on the coagulation cascade via mixing studies. Coagulation factors were significantly depleted in hemothorax blood compared with venous blood: international normalized ratio (>9 vs. 1.1, $p < 0.001$) and activated partial thromboplastin time (>180 vs. 24.5 s, $p < 0.001$). Mixing studies showed a dose-dependent increase in coagulation dilutions through 1:8 ($p < 0.05$). The authors concluded that an evacuated hemothorax does not vary in composition significantly with time and is incoagulable alone. Mixing studies with hemothorax plasma increased coagulation, raising safety concerns if the hemothorax blood were to be autotransfused [35].

Carless conducted a Cochrane review [26] in 2010 to examine the evidence for the efficacy of cell salvage in reducing allogeneic blood transfusion and the evidence for any effect on clinical outcomes. They selected randomized controlled trials with a concurrent control group in which adult patients, scheduled for nonurgent surgery, were randomized to cell salvage (autotransfusion) or to a control group who did not receive the intervention. Data were independently extracted and the risk of bias assessed. The primary outcomes were the number of patients exposed to allogeneic red cell transfusion and the amount of blood transfused. Overall, the use of cell salvage reduced the rate of exposure to allogeneic RBC transfusion by a relative 38% (RR 0.62; 95% CI, 0.55–0.70). The absolute reduction in risk of receiving an allogeneic RBC transfusion was 21% (95% CI, 15%–26%). In orthopedic procedures, the RR of exposure to RBC transfusion was 0.46 (95% CI, 0.37–0.57) compared with 0.77 (95% CI, 0.69–0.86) for cardiac procedures. The use of cell salvage resulted in an average saving of 0.68 units of allogeneic RBC per patient (weighted mean difference [WMD] −0.68; 95% CI, −0.88 to −0.49). Cell salvage did not adversely impact clinical outcomes. The authors concluded that cell salvage is efficacious in reducing the need for allogeneic red cell transfusion in adult elective cardiac and orthopedic surgery [26]. Although this review is quite comprehensive, especially regarding the cardiac and orthopedic literature, it does not specifically address trauma patients with autotransfused hemothoraces.

*Recommendation*: Current evidence does not support the routine autotransfusion of traumatic hemothorax. However, because of the paucity of evidence, we cannot recommend against this practice either. Studies suggest several theoretical advantages and disadvantages to autotransfusion of hemothorax blood. We recommend that in the clinical scenario where transfusion is required and a significant traumatic hemothorax exists, the clinician should consider the urgency of the situation and balance the risks and benefits to each patient on an individual basis. These are grade C recommendations.

## 17.3 Should Small-Bore Chest Drainage Catheters Be Used rather than Large-Bore Tubes for Traumatic Hemothorax?

In elective cardiac surgery, blood accumulating inside chest cavities can lead to serious complications if it is not drained properly [36]. In trauma patients, a similar argument could be made. The optimal chest tube size for the drainage of traumatic hemothoraces and pneumothoraces is unknown [37,38]. Patients experience increasing discomfort with increasing drain size [36]. Smaller tube sizes may cause less pain and possibly result in improved respiratory effort and pulmonary toilet. The concern with smaller tubes is whether or not they will adequately drain a hemothorax. Because life-threatening conditions can result from chest tube occlusion after thoracic surgery, large-bore tubes are generally employed to optimize patency [36].

Shalli et al. [36] conducted a survey of cardiothoracic surgeons and specialized cardiac nurses. Of surgeons responding, 106 of 106 (100%) had observed chest tube clogging, and 93 of 106 (87%) reported adverse patient outcomes from a clogged tube. The major reason surgeons choose large-diameter chest tubes is linked to concern about the suboptimal available methods to avoid and treat chest tube clogging. Even though larger tubes are thought to be associated with more pain, physicians generally err on the side of caution to avoid clogging and insert tubes with larger diameters [36]. This is valuable in that it quantifies the clinical dilemma and highlights that the decision about tube size is not necessarily evidence based.

Rahman et al. [39] studied the effect of tube size on the management empyema. They prospectively enrolled a total of 405 patients with pleural infection into a multicenter study investigating the utility of fibrinolytic therapy. The combined frequency of death and surgery, and secondary outcomes (hospital stay, change in chest radiograph, and lung function at 3 months) were compared in patients receiving different size chest tubes. Tubes were stratified according to size as follows: <10fr, 10–14fr, 15–20fr, and >20fr. They did find that smaller, guide-wire-inserted chest tubes cause substantially less pain than blunt dissection-inserted larger tubes, without any impairment in clinical outcome in the treatment of pleural infection. The authors concluded that smaller size tubes may be the initial treatment of choice for pleural infection, and randomized studies are now required [39].

Rivera et al. [40] conducted a retrospective trauma registry review of tube thoracostomies at a level 1 trauma center after the center adopted the practice of using small catheter tube thoracostomy (SCTT) as a less invasive method to manage nonemergent chest injuries. The investigators collected data that included age, sex, indications and timing for chest tube placement, use of antibiotics, length of stay, complications, and outcomes. Large catheter tube thoracostomy (LCTT) not performed in the operating room or trauma room and all SCTT were considered nonemergent. During their study period, 565 tube thoracostomies were performed in 359 patients and 252 were deemed emergent and 157 were nonemergent. Of the patients receiving nonemergent tubes, 63 received LCTT and 107 received SCTT. The average duration of SCTT was shorter than nonemergent LCCT (5.5 days vs. 7 days, $p < 0.05$). Rates of hemothoraces were similar for SCTT versus nonemergent LCTT (6.1% vs. 4.2%, $p$ = NS) and rates of residual/recurrent pneumothoraces were not significantly different (8% vs. 14%, $p$ = NS). The rate of occurrence of fibrothorax was significantly lower for SCTT compared with nonemergent LCTT (0% vs. 4.2%, $p < 0.05$). These results led the authors to conclude that SCTT was effective in managing chest trauma and was comparable with LCTT in stable trauma patients. The investigators felt the study supported their institutional practice of adopting image-guided small catheter techniques in the management of chest trauma in stable patients [40].

Kulvatunyou et al. [38] hypothesized that 14fr pigtail catheters (PCs) could drain blood as well as large-bore 32fr to 40fr chest tubes. They prospectively collected data on all bedside-inserted PCs in patients with traumatic hemothorax or hemopneumothorax during a 30-month period (July 2009 through December 2011) at a level 1 trauma center. They compared their PC prospective data with trauma registry-derived retrospective chest tube data (January 2008 through December 2010). In the study population, they found that 36 patients received PCs and 191 received chest tubes. The primary outcome was the initial drainage output. Secondary outcomes were tube duration, insertion-related complications, and failure rate. The mean initial output was similar between the PC group the chest tube group. Tube duration, rate of insertion-related complications, and failure rate were all similar between groups. This led Kulvatunyou et al. to conclude that 14fr PCs drained blood as well as large-bore chest tubes. They also stated that to make any definitive clinical recommendations, they would need a larger sample size and possibly a well-designed prospective study [38].

Inaba et al. [37] attempted to address the specific issues of adequate drainage and pain as they relate to chest tube size in trauma patients by conducting a prospective observational trial between 2007 and 2010. They collected demographic and outcome data including efficacy of drainage, complications, retained hemothoraces, residual pneumothoraces, need for additional tube insertion, video-assisted thoracoscopy, and thoracotomy. The data were then analyzed by tube size stratified as either small (28–32fr) or large (36–40fr). A total of 353 chest tubes (small, 186; large, 167) were placed in 293 patients. Of the 275 chest tubes inserted for a hemothorax, 144 were small (52.3%) and 131 were large (47.7%). The volume of blood drained initially and the total duration of tube placement were similar for both groups (small 6.3 ± 3.9 days vs. large 6.2 ± 3.6 days; adjusted [adj.] $p = 0.427$). No statistically significant difference in tube-related complications, including pneumonia (4.9% vs. 4.6%; adj. $p = 0.282$), empyema (4.2% vs. 4.6%; adj. $p = 0.766$), or retained hemothorax (11.8% vs. 10.7%; adj. $p = 0.981$), was found. The need for tube reinsertion, image-guided drainage, video-assisted thoracoscopy, and thoracotomy was the same (10.4% vs. 10.7%; adj. $p = 0.719$). For patients with a pneumothorax requiring chest tube drainage ($n = 238$), there was no difference in the number of patients with an unresolved pneumothorax (14.0% vs. 13.0%; adj. $p = 0.620$) or those needing reinsertion of a second chest tube. The mean visual analog pain score was similar for small and large tubes (6.0 ± 3.3 and 6.7 ± 3.0; $p = 0.237$). These findings led the investigators to conclude that tube size did not affect efficacy of drainage. They also concluded that tube size did not impact tube-associated complication rates or pain [37].

*Recommendation*: The available evidence suggests that small-bore chest tubes may be as effective as large-bore drains in patients with traumatic hemothoraces. The published data also suggest that there is no increase in tube-associated complications. The body of evidence, however, is insufficient to recommend a change in practice. This is a grade C recommendation.

## References


1. Bergeron E, Lavoie A, Clas D, Moore L, Ratte S, Tetreault S, Lemaire J, Martin M. Elderly trauma patients with rib fractures are at greater risk of death and pneumonia. *J Trauma.* 2003;54:478–485.
2. Holcomb JB, McMullin NR, Kozar RA, Lygas MH, Moore FA. Morbidity from rib fractures increases after age 45. *J Am Coll Surg.* 2003;196:549–555.
3. Sirmali M, Türüt H, Topcxu S, Gülhan E, Yazici U, Kaya S, Tasxtepe I. A comprehensive analysis of traumatic rib fractures: Morbidity, mortality and management. *Eur J Cardiothorac Surg.* 2003;24:133–138.
4. Brasel KJ, Guse CE, Layde P, Weigelt JA. Rib fractures: Relationship with pneumonia and mortality. *Crit Care Med.* 2006;34:1642–1646.
5. Ciraulo DL, Elliott D, Mitchell KA, Rodriguez A. Flail chest as a marker for significant injuries. *J Am Coll Surg.* 1994;178:466–470.
6. Kent R, Woods W, Bostrom O. Fatality risk and the presence of rib fractures. *Annu Proc Assoc Adv Automot Med.* 2008;52:73–82.
7. Landercasper J, Cogbill TH, Lindesmith LA. Long-term disability after flail chest injury. *J Trauma.* 1984;24:410–414.
8. Bulger EM, Arneson MA, Mock CN, Jurkovich GJ. Rib fractures in the elderly. *J Trauma.* 2000;48:1040–1047.
9. Ahmed Z, Mohyuddin Z. Management of flail chest injury: Internal fixation versus endotracheal intubation and ventilation. *J Thorac Cardiovasc Surg.* 1995;110:1676–1680.
10. Lardinois D, Krueger T, Dusmet M, Ghisletta N, Gugger M, Ris HB. Pulmonary function testing after operative stabilization of the chest wall for flail chest. *Eur J Cardiothorac Surg.* 2001;20:496–501.
11. Tanaka H, Yukioka T, Yamaguti Y, Shimizu S, Goto H, Matsuda H, Shimazaki S. Surgical stabilization of internal pneumatic stabilization? A prospective randomized study of management of severe flail chest patients. *J Trauma.* 2002;52:727–732.
12. Cacchione RN, Richardson JD, Seligson D. Painful nonunion of multiple rib fractures managed by operative stabilization. *J Trauma.* 2000;48:319–321.
13. Slater MS, Mayberry JC, Trunkey DD. Operative stabilization of a flail chest six years after injury. *Ann Thorac Surg.* 2001;72:600–601.
14. Nirula R, Diaz JJ, Jr., Trunkey DD, Mayberry JC. Rib fracture repair: Indications, technical issues, and future directions. *World J Surg.* 2009;33:14–22.
15. Voggenreiter G, Neudeck F, Aufmkolk M, Obertacke U, Schmit-Neuerburg KP. Operative chest wall stabilization in flail chest—Outcomes of patients with or without pulmonary contusion. *J Am Coll Surg.* 1998;187:130–138.
16. Karev DV. Operative management of the flail chest. *Wiad Lek.* 1997;50(Suppl 1):205–208.
17. Velmahos GC, Vassiliu P, Chan LS, Murray JA, Berne TV, Demetriades D. Influence of flail chest on outcome among patients with severe thoracic cage trauma. *Int Surg.* 2002;87:240–244.
18. Simon B, Ebert J, Bokhari F et al. EAST Practice Management Workgroup for Pulmonary Contusion—Flail Chest. Practice management guideline for "pulmonary contusion—flail chest." *J Trauma Acute Care Surg.* 2012;73: S351–S361.
19. Granetzny A, Abd El-Aal M, Emam E, Shalaby A, Boseila A. Surgical versus conservative treatment of flail chest. Evaluation of the pulmonary status. *Interact Cardiovasc Thorac Surg.* 2005;4:583–587.
20. Mayberry JC, Kroeker AD, Ham LB, Mullins RJ, Trunkey DD. Long-term morbidity, pain, and disability after repair of severe chest wall injuries. *Am Surg.* 2009;75:389–394.
21. Nirula R, Allen B, Layman R, Falimirski ME, Somberg LB. Rib fracture stabilization in patients sustaining blunt chest injury. *Am Surg.* 2006;72:307–309.

22. Doben AR, Eriksson EA, Denlinger CE et al. Surgical rib fixation for flail chest deformity improves liberation from mechanical ventilation. *J Crit Care*. 2013;29:139–143.
23. Symbas PN. Autotransfusion from hemothorax: Experimental and clinical studies. *J Trauma*. 1972;12(8):689–695.
24. Ferrara, BE. Autotransfusion: Its use in acute hemothorax. *South Med J*. 1957;50:516–519.
25. Lassié P, Sztark F, Petitjean ME. Autotransfusion, with blood drained from a hemothorax, using the ConstaVac device. *Ann Fr Anesth Reanim*. 1994;13(6):781–784.
26. Carless PA, Henry DA, Moxey AJ, O'Connell D, Brown T, Fergusson DA. Cell salvage for minimising perioperative allogeneic blood transfusion. *Cochrane Database Syst Rev*. 2010;(4):CD001888.
27. Body SC, Birmingham J, Parks R et al. Safety and efficacy of shed mediastinal blood transfusion after cardiac surgery: A multicenter observational study. Multicenter Study of Perioperative Ischemia Research Group. *J Cardiothorac Vasc Anesth*. 1999;13(4):410–416.
28. Helm RE, Klemperer JD, Rosengart TK et al. Intraoperative autologous blood donation preserves red cell mass but does not decrease postoperative bleeding. *Ann Thorac Surg*. 1996;62:1431–1441.
29. Eng J, Kay PH, Murday AJ et al. Postoperative autologous transfusion in cardiac surgery. A prospective, randomised study. *Eur J Cardiothorac Surg*. 1990;4(11):595–600.
30. Ward HE, Smith RR, Landis KP et al. Prospective, randomized trial of autotransfusion after routine cardiac operations. *Ann Thorac Surg*. 1993;56(1):137–141.
31. Barriot P, Riots B, Viarst P. Prehospital autotransfusion in life-threatening hemothorax. *Chest*. 1988;93(3):522–526.
32. Broadie TA, Glover JL, Bang N et al. Clotting competence of intracavitary blood in trauma victims. *Ann Emerg Med*. 1981;10(3):127–130.
33. Ahmed AM, Riye MH, Baldan M, Autotransfusion in penetrating chest war trauma with haemothorax: The Keysaney hospital experience. *East Cent Afr J Surg*. 2003;8(1):51–54.
34. Salhanick M(1), Corneille M, Higgins R et al. Autotransfusion of hemothorax blood in trauma patients: Is it the same as fresh whole blood? *Am J Surg*. 2011;202(6):817–821.
35. Smith WZ(1), Harrison HB, Salhanick MA et al. A small amount can make a difference: A prospective human study of the paradoxical coagulation characteristics of hemothorax. *Am J Surg*. 2013;206(6):904–909.
36. Shalli S, Saeed D, Fukamachi K et al. Chest tube selection in cardiac and thoracic surgery: A survey of chest tube related complications and their management. *J Card Surg*. 2009;24(5):503–509.
37. Inaba K, Lustenberger T, Recinos G et al. Does size matter? A prospective analysis of 28–32 versus 36–40 French chest tube size in trauma. *J Trauma*. 2012;72:422–427.
38. Kulvatunyou K, Joseph B, Friese RS et al. 14 French pigtail catheters placed by surgeons to drain blood on trauma patients: Is 14-Fr too small? *J Trauma Acute Care Surg*. 2012;6:1423–1427.
39. Rahman NM, Maskell NA, Davies CW et al. The relationship between chest tube size and clinical outcome in pleural infection. *Chest*. 2010;137(3):536–543.
40. Rivera L, O'Reilly EB, Sise MJ et al. Small catheter tube thoracostomy: Effective in managing chest trauma in stable patients. *J Trauma*. 2009;66:393–399.

## Commentary on Chest Wall Trauma

*Tom Scalea*

Chest wall injuries are very common and accompany virtually all patients with polysystem injury. The chest wall represents a great deal of the surface area of the body.

Thirty years ago, when I was a fellow, we believed that the chest wall deformity was in fact, physiologically important. I can remember being a fellow making rounds on patients in the ICU with flail chest. At that time, we believed that all patients required mechanical ventilation until the flail segment healed. Each morning, I would allow the patients to wake up. If the patients still had paradoxical chest wall motion, I again paralyzed them, sedated them, and repeated that assessment each day. Not surprisingly, virtually all of these patients ended up on long-term mechanical ventilation. Virtually all of them also came to tracheostomy.

At some point, we realized that the chest wall deformity was physiologically unimportant. It was the underlying pulmonary contusion that determined whether patients required mechanical ventilation or not. This saved innumerable patients from many ventilator days and obviated the need for tracheostomy in such patients.

When autotransfusion became available, virtually everyone embraced this. This was of course in the early days of HIV and AIDS was a death sentence. When we realized that HIV was a blood-borne disease, the ability to use the patient's own blood became incredibly attractive. This was never subjected to any scientific rigor. Autotransfusion had to be better than the use of banked blood. We knew it was true, thus we never studied it.

The use of tube thoracostomy was also very common. Even small pneumothoraces or hemothoraces were thought to require drainage. Large bore tubes were always used for hemothoraces. The mantra was "small tubes evacuate air, but big tubes evacuate blood."

Our understanding of chest wall injury has evolved substantially over the past 30 years. Practice has migrated and we now are better at studying these problems. However, this chapter by Dr. Bini illustrates that we have much yet to learn.

Many people have embraced the notion that rigid stabilization of the flail chest is wise. It makes perfect sense that restoring stability to the damaged chest wall should reduce the pain associated with multiple rib fractures and should liberate patients from the ventilator more quickly. In fact, if one wishes to spark "spirited discussions" among a group of physicians caring for injury, one needs to simply introduce the concept of rib fracture fixation. In fact, the same exists in our own surgery group. Several of our partners believe strongly that rib fixation is wise. When they rotate onto a trauma service, many patients *need* the operation. When they leave, that *need* seems to leave with them. If chest wall stability is not the problem, but the pulmonary injury underneath is, it is not surprising that we have been unable to demonstrate that blanket use of rib fracture fixation in patients with flail chest simply does not work. The key here seems to be patient selection. I am sure that some patients do benefit from rigid chest wall stabilization. Defining who those patients are have eluded us up to this point.

Other techniques such as innovative strategies for pain control, early mobilization out of bed, and crisp attention to all other facets of the patients care may be as important as fixing the ribs. Rib fracture fixation is a technique that must exist in a comprehensive patient care package. Simply doing an operation is unlikely to be the difference between success and failure.

Likewise, autotransfusion has not been demonstrated to be efficacious. While risk of disease transmission exists, it is much lower with better blood bank screening[*]. In addition, transfusion triggers continue to change. When I was a resident, everybody with a hemoglobin less than 10 mg/dL got blood. Now we have become far more selective and rarely transfuse patients until hemoglobins are 7 mg/dL or less[†]. Younger people can likely do well with hemoglobin levels that are much lower.

In addition, the simple act of autotransfusion raises some concerns. Blood dwells in the chest cavity for some period of time. It is then rapidly evacuated via a tube into a pleur-evac, where the blood is again collected and reinfused. How injurious is the process to the red cells. One might rationally think that red cells that sit in the chest for a while and undergo the trauma of evacuation and reinstallation are certainly not normal.

Finally, the issues of size of chest tube seem to be unimportant. At least, if it is important, we have been unable to demonstrate that. For years, we taught that blood did not clot in the pleura space. Anyone who cares for trauma patients knows blood clots all of the time in the chest cavity. A clotted hemothorax will

* Sander SG, Yu H, Rassai N. Risks of blood transfusions and their prevention. *Clin Adv Hematol Oncol.* 2003;1:307–313.

† Carless PA, Henry DA, Carson J et al. Transfusion threshold and other strategies for guiding allogenic red blood cell transfusion. *Cochrane Database Syst Rev.* 2010;10:CD002042.

not come out via a chest tube, regardless of the size. Likewise, free-flowing blood may actually come out of a small tube as easily as it comes out of a larger bore chest tube.

Injury to the chest wall is common. There is little question in my mind that we are better for caring for this than we were 30 years ago when I was in training. However, this chapter makes it clear that we still have much left to discover. This evidence-based chapter demonstrates that blanket application of rigid chest wall fixation is not wise. In addition, autotransfusion may be no better than using banked blood. Finally, evacuating blood from the chest seems to make sense. The size of the tube is probably unimportant. Retained hemothoraces should be identified and dealt with. However, it is unlikely that the size of the tube matters.

# 18

# *Evidence-Based Surgery: Injury to the Thoracic Great Vessels*

**Mark Cockburn and Ali Salim**

**CONTENTS**



## 18.1 Introduction

Chest injury from blunt trauma is a significant cause of morbidity and mortality. Most of the literature published on injury to the thoracic great vessels has focused on the aorta and on blunt thoracic aortic injury (BTAI), which is a devastating injury that requires early recognition to minimize morbidity and mortality. It has been estimated that there are about 8000 cases of blunt aortic injury (BAI) each year in the United States [1]. Approximately 80%–85% die at the scene or in transport [2]. This injury most commonly results from motor vehicle collisions [3], but we have seen an increase in fatality from this injury among pedestrians hit by cars [4]. The remaining mechanisms for this injury include falls from heights and crushing chest injuries. In 2000, the Eastern Association for the Surgery of Trauma (EAST) Practice Management Groups published their guidelines for the diagnosis and management of BAI [3]. This group reviewed 137 articles from a MEDLINE search of English language citations published between 1966 and 1997. They analyzed these papers and produced recommendations based on Level 1, Level 2, and Level 3 data. Since 2000, a number of other studies have been published looking at the diagnosis and management of BAI (Table 18.1).

## 18.2 Diagnosis of BAI

### 18.2.1 What Is the Ultimate Imaging Modality for Diagnosing BTAI?

The EAST guidelines stated that Level 2 data supported chest x-ray as a good screening tool and angiography as the standard by which most other diagnostic tests are compared. The Level 2 data also supported that helical or spiral computed tomographic scanners have an extremely high negative predictive value and may be used to rule out BAI [3]. Since the EAST guidelines, other studies have been done looking at the ability of the newer-generation computed tomography (CT) scanners to diagnose BAI. In 2004, Chen et al. published their data looking at the use of helical CT (HCT) to detect acute thoracic aortic and branch vessel injury after blunt thoracic trauma. This was a retrospective study of 85 patients who had BAI diagnosed by chest CT, aortography, or both. Isolated aortic, branch vessel, or combined injuries were found in 71 (84%), 11 (13%), and 3 (4%) patients, respectively. All patients with branch vessel injuries were diagnosed by aortography. Ninety-eight percent of patients with aortography were true positives, and 20% with chest CT had indirect signs of aortic injury. They concluded that patients with indirect signs on chest CT require further evaluation and that angiography remains the optimal diagnostic modality for evaluating aortic branch vessel injuries [5]. Melton et al. also looked at the evolution of chest CT for the definitive diagnosis of BAI. Their study was also retrospective and they performed 113 aortograms that confirmed 28 BAI cases. Twenty-seven of these were congruently diagnosed by CT. Only one CT scan diagnostic for BAI had a negative aortogram. Seventeen BAIs were diagnosed with CT alone. Ten BAIs were confirmed operatively and seven were treated nonoperatively because of age, comorbid conditions, severity of injury, or presence of small intimal defects. They concluded that CT has evolved to allow for the definitive diagnosis and treatment of BAI [6].

There has been an increase in the use of CT scans for trauma and for diagnosing thoracic aortic injuries. Demetriades et al. [7] published in 2008 a prospective observational multicentre study with 50 participating centers over a 30 month period as part of an American Association for the Surgery of Trauma (AAST) study and compared the mode used for diagnosing BAI with a previous AAST study by Fabian, published in 1997. He noted that diagnostic aortogram was performed in 8.3% of patients compared to 87% of patients in Fabian's study [17]. Similarly, Demetriades noted a 1% use of transesophageal echocardiography (TEE) compared to 11.9% use in Fabian's study.

Chest CT is a highly sensitive and specific test for thoracic aortic injury and is the diagnostic test of choice. Thoracic aortography is no longer routinely used to identify BAI because it is invasive and associated with delays related to the need to set up the interventional suite and call in appropriate personnel. However, aortography may be needed where newer-generation CT scanning is not available. In a study of 494 patients of whom 71 had BTAI, the sensitivity of CT approached 100% compared with 92% for aortography [8A]

*Recommendation*: Angiography remains the gold standard modality for making the diagnosis of BTAI.

*Level of evidence*: 2b

HCT has become the diagnostic test of choice [7,8].

*Level of evidence*: 2b

*Grade of recommendation*: B

## 18.3 Minimal Aortic Injuries

### 18.3.1 What Modality Should Be Used to Follow Minimal Aortic Injuries (MAIs) from Blunt Trauma?

#### *18.3.1.1 What Medications Should We Use in the Medical Management of These Injuries and for How Long Should Patients Be Required to Take These Medications?*

As a direct result of the improvement in the diagnostic techniques, MAIs are being recognized more frequently. The management of such injuries has created some anxiety among surgeons and has left some questions unanswered. What modalities should be used to follow these injuries? How often should follow-up studies be obtained? What medications should be used in the medical management of these injuries and for how long should patients be required to take these medications? What should the target blood pressure be?

Malhotra et al. published their paper in 2001 describing their experience with MAIs. They conducted a retrospective review of all patients suspected of BAI seen on screening HCT over the study period July 1994 to June 2000. For their discussion, MAI was defined as a small (<1 cm) intimal flap with minimal to no periaortic hematoma, estimated to occur in 10% of patients with BAI. These patients underwent confirmatory aortography with or without intravascular ultrasound. All patients were admitted to the trauma intensive care unit and all received short-acting β-blockade infusion (esmolol or labetalol) to control heart rate (<90 beats/min) and blood pressure (systolic blood pressure <120 mmHg). Sodium nitroprusside was added to the regimen when β-blockade alone did not adequately control blood pressure. Patients were changed to oral antihypertensive therapy over the following 5–7 days. BAI was suspected in 198 (1.3%) of the 15,000 patients evaluated with screening HCT and confirmed in 87 (0.6%) of these. Nine of these 87 patients met the criteria for MAI, as defined earlier, and the remaining 78 patients had significant aortic injuries. Aortography was performed in 189 patients who had suspicious HCT. The initial aortogram was positive in 77 patients, and of these, 71 were true positives. Of the 112 negative aortograms, 105 were true negatives and 7 were false negatives. Of the seven patients with false-negative initial aortogram, five had MAI and two had significant aortic injuries. The correct diagnosis in patients with false-negative aortograms was established by further tests including intravascular ultrasound (five patients), repeat aortography (one patient), and video angiography (one patient). Although the overall sensitivity and specificity of the initial aortogram were 91% and 94.6%, respectively, the actual sensitivity of the initial aortogram for MAI was 37.5% and that for significant aortic injury was 97.1%. Eight of the nine patients with MAI were managed nonoperatively. One patient refused nonoperative management and was operated upon 5 days after injury. Aortotomy at the time of surgery revealed an intimal defect that was repaired by incorporating it into the aortotomy closure using three pledgeted prolene sutures [9].

The earlier study demonstrated the low sensitivity of aortograms in making the diagnosis of MAI. Kepros et al. reviewed their experience with MAIs [10]. In their report, five blunt trauma patients treated for an aortic injury demonstrated by TEE to be limited to the intima with or without thrombus were reviewed. All were managed nonoperatively on the basis of the limited and superficial nature of their aortic injury. They used a management strategy that included serial TEE studies to visualize and monitor the progression or resolution of injury, hypotension (systolic blood pressure between 80 and 90 mmHg), and prevention of tachycardia (heart rate between 60 and 80 beats/min) using β-blockade, close invasive monitoring in the surgical intensive care unit, and standard intravenous fluid resuscitation using serum lactate levels and base deficit as endpoints of adequate tissue perfusion. They noted that TEE was more sensitive in diagnosing aortic intimal injuries compared with aortic arch angiography or HCT of the chest, as the latter two studies failed to identify any of the intimal injuries. Nonoperative management was successfully completed in all cases. Complete resolution of all intimal tears was documented by TEE within 3–19 days (mean = 9.4 ± 6.6 days). In one patient, the intimal tear extended during the first 48 h. This patient was still managed nonoperatively, as there was no sonographic evidence of transmural involvement and/or dissection. There was complete resolution of injury by 11 days. There were no complications related to the aortic injuries in any of the patients during a mean follow-up of 16.8 months. Thus, TEE appears to be a good modality in diagnosing and following these MAIs.

Kidane et al. performed a retrospective review of their Level 1 trauma center's database to identify patients who had a BAI between October 1998 and March 2010. CT scans of those who were initially treated nonoperatively were reviewed to determine the extent of BAI as either MAI (intimal flap with minimal or no periaortic hematoma) or more severe injuries (pseudoaneurysm and greater periaortic hematomas). They reviewed follow-up CT scans and clinical information to determine the natural history of these lesions and the clinical outcomes related to their nonoperative management. All CT scans were assessed by two reviewers, and there was 100% agreement between them. They identified 69 patients with a BTAI during the study period; 10 were initially untreated and were included in this study. Degree of injury included intimal flaps ($n = 7$, 70%), pseudoaneurysms with minimal hematoma ($n = 2$, 20%), and circumferential intimal tear ($n = 1$, 10%). Six (60%) patients were male, and the median age was 40 years. Duration of clinical follow-up ranged from 1 month to 6 years (median = 2 months) after discharge, whereas CT radiologic follow-up ranged from 1 week to 6 years (median = 6 weeks). Seven (70%) patients had complete resolution or stabilization of their MAI, 1 (10%) with circumferential intimal tear showed extension of the injury at 8 weeks postinjury and underwent successful repair, and 2 (20%) were lost to follow-up. They concluded that there appears to be a subset of patients with BTAI who require no surgical intervention. This includes those with limited intimal flaps, which often resolve. Radiologic surveillance is mandatory to ensure MAI resolution and identify any progression that might prompt repair [11].

*Recommendations*:

1. TEE appears to be a good modality in following MAIs.

   *Level of evidence*: 2b

   *Grade of recommendation*: B

2. β-Blockade and intravenous vasodilator therapy should be used for the medical management of MAIs. There is no study answering the question as to how long these medications should be used.

   Controlling the heart rate and blood pressure (systolic between 100 and 120 mmHg) using β-blockade and intravenous vasodilator is effective in treating patients with MAIs.

   *Level of evidence*: 2b

   *Grade of recommendation*: B

## 18.4 Nonoperative Management of Blunt Traumatic Aortic Injuries

### 18.4.1 When Is Nonoperative Management to Be Considered?

#### *18.4.1.1 What Is the Target Blood Pressure to Maintain When Nonoperative Management or Delayed Surgical Therapy Is Considered?*

The nonoperative management of blunt aortic injuries stemmed out of studies reporting the use of medical management of these injuries in patients who were poor operative candidates due to advanced age or comorbidities that prohibit emergency thoracic surgery [12,13]. Another subset of patients that are treated medically and in whom immediate repair is not possible is those patients unstable from intra-abdominal injuries who require laparotomy or patients with severe closed head injuries who require craniotomies [14–16]. The use of pharmacologic treatment to decrease wall stress in acute aortic dissection and thereby reduce the risk of rupture was originally introduced by Wheat et al. in 1965 [17]. Nonoperative management of BAI was first described by Akins in 1981 when five patients were managed with antihypertensive therapy and all survived [18]. Most of these nonoperative cases had surgery purposefully delayed or indefinitely postponed because of severe comorbidities.

The concerns with the nonoperative management of BAIs are risks of subsequent rupture of the aorta and the development of chronic thoracic aneurysms. Reports estimate that the risk of aortic rupture is less than 4% in patients presenting to the emergency room with stable hemodynamics during the initial workup; however, once rupture occurred, survival is rare [19,20]. A recent literature search by Hirose et al. [21] showed that only 1.5% of patients died of aortic rupture if they survived the initial few hours. Pate's study showed that only 7% of patients with a history of acute aortic injury developed chronic thoracic aneurysm over 7–48 years [19]. Interestingly, some patients have regression of the aortic injury with antihypertensive management.

The use of antihypertensives for BAI was based on the successful management of type B dissection [18,19]. In 1995, Pate described two cases of aortic rupture during nonoperative management when blood pressure was not adequately managed [19]. Pate later published follow-up results in 1997 and 1999, showing that there was no aortic rupture using a blood pressure control strategy during a waiting period for delayed surgery or among medically managed patients [12,22]. In his study, Pate used the β-blockade when the cardiac rate was >90 beats/min and the systolic blood pressure was >100 mmHg. When the systolic blood pressure persisted at levels of >100 mmHg after β-blockade, an intravenous vasodilator (usually nitroprusside) was used to control the pressure.

*Recommendations*:

1. MAIs can be managed nonoperatively with specific medical treatment protocols to control heart rate and blood pressure. Similarly, patients who are poor operative candidates can have their injuries managed nonoperatively with the same treatment protocols (β-blockade and intravenous vasodilator). Patients who are initially managed nonoperatively because of concerns of concomitant injuries and whose follow-up studies reveal resolution of the aortic injury can continue to be managed nonoperatively on β-blockade and intravenous vasodilator.
2. There are no Level 1 data that have answered this question specifically. Pate's study provides Level 2b data. There are also references to a target systolic blood pressure quote between 100 and 110 mmHg [Pate], 110 mmHg [Hirose], less than a systolic blood pressure of 120 mmHg [Malhotra], and between 80 and 90 mmHg [Kepros].

Controlling the heart rate and blood pressure (systolic between 100 and 120 mmHg) using β-blockade and intravenous vasodilator is effective in preventing rupture of BTAI.

*Level of evidence*: 2b

*Grade of recommendation*: B

## 18.5 Operative Technique for Repair of Blunt Traumatic Thoracic Aortic Injuries

### 18.5.1 Which Operative Technique Should Be Used for Repair of Descending Thoracic Aortic Injuries? Is Any Technique Superior?

The optimal intraoperative technique for the repair of BAIs remains controversial. The EAST management guidelines stated that there were Level 3 data to support that the repair of aortic injury is best accomplished with some form of distal perfusion, either bypass or shunt [3].

Cardarelli et al. looked at the University of Maryland's 30 years of experience with traumatic aortic rupture [23]. There were 219 patients with a diagnosis of traumatic aortic rupture between 1971 and 2001. Patients were divided according to surgical technique. There were 82 patients in the clamp-and-sew technique group (Group A), 64 patients in the passive shunt group (Group B), and 73 patients in the heparin-less partial cardiopulmonary bypass (Group C). Mortality was 18 patients for Group A (21.9%), 23 patients for Group B (35.9%), and 13 patients for Group C (17.8%) ($p = 0.03$). Paraplegia occurred in 15 of the 64 survivors in Group A (23.4%), 7 of the 41 survivors in Group B (17%), and 0 of the 60 survivors in Group C ($p = 0.0005$). Aortic occlusion without lower body perfusion for longer than 30 min ($p = 0.004$) and surgical technique without lower body bypass support ($p = 0.0005$) were associated with paraplegia. They concluded that the use of heparin-less distal cardiopulmonary bypass in the authors' hands is safe and is associated with a reduced incidence of paraplegia.

Whitson et al. describe their experience with the repair of this injury [24]. They did a retrospective review (1991–2004) of patients with traumatic thoracic aortic injuries to evaluate whether or not an individualized approach to operative management provides acceptable neurologic outcomes. Ninety-one percent of the 67 patients who met the study criteria had concomitant injuries. Distal aortic perfusion was used in 81% of cases (75% left heart bypass, 6% cardiopulmonary bypass), and 19% underwent clamp-and-sew technique without heparinization. There were no spinal cord deficits or adverse cerebral events related to repair. If definitive repair was completed, the mortality was 16%. They concluded that judicious use of clamp-and-sew techniques can achieve excellent neurologic outcomes, equivalent to distal aortic perfusion.

*Recommendation*: Distal perfusion has been shown to decrease the incidence of paraplegia compared to clamp-and-sew technique when the aortic cross clamp time exceeds 30 min.

Some form of distal perfusion should be used since neurologic complications seem to correlate with ischemia time.

*Level of evidence*: 2a

*Grade of recommendation*: B

## 18.6 Endovascular Treatment of Blunt Traumatic Thoracic Aortic Injuries

### 18.6.1 Are Endovascular Stent Procedures Superior to Open Vascular Procedures?

Patients with blunt aortic injuries frequently have significant associated injuries that can preclude them from immediate surgical repair. Some of these associated injuries were described earlier in this chapter. Endovascular grafts have been used since 1991 for the repair of abdominal aortic aneurysms, and this approach was first described as an alternative to open repair by Parodi et al. [25]. Since then, there has been improvement in the stent graft technology, which has led to the use of stent grafts for the treatment of traumatic BAIs. Most of the studies published on the use of this technology for the treatment of blunt aortic injuries have been retrospective. In 2001, Fujikawa et al. published the first prospective case study on the use of endovascular stent grafting for the treatment of traumatic BAIs [26]. They treated six patients who had sustained blunt thoracic aortic injuries confirmed by digital subtraction angiogram with stent grafts. All patients had injury of the aortic isthmus. All patients except one had an event-free clinical course. One patient died because of rupture of the ascending aorta. They concluded that an endovascular stent graft is a valid therapeutic option with minimal surgical invasion for patients with acute-phase aortic injury.

In 2004, Ott et al. published their review of 18 patients who underwent repair of a BTAI over an 11-year period, comparing the outcomes of patients treated with endovascular repair and open repair. Six of these patients had an endovascular repair and 12 an open repair. There were no significant differences in demographics, injury, or crash statistics between the two groups. The open group had a 17% early mortality rate, a paraplegia rate of 16%, and an 8.3% incidence of recurrent laryngeal nerve injury compared to a 0% rate of mortality, paraplegia, and recurrent laryngeal nerve injury in the endovascular group. A definite trend toward decreased morbidity, mortality, intensive care unit length of stay, and number of ventilator days was seen with endovascular repair. They concluded that there was a clear trend toward improved outcomes after endovascular repair of thoracic aortic injuries compared with the standard open repair in the setting of trauma [27]. In 2004, Dunham et al. also published their retrospective review of 28 patients treated with endovascular stent grafts for blunt thoracic aortic injuries. Twelve patients were excluded because injuries occurred more than 30 days before grafting or under a different protocol, or the procedure was performed in a different center, leaving 16 patients for review. Technical success was achieved in all patients, no graft-related complications were detected during follow-up, and no patient developed postoperative paraplegia. There was one postoperative mortality secondary to comorbid injury. There was one patient with a preoperative traumatic carotid dissection who demonstrated a postoperative stroke and another patient who required thoracentesis for a pleural effusion. They concluded that endovascular stent graft repair of blunt thoracic aortic injuries can be performed safely [28].

In 2006, Andrassy et al. published their retrospective review of all patients treated for acute and chronic traumatic injury of the thoracic aorta and compared the outcome of the endovascular approach versus surgery [29]. In the study period of 14 years, 46 patients were treated. The overall 30-day mortality was 16% in patients treated for acute or contained rupture ($n = 31$) and not significantly different after endovascular versus open repair (13.3% vs. 18.8%). There was no mortality in the patients undergoing elective stent grafting or open surgery for chronic posttraumatic aortic aneurysms ($n = 15$). Conversion and/or operative revision following stent graft implantation occurred in three patients (12.5%). Neurologic complications were absent in the stent graft group (0 of 24), whereas paraplegia ($n = 2$) or minor neurologic deficits ($n = 3$) developed following open surgery (5 of 22; 22.7%; $p = 0.013$). The length of intensive care and overall hospital stay was significantly shorter for patients after elective stent graft treatment compared to open surgery ($p = 0.045$). They concluded that minimally invasive endovascular repair for patients with acute and chronic posttraumatic aneurysms is an equally effective treatment option compared with open surgery, with advantages regarding perioperative neurologic complications and duration of hospital stay under elective circumstances.

Demetriades et al. published the results of a prospective, multicenter study assessing the early efficacy and safety of endovascular stent grafts in traumatic thoracic aortic injuries and comparing outcomes with standard operative repair [30]. The decision for open or endovascular repair was surgeon's preference. One hundred and twenty-five patients (64.9%) were selected for stent grafts and 68 (35.2%) for operative repair. Stent grafts were selected in 71.6% of the 74 patients with major extrathoracic injuries and in 60% of the 115 patients with no extrathoracic injuries. Twenty-five patients in the stent graft group (20%) developed 32 device-related complications. There were 18 endoleaks (14.4%), of which 6 needed open repair. Procedure-related paraplegia developed in 2.9% in the open repair group and 0.8% in the stent graft group ($p = 0.28$). Multivariate analysis adjusting for severe extrathoracic injuries, hypotension, Glasgow Coma Scale (GCS), and age revealed that the stent graft group had a significantly lower mortality (adjusted odds ratio, 8.42; 95% confidence interval [CI], 2.76–25.69; adjusted $p$ value, <0.001) and fewer blood transfusions (adjusted mean difference, 4.98; 95% CI, 0.14–9.82; adjusted $p$ value, 0.046) than the open repair group. Among the 115 patients without major extrathoracic injuries, higher mortality and higher transfusion requirements were also found in the open repair group (adjusted odds ratio for mortality, 13.08; 95% CI, 2.53–67.53; adjusted $p$ value, 0.002; and adjusted mean difference in the transfusion units, 4.45; 95% CI, 1.39–7.51; adjusted $p$ value, 0.004). Among the 74 patients with major extrathoracic injuries, significantly higher mortality and pneumonia rates were found in the open repair group (adjusted $p$ values 0.04 and 0.03, respectively). Multivariate analysis also showed that centers with high volume of endovascular procedures had significantly fewer systemic complications (hospital length of stay [adjusted $p$ value = 0.005]) than low-volume centers. They concluded that most surgeons at the centers in the study select stent grafts for traumatic thoracic aortic ruptures, irrespective of associated injuries, injury severity, and age. Stent graft repair is associated with significantly lower mortality and fewer blood transfusions, but there is a considerable risk of serious device-related complications.

Estrera et al. reviewed their experience between January 1, 1997, and January 1, 2012, on the data regarding 338 patients who presented with suspected BTAI that were entered into the University of Texas Medical School at Houston Trauma Center Registry [31A]. A total of 175 patients (52%) underwent thoracic aortic repair; 29 (17%) had open repair with aortic cross clamping, 77 (44%) had open repair with distal aortic perfusion, and 69 (39%) had thoracic endovascular aortic repair. Outcomes were determined, including early mortality, morbidity, length of stay, and late survival. Multiple logistic regression analysis was used to compute adjusted estimates for the effects of the operative technique. The early mortality for all patients with BTAI was 41% (139/338). Early mortality rate was 17% (27/175) for operative aortic interventions, 4% (3/69) for thoracic endovascular aortic repairs, 31% (11/29) for open repairs with aortic cross clamping, and 14% (11/77) for open repairs with distal aortic perfusion. The survival rate for thoracic endovascular aortic repair at 1 and 5 years were 92% and 87%, respectively. The survival rate for open repair at 1, 5, 10, and 15 years were 76%, 75%, 72%, and 68%, respectively. They concluded that BTAI remains associated with significant early mortality. Delayed selective management, when applied with open repair with distal aortic perfusion and the use of thoracic endovascular aortic repair, has been associated with improved early outcomes. The long-term durability of thoracic endovascular aortic repair is unknown, necessitating close radiographic follow-up [31].

*Recommendation*: Endovascular stent grafts are associated with less mortality, less postoperative neurologic complications including paraplegia, and fewer systemic complications than open procedures.

Endovascular stent grafts can be safely used in the treatment of acute and chronic posttraumatic thoracic aortic aneurysms as an alternative to open repair.

*Level of evidence*: 2a

*Grade of recommendation*: B

## 18.7 Penetrating Injuries of the Aorta

There are fewer numbers of studies published on penetrating injury to the aorta compared to BAI. Penetrating injury to the thoracic aorta accounts for approximately 1% of traumatically injured aortas [32]. Mortality from such injuries has not changed in the past decade, and open surgical repair remains the gold standard in emergent situations. Endovascular stent grafts have been used successfully for the management of BAIs, and

**TABLE 18.1**

Clinical Questions

| Question | Answer | Grade of Recommendation |
|---|---|---|
| What is the ultimate imaging modality for diagnosing BTAI? | Angiography is the ultimate modality for making the diagnosis of BTAI. | B |
| What modality should be used to follow MAIs from blunt trauma? | TEE appears to be a good modality in following MAIs. | B |
| What medications should we use in the medical management of MAI and for how long should patients be required to take these medications? | β-Blockade and intravenous vasodilator therapy should be used for the medical management of MAIs. There is no study answering the question as to how long these medications should be used. | B |
| When is nonoperative management to be considered? | MAIs can be managed nonoperatively with specific medical treatment protocols to control heart rate and blood pressure. Similarly, patients who are poor operative candidates can have their injuries managed nonoperatively with treatment protocols (β-blockade and intravenous vasodilator). Patients who are initially managed nonoperatively because of concerns of concomitant injuries and whose follow-up studies reveal resolution of the aortic injury can continue to be managed nonoperatively on β-blockade and intravenous vasodilator. | B |
| What is the target blood pressure to maintain when nonoperative management or delayed surgical therapy is considered? | Controlling the heart rate and blood pressure (systolic between 100 and 120 mmHg) using β-blockade and intravenous vasodilator is effective in preventing rupture of BTAI. | B |
| Which operative technique should be used for repair of descending thoracic aortic injuries? Is any technique superior? | Some form of distal perfusion should be used because neurologic complications seem to correlate with ischemia time. | B |
| Are endovascular stent procedures superior to open vascular procedures? | Endovascular stent grafts are associated with less mortality, less postoperative neurologic complications including paraplegia, and fewer systemic complications than open procedures. | B |

there are case reports in the literature describing the use of endovascular stent grafts in penetrating injuries to the aorta [33].

Demetriades et al. conducted a retrospective analysis of all patients with penetrating aortic injuries admitted over a 5-year period [34]. The abdominal aorta was injured in 72% of 93 patients and the thoracic aorta in 28%. Eighty-two percent of the patients were admitted in shock and 41% with unrecordable blood pressures. Victims with thoracic aortic injuries were more likely to have an unrecordable blood pressure on admission than patients with abdominal aortic injuries (73% vs. 28.4%), and more likely to require an emergency room thoracotomy (76.9% vs. 20.9%). There were no survivors among the 36 patients who required an emergency room thoracotomy. The overall mortality was 80.6% (87.5% for gunshot wounds and 64.7% for knife wounds). Patients with abdominal aortic injuries were three times more likely to survive than those with thoracic aortic injuries (23.9% vs. 7.7%) [34].

Injury to the thoracic aorta, gunshot wounds, unrecordable blood pressure on admission, and the need for emergency room thoracotomy are important predictors of mortality.

*Level of evidence*: 2b

## 18.8 Injury to the Thoracic Vena Cava

Injury to the thoracic vena cava is extremely rare and is usually fatal. Most of the literatures published on these injuries are case studies and describe experience in the management of these injuries. Management involves surgical repair, and there are not enough papers to render any Levels 1, 2, or 3 data.

## References

### Diagnosis of BAI


1. Jackson DH. Of TRAs and ROCs. *Chest*. 1984;85:585–587.
2. Smith RS, Chang FC. Traumatic rupture of the aorta: Still a lethal injury. *Am J Surg*. 1986;152:660–663.
3. Nagy K, Fabian T, Rodman G et al. Guidelines for the diagnosis and management of blunt aortic injury: An EAST practice management guidelines work group. *J Trauma*. 2000;48(6):1128–1143.
4. Burkhart HM, Gomez GA, Jacobson LE et al. Fatal blunt aortic injuries: A review of 242 cases. *J Trauma*. 2001;50:113–115.

5. Chen MY, Miller PR, McLaughlin CA et al. The trend of using computed tomography in the detection of acute thoracic aortic and branch vessel injury after blunt thoracic trauma: Single-center experience over 13 years. *J Trauma*. 2004;56:783–785.
6. Melton SM, Kerby JD, McGiffin D et al. The evolution of chest computed tomography for the definitive diagnosis of blunt aortic injury: A single-center experience. *J Trauma Inj Infect Crit Care*. 2004;56:243–250.
7. Demetriades D, Velhamos G, Scalea T et al. Diagnosis and treatment of blunt thoracic aortic injuries: Changing perspectives. *J Trauma*. 2008;64(6):1415–1419.
8. Fabian T, Davis K, Gavant M et al. Prospective study of blunt aortic injury: Helical CT is diagnostic and antihypertensive therapy reduces rupture. *Ann Surg*. May 1998;227(5):666–676 discussion 676–677.


### Minimal Aortic Injuries


9. Malhotra AK, Fabian TC, Croce MA et al. Minimal aortic injury: A lesion associated with advancing diagnostic techniques. *J Trauma*. 2001;51:1042–1048.
10. Kepros J, Angood P, Jaffe CC et al. Aortic intimal injuries from blunt trauma: Resolution profile in nonoperative management. *J Trauma*. 2002;52:475–478.
11. Kidane B, Abramowitz D, Harris JR, DeRose G, Forbes TL. Natural history of minimal aortic injury following blunt thoracic aortic trauma. *Can J Surg*. December 2012;55(6):377–381.


### Nonoperative Management of Blunt Traumatic Aortic Injuries


12. Camp PC, Shackford SR. Outcome after blunt traumatic aortic laceration: Identification of a high risk cohort. *J Trauma*. 1997;43:413–422.
13. Camp PC, Rogers RB, Shackford SR et al. Blunt traumatic thoracic aortic lacerations in the elderly: An analysis of outcome. *J Trauma*. 1994;37:418–423.
14. Borman KR, Aurbakken CM, Weigelt JA. Treatment priorities in combined blunt abdominal and aortic trauma. *Am J Surg*. 1982;144:728–732.
15. Hudson HM, Woodson J, Hirsch E. The management of traumatic aortic tear in the multiply-injured patient. *Ann Vasc Surg*. 1991;5:445–448.
16. Maggisano R, Nathens A, Alexandrova NA et al. Traumatic rupture of the thoracic aorta: Should one always operate immediately? *Ann Vasc Surg*. 1995;9:44–52.
17. Wheat MW, Palmer FF, Bartley TD et al. Treatment of dissecting aneurysms of the aorta without surgery. *J Thorac Cardiovasc Surg*. 1965;50:364–373.
18. Akins CW, Buckley MJ, Daggett W et al. Acute traumatic disruption of the thoracic aorta: A ten year experience. *Ann Thorac Surg*. 1981;31:305–309.
19. Pate JW, Fabian TC, Walker W. Traumatic rupture of the aortic isthmus: An emergency? *World J Surg*. 1995;19:119–126.
20. Fabian TC, Richardson JD, Croce MA et al. Prospective study of blunt aortic injury: Multicenter trial of the American association for the surgery of trauma. *J Trauma*. 1997;42:374–383.
21. Hirose H, Gill IS, Malangoni MA. Nonoperative management of traumatic aortic injury. *J Trauma*. 2006;60:597–601.
22. Pate JW, Gavant ML, Weiman DS, Fabian TC. Traumatic rupture of the aortic isthmus: Program of selective management. *World J Surg*. 1999;23:59–63.


### Operative Technique for Repair of Blunt Traumatic Thoracic Aortic Injuries


23. Cardarelli MG, McLaughlin JS, Downing SW et al. Management of traumatic aortic rupture: A 30-year experience. *Ann Surg*. 2002;236(4):465–469.
24. Whitson BA, Nath DS, Knudtson JR et al. Is Distal aortic perfusion in traumatic thoracic aortic injuries necessary to avoid paraplegic postoperative outcomes? *J Trauma*. 2008;64:115–120.


### Endovascular Treatment of Blunt Traumatic Aortic Injuries


25. Parodi JC, Palmaz JC, Barone HD. Transfemoral intraluminal graft implantation for abdominal aortic aneurysms. *Ann Vasc Surg*. 1991;5:491–499.
26. Fujikawa T, Yukioka T, Ishimaru S et al. Endovascular stent grafting for the treatment of blunt thoracic aortic injury. *J Trauma*. February 2001;50(2):223–229.
27. Ott MC, Stewart TC, Lawlor DK et al. Management of blunt thoracic injuries: Endovascular stents versus open repair. *J Trauma*. 2004;56:565–570.
28. Dunham MB, Zygun D, Petrasek P et al. Endovascular stent grafts for acute blunt aortic injury. *J Trauma*. 2004;56:1173–1178.
29. Andrassy J, Weidenhagen R, Meimarakas G et al. Stent versus open surgery for acute and chronic traumatic injury of the thoracic aorta: A single-center experience. *J Trauma*. 2006;60:765–772.
30. Demetriades D, Velhamos GC, Scalea TM et al. Operative repair or endovascular stent graft in blunt traumatic thoracic aortic injuries: Results of an American association for the surgery of trauma multicenter study. *J Trauma*. 2008;64:561–571.
31. Estrera A, Miller C, Guajardan-Salinas G, Coogan S, Charlton-Ouw K, Safi H, Azizzadeh A. Update on blunt thoracic aortic injury: Fifteen-year single-institution experience. *J Thorac Cardiovasc Surg*. March 2013;145(3):S154–S158.


### Penetrating Injuries of the Aorta


32. Cornwell EE III, Kennedy F, Berne TV et al. Gunshot wounds to the thoracic aorta in the '90s: Only prevention will make a difference. *Am Surg*. 1995;61:721–723.
33. Fang TD, Peterson DA, Kirilcuk NN et al. Endovascular management of a gunshot wound to the thoracic aorta. *J Trauma*. 2006;60:204–208.
34. Demetriades D, Theodorou D, Murray J et al. Mortality and prognostic factors in penetrating injuries of the aorta. *J Trauma*. 1996;40:761–763.

## Commentary on Evidence-Based Surgery: Injury to the Thoracic Great Vessels

*J. Wayne Meredith*

The management of a torn thoracic aorta has dramatically changed over the course of my career. Advancements over the last two decades in the understanding of the etiology, diagnosis, and timing of operation have led to radical changes in the management of this injury.

The fundamental etiology has been recognized to not be exclusively brought on by frontal collisions, but to include a significant proportion of patients injured obliquely. The manner in which the diagnosis is made has changed dramatically. When I began treating patients with torn thoracic aortas, we were teaching residents the signs on chest x-ray that would alert one of the possible presence of a torn thoracic aorta. We went through considerable manipulations in many patients to try to get upright chest x-rays to exclude the widened mediastinum, etc. This obviously has been totally replaced by CT angiography of the chest, which has dramatically simplified and improved diagnosis of the injury. The timing of treatment has changed with the recognition that a wide mediastinum in the presence of a torn thoracic aorta is not, as we used to say, "a ticking time bomb" awaiting rupture, necessitating a sense of urgency to get the patient to the operating room before the pseudoaneurysm ruptured. In fact, the place on the list of priorities for management of this injury has changed, since it has been demonstrated that it is safe to manage the patient's blood pressure and DP/PT, allowing a more measured approach to diagnosis and treatment of other injuries.

The controversy over operative management with clamp and sew versus some sort of protected repair has never been completely resolved, but as by-pass techniques have improved, it has definitely moved in the direction of greater utilization of protection with some sort of distal perfusion. However, the advent of endovascular repair has completely revolutionized the management of this injury and dramatically reduced traditional operative morbidity and mortality.

So what does a surgeon really need to know about the management of torn thoracic aorta?

### Diagnosis of BAI

As soon as the diagnosis is suspected, one should manage the patient's blood pressure and DP/DT with beta-blockers, preferably short-acting intravenous beta-blockers. The diagnosis can then be confirmed or excluded in the vast majority of patients with chest CT angiography (CTA). CTA technology has improved to the point that it is not only sufficient to make or exclude the diagnosis of blunt aortic injury, but allows the experienced surgeon to plan and prepare the operation. In many cases, chest CTA provides superior information for operative planning, in my opinion, than that available from aortography. Furthermore, with the advent of endovascular repair, those images that need intra-aortic contrast for delineation of specific anatomic components can be obtained at the time of stent graft therapy in the vast majority of patients. Aortography remains the gold standard for diagnosis of blunt aortic injuries but has largely been replaced by CT angiography. As the chapter describes, chest CTA is a highly sensitive and specific test for the diagnosis of thoracic aortic injuries. In my opinion, it is the diagnostic test of choice for both confirmation/exclusion of the injury and operative planning.

### Minimal Aortic Injuries

Minimal aortic injury is a creature of the modern era and improved imaging techniques. Most minimal aortic injuries are best recognized with transesophageal echocardiography (TEE) technology, which is much more capable of showing small intimal tears than other imaging modalities although CT angiography is ever increasing in sensitivity for these injuries. These injuries have probably been occurring and gone untreated for the history of medicine prior to the advent of these advanced imaging technologies in the last two decades. In the period of time between the development of high-speed motor vehicle crashes and the advent of these high-definition imaging technologies, these were not identified, resulting in a plethora of latent blunt injuries of the aorta discovered months and weeks after the time of the crash. There were cases of patients undiagnosed who suddenly exsanguinated in whom there were minimal injuries that subsequently developed pseudoaneurysms and ruptured. I think the minimal aortic injuries are a definitely diagnosable phenomenon; they simply need blood pressure control, typically beta-blockers and observation. They can be followed with TEE or chest CTA.

### Nonoperative Management of Blunt Traumatic Aortic Injuries

The role for nonoperative management of blunt aortic injuries, in my estimation, is for those patients in whom the comorbidities or concomitant injuries are so significantly morbid and life-threatening that delay of treatment is warranted in the context of expected management of the patient. Otherwise, nonoperative management of blunt traumatic aortic injuries should be confined to those minimal injuries discussed earlier, which likely have always occurred and healed on their own without treatment and are likely to continue to do so.

### Operative Technique for Repair of Blunt Traumatic Thoracic Aortic Injuries

There are many salient points and elegant nuances of the proper open technique for torn thoracic aorta. I would counsel those preparing to attempt this that they should be individuals who have some experience in operating in this region. I think a generous exposure is valuable and necessary to approach the site of injury from outside the hematoma. Then, working into the hematoma, one should make every effort to open the aorta only at the site of injury so as to not create another aortotomy, resulting in two defects in the wall of the aorta. Following this plan of attack, a great many torn thoracic aortas can be repaired primarily. Care should be taken to exclude as few intercostal vessels as possible so as to reduce the incidence of spinal ischemia. If primary repair is not feasible, a graft is required. It generally requires a smaller graft than one would think. Except in the most simple and straightforward operation, distal bypass is preferred and has been shown to reduce the likelihood of major complications, including death and paraplegia. My preference is full cardiopulmonary bypass under the logic that those patients who most need it are those who have injury that spirals proximal to the subclavian artery and in those who rupture before proximal and distal control can be obtained. These situations are best managed with the capability of cooling the patient on full bypass. This approach does require heparin and this needs careful consideration in terms of the patient's concomitant injuries, etc. and is not always possible. A nonheparinized distal bypass is a sound second choice.

### Endovascular Treatment of Blunt Traumatic Thoracic Aortic Injuries

Endovascular repair has become the most prevalent treatment for blunt traumatic thoracic aortic injuries in the modern era. It has been shown to be safe and effective and to have a lower incidence of major complications and mortality. The long-term durability of this repair has not yet been shown, but it is clearly efficacious for at least months to years. I would argue, given our current state of knowledge, that this would be, if it is possible, the proper initial approach for most patients with blunt aortic injury. If indeed it has long-term failure, I think it is probably safer to electively repair a pseudoaneurysm or endoleak many years after injury. Even if it requires an open operation, it is safer to perform that operation months to years following the injury once the patient has completely rehabilitated rather than operating on them during the throws of early resuscitation and metabolic, nutritional, coagulation, and immune changes that occur from a major injury and resuscitation.

# 19

# Cardiac Trauma

**Dror Soffer and Adam Lee Goldstein**

**CONTENTS**



## 19.1 Introduction

Cardiac injury comprises a small percentage of trauma patients being received at emergency centers, with the majority of patients dying in the prehospital setting [1,2]. Despite the rarity of these cases, the importance of a high index of suspicion, precise diagnosis, and rapid intervention is vital in order to optimize survival. There are major differences between penetrating cardiac injury and blunt cardiac injury (BCI) with regard to the presentation of the patient, associated injuries, diagnostic methods, and therapeutic interventions. Depending on the mechanism of injury and management of these patients, a low mortality is obtainable [3]. There is a paucity of recommendations and guidelines in the management of traumatic cardiac injury. This chapter focuses on relevant topics of debate while reviewing the current evidence-based knowledge in the management of penetrating cardiac injury and BCI from their presentation to definitive care in the hospital setting (Table 19.1).

## 19.2 How Do You Rule Out a Significant BCI?

BCI in a stable patient seems an elusive diagnosis and is easily missed because of a high incidence of associated injuries. In an autopsy-based study looking at 1597 fatalities due to blunt trauma, 11.9% were found to have cardiac injury. In the subset with cardiac trauma, motor vehicle crashes were the cause of 56% of the BCIs, followed by falls from a significant heights (38%) and crush injuries (4%) [2]. The majority of BCI patients had associated injuries that include the thorax, abdominal cavity, and spine [4]. Another postmortem study found that sternal fractures were found in 76% of patients with BCI due to falls from a certain height, and the conclusion was made that any fall greater than 6 m (20 ft) with sternal fracture should undergo an immediate and thorough cardiac evaluation [5]. Of note, sternal fractures alone were not significantly associated with BCI [6]. Even with suggested clinical signs, laboratory tests, and imaging modalities that aid in diagnosing BCI, there remains a lack of evidence in the literature to support evidence-based clinical practice. Commonly used diagnostic modalities for BCI are electrocardiogram (ECG), cardiac enzymes (CPK-MB and troponin I), echocardiography, and most recently chest computed tomography (CCT).

Currently, the only Level 1 evidence for diagnosing BCI is the use of ECG [6]. For clinically significant BCI, a normal ECG has been found to have a negative predictive value (NPV) of 98% and a sensitivity of 89% [7]. However, further evidence has shown that ECG alone is not sufficient in ruling out significant BCI and that a number of patients with normal ECG were further diagnosed as having significant BCI within 24 h of observation [8]. A prospective study of 333 patients presenting after blunt thoracic trauma was able to demonstrate a NPV of 100% when combining a normal ECG and the cardiac-specific serum troponin I (cTnI) at admission and after 8 h to rule out significant BCI. This study concluded that in the absence of other reasons for hospitalization, such patients may be safely discharged from the emergency room [6,7].

A prospective study evaluated 187 patients with blunt cardiac trauma and concluded that cTnI levels below 1.05 μg/L in asymptomatic patients at admission and within the first 6 h after admission ruled out myocardial injury, whereas positive cTnI levels more than 1.05 μg/L mandate further cardiologic workup for the detection and management of myocardial injury. This study further described how the peak levels of pathologic cTnI correlated with the occurrence of (and severity of) ventricular arrhythmias [9].

A formal transthoracic echocardiogram (TTE) has not been found useful and is, therefore, not recommended in the initial diagnosis of BCI. No correlation was found between significant BCI and pathologic findings during TTE [10]. An analysis of 213 patients with significant BCI and a positive cTnI found only 49% to have evidence of heart injury on TTE [11]. The only current utilization of TTE has been found in patients with clinically established significant BCI who have persistent dysrhythmias and/or are hemodynamically unstable (i.e., hypotension and/or unexplained depressed cardiac index) [12].

A recent study from the United States found the cardiac portion of the focused assessment with sonography in trauma (FAST) exam to have limited utility in the majority of blunt trauma patients. This study evaluated 777 FAST exams and found blunt hemopericardium to be extremely rare and that the rate of incidental effusion was higher, thus leading to a significant amount of false positive results. Hemopericardium or cardiac rupture was only present if at least one of three identified high-acuity variables was present: major mechanism of injury, hypotension, or emergency intubation [13].

*Recommendation*: Significant BCI may be ruled out with a normal ECG and two normal serum cTnI measurements at the time of admission and after 8 h. There is no role for a TTE in the initial diagnosis for BCI in asymptomatic patients, but may be useful in patients with dysrhythmias or hemodynamic instability. The cardiac component of the FAST exam is not diagnostic in these patients.

*Level of evidence*: 1, 2

*Grade of recommendation*: B

## 19.3 What Is the Role of CCT in Cardiac Trauma?

The diagnostic workup for the hemodynamically stable patient with penetrating chest injury has changed over the years with the increased use of CCT during the initial evaluation despite inconclusive evidence. The utilization of CCT in this patient population has increased up to 3.5-fold without a clear benefit when compared to delayed follow-up chest x-ray (CXR) and/or FAST exam. CXR and FAST when combined had an equal sensitivity and increased specificity compared to CCT in identifying penetrating cardiac injuries needing intervention [14]. In the 1990s, trauma centers begin questioning the value of CCT in the management of stable thoracic trauma patients with suspected cardiac injury. A group led by Kimberly Nagy at Cook County Hospital advocated the use of CCT when ultrasound (US) was not immediately available [15]. This report identified the benefits of being able to identify trajectories and retained missile locations, while balancing the disadvantage of having to transport the patient. Similar sensitivities, specificities, and accuracy in identifying penetrating cardiac trauma were reported between US (90%–96%, 96%–97%, and 96%) and CCT (100%, 96.6%, and 96.7%). In 2012, the question of the potential use of CCT in penetrating cardiac injury was still unanswered, and another study examined the utility of CCT in stable patients and the potential diagnostic value of hemo- and/or pneumopericardium seen on CCT. They found CCT to have a sensitivity of 76.9%, specificity of 99.7%, positive predictive value of 90.9%, and NPV of 99.1%. They concluded that CCT is a potentially useful modality for the evaluation of cardiac injuries in stable patients, and that hemo- and/or pneumopericardium on CCT is highly specific for significant cardiac injury [16]. In CCT, cardiac penetrating injury is found as hemopericardium, pneumopericardium, intracardiac foreign bodies, extravasation of contrast material from the cardiac chambers, or coronary artery/cardiac vein/valvular injury [17]. CCT in the setting of cardiac penetrating trauma in the stable patient still has not been proven superior to a competent FAST of the pericardium, specifically when dealing with cardiac injuries. Nevertheless, CCT has gained popularity in this setting and has been found beneficial and cost-efficient in identifying cardiac injury in a manner equivalent to US while being able to provide additional information regarding injuries to other thoracic organs [18].

As in penetrating trauma, CCT is being used more frequency as a diagnostic modality in the stable blunt trauma patient. More specifically, CCT using ECG-gating techniques have been able to improve resolution by minimizing imaging artifacts caused by cardiac motion [19]. Despite being rarely utilized in the emergency setting, the ECG-gating scans have been shown not to slow down the diagnostic workup, have better resolution of the cardiac thoracic aorta, yet have inferior resolution of the lung parenchyma, spine, and ribs but without compromising the detection of lesions or fractures [20]. An advantage of gated CCT is that ability to visualize the coronary vessels and aid in the diagnosis of acute myocardial infarction (AMI) together with the clinical and biochemical picture

[21]. This is important in ruling out an AMI in the symptomatic patient as the primary event leading to the blunt trauma (e.g., a driver having an AMI leading to an automobile accident) or secondary to the BCI (e.g., a myocardial hematoma compressing a coronary vessel). CCT is capable of identifying hemopericardium and diagnosing cardiac tamponade, rupture, septal tears, valvular injury, herniation, cardiovascular injury, and other pathologies in the chest affecting the heart (such as extrapericardial mediastinal hematomas) after blunt trauma [22].

*Recommendation*: For penetrating trauma, CCT has not been found to be more accurate or useful than FAST together with CXR in identifying cardiac injury. Nevertheless, CCT has been found to be of value, with an increased advantage from FAST/TTE and CXR, in diagnosing other injuries in the chest cavity, while also being able to diagnose cardiac injury with a high specificity and sensitivity. CCT in blunt trauma is more specific than the FAST exam and useful in identifying hemopericardium. Evidence for the utility of gated CCT has begun to surface, especially in its ability to visualize the coronary vessels, and appears to be a useful combined modality for cardiac imaging.

*Level of evidence*: 2

*Grade of recommendation*: B

## 19.4 When Does the Stable BCI Patient Need Continuous ECG Monitoring, and for How Long?

A large number of stable patients after BCI, who are in no need for emergent surgery, will present to the emergency room symptomatic with, or without, changes in the ECG and/or a rise in cTnI. As noted earlier, cardiac arrhythmias are considered to be one of the most common manifestations of BCI, and the question remains on how to proceed with these patients by either discharging them or admitting them for observation ± further workup.

A classic review from 1989 determined that patients who will develop life-threatening arrhythmias, or relative complications, are identified in the emergency room by conduction abnormalities in the initial ECG. This group recommended that stable patients should be triaged (e.g., need for monitored/unmonitored bed, or to be discharged) based on the initial ECG, and if there are abnormalities and no other injury requiring intensive care, patients should be monitored for at least 48 h [23]. The reason behind a 48 h "window" was not clear from this study. In a prospective study of 336 patients, Cachecho et al. concluded that young patients with minor blunt thoracic trauma and normal or minimally abnormal ECG did not benefit from cardiac monitoring [24]. Another prospective study from Toronto, Canada, followed 312 patients after BCI for new cardiac arrhythmias, and found that all arrhythmias were present on admission, and that the majority were of atrial fibrillation type. They had no recommendations regarding the need and length or continuous ECG monitoring [25].

The trauma group from Cook County in Chicago, Illinois, identified a group of BCI patients—hemodynamically stable, no history of cardiac disease, a normal baseline ECG, did not require surgery or neurological observation for other injuries, and who were less than 55 years old—as being able to have a limited cardiac evaluation by admitting and monitoring for only 24 h without the development of arrhythmias or other complications related to the BCI [26].

*Recommendation*: There is clear evidence for those needing continuous monitoring when an arrhythmia is present in the emergency room and/or cardiac enzymes are abnormal. For patients without these findings, there is no evidence for the need of continuous ECG monitoring; however, in certain patient populations, 24 h of observation and monitoring has been found adequate and safe.

*Level of evidence*: 2

*Grade of recommendation*: C

## 19.5 Is There an Advantage of Using Pledgets When Suturing the Heart?

The role of pledgets in cardiac surgery is a widely debated yet hardly researched topic. A search over the past several decades yielded few published studies on cardiac suturing techniques. Despite other techniques, such as a prolene suture buttressed with polytetrafluoroethylene [27], there are no comparison studies allowing for evidence-based recommendations. In 1981, a study was conducted between nonpledgeted sutures and pledget-supported sutures and the potential for dehiscence of sutured atrioventricular valves. Pledget-supported sutures were found to be advantageous with higher suture line strength than nonpledgeted stitches [28]. In 1984, the role of pledgets in mitral valve replacements was evaluated. A prospective cohort study found the yield force of initial disruption of pledgeted sutures to be comparable to that of nonpledgeted sutures and recommended their use for mitral valve surgery [29]. In 1996, a study on cardiac suturing was conducted on canines, comparing pledget sutures to a stapling device for the rapid closure of cardiac wounds. The authors compared gross blood loss, hemodynamic instability, and the

**TABLE 19.1**

Cardiac Trauma: Question Summary

| No. | Question | Answer | Level of Evidence | Grade | References |
|---|---|---|---|---|---|
| 1 | How do you rule out a significant BCI? | The combination of repeated normal cTnI levels with a normal ECG | 1B | B | [2–13] |
| 2 | What is the role of computer tomography in cardiac trauma? | It is useful in both penetrating and blunt trauma for diagnosis of cardiac injury along with associated chest injuries, but in penetrating trauma, it is not more sensitive or specific than US. | 1 | B | [14–22] |
| 3 | When does the stable BCI patient need a continuous ECG monitoring, and for how long? | When there are changes in the ECG and/or elevated cardiac enzymes. Patients admitted for monitoring with neither ECG or enzyme abnormalities may be monitored for only 24 h. | 2 | C | [23–26] |
| 4 | Must one use pledgets when suturing the heart? | There are not enough data to show that pledgets are beneficial in cardiac trauma surgery. | 4 | C | [27–32] |
| 5 | How do you manage a foreign body in the heart? | Nonoperable and noninvasive conservative therapy is safe when the foreign object does not cause hemodynamic compromise or has a clear risk of causing embolization, infection, or fistulization. | 3 | C | [32–34] |

integrity of the repair. They concluded that stapling was faster, had similar integrity, and carried less risk of accidental needle stick than traditional repair [30]. In other somewhat-dated reports, the potential fatal complications of pledget suturing have been described. Two deaths occurred as a result of embolization of cotton pledgets following aortic valve replacement [31], and another case reporting an embolization to the pulmonary arteries [32].

*Recommendation*: There is minimal evidence available suggesting that pledget usage in elective cardiac valve surgery is beneficial, and there are few studies examining the use in the repair of traumatic cardiac injury. In contrast, there have also been several reports showing how complications directly from the pledget use may be life threatening. Despite their popularity, there is no evidence that pledget use is beneficial in suture repair of cardiac injuries.

*Level of evidence*: 4

*Grade of recommendation*: C

## 19.6 How Do You Manage a Foreign Body in the Heart?

There are multiple approaches and techniques to treat a foreign body in the heart, depending on the characteristics of the impaled or retained object and the resources available at the hospital. Over the past decade, advances in interventional radiologic techniques have been able to replace previously mandatory open-heart procedures and successfully retrieve retained intracardiac objects [32]. Reviews of case reports, editorials, and case-related analysis have formed current recommendations for these traumatic events that are not infrequent at major trauma centers.

One common theme in the past decades has been the observation that many cases of retained foreign bodies in the heart may be treated conservatively, nonoperatively, and without retrieval if it is asymptomatic and unlikely to cause problems. Complications that would require removal are perceived likelihood of embolization (due to size and location), erosion (into the bronchial system or cause fistulas within the heart), or infection (nonmetal objects) [27]. In a 1989 study, Symbas et al. retrospectively analyzed 24 gunshot patients with bullets retained in the heart, in which 14 were managed successfully without surgical intervention. Their results suggest that the management of bullets in the heart should be "individualized according to the patient's clinical course" and that bullets left in the heart are tolerated well if they remain asymptomatic [34].

*Recommendation*: Foreign bodies in the heart may be treated conservatively in stable, asymptomatic patients if there is determined to be little risk of embolization, infection, or fistula formation.

*Level of evidence*: 3

*Grade of recommendation*: C

## References

1. Campbell NC, Thomsen SR, Murkart DJ et al. Review of 1198 cases of penetrating cardiac trauma. *Br J Surg*. 1997;84:1737–1740.

2. Turan AA, Karayel FA, Akyildiz E et al. Cardiac injuries caused by blunt trauma: An autopsy based assessment of the injury pattern. *J Forensic Sci.* 2010;55:82–84.
3. Degiannis E, Loogna P, Doll D et al. Penetrating cardiac injuries: Recent experiences in South Africa. *World J Surg.* 2006;30(7):1258–1264.
4. Teixeira PG, Georgiou C, Inaba K et al. Blunt cardiac trauma: Lessons learned from the medical examiner. *J Trauma.* 2009;67(6):1259–1264.
5. Turk EE, Tsokos M. Blunt cardiac trauma caused by fatal falls from height: An autopsy-based assessment of the injury pattern. *J Trauma.* 2004;57:301–304.
6. Clancy K, Velopulos C, Bilaniuk JW et al. Eastern Association for the Surgery of Trauma. Screening for blunt cardiac injury: An eastern association for the surgery of trauma practice management guideline. *J Trauma Acute Care Surg.* 2012;73:S301–S306.
7. Velmahos GC, Karaiskakis M, Salim A et al. Normal electrocardiography and serum troponin I levels preclude the presence of clinically significant blunt cardiac injury. *J Trauma.* 2003;54:45–51.
8. Salim A, Velmahos GC, Jindal A et al. Clinically significant blunt cardiac trauma: Role of serum troponin levels combined with electrocardiographic findings. *J Trauma.* 2001;50(2):237–243.
9. Rajan GP, Zellweger R. Cardiac troponin I as a predictor of arrhythmia and ventricular dysfunction in trauma patients with myocardial contusion. *J Trauma.* 2004;57(4):801–808.
10. Nagy KK, Krosner SM, Robert RR et al. Determining which patients require evaluation for blunt cardiac injury following blunt chest trauma. *World J Surg.* 2001;25(1):108–111.
11. Yousef R, Carr JA. Blunt cardiac trauma: A review of the current knowledge and management. *Ann Thorac Surg.* 2014;98:1134–1140.
12. Joos E, Tadloc MD, Inaba K. Diagnosis, work-up and management of blunt cardiac injuries. *J Trauma.* 2014;16(2):93–98.
13. Press GM, Miller S. Utility of the cardiac component of FAST in blunt trauma. *J Emerg Med.* 2013;44(1):9–16.
14. Mollberg NM, Wise SR, De Hoyos AL et al. Chest computed tomography for penetrating thoracic trauma after normal screening chest roentgenogram. *Ann Thorac Surg.* 2012;93(6):1830–1835.
15. Nagy KK, Gilkey SH, Roberts RR et al. Computed tomography screens stable patients at risk for penetrating cardiac injury. *Acad Emerg Med.* 1996;3(11):1024–1027.
16. Plurad DS, Bricker S, Van Natta TL et al. Penetrating cardiac injury and the significance of chest computed tomography findings. *Emerg Radiol.* 2013;20(4):279–284.
17. Gunn ML, Clark RT, Sadro CT et al. Current concepts in imaging evaluation of penetrating transmediastinal injury. *Radiographics.* 2014;34(7):1824–1841.
18. Stassen NA, Lukan JK, Spain DA et al. Reevaluation of diagnostic procedures for transmediastinal gunshot wounds. *J Trauma Inj Infect Crit Care.* 2002;53(4):635–638.
19. Desjardins B, Kazerooni EA. ECG-gated cardiac CT. *Am J Roentgenol.* 2004;182(4):993–1010.
20. Schertler T, Glücker T, Wildermuth S et al. Comparison of retrospectively ECG-gated and nongate chest in an emergency setting regarding workflow, image quality, and diagnostic certainty. *Emerg Radiol.* 2005;12:19–29.
21. Restrepo CS, Gutierrez FR, Marmol-Velez JA et al. Imaging patients with cardiac trauma. *Radiographics.* 2012;32(3):633–649.
22. Malbranque G, Serfaty JM, Himbert D et al. Myocardial infarction after blunt chest trauma: Usefulness of cardiac ECG-gated CT and MRI for positive and aetiologic diagnosis. *Emerg Radiol.* June 2011;18(3):271–274.
23. Wisner DH, Reed WH, Riddick RS. Suspected myocardial contusion: Triage and indications for monitoring. *Ann Surg.* 1990;212(1):82.
24. Cachecho R, Grindlinger GA, Lee VW. The clinical significance of myocardial contusion. *J Trauma.* 1992;33(1):68–71.
25. McLean RF, Devitt JH, Dubbin J et al. Incidence of abnormal RNA studies and dysrhythmias in patients with blunt chest trauma. *J Trauma.* 1991;31(7):968–970.
26. Fildes JJ, Betlej TM, Manglano R et al. Limiting cardiac evaluation in patients with suspected myocardial contusion. *Am Surg.* 1995;61(9):832–835.
27. Beattie R, Mhandu PC, McManus K. Penetrating thoracic trauma. *Surgery.* 2014;32(5):249–253.
28. Katz NM, Blackstone EH, Kirklin JW et al. Suture techniques for atrioventricular valves: Experimental study. *J Thorac Cardiovasc Surg.* 1981;81(4):528–536.
29. Newton JR, Jr., Glower DD, Davis JW et al. Evaluation of suture techniques for mitral valve replacement. *J Thorac Cardiovasc Surg.* 1984;88(2):248–252.
30. Bowman MR, King RM. Comparison of staples and sutures for cardiorrhaphy in traumatic puncture wounds of the heart. *J Emerg Med.* 1996;14(5):615–618.
31. Lifschultz BD, Donoghue ER, Leestman RA et al. Embolization of cotton pledgets following insertion of porcine cardiac valve bioprostheses. *J Forensic Sci.* 1987;32(6):1796–1800.
32. Weingarten J, Kauffman SL. Teflon embolization to pulmonary arteries. *Ann Thorac Surg.* 1977;23(4):371–373.
33. Gilchrist IC. Foreign body in the heart: Be careful how you remove it. *Cathet Cardiovasc Interv.* 2012;80(3):497.
34. Symbas PN, Vlasis-Hale SE, Picone AL et al. Missiles in the heart. *Ann Thorac Surg.* 1989;48(2):192–194.

## Commentary on Cardiac Trauma

*Demetrios Demetriades*

Following penetrating trauma to the chest, about 10% of patients reaching hospital care have cardiac injuries. However, the majority of patients with penetrating cardiac injuries, especially due to gunshot wounds, die at the scene and never reach hospital care.

Blunt cardiac injury includes a wide spectrum of pathologies, ranging from asymptomatic myocardial contusion to cardiac rupture. The incidence of symptomatic blunt cardiac contusion requiring treatment (arrhythmias or cardiogenic shock) after significant chest trauma resulting in chest wall fractures or intrathoracic injuries is about 13%. The reported incidence of cardiac rupture in patients reaching hospital care is about 0.05%. However, this is the tip of the iceberg, because the vast majority of cases are declared dead at the scene. In a recent autopsy study of 304 deaths after traffic injuries in the County of Los Angeles, 20% had cardiac rupture; 85% of deaths occurred at the scene and only 15% reach medical care.

### How Do You Rule Out a Significant Blunt Cardiac Injury?

The diagnosis of blunt cardiac trauma in the multitrauma patient is not always easy. Every patient with significant chest trauma (defined as rib, sternal or scapular fractures, pulmonary contusion, hemo-pneumothorax, or anterior seatbelt mark) should always be evaluated for cardiac trauma. The presence of a left flail chest or sternal fracture is a strong marker of underlying blunt cardiac injury.

Patients with cardiac rupture due to blunt trauma who reach hospital care are almost always in extremis or cardiac arrest on arrival to the emergency room. A FAST (focused assessment with sonography for trauma) exam and/or resuscitative thoracotomy are the only useful diagnostic or therapeutic procedures. On rare occasions with small atrial ruptures and short prehospital times, the patient might be alive and occasionally stable on arrival and the diagnosis is made by FAST or CT scan.

The majority of patients with cardiac contusions are asymptomatic and the diagnosis is made by ECG or elevated troponins. Symptomatic cardiac arrhythmias or cardiogenic shock requiring treatment are diagnosed in approximately 13% of patients with significant chest trauma

Stable patients with suspected blunt cardiac trauma should be evaluated by FAST exam, EKG, and cardiac biomarkers. Several studies have demonstrated the superiority of troponin-I as a biomarker of traumatic myocardial injury when compared to CK-MB. A formal echocardiogram should be performed in all patients with abnormal clinical, EKG, or troponin level findings. ECG abnormalities may include arrhythmias, elevated ST, inverted T-waves, and low QRS complexes.

Admission ECG and troponin-I levels may predict which patients are likely to develop a cardiac-related complication. In a Los Angeles large prospective study of 333 consecutive patients with severe chest trauma, the diagnostic role of the initial and serial troponin and ECG evaluation was evaluated. The sensitivity and specificity of the initial troponin-I alone were about 75% and 60%, respectively, and those of ECG alone about 90% and 70%, respectively. However, when the two investigations were combined, the sensitivity and specificity increased to 100% and 70%, respectively. From a different angle, if the troponin-I alone was abnormal, the incidence of significant blunt cardiac trauma was 7%; if only the ECG was abnormal, the incidence was 22%; and if both were abnormal, the rate increased to 36%. Most importantly, if both investigations were normal, no clinically significant blunt cardiac trauma was observed.

On the basis of the available evidence, it is suggested that all asymptomatic patients with severe chest trauma should be evaluated for blunt cardiac trauma, by means of routine EKG and troponin levels. Those with abnormal findings should undergo formal echocardiography evaluation, admission to a monitored area, and serial EKG and troponin tests until normalization. Patients with normal initial EKG and troponins do need further evaluation or monitoring for cardiac trauma (Figure C19.1).

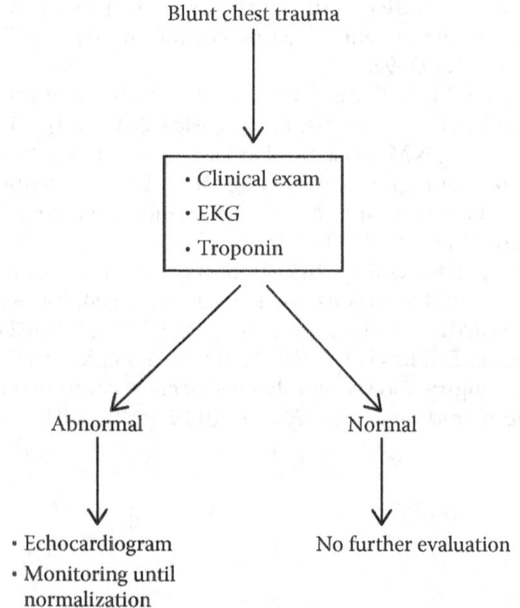


**FIGURE C19.1**

### What Is the Role of Computed Tomography in Cardiac Trauma?

Although computed tomography has a major role in the evaluation of blunt or penetrating chest trauma, it has a very limited role in the evaluation of suspected cardiac trauma. However, it has a definitive role in the evaluation of suspected retained missiles or other foreign bodies in the heart. In all other cases, a CT scan should be used mainly as part of the general evaluation of chest trauma.

### When Does the Stable BCI Patient Need a Continuous ECG Monitoring, and for How Long?

Symptomatic BCI patients with arrhythmias or cardiogenic shock should be admitted in the intensive care unit for continuous clinical, EKG, and troponin monitoring, until resolution of the symptoms or abnormal findings. A formal echocardiogram should be performed to evaluate for any underlying functional or anatomical cardiac abnormalities.

Asymptomatic patients with abnormal EKG or troponins should be observed in a monitored area until normalization. There is no need for any specific treatment in this group of patients. Transthoracic echocardiography (TTE) should be performed.

In patients with myocardial contusion requiring early surgery for other associated injuries, general anesthesia and operation are safe, although more aggressive intraoperative hemodynamic monitoring is advisable.

### Is There an Advantage to Using Pledgets When Suturing the Heart?

The vast majority of cardiac wounds can safely be repaired with figure-of-eight, horizontal mattress or running sutures, using nonabsorbable 2/0 or 3/0 sutures on a large tapered needle. Routine use of pledgets is time consuming and unnecessary in the majority of cases and should be reserved for cases where the myocardium tears during tying the sutures.

### How Do You Manage a Foreign Body in the Heart?

Foreign bodies in the pericardial sac, myocardium, or the cardiac chambers may be due to direct penetrating trauma. However, a significant number of cardiac intracavitary foreign bodies are due to embolization, secondary to a peripheral or pulmonary vascular injury.

Retained cardiac missiles or foreign bodies in the heart may lead to serious complications, including embolization, transmural erosion resulting in cardiac tamponade, delayed pericardial effusion, dysrhythmias, valve dysfunction, and endocarditis.

The management of retained cardiac foreign bodies should be individualized, taking into account the timing of diagnosis, the presence of symptoms, the anatomical location, and the type and size of the foreign body.

As a general rule, all foreign bodies in the heart diagnosed at the time of injury should be removed, because of the risks described earlier. The exact location of the foreign body and planning of the procedure are determined by CT scan and echocardiography.

Intracavitary foreign bodies may embolize and should be removed without any delay. Removal by interventional cardiology, using catheterization and a wire basket or a snare, is possible in many cases. Open heart surgery with cardiac bypass may be necessary if the endovascular approach fails or is not available.

The management of foreign bodies embedded in the myocardium or in the pericardial sac depends on the timing of diagnosis, symptomatology, size of the foreign body, and the echocardiogram or CT scan findings. Generally, asymptomatic foreign bodies fully embedded in the myocardium or in the pericardial sac, identified long after the injury, can safely be managed without removal. However, if the diagnosis is made soon after the injury, the foreign bodies should be removed, except in cases with very small objects, such as shotgun pellets. The removal is performed operatively, almost always without the need for cardiac bypass. The foreign body can usually be palpated and a 3-0 non absorbable figure-of-8 suture is placed underneath the bullet, followed by cardiotomy and enucleation of the foreign body. The suture is tied immediately after the removal.

# 20

# *Injury to the Esophagus, Trachea, and Bronchus*

**Deborah L. Mueller**

## CONTENTS



David Hume, a Scottish philosopher, remarked that a wise man proportions his belief to the evidence. In the case of traumatic injuries to the esophagus and tracheobronchial tree, the evidence consists mostly of case reports, retrospective analyses, and opinions. The rarity of these injuries has prevented the accumulation of significant prospective data. This brief synopsis will cover incidence, mechanism of injury, and current practices in the diagnosis and management of these rare injuries. It may not strengthen the wise physician's beliefs, but it accurately reflects the current evidence (Table 20.1).

## 20.1 Trachea and Bronchus

### 20.1.1 What Is the Incidence of Blunt and Penetrating Tracheobronchial Injuries?

Dated autopsy studies of blunt trauma patients reveal an incidence of tracheobronchial injury in 1%–2.8% of fatalities [1,2]. In a more recent review spanning 9 years including blunt and penetrating mechanisms of injury, the incidence rate of tracheobronchial injury was only 0.13% [3].

Penetrating cervical tracheal injury is more common occurring in up to 7.5% of patients [4]. In contrast, penetrating thoracic tracheobronchial injury is rare occurring in less than 1% of patients even with transmediastinal trajectories [5,6].

### 20.1.2 What Is the Mechanism for Penetrating and Blunt Tracheobronchial Injuries?

While most penetrating injuries from knives and bullets require no explanation, the clothesline injury pattern is more unique. An obvious penetrating or subtle closed injury to the trachea can occur when a patient strikes an unseen wire while on a moving vehicle. Blunt cervical tracheal injury can occur from hyperextension or flexion and contact of the neck with the dashboard or steering wheel in a motor vehicle crash. It has also been described after a blow to the neck from a table corner, a knee, and bicycle handlebars in children [7]. Blunt thoracic tracheobronchial injury has been reported more commonly after forceful anterior–posterior compression of the thoracic cage with presumed lateral traction causing injury at the carina or by shearing forces exerted at the fixed carina [8]. Additional reports suggest a closed glottis with high airway pressures may also lead to injury [9]. In an analysis of 88 cases with the site of blunt tracheobronchial injury recorded, 76% occurred within 2 cm of the carina, lending credibility to the postulated mechanisms [10].

### 20.1.3 What Are the Most Reliable Initial Symptoms and Signs of Traumatic Tracheobronchial Injury?

Series that include data on symptomatology and physical findings report the most common symptom as respiratory distress in 59% of patients and the most common physical finding as subcutaneous emphysema in 81% of patients [7,11–14]. The initial chest x-ray (CXR) findings of patients in one of these series demonstrated subcutaneous emphysema in 81%, pneumothorax in 56%, and pneumomediastinum in 37% [13]. In most case series in the literature, there are occasional patients with a delay in diagnosis due to minimal symptoms and findings or due to findings being attributed to other etiologies [8].

*Recommendation*: Respiratory distress and subcutaneous emphysema/crepitus

Grade *of recommendation*: B

### 20.1.4 What Is the Best Diagnostic Test for Traumatic Tracheobronchial Injury?

Certain patients with airway injury will have obvious findings on physical exam such as air bubbling from a penetrating neck wound. An additional subset of patients will require operative intervention immediately for injury to adjacent vascular structures, leading to the discovery of airway injury. Patients with a blunt mechanism of injury can be more difficult to diagnose.

While an initial CXR may demonstrate an abnormality, it can be normal in 12% of patients on presentation [13]. In addition, the findings on CXRs such as subcutaneous emphysema, pneumothorax, and pneumomediastinum are not specific for tracheobronchial injury. In a review of 51 blunt thoracic trauma patients who had a CXR followed by chest computed tomography (CT) demonstrating pneumomediastinum, only 10% had tracheobronchial injury [15]. More often pneumomediastinum was ascribed to the Macklin effect originally described in 1939 when blunt alveolar rupture leads to air dissection along bronchovascular sheaths and into the mediastinum.

In this era of high-quality rapid imaging with CT, many patients will undergo CT as part of their trauma evaluation. In a prospective trial of multidetector computed tomographic angiography (MDCTA) for penetrating cervical wounds, MDCTA was 100% sensitive for aerodigestive injury [16]. Overall specificity was 97.5% with three of the five false-positive studies demonstrating air tracking suspicious for aerodigestive injury that was subsequently ruled out by other diagnostic modalities. In a retrospective review of 18 patients with either blunt or penetrating tracheobronchial injury who underwent both chest CT and bronchoscopy, Scaglione et al. described radiologic findings that showed the site of injury was detectable by CT in 94% of cases [17]. Findings included over distension of the endotracheal cuff (>4 cm), endotracheal cuff herniation through a tracheal wall defect, displacement of the endotracheal tube, tracheal/bronchial wall discontinuity, enlargement of the bronchus, and the "fallen lung" sign. There was no control group in this retrospective review, and scans were extensively reformatted and read by experienced radiologists.

Bronchoscopy with direct visualization of the airway remains a good diagnostic tool for tracheobronchial injury. While most injuries are obvious, a few can be subtle to the eye. Peribronchial tissue can make the airway tree seem intact with only slight distraction of the cartilaginous rings [8,18]. Kiser et al. found reports of 46 patients with repair of chronic tracheobronchial obstruction from 3 months to 34 years after injury [10]. Repeat bronchoscopy may be necessary if suspicion for the injury is high, but initial bronchoscopy appeared normal.

*Recommendation*: Bronchoscopy; CT that may be used as a screening study

*Grade of recommendation*: C

### 20.1.5 What Are the Surgical Management Options for Tracheobronchial Injuries?

The principles of surgical repair are for the most part consistent throughout the literature [3,11–13]. The cervical trachea is approached through a collar or anterior sternocleidomastoid incision, while the mediastinal trachea and right mainstem bronchus are best approached through a right posterolateral thoracotomy at the level of the fifth rib to avoid the aorta. The left mainstem bronchus is best approached through a left posterolateral thoracotomy. The high mediastinal tracheal injury with associated vascular injury may also be approached through a sternotomy incision [13]. Debridement of devitalized tissue is recommended with the use of absorbable sutures with knots secured exterior to the airway to prevent granulation tissue formation in the airway. Minimal dissection of the lateral aspects of the trachea will prevent ischemia to the repair. The use of a tracheostomy, while touted by some authors, is discouraged by others who suggest that extubation and avoidance of positive pressure ventilation in the postoperative period is best for healing of the injury [11].

In the setting of larger destructive wounds, several centimeters of trachea can be resected and primary anastomosis performed. More length can be obtained if spine fracture has been eliminated and the neck can be flexed. There are additional maneuvers to gain length for tracheal repair that are beyond the scope of this chapter. Most authors recommend buttressing of complex repairs with flaps of pericardium or intercostal muscle in the chest or strap muscles or the sternocleidomastoid in the neck [3,11–13]. Alternatively, the use of a silicone T-tube placed in the trachea to extend from below the vocal cords to the carina with an airway maintained by cannulating the horizontal exteriorized limb with an endotracheal tube has been described in at least 16 traumatic tracheal injuries [19]. This maneuver allows damage control in an unstable patient with repair of the airway in a more elective manner or the T-tube can serve as a stent while healing by secondary intention occurs.

### 20.1.6 What Is the Role of Nonoperative Management for Tracheobronchial Injuries?

Nonoperative management of small iatrogenic injuries of the trachea sustained during endotracheal intubation has been described by multiple authors [20–22]. The largest of these types of injuries managed nonoperatively was 4 cm [21]. Duval et al. described five children with noniatrogenic traumatic tracheobronchial injuries that were successfully managed nonoperatively with intubation and antibiotics [7]. A retrospective review of adults at one institution over 10 years described a nonoperative approach for both iatrogenic and traumatic tracheobronchial injuries [11]. While 89% of iatrogenic intubation injuries in these adults were managed nonoperatively, only 27% of traumatic injuries met their criteria to be managed nonoperatively. Surgical management was performed if patients had concomitant esophageal injury, progressive subcutaneous or mediastinal emphysema, severe dyspnea requiring intubation, difficulty with mechanical ventilation, pneumothorax with a persistent air leak, the presence of an open tracheal injury or mediastinitis. The traumatic injuries managed nonoperatively were all blunt mechanism small (<2 cm) injuries. All patients were followed up for 2 years with repeat bronchoscopy, and the incidence of scarring, granuloma formation, and stenosis did not appear significantly different between the nonoperative and operative groups.

It may be reasonable to allow some tracheobronchial injuries to heal by secondary intention if the patient has no associated injuries requiring surgical repair, no significant respiratory difficulty, no persistent air leak, and well-opposed edges at the site of injury. Antibiotic utilization to prevent mediastinitis is described in all of these nonoperative approaches. It is important to remember that the numbers of patients in all of these reports whether operative or nonoperative is incredibly small, and therefore, the only evidence we have is past experience.

*Recommendation*: Yes, in patients with small (<2 cm) tears and a benign clinical presentation

*Grade of recommendation*: C

## 20.2 Esophagus

### 20.2.1 What Is the Incidence of Blunt and Penetrating Esophageal Injuries?

Autopsies from all fatal traffic accidents in one metropolitan area demonstrated that blunt esophageal injury is rarer than tracheobronchial injury, occurring in only 1 of the 585 victims or 0.2% [2]. In blunt trauma patients arriving at a hospital, Beal et al. found three esophageal injuries in 2560 patients for an incidence of 0.001% [23]. Not surprisingly, in studies of penetrating trauma, the incidence of esophageal injury, both cervical and thoracic, is nearly identical to the incidence of penetrating tracheobronchial injury. Cervical esophageal injuries occurred in 8.5% of penetrating neck wounds, and thoracic esophageal injuries occurred in 1.2% of penetrating thoracic wounds [24,25].

### 20.2.2 What Is the Mechanism for Penetrating and Blunt Esophageal Injuries?

The most common mechanism for penetrating esophageal injury is iatrogenic endoscopic perforation with rates escalating significantly when therapeutic interventions such as dilation are undertaken [26]. While many articles in the literature lump iatrogenic and noniatrogenic injuries together to achieve a better number of esophageal injuries to analyze, the average trauma patient has significant other associated injuries that may affect the presentation, management, and outcome. The focus of this chapter will remain strictly noniatrogenic traumatic esophageal injuries to allow a more narrow focus on the true presentation, diagnosis, and management of these specific types of injuries.

Blunt cervical esophageal injury is thought to occur from a sudden blow to a hyperextended neck similar to cervical tracheal injury with the esophagus stretched against the cervical spine [27]. In the most extensive review published of 63 patients with blunt esophageal injury, Beal et al. demonstrated 82% of the injuries occurred in the cervicothoracic esophagus defined as the esophagus from origination to the tracheal carina [23]. Interestingly, in this same series, 56% had concomitant tracheal injuries. When both the trachea and esophagus are injured at the level of the carina, Martel et al. suggest this disruption is best described as "acute tracheoesophageal burst injury," resulting from an acute increase in tracheal intraluminal pressure after rapid compression of the thoracic cavity with a closed glottis leading to rupture of the membranous trachea and the adjacent esophagus [28]. This mechanism was delineated clearly in a case report of a 14-year-old boy struck abruptly in the chest while lying flat and sustaining a tracheoesophageal injury [9]. The majority of these combined tracheoesophageal injuries occur in young patients without accompanying rib fractures, which, as Martel et al. suggest, demonstrates that the rapid compressive force to an elastic chest cavity causes a pneumatic blast in the distal trachea as the pulmonary alveoli empty rupturing the trachea and then the esophagus [28].

### 20.2.3 What Are the Most Reliable Initial Symptoms and Signs of Traumatic Esophageal Injury?

In a large retrospective series of 405 penetrating esophageal injuries, Asensio et al. state that most patients had no symptoms or signs on initial presentation [29]. However, if one looks closely at the hospital course of these patients, the early mortality defined as death in the emergency room or operating room was 14.6%. These patients may have had symptoms or signs of esophageal injury, but the urgency of other injuries probably superseded any detailed examination or documentation. Another 175 patients went directly to the operating room, and careful evaluation for symptoms or signs may have been appropriately abbreviated. Delving into single-center studies of penetrating cervical trauma, several authors report that symptoms or signs were present in 70%–100% of patients with esophageal injury [14,30–32]. The symptoms in these studies include dysphagia, odynophagia, dysphonia, hoarseness, and hematemesis. Beal et al. also demonstrated that 66% of patients with blunt esophageal injury had symptoms including neck pain, chest pain, dyspnea, dysphagia, and/or hoarseness [23].

The most reliable physical exam finding was subcutaneous emphysema in both blunt and penetrating esophageal injuries. This sign was found in 33% of patients with blunt injury and 45% of patients with penetrating injury [23,33]. The most likely etiology for crepitus on palpation is a concomitant tracheal injury, as the incidence of this finding drops to 13% in blunt trauma patients and 28% in penetrating trauma patients when only the esophagus is injured [23,34]. The presence of subcutaneous emphysema or pneumomediastinum was also the most common finding on CXR, occurring in 30%–40% of patients with both mechanisms of injury [23,33]. It is important to note that based on these more detailed studies in regard to signs and symptoms, 25% of patients may still be completely asymptomatic with minimal physical findings and a normal CXR.

*Recommendation*: Pain (neck, chest, or on swallowing) and crepitus on physical exam

*Grade of recommendation*: B

### 20.2.4 What Is the Best Diagnostic Test for Traumatic Esophageal Injury?

The overall mortality rates for blunt and penetrating esophageal injuries in the literature are high at 17% and 19%, respectively [23,29]. The majority of the deaths in the penetrating group occur early from associated injuries [29,35]. In patients stable enough to undergo diagnostic studies, it appears that infectious morbidity is increased secondary to the delay in operative repair that occurs with a lengthy diagnostic workup. Evaluation for injury took a mean of 13 h in the largest retrospective review of penetrating injuries [29]. Although this large study did not demonstrate a difference in mortality secondary to delays in diagnosis, several single-center reviews of esophageal perforation have [32,34,36,37].

CT scan has emerged as a rapidly available screening test for esophageal injury in both blunt and penetrating trauma. In blunt trauma patients, there are often other indications for CT of the neck and chest. In stable penetrating injury patients, CT can be obtained much more rapidly than traditional studies such as esophagography and endoscopy. Indeed, Patel et al. found median times to first CT for diagnosis of 1.1 h with an interquartile range of 0.6–3 h in a contemporary analysis of penetrating esophageal injury utilizing the National Trauma Data Bank [35]. Information about confirmatory diagnostic studies was not provided, but time to operative intervention appeared to be less than 4 h for the majority of patients. Castelguidone et al. have described retrospectively the CT findings in six patients with traumatic esophageal injuries [38]. The most common findings were periesophageal air and fluid in 83% and esophageal wall thickening in 66%. Other nonspecific findings included pneumothorax, pleural effusion, and subcutaneous emphysema. In a recent study of neck CTA for detecting significant vascular or aerodigestive injuries from penetrating trauma, sensitivity was 100% and specificity was 97.5% [16]. Three false-positive findings in this study were for air tracking that was highly suspicious for aerodigestive injury. Esophageal injury was ruled out using endoscopy and esophagography. Notably, 98% of patients screened with CTA avoided further esophageal diagnostic studies with no missed injuries. CT has emerged as a tool to quickly screen for esophageal injury. It can potentially be definitive for diagnosis, but more often may show nonspecific yet concerning findings that should be further evaluated with esophagography and/or endoscopy.

The most methodologically sound study of traditional diagnostic techniques for esophageal injuries remains a prospective study in 118 stable patients with penetrating zone II and III injuries performed in the early 1980s [30]. After consent, patients underwent angiography and barium esophagography, followed by operative exploration. Prior to surgical exploration, both fiber optic and rigid endoscopy were performed by an endoscopist unaware of the esophagography results. Sensitivity and specificity were calculated for each diagnostic technique. Barium esophagography had a sensitivity of 89% and a specificity of 100%, flexible esophagoscopy had a sensitivity of 37% and a specificity of 99%, and rigid esophagoscopy a sensitivity of 89% and specificity of 95%. Therefore, Weigelt et al. summarized that patients should undergo barium esophagography initially. If an injury is seen, the patient should proceed to neck exploration, but if the study is equivocal, a rigid esophagoscopy should be performed.

Subsequently, several small retrospective studies evaluating the role of flexible endoscopy in the diagnosis of esophageal trauma have been published. The sensitivity of flexible endoscopy reported in these trials ranged from 67% to 100% with specificities also of 67%–100% [32,39,40]. Perhaps the improvement in sensitivity was secondary to technologic advances in the equipment with substantial improvement in resolution and magnification over time, or perhaps it is just a sequela of weaker study design. There are clearly some advantages to flexible endoscopy, one of which is the ability to perform it in any location. Flowers et al. performed 65% of their endoscopies in the emergency room with an average time between presentation and procedure of 2.6 h [39]. While rigid esophagoscopy can probably be performed as expediently, it requires endotracheal intubation and general anesthesia. In addition, in blunt trauma patients with unclear cervical spine status, the procedure cannot be performed.

CT appears to be a reasonable screening exam in stable patients with either blunt or penetrating mechanisms who do not require immediate operative intervention for other injuries. If the CT is suggestive of but not diagnostic for esophageal injury, a confirmatory diagnostic test should be undertaken. The best confirmatory test should probably be the one that can be performed most expediently at any individual institution and is most appropriate for the clinical scenario of the patient. Both flexible esophagoscopy and esophagography are reasonable confirmatory studies if readily available. In either case, if one test is equivocal, the second study should be undertaken to try to ensure minimization of missed injuries. Since rigid esophagoscopy requires general anesthesia and intubation, it does not seem logical as the first confirmatory diagnostic study. While prior studies demonstrated a higher incidence of false-negative exams using flexible endoscopy as compared to rigid endoscopy in the proximal esophagus due to blind passage of the flexible scope at this location, contemporary studies dispute those data [32,41].

*Recommendation*: CT for initial screening with confirmation endoscopy and/or esophagography.

*Grade of recommendation*: C

### 20.2.5 What Are the Surgical Management Options for Esophageal Injuries?

The surgical options described in the literature range from primary repair to multiple variations on diversion with drainage [32,33,36,37,42]. Approaches to the esophagus like the trachea vary based on anatomic location of the injury. The cervical esophagus is approached through a cervical incision. The upper thoracic esophagus is approached through a right fourth interspace posterolateral thoracotomy, and the lower esophagus is approached through the left fifth or sixth interspace posterolateral thoracotomy [43]. Primary repair has been described with both single-layer and two-layer closures of the esophagus after debridement of devitalized tissue [33,37,42]. Drainage as an adjunct to primary repair was used in the majority of patients in the largest studies of noniatrogenic penetrating esophageal injuries [29,42]. Buttressing of repairs with flaps of muscle, pleura, pericardium, omentum, and stomach have all been described, and their use seems predicated on the amount of local tissue destruction, injuries to adjacent structures such as the trachea, and the location of the primary injury [24,28,29,33,36,37,42]. After primary repair, the most common procedure performed in the largest studies of both penetrating and blunt esophageal injury was drainage alone [23,29]. More complex esophageal resection, exclusion, or diversion only occurred in 7% of penetrating esophageal injuries and 9% of blunt esophageal injuries. Instead of resection, Richardson et al. suggest that patients with large defects not amenable to primary repair are candidates for primary muscle flap closure [37]. In his review of factors that affected mortality, surgical management with esophageal exclusion and diversion was statistically significant for an increase in mortality. These patients in all likelihood had more severe injuries, but that is difficult to elucidate from the article.

Past experience would, therefore, suggest that primary repair with drainage is appropriate in most patients. Primary repair without drainage for simple stab wounds with minimal tissue destruction is also reasonable. Drainage alone, if the injury is difficult to identify or the patient's condition warrants abbreviated surgery, is a reasonable choice as well. Finally, more extensive esophageal surgery such as diversion, resection with or without anastomosis, or exclusion may be necessary but portends a poor prognosis similar to delays in diagnosis.

**TABLE 20.1**

Clinical Question Summary

| Question | Answer | Levels of Evidence | Grade of Recommendation | References |
|---|---|---|---|---|
| What are the most common symptoms and signs of tracheobronchial injury? | Respiratory distress and subcutaneous emphysema/crepitus | IIIb, IIIb, IIIb, IIIb, Ib | B | [7,11–14] |
| What is the best diagnostic test for tracheobronchial injury? | Bronchoscopy; CT that may be used as a screening study | IIb, IV, IV, IV, IV, IIb, IV | C | [4,7,11–13,16,17] |
| Is there a role for nonoperative management of traumatic tracheobronchial injuries? | Yes, in patients with small (<2 cm) tears and a benign clinical presentation | IV, IV, IV, IV | C | [7,11,21,22] |
| What are the most common symptoms and signs of esophageal injury? | Pain (neck, chest, or on swallowing) and crepitus on physical exam | Ib, IIIa, IIb, Ib, IIb | B | [14,23,29–31] |
| What is the best initial diagnostic test for esophageal injury? | CT for initial screening with confirmation endoscopy and/or esophagography | IIb, IV, IIb, V, IV, IV, IIb | C | [30,32,35,38–41] |
| Is there a role for nonoperative management of traumatic esophageal injury? | Not enough evidence to recommend for traumatic injuries at this time | IV, IV | D | [42,44] |

### 20.2.6 Is There Any Role for Nonoperative Management in Traumatic Esophageal Injury?

In some reviews of esophageal perforation, there seems to be a category of conservative or nonoperative management [26,32,36]. Looking closely at these reviews, most articles have a mix of etiologies for the perforation including iatrogenic, external trauma, emetogenic, and foreign body ingestion. Upon further inspection, almost none of the external trauma patients were managed nonoperatively except in a few studies [42,44].

Smakman et al. reported on two patients managed nonoperatively [42]. One patient had arrived in a delayed fashion with nonoperative management instituted at another facility and appeared to be doing well so it was continued. The second patient had what appeared to be a sealed off small thoracic perforation at endoscopy. It is impossible to discern whether this was a false-positive endoscopy or a true injury. These patients were hospitalized an average of 22 days for unclear reasons. Madiba and Muckart reported on 17 patients with esophageal injury managed nonoperatively after penetrating cervical trauma, which represented 61% of patients, identified with this injury in a 5-year retrospective review [44]. Criteria for nonoperative management included a contained extravasation on esophagography with no other indication for operative intervention. These patients were managed with enteral tube feeds and antibiotics. The median hospital stay was 18 days for all patients, but any difference between the operative and nonoperative groups in regard to length of stay was not discussed. One patient (6%) of those managed conservatively subsequently developed local sepsis, requiring operative intervention. Although this approach was relatively effective for this subset of esophageal injuries, it may not be very efficient (Table 20.1).

*Recommendation*: Not enough evidence to recommend for traumatic injuries at this time

*Grade of recommendation*: D

## References

1. Bertelsen S, Howitz P. Injuries of the trachea and bronchi. *Thorax*. 1972;27:188–194.
2. Kemmerer WT, Eckert WG, Gathright JB et al. Patterns of thoracic injuries in fatal traffic accidents. *J Trauma*. 1961;1:595–599.
3. Huh J, Milliken JC, Chen JC. Management of tracheobronchial injuries following blunt and penetrating trauma. *Am Surg*. 1997;63(10):896–899.
4. Inaba K, Munera F, McKenney M et al. Prospective evaluation of screening multislice helical computed tomographic angiography in the initial evaluation of penetrating neck injuries. *J Trauma*. 2006;61:144–149.
5. Inci I, Ozcelik C, Tacyildiz I et al. Penetrating chest injuries: Unusually high incidence of high-velocity gunshot wounds in civilian practice. *World J Surg*. 1998;22:438–442.
6. Okoye OT, Talving P, Teixeira PG et al. Transmediastinal gunshot wounds in a mature trauma centre: Changing perspectives. *Injury*. 2013;44(9):1198–1203.
7. Duval EL, Geraerts SD. Management of blunt tracheal trauma in children: A case series and review of the literature. *Eur J Pediatr*. 2007;166:559–563.
8. Kirsh MM, Orringer MB, Behrendt DM et al. Management of tracheobronchial disruption secondary to nonpenetrating trauma. *Ann Thorac Surg*. 1976;22(1):93–101.
9. Martin de Nicolas JL, Gamez AP, Cruz F et al. Long tracheobronchial and esophageal rupture after blunt chest trauma: Injury by airway bursting. *Ann Thorac Surg*. 1996;62:269–272.

10. Kiser AC, O'Brien SM, Detterbeck FC. Blunt tracheobronchial injuries: Treatment and outcomes. *Ann Thorac Surg.* 2001;71:2059–2065.
11. Gomez-Caro A, Ausin P, Moradiellos FJ et al. Role of conservative medical management of tracheobronchial injuries. *J Trauma.* 2006;61:1426–1435.
12. Cassada DC, Munyikwa MP, Moniz MP et al. Acute injuries of the trachea and major bronchi: Importance of early diagnosis. *Ann Thorac Surg.* 2000;69:1563–1567.
13. Rossbach MM, Johnson SB, Gomez MA et al. Management of major tracheobronchial injuries: A 28-year experience. *Ann Thorac Surg.* 1998;65:182–186.
14. Demetriades D, Theodorou D, Cornwell E et al. Evaluation of penetrating injuries of the neck: Prospective study of 223 patients. *World J Surg.* 1997;21:41–48.
15. Wintermark M and Schnyder P. The Macklin Effect: A frequent etiology for pneumomediastinum in severe blunt chest trauma. *Chest.* 2001;120:543–547.
16. Inaba K, Branco B, Menaker J et al. Evaluation of multidetector computed tomography for penetrating neck injury: A prospective multicenter study. *J Trauma.* 2012;72(3):576–584.
17. Scagilone M, Romano S, Pinto A et al. Acute tracheobronchial injuries: Impact of imaging on diagnosis and management implications. *Eur J Radiol.* 2006;59:336–343.
18. Allan PF, Kelley TC, Taylor TL et al. Bronchial transection: Diagnosis and management. *Clin Pulm Med.* 2006;13(3):203–208.
19. Miller BS, Shafi S, Thal ER. Damage control in complex penetrating tracheal injury and silicone t-tube. *J Trauma.* 2008;64:E18–E20.
20. Ross HM, Grant FJ, Wilson RS et al. Nonoperative management of tracheal laceration during endotracheal intubation. *Ann Thorac Surg.* 1997;63:240–242.
21. Conti M, Pougeoise M, Wurtz A et al. Management of postintubation tracheobronchial ruptures. *Chest.* 2006;130:412–418.
22. Jougon J, Ballester M, Choukroun E et al. Conservative treatment for postintubation tracheobronchial rupture. *Ann Thorac Surg.* 2000;69:216–220.
23. Beal SL, Pottmeyer EW, Spisso JM. Esophageal perforation following external blunt trauma. *J Trauma.* 1988;28(10):1425–1432.
24. Winter RP and Weigelt JA. Cervical esophageal trauma incidence and cause of esophageal fistulas. *Arch Surg.* 1990;125:849–851.
25. Cornwell EE, Kennedy F, Ayad IA et al. Transmediastinal gunshot wounds a reconsideration of the role of aortography. *Arch Surg.* 1996;131:949–953.
26. Plott E, Jones D, McDermott D et al. A state-of-the-art review of esophageal trauma: Where do we stand? *Dis Esophagus.* 2007;20:279–289.
27. Stringer WL, Kelly DL Jr, Johnston FR et al. Hyperextension injury of the cervical spine with esophageal perforation. Case report. *J Neurosurg.* 1980;53(4):541–543.
28. Martel G, Al-Sabti H, Mulder D et al. Acute tracheoesophageal burst injury after blunt chest trauma: Case report and review of the literature. *J Trauma.* 2007;62:236–242.
29. Asensio JA, Chahwan S, Forno W et al. Penetrating esophageal injuries: Multicenter study of the American Association for the Surgery of Trauma. *J Trauma.* 2001;50(2):289–296.
30. Weigelt JA, Thal ER, Snyder WH et al. Diagnosis of penetrating cervical esophageal injuries. *Am J Surg.* 1987;154:619–622.
31. Vassiliu P, Baker J, Henderson S et al. Aerodigestive injuries of the neck. *Am Surg.* 2001;67(1):75–79.
32. White RK, Morris DM. Diagnosis and management of esophageal perforations. *Am Surg.* 1992;58:112–119.
33. Glatterer MS, Toon RS, Ellestad C et al. Management of blunt and penetrating external esophageal trauma. *J Trauma.* 1985;25(8):784–792.
34. Sheely CH, Mattox KL, Beall AC et al. Penetrating wounds of the cervical esophagus. *Am J Surg.* 1975;130:707–710.
35. Patel MS, Malinoski DJ, Neal ML, Hoyt DB. Penetrating oesophageal injury: A contemporary analysis of the National Trauma Data Bank. *Injury.* 2013;44(1):48–55.
36. Goldstein LA and Thompson WR. Esophageal perforations: A 15 year experience. *Am J Surg.* 1982;143:495–503.
37. Richardson JD, Martin LF, Borzotta AP et al. Unifying concepts in treatment of esophageal leaks. *Am J Surg.* 1985;149:157–162.
38. Castelguidone E, Merola S, Pinto A et al. Esophageal injuries: Spectrum of multidetector row CT findings. *Eur J Radiol.* 2006;59:344–348.
39. Flowers JL, Graham SM, Ugarte MA et al. Flexible endoscopy for the diagnosis of esophageal trauma. *J Trauma.* 1996;40(2):261–266.
40. Srinivasan R, Haywood T, Horwitz B et al. Role of flexible endoscopy in the evaluation of possible esophageal trauma after penetrating injuries. *Am J Gastroenterol.* 2000;95:1725–1729.
41. Ahmed N, Massier C, Tassie J et al. Diagnosis of penetrating injuries of the pharynx and esophagus in the severely injured patient. *J Trauma.* 2009;67(1):152–154.
42. Smakman N, Nicol AJ, Walther G et al. Factors affecting outcome in penetrating oesophageal trauma. *Br J Surg.* 2004;91:1513–1519.
43. Mattox KL. The injured esophagus. *Tex Heart Inst J.* 2010;37(6):683–684.
44. Madiba TE, Muckart DJJ. Penetrating injuries to the cervical oesophagus: Is routine exploration mandatory? *Ann R Coll Surg Engl.* 2003;85:162–166.

## Commentary on Injury to the Esophagus, Trachea, and Bronchus

*Scott B. Johnson*

Injuries to the tracheobronchial tree can be challenging to successfully manage even for the most experienced surgeon. Airway and anesthetic management need to be carefully planned and coordinated, and good intraoperative communication is essential. Esophageal injuries often require a high index of suspicion to accurately and timely diagnose. Missed injuries, or breakdown of ill-conceived repairs, can be fatal. Management of tracheobronchial and esophageal injuries is often learned through experience or retrospective studies rather than on sound, evidence-based medicine, as the chapter rightly points out secondarily to the relative rarity of these injuries. Having said this, there are a few management strategies that I have learned during my career that I think are worth sharing.

### What Are the Surgical Management Options for Tracheobronchial Injuries?

Collapsed lung beyond a chronically obstructed, injured bronchus has been known to re-expand when repaired even when many years out from injury. Therefore, repair of injured tracheobronchial injuries should not be discouraged regardless of time from injury. If the injury is relatively distal in the tracheobronchial tree, often times resection with bronchial stump stapling is the most expeditious and durable operative repair. Obviously the decision to repair versus resect should be based on many factors, with perhaps the main one being the amount of lung parenchyma distal to the injury. Performing lung transplants and elective tracheal resections at our institution has given us considerable experience performing primary tracheobronchial anastomoses and reconstructions. We generally use absorbable 4-0 monofilament suture (e.g., PDS [TM]): interrupted figure-of-8 sutures for the anterior, cartilaginous side; and simple running for the posterior membranous side, with the knots tied on the outside. It should be noted that with proper retraction and visualization, a large portion of the intrathoracic trachea can be reached from a cervical incision alone, especially with extension of the neck (after a C-spine injury has been ruled out). I once primarily repaired a membranous tracheal injury near the carina that I caused while performing a transhiatal esophagectomy through a left neck incision.

### What Is the Best Diagnostic Test for Traumatic Esophageal Injury?

With regard to which study is best to diagnose and locate esophageal injuries—i.e., swallow study versus endoscopy?—I believe the tests are not mutually exclusive but rather complementary, each having their own strengths and weaknesses. To illustrate this point, I remember one case in which I was called to the endoscopy suite by an experienced endoscopist who was performing an ERCP in a 99-year-old frail lady who had some difficulty, made a "wrong turn," and saw her lung and the inside of her pleural space (incidentally, this case also illustrates the fact that the vast majority of esophageal "injuries" that you will be called upon to manage will in fact be secondary to iatrogenic causes, most likely from an endoscopic procedure or from a misguided tracheostomy). In addition, the patient had a left hydropneumothorax on chest radiograph in the recovery room, and a subsequent swallow study that confirmed extravasation of contrast distally into her left chest. After taking her to the operating room and putting her to sleep—but prior to any skin incision—I performed my own endoscopy that showed a double barrel configuration just beyond her cricopharyngeus—one was a true lumen, and the other a false lumen. Passing down the true lumen, her esophagus appeared pristine beyond the cervical injury. I reasoned that most likely the cervical esophageal mucosa was perforated with the ERCP scope, which then dissected a false lumen down through the muscularis propria, eventually perforating freely through the mediastinal pleura distally into her left chest. What had been planned as a left thoracotomy was now changed to a left neck incision, in which I was able to locate and primarily close the mucosal defect and drain the mediastinum. I can only imagine having been tricked into performing a left thoracotomy on a frail 99-year-old solely based on the swallow study alone. As it was, the patient did well from a relatively low-risk incision, and went on to invite me to her 100th birthday party.

### What Are the Surgical Management Options for Esophageal Injuries?

Whether an esophageal injury should be treated operatively or nonoperatively should be based on multiple factors, including the extent of the injury, the underlying pathology (if any), and the clinical condition of the patient. When the decision is made to operate, primary repair should be performed when possible. This decision should be based on the extent of the injury and the condition of the tissues after debridement, rather than the time from injury. If the tissues are poor and non-pliable, primary repair is risky. Likewise, if the patient is septic appearing, a reconstruction with primary anastomoses probably should not be attempted since gut perfusion diminishes during periods of sepsis. Performing too much surgery in an otherwise unstable patient—thinking that the best (and perhaps only) chance to reconstruct is immediate—can make a bad situation worse. Even if one is unfamiliar or uncomfortable in the techniques of delayed esophageal reconstruction, one can always resect, bail out with an end cervical esophagostomy, and then transfer the patient to a tertiary referral center later for reconstruction once the patient recovers from the initial injury. Performing an intrathoracic anastomosis in a septic patient is risky, and may jeopardize a reconstructive conduit that could have otherwise been used later. However, if the quality of the tissues appears healthy—regardless of time from injury or degree of sepsis—it is my opinion to perform a primary repair when possible (rather than reconstruct or resect). In these cases I endoscope postrepair with the chest (incision) still open, and test the repair underwater with insufflation to confirm closure. I avoid using methylene blue—it will only end up staining everything blue in your operative field if there is in fact a leak. However, if the tissues are friable, stiff, or necessarily debrided nearly circumferentially, resection is probably your best bet. It is important that while performing a resection with an end cervical esophagostomy, one needs to try and leave as much proximal esophagus as possible, which will later aid in swallowing function once the patient has been reconstructed via the substernal tunnel. It is always amazing to me as to how short the esophagus really is after dividing it distally in the chest and bringing it out through a separate neck incision as an end stoma. It is my experience that trying to perform a loop cervical esophagostomy (as opposed to an end esophagostomy) is usually very difficult secondary to the length of esophagus required to reach the skin. I have only performed a handful of these during my career—necessarily—and all were a struggle.

One type of traumatic injury to the esophagus that was not discussed in the chapter but is probably worth mentioning is that of caustic injuries, usually as the result of either accidental ingestion (in the very young) or as a suicide attempt (in adults). The main role of the surgeon in these cases is usually damage control. I have seen cases where esophagectomies, splenectomies, gastrectomies, and even colectomies were necessarily performed secondary to extensive liquefaction necrosis. Convincing evidence lacks that either early dilation or steroid use plays any major role in improving outcomes with regard to healing or subsequent stricture formation, although I do believe that in cases where perforation is even slightly suspected that antibiotics (and perhaps antifungals, since many foregut perforations involve *Candida*) should be administered. An argument can also be made to endoscope these patients early, mainly to document the proximal extent of the injury. If there are obvious burns to the mouth and/or posterior pharynx on visual examination, there is no need to go any further. Judgment can also be made as to how the mucosa appears at the time of endoscopy; however, any decision to operate should be made on multiple factors and not just on visual inspection of the mucosa, since mucosal sloughing can be part of the initial injury without full-thickness perforation or necrosis, especially in the case of acidic burns. Conservatism rather than overzealous treatment is the key to success. Later stricture formation and need for late operative intervention is not uncommon in these often very troubled and challenging individuals.

I think it is also worth mentioning that I do not find pleural or intercostal muscle flaps to be very useful. Intercostal muscle flaps are not reliable and when placed circumferentially can cause stricturing. If a viable intrathoracic muscle flap is truly deemed necessary, I recommend performing a Latissimus Dorsi muscle sparing incision, mobilizing the muscle completely anteriorly and posteriorly to its insertion and origin sites (being careful not to disturb its blood supply on the posterior aspect of the muscle), and then dividing its origins from the iliac wing and transverse processes of the vertebral column. It can then be inserted through a separate thoracotomy site based on its superior (i.e., thoracoacromial artery) blood supply, usually superior to the thoracotomy approach site, and then brought posteromedially to reach the trachea and/or esophagus. I find this to be an excellent, robust muscle flap especially when separation of a combined intrathoracic esophageal and tracheal repair is desired. Likewise, when a cervical muscle flap is needed, I find the sternal portion of the sternocleidomastoid muscle to be robust and easy to harvest. This muscle has two portions, and the sternal portion can be divided off the manubrium and bluntly separated from its clavicular portion. I find that the strap muscles are generally flimsy and not helpful.

# 21

# *An Evidence-Based Approach to Spleen Injury*

Mark Muir

CONTENTS



## 21.1 Introduction

Blunt and penetrating injuries to the spleen are common in trauma, resulting in a significant number of hospital admissions, morbidity, and occasionally death. The spleen is the second most commonly injured organ in blunt abdominal trauma, and penetrating injury also accounts for 15% of splenic injuries [1,2]. Between 1989 and 2012, rates of successful nonoperative management (NOM) of splenic injury increased from 12% to 76% [3,4]. Over the same time frame, estimated costs associated with treatment of splenic trauma fell by 29% and hospital length of stay decreased by an average of 2 days. Mortality for high-risk splenic trauma patients (expected mortality greater than 30%) fell from 30% to 20% for those managed nonoperatively, and from 46% to 38% for those undergoing emergency surgery [5]. Overwhelming postsplenectomy infection (OPSI) was originally described in the 1950s in asplenic children; since that time, a greater appreciation of the immunologic role of the spleen and case series reporting an incidence of OPSI of 3%–7% with a case fatality rate of 50%–70% created an impetus for splenic salvage whenever possible [6]. NOM of splenic trauma has been enabled by the widespread availability of rapid, high-resolution computed tomography (CT) scanning, and by the frequent success of angiographic embolization of the spleen. This chapter will attempt to answer some of the current management controversies involving traumatic spleen injury by evaluating the relevant data and developing evidence-based recommendations (Table 21.1).

## 21.2 Which Patients Are Candidates for Nonoperative Management of Blunt Spleen Injury?

Over the past 20 years, selective NOM of blunt splenic injuries has become standard for hemodynamically stable patients and those who respond rapidly to initial resuscitation [7]. Properly identifying patients for NOM may alleviate the risks of unnecessary laparotomy or subsequent OPSI [1,8]. The minimal criteria for NOM of blunt spleen injuries have been identified as hemodynamic stability and the absence of generaslized peritonitis in the setting of a reliable and reproducible exam [8]. The risk of failure of NOM increases with increasing injury grade: grade 3%–19%, grade 4%–33%, and grade 5%–75%. Increasing injury grade is directly proportional to the amount of hemoperitoneum, and this combination (high grade with large hemoperitoneum) is the most predictive of failure [8].

A recent meta-analysis by Bhangu et al. evaluated other risk factors for failure of NOM of blunt splenic injury [7]. Reported failure rates for NOM (patients undergoing surgical exploration for continuing hemorrhage) ranged from 4% to 52% with a mean failure rate of 12%. The factors associated with failure of NOM were The American Association for the Surgery of Trauma (AAST) injury grade of 3 or greater, age over 55 years, and moderate or large hemoperitoneum (compared with small or absent hemoperitoneum). Large hemoperitoneum is defined as abdominal free fluid extending from the splenic recess to the pelvis, whereas small and moderate hemoperitoneum is free fluid contained in the splenic recess and free fluid extending into the pericolic gutters, respectively. Patients who failed NOM had a 5-day longer hospital stay, higher mortality, and were transfused more blood in the first 24 h. In a subset of five studies from this meta-analysis, introduction of an angioembolization protocol decreased rates of failure of NOM, but 10% of patients who underwent embolization ultimately required operation. Another recent systematic review found strong evidence that age of 40 years or greater, injury severity score of 25 or greater, and injury grade 3 or greater were associated with higher failure rates of NOM [9]. Of note, Haan et al. have reported that a traumatic splenic arteriovenous fistula is associated with a 40% failure rate of NOM, even with angiography [10]. Patients who fail NOM are more likely to have other associated injuries on CT scan or physical exam (52% vs. 20%) [11].

Although increasing transfusion requirements within the first 24 h have been shown to be associated with increasing failure rates of NOM, the exact transfusion level that should trigger concern is not clear. Transfusion of just one unit of packed red blood cells is associated with increased rates of failure of NOM [9,12]. Conversely, patients who failed NOM were reported to have received anywhere from 1.5 to 4 units of blood more than those who were successfully managed nonoperatively [7,12].

*Recommendations*:

1. Selective NOM of patients with blunt splenic trauma has a high rate of success. Criteria include hemodynamic stability and absence of peritonitis. Age, injury grade, degree of hemoperitoneum, Injury Severity Score, transfusion requirements, and CT evidence of extravasation or other vascular injury portend higher failure rates of NOM.

   *Level of evidence*: 2A

   *Grade of recommendation*: B

2. Need for transfusion of just 1 unit of blood is associated with failure of NOM. The available data can neither justify nor refute a specific transfusion threshold for nonoperative failure (such as the traditional 2 units of blood). Clinical judgment must be exercised. (No recommendation)

## 21.3 What Is the Role of Nonoperative Management in Penetrating Spleen Injury?

As the role of NOM of penetrating abdominal injuries has increased in general, the rate of successful NOM of penetrating splenic injuries has increased as well. In 2006, Demetriades et al. published a protective study of patients with penetrating injuries to solid abdominal organs, following a protocol mandating surgical exploration for hemodynamic instability, peritonitis, unreliable exam, or CT scan suggestive of perforated hollow viscus [13]. Of the 28 patients with a penetrating splenic injury, 23 underwent immediate operation. Seventeen of those underwent splenectomy and six underwent splenic repair. Of the five patients not undergoing immediate surgery, four underwent surgery either based on subsequent CT findings, development of peritonitis, or laparoscopy for evaluation of the diaphragm. Only one patient (3.6% of all penetrating splenic injuries) was managed entirely nonoperatively. Of note, none of the splenic injury patients in this series underwent angiography. Berg et al. recently published a larger series exclusively of penetrating splenic injury patients [14]. In this cohort of 255 patients, 177 (79%) underwent immediate laparotomy and an additional 10 patients underwent laparotomy immediately after CT scan based on the CT findings. Thirty-eight patients underwent attempted NOM, with 14 (37%) of these patients ultimately undergoing laparotomy and 24 patients (9% of all penetrating splenic injuries) successfully managed nonoperatively. Gunshot wounds and increasing AAST injury score were associated with early laparotomy, but not with laparotomy in patients undergoing attempted NOM. No patients were reported to have undergone angiography. Selective NOM of penetrating splenic injuries seems feasible in hemodynamically stable patients with a reliable exam and no peritonitis or CT evidence of hollow viscus injury, with reported rates of successful NOM ranging from 3.6% to 9%. The role of angiography in the management of penetrating splenic injuries has yet to be defined.

*Recommendation*: The current evidence suggests that in appropriately selected patients, NOM of penetrating spleen injury can be successful in more than 50% of patients, but the total percentage of penetrating splenic injury patients meeting these criteria is small (3%–9%). Patients with hemodynamic instability, peritonitis, unreliable exam, or CT evidence of hollow viscus injury should undergo immediate exploration. The role of angiography in penetrating splenic injury is unknown.

*Level of evidence*: 2B

*Grade of recommendation*: B

## 21.4 Which Patients Should Undergo Splenic Angiography?

Splenic artery embolization was first introduced in 1981 by Sclafani [15]. Splenic artery embolization (SAE) has become an important adjunct in patients at highest risk for NOM failure. If a contrast blush or pseudoaneurysm is confirmed on diagnostic angiography, the physician will deploy a coil or gelfoam to occlude the proximal splenic artery, selective distal arteries, or a combination thereof [16,17]. Although many institutions have instituted splenic angiogram protocols, controversy remains concerning which patients benefit from this technique.

Haan et al. performed a large retrospective study of 645 patients, 368 of whom were managed nonoperatively. The study was protocol driven; patients with Grade 3, 4, or 5 injury and a blush on CT scan qualified for angiography and embolization. The overall nonoperative success rate was 94%. One hundred and thirty-two patients underwent embolization with a salvage rate of 90%. However, patients with Grades 4 and 5 injury had a success rate of 80%. The failure rate for arteriovenous fistulas was 40%. Patients with a moderate/large hemoperitoneum or pseudoaneurysm had a failure rate of 10% and 12%, respectively. Individual Grades 3, 4, and 5 salvage rates were 92%, 83%, and 83%, respectively, which was significantly higher than the salvage rates of 80%, 66%, and 25%, reported by Peitzman et al. [8,10]. They document 167 negative angiographies, but there is no report of grade or size of hemoperitoneum to which negative findings correlate. A meta-analysis by Requarth et al. found the overall failure rate for patients undergoing SAE to be 15.7%, and there was no significant difference in the failure rate with splenic injury Grades 1–5 [18]. However, for Grades 4 and 5 injuries, the failure rate was higher for patients managed without SAE compared to patients undergoing SAE (43.7% vs. 17.3% for Grade 4 and 83.1% vs. 25% for Grade 5). A retrospective review of 1039 patient with blunt splenic injury found no difference in rates of failure of NOM for Grade 1–3 injury, but significantly lower failure rates in Grade 4 and 5 injuries in those patients undergoing SAE [19]. NOM failure rates with and without SAE were 23% versus 3% for Grade 4 and 63% versus 9% for Grade 5 injuries. A recent prospective study by Miller et al. employed a protocol by which all hemodynamically stable AAST Grades 3–5 injuries underwent mandatory angiography regardless of other associated imaging features (i.e., blush, pseudoaneurysm) [20]. Failure rates for NOM after implementation of the protocol were 5%, compared with 25% for managed, in whom the protocol was violated (no angiography despite Grades 3–5 injury), and a failure rate of 15% for a historical control group prior to implementation of the protocol.

Finally, there is controversy concerning factors predicting failure of embolization. Another group performed a large retrospective study which revealed that patients with arteriovenous fistulas failed embolization 40% of the time. They also found that pseudoaneurysm and high-grade injuries were not associated with a significant failure rate [10]. Other institutions published conflicting data. These institutions' embolization failure rates were 43% for high-grade injuries, 56% for large hemoperitoneum, and 59% for extravasation [17,21]. This discrepancy may be accounted for by the frequency and familiarity that each institution has concerning embolization. In addition, different embolization protocols may produce different outcomes.

*Recommendation*: Hemodynamically stable patients with Grade 4 or 5 blunt splenic injuries, or with contrast extravasation, pseudoaneurysm, or arteriovenous fistula on CT scan, should routinely undergo SAE. SAE in these patients decreases the failure rate of NOM. Routine angiography in Grade 3 injuries without contrast extravasation is controversial, as failure rates of NOM of Grade 3 injuries are low (5%) and negative angiography rate is high (70%). Further study is needed regarding indications for SAE in Grade 3 injuries.

*Level of evidence*: 2A

*Grade of recommendation*: B

## 21.5 What Imaging Studies Should Be Obtained in Patients with Splenic Injuries?

The focused abdominal sonography for trauma (FAST) is often the initial imaging study performed for blunt trauma patients. It has the advantage of being rapid, noninvasive, bedside, and easy to repeat. It has 90%–93% sensitivity for the presence of hemoperitoneum [22]. FAST is limited by the inability to detect the presence of active hemorrhage and has a reported sensitivity of only 46% for detection of solid organ injury [23]. A positive FAST in a hemodynamically stable patient should prompt follow-up CT scan, as abdominal ultrasound has limited utility in identifying specific solid organ injuries and characterizing the extent of the injury [23]. There is debate about the role of CT in a stable patient with a negative FAST, but the rate of additional injuries in the abdomen found exclusively on CT after a negative FAST is 15%, leading to a change in management in 6.4% [24]. This suggests that CT should be routine even with a negative FAST in significant blunt force injury to the abdomen.

CT scan has long been the "gold standard" for diagnosing and characterizing spleen injuries in hemodynamically stable patients. Benefits of CT scan include the ability to reliably determine the severity or grade of injury; evaluate for contrast extravasation, pseudoaneurysm, or arteriovenous fistula; quickly estimate the degree of hemoperitoneum; and identify other significant injuries [25].

With CT scan already established as the gold standard for determining the extent of splenic injury, recent literature has sought to answer questions pertaining to follow-up scans and their indications. When Haan looked at patients with Grade 1 or 2 blunt splenic injuries, he found that repeat CT scan at 24–48 h postinjury showed progression of injury in only 2/140 patients [26]. Both patients had clinical symptoms of worsening injury. Uecker et al. had published similar findings; the three patients who had radiologic evidence of injury progression also had clinical symptoms. The 10 asymptomatic patients had no radiologic evidence of injury progression [27]. Weinburg et al. have published results from a retrospective review in which all patients with blunt splenic injury Grade 2 or higher underwent follow-up CT at 24–48 h [28]. They report a 2.7% incidence of delayed pseudoaneurysm (11/411 patients). Splenic injury grade on admission CT scan was not associated with the presence of a latent pseudoaneurysm, but no information regarding the clinical status of the patients is presented. Only 3 of the 11 latent pseudoaneurysms were in Grade 1 or 2 injuries. A retrospective review in pediatric patients by Safavi et al. revealed similar findings, with an incidence of delayed pseudoaneurysm of 5.4%, all in Grade 3 or 4 injuries [29]. Based on these studies, repeat imaging of Grade 3 or higher injuries or patients with a change in exam/clinical status prior to discharge appears justified.

Several studies have followed patients with splenic injuries after discharge and noted that patients who had injury progression usually also had clinical symptoms [30,31]. There is no evidence to recommend repeat radiologic imaging of outpatients due to the low incidence of delayed complications and complications without clinical symptoms.

*Recommendations*:

1. FAST may play a role as a screening tool in blunt trauma patients, but CT scan is the diagnostic tool of choice for splenic injury in stable trauma patients.

   *Level of evidence*: 2A

2. Repeat imaging with CT scan should be considered prior to hospital discharge in patients with Grades 3–5 injuries or patients with a change in physical exam or clinical status.

   *Level of evidence*: 2B

3. There is no evidence to support repeat imaging after hospital discharge in absence of clinical symptoms.

   *Level of evidence*: 2B

   *Grade of recommendation*: B

## 21.6 What Steps Can Be Taken to Prevent Overwhelming Postsplenectomy Sepsis?

OPSI is rare (3%–7%) but carries a high mortality rate (40%–70%) [6]. This heightened susceptibility to infection was described by King and Schumacker in 1952 in asplenic infants, and causative organisms were later identified as encapsulated bacteria (*S. pneumoniae* is the causative agent 50%–90% of the time) [6,32]. Vaccinations against encapsulated organisms, antibiotic prophylaxis against encapsulated organisms, and attempts at splenic salvage have been used to prevent OPSI. Determining the relative effect of each of these interventions on rates of OPSI is difficult because of the long follow-up and low incidence of the disease [6].

As an intact spleen is the best defense against OPSI, and even Grades 4 and 5 injuries may now be managed nonoperatively, it is important to know whether a severely injured spleen retains the same immunologic function as a healthy spleen. There are no data regarding immunologic clinical outcomes (rates of infection or OPSI) in patients with severe spleen injury and splenic preservation, but studies evaluating immunologic surrogates of splenic function show patients with injured spleens to have higher levels of immune function than asplenic patients [33,34]. Resende found Howell-Jolly bodies in all patients who underwent splenectomy for trauma, but none in noninjured controls or patients with subtotal splenectomy [33]. Another study showed that the immunologic profile of nonoperatively managed Grade 4 or 5 injuries more closely resembled patients with spleens than those without spleens [34].

Current recommendations from the Centers for Disease Control and Prevention (CDC) recommend immunization for *S. pneumoniae* (pneumococcus), *N. meningitidis* (meningococcus), and *H. influenzae* type b (Hib) following splenectomy [35]. The two available pneumococcal vaccines are the pneumococcal conjugate (PCV13) vaccine and the pneumococcal polysaccharide (PPSV23) vaccine. The CDC recommends that PCV13 be administered first, followed by PPSV23 8 weeks later. A one-time revaccination with PPSV23 should be given 5 years after the first dose (in patients younger than 65 at the time of initial vaccination), and an additional dose given after age 65 if at least 5 years have elapsed since the last vaccination. The quadrivalent meningococcal conjugate vaccine should be administered in two doses 2 months apart, with revaccination every 5 years. Hib vaccine is administered as a single one-time dose. Timing of vaccination may depend on practical considerations, but studies have shown higher antibody titers in response to vaccination when the vaccine is administered at least 14 days postsplenectomy, with no further improvement in titers when comparing 14 and 28 days [36,37]. Thus, it is ideal to administer the vaccines at least 14 days after splenectomy, even if that means administering the vaccines at an outpatient follow-up visit. However, if the patient is at risk for being lost to follow-up, vaccination prior to hospital discharge, even if prior to 14 days, seems prudent.

*Recommendations*:

1. Even after severe splenic trauma, injured spleens retain most of their immune function. Therefore, splenic preservation should be the most effective prevention of OPSI.
2. Pneumococcus (PCV13 followed by PPSV23 8 weeks later), meningococcus (two doses 2 months apart), and Hib vaccine should be given at least 14 days postsplenectomy, but patients who are at high risk for loss to follow-up should be immunized prior to discharge. The most up-to-date guidelines for postsplenectomy vaccinations are available through the CDC Advisory Committee for Immunization Practices.

   *Level of evidence*: 2B (retrospective studies and small prospective studies)

   *Grade of recommendation*: B

## 21.7 When Is It Safe to Resume Activities after Splenic Injuries?

Evidence in support of specific time frames for observation of blunt splenic injuries and duration of restriction of physical activity is limited to guidelines devised from retrospective data, although with prospective validation of guidelines in pediatric patients. A large retrospective review by Smith et al. found that 95% of failures of NOM occurred in the first 72 h, with only 1.5% more detected with an additional 2 days of observation [2]. They conclude that blunt splenic injury patients should be observed for 3–5 days. For pediatric patients, the American Pediatric Surgical Association Trauma Committee published recommendations regarding length of hospitalization and return to activity based on grade of splenic injury [38]. In 2002, Stylianos published a prospective series based on the guidelines, with resultant decreases in hospital length of stay, intensive care unit length of stay, and duration of physical activity restriction without adverse outcomes [39]. The guidelines can be easily remembered, as hospital length of stay (in days) equals one more than the injury grade (e.g., 3 days for a Grade 2 injury), and restriction of activity (in weeks) equals two more than injury grade (e.g., 6 weeks for a Grade 4 injury) [38]. St Peter et al. recently published a protocol-driven prospective series in which pediatric patients with Grade 1 or 2 injuries underwent one night of bed rest, and all Grade 3 or higher injuries underwent two nights of bed rest, resulting in significant reductions in hospital stay without any readmissions related to the spleen injury [40].

*Recommendations*:

1. The American Pediatric Surgical Association Trauma Committee's guidelines for management of splenic injury have been prospectively validated and provided specific recommendations for hospital stay and physical activity restriction based on grade of injury. Shorter duration of hospital stay may be feasible, but more data are needed.

   *Level of evidence*: 2A

   *Grade of recommendation*: B
2. Adult patients with blunt splenic injury undergoing NOM should be observed for 3–5 days. Determinants of hospital stay should be clinical, as no specific data regarding length of stay relative to grade of injury are available (unlike pediatric patients). Activity restrictions similar to those recommended for children are reasonable, but supporting data are lacking.

   *Level of evidence*: 4

   *Grade of recommendation*: C

## 21.8 Special Circumstances in Splenic Injury

Recommendations for hospital admission and resuming activities in pediatric patients have been discussed earlier. There are data indicating that the type of treatment facility may influence treatment decisions in pediatric blunt spleen injury patients, with children having a lower splenectomy rate when they are treated at pediatric specialty centers compared to adult trauma centers or rural hospitals [41]. Other risks for splenectomy in the

**TABLE 21.1**

Clinical Questions

| Questions | Answers | Level of Evidence | Grade of Recommendation | References |
|---|---|---|---|---|
| Which patients are candidates for NOM of blunt spleen injury? | Hemodynamically stable patients without peritonitis | 2A | B | [7–11] |
| | Increasing age, injury grade, size of hemoperitoneum, ISS, extravasation, or vascular abnormality on CT portend higher NOM failure. | | | |
| | Any transfusion of PRBCs increases chances of NOM failure. A "transfusion threshold" for failure of NOM has not been defined. | | No recommendation | [7,9,12] |
| What is the role of NOM in penetrating spleen injury? | In selected patients (hemodynamically stable, no peritonitis, reliable exam), up to two-thirds of patients are managed successfully nonoperatively. | 2B | B | [13,14] |
| | Role of SAE in penetrating injury is unknown. | | No recommendation | |
| Which patients should undergo splenic angiography? | Hemodynamically stable patients with blunt splenic injury with either: | 2A | B | [10,18–21] |
| | CT evidence of contrast extravasation or other vascular injury (pseudoaneurysm or arteriovenous fistula) | | | |
| | AAST Grades 4 and 5 injury | | No recommendation | |
| | Role of routine SAE in Grade 3 injury (without extravasation or vascular abnormality) is unknown. | | | |
| What radiologic studies should be obtained in patients with splenic injuries? | CT scan is the imaging modality of choice for splenic injury. | 2A | B | [24,25] |
| | Repeat CT scan should be considered prior to discharge for Grades 3–5 injuries or for change in clinical status. | 2B | B | [26–29] |
| | Outpatient imaging is of little use in asymptomatic patients. | 2B | B | [30,31] |
| What are the steps to prevent OPSI | OPSI is best prevented by splenic preservation, when possible. | 2B | B | [6,33,34] |
| | Pneumococcus, meningococcus, and Hib vaccine should be given >14 days postsplenectomy, if feasible. They may be given earlier if follow-up is a concern. | 2B | B | [6,35–37] |
| | Specific vaccine recommendations are available through the CDC. | | | |
| When is it safe to resume activities after splenic injuries? | Pediatric patients: Manage according to APSA 2000 guidelines. | 2A | B | [38–40] |
| | Adult patients: Hospital observation for 3–5 days. Activity restriction similar to pediatric patients. | 4 | C | [2] |
| How are patients with special circumstances managed nonoperatively? | Pediatric patients: see earlier text | | | |
| | Patients over age 55 years: Likely have a higher failure rate of NOM. Age alone does not preclude NOM. | 2B | B | [7,9,45–49] |
| | Cirrhotic patients: Worse prognosis, but still high success rate for NOM. | 2B | B | [50] |
| | Anticoagulation: Treat as all other trauma patients once acute bleeding has resolved. | 4 | C | [51,52] |

*Abbreviations:* APSA, American Pediatric Surgical Association; CDC, Centers for Disease Control and Prevention; ISS, Injury Severity Score; CT, computed tomography; Hib, haemophilus influenza B; OPSI, overwhelming postsplenectomy infection; PRBCs, packed red blood cells; SAE, splenic artery embolization.

pediatric patient include Glasgow Coma Scale score ≤8, Grades 3–5 injury, older age, and associated injuries [41–43]. The role of angiography in pediatric splenic injury is not as well defined as it is in adult patients. A systematic review by van der Vlies et al. showed that the failure rate of NOM in pediatric patients with contrast extravasation and without angioembolization was 28%. The studies they analyzed that included angiography as an adjunct showed a failure rate of only 6.5%; however, those studies included a large number of adolescent patients, so the role of angiography in younger pediatric patients remains unclear [44].

Older patients have worse outcomes than younger patients with splenic injuries, regardless of the management strategy employed. The mortality rate of those older patients who have successful NOM is 8%, whereas younger patients have a mortality rate of 4%. For those patients over 55 years old who failed NOM, the mortality rate was 29% compared to 12% of those younger than 55 years of age [45]. In fact, elderly patients who failed NOM had a lower mortality rate than those elderly patients who had immediate laparotomy [46,47]. Nix found that the elderly had 40% mortality with immediate laparotomy, 13% mortality with failed NOM, and 14% mortality with successful NOM [47].

The data are conflicting regarding the effect of age on success of NOM of blunt splenic injuries. Bee et al. found that 22% of patients over 55 years old failed NOM compared to 6% of those younger than 55 years of age [48]. However, a more recent retrospective review of blunt splenic injuries comparing patients younger than 55 years of age to those aged 55 years or older found no differences in success rates of NOM overall or for any grade of injury [49]. Angiography was successful in increasing the success rate of NOM in both age groups. This contrasts with two systematic reviews that found that age greater than either 55 or 40 years was associated with higher rates of NOM [7,9].

A large retrospective review comparing cirrhotic patients with blunt splenic injury to noncirrhotic patients found that cirrhotic patients had a higher failure rate of NOM (83% vs. 90%), higher mortality (22% vs. 6%), and longer intensive care unit and hospital length of stay [50]. In addition to high injury grade (Grades 4 and 5), preexisting coagulopathy was found to predict failure of NOM.

Timing of administration of chemical thromboembolic prophylaxis does not seem to influence the rate of bleeding complications or failure of NOM. Alejandro et al. showed no difference in failure of NOM or mortality between early (less than 48 h) and late (over 48 h) initiation of low molecular weight heparin [51]. Similarly, Joseph et al. demonstrated no differences in rates of bleeding complications, operative interventions, or blood transfusion in early versus late thromboembolic chemoprophylaxis with enoxaparin [52].

*Recommendations*:

1. Level 2A evidence supports the previously stated American Pediatric Surgical Association guidelines for NOM of blunt spleen injuries in children.
2. The data are conflicting on the impact of age on success of NOM of blunt spleen injury, but the higher quality evidence suggests that older age is associated with higher NOM failure rates. Age should not preclude NOM.

   *Level of evidence*: 2B

   *Grade of recommendation*: B
3. Based on limited retrospective data, patients with cirrhotic have worse outcomes than noncirrhotic patients with blunt spleen injury.

   *Level of evidence*: 2B

   *Grade of recommendation*: B
4. Retrospective studies show no adverse effects of early anticoagulation in blunt spleen injury. Once acute bleeding has stopped, thromboembolic chemoprophylaxis should proceed as with any other trauma patient.

   *Level of evidence*: 4

   *Grade of recommendation*: C

## Acknowledgments

Robert Benjamin, MD, FACS, and Anne Saladyga, MD, who authored the first edition of this chapter, "An Evidence-Based Approach to Spleen Trauma: Management and Outcomes."

## References

1. Richardson JD. Changes in the management of injuries to the liver and spleen. *J Am Coll Surg*. 2005;200(5):648–669.
2. Smith J, Armen S, Cook CH, Martin LC. Blunt splenic injuries: Have we watched long enough? *J Trauma*. 2008;64(3):656–663.
3. Cogbill TH, Moore EE, Jurkovich GJ et al. Nonoperative management of blunt splenic trauma: A multicenter experience. *J Trauma*. 1989;29(10):1312–1317.
4. Leeper WR, Leeper TJ, Ouellette D, Moffat B, Sivakumaran T, Charyk-Stewart T, Kribs S, Parry NG, Gray DK. Delayed hemorrhagic complications in the nonoperative management of blunt splenic trauma: Early screening leads to a decrease in failure rate. *Trauma Acute Care Surg*. 2014;76(6):1349–1353.
5. Hafiz S, Desale S, Sava J. The impact of solid organ injury management on the US health care system. *J Trauma Acute Care Surg*. 2014;77(2):310–314.
6. Di Sabatino A, Carsetti R, Corazza GR. Post-splenectomy and hyposplenic states. *Lancet*. 2011;378(9785):86–97.
7. Bhangu A, Nepogodiev D, Lal N, Bowley DM. Meta-analysis of predictive factors and outcomes for failure of nonoperative management of blunt splenic trauma. *Injury*. 2012;43(9):1337–1346.
8. Peitzman AB, Heil B, Rivera L et al. Blunt splenic injury in adults: Multi-institutional Study of the Eastern Association for the Surgery of Trauma. *J Trauma*. 2000;49(2):177–189.

9. Olthof DC, Joosse P, van der Vlies CH, de Haan RJ, Goslings JC. Prognostic factors for failure of nonoperative management in adults with blunt splenic injury: A systematic review. *J Trauma Acute Care Surg.* 2013;74(2):546–557.
10. Haan JM, Bochicchio GV, Kramer N et al. Nonoperative management of blunt splenic injury: A 5-year experience. *J Trauma.* 2005;58(3):492–498.
11. Meguid AA, Bair HA, Howells GA et al. Prospective evaluation of criteria for the nonoperative management of blunt splenic trauma. *Am Surg.* 2003;69(3):238–243.
12. Velmahos GC, Toutouzas KG, Radin R et al. Nonoperative treatment of blunt injury to solid abdominal organs: A prospective study. *Arch Surg.* 2003;138(8):844–851.
13. Demetriades, D, Hadjizacharia, P, Constantinou, C et al. Selective nonoperative management of penetrating abdominal solid organ injuries. *Ann Surg.* 2006;244(4):620–628.
14. Berg RJ, Inaba K, Okoye O, Pasley J, Teixeira PG, Esparza M, Demetriades D. The contemporary management of penetrating splenic injury. *Injury.* 2014;45(9):1394–1400.
15. Sclafani SJ. The role of angiographic hemostasis in salvage of the injured spleen. *Radiology.* 1981;141(3):645–650.
16. Haan J, Ilahi ON, Kramer M et al. Protocol-driven nonoperative management in patients with blunt splenic trauma and minimal associated injury decreases length of stay. *J Trauma.* 2003;55(2):317–322.
17. Smith HE, Biffl WL, Majercik SD et al. Splenic artery embolization: Have we gone too far? *J Trauma.* 2006;61(3):541–546.
18. Requarth JA, D'Agostino RB, Jr., Miller PR. Nonoperative management of adult blunt splenic injury with and without splenic artery embolotherapy: A meta-analysis. *J Trauma.* 2011;71(4):898–903.
19. Bhullar IS, Frykberg ER, Siragusa D, Chesire D, Paul J, Tepas JJ 3rd, Kerwin AJ. Selective angiographic embolization of blunt splenic traumatic injuries in adults decreases failure rate of nonoperative management. *J Trauma Acute Care Surg.* 2012;72(5):1127–1134.
20. Miller PR, Chang MC, Hoth JJ, Mowery NT, Hildreth AN, Martin RS, Holmes JH, Meredith JW, Requarth JA. Prospective trial of angiography and embolization for all grade III to V blunt splenic injuries: Nonoperative management success rate is significantly improved. *J Am Coll Surg.* 2014;218(4):644–648.
21. Gaarder C, Dormagen JB, Eken T et al. Nonoperative management of splenic injuries: Improved results with angioembolization. *J Trauma.* 2006;61(1):192–198.
22. Rozycki GS, Ochsner MG, Schmidt JA et al. A prospective study of surgeon-performed ultrasound as the primary adjuvant modality for injured patient assessment. *J Trauma.* 1995;39:492–498.
23. Rozycki GS, Knudson MM, Shackford SR et al. Surgeon-performed bedside organ assessment with sonography after trauma (BOAST): A pilot study from the WTA Multicenter Group. *J Trauma.* 2005;59(6):1356–1364.
24. Deunk J, Brink M, Dekker HM et al. Routine versus selective computed tomography of the abdomen, pelvis, and lumbar spine in blunt trauma: A prospective evaluation. *J Trauma.* 2009;66:1108–1117.
25. van der Vlies CH, Otto M. van Delden OM, Punt BJ, Ponsen KJ, Reekers JA, Goslings JC. Literature review of the role of ultrasound, computed tomography, and transcatheter arterial embolization for the treatment of traumatic splenic injuries. *Cardiovasc Intervent Radiol.* 2010;33(6):1079–1087.
26. Haan JM, Boswell S, Stein D et al. Follow-up abdominal CT is not necessary in low-grade splenic injury. *Am Surg.* 2007;73(1):13–18.
27. Uecker J, Pickett C, Dunn E. The role of follow-up radiographic studies in nonoperative management of spleen trauma. *Am Surg.* 2001;67(1):22–25.
28. Weinberg JA, Lockhart ME, Parmar AD, Griffin RL, Melton SM, Vandromme MJ, McGwin G, Jr., Rue LW III. Computed tomography identification of latent pseudoaneurysm after blunt splenic injury: Pathology or technology? *J Trauma.* 2010;68(5):1112–1116.
29. Safavi A, Beaudry P, Jamieson D, Murphy JJ. Traumatic pseudoaneurysms of the liver and spleen in children: Is routine screening warranted? *J Pediatr Surg.* 2011;46(5):938–941.
30. Minarik L, Slim M, Rachlin S et al. Diagnostic imaging in the follow-up of nonoperative management of splenic trauma in children. *Pediatr Surg Int.* 2002;18(5–6):429–431.
31. Thompson SR, Holland AJ. Current management of blunt splenic trauma in children. *ANZ J Surg.* 2006;76(1–2):48–52.
32. King H, Schumacker HB, Jr. Splenic studies. I. Susceptibility to infection after splenectomy performed in infancy. *Ann Surg.* 1952;136(2):239–242.
33. Resende V, Petroianu A. Functions of the splenic remnant after subtotal splenectomy for treatment of severe splenic injuries. *Am J Surg.* 2003;185(4):311–315.
34. Falimirski M, Syed A, Prybilla D. Immunocompetence of the severely injured spleen verified by differential interference contrast microscopy: The red blood cell pit test. *J Trauma.* 2007;63(5):1087–1092.
35. Bennett NM, Whitney CG, Moore M, Pilishvili T, Dooling KL. Use of 13-valent pneumococcal conjugate vaccine and 23-valent pneumococcal polysaccharide vaccine for adults with immunocompromising conditions: Recommendations of the Advisory Committee on Immunization Practices (ACIP). *CDC MMWR.* 2012;61(40):816–819.
36. Shatz DV, Romero-Steiner S, Elie CM et al. Antibody responses in postsplenectomy trauma patients receiving the 23-valent pneumococcal polysaccharide vaccine at 14 versus 28 days postoperatively. *J Trauma.* 2002;53(6):1037–1042.
37. Shatz DV, Schinsky MF, Pais LB et al. Immune responses of splenectomized trauma patients to the 23-valent pneumococcal polysaccharide vaccine at 1 versus 7 versus 14 days after splenectomy. *J Trauma.* 1998;44(5):760–766.
38. Stylianos S. Evidence-based guidelines for resource utilization in children with isolated spleen or liver injury. The APSA Trauma Committee. *J Pediatr Surg.* 2000;35(2):164–169.
39. Stylianos S. Compliance with evidence-based guidelines in children with isolated spleen or liver injury: A prospective study. *J Pediatr Surg.* 2002;37(3):453–456.

40. St Peter SD, Aguayo P, Juang D, Sharp SW, Snyder CL, Holcomb GW III, Ostlie DJ. Follow up of prospective validation of an abbreviated bedrest protocol in the management of blunt spleen and liver injury in children. *J Pediatr Surg.* 2013;48(12):2437–2441.
41. Stylianos S, Egorova N, Guice KS et al. Variation in treatment of pediatric spleen injury at trauma centers versus nontrauma centers: A call for dissemination of American Pediatric Surgical Association benchmarks and guidelines. *J Am Coll Surg.* 2006;202(2):247–251.
42. Holmes JH, Wiebe DJ, Tataria M et al. The failure of nonoperative management in pediatric solid organ injury: A multi-institutional experience. *J Trauma.* 2005;59(6):1309–1313.
43. Potoka DA, Schall LC, Ford HR. Risk factors for splenectomy in children with blunt splenic trauma. *J Pediatr Surg.* 2002;37(3):294–299.
44. van der Vlies CH, Saltzherr TP, Wilde JC, van Delden OM, de Haan RJ, Goslings JC. The failure rate of nonoperative management in children with splenic or liver injury with contrast blush on computed tomography: A systematic review. *J Pediatr Surg.* 2010;45(5):1044–1049.
45. Harbrecht BG, Peitzman AB, Rivera L et al. Contribution of age and gender to outcome of blunt splenic injury in adults: Multicenter study of the eastern association for the surgery of trauma. *J Trauma.* 2001;51(5):887–895.
46. Albrecht RM, Schermer CR, Morris A. Nonoperative management of blunt splenic injuries: Factors influencing success in age >55 years. *Am Surg.* 2002;68(3):227–231.
47. Nix JA, Costanza M, Daley BJ et al. Outcome of the current management of splenic injuries. *J Trauma.* 2001;50(5):835–842.
48. Bee TK, Croce MA, Miller PR et al. Failures of splenic nonoperative management: Is the glass half empty or half full? *J Trauma.* 2001;50(2):230–236.
49. Bhullar IS, Frykberg ER, Siragusa D, Chesire D, Paul J, Tepas JJ III, Kerwin AJ. Age does not affect outcomes of nonoperative management of blunt splenic trauma. *J Am Coll Surg.* 2012;214(6):958–964.
50. Bugaev N, Breeze JL, Daoud V, Arabian SS, Rabinovici R. Management and outcome of patients with blunt splenic injury and preexisting liver cirrhosis. *J Trauma Acute Care Surg.* 2014;76(6):1354–1361.
51. Alejandro KV, Acosta JA, Rodriguez PA. Bleeding manifestations after early use of low-molecular-weight heparins in blunt splenic injuries. *Am Surg.* 2003;69(11):1006–1009.
52. Joseph B, Pandit V, Harrison C et al. Early thromboembolic prophylaxis in patients with blunt solid abdominal organ injuries undergoing nonoperative management: Is it safe? *Am J Surg.* May 4, 2014;209:194–198.

## Commentary on Evidence-Based Approach to Spleen Injury

*Andrew B. Peitzman*

Injury to the spleen has evolved dramatically over the past three decades. The availability of high-definition computed tomography (CT) has allowed accurate diagnosis of blunt abdominal injury. Nonoperative management of blunt splenic injury is safe in over 95% of children; decision-making/management in adults is more complex.

1. Nonoperative management of penetrating injury to the spleen. The author presents the available data, but I would interpret these differently. The author states that "selective nonoperative management of penetrating splenic injuries seems feasible in hemodynamically stable patients with a reliable exam and no peritonitis or CT evidence of hollow viscus injury." As the author states, the vast majority of patients with penetrating injury to the spleen underwent immediate laparotomy and substantial failure rate in the patients initially observed. Successful observation of penetrating splenic injury was documented in only 3.6% and 9% of patients in the series with penetrating injury to the spleen. Clearly, the data suggest the safest approach is laparotomy for patients with penetrating splenic injury.
2. Which patients (adults) are candidates for nonoperative management of blunt splenic injury? As the author states, hemodynamic stability is essential for safe observation. Several reviews discussed by the author document higher rate of failure of nonoperative management with AAST splenic injury grade 3 or higher, moderate or large hemoperitoneum, or ISS > 25. Two studies referenced suggest age (greater than 40 years or greater than 55 years) have higher rates of failure of observation.

   Importantly, the author did not reference the EAST multicenter study, which reviewed complete charts on adult patients who failed nonoperative management of splenic injury*. This study documented that of the deaths which occurred in patients who failed observation, 60% were preventable deaths, demonstrating that the risk of failure of observation of blunt injury to the spleen will include preventable deaths.

   Two studies utilizing the National Trauma Data Bank†‡ have confirmed that the risk of observation of grade 4 and 5 splenic injuries incurs a failure rate greater than 50%. The ReCONECT study from the New England Trauma centers corroborates that only 40% of grade IV and 14% of grade V adult splenic injuries ultimately kept their spleens§. Does it make sense to observe an adult with a grade V splenic injury—I think not; grade IV injury is less clear.
3. Which patients should undergo splenic angiography? The author has outlined this literature well and made appropriate conclusions. Empiric use of angiography/embolization seems to decrease the high risk of observation alone for grade IV and V splenic injuries in adults. Contrast extravasation, pseudoaneurysm, or arteriovenous fistula have lower incidence of failure with angiography/embolization.
4. What imaging studies should be obtained in patients with splenic injuries? Technique and timing of contrast extravasation are critical to optimize the utility of CT. A properly timed arterial phase is essential for the diagnosis of splenic artery pseudoaneurysm or arteriovenous fistula. A correctly timed venous phase image is needed for accurate confirmation of active hemorrhage or parenchymal injury.
5. My additional comments are related to the risks of overwhelming postsplenectomy sepsis in relation to the patient with splenic injury managed nonoperatively or who has undergone angiography embolization. First, the

* Peitzman AB, Harbrecht BG, Rivera L et al. Failure of observation of blunt splenic injury in adults: Variability in practice and adverse consequences. *J Am Coll Surg*. 2005;201:179–187.

† Smith J, Armen S, Cook CH, Martin LC. Blunt splenic injuries: Have we watched long enough? *J Trauma*. 2008;64(3):656–663.

‡ Watson GA, Rosengart MR, Zenati MS et al. Nonoperative management of severe splenic injury: Are we getting better? *J Trauma Acute Care Surg*. 2006;61:1113–1119.

§ Velmahos GC, Zacharias N, Emhoff TA et al. Management of the most severely injured spleen: A multicenter study of the Research Consortium of the New England Centers for Trauma. *Arch Surg*. 2010;145:456–460.

absence of Howell–Jolly bodies does not confirm immunocompetence, simply the presence of some functioning splenic tissue. Addressing immunocompetence after angiography/embolization, Skattum et al. compared 15 patients embolized patients with 14 patients who underwent splenectomy and 30 control subjects. Both embolized and asplenic patients had higher platelet and white blood cell counts compared to controls. Immunoglobulin titers were comparable between controls and embolized patients*. On the other hand, Nakae et al. reported no advantage in immunologic function comparing embolization over splenectomy†. The immunologic effects of angiography/embolization of the spleen are still undefined.

* Skattum J, Titze TL, Dormagen JB et al. Preserved splenic function after angioembolization of high grade injury. *Injury*. 2012;43:62–66.

† Nakae H, Shimazu T, Miyauchi H et al. Does splenic preservation treatment improve immunologic function and longterm prognosis after splenic injury? *J Trauma Acute Care Surg*. 2009;67:557–564.

# 22

# Injury to the Liver

**Daniel J. Bonville, Lori A. DeFreest, Marcel Tafen, and Andrew DeRoo**

**CONTENTS**



The liver is the most commonly injured organ in patients with abdominal trauma [1]. The diagnosis and treatment of liver injuries have evolved significantly over the past five decades. In the 1960s and 1970s, the main treatment was liberal use of exploratory laparotomy with repair, resection, or liver packing to achieve hemostasis. This approach resulted in a death rate from 20% to over 50% including all grades of injury [2]. Currently, less than 20% of the blunt injury patients undergo surgery. Over the past 25 years, nonoperative management (NOM) has become the mainstay of the treatment for stable patients with blunt liver injuries [3]. In penetrating trauma, the liver may be severely damaged, and the operative management of hepatic injuries remains one of the greatest technical challenges in trauma surgery; however, recent trends increasing NOM for penetrating trauma have been reported as well. These are just a few factors that have contributed to improved mortality over the past 40 years. However, despite these advances, many questions regarding best practices in patients with liver injuries remained unanswered.

## 22.1 What Are the Criteria for Selecting Blunt Trauma Patient for NOM?

For over 25 years, there has been an increasing quantity of data validating NOM, with or without adjuncts, as the gold standard for the management of blunt hepatic injuries [3,4]. This includes the evidence compiled by the latest iteration of the Eastern Association for the Surgery of Trauma (EAST) guide on NOM of hepatic injuries in 2012 [5]. There are no controlled randomized trials comparing efficacy of operative versus NOM. Three prospective cohort trials on NOM of liver injuries are published to date [6–8], but the bulk of evidence emanates from Class III references. Currently available data suggest that every hemodynamically stable patient should be treated initially by NOM [4–10,16,18,21]. The suitability for NOM should no longer be based on the amount of hemoperitoneum, the grade of injury [11], the presence of head injury [9], Injury Severity Score, the patient's age, or even contrast extravasation [12,13]. Concomitant or combined injuries increase the failure rate of NOM but do not preclude implementation [4].

Less than 20% of patients with blunt liver injury will require emergent laparotomy because of either the liver or associated intra-abdominal injuries [14]. Associated intra-abdominal injuries necessitating laparotomy, peritonitis, and hemodynamic instability constitute the three absolute contraindications to NOM [4,15–17]. Based on the aforementioned criteria, close to 80% of blunt trauma patients are candidates for NOM, with a success rate ranging between 82% and 100% [6,18,19].

*Recommendation*: Patients with blunt liver trauma who are hemodynamically stable are the best candidates for successful NOM (level of evidence Class IIb–III, grade of recommendation grade B). Patients with a combination of injuries are more likely to fail NOM but should be given a trial if they are hemodynamically normal and do not have other indications for exploratory laparotomy.

*Level of evidence*: Class III

*Grade of recommendation*: B

## 22.2 When Should NOM Patients Be Allowed Out of Bed after Sustaining a Liver Injury?

Historically, an integral part of the NOM of liver injuries is bed rest. The optimal duration of this measure is unknown, and protocols are highly variable among practitioners even within the same institution [17]. Only retrospective studies have addressed the question in the adult population. London et al. showed no failure of NOM in patients mobilized before the third hospital day postinjury and concluded that bed rest was unnecessary [20,21]. Studies in the pediatric population including a prospective study have shown it to be safe to lift bed rest restrictions after 24 h for low-grade injuries and 48 h for greater than grade III injuries [22,23].

*Recommendation*: The available evidence suggests that patients can safely ambulate after 48 h of bed rest, but this literature is not sufficient to make a recommendation regarding duration of bed rest limitations for hepatic trauma.

*Level of evidence*: Class III–IV

*Grade of recommendation*: C

## 22.3 Does Drainage Prevent Complications in Surgically Treated Hepatic Injuries and Should Routine Endoscopic Retrograde Cholangiopancreatography (ERCP) and Stenting Be Used for Bile Leaks?

Multiple studies have evaluated the need for systemic biliary tract drainage via T-tube choledochostomy, cholecystostomy tube, or perihepatic drains in surgically treated hepatic trauma. These studies showed an increase risk of infectious complications and abscess formation in those managed with drains. Therefore, the routine use of drains in surgically treated hepatic trauma has not been recommended [24,25].

At the same time, the trend in the management of complex traumatic hepatic injuries is the use of damage control surgery (DCS) and perihepatic packing. With DCS, there is the potential to have severe parenchymal damage left untreated with the risk of having a larger and more complex postoperative bile leak with rates reported in 0.5%–21% of patients [26,27]. Of particular concern are infectious complications arising from a biliary source and the significant morbidity associated with reoperation [27].

The use of ERCP for diagnosis and management of biliary complications in surgically managed hepatic trauma has developed out of the use of ERCP in iatrogenic causes of biliary leaks. ERCP with transpapillary stenting or sphincterotomy is used to promote flow of bile into the duodenum, allowing for transhepatic and intrahepatic biliary injuries to heal [27]. ERCP in the management of traumatic hepatic biliary injuries has been mostly limited to small case series and case reports with a reported success rate of 85% [26,27]. Its use in traumatic biliary complications by Bajaj et al. identified 11 case series published between 1999 and 2007. In this study, 69 out of the 73 patients were resolved with ERCP maneuvers [27]. Furthermore, a retrospective study by Anand et al. showed a 100% success rate in the management of biliary leaks in 26 patients with traumatic associated biliary leaks. Of the 26 patients, 23 had resolution within 3 months with an average of 47 days with the remaining leaks closing by 7 months [28].

Hommes and Nicol evaluated the role of conservative management of intrahepatic biliary leaks and questioned the need for routine ERCP and sphincterotomy/stenting for all trauma-associated biliary injuries. In their prospective study of 412 patients, 14 patients had major bile leaks (>400 mL/day or leak >14 days) and 26 had minor leaks. The major leaks underwent ERCP with stenting, and the minor leaks were treated conservatively. All bile leaks resolved, and there was no significant difference in septic complications, ICU length of stay, and mortality between the groups treated with ERCP (major leak) and those managed conservatively (minor leak) [26]. In summary, ERCP has been found to be effective in managing posttraumatic biliary leaks. However, it needs to be determined which biliary leaks benefit from ERCP management versus those that will resolve spontaneously.

*Recommendations*: The routine use of drains after surgical treatment of liver injuries is not supported.

*Level of evidence*: Class IIb

*Grade of recommendation*: B

Selective use of ERCP in the management of posttraumatic biliary complications is effective.

*Level of evidence*: Class IV

*Grade of recommendation*: C

## 22.4 Can Gunshot Wounds (GSWs) to the Liver of Stable Patients Be Managed Nonoperatively on Clinical Exam?

Can computed tomography (CT) scan be safely used as an adjunct to determine who can be managed nonoperatively? Although the policy of selective NOM (sNOM) of stab wounds (SW) to the liver has gained acceptance, utilization of this strategy for GSWs still remains controversial. At its conception [29], it was based on serial physical examination by skilled practitioners, but this has now been augmented by the use of contrast-enhanced CT to aid in determining which trauma patients are candidates for sNOM.

In March 2010, the EAST published practice management guidelines for sNOM of penetrating abdominal trauma, which specifically addressed the indications for laparotomy for GSW, postinjury imaging, and specific recommendations for sNOM [30]. It is generally agreed that all hemodynamically unstable patients or those with diffuse abdominal tenderness should undergo emergent laparotomy for penetrating abdominal injuries. Furthermore, those who are hemodynamically stable but have an unreliable clinical exam because of concomitant injuries or altered mental status require further diagnostic evaluation or should undergo exploratory laparotomy [30]. In 1991, Demetriades et al. [31] prospectively evaluated 146 patients with abdominal GSW. One hundred and five patients had peritoneal signs and underwent laparotomy, but 41 who presented with minimal peritoneal signs were managed nonoperatively, with serial abdominal exams. Seven of these (17%) required delayed laparotomy, and there were surgical complications in two of these patients but no reported morbidity. The authors concluded that sNOM was safe and, furthermore, theoretically reduced the negative or nontherapeutic laparotomy rate for these patients from 27 to 5. A number of studies, reviewed by Navsaria et al. [32], evaluating sNOM of thoracoabdominal or abdominal GSW were subsequently published, which specifically evaluated hepatic injury. The majority of these had a small sample size, but reported success rates for sNOM of liver injuries of 69%–100% and sNOM included angioembolization for active bleeding in two of these patients. Demetriades et al. [33] retrospectively reported on 928 patients with abdominal GSWs, of which 152 had liver injuries. Of the 52 with isolated liver injuries, 16 underwent sNOM. Five in this group required delayed laparotomy, four for signs of peritonitis and one for abdominal compartment syndrome. The remaining 11 patients were successfully treated nonoperatively (69%), although one patient developed a biloma requiring percutaneous drainage.

Demetriades et al. [34] subsequently published a prospective series of 152 patients with penetrating abdominal wounds, 70.4% GSW and 29.6% SW; 73.0% of these patients had hepatic injury. Of the 61 stable patients who underwent CT scan, 42 had liver injury from either SW or GSW. Based on CT findings, 39 patients (67.2%) with abdominal injury were managed nonoperatively. Overall, of all injured patients, 28.4% of those with liver injuries were successfully managed nonoperatively, although it was not clear what percentage were from GSW. DuBose et al. [35] retrospectively studied 644 patients with abdominal GSW, of which 144 were managed nonoperatively. Ten of these had isolated liver injury, one of whom required delayed laparotomy. The remaining nine underwent sNOM for an overall success rate of 90%.

Subsequent to the EAST guidelines [30], there have been a number of studies further supporting sNOM of abdominal GSW, and four of these specifically discuss hepatic injury. Navsaria et al. [32] published a prospective, protocol-driven study of all liver GSW injuries presenting to a Level I trauma center over a 4-year period. All hemodynamically stable, nonperitoneal, and neurologically intact patients with right upper quadrant or right thoracoabdominal GSW injury, even if focally tender, underwent contrast CT scan for evaluation of the extent of their injuries. Of the 63 patients (33.3%) with liver injury that did not meet criteria for emergent laparotomy, all but five were successfully managed nonoperatively (92.1%). Two of these 58 subsequently developed short-term complications; one developed pleurobiliary fistula and two patients experienced an infected tract hematoma.

In a retrospective series of 133 injured military personnel with penetrating abdominal injury, 32 were identified as having hepatic injury at laparotomy (24 patients) or by CT scan (8 patients). Seven of those undergoing CT scan were successfully managed nonoperatively [36]. Starling et al. [37] published a prospective study of 115 patients over a 7-year period with right thoracoabdominal GSW who met inclusion criteria for sNOM. All but 6 of these had injury to the liver, and 81 also had injury to kidney or diaphragm determined by CT scan. Four patients, all with liver and associated injuries, failed NOM (3.5%) and underwent laparotomy, two for fecal peritonitis and one for hemoperitoneum. The remaining laparotomy was nontherapeutic.

In 2014, Navsaria et al. [38] performed a prospective trial of NOM of abdominal GSW. Of the 1106 patients admitted, 272 were selected for NOM. Of these, 82 (30.1%) were followed by serial abdominal examination alone and 190 (69.9%) underwent CT scan based on trajectory as well as serial examination. Within this latter group, hepatic injuries were seen in 79 (41.6%). The success rate of sNOM was 95.2% overall with only 13 patients requiring delayed laparotomy, of which only 10 were therapeutic.

Much of the data supporting the use of sNOM for hepatic GSW have come from two groups, and the numbers of those specifically with hepatic injury have been small or not clearly stated. However, overall, and notably in the more recent studies [38,39], the trend has been toward successful sNOM for those hemodynamically stable patients with hepatic GSW. Thus, the conclusions reached by the EAST Practice Management Group [30] stand and support that sNOM of hepatic GSW can be safely pursued. Furthermore, they concluded that serial physical examination is reliable in detecting significant injuries after penetrating trauma to the abdomen if performed by experienced clinicians and preferably by the same team.

Although choice of patients for sNOM was initially based on clinical examination, this has largely been replaced by CT scan. In 1998, two retrospective studies were published that sought to evaluate the role of CT in the management of torso GSW. Grossman et al. [39] reviewed the CT scans of 50 patients with torso GSW over 6 years that had been performed in hemodynamically stable patients to assess missile trajectory. Of the 37 abdominal/pelvic and 15 thoracic CT, 23 were positive for transabdominal, transpelvic, or proximity to vascular structures. Of the 17 positive in the former group, 9 laparotomies were performed and 8 patients were successfully managed nonoperatively. The remaining 20 patients with negative CT were also managed nonoperatively. Three of the positive abdominal CT showed a transhepatic tract, and in these cases, they were managed nonoperatively without complications.

The EAST Practice Guidelines [30] strongly recommended the use of abdominopelvic CT scan as a diagnostic tool. Three studies published since the release of the EAST guidelines further support this. As noted previously, Morrison et al. [36] utilized CT scanning as an aid in the initial decision to triage the hemodynamically stable patients within the study. In this study of 133 patients with battlefield penetrating trauma, which included 32 patients with hepatic injury, the mechanism of injury was predominantly by missile. Overall, CT had a sensitivity of 92%, specificity of 89%, positive predictive value of 71%, and negative predictive value of 98%. A retrospective study of all patients with penetrating liver injures was undertaken and reported in 2011 [40]. One hundred and seventy-eight patients with penetrating liver injuries, 70.2% as a result of GSW, were admitted over the period studied. Of the 55 hemodynamically stable patients who then underwent CT at admission, 54.5% were selected for NOM. Sensitivity and specificity of the admission CT to predict a positive laparotomy was 95.7% and 90.6%, respectively. Overall, 80.6% of isolated liver injuries were successfully managed nonoperatively. However, they recommended follow-up CT because of the high percentage of liver-related complications that they saw subsequently in both the laparotomy and sNOM groups.

*Recommendations*: NOM based on clinical evaluation, complemented with early IV contrast CT, can be implemented safely for hepatic injury secondary to GSW.

*Level of evidence*: Class IIb

*Grade of recommendation*: B

CT with IV contrast discriminates the stable GSW patients who do not need operative management.

*Level of evidence*: Class IIb

*Grade of recommendation*: B

## 22.5 Is Arterial Embolization Effective in the Management of Penetrating and Blunt Hepatic Injuries?

The use of hepatic angiography (HA) and hepatic arterial embolization (HAE) in trauma centers appears quite variable. According to Richardson et al., the use of HA and HAE to treat injuries to the liver has increased from 1% to 9% over three decades [3]. This trend has continued to rise over the last decade at some centers [18,41]. However, in a recent report of the National Trauma Data Bank, HAE was only reported in 3% of nonoperatively managed isolated liver trauma patients with American Association for the Surgery of Trauma (AAST) grade liver injuries ≥4 [42]. Over the last decade, there have been several studies advocating HAE as an important part of NOM of liver trauma as well as an important adjunct to achieving hemorrhage control in patients that require emergent laparotomy.

Emergent laparotomy is undertaken on the basis of hemodynamic status and response to initial resuscitation more than the severity grade of the injury. All experts agree that unresponsive shock and the presence of findings suggestive of associated injuries (i.e., peritonitis) are absolute indications for exploratory laparotomy and possible DCS. The efficacy for hemorrhage control of HAE in severe liver trauma has been reported as high as 75%–100% [43–46]. Thus, mortality from severe liver injuries has been reportedly decreased with the use of HAE [41,47]. The level of morbidity, however, has been reported with significant variability by several authors. In some series, it is unclear whether the morbidity experienced in patients treated with HAE is related to the HAE or to the liver trauma itself. A large series by Kozar et al. [48] of 453 liver injuries (Grades III–V) treated with NOM revealed an HAE rate of 8% but overall high complication rate in patients with injury Grades IV and V as well as in patients with requiring blood products. Complications, in this study, did not appear to correlate with the use of HAE.

Normotensive patients who have active extravasation or pooling of IV contrast within the liver parenchyma on CT scan are candidates for HAE. Gaarder et al. [43] observed a reduction in the number of laparotomies when comparing outcomes of patients with or without use of HA and HAE for the treatment of liver injuries (Abbreviated Injury Scale score >3) after the implementation of angiography protocol in hemodynamically stable patients. Their nonoperative rate increased from 51% to 76% ($p > 0.05$) without increasing failure rate, mortality, transfusion, or liver-related complications.

Asencio et al. [47] showed a mortality benefit with HAE alone in NOM patients as well as an adjunct to operative management in a prospective study of patients with AAST Grades IV and V from both blunt and penetrating mechanisms of injury. Hagiwara et al. [44], in a case-control study, suggested that a combination of a CT scan Grades IV and V lesion and fluid requirements of >2000 mL/h to maintain normotension are indications for laparotomy. However, this study also revealed that many stable patients with high-grade injuries had bleeding on angiography regardless of the presence of a contrast blush on CT scan. Nearly half of Grade III injuries and nearly all Grade IV injuries had bleeding on HA. Furthermore, Monnin et al. [45] used a multidisciplinary approach (surgeon, interventional radiologist, and anesthetist) to perform HAE in unstable patients of high-grade injuries with hemorrhage control rate of 100% and only two HAE-related complications. They recommend this approach to avoid immediate surgery and consider embolization to be more effective to stop arterial bleeding than surgery without a concomitant increase in failure rate or mortality.

More recently, other authors have reported high success rates with HAE but with variable rates of morbidity [18,41,46,49]. Mitsusada et al. [50] in Tokyo, Japan, studied 77 patients with AAST Grades III–V liver injuries before and after changing the *target systolic blood pressure* from >90 to >80 mmHg after initial intravenous fluid resuscitation to trigger the decision for immediate laparotomy. They showed increased use of HAE and decreased urgent and overall laparotomy rate as well as decreased 24 h transfusion requirements in the group with a target for laparotomy of 80 mmHg. There was no change in mortality or liver-related morbidity during this study.

The use of mandatory HA after a DCS in patients with severe liver injuries is based on the concept that ongoing arterial bleeding is difficult to rule out at the end of DCS. This role of HAE following damage control laparotomy is to control hemorrhage in inaccessible hepatic deep parenchyma regions. This approach, which has been demonstrated to be a safe adjunct procedure to perihepatic packing with a therapeutic success for HAE, has been studied by several groups [41,47,49].

Liver-related complications in patients who were treated with HAE have been reported: hepatic necrosis, bile leak, gallbladder infarction, and hepatic abscesses. These rates vary significantly in different published reports. They appear to correlate mostly with severity of injury grade, hemodynamic status, and transfusion requirements [18,41,48,49]. In 2012, the EAST published guidelines on the NOM of blunt hepatic injury [5]. In this guideline, the authors recommend HAE be considered as a first-line intervention for patients who are transient responders to resuscitation and as adjunct to potential operative intervention. The authors also concluded that HAE be considered following laparotomy in unstable patients (Table 22.1).

In summary, HAE should be the treatment of choice for managing hemodynamically stable patients in whom CT scan shows extravasation of contrast medium

**TABLE 22.1**

Clinical Questions

| Question | Answer | Grade of Recommendation | Levels of Evidence | References |
|---|---|---|---|---|
| What are the criteria for selecting blunt liver trauma patient for NOM? | Hemodynamic stability regardless of CT findings (including grade, amount of hemoperitoneum, age, and TBI). These findings, however, may dictate use of adjuncts in NOM. NOM is the standard of care for hemodynamically stable patients. | B | IIb–III | [4–19] |
| When patients undergoing NOM should be allowed to ambulate? | After 48 h for higher-grade liver injuries and after 24 h for injuries Grade III or less. | C | III–IV | [17,20–23] |
| Does drainage prevent complications in surgically treated hepatic injuries? | The systematic or routine use of drainage of the biliary tract does not benefit hepatic trauma patients and is associated with increased infection risk and septic complications. | B | IIb | [24,25] |
| Should routine ERCP and stenting be used for bile leaks? | ERCP is a useful adjunct in management of traumatic associated bile leaks but its routine use is not warranted. | C | IV | [26–28] |
| Can GSWs to the liver of stable patients be managed nonoperatively based on clinical exam? | NOM based on clinical evaluation, complemented with early IV contrast CT, can be implemented safely for hepatic injury secondary to GSW. | B | IIb | [30–40] |
| Is CT scan an adjunct to determine who can be NOM? | CT with IV contrast discriminates the stable GSW patients who do not need to be operated. | B | IIb | [34–40] |
| Is hepatic angioembolization effective in controlling hemorrhage in liver trauma? | HAE is safe and effective in the management of severe hepatic trauma as part of NOM as well as when performed as an adjunct to the principles of damage control. | B | IIc–III | [41–50] |

when the injury is severe (AAST Grade IV or greater) (grade of recommendation B). More recent reports suggest the first-line use of HAE in transient responders as well. HAE has a high success rate in controlling hemorrhage and provides a safe adjunct to the principles of damage control regardless of whether bleeding appears to be controlled with perihepatic packing (grade of recommendation B).

*Recommendation*: HAE is safe and effective in the management of severe hepatic trauma as a key component of nonoperative treatment of severe liver trauma. It can also be safely performed as an adjunct to the principles of DCS.

*Level of evidence*: Class IIc–III

*Grade of recommendation*: B

## References

1. Trunkey DD. Hepatic trauma: Contemporary management. *Surg Clin North Am.* 2004;84(2):437–450.
2. Peitzman AB, Richardson JD. Surgical treatment of injuries to the solid organs: A 50-year perspective from the Journal of Trauma. *J Trauma.* November 2010;69(5):1011–1121.
3. Richardson J, Franklin GA, Lukan JK et al. Evolution in the management of hepatic trauma: A 25-year perspective. *Ann Surg.* 2000;232(3):324–330.
4. Malhotra AK, Fabian TC, Croce MA et al. Blunt hepatic injury: A paradigm shift from operative to nonoperative management in the 1990s. *Ann Surg.* 2000;231:804–813.
5. Stassen NA, Bhullar I, Cheng JD et al. Nonoperative management of blunt hepatic injury: An Eastern Association for the Surgery of Trauma practice management guideline. *J Trauma Acute Care Surg.* 2012;73:S288–S293.
6. Velmahos GC, Toutouzas K, Radin R et al. High success with nonoperative management of blunt hepatic trauma: The liver is a sturdy organ. *Arch Surg.* 2003;138:475–481.
7. Sherman HF, Savage BA, Jones LM et al. Nonoperative management of blunt hepatic injuries: Safe at any grade? *J Trauma.* 1994;37:616–621.
8. Croce MA, Fabian TC, Menke PG et al. Nonoperative management of blunt hepatic trauma is the treatment of choice for hemodynamically stable patients. Results of a prospective trial. *Ann Surg.* 1995;221:744–753; discussion 753–755.
9. Archer LP, Rogers FB, Shackford SR. Selective non-operative management of liver and spleen injuries in neurologically impaired adult patients. *Arch Surg.* 1996;131:309–315.
10. Petrowsky H, Raeder S, Zuercher L et al. A quarter century experience in liver trauma: A plea for early computed tomography and conservative management for all hemodynamically stable patients. *World J Surg.* February 2012;36(2):247–254.
11. Cohn SM, Arango JI, Myers JG. Computed tomography grading systems poorly predict the need for intervention after spleen and liver injuries. *Am Surg.* 2009;8:133–139.
12. Fang JF, Chen RJ, Wong YC et al. Pooling of contrast material on computed tomography mandates aggressive management of blunt hepatic injury. *Am J Surg.* 1998;176:315–319.
13. Pachter HL, Knudson MM, Esrig B et al. Status of nonoperative management of blunt hepatic injuries in 1995: A multicenter experience with 404 patients. *J Trauma.* 1996;40:31–38.
14. Galvan DA, Peitzman AB. Failure of nonoperative management of abdominal solid organ injuries. *Curr Opin Crit Care.* 2006;12:590–594.
15. Wallis A, Kelly MD, Jones L. Angiography and embolization for solid abdominal organ injury in adults—A current perspective. *World J Emerg Surg.* 2010;5:18.
16. Prichayudh S, Sirinawin C, Sriussadaporn S et al. Management of liver injuries: Predictors for the need of operation and damage control surgery. *Injury.* September 2014;45(9):1373–1377.
17. Stein DM, Scalea TM. Nonoperative management of spleen and liver injuries. *J Intensive Care Med.* September–October 2006;21(5):296–304.
18. Li M, Yu WK, Wang XB et al. Non-operative management of isolated liver trauma. *Hepatobiliary Pancreat Dis Int.* October 2014;13(5):545–550.
19. Coimbra R, Hoyt DB, Engelhart S et al. Non-operative management reduces the overall mortality of grades 3 and 4 blunt liver injuries. *Int Surg.* 2006;91:251–257.
20. London JA, Parry L, Galante J et al. Safety of early mobilization of patients with blunt solid organ injuries. *Arch Surg.* October 2008;143(10):972–976; discussion 977.
21. Parks NA, Davis JW, Forman D et al. Observation for nonoperative management of blunt liver injuries: How long is long enough? *J Trauma.* March 2011;70(3):626–629.
22. St Peter SD, Sharp SW, Snyder CL Prospective validation of an abbreviated bedrest protocol in the management of blunt spleen and liver injury in children. *J Pediatr Surg.* January 2011;46(1):173–177.
23. Dodgion CM, Gosain A, Rogers A et al. National trends in pediatric blunt spleen and liver injury management and potential benefits of an abbreviated bed rest protocol. *J Pediatr Surg.* June 2014;49(6):1004.
24. Lucas CE, Walt AJ. Analysis of randomized biliary drainage for liver trauma in 189 patients. *J Trauma.* 1972;12(11):925–930.
25. Noyes LD Doyle DJ, McSwain NE, Jr. Septic complications associated with the use of peritoneal drains in liver trauma. *J Trauma.* 1988;28(3):337–346.
26. Hommes M, Nicol AJ. Management of biliary complications in 412 patients with liver injuries. *J Trauma Acute Care Surg.* 2014;77(3):448–451.
27. Bajaj JS, Dua, KS. The role of endoscopy in noniatrogenic injuries of the liver. *Curr Gastroenterol Rep.* 2007;9:147–150.
28. Anand RJ, Farrada PA. Endoscopic retrograde cholangiopancreatography is an effective treatment for bile leak after severe liver trauma. *J Trauma.* 2011;71(2):480–485.
29. Shaftan GW. Indications for operation in abdominal trauma. *Am J Surg.* 1960;99:657–664.
30. Como JJ, Bokhari F, Chiu WC et al. Practice management guidelines for selective nonoperative management of penetrating abdominal trauma. *J Trauma.* 2010;68(3):721–733.

31. Demetriades D, Charalambides D, Lakhoo M, Pantanowitz D. Gunshot wound of the abdomen: Role of selective conservative management. *Br J Surg.* 1991;78(2):220–222.
32. Navsaria PH, Nicol AJ, Krige JE, Edu S. Selective nonoperative management of liver gunshot injuries. *Ann Surg.* 2009; 249:653–656.
33. Demetriades D, Velhamos G, Cornwell E III et al. Selective nonoperative management of gunshot wounds of the anterior abdomen. *Arch Surg.* 1997;132:178–183.
34. Demetriades D, Hadjizacharia P, Constantinou C et al. Selective nonoperative management of penetrating abdominal solid organ injuries. *Ann Surg.* 2006;244(4):620–628.
35. DuBose J, Inaba K, Teixeira PG, Pepe A, Dunham MB, McKenney M. Selective non-operative management of solid organ injury following abdominal gunshot wounds. *Injury.* 2007;38(9):1084–1090.
36. Morrison JJ, Clasper JC, Gibb I, Midwinter M. Management of penetrating abdominal trauma in the conflict environment: The role of computer tomography scanning. *World J Surg.* 2011;35:27–33.
37. Starling SV, Rodrigues BDL, Martins NPR et al. Nonoperative management of gunshot wounds on the right thoracoabdomen. *Rev Col Bras Cir.* 2012;39(4):286–294.
38. Navsaria PH, Nicol AJ, Edu S et al. Selective nonoperative management in 1106 patients with abdominal gunshot wounds: Conclusions of safety, efficacy, and role of selective CT imaging in a prospective single-center study. *Ann Surg.* 2015;261:760–764.
39. Grossman MD, May AK, Schwab CW et al. Determining anatomic injury with computed tomography in selected torso gunshot wounds. *J Trauma.* 1998;45(3):446–456.
40. Schnuriger B, Talving P, Barbarino R et al. Current practice and the role of the CT in the management of penetrating liver injuries at a level I trauma center. *J Emerg Trauma Shock.* 2011;4(1):53–57.
41. Dabbs D, Stein D, Scalea TM. Major hepatic necrosis: A common complication after angioembolization for treatment of high-grade liver injuries. *J Trauma.* 2009;66:621–629.
42. Polanco PM, Brown JB, Puyana JC et al. The swinging pendulum: A national perspective of nonoperative management in severe blunt liver injury. *J Trauma Acute Care Surg.* 2013;75:590–595.
43. Gaarder C, Naess PA, Eken T et al. Liver injuries—Improved results with a formal protocol including angiography. *Injury.* 2007;38(9):1075–1083.
44. Hagiwara A, Murata A, Matsuda T, Matsuda H, Shimazaki S. The efficacy and limitations of transarterial embolization for severe hepatic injury. *J Trauma.* 2002;52(6):1091–1096.
45. Monnin V, Sengel C, Thony F et al. Place of arterial embolization in severe blunt hepatic trauma: A multidisciplinary approach. *Cardiovasc Intervent Radiol.* 2008;31(5):875–882.
46. Misselbeck TS, Teicher EJ, Cipolle MD et al. Hepatic angioembolization in trauma patients: Indications and complications. *J Trauma.* 2009;67:769–773.
47. Asencio JA, Petrone P, Garcia-Nunez L, Kimbrell B, Kuncir E. Multidisciplinary approach for the management of complex hepatic injuries AAST-OIS grades IV–V: A prospective study. *Scand J Surg.* 2007;96(3):214–220.
48. Kozar RA, Moore FA, Cothern CC et al. Risk factors for hepatic morbidity following nonoperative management. *Arch Surg.* 2006;141:451–459.
49. Letoublon C, Morra I, Chen Y et al. Hepatic arterial embolization in the management of blunt hepatic trauma: Indications and complications. *J Trauma Acute Care Surg.* 2011;70:1032–1037.
50. Mitsusada M, Nakajima Y, Shirokawa M, Takeda T, Honda H. Nonoperative management of blunt liver injury: A new protocol for selected hemodynamically unstable patients under hypotensive resuscitation. *J Hepatobiliary Pancreat Sci.* 2014;21:205–211.

## Commentary on Injury to the Liver

*H. Leon Pachter*

The more things change, the more they stay the same, or so goes the age old phrase of wisdom. To a certain extent, the aforementioned sagacious declarative sentence rings true when it comes to traumatic injuries to the liver. The incidence of complex hepatic injuries remains at a steady state of 12%–15%, and fortunately has not increased over the last two decades. In the past, most of these complex injuries required operative intervention, and some even today continue to do so. The game changer, however, responsible for a decrease in operative intervention while concomitantly lowering the mortality in these complex injuries has been, for the most part, the advent of a nonoperative approach, in its most basic form. Over the years, however, the nonoperative approach has employed T-helper cells, so to say, in the form of angioembolization, insertion of vascular stents, ERCP, and biliary tract stents to expand its horizon and bring us to where we are today. Moreover, when operative intervention is required, a multidisciplinary approach consisting of early damage control with perihepatic packing, adjunctive interventional procedures, and subsequent radical debridement of nonviable hepatic tissue has contributed to the lowering what was in the past prohibitive mortalities.

Additionally, two myths that have persisted for decades have recently been dispelled through evidence-based data. The first myth was that hepatic resection for traumatic injuries carried a mortality in excess of 50%, thus limiting its use (an issue not discussed in this chapter, but relevant, nevertheless). The second myth commonly touted about was that gunshot wounds of the liver could never be managed nonoperatively. As with all myths, once disproven, new vistas open which have in the aforementioned two instances proven highly beneficial to patients sustaining complex hepatic injuries.

Finally, there are always questions that surgeons wanted the answers to when dealing with complex liver injuries, but despite a wide body of literature, could never convince themselves on exactly which approach was best suited for the individual patient.

The authors, in this chapter, provide the reader with a series of commonly asked questions to which they provide reasonable, and cogent answers to. This format and the data therein can readily be adapted to any surgical armamentarium or algorithm with confidence.

My role is to interject my own thoughts on the approaches the authors have suggested.

### What Are the Criteria for Selecting Blunt Trauma Patients for Nonoperative Management (NOM)?

In the new millennium, 80%–90% of patients sustaining blunt hepatic injuries are candidates for NOM with uniformly reported success rates in excess of 90%. When all opinions are considered, only four requirements for NOM remain.

1. Hemodynamic stability
2. CT scan delineation of the injury
3. CT documentation of the absence of concomitant injuries requiring immediate operative intervention
4. Limited need for hepatic related blood transfusions.

I would agree with authors that neither grade of injury, amount of hemoperitoneum, ISS, nor patient age should deter one from pursuing a nonoperative approach, if the aforementioned listed criteria are met.

I would, however, differ on the concept that "contrast extravasation" should not preclude a nonoperative approach. There are "contrast blushes" and there are "contrast blushes." Examining the "fine print," it becomes readily apparent that not all "contrast blushes" are alike and further clarification is therefore warranted as are certain caveats. There are three types of contrast extravasation as delineated by Fang. Those with extravasation confined within the liver are most amenable to being controlled with angioembolization and remain, all things being equal, prime candidates for a nonoperative approach. Those with free extravasation of contrast material into the peritoneal cavity are unlikely to avoid surgery even with the adjunct of angioembolization, and thus are by no stretch of the imagination candidates for nonoperative therapy. Those with a combination of intraparenchymal and peritoneal extravasation may be candidates for nonoperative management if angioembolization can arrest the bleeding, and the patient remains hemodynamically stable

*Combined hepatic and splenic injuries*

It would stand to reason that a combined splenic and hepatic injury managed nonoperatively increases the failure rate of nonoperative management to 12% as noted by the authors. I would, however, submit that the failure rate would most likely be as a result of the splenic injury, and not the hepatic injury. That having been said, I would never hesitate to manage a combined hepatic and splenic injuries nonoperatively if the patients remain hemodynamically stable, and meet all other accepted criteria.

One caveat, however, is the presence of a combined blunt splenic, and hepatic injury renders that patient as having a twofold increase in sustaining a hollow viscus injury as opposed to either an isolated splenic or hepatic injury alone. In this clinical setting, it is incumbent on the trauma surgeon to have a heightened awareness of a greater possibility of a concomitant bowel injury.

### When Should NOM Patients Be Allowed Out of Bed after Sustaining a Liver Injury?

This question has plagued surgeons from the very first day that a nonoperative management strategy was adopted precisely, because there is no right or wrong answer. At present, it is unknown whether a lack of bed rest contributes to delayed rupture of a stable hematoma or prevents slow but persistent hemorrhage from the liver that would otherwise have ceased.

The authors cite four papers. The two papers in the pediatric literature, in my view, cannot be extrapolated to the adult patient as the fibrous consistency of hepatic tissue of a child may be greater than that of an adult, and thus allows for earlier mobilization without the risks of "stirring up" a hemorrhagic event. The two citations in the adult population merit comment. In my experience, as well as others who have managed a great number of patients nonoperatively, failure of this approach usually occurs within the first 24–48 h. Both London and Davis, in their retrospective studies, confirm this observation. It would therefore seem prudent that an intense protocol-driven observation period, which includes the patient's clinical status as well monitoring serial hemoglobins, be employed during, what appears to be, this vulnerable period. Whether such an approach can be routinely be extrapolated to Grades IV–V injuries is unknown as the number of these patients in both studies is not sufficient enough to draw any hard and fast conclusions.

### Does Drainage Prevent Complications in Surgically Treated Hepatic Injuries and Should Routine ERCP and Stenting Be Used for Bile Leaks?

External drains are a two-way street, and if left in long enough serve as a portal for bacterial entry, and thus increase the risk of infectious complications, not the least of which is abscess formation. In my estimation, there is not a shred of evidence to support the concept that prophylactic drain placement can avert septic or bile leak complications in patients sustaining hepatic trauma. What is also clear is that Grades I–III hepatic injuries require no drainage at all. In instances where a Grade IV or V injury has occurred, a serious parenchymal injury was most certainly sustained. I believe in those instances closed suction drainage is warranted for a short period of time. These drains serve as an egress to bile and liquefaction necrosis of the damaged liver. Were drains not placed, under these circumstances, I have no doubt that a greater incidence of septic complications would ensue, requiring subsequent percutaneous drainage. Likewise, data derived from major elective hepatic resections that routine drainage may be superfluous, cannot be applied to those patients sustaining complex hepatic trauma.

In patients requiring damage control surgery (DCS) and perihepatic packing, the source of sepsis is twofold: (1) The timing of pack removal, as packs left in for over 72 h are associated with an increased incidence of sepsis; (2) The damaged parenchyma left behind at reoperation. If nonviable parenchyma is not adequately debrided, then septic complications are sure to follow. It is quite understandable that there is a natural reluctance to be too aggressive at this point, for fear of inciting bleeding and thus the need exists for, in my opinion, external closed suction drainage.

Regarding the role of ERCP, and stenting, I agree with the authors that minor bile leaks will resolve on their own with conservative therapy. Major bile leaks, on the other hand, will not, and ERCP with stenting has become an essential tool in dealing with this potentially difficult problem.

What to do with a stable intrahepatic "biloma"? That depends on the clinical situation. Those exhibiting no clinical signs of sepsis, pain, or derangements of liver function test can be followed with simple serial sonograms. Those that do not meet these criteria can be managed with an ERCP and internal drainage if connected to the ductal system or by the placement of an external percutaneous drain if communication with the biliary system is lacking.

### Can Gunshot Wounds to the Liver of Stable Patients Be Managed Nonoperatively Based on Clinical Exam? Can CT Scan Be Safely Used as an Adjunct to Determine Who Can Undergo NOM?

It has been known for some time that patients sustaining stab wounds to the abdomen, if hemodynamically stable, without signs of abdominal tenderness or peritonitis, and the ability to be evaluated by "skilled" physicians, and the same trauma team can successfully be managed nonoperatively. Can this approach be extrapolated to gunshot wounds to the liver is a question that begs asking, particularly in age where "sign-outs" are often conveyed by text messages, and continuity of care by a single experienced trauma surgeon can be a rarity. Nevertheless, there is a body of literature, albeit concentrated in reports from a small number of groups both national and international, that in select hemodynamically stable patients particularly those with right upper quadrant of right thoracoabdominal injuries can safely be managed nonoperatively. It would appear that 25%–30% of gunshot wounds to the liver, if criteria are met, can be managed nonoperatively with reported success rates of 90%–95%. In the new millennium, CT imaging seems to be a critical triage component in the NOM of these patients as the missile tract and its trajectory can be delineated, concomitant solid and hollow viscus injuries can at the same time be identified, and often diaphragmatic injuries may be detected. However, if one is to embark on this management stratagem, one must be equally cognizant of the possibility of delayed hepatic related complications. Biliary fistulas, intrahepatic bilomas, hepatic abscess, and arterial pseudoaneurysms, retained hemothorax have all been reported. The good news is that almost all of these can often be managed with the help of an experienced interventional radiologist.

Can successful NOM of GSW s of the liver be accomplished? Of course, it can. Is the NOM of GSW of the abdomen for everyone? Probably not despite criteria delineated by august societies such as the Eastern Association for the Surgery of Trauma (EAST). This approach should be undertaken only in high volume Level I trauma Centers with a broad array of experts conversant in dealing with these patients, and the ready availability of instituting multidisciplinary maneuvers, if necessary, in ensuring the success of this approach.

### Is Arterial Embolization Effective in the Management of Penetrating and Blunt Hepatic Injuries?

Despite the information stemming from the National Trauma Data Bank of the paucity of using hepatic arterial embolization in patients managed nonoperatively with injury grades > 4, this technique has become, in of itself or as part of a multidisciplinary approach, a crucial treatment modality in avoiding operative intervention. As noted by the authors, operative rates with use of HAE have been reported to be decreased, and in some reports by 25%. Moreover, in those patients with blunt and penetrating hepatic injuries requiring operative intervention because of hemodynamic instability, and the subsequent need for damage control, angioembolization has played a crucial role as an adjunctive approach in arresting ongoing hemorrhage, both in the immediate postoperative period or several days later.

The technical success rate achieved with HAE, in expert hands, is over 90%, and in some reports as high as 100%. It would stand to reason that depriving the damaged portion of liver of arterial inflow, often in a setting of intermittent hypotension, has consequences in the form of septic complications and bile leaks.

Reports of these complications, however, are variable in the literature, and may be due to the fact that HAE has to date been employed in less than 10% of hepatic injuries in many large series. Nevertheless, HAE is a *must* maneuver as it has been shown to be highly effective in arresting hemorrhage, decreasing units of blood transfused, and avoiding unnecessary surgical intervention.

An unresolved issue to date is whether high-grade injuries, Grades III–V, should undergo angiography irrespective of the lack of a CT blush. Likewise the question of whether all patients undergoing a damage control laparotomy for hepatic injury should undergo routine angiography. Further investigational data will be required before either of these questions can rationally be answered.

At the end of the day, all patients need to be individualized, and surgical experience in the management of these patients becomes paramount as many intangible clinical scenarios continue to challenge trauma surgeons.

# 23

# Small Bowel and Colon Injuries

**Daniel L. Dent**

**CONTENTS**



Injuries to the small intestine and colon are found in less than 5% of victims of blunt abdominal trauma, but are the most common injuries sustained after penetrating abdominal trauma. Despite a large experience with these injuries in both military and civilian environments, management of hollow viscus injuries remains controversial.

Important questions to consider in the care of a patient with a hollow viscus injury includes the need for ostomy in colon trauma, management of resected bowel after damage control surgery, consideration for stapled versus hand-sewn anastomosis, abdominal skin management, duration of antibiotics, and presacral drainage of rectal injuries.

## 23.1 When Is an Ostomy Preferred over an Anastomosis in Colon Trauma?

Multiple prospective randomized trials have been performed to answer the question of repair versus anastomosis in colon trauma. For partial circumference colon injuries that do not require resection and full anastomosis, it is clear that primary repair is preferred. It is also clear that the majority of penetrating civilian colon injuries do not require resection. For this reason, many trials that have been done have not accrued enough patients with destructive colon wounds to definitively answer the question of what to do after resection for colon trauma [1–4]. It is also unclear if blunt, destructive colon injuries should be managed in the same manner as penetrating injuries. One prospective and two retrospective studies have evaluated a relatively large number of patients with destructive colon wounds requiring resection [5–7]. In all series, management was left to surgeon discretion. Risk factors that may be related to anastomotic leak—and therefore may lead one to manage a patient with a colostomy—include underlying medical condition, transfusion requirement of four or more units of packed red blood cells, hypotension on presentation, or Abdominal Trauma Index >25. It is also generally not recommended that anastomosis be performed in the case of severe bowel wall edema or poor perfusion to the segments of colon in question. It is clear that regardless of how a colon injury is managed, the risk of abdominal septic complications exceeds 20% in this patient population.

*Recommendation*: Nondestructive or partial circumference wounds that do not require resection should be closed primarily. Destructive wounds that require resection may usually be managed with anastomosis, although the following factors may lead to increased risk of anastomotic leak—hypotension on presentation, transfusion requirement of four or more units of packed red blood cells, underlying medical condition, or Abdominal Trauma Index >25. Colostomy may be considered if one or more of these risk factors is present or if the edges of the resected colon do not appear optimal for anastomosis.

*Grade of recommendation*: B

## 23.2 Is It Safe to Do a Colon Anastomosis after Damage Control Laparotomy?

Several publications have addressed this issue, none of which are large, prospective, or randomized [8–13]. In each study, low-risk patients were selected for colonic anastomosis at the time of a repeat laparotomy after an initial damage control procedure. Depending on the study, this ranged from 46% to 82% of the patients who had initial colon resection. Factors that are deemed to make a patient at "high risk" include bowel edema, medical comorbidity, recent shock, and prolonged interval from injury to operation. In patients who were deemed to be at low risk for anastomotic leak, both Ott et al. and Anjaria et al. identified that if anastomosis and abdominal closure were not performed at the first relaparotomy, the risk of anastomotic leak was unacceptably high at 27% and 19%, respectively.

*Recommendation*: It appears to be safe to perform colon anastomosis at the first relaparotomy in selected patients in whom the abdominal fascia will also be closed at that time. Factors that may influence the decision to manage the patient with a colostomy include bowel edema, medical comorbidity, recent shock, and prolonged interval between injury and definitive operation.

*Grade of recommendation*: C

## 23.3 When is Hand-Sewn Anastomosis Preferable to Stapled Anastomosis—If Ever?

This question has been debated since the invention of intestinal stapling devices. In the setting of elective surgical procedures, the literature can best be summarized by stating that no outcome difference between stapled and hand-sewn anastomoses have been identified [14]. However, when this question has been raised in trauma patient populations, there has been a slight, but sometimes statistically significant, increase in anastomotic leak in trauma patients who received stapled anastomoses [14–18]. The postulated mechanism for an increased leak rate in patients with stapled anastomoses is bowel edema. A stapler does not alter its depth based on bowel wall thickness, although in a hand-sewn anastomosis, the surgeon can do so.

*Recommendation*: There is no consensus on the issue of stapled versus hand-sewn anastomosis after small bowel or colon resection for trauma. Some data suggest that hand-sewn anastomosis is associated with a lower rate of anastomotic leak in trauma patients. Hand-sewn anastomosis may be preferable in situations where the portion of intestine under consideration for anastomosis is edematous or is at risk for becoming edematous, such as a patient requiring a large-volume resuscitation.

*Grade of recommendation*: D, due to nonconsensus of the literature

## 23.4 Should the Skin Be Closed after Laparotomy for Colon Injury?

Injury to the small intestine has not been shown to result in a high rate of infectious complications and skin closure after small bowel trauma is generally recommended [19]. However, surgical site infection rates have been shown to range from 2.7% to over 50% after colonic trauma [19–25]. This has led some authors to recommend closing only abdominal fascia and leaving the skin open. The best study on this topic is a prospective, randomized trial published by Velmahos et al. [24]. In this trial, the infection rate for open wounds was noted to be 36%, whereas the infection rate in closed wounds was seen to be 65%. Wound infection was predictive of risk for wound dehiscence and necrotizing soft tissue infection. Subjecting patients to this increased risk of major complications in an effort to avoid the need to care for an open wound does not seem prudent.

*Recommendation*: Skin should be left open after laparotomy for colon trauma.

*Grade of recommendation*: B

## 23.5 What Is the Appropriate Duration of Antibiotics after Colon Injury?

Three double-blind, prospective, randomized trials have compared 24 h versus longer antibiotic coverage in patients with abdominal trauma. All studies found no significant difference in infectious complications between patients randomized to 1 day versus 5 days of perioperative antibiotics [26–28]. Specifically, in 1992, Fabian et al. published a double-blind, prospective, randomized trial in 515 patients. After sustaining penetrating abdominal trauma, the patients were randomized to receive either 5 days of a broad-spectrum antibiotic postoperatively, or 1 day of the same antibiotic plus 4 days of saline placebo. The patients who received 5 days of antibiotics had a slightly, but statistically insignificant, higher rate of abdominal infections and were more likely to develop infection from multidrug-resistant organisms. In 1999, Cornwell et al. published the results of a study in which they randomized 63 patients to 5 days versus 1 day of antibiotics

**TABLE 23.1**

Levels of Evidence

| Question | Answer | Level of Evidence | Grade of Recommendation | References |
|---|---|---|---|---|
| Anastomosis or ostomy after colon resection for trauma? | Anastomosis, except in selected patients | 2A | B | [1–7] |
| Is it safe to perform colon anastomosis after damage control laparotomy? | Yes, in selected patients | 4 | C | [8–13] |
| Stapled or hand-sewn anastomosis after hollow viscus injury for trauma? | Either, although hand-sewn may be better in patients with edematous bowel | 4 | D | [14–18] |
| Should the skin be closed after laparotomy for colon trauma? | No | 1B | B | [19–25] |
| How long should antibiotics be continued after repair of hollow viscus injury? | No more than 24 h | 1A | A | [26–28] |
| Should presacral drains be used in the management of rectal trauma? | No, except in selected cases | 2A | D | [29–32] |

after penetrating abdominal trauma. They also found a higher infection rate (38% versus 19%) in the patients who received a longer duration of antibiotics, although statistical significance was not reached, possibly due to the small sample size. In a trial of similar design involving 317 patients, published in 2000, Kirton et al. found similar results, although the infection rate was slightly higher in the patients who received antibiotics for 1 day as opposed to 5 days. This difference was not statistically significant.

From the data in these well-designed and executed trials, it is safe to conclude that in patients with penetrating abdominal trauma, the duration of postoperative antibiotics should be limited to a maximum of 24 h.

*Recommendation*: Antibiotic prophylaxis should be limited to no more than 24 h after laparotomy for intestinal injury.

*Grade of recommendation*: A

## 23.6 Should Presacral Drains Be Used in the Management of Rectal Injuries?

Placement of presacral drains has been thought to be a useful adjunct to colonic diversion to prevent development of pelvic sepsis in the management of rectal injuries. Although the concept has theoretical merit, at the time of placement there, it is difficult to ensure that the drains are placed in a position that drains the space directly adjacent to the injury. This is especially true for anterior injuries. Gonzalez et al. [29] reported their results from a prospective randomized trial and found that presacral drainage did not reduce the incidence of pelvic sepsis. As this is the only prospective randomized trial on this topic in the literature and as only 48 patients were included in the study, it is difficult to consider this question as having a definitive answer. Two reports have suggested that pelvic sepsis is relatively rare in patients with penetrating rectal trauma, even in the absence of presacral drains, suggesting that they are of little utility [30,31]. Other authors, such as Weinberg et al. [32], have argued that having a pelvic infection that is decompressed by a presacral drain is preferable to having undrained pelvic sepsis. Based on this review of the literature, it appears that presacral drainage is not routinely necessary for rectal injuries. These data are derived almost exclusively from low velocity, penetrating trauma patients. This may not apply to patients with blunt injury or significant perirectal soft tissue damage. The author's personal practice is to selectively place a presacral drain(s) in patients who have obvious extraperitoneal tissue destruction with perirectal hematoma and/or soilage that is accessible via presacral drainage (Table 23.1).

*Recommendation*: In general, presacral drains should not appear to be necessary in the management of civilian penetrating rectal injuries. In the case of a destructive wound with significant hematoma and tissue destruction that is in direct communication with a rectal injury, presacral drainage may be considered.

*Grade of recommendation*: D

## References

1. Stone HH, Fabian TC. Management of perforating colon trauma: Randomization between primary closure and exteriorization. *Ann Surg*. 1979;190:430–436.
2. Chappuis CW, Frey DJ, Dietzen CD, Panetta TP, Buechter KJ, Cohn I. Management of penetrating colon injuries. A prospective randomized trial. *Ann Surg*. 1991;213:492–497.
3. Sasaki LS, Allaben RD, Golwala R, Mittal VK. Primary repair of colon injuries: A prospective randomized study. *J Trauma*. 1995;39:895–901.

4. Gonzalez RP, Falimirsky ME, Holevar MR. Further evaluation of colostomy in penetrating colon injury. *Am Surg.* 2000;66:342–347.
5. Murray JA, Demetriades D, Colson M et al. Colonic resection in trauma: Colostomy versus anastomosis. *J Trauma.* 1999;46:250–254.
6. Stewart RM, Fabian TC, Croce MA, Pritchard FE, Minard G, Kudsk KA. Is resection with primary anastomosis following destructive colon wound always safe? *Am J Surg.* 1994;168:316 319.
7. Demetriades D, Murray JA, Chan L, Ordoñez C, Bowley D, Nagy K. Penetrating colon injuries requiring resection: Diversion or primary anastomosis? An AAST prospective multicenter study. *J Trauma.* 2001;50:765–775.
8. Miller PR, Chang MC, Hoth JJ, Holmes JH IV, Meredith JW. Colonic resection in the setting of damage control laparotomy: Is delayed anastomosis safe? *Am Surg.* 2007;73:606–609; discussion 609–610.
9. Kashuk JL, Cothren CC, Moore EE, Johnson JL, Biffl WL, Barnett CC. Primary repair of colon injuries is safe in the damage control scenario. *Surgery.* 2009;146:663–668; discussion 668–670.
10. Weinberg JA, Griffin RL, Vandromme MJ, Melton SM, George RL, Reiff DA, Kerby JD, Rue LW III. Management of colon wounds in the setting of damage control laparotomy: A cautionary tale. *J Trauma.* 2009;67:929–935.
11. Ott MM, Norris PR, Diaz JJ, Collier BR, Jenkins JM, Gunter OL, Morris JA, Jr. Colon anastomosis after damage control laparotomy: Recommendations from 174 trauma colectomies. *J Trauma.* 2011;70:595–602.
12. Georgoff P, Perales P, Laguna B, Holena D, Reilly P, Sims C. Colonic injuries and the damage control abdomen: Does management strategy matter? *J Surg Res.* 2013;181:293–299.
13. Anjaria DJ, Ullmann TM, Lavery R, Livingston DH. Management of colonic injuries in the setting of damage-control laparotomy: One shot to get it right. *J Trauma Acute Care Surg.* 2014;76:594–598.
14. Neutzling CB, Lustosa SA, Proenca IM, da Silva EM, Matos D. Stapled versus handsewn methods for colorectal anastomosis surgery. *Cochrane Database Syst Rev.* February 2012;2:CD003144.
15. Brundage SI, Jurkovich GJ, Grossman DC et al. Stapled versus sutured gastrointestinal anastomoses in the trauma patient. *J Trauma.* 1999;47:500–507.
16. Brundage SI, Jurkovich GJ, Hoyt DB et al. Stapled versus sutured gastrointestinal anastomoses in the trauma patient: A multicenter trial. *J Trauma.* 2001;6:1054–1061.
17. Demetriades D, Murray JA, Chan LS et al. Handsewn versus stapled anastomosis in penetrating colon injuries requiring resection: A multicenter study. *J Trauma.* 2002;52:117–121.
18. Behrman SW, Bertken KA, Stefanacci HA, Parks SN. Breakdown of intestinal repair after laparotomy for trauma: Incidence, risk factors, and strategies for prevention. *J Trauma.* 1998;45:227–231; discussion 231–233.
19. Borlase BC, Moore EE, Moore FA. The Abdominal Trauma Index: A critical reassessment and validation. *J Trauma.* 1990;30:1340–1344.
20. Adkins RB, Zirkle PK, Waterhouse G. Penetrating colon trauma. *J Trauma.* 1984;24:491–499.
21. Voyles CR, Flint LM, Jr. Wound management after trauma to the colon. *South Med J.* 1977;70:1067–1069.
22. Demetriades D, Charalambides D, Pantanowitz D. Gunshot wounds of the colon: Role of primary repair. *Ann R Coll Surg Engl.* 1992;74:381–384.
23. Velmahos GC, Souter I, Degiannis E et al. Primary repair for colonic gunshot wounds. *Aust N Z J Surg.* 1996;66:344–347.
24. Velmahos GC, Vassiliu P, Demetriades D et al. Wound management after colon injury: Open or closed? A prospective randomized study. *Am Surg.* 2002;68:795–801.
25. Seamon MJ, Smith BP, Capano-Wehrle L, Fakhro A, Fox N, Goldberg M, Martin NM, Pathak AS, Ross SE. Skin closure after laparotomy in high-risk trauma patients: Opening opportunities for improvement. *J Trauma Acute Care Surg.* 2013;74:433–440.
26. Fabian TC, Croce MA, Payne LW et al. Duration of antibiotic therapy for penetrating abdominal trauma: A prospective trial. *Surgery.* 1992;112:788–794; discussion 794–795.
27. Cornwell EE III, Dougherty WR, Berne TV et al. Duration of antibiotic prophylaxis in high-risk patients with penetrating abdominal trauma: A prospective randomized trial. *J Gastroint Surg.* 1999;3:648–653.
28. Kirton OC, O'Neill PA, Kestner M, Tortella BJ. Perioperative antibiotic use in high-risk penetrating hollow viscus injury: A prospective randomized, double-blind, placebo-control trial of 24 hours versus 5 days. *J Trauma.* 2000;49:822–832.
29. Gonzalez RP, Falimirski ME, Holevar MR. The role of presacral drainage in the management of penetrating rectal injuries. *J Trauma.* 1998;45:656–661.
30. Navasaria P, Edu S, Nicol AJ. Civilian extraperitoneal rectal gunshot wounds: Surgical management made simpler. *World J Surg.* 2007;31:1345–1351.
31. Navsaria PH, Shaw JM, Zellweger R et al. Diagnostic laparoscopy and diverting sigmoid loop colostomy in the management of civilian extraperitoneal rectal gunshot injuries. *Br J Surg.* 2004;91:460–464.
32. Weinberg JA, Fabian TC, Magnotti LJ et al. Penetrating rectal trauma: Management by anatomic distinction improves outcome. *J Trauma.* 2006;60:508–514.

## Commentary on Small Bowel and Colon Injuries

*Timothy C. Fabian*

Commenting on this chapter details areas of clinical research that I have been fairly heavily involved with since my trauma fellowship with Dr. H. Harlan Stone at Grady Memorial Hospital in Atlanta several years ago. Dr. Stone was many years ahead of the academic crowd relative to clinical research. He was one of the earliest surgeons in this country to perform prospective, randomized controlled trials (RCTs). RCTs are the major foundation upon which evidence-based medicine is developed. I consider myself extremely fortunate to have been mentored in "evidence-based medicine" before the moniker was developed and the process was established. I was introduced to this research methodology in Atlanta by undertaking the first prospective, randomized trial regarding the management of penetrating colon wounds. Make no mistake, the brains behind the rationale and conduct of the trial were those of Dr. Stone.

Briefly, exteriorization or proximal diversion of colonic wounds was the standard of care for many years primarily based on the military experience from World War II, but those conditions and the wounding mechanisms were different than civilian trauma. A few surgeons around the country began question whether the dictum of obligatory exteriorization was always necessary. Hence, we performed the RCT in patients with nondestructive colon wounds for the evaluation of primary repair versus exteriorization or diversion. That trial demonstrated clearly better results with primary repair. Those results led to a major shift in the management of colonic wounds in this country and ultimately throughout the world.

Following my time in Atlanta, we continued to pursue areas associated with colon wound management that attempted to tackle many of the questions addressed in Dr. Dent's chapter. Those questions have included optimal management of destructive colon wounds relative to safety of anastomosis versus exteriorization, the use of retrorectal drains for rectal injuries, colon wound management in the open abdomen, and appropriate use of antibiotics in the scenario of colon wounding. My commentary will focus on each of the six questions entertained by Dr. Dent.

### When Is an Ostomy Preferred over an Anastomosis in Colon Trauma?

An ostomy is almost never indicated for management of penetrating nondestructive wounds. My definition of a destructive colon wound is one that involves over 50% of the circumference of the bowel and/or destruction of the mesentery such that the colon is ischemic or necrotic due to the loss of blood supply. It is appropriate to point out here that the overwhelming majority of colonic wounds are caused by penetrating trauma and for many years, the appropriate management of blunt colon injuries was not well addressed in the literature due to the relatively small number seen. In recent years, we have begun looking specifically at blunt colonic injuries in Memphis and found that applying the same algorithm for blunt colon injury as has been applied for many years for penetrating trauma is appropriate.

While Ronny Stewart, current Chairman of the American College of Surgeons Committee on Trauma, was a fellow in Memphis, he became interested in defining when primary anastomosis might be safe in the face of destructive colon injury. At that time, we noted that patients who received a significant transfusion in the preoperative and intraoperative period (≥6 units) were at significant risk of anastomotic failure as were patients with significant underlying comorbidities. Based on that early retrospective study, we began applying those criteria. And up to today, we continue to follow those risks as indications for when to perform colostomy or exteriorization. We have re-evaluated our results several times over the years and found that they have held true and that, in the absence of the risk factors, primary anastomosis of destructive wounds is safe.

We have relied on the same risk factors in management of blunt colon wounds. Although the number of colon injuries is lower than the number of penetrating wound, the results have trended in the same direction. Hence, we use the same algorithm for management of both blunt and penetrating colon injuries. What is the picture of the patient whom I would continue to exteriorize today? Any patient who requires six or more units of blood, requires intraoperative vasopressors, is in an advanced physiologic age (might be 40 or could be 90), those with significant chronic disease including diabetes mellitus or significant cardiovascular disease. Using those parameters today, approximately half of our destructive wounds receive primary anastomosis, with the remainder requiring either end-ostomy or proximal diversion.

### Is It Safe to Do a Colon Anastomosis after Damage Control Laparotomy?

This remains a controversial issue. Widespread use of damage control has a relatively brief history. The rationale and indications for the current extensive use has only developed over the past 15 years. Hence, there is not a large experience with destructive colonic injuries associated with the application of damage control laparotomy principles. When the safety of anastomosis was first brought up approximately a decade ago, I was quite skeptical that it was safe. Over time there have been publications, as detailed by Dr. Dent, that have supported a more liberal approach to anastomosis. Base on those retrospective studies as well as data from our institution and my own experience, I have had a change of heart. I believe there is little indication for doing primary anastomosis at the initial laparotomy for damage control. The very definition of damage control includes avoidance of anastomoses and rapid termination of laparotomy following control of surgical hemorrhage. To me the question becomes: is it safe on follow-up laparotomy to do an anastomosis? In general, I believe it is appropriate. My rationale is based on the fact that, of those cases I have seen leak in this scenario, there are patients who are not ready for fascial closure and the colonic leak becomes apparent very early and I do not believe that really causes any problem, assuming there has been appropriate attention paid to the open abdominal wound in the intensive care unit. If the anastomosis fails, an ostomy can be done and I do not believe that the minimal amount of contamination when discovered early significantly harms the patient. I think it is a completely different scenario compared to the patient who leaks following primary anastomosis at the initial operation or follow-up operation in which the fascia has been closed. Those patients, as we all know, have significant morbidity and occasional mortality associated with intraperitoneal sepsis from a colonic leak. This is a very difficult arena in which to do RCTs due to heterogeneity of patients, wounding, wound management, and a paucity of cases.

### When Is Hand-Sewn Anastomosis Preferable to Stapled Anastomosis: If Ever?

For emergency procedures, I almost always prefer hand-sewn anastomoses. The rationale for such is actually delineated by Dr. Dent, including the concern for inflamed or edematous bowel. I believe the hand-sewn technique allows one to place the sutures at appropriate depth within the tissue and carries a lower risk of failure. I feel the same about both small bowel and colon. However, as a practical consideration, I believe the experience of the surgeon should be considered. In many training programs, residents are instructed primarily on stapled anastomosis and may have a relatively scant experience with hand-sewn anastomoses. I think it is clear that stapled anastomoses are quite safe for nearly all elective intestinal reconstructions. I may be considered a dinosaur, but I believe that there is a slightly increased risk of suture line dehiscence with stapling for emergency anastomosis and therefore continue to believe that hand-sewn anastomosis is preferred. As with colonic anastomosis in the scenario of damage control laparotomy, the heterogeneity of these injuries is such that outside of a large RCT, it is doubtful that we will ever have solid evidence-based approached developed around this question.

### Should the Skin Be Closed after Laparotomy for Colon Injury?

I think the skin should nearly routinely be left open following colon injury. In the very occasional circumstance where there is almost no fecal contamination, I suppose skin closure would be appropriate. Though the infection may be modest relative to the number of infections, occasionally, outcomes are catastrophic related to delay in recognition of infection. Obese patients develop can develop extensive soft-tissue infections that are not clinically apparent until late, and occasionally progress to life-threatening necrotizing fasciitis. I believe that with simple wound care management when the skin is left open, there is very little morbidity associated with those wounds and cosmetically, they look as good in 6 months as those who have had meticulous skin closure. The short story: if there is more than flatus in the peritoneal cavity, leave the skin open.

### What Is the Appropriate Duration of Antibiotics after Colon Injury?

Dr. Dent nicely outlined the evidence for this query. Over my career, I have had significant interest in research with surgical infection and appropriate use of antibiotics. In the large trial that was referred to with over 500 patients, it became immediately clear to me that prolongation of antibiotics served no purpose other than increasing hospital expenses. With more contamination, patients indeed have an increase of infections, but the prolongation of antibiotics does not reduce the infection incidence. I believe there is enough high-quality prospective, randomized data in this area to support Dr. Dent's Grade A recommendation that prophylaxis should be limited to no more than 24 h after laparotomy for intestinal injury.

### Should Presacral Drains Be Used in the Management of Rectal Injuries?

This is another area where all institutions have relatively small numbers in order to address the question and again the heterogeneity of both the patient and the injury make it difficult to address with solid evidence. Nonetheless, I have been interested in this question for many years since completing my residency. I think I understand the appropriate use of presacral drains today. Everybody with a rectal injury does not need a presacral drain. The entire issue revolves around the anatomy of the injury. If the portion of the rectum involves the intraperitoneal portion, I do not believe the colon wound should be managed any differently than any other more proximal part of the colon. However, if there is a retroperitoneal component, it changes things considerably. As we all learned in the anatomy lab as medical students, there is no serosa in the retroperitoneal portion of the rectum. Thus, there are higher leak rates with low anterior anastomosis not only due to the difficulty with resection but also the fact that there is no posterior serosal surface. While retroperitoneal infections are quite uncommon with rectal injuries, when they occur, they are disastrous. Retroperitoneal sepsis develops and spreads cephalad, a very morbid complication that not uncommonly leads to death. I believe placement of a presacral drain guided to the area of rectal perforation significantly decreases the likelihood of developing ascending retroperitoneal sepsis: My rationale somewhat parallels that of leaving the skin open for colon wounds. I can see almost no morbidity associated with the placement of a retrorectal drain but significant risk of catastrophe should an infection develop.

## Bibliography

George SM, Fabian TC, Voeller GR, Kudsk KA, Mangiante EC, Britt LG. Primary repair of colon wounds: A prospective trial in nonselected patients. *Ann Surg.* 1989;209(6):728–734.

Sharpe JP, Magnotti LJ, Weinberg JA, Parks NA, Maish GO, Shahan CP, Fabian TC, Croce MA. Adherence to a simplified management algorithm reduces morbidity and mortality after penetrating colon injuries: A 15-year experience. *J Am Coll Surg.* 2012;214(4):591–598.

Sharpe JP, Magnotti LJ, Weinberg JA, Shahan CP, Cullinan DR, Fabian TC, Croce MA. Applicability of an established management algorithm for colon injuries following blunt trauma. *J Trauma Acute Care Surg.* 2013;74(2):419–425.

Sharpe JP, Magnotti LJ, Weinberg JA, Shahan CP, Cullinan DR, Marino KA, Fabian TC, Croce MA. Applicability of an established management algorithm for destructive colon injuries after abbreviated laparotomy: A 17-year experience. *J Am Coll Surg.* 2014;218:636–643.

Stewart RM, Fabian TC, Croce MA, Pritchard FE, Minard G, Kudsk KA. Is resection with primary anastomosis following destructive colon wounds always safe? *Am J Surg.* 1994;168(4):316–319.

Stone HH, Fabian TC. Management of perforating colon trauma. *Ann Surg.* 1979;4:430–436.

# 24

# *Diaphragmatic Injuries*

**Fahim Habib**

**CONTENTS**



Traumatic diaphragmatic injuries (TDIs) are uncommon injuries, resulting more often from penetrating trauma, occurring usually in the context of multiple injuries, and carry high mortality rates largely due to the severity of the associated injuries [1].

The optimal approach to the evaluation and management of these TDI remains poorly defined and is particularly challenging. Several factors are responsible for this. First, the diaphragm is a thin musculoaponeurotic layer at the junction of the thoracic and peritoneal cavities. As a result, it may be involved in traumatic injuries involving either or both of these cavities. Second, associated injuries are frequent. These may dominate the clinical pictures and dictate the course of management making the issue of diaphragm injury secondary. Third, when isolated, these injuries usually have no pathognomic features; hence, they require a high index of suspicion if the diagnosis is to be made in a timely manner. This is becoming increasingly important as nonoperative strategies are being more commonly employed in select cases of thoracoabdominal trauma. Also, key differences exist in injuries due to blunt and penetrating trauma and in injuries to the left and right sides of the diaphragm. This effectively precludes a universal algorithm for the management of all diaphragmatic injuries. Finally, while some of these missed injuries may never manifest, the potential for an adverse outcome with its attendant increase in morbidity and mortality makes prompt diagnosis and management desirable.

Adding to the aforementioned challenges is a paucity of scientific evidence to guide clinical decision-making. The overwhelming majority of publications involve case reports and case series. These usually describe the unusual and often dramatic presentation of isolated cases. Few retrospective reviews are available that summarize the practices of individual institutions. Prospective studies are even fewer and are mostly observational in nature, directed largely toward establishing the diagnosis. The relative infrequency of these injuries makes it unlikely that a single center will be able to address the key issues in a timely manner. A multicenter study is more likely to be able to generate the required evidence to answer some of the key questions. At the present time, there is no level I or level II evidence on any aspect of the diagnosis or management of TDI. As the available evidence is limited, much of what is presented in this chapter represents a summary of the current body of the knowledge and the opinions of the author.

The key questions include the following: (1) What is the optimal diagnostic modality for the diagnosis of TDI in blunt trauma? (2) What is the optimal diagnostic modality for the diagnosis of TDI in penetrating trauma? (3) What is the clinically useful classification system that guides operative management? (4) What is the optimal approach to the operative management of TDI? (5) What is the ideal suture material/prosthesis for repair of diaphragmatic injuries? (6) What are the differences in the approach to left- versus right-sided injuries? (7) What are the consequences of missed injuries?

## 24.1 What Is the Optimal Diagnostic Modality for the Diagnosis of Diaphragmatic Injury in Blunt Trauma?

The gold standard for establishing the diagnosis of TDI is direct visualization of the diaphragm by using either laparotomy or the minimally invasive techniques of laparoscopy or thoracoscopy. However, given the relative rarity of the injury, the highly invasive nature of techniques for direct visualization, their need for general anesthesia, and the high resource use and resultant costs, the routine use of this approach cannot be advocated. Instead, it is more prudent to maintain a high index of suspicion in patients whose trauma mechanism and physical findings are suggestive. In these patients, imaging studies can be undertaken starting with the simplest, most readily available and cheapest: the chest x-ray, and proceeding in a sequential manner with more complex and relatively invasive studies until the diagnosis has either been suspected to a degree where operative intervention is warranted or excluded beyond reasonable doubt.

Maintaining a high index of suspicion is the first key step. Mechanisms of blunt trauma most commonly associated with diaphragmatic injury (DI) are motor vehicle collisions, falls from heights, and crush injury to the thoracoabdominal region [2]. Among vehicular crashes, those with a near lateral principal direction of force and those associated with a significant abrupt change on velocity of 40 km/h or greater are most likely to result in TDI [3]. In cases of penetrating trauma, wounds in the thoracoabdominal region, defined as extending from the nipple lines to the costal margins, necessitate additional evaluation.

Physical examination is notoriously unreliable. Signs and symptoms depend on the stage of presentation, which may be divided into the acute, latent, and obstructive phases [4]. In the acute phase, variable degrees of respiratory distress occur. This is accompanied by chest and/or abdominal tenderness, reduced breath sounds in the chest, and possibly bowel sounds in the chest [5,6]. Alternatively, the presentation may be masked by that of the associated injuries and be discovered incidentally or not at all. The latent phase is usually asymptomatic, with the diagnosis being made incidentally when bowel sounds are heard in the chest or the patient undergoes imaging for unrelated reasons. In the obstructive phase, intra-abdominal contents herniate into the thoracic cavity. This may result in obstruction of the gastrointestinal tract, ischemia of the herniated organ, or compression of thoracic structures with possible mediastinal shift. The patient may, therefore, present with bowel obstruction, an acute abdomen, or even features suggestive of a tension pneumothorax [6,7], a condition to which the term tension gastrothorax is applied.

The chest x-ray is usually the initial diagnostic modality employed. When present, the abnormal course of the nasogastric tube with the tip in the left chest, elevation of the hemidiaphragm over 6 cm when compared to the contralateral side, a gas-containing hollow viscera within the thoracic cavity, a visceral fluid level in the pleural space, and obscuring of the diaphragmatic shadow are highly suggestive [8,9]. Nonspecific findings on the chest x-ray that should prompt additional work-up include obliteration of the diaphragmatic contour, mild elevation of the injured diaphragm, shift of the mediastinum to the contralateral side, or evidence of additional thoracic injuries, such as a pneumothorax, pleural effusions, or rib fractures [10]. Increase in the elevation of the hemidiaphragm on the right on a repeat x-ray is another reported finding. Having the film reviewed by a radiologist increases accuracy. In a retrospective review, the accuracy of diagnosis of chest x-ray increased from 23% when read by the trauma team leader in the trauma bay to 44% when interpreted by a radiologist [2]. Limitations of the technique include the fact that the film is almost always obtained in the supine position, is portable hence often of suboptimal quality, patient cooperation is usually limited, may be influenced by associated injuries and by use of positive pressure ventilation [11].

Ultrasonography is most useful for right-sided injuries where the "lung sliding sign," visualization of the hepatic veins in the chest, and loss of the hepatorenal interface have been reported [12]. Other findings include movement of the free edge of the diaphragm in pleural fluid, splenic herniation into the thorax, inability to visualize the diaphragm, and the identification of bowel loops in the chest. Using "m-mode" imaging, failure to identify rise of the diaphragm tracing with respiratory movements is considered diagnostic [13]. It must be remembered, however, that even a ruptured diaphragm will move in mechanically ventilated patients, limiting the use of this technique to spontaneously breathing patients alone.

Computed tomography (CT) performed using conventional techniques has low sensitivity and moderate specificity in identifying the presence of a DI. The invention of multidetector CT (MDCT) with multiplanar reformations has redefined the role of this modality in the diagnosis of TDI. Acquired images can be reformatted in the axial, coronal, and sagittal planes. A number of radiographic features are suggestive of TDI. A "segmental diaphragmatic defect" may be observed with abrupt loss of diaphragmatic continuity [14]. While this is highly specific, it is not very sensitive for TDI. It is most useful in blunt trauma where the resultant defect is large and on the left side where there is a significant difference in the appearance of the diaphragm and adjacent structures. A false positive reading may result in cases of congenital defects or other nontraumatic causes of diaphragmatic discontinuity. Here, the absence of other features of acute injury, such as accompanying bleeding may be useful. The "dangling diaphragm sign" is the inward curling of the free edge of the torn diaphragm toward the center of the body, and is best visualized on coronal images [15]. The "collar sign" is a waist-like constriction of herniated viscera at the site of the diaphragmatic tear. The "contiguous injury sign," initially described by Shanmuganathan et al. is positive when there is injury immediately adjacent to both sides of the diaphragm [16]. The "dependent viscera sign" represents the loss of the normal costophrenic sulcus by the DI, which then allows the intra-abdominal viscera to lie in direct contact with the toe posterior ribs [17]. Thickening of the diaphragm to more than 10 mm which represents retraction of the injured diaphragm and the simultaneous presence of a hemothorax associated with hemoperitoneum are other suggestive findings [18]. Additional tomographic signs specific to injuries to the right side of the diaphragm include the "hump sign" and the "band sign." The hump sign is the rounded herniation of hepatic tissue into the thoracic cavity through the diaphragmatic defect [9]. The band sign is the linear area of hypodensity through the liver at the level of the torn diaphragm. It represents reduced perfusion at the site of compression by the torn diaphragm and is best visualized on the portal venous phase [19].

In a retrospective case-control study using a single detector helical CT with coronal and sagittal reconstruction, the sensitivity and specificity of the technique were 82% and 75%, respectively [20]. The dependent viscera sign was the most sensitive and the collar sign and active extravasation of contrast were the most specific [21]. The presence of pleural effusions and perisplenic hematomas was the most common reason for false negative examination [21]. In right-sided injuries, the presence of an associated hemothorax may limit the ability to make a diagnosis. Here the high position of the liver may suggest the diagnosis [22]. More recent studies have validated the use of MDCT in establishing the diagnosis [23].

Nuclear medicine scan techniques have been described, where 2.1 mCi of technetium-99 m sulfur colloid in 500 mL of sterile saline are injected into the peritoneal cavity. Imaging is performed immediately and at 2 and 4-h intervals. The appearance of a large amount of radioactivity in the chest confirms the presence of a diaphragmatic defect [24].

Intraoperative evaluation of the diaphragm remains the gold standard against which all other modalities have been compared. The operative approach selected is guided by two key principles: hemodynamic stability and clinical or radiologic evidence of associated injury. In unstable patients, emergent operative intervention is undertaken. The presence of peritoneal signs, abdominal distention, chest tube output, and radiologic evidence of a significant hemothorax guide the decision whether to perform a laparotomy, a thoracotomy, or both and the sequence in which these interventions should be undertaken [25]. The diaphragm is directly evaluated during these interventions. In the hemodynamically stable patient with no indication for immediate operative intervention, a minimally invasive approach may be adopted. This may be achieved by using either laparoscopy or thoracoscopy. Irrespective of the modality selected, the intervention must be delayed at least 24 h after the initial injury. This allows associated injuries to declare themselves. In patients remaining asymptomatic after this interval, the intervention can be directed solely toward the evaluation and management of the diaphragm. Laparoscopy for the diagnosis of traumatic diaphragmatic lacerations was initially demonstrated by Adamthwaite [26], and subsequently confirmed by Ivatury et al. [27], especially for the identification of injury in asymptomatic cases [28]. As trauma surgeons are becoming more facile with the use of laparoscopic techniques, their use in the repair of TDI is increasing [29–31]. Laparoscopy has the advantage of both diagnostic and potentially therapeutic. Majority of trauma surgeons have developed an adequate comfort level with its use for therapeutic interventions. Additional advantages of laparoscopy include shorter hospital stay, faster recovery, earlier return to normal activities, less analgesic requirements, less wound complications, and lower long-term sequelae, such as adhesions and development of incisional hernias when compared to open surgery. Although technically feasible, several disadvantages of laparoscopic approach must be recognized. The most common complication following any laparoscopic surgery is the development of a trocar site hernia. Frequently underdiagnosed, its true incidence remains unknown. With careful long-term follow up, and the use of a combination of physical examination and imaging studies, such as ultrasound and CT, incidences of >30% have been reported, especially in high-risk patients. These include those with diabetes mellitus, obesity, postoperative wound infection, need for enlargement of the fascia at the trocar site, and the presence of chronic pulmonary disease [32,33]. Additionally, the need for creation of a pneumoperitoneum carries the potential to induce cardiopulmonary compromise as the carbon dioxide traverses across the injury into the thoracic cavity. Other disadvantages include potential for inadvertent injury to intra-abdominal structures, inadequate visualization of portions of the diaphragm, risk for subsequent formation of adhesions, and the inability to evacuate an associated hemothorax. For these reasons, it is the authors' preference to utilize video-assisted thoracoscopic surgery (VATS) for the diagnosis and management of diaphragmatic injuries in asymptomatic hemodynamically stable patients with thoracoabdominal injury without indication for immediate operative indication. Like laparoscopy, VATS is performed at least 24 h after the initial injury to allow any intra-abdominal injury to declare itself. Advantages that favor the use of VATS over laparoscopy include excellent visualization of the entire hemidiaphragm, the ability to evacuate a retained hemothorax, the ability to evaluate the lung and other mediastinal structures for injury, and avoidance of trocar site hernias and postoperative adhesions. VATS requires the patient to be placed in the lateral decubitus position, requires the ability to tolerate single lung ventilation, and limits the evaluation to one hemidiaphragm. A number of retrospective series have validated the clinical utility of VATS in the diagnosis and management of TDI [34,35]. Ultimately, the surgeon must select the procedure that they are most adept at applying to the particular patient based on which side of the diaphragm the preponderance of injury lies.

*Recommendation*: In at-risk patients, begin with a chest x-ray followed by an MDCT reformatted in the axial, coronal, and sagittal planes. If the MDCT findings are suggestive of TDI, thoracoscopy is performed to confirm the diagnosis with the possible thoracoscopic repair if expertise is available or conversion to thoracotomy if not. Laparoscopy may be similarly employed if the patient cannot be placed in the lateral decubitus position or will not tolerate single lung ventilation.

*Grade of recommendation*: D

## 24.2 What Is the Optimal Diagnostic Modality for the Diagnosis of DI in Penetrating Trauma?

Diaphragmatic injuries due to penetrating trauma result most often from stab wounds and gunshot wounds to the thoracoabdominal region. For purposes of definition, this region extends from the nipples cranially to the costal margin caudally. The initial approach to these patients is determined by the hemodynamic stability of the patient. In unstable patients, urgent operative intervention is indicated. Evaluation of the diaphragm is then performed intraoperatively. In the stable patient, work-up progresses from simple noninvasive modalities to more invasive methods until the injury has been ruled out or ruled in. A thorough work-up for all patients with penetrating trauma to the thoracoabdominal region is essential, since over 40% of pericostal wounds are associated with injury to the diaphragm [36]. In contrast to blunt trauma, the resultant DI is often small and may easily be missed. While gunshot wounds may occur on either side, stab wounds are more likely to occur on the left as most assailants are right handed.

The chest x-ray is once again the initial imaging modality of choice. Radio-opaque markers must be used to mark the site of the external injury. Determination of the resultant trajectory allows estimation of the likelihood of diaphragmatic involvement. Findings may however be subtle or masked by associated injuries making diagnosis difficult. As was seen in a prospective study, 21% of patients with diaphragmatic injuries had a normal chest x-ray [16]. In another retrospective series, the chest x-ray was normal in 68% and showed only a nonspecific hemopneumothorax in the remaining 32% of patients with TDI confirmed at laparoscopy.

Computed tomography, especially with multidetector row scanners and appropriate reformatting has over 90% accuracy in detecting the presence of DI when the wound tract is seen extending to the diaphragm. In a retrospective series of 803 patients with penetrating torso injury over a 4 year period, CT had a sensitivity, specificity, and accuracy of 76%, 98%, and 91%, respectively, to detect injury and 92%, 89%, and 90%, respectively to exclude injury [20]. Equivocal findings necessitate use of additional diagnostic techniques. In a more recent retrospective study the accuracy of the 64-section MDCT with trajectography has been described. Here images are acquired in nonstandard planes aligned with the knife or gunshot track. Contiguous injury on CT trajectography was found to be a very sensitive sign (80%–93%) and its absence can be used to reliably forego further work-up with laparoscopy or thoracoscopy [17].

Digital exploration has been described for stab wounds to the left thoracoabdominal region [37]. In the acute setting in patients with a left thoracoabdominal stab wound and no indication for immediate exploration, the stab wound was cleansed, infiltrated with local anesthetic and digital exploration carried out to assess the integrity of the diaphragm. Of the 82 patients evaluated, 51 patients had a positive digital exploration in which 50 of them had a DI confirmed at laparotomy. In 25 patients with negative digital explorations, the absence of diaphragmatic injuries was confirmed by laparotomy or thoracoscopy in all 25. An equivocal digital exam was noted in 6, of which a DI was present in 2. Digital exploration thus had a sensitivity of 96%, specificity of 83.3%, a positive predictive value of 91%, and a negative predictive value of 93.7%.

Magnetic resonance imaging allows superior delineation of the anatomy, but is challenging to employ in the acute setting. It may not always be readily available, requires transport of a quasi-stable patient to a remote location, and places the patient in a situation where adequate monitoring and access to the patient for ongoing resuscitation may not be optimal. Its use is mostly restricted to cases that are identified in the latent or obstructive phases.

Intraoperative evaluation of the diaphragm during laparotomy or thoracotomy remains the gold standard. Laparoscopy is a useful diagnostic modality, especially in injuries involving the left side. Improved image quality and routine availability of angled scopes has allowed almost all areas of the diaphragm to be visualized. Identification of injuries of the posterior right diaphragm may however still prove challenging. Utility of this technique was prospectively studied for penetrating trauma involving the left thoracoabdominal region. Of 110 patients studied, diaphragmatic injuries were identified in 26 (24%). Similar incidences were detected for anterior, lateral, and posterior wounds (22%, 27%, and 22%, respectively) [38]. A similar incidence, 22 of 108 (20%) was reported in another retrospective series [39]. As with blunt diaphragmatic injuries, it is the preferred technique when a VATS is not possible or feasible.

Thoracoscopy is an alternative approach to the identification of TDI [40]. The patient must, however, be hemodynamically stable, be able to tolerate single lung ventilation, and be able to be placed in a lateral decubitus position. There must also be the absence of any indication for emergent laparotomy or thoracotomy. In a prospective study of 28 patients who met the earlier criteria, TDI was found in 9 of the 28 (32%) [41]. All injuries were confirmed and repaired at laparotomy. Associated intra-abdominal injuries were present in 89%. VATS is the preferred minimally invasive approach in the asymptomatic hemodynamically stable patient.

*Recommendation*: In unstable patients, diagnosis is established at operation. In stable patients, obtain a chest x-ray and CT scan. If stab wound to the left thoracoabdominal region, perform a careful digital exploration through the stab wound. If equivocal, proceed with thoracoscopy. Laparoscopy is performed if thoracoscopy is not possible or not feasible.

*Grade of recommendation*: D

## 24.3 What Is the Clinically Useful Classification System That Guides Operative Management?

The most popular current classification system for diaphragmatic injuries is that of the American Association for the Surgery of Trauma. Here a contusion is classified as grade I, lacerations <2 cm as grade II, laceration 2–10 cm as grade III, laceration ≥10 cm with tissue loss <25 cm$^2$ as grade IV, and lacerations with tissue loss >25 cm$^2$ as grade V. The clinical significance of this classification system remains unclear [42].

In reviewing the operative techniques described in a number of case reports and case series [43–46], a common theme emerges. Using this, the author proposes the following classification system:

*Grade I*: Contusion: No acute intervention is required, maintain high index of suspicion for progression.

*Grade II*: Linear tears with viable tissue on either side of the defect that can be primarily approximated without significant tension.

*Grade III*: Avulsion of the diaphragm off the chest wall, reattachment is however possible.

*Grade IV*: Significant tissue loss that precludes primary repair necessitating the use of a prosthesis for repair.

*Recommendation*: Diaphragmatic injuries are best classified as contusions requiring no intervention, lacerations than can be primarily repaired, avulsions that can be reattached, or associated with significant tissue loss where prosthetics have to be used for adequate repair.

*Grade of recommendation*: D

## 24.4 What Is the Optimal Approach to the Operative Management of Diaphragmatic Injuries?

The need for operative intervention in all cases of TDI has been questioned by several animal studies that suggest the potential for spontaneous healing [47–49]. In all studies, the left diaphragm protected by the relatively fixed left lobe of the animal liver prevented herniation of abdominal contents and allowed healing of the defect. In humans, this implies that a nonoperative approach may be adopted for small defects on the right side, such as those caused by knife wounds and low-velocity gunshot wounds. In contrast, on the left side the pressure gradient between the pleural and peritoneal cavities and the constant motion of the diaphragm will likely prevent spontaneous healing and preclude nonoperative management strategies.

As the diaphragm borders the thoracic and abdominal cavities, it can be adequately approached from either side. The optimal approach is determined by the timing of injury identification, the presence of associated injuries, and the side of the injury.

For injuries identified in the acute phase, the incidence of associated intra-abdominal injuries most common to the liver and spleen requiring operative intervention is as high as 89% [30]. Here the injury is best approached via a laparotomy.

If the injury presents in the latent phase, a thoracic approach is preferred. Here, compromise of intra-abdominal contents is much less likely and the need for formal abdominal exploration is minimal. An abdominal component may become necessary if the herniated contents cannot be adequately reduced through the chest alone.

For injuries presenting in the obstructive phase, the initial approach can be made through the chest. If the herniated organs are viable and can easily be reduced into the abdominal cavity the repair can be completed through the chest. If, however, there is the need to resect nonviable or marginally viable intra-abdominal organs or adhesions preclude effective reduction, a combined thoracic and subcostal approach may be employed.

Left-sided injuries can be visualized well from the abdominal cavity and can be approached as such. The liver may preclude adequate visualization on the right especially in posteriorly located injuries. A thoracic approach is then more appropriate in this circumstance [8,9].

In experienced hands, laparoscopy can be employed as both a diagnostic and a therapeutic modality (22%, 27%, 34%, 35%) and is increasingly being reported [50–52]. Modifications of the laparoscopic approach with laparoscopically assisted minithoracotomy have been described [53].

*Recommendation*: In the acute phase, approach the injury abdominally. In the latent phase, use a thoracic approach. In the obstructive phase, use an abdominal approach for the left side and a combined approach for the right side is preferred.

*Grade of recommendation*: D

## 24.5 What Is the Ideal Suture Material/Prosthesis for Repair of Diaphragmatic Injuries?

In 13 of 105 patients available for long-term follow-up [2], two recurrences were noted. In both cases, absorbable suture was used for repair. In all other reported cases, nonabsorbable suture has been used. As the diaphragm is a thin muscle, in constant motion, healing of injuries is likely slow. The use of nonabsorbable material therefore appears justified. Polypropylene, nylon, or polyester applied as simple interrupted; continuous or figure-of-eight sutures have all been reported. It is the author's preference to use polypropylene in the presence of contamination from associated intra-abdominal injuries and braided polyester when such contamination is absent. The sutures are placed in a horizontal mattress manner. For all defects requiring more than one or two sutures, the resultant ridge of approximated tissue is over sewn with a running simple continuous stitch. In cases where the edges of the diaphragm could not be brought together primarily, the use of expanded polytetrafluoroethylene has been described [8,22]. More recently, biologic prostheses are being used increasingly for the repair of large abdominal wall defects. Their use has also been reported in the repair of paraesophageal hernia. While the use of biologics in repair of DI has not yet been reported, this offers an attractive option especially in cases with associated contamination from intra-abdominal injuries.

*Recommendation*: Nonabsorbable material applied as simple interrupted, continuous, or horizontal mattress sutures are appropriate. Prosthetics, possibly biologics, should be used when the defect cannot be closed primarily.

*Grade of recommendation*: D

## 24.6 What Are the Differences in the Approach to Left- versus Right-Sided Injuries?

Injuries to the left side are three times more frequent than those on the right. This is believed to be a result of the left side being congenitally weaker and lacking the protective effect of the liver. These factors make it less resistant to pressure. The incidence of right-sided injuries is however increasing due to increasing number of automobile accidents and improvements in CT technology.

All injuries on the left, both those due to blunt and penetrating trauma must be sought and repaired early. Even small defects will likely progress over time as the diaphragm is a thin muscle, in constant motion that is subject to differential pressure gradients between the peritoneal and pleural cavities. This pressure gradient eventually causes intra-abdominal contents to herniate through placing them at risk for obstruction or strangulation.

For right-sided injuries, the mechanism must be taken into account. In penetrating injuries, especially due to stab wounds, the defect is often small, is sealed by the liver, and prevents the herniation of bowel. In blunt injuries, on the other hand, there is a significant transfer of force causing a larger defect with progressive herniation of the liver [8,22]. This may occur years after the initial injury [54,55].

**TABLE 24.1**

Current Evidence-Based Recommendations for the Evaluation and Management of Diaphragmatic Injuries

| Question | Answer | Levels of Evidence | Grade of Recommendation |
|---|---|---|---|
| What is the optimal diagnostic modality for the diagnosis of DI in blunt trauma? | There is no single diagnostic modality of choice. The optimal approach is to utilize the earlier studies in a sequential manner until the diagnosis has either been suspected to a degree where operative intervention is warranted or excluded beyond reasonable doubt. Thoracoscopy is the preferred minimally invasive approach in the asymptomatic hemodynamically stable patient when performed at least 24 h after the initial injury. | 3b | D |
| What is the optimal diagnostic modality for the diagnosis of DI in penetrating trauma? | In unstable patients, diagnosis is established at operation. In stable patients, obtain a chest x-ray and CT scan. If equivocal proceed with laparoscopy or thoracoscopy. | 3b | D |
| What is a clinically useful classification system that guides operative management? | Diaphragmatic injuries are best classified as contusions requiring no intervention, lacerations than can be primarily repaired, avulsions that can be reattached, or associated with significant tissue loss where prosthetics have to be used for adequate repair. | 5 | D |
| What is the optimal approach to the operative management of diaphragmatic injuries? | In the acute phase, approach the injury abdominally. In the latent phase, use a thoracic approach. In the obstructive phase, use an abdominal approach for the left side and a combined approach for the right side is preferred. | 2b | D |
| What is the ideal suture material/prosthesis for repair of diaphragmatic injuries? | Nonabsorbable material applied as simple interrupted, continuous, or horizontal mattress sutures are appropriate. Prosthetics, possibly biologics, should be used when the defect cannot be closed primarily. | 3b | D |
| What are the differences in the approach to left- versus right-sided injuries? | On the left side, repair all injuries irrespective of the mechanism. On the right side, repair those due to blunt trauma and penetrating trauma only if large. | 3b | D |
| What are the consequences of missed injuries? | A wide spectrum of often-dramatic consequences may result. These make early diagnosis and repair desirable. | 4 | D |

*Recommendation*: On the left side, repair all injuries irrespective of the mechanism. On the right side, repair those due to blunt trauma and penetrating trauma only if large.

*Grade of recommendation*: D

## 24.7 What Are the Consequences of Missed Injuries?

Literature is replete with cases describing the delayed presentation of TDI that were missed at initial evaluation. Latent periods of up to 28 years have been reported. The presentation depends on the herniation organ. Right-sided injuries are associated with progressive herniation of the liver, which compresses the lung causing progressive respiratory embarrassment. On the left, gastrothorax, gastrointestinal bleeding from splenic vein thrombosis due to herniation of the spleen, tension fecopneumothorax from acute rupture of a herniated colon, and symptoms of bowel obstruction have all been reported. Yet, the true number of patients with unidentified diaphragmatic injuries that remain asymptomatic remains unknown. It is unlikely that this number will ever be known. The consequence of missed injuries will therefore remain anecdotal. It does seem prudent, however, to aggressively seek out these injuries with early repair (Table 24.1).

*Recommendation*: A wide spectrum of often-dramatic consequences may result. These make early diagnosis and repair desirable.

*Grade of recommendation*: D

## References


1. Zarour AM, El-Menyar A, Al-Thani H, Scalea TM, Chiu WC. Presentations and outcomes in patients with traumatic diaphragmatic injury: A 15-year experience. *J Trauma Acute Care Surg*. 2013;74:1392–1398.
2. Hanna WC, Ferri LE, Fata P, Razek T, Mulder DS. The current status of traumatic diaphragmatic injury: Lessons learned from 105 patients over 13 years. *Ann Thorac Surg*. March 2008;85(3):1044–1048.
3. Ryb GE, Dischinger PC, Ho S. Causation and outcomes of diaphragmatic injuries in vehicular crashes. *J Trauma Acute Care Surg*. 2013;74:835–838.
4. Grimes OF. Traumatic injuries of the diaphragm. *Am J Surg*. February 1975;38(2):OR8, OR10, OR12.
5. Howard R, Alijani A, Munshi IA. Right-side diaphragm injury resulting from blunt trauma. *J Emerg Med*. January 2008;34(1):85–87.

6. Matsevych OY. Blunt diaphragmatic rupture: Four year's experience. *Hernia*. February 2008;12(1):73–78.
7. Nishijima D, Zehbtachi S, Austin RB. Acute posttraumatic tension gastrothorax mimicking acute tension pneumothorax. *Am J Emerg Med*. July 2007;25(6):734.e5–e6.
8. Igai H, Yokomise H, Kumagai K, Yamashita S, Kawakita K, Kuroda Y. Delayed hepatothorax due to right-sided traumatic diaphragmatic rupture. *Gen Thorac Cardiovasc Surg*. October 2007;55(10):434–436.
9. Dineen S, Schumacher P, Thal E, Frankel H. CT reconstructions of right-sided blunt diaphragm rupture. *J Trauma*. May 2008;64(5):1412.
10. Patlas MN, Leung VA, Romano L, Gagliardi N, Ponticiello G, Scaglione M. Diaphragmatic injuries: Why do we struggle to detect them? *Radiol Med*. January 2015;120(1):12–20.
11. Iochum S, Ludig T, Walter F, Sebbag H, Grosdidier G, Blum AG. Imaging of diaphragmatic injury: A diagnostic challenge? *Radiographics*. October 2002;22:S103–S116; discussion S116–S118.
12. Kirkpatrick AW, Ball CG, Nicolaou S, Ledgerwood A, Lucas CE. Ultrasound detection of right-sided diaphragmatic injury; the "liver sliding" sign. *Am J Emerg Med*. March 2006;24(2):251–252.
13. Blaivas M, Brannam L, Hawkins M, Lyon M, Sriram K. Bedside emergency ultrasonographic diagnosis of diaphragmatic rupture in blunt abdominal trauma. *Am J Emerg Med*. November 2004;22(7):601–604.
14. Hammer MM, Flagg E, Mellnick VM, Cummings KW, Bhalla S, Raptis CA. Acute rupture of the diaphragm due to blunt trauma: Diagnostic sensitivity and specificity of CT. *Emerg Radiol*. 2013;1:143–149.
15. Desser TS, Edwards B, Hunt S, Rosenberg J, Purtill MA, Jeffrey RB. The dangling diaphragm sign: Sensitivity and comparison with existing CT signs of blunt traumatic rupture. *Emerg Radiol*. January 2010;17(1):37–44.
16. Shanmuganathan K, Mirvis SE, Chiu WC, Killeen KL, Hogan GJF, Scalea TM. Penetrating torso trauma: Triple-contrast helical CT in peritoneal violation and organ injury—A prospective study in 200 patients. *Radiology*. 2004;231:775–784.
17. Dreizin D, Borja MJ, Danton GH, Kasakia K, Caban K, Rivas LA, Munera F. Penetrating diaphragmatic injury: Accuracy of 64-section multidetector CT with trajectography. *Radiology*. 2013;268:729–737.
18. Nchimi A, Szapiro D, Ghaye B, Willems V, Khamis J, Haquet L, Noukoua C, Dondelinger RF. Helical CT of blunt diaphragmatic rupture. *AJR*. January 2005;184(1):24–30.
19. Rees O, Mirvis SE, Shanmuganathan K. Multidetector-row CT of right hemidiaphragmatic rupture caused by blunt trauma: A review of 12 cases. *Clin Radiol*. 2005;60:1280–1289.
20. Stein DM, York GB, Boswell S, Shanmuganathan K, Haan JM, Scalea TM. Accuracy of computed tomography (CT) scan in the detection of penetrating diaphragm injury. *J Trauma*. September 2007;63(3):538–543.
21. Larici AR, Gotway MB, Litt HI, Reddy GP, Webb WR, Gotway CA, Dawn SK, Marder SR, Storto ML. Helical CT with sagittal and coronal reconstructions: Accuracy for detection of diaphragmatic injury. *AJR*. August 2002;179(2):451–457.
22. Mintz Y, Easter DW, Izhar U, Edden Y, Talamini MA, Rivkind AI. Minimally invasive procedures for diagnosis of traumatic right diaphragmatic tears: A method for correct diagnosis in selected patients. *Am Surg*. April 2007;73(4):388–392.
23. Magu S, Agarwal S, Singla A. Computed tomography in the evaluation of diaphragmatic hernia following blunt trauma. *Indian J Surg*. July–August 2012;74:288–293.
24. May AK, Moore MM. Diagnosis of blunt rupture of the right hemidiaphragm by technetium scan. *Am Surg*. August 1999;65(8):761–765.
25. Asensio JA, Arroyo H, Jr., Veloz W, Forno W, Gambaro E, Murray J, Velmahos G, Demetraides D. Penetrating thoracoabdominal injuries: Ongoing dilemma-which cavity and when ? *World J Surg*. 2002;28:539–543.
26. Adamthwaite DN. Traumatic diaphragmatic hernia: A new indication for laparoscopy. *Br J Surg*. 1984;71:315.
27. Ivatury RR, Simon RJ, Weksler B, Bayard V, Stahl WM. Laparoscopy in the evaluation of the intrathoracic abdomen after penetrating injury. *J Trauma*. 1992;33:101–108.
28. Murray JA, Demetriades D, Asensio JA, Cornwell EE III, Velmahos GC, Beizberg H, Berne TV. Occult injuries to the diaphragm: Prospective evaluation of laparoscopy in penetrating injuries to the left lower chest. *J Am Coll Surg*. 1998;187:626–630.
29. Cooper C, Brewer J. Laparoscopic repair of acute penetrating diaphragm injury. *Am Surg*. 2012;78:490–492.
30. Yahya A, Shuweiref H, Thoboot A, Ekhail M, Ali AA. Laparoscopic repair of penetrating injury to the diaphragm: An experience from a district hospital. *Libyan J Med*. 2008;3:138–139.
31. Mjoli M, Oosthuizen G, Clarke D, Madiba T. Laparoscopy in the diagnosis and repair of diaphragmatic injuries in left-sided penetrating thoracoabdominal trauma. *Surg Endosc*. March 2015;29(3):747–752.
32. Armananzas L, Ruiz-Tovar J, Arroyo A, Garcia-Peche P, Armananzas E, Diez M, Galindo I, Calpena. Prophylactic mesh vs. suture in the closure of umbilical trocar site after laparoscopic cholecystectomy in high-risk patients for incisional hernia: A randomized clinical trial. *J Am Coll Surg*. 2014;218:960–968.
33. Comajuncosas J, Hermosa J, Gris P, Jimeno J, Orbeal R, Vallverdu H, Negre JLL, Urgelles J, Estalella L, Pares D. Risk factors for umbilical trocar sites incisional hernia in laparoscopic cholecystectomy: A prospective 3-year follow-up study. *Am J Surg*. 2014;207:1–6.
34. Martinez M, Briz JE, Carillo EH. Video thoracoscopy expedites the diagnosis and treatment of penetrating diaphragmatic injuries. *Surg Endosc*. 2001;15:28–32.
35. Freeman RK, Al-Dossari G, Hutcheson KA, Huber L, Jessen ME, Meyer DM, Wait MA, DiMaio JM. Indications for using video-assisted thoracoscopic surgery to diagnose diaphragmatic injuries after penetrating chest trauma. *Ann Thorac Surg*. 2001;72:342–347.
36. Bodanapally UK, Shanmuganathan K, Mirvis SE, Silker CW, Fleiter TR, Sarada K, Miller LA, Stein DM, Alexander M. MDCT diagnosis of penetrating diaphragm injury. *Eur Radiol*. 2009;19:1875–1881.

37. Morales CH, Villegas MI, Angel W, Vasquez. Value of digital exploration for diagnosing injuries to the left side of the diaphragm caused by stab wounds. *Arch Surg.* 2001;136:1131–1135.
38. Murray JA, Demetriades D, Asensio JA, Cornwell EE III, Velmahos GC, Belzberg H, Berne TV. Occult injuries to the diaphragm: Prospective evaluation of laparoscopy in penetrating injuries to the left lower chest. *J Am Coll Surg.* December 1998;187(6):626–630.
39. Powell BS, Magnotti LJ, Schroeppel TJ, Finnell CW, Savage SA, Fischer PE, Fabian TC, Croce MA. Diagnostic laparoscopy for the evaluation of occult diaphragmatic injury following penetrating thoracoabdominal trauma. *Injury.* May 2008;39(5):530–534.
40. Bagheri R, Tavassoli T, Sadrizadeh A, Mashhadi MR, Shahri F, Shojaeian R. The role of thoracoscopy for the diagnosis of hidden diaphragmatic injuries in penetrating thoracoabdominal trauma. *Interact Cardiovasc Thorac Surg.* 2009;9:195–197.
41. Paci M, Ferrari G, Annessi V, de Franco S, Guasti G, Sgarbi G. The role of diagnostic VATS in penetrating thoracic injuries. *World J Emerg Surg.* October 2006;1:30.
42. Asensio JA, Demetriades D, Rodriguez A. 1996. Injury to the diaphragm. In: Feliciano DV, Moore EE, Mattox KL, eds. *Trauma,* 3rd edn. Appleton and Lange: Stamford, CT, pp. 461–485.
43. Konstantinos S, Georgios I, Christos C, Vasilissa K, Nikolaos K, Fred L, John H, Frank S. Traumatic avulsion of kidney and spleen into the chest through a ruptured diaphragm in a young worker: A case report. *J Med Case Rep.* December 2007;1:178.
44. Haciibrahimoglu G, Solak O, Olcmen A, Bedirhan MA, Solmazer N, Gurses A. Management of traumatic diaphragmatic rupture. *Surg Today.* 2004;34(2):111–114.
45. Baldassarre E, Valenti G, Gambino M, Arturi A, Torino G, Porta IP, Barone M. The role of laparoscopy in the diagnosis and the treatment of missed diaphragmatic hernia after penetrating trauma. *J Laparoendosc Adv Surg Tech A.* June 2007;17(3):302–306.
46. Matz A, Landau O, Alis M, Charuzi I, Kyzer S. The role of laparoscopy in the diagnosis and treatment of missed diaphragmatic rupture. *Surg Endosc.* June 2000;14(6):537–539.
47. Zierold D, Perlstein J, Weidman ER, Wiedeman JE. Penetrating trauma to the diaphragm: Natural history and ultrasonographic characteristics of untreated injury in a pig model. *Arch Surg.* 2001;136:32–37.
48. Rivaben AH, Junior RS, Neto VD, Botter A, Goncalves R. Natural history of extensive diaphragmatic injury of the right side: Experimental study in rats. *Rev Col Bras Cir.* 2014;41:267–271.
49. Gamblin TC, Wall CE, Morgan JH, Erickson DJ, Dalton ML, Ashley DW. The natural history of untreated penetrating diaphragm injury: An animal model. *J Trauma.* 2004;57:989–992.
50. Baldwin M, Dagens A, Sgromo B. Laparoscopic management of a delayed traumatic diaphragmatic rupture complicated by bowel strangulation. *J Surg Case Rep.* July 2014;2014(7):pii.
51. Kuy S, Juern J, Weigelt JA. Laparoscopic repair of a traumatic intrapericardial diaphragmatic hernia. *JSLS.* April–June 2014;18(2):333–337.
52. Ties JS, Peschman JR, Moreno A, Mathiason MA, Kallies KJ, Martin RF, Brasel KJ, Cogbill TH. Evolution in the management of traumatic diaphragmatic injuries: A multicenter review. *J Trauma Acute Care Surg.* April 2014;76(4):1024–1028.
53. Amini A, Latifi R. Laparoscopic-assisted minithoracotomy for repair of diaphragmatic penetrating trauma. *Surg Laparosc Endosc Percutan Tech.* 2013;23:406–409.
54. Christie DB III, Chapman J, Wynne JL, Ashley DW. Delayed right-sided diaphragmatic rupture and chronic herniation of unusual abdominal contents. *J Am Coll Surg.* January 2007;204(1):176.
55. Peker Y, Tatar F, Kahya MC, Cin N, Derici H, Reyhan E. Dislocation of three segments of the liver due to hernia of the right diaphragm: Report of a case and review of the literature. *Hernia.* February 2007;11(1):63–65.

## Commentary on Diaphragmatic Injury

*Erik Barquist*

Despite the near-ubiquitous use of CT scanning in trauma patients, almost always with sagittal and coronal reconstruction, the diagnosis and treatment of diaphragmatic herniation due to injury seems to have changed little over two and a half decades that I have been involved in the care of this injury. In some respects, we may have taken a step backward as the decreased use of diagnostic peritoneal lavage (DPL) has decreased the number of occasions in which the diagnosis of a diaphragmatic defect was made by the appearance of DPL fluid in the chest tube output! In order to care for these injuries, I divide them into four categories: those found during the initial hospitalization or at least shortly after injury versus those found more than 2 months after injury and those that require mesh to complete the repair versus those that do not require any use of prosthetic material. A fifth category that could be considered, although increasingly rare, are those hernias presenting with feculent pleuritis due to gangrenous intestine in the thoracic space.

In the past 15 years, many case reports have described a laparoscopic approach to repair of these hernias. While there is no class one data to support a minimally invasive approach to the repair of these hernias, it seems almost self-evident that the minimally invasive repair of diaphragmatic hernias, which are discovered in the late stage, would be less stressful for the patient. Since these hernias are usually associated with other intra-abdominal injuries, the repair of hernias found in the early stage is much more likely to be repaired via an open approach during laparotomy for concomitant injury. While not commonly described in the literature, a combined laparoscopic and thoracoscopic approach could also be entertained. While thoracoscopy is very useful in the diagnosis of diaphragmatic defects, the repair via this approach is challenging because of the difficulty of reducing the abdominal content. As such, laparoscopic repair is more often discussed in the published case reports.

The preferred approach to closure of these defects is well described in the chapter. Nonabsorbable suture is used to provide primary reapproximation and the suture line can be reinforced as needed with additional suture material. Some care must be taken to assure viability of the possibly compromised diaphragmatic tissue, but in most cases, this leads to a satisfactory result. In cases where mesh is used, it appears that Gortex is most commonly selected, but this is based on the reading of case reports and small series, rather than any concrete scientific evidence. Biologics have their place as well, but tend to be expensive and are similarly not supported by any evidence other than reports of single successful repairs. The rare case of feculent pleuritis caused by incarceration of intestine in the thoracic cavity creates its own unique challenges and may require a multistep approach to the operation especially since the possibility of mesh becomes less palatable in these cases. Usually, however, it is the smaller defects that cause strangulation; thus, simple suture repair is likely to be successful.

### What Is the Optimal Diagnostic Modality in the Diagnosis of Diaphragmatic Injury in Blunt Trauma?

For those patients undergoing laparotomy, or less commonly thoracotomy, I concur with the author that visualization via a complete abdominal exploration is the optimal technique. The diaphragm should be explored in all trauma laparotomies and the hand of the operating surgeon should be passed on both the right and left sides of the cavity to assure diaphragmatic integrity or lack thereof. This injury can also be diagnosed in the unusual case of a patient undergoing diagnostic laparoscopy, although patient positioning, an angled scope, and retraction of upper abdominal content make this more complex than in the open laparotomy. For those patients who do not undergo surgical exploration, the CT with reconstruction should give visualization of the lesion, or at least allow for a high level of suspicion, which can be dealt with by serial chest X-rays (CXRs). For the patient who is intubated and therefore being ventilated with positive intrathoracic pressure, there may be no movement of abdominal content until after extubation. If a high level of suspicion exists, a late CXR just prior to discharge should be considered. While the plain CXR in the trauma bay in a patient with a previously inserted nasogastric (NG) tube is well described, this is an uncommon finding. MRI scans, ultrasound, and nuclear medicine scans are infrequently used. Lastly, for those patients with a high-risk penetrating injury, who have been treated with nonoperative observation for the first 24 h, I prefer to rule out a diaphragmatic injury via thoracoscopy rather than laparoscopy, as this is technically easier, allows removal of any retained pleural blood, and avoids periumbilical incisions. On the other hand, it does require placement of a small 9 French chest tube/drain, which can be removed in the same day if no air leak is found and the CXR is acceptable.

### What Is the Optimal Diagnostic Modality in Penetrating Trauma?

Again, operative localization of the defect is preferred, although digital probing of the wound or infusion of DPL fluid is an alternative method of diagnosis. If these methods are inconclusive, thoracoscopy in the stable patient is definitive.

### What Is a Clinically Useful Classification System That Guides Operative Management?

As the author states, the AAST grading scale is useful especially for those injuries that are found early. For those found well after the traumatic event, the operative decisions depend on the ability to reduce the abdominal content via laparoscopy, the need for mesh material to bridge any gap, and the presence of feculent or infected material in the chest cavity that may preclude mesh placement or be better treated with a "damage control" multistep operation.

### What Is the Optimal Approach to Operative Management of Diaphragmatic Injuries?

In the acute phase, the repair should be performed as part of the initial laparotomy or thoracoscopy for other injuries. If this is not possible, or the injuries were managed in a nonoperative fashion, the surgeon frequently finds himself or herself making the diagnosis via thoracoscopy. While a thoracoscopic repair is feasible, a combined laparoscopic/thoracoscopic technique is more often successful due to the need to reduce the abdominal content, particularly on the left side. Hand ports or even open surgery may be needed to complete these sometimes difficult operations. Angled tacking devices are useful if mesh is needed in minimally invasive repairs.

### What Is the Ideal Suture Material/Prosthesis for Repair of Diaphragmatic Injuries?

There is no data in this subject. I agree with the author that nonabsorbable suture should be used. If mesh must be placed, I prefer biologic prosthetics, but there is no data to support this approach and many authors have reported good results with the use of Gortex prosthetic.

### What Are the Differences in the Approach to Left Versus Right Sided Injuries?

Because of the size of the liver, right-sided injuries are more amenable to thoracoscopic repair, since the liver can usually be reduced into the abdomen, allowing for primary repair with nonabsorbable suture. If there are deep lacerations to the liver, abdominal counter traction to gently reduce the liver into the abdominal cavity may be needed to prevent new bleeding from the liver injuries. In left-sided injuries, a combined thoracoscopic/laparoscopic approach is more likely to be needed.

### What Are the Consequences of Missed Injuries?

The author correctly states that the literature is replete with injuries that were missed for up to 50 years. Pleuritic pain, which is worked up with a CXR, is a common presentation of these missed injuries, but respiratory insufficiency may result from abdominal content pushing against the lung tissue. While unusual, feculent pleuritis from incarcerated organs progressing to gangrene and perforation is reported.[*†‡]

---

* Mintz Y, Easter DW, Izhar U Edden Y, Talanmani MA, Rivkind A. Minimally invasive procedure for diagnosis of traumatic right diaphragm tears: A method for correct diagnosis in selected patients. *Am Surg.* 2007;73:388–392.

† Campanelli G, Catena F, Ansaloni L. Prosthetic abdominal wall hernia repair in emergency surgery: From polypropylene to biologic meshes. *World J Emerg Surg.* 2008;3:33–34.

‡ Singh S, Kalan MM, Moreyra CE, Buckman RF Jr. Diaphragmatic rupture presenting 50 year after the traumatic event. *J Trauma.* 2000;49:156–159.

# 25

## *Pancreatic and Duodenal Injuries*

**Firas G. Madbak and Adrian W. Ong**

**CONTENTS**



### 25.1 History and Epidemiology

Injures to the pancreas and duodenum are uncommon but challenging because their retroperitoneal location may confound injury detection. Delays in diagnosis therefore are not infrequent. Moreover, these injuries are associated with significant complication rates of up to 40% [1–3].

Depending on the prevalence of penetrating trauma and the age group, the incidence of pancreatic and duodenal injuries seen in trauma centers may vary, and ranges from 0.004% to 5% of all trauma admissions [1–6]. Particularly in penetrating trauma, pancreatic and duodenal injuries are frequently associated with injuries to other organs [1,7]. Combined pancreatic and duodenal injuries seem to have a higher mortality rate than either injury alone [8].

### 25.2 Injury Classification

The organ injury scaling systems of the American Association for the Surgery of Trauma (AAST) [9] are widely used in the published literature describing these injuries. They will be used in this chapter for discussion (Tables 25.1 and 25.2).

### 25.3 Diagnosis and Management

#### 25.3.1 Questions

1. What is the accuracy of computed tomography (CT) in the diagnosis of main pancreatic duct (MPD) injury?

**TABLE 25.1**

Pancreas Injury Scale

| Grade[a] | Type of Injury | Description of Injury | ICD-9 | AIS-90 |
|---|---|---|---|---|
| I | Hematoma | Minor contusion without duct injury | 863.81–863.84 | 2 |
| | Laceration | Superficial laceration without duct injury | | 2 |
| II | Hematoma | Major contusion without duct injury or tissue loss | 863.81–863.84 | 2 |
| | Laceration | Major laceration without duct injury or tissue loss | | 3 |
| III | Laceration | Distal transection or parenchymal injury with duct injury | 863.92/863.94 | 3 |
| IV | Laceration | Proximal[b] transection or parenchymal injury involving ampulla | 863.91 | 4 |
| V | Laceration | Massive disruption of pancreatic head | 863.91 | 5 |

*Source:* Moore, EE et al., *J Trauma*, 30, 1427, 1990.

[a] Advance one grade for multiple injuries up to grade III. 863.51,863.91—head; 863.99,862.92—body; 863.83,863.93—tail.

[b] Proximal pancreas is to the patients' right of the superior mesenteric vein.

**TABLE 25.2**

Duodenum Injury Scale

| Grade[a] | Type of Injury | Description of Injury | ICD-9 | AIS-90 |
|---|---|---|---|---|
| I | Hematoma | Involving single portion of duodenum | 863.21 | 2 |
| | Laceration | Partial thickness, no perforation | 863.21 | 3 |
| II | Hematoma | Involving more than one portion | 863.21 | 2 |
| | Laceration | Disruption <50% of circumference | 863.31 | 4 |
| III | Laceration | Disruption 50%–75% of circumference of D2 | 863.31 | 4 |
| | | Disruption 50%–100% of circumference of D1, D3, D4 | 863.31 | 4 |
| IV | Laceration | Disruption >75% of circumference of D2 | 863.31 | 5 |
| | | Involving ampulla or distal common bile duct | | 5 |
| V | Laceration | Massive disruption of duodenopancreatic complex | 863.31 | 5 |
| | Vascular | Devascularization of duodenum | 863.31 | 5 |

*Source:* Moore, EE et al., *J Trauma*, 30, 1427, 1990.

[a] Advance one grade for multiple injuries up to grade III. D1, first position of duodenum; D2, second portion of duodenum; D3, third portion of duodenum; D4, fourth portion of duodenum.

2. What is the accuracy of CT in the diagnosis of duodenal perforation?
3. Does the addition of pyloric exclusion (PE) to primary repair (PR) of a duodenal perforation decrease the likelihood of duodenal leak?
4. When blunt pancreatic injury is suggested or diagnosed on CT, under what circumstances is initial nonoperative management (NOM) acceptable?
5. For patients with distal major pancreatic duct (MPD) injury undergoing operative management, is resection preferred over simple drainage?
6. In hemodynamically stable patients undergoing distal pancreatectomy (DP) for trauma, is splenic preservation associated with better outcomes than splenectomy?
7. Does octreotide reduce postoperative pancreatic-related complications after trauma?
8. Should pancreaticoduodenectomy (PDT) be done for duodenal injuries involving the ampulla or distal common bile duct or massive disruption of the pancreaticoduodenal complex (AAST Grade IV and V injuries)?

#### *25.3.1.1 What Is the Accuracy of CT in the Diagnosis of an MPD Injury?*

Advances in multidetector CT (MDCT) technology have shortened acquisition times, increased spatial resolution, and allowed for better multiplanar reconstruction of acquired images. Recent studies utilizing MDCT show varying sensitivities for detecting pancreatic injury. A recent AAST multicenter study examined the use of 16- and 64-detector row CT. The criteria used on this study were "hard signs" of injury to the gland itself, namely, active pancreatic bleeding, pancreatic hematoma or laceration, focal or diffuse enlargement or edema of the gland, or low pancreatic attenuation. The findings were correlated with laparotomy findings as the "gold standard," which meant that patients who were successfully managed nonoperatively were excluded. Although specificity was high (>90%), sensitivities for diagnosing an MPD using both 16- and 64-slice MDCTs were only 47%–60% [10]. Gordon et al. similarly examined the accuracy of MDCT for detecting duct injury: the "hard signs" of pancreatic laceration, pancreatic laceration >50%, active hemorrhage, pancreatic contusion each had a sensitivity of 50%. Specificities ranged from 73% to 100% for these criteria. In their study, however, patients who were successfully managed nonoperatively were considered to have no duct injury, which could have potentially even reduced the computed sensitivities [11]. The low sensitivity of CT in diagnosing MPD injury is also supported by a prospective study comparing CT to endoscopic retrograde cholangiopancreatography (ERCP) in 23 patients [12].

On the other hand, in another retrospective study evaluating 50 patients with blunt pancreatic injury, 33 had both preoperative CT followed by laparotomy. The authors found that CT was 91% sensitive and 91% specific for identifying pancreatic ductal injury [13]. Further, in a prospective study of 95 patients with blunt abdominal trauma, MDCT was utilized with multiphasic scanning (parenchymal phase, portal venous phase, and equilibrium phase). Of nine patients found to have pancreatic injuries confirmed on ERCP or laparotomy, six had MPD injury. The sensitivities of CT were 100% for the first two phases and only 50% for the equilibrium phase. The authors concluded that multiphasic CT showed great promise for the detection of MPD injury [14].

Comparison of these studies is limited by small sample sizes and the use of MDCTs of different slice widths. Clinicians should be cognizant of the fact that while pancreatic injuries are often associated with abnormalities on CT, the confirmation of MPD injury based on CT alone remains difficult. Management decisions after concerning CT findings could include additional modalities, such as ERCP, magnetic resonance cholangiopancreatography (MRCP), or close observation.

*Recommendation*: For MPD injury, CT signs of pancreatic gland injury have a low sensitivity, but high specificity (level 3)

*Grade of recommendation*: C

### 25.3.1.2 What Is the Accuracy of CT in the Diagnosis of Duodenal Perforation?

Signs of duodenal perforation include free air and oral contrast extravasation. More subtle findings, such as bowel wall thickening, surrounding retroperitoneal fluid, fat stranding should also raise suspicion of duodenal injury. A crucial distinction between perforation and contusion or wall hematoma should be made since, in the absence of perforation, these duodenal injuries may be managed nonoperatively.

Limited studies exist evaluating the accuracy of CT in diagnosing duodenal perforation. A retrospective study involving pediatric patients [15] examined the results of CT which was performed on 19 patients (9 with perforation, 10 with hematoma). All patients with duodenal perforation had either retroperitoneal air (8/9) and/or retroperitoneal contrast (4/9). In 10 patients with duodenal hematoma, none had retroperitoneal contrast or air. Retroperitoneal fluid did not reliably distinguish the two conditions. The authors concluded that CT will show some sort of abnormality in all of the patients with duodenal perforation, but that only retroperitoneal air or contrast could reliably distinguish perforation from duodenal hematoma. Ballard et al. [6] studied 30 cases of blunt duodenal rupture; 18 underwent CT, with 15 done within 4 h of admission. CT was normal in 4 (27%). Retroperitoneal air was seen in only 2 (13%), contrast extravasation in 2 (13%) and free air seen in 5. Patients had other findings suggestive of intra-abdominal injury, but not specifically duodenal perforation. The authors concluded that CT for the diagnosis of blunt duodenal perforation was inaccurate, as the classic findings were often absent when the CT was performed within 4 h after admission. It was unclear how many patients received oral contrast.

*Recommendation*: There are insufficient data evaluating the accuracy of CT in diagnosing traumatic duodenal perforation (level 3).

### 25.3.1.3 Does the Addition of PE to PR of a Duodenal Perforation Decrease the Likelihood of Duodenal Leak?

There are no randomized trials addressing this question. Jansen et al. [16] studied retrospectively their experience of management of duodenal injuries, where 18 patients underwent PR and 11 patients underwent PE. No analysis of injury severity between the two groups was available for comparison. No duodenal leaks were seen. The authors concluded that PE should be used liberally to minimize duodenal-related morbidity.

Velmahos et al. [17] analyzed 50 patients with high-grade (>III) duodenal injuries. PR was performed in 34 (68%) and PE in 16 (32%) of patients. The two groups were similar for age, injury severity, abdominal Abbreviated Injury Score (AIS), and time to operation. However, the PE group had more pancreatic injuries (63% vs. 24%, $p = 0.01$) and more Grade IV or V injuries (although not statistically significant). The duodenal leak rate was not significantly different (PR, 18% vs. PE, 24%) and there was no difference in mortality, intensive care unit or hospital lengths of stay.

Seamon et al. [18] also retrospectively analyzed the outcome of PE ($n = 15$) versus PR ($n = 14$) after penetrating injuries to the duodenum and combined pancreaticoduodenal injuries, with >Grade II duodenal injuries. Both groups were well matched for age, sex, presence of shock, vascular injuries, and injury severity score. However, the PE group had a higher incidence of Grades III and IV duodenal injuries (but not statistically significant) and combined injuries (71% vs. 20%). Outcomes were similar between both groups, with a 0% duodenal fistula rate, similar length of stay and mortality. The fact that there were more patients with combined injuries and higher grade duodenal injuries in the PE group makes it difficult to accurately compare outcomes.

Using the American College of Surgeons National Trauma Data Bank (NTDB v 5.0), Dubose et al. [19] evaluated 147 adult patients with severe duodenal injuries [Grade ≥III] undergoing PR only or repair with a PE within 24 h of admission. The majority (81%) of the patients did not undergo PE. The proportions in each group with associated pancreatic injury, hepatic injury, admission hypotension, Grade IV or V duodenal injuries, ISS >20 were statistically similar. PE was found to be associated with a longer mean hospital stay. After multivariable analysis using propensity scoring, no statistically significant differences in mortality or occurrence of septic abdominal complications was noted between those patients undergoing PR only or PE. The authors concluded that the use of PE in patients with severe duodenal injuries may contribute to longer hospital stay and confers no survival or outcome benefit.

There is a lack of adequately powered studies examining the role of PE controlled for duodenal injury severity. Whereas the use of PE may have a role in a subset of patients with duodenal injuries, the specific circumstances where this is applicable has not been clearly elucidated.

*Recommendation*: PE does not decrease the likelihood of duodenal leak after PR of a duodenal perforation (level 3).

*Grade of recommendation*: B

#### 25.3.1.4 When Blunt Pancreatic Injury Is Suggested or Diagnosed on CT, under What Circumstances Is Initial NOM Acceptable?

Recognizing that most of the morbidity in blunt pancreatic trauma is related to MPD injury, NOM has been advocated for low-grade blunt injuries. Velmahos et al. [8] retrospectively analyzed 230 patients with blunt pancreatic and/or duodenal injuries in a multicenter study, and found that 97 (42%) had initial NOM. Of the 158 patients with Grades I and II blunt pancreatic and/or duodenal injuries, 93 (58%) underwent NOM with 8 (8.6%) failures. Of the higher grade injuries ($n$ = 72), only four underwent NOM, with two (50%) failures. The NOM strategy had a complication rate of 10/97 (10.3%), of which three required delayed operative intervention (one for a missed duodenal perforation and two for obstructing duodena hematoma). The mortality rate for NOM patients was 7/97 (6.7%), all of whom died due to unrelated severe brain injuries. The authors concluded that NOM of selected lower grade pancreatic and duodenal injuries diagnosed by CT was safe. However, a limitation of this study was that there were no data on ERCP.

Wood et al. [20] studied 43 pediatric patients with an average age of 7.1 years sustaining blunt pancreatic injury. For Grades II–IV injuries, patients managed operatively ($n$ = 14) and nonoperatively ($n$ = 11) had similar lengths of stay and rates of readmission, despite increased pancreatic complications in the nonoperative cohort (21% vs. 73%). For patients who underwent resection, there was a trend toward complications that were not pancreas related. Twelve patients underwent successful diagnostic ERCP in which duct injury was identified. In this group, NOM was pursued in six patients but was associated with increased rates of pancreatic complications (86% nonoperative vs. 29% operative). The authors concluded that operative management of children with Grades II–IV pancreatic injury resulted in significantly decreased rates of pancreatic complications, but failed to decrease length of stay in the hospital, possibly as a result of other complications. They also suggested that ERCP be used to guide management.

Duchesne et al. [21] examined 63 patients with Grades I and II blunt pancreatic injuries of which 35 were selected for NOM. Five (14%) failed NOM due to pancreas-related complication ($n$ = 3) and missed bowel injuries ($n$ = 2), with no mortality among the five patients. They concluded that NOM of low-grade blunt pancreatic injuries was feasible with low morbidity and/or mortality.

In a multicenter study [22], 167 patients from 14 pediatric trauma centers with Grades II or III pancreatic injuries were studied. Of the 167, 57 underwent DP and 95 (57%) were managed nonoperatively. For Grade III injuries ($n$ = 80), patients undergoing NOM ($n$ = 26) were found to have a higher rate of pseudocyst formation (44% vs. 0%), higher rate of repeat interventions (46% vs. 2%), longer times to initial feeds and goal feeds, and a longer length of stay, than those managed with operation. When Grade II injuries managed nonoperatively were compared to all patients undergoing resection, the rate of pseudocyst formation was only 7%. The authors concluded that for patients with MPD injury, operative intervention in the form of resection had better outcomes than NOM.

Another multicenter study involving pediatric patients by Mattix et al. [5] found that of 173 patients with pancreatic injuries, 53 had Grade III and earlier injuries. There was a 43% rate of failure of NOM among those with ductal injuries. The corresponding failure rate for injuries of lesser severity was 22%. For ductal injuries managed nonoperatively, the length of stay, rate of pseudocyst formation and pancreatitis were similar when compared to patient managed operatively.

*Recommendation*: It is acceptable to manage selected patients without MPD disruption nonoperatively (level 3, grade B).

Patients with ductal injuries or who have more severe injuries (Grade III and higher) should be managed operatively (level 3, grade B).

#### 25.3.1.5 For Patients with MPD Injury Undergoing Operative Management, Is Resection Preferred over Simple Drainage?

Studies comparing resection with drainage for distal pancreatic trauma that are well matched for degree of shock, pancreatic injury severity, and associated injuries are lacking. An alternative to DP—pancreaticojejunostomy is also described in several series. The small numbers undergoing each treatment modality and the retrospective nature in each study makes it difficult to compare outcomes among studies.

Lin et al. [23] analyzed the outcomes of 48 cases of blunt major pancreatic injury treated during a 10-year period: Of the 32 Grade III and 14 Grade IV patients, the majority ($n$ = 22) underwent DP with splenic preservation while only five had simple drainage. These five died due to hemodynamic instability. While the authors suggested DP with spleen preservation for Grade III and Grade IV injuries, there was no rigorous comparison with simple drainage.

Wind et al. [24] examined their experience with distal pancreatic trauma, and found that of 19 patients with MPD injury that did not undergo resection, 14 had external drainage and ultimately, 10 of the 14 underwent DP for persistent pancreatic fistula ($n$ = 7), pseudocyst ($n$ = 2), and persistent pain ($n$ = 1). The other five patients who underwent laparotomy or no surgery instead of external drainage all developed pseudocysts that eventually required surgery. Of the six with MPD injury who underwent DP initially, three developed subphrenic abscesses requiring drainage. The authors concluded that much of the morbidity was related to inadequate treatment for distal MPD injuries and therefore recommended DP in this situation.

*Recommendation*: For distal pancreatic trauma with MPD injury, resection is preferred over simple drainage (level 3, grade C).

#### 25.3.1.6 In Hemodynamically Stable Patients Undergoing DP for Trauma, Is Splenic Preservation Associated with Better Outcomes Than Splenectomy?

Several studies [25–28] have compared outcomes of DP with or without splenic preservation in patients with benign or low-grade malignant pancreatic diseases. DP with splenic preservation had been found to be safe with equivalent or better outcomes in terms of infectious complications. However, rates of pancreatic fistula after DP with splenic preservation have been either equivalent [26–28] or higher compared to DP with splenectomy [25]. Controlled studies comparing DP with splenic preservation and DP with splenectomy in the trauma setting have been limited to case reports involving the pediatric age group. However, the retrospective study by Lin et al. [23] of major blunt pancreatic injury (Grades III–V) found a complication rate of 72% in 22 patients treated with DP and splenectomy versus 22% in 9 patients with DP and splenic preservation [23].

*Recommendation*: There is insufficient evidence to determine if DP with splenic preservation is associated with better outcomes compared to DP with splenectomy (level 3).

#### 25.3.1.7 Does Octreotide Reduce Postoperative Pancreatic-Related Complications after Trauma?

Nwariaku et al. [29] retrospectively analyzed patients who were treated with octreotide postoperatively ($n$ = 21) versus no octreotide ($n$ = 96). Matched for age, mechanism, and ISS, the octreotide group had higher injury grades and longer hospital stay. Fistula rates were statistically similar when stratified by grade of pancreatic injury (Grades I, II: octreotide vs. no octreotide, 46% vs. 35%; Grades III–V: 50% vs. 56%). The authors concluded that the incidence of pancreatic complications was not reduced with octreotide administration. On the other hand, Amirata et al. [30] retrospectively studied 28 patients, seven of whom were given octreotide postoperatively. The majority of the cases in both groups were Grade II injuries (6/7 vs. 18/21). There were 0/7 pancreatic complications in the octreotide group versus 6/21 (29%) in the no octreotide group. The cases were "well matched" for age, mechanism of injury, and ISS. The authors concluded that octreotide use was associated with fewer postoperative pancreatic-related complications.

In a systematic review, the use of octreotide after pancreatic surgery was associated with a lower risk of all pancreatic fistulae, but a similar risk of "clinically significant" pancreatic fistula [31]. However, the randomized studies in the review were done mainly in patients undergoing elective PDT, which is rarely done for trauma. It is unclear whether the conclusions can be extrapolated to the trauma setting.

*Recommendation*: There is insufficient evidence for or against the prophylactic use of octreotide to reduce postoperative pancreatic-related complications (level 3).

#### 25.3.1.8 Should PDT Be Done for Duodenal Injuries Involving the Ampulla or Distal Common Bile Duct or Massive Disruption of the Pancreaticoduodenal Complex (AAST Grades IV and V Injuries)?

There is a paucity of literature and no guidelines for optimal surgical therapy. Van der Wilden et al. [32] examined the National Trauma Data Bank and compared outcomes of PDT patients ($n$ = 39) to similarly injured patients who did not undergo PDT ($n$ = 38), but with

**TABLE 25.3**
Evidentiary Table

| Question | Answer | Level of Evidence | Grade of Recommendation | References |
|---|---|---|---|---|
| What is the accuracy of computed tomography (CT) in the diagnosis of a main pancreatic duct injury? | For MPD injury, CT signs of pancreatic gland injury have a low sensitivity, but high specificity | 3 | C | [10–14] |
| What is the accuracy of CT in the diagnosis of duodenal perforation? | There is insufficient data evaluating the accuracy of CT in diagnosing traumatic duodenal perforation | 3 | — | [6,15] |
| Does the addition of pyloric exclusion to primary repair of a duodenal perforation decrease the likelihood of duodenal leak? | Pyloric exclusion does not decrease the likelihood of duodenal leak after primary repair of a duodenal perforation (level 3) | 3 | B | [16–19] |
| When blunt pancreatic injury is suggested or diagnosed on CT, under what circumstances is initial nonoperative management acceptable? | It is acceptable to manage selected patients without main pancreatic duct disruption nonoperatively | 3 | B | [5,8,20–22] |
| | Patients with ductal injuries or who have more severe injuries (Grade III and earlier) should be managed operatively | 3 | B | |
| For patients with distal major pancreatic duct injury undergoing operative management, is resection preferred over simple drainage? | For distal pancreatic trauma with MPD injury, resection is preferred over simple drainage | 3 | C | [23,24] |
| In hemodynamically stable patients undergoing distal pancreatectomy for trauma, is splenic preservation associated with better outcomes than splenectomy? | There is insufficient evidence to determine if distal pancreatectomy with splenic preservation is associated with better outcomes compared to distal pancreatectomy with splenectomy | 3 | — | [23] |
| Does octreotide reduce postoperative pancreatic-related complications after trauma? | There is insufficient evidence for or against the prophylactic use of octreotide to reduce postoperative pancreatic-related complications | 3 | — | [29,30] |
| Should pancreaticoduodenectomy be done for duodenal injuries involving the ampulla or distal common bile duct or massive disruption of the pancreaticoduodenal complex (AAST Grades IV and V injuries)? | There is insufficient evidence for or against pancreaticoduodenectomy for Grades IV and V injuries | 3 | — | [32–34] |

severe combined pancreaticoduodenal injuries (at least grade IV in both organs). The PDT sample included any patient who underwent PDT within 4 days of admission. The non-PDT group had a significantly lower systolic blood pressure and Glasgow Coma Scale values at baseline and more severe duodenal, pancreatic, and liver injuries. There were no significant differences in outcomes between the two groups in terms of length of stay, complications, and mortality. The Injury Severity Score was the only independent predictor of mortality. The authors concluded that PDT did not result in improved outcomes despite a lower physiologic burden among PDT patients.

Uncontrolled case series have demonstrated good survival rates after PDT, particularly if PDT was done as a staged procedure in conjunction with an initial damage control procedure [33,34]. Controlled studies are needed to assess the indications and timing of this procedure especially for patients with associated massive hemorrhage (Table 25.3).

*Recommendation*: There is insufficient evidence for or against PDT for AAST Grade IV or V injuries.

## References

1. Blocksom JM, Tyburski JG, Sohn RL et al. Prognostic determinants in duodenal injuries. *Am Surg.* 2004;70:248–255.
2. Kao LS, Bulger EM, Parks DL et al. Patterns of morbidity after traumatic pancreatic injury. *J Trauma.* 2003;55:898–905.
3. Akhrass R, Yaffe MB. Pancreatic trauma: A ten-year multi-institutional experience. *Am Surg.* 1997;63:598–605.

4. Duchesne JC, Schmieg R, Islam S et al. Selective nonoperative management of low-grade blunt pancreatic injury: Are we there yet? *J Trauma*. 2008;65:49–53.
5. Mattix KD, Tataria M, Holmes J et al. Pediatric pancreatic trauma: Predictors of nonoperative management failure and associated outcomes. *J Pediatr Surg*. 2007;42:340–344.
6. Ballard RB, Badellino MM, Eynon CA et al. Blunt duodenal rupture: A 6-year statewide experience. *J Trauma*. 1997;43:229–233.
7. Madiba TE, Mokoena TR. Favourable prognosis after surgical drainage of gunshot, stab or blunt trauma of the pancreas. *Br J Surg*. 1995;82:1236–1239.
8. Velmahos GC, Tabbara M, Gross R et al. Blunt pancreatoduodenal injury: A multicenter study of the research consortium of New England centers for trauma (ReCONECT). *Arch Surg*. 2009;144:413–419.
9. Moore EE, Cogbill TH, Malangoni MA et al. Organ injury scaling, II: Pancreas, duodenum, small bowel, colon, and rectum *J Trauma*. 1990;30:1427–1429.
10. Phelan HA, Velmahos GC, Jurkovich GJ. An evaluation of multidetector computed tomography in detecting pancreatic injury: Results of a multicenter AAST study. *J Trauma*. 2009;66:641–646.
11. Gordon RW, Anderson SW, Ozonoff A et al. Blunt pancreatic trauma: Evaluation with MDCT technology. *Emerg Radiol*. 2013;20:259–266.
12. Kim HS, Lee DK, Kim IW et al. The role of endoscopic retrograde pancreatography in the treatment of traumatic pancreatic duct injury. *Gastrointest Endosc*. 2001;54:49–55.
13. Teh S, Sheppard BC, Mullins RJ et al. Diagnosis and management of blunt pancreatic ductal injury in the era of high-resolution computed axial tomography. *Am J Surg*. 2007;193:641–643.
14. Wong YC, Wang LJ, Fang JF et al. Multidetector-row computed tomography (CT) of blunt pancreatic injuries: Can contrast-enhanced multiphasic CT detect pancreatic duct injuries? *J Trauma*. 2008;64:666–672.
15. Shilyansky J, Pearl RH, Kreller M et al. Diagnosis and management of duodenal injuries in children. *J Pediatr Surg*. 1997;32:880–886.
16. Jansen M, DuToit DF, Warren BL. Duodenal injuries: Surgical management adapted to circumstances. *Injury*. 2002;33:611–615.
17. Velmahos GC, Constantinou C, Kasotakis G. Safety of repair for severe duodenal injuries. *World J Surg*. 2008;32:7–12.
18. Seamon MJ, Pieri PG, Fisher CA et al. A ten-year retrospective review: Does pyloric exclusion improve clinical outcome after penetrating duodenal and combined pancreaticoduodenal injuries? *J Trauma*. 2007;62:829–833.
19. DuBose JJ, Inaba K, Teixeira PG et al. Pyloric exclusion in the treatment of severe duodenal injuries: Results from the National Trauma Data Bank. *Am Surg*. 2008;74: 925–929.
20. Wood JH, Partrick DA, Bruny JL et al. Operative vs nonoperative management of blunt pancreatic trauma in children. *J Pediatr Surg*. 2010;45:401–406.
21. Duchesne JC, Schmieg R, Islam S et al. Selective nonoperative management of low-grade blunt pancreatic injury: Are we there yet? *J Trauma*. 2008;65:49–53.
22. Iqbal CW, St Peter SD, Tsao K et al. Operative vs nonoperative Management for blunt pancreatic transection in children: Multi-institutional outcomes. *J Am Coll Surg*. 2014;218:157–162.
23. Lin BC, Chen RJ, Fang JF et al. Management of blunt major pancreatic injury. *J Trauma*. 2004;56:774–778.
24. Wind P, Tiret E, Cunningham C et al. Contribution of endoscopic retrograde pancreatography in management of complications following distal pancreatic trauma. *Am Surg*. 1999;65:777–783.
25. Tsiouris A, Cogan CM, Velanovich V. Distal pancreatectomy with or without splenectomy: Comparison of postoperative outcomes and surrogates of splenic function. *HPB*. 2011;13:738–744.
26. Lee SE, Jang JY, Lee KU, Kim SW. Clinical comparison of distal pancreatectomy with or without splenectomy. *J Korean Med Sci*. 2008;23:1011–1014.
27. Shoup M, Brennan MF, McWhite K et al. The value of splenic preservation with distal pancreatetomy. *Arch Surg*. 2002;137:164–168.
28. Goh BKP, Tan YM, Chung YA et al. Critical appraisal of 232 consecutive distal pancreatectomies with emphasis on risk factors, outcome, and management of the postoperative pancreatic fistula. *Arch Surg*. 2008;143:956–965.
29. Nwariaku FE, Terracina A, Mileski WJ et al. Is octreotide beneficial following pancreatic injury? *Am J Surg*. 1995;170:582–585.
30. Amirata E, Livingston DH, Elcavage J. Octreotide acetate decreases pancreatic complications after pancreatic trauma. *Am J Surg*. 1994;168:345–347.
31. Gurusamy KS, Koti R, Fusai G, Davidson BR. Somatostatin analogues in for pancreatic surgery. *Cochrane Database Syst Rev*. Apr 2013;4:CD008370.
32. van der Wilden GM, Yeh D, Hwabejire JO et al. Trauma Whipple: Do or don't after severe pancreaticoduodenal injuries? An analysis of the National Trauma Data Bank (NTDB). *World J Surg*. 2014;38:335–340.
33. Asensio JA, Petrone P, Roldan G et al. Pancreaticoduodenectomy: A rare procedure for the management of complex pancreaticoduodenal injuries. *J Am Coll Surg*. 2003; 197:937–942.
34. Thompson CM, Shalhub S, DeBoard ZM, Maier RV. Revisiting the pancreaticoduodenectomy for trauma: A single institution's experience. *J Trauma Acute Care Surg*. 2013;75:225–228.

## Commentary on Pancreatic and Duodenal Injuries

*Chad G. Ball*

Despite their relative rarity, injuries to the pancreas and duodenum are always challenging, and often deadly. More specifically, they can be difficult to expose, temporize, and/or repair for any surgeon who does not make their living in this region of the upper abdomen. In the context of trauma, the pancreas and duodenum are also components of the anatomical region commonly referred to as the "surgical soul." Whether you are a trauma, acute care, or hepato-pancreato-biliary (HPB) surgeon, these injuries will engage all of your senses, test your technical skills, require the utmost focus, and demand great teamwork from you and your colleagues.

One of the most dominant issues that surrounds the current literature, and therefore our understanding of optimal therapies for both pancreas and duodenal injuries, is the glaring lack of high-level evidence. Conclusions with regard to treating these injuries generally remain based on small to medium case series, nonrandomized treatment arms, and significant bias due to their ubiquitous retrospective nature. More specifically, the mean number of subjects within pancreas and duodenal peer-reviewed publications is 18 and 22, respectively. As a result, our current understanding of the best care for patients with pancreas and duodenal injuries remains based on expert opinion that is typically built by low volume experiences. Unfortunately, one of the most continually underutilized sources of additional wisdom remains peer-reviewed publications within the elective HPB arena. Many of these lessons are applicable to both critically ill, as well as stable severely injured patients.

### What Is the Accuracy of Computed Tomography (CT) in the Diagnosis of Main Pancreatic Duct (MPD) Injury?

The authors have eloquently and thoroughly discussed the current evidence for the utility of CT as the primary diagnostic tool in diagnosing MPD injuries. More specifically, based on the available literature, CT is highly specific, but variably sensitive. The dominant issue when discussing a technology-based question remains the evolution of the technology itself. As described, the majority of the literature utilizes relatively low fidelity CT scanners with 64 or less detector rows. Numerous institutions now have 256, or even 512-slice scanners with the ability to offer 3-dimensional reconstructions that are staggering in fidelity and visualization. We must keep in mind that a busy elective pancreatic surgeon uses nothing more than a high-quality pancreas-protocol CT for virtually all preoperative decision making and planning. The exception remains patients with chronic pancreatitis, where main ductal anatomy can be so distorted that an MRCP is needed. The second issue falls upon the specific experience level of the person(s) interpreting the CT images themselves. A tremendous variability is noted between body imaging radiologists who read CT scans of the pancreas on a daily basis versus most other radiologists. The same can be said about members of the surgical team evaluating CT imaging in real time. As a result, both the quality of the technology itself and the experience of the interpreter make comparisons and conclusions very difficult across studies, and therefore the literature of limited value in their application to a specific facility. The other topic proposed by the authors surrounds the utility of ancillary tests such as MRI/MRCP. The clear take-home message remains that defining the integrity of the MPD is essential. Nearly all subsequent management decisions in these patients should revolve around confirming MPD status (i.e., leaks from side branch/ducts almost always seal with time and good nutrition). If a patient's MPD is unclear on CT (inadequate CT technology or interpreter inexperience), then an MRCP should be the next investigative step. On the extremely rare occasion that MR does not confirm a diagnosis, ERCP may be of value despite a significant risk of associated complications. It should also be stated that despite a litany of described impractical options for the intraoperative delineation of MPD integrity, ultrasound evaluation by a trained surgeon remains easy and reliable.

### What Is the Accuracy of CT in the Diagnosis of Duodenal Perforation?

This segment nicely highlights the lack of obvious conclusions from the literature with regard to the utility of CT for diagnosing duodenal injuries. Unfortunately, the 2 dominant issues surrounding technology discussed earlier remain relevant for the duodenum as well (scanner technology and interpreter experience). Similarly, we can also learn from our elective colleagues in the context of duodenal perforations secondary to ERCP. More specifically, type II perforations (retroperitoneal duodenal) are most akin to injuries of questionable diagnosis within the trauma arena. It is clear that the presence and volume of retroperitoneal air does not predict the need for operative exploration. Retroperitoneal fluid and/or free intraperitoneal air (type I) do reliably mandate intervention however.

### Does the Addition of Pyloric Exclusion (PE) to Primary Repair (PR) of a Duodenal Perforation Decrease the Likelihood of Duodenal Leak?

Although the retrospective Dubose project outlining the use of pyloric exclusion among 147 patients within the NTDB remains our best study, the use of pyloric exclusion has been anecdotally decreasing for years. This is based on a number of realities including young surgeons' lack of familiarity with this technique, an unclear benefit across the literature, and the avoidance of this occlusion among our elective duodenal surgeons during duodenoplasty- and/or ampulloplasty-based cases. In the scenario where a surgeon feels absolutely compelled to utilize an exclusion technique however, another option remains the "Cali variant." This modification is distinguished by placing a small transnasal feeding tube through the pylorus itself and then completing the exclusion around it. The other advancement to remember surrounds the evolution of safety and efficacy using serial endoscopic dilation. More specifically, narrowing the antipancreatic duodenum via primary closure can typically be addressed later using endoscopic methods. It should also be noted that the utility of a roux-en-y duodeno-jejunostomy (i.e., large hole in the duodenum) is a rapid and superb technique. Additional descriptions of serosal patches and triple tube decompressions should be viewed as relics.

### When Blunt Pancreatic Injury Is Suggested or Diagnosed on CT, under What Circumstances Is Initial Nonoperative Management (NOM) Acceptable?

The authors have provided us with a masterful description of the current literature surrounding NOM of blunt pancreatic injuries. It remains reliant on common sense, frequent patient re-evaluations, and high fidelity imaging. It must be reiterated, however, that injuries to the MPD (grade III and above) mandate reasonably early intervention. More to the point, planned acceptance of the occurrence of either a pseudocyst or walled-off pancreatic necrosis (WOPN) should be viewed with skepticism and as a failure in management. Although the literature reports a number of grade III injuries that were managed nonoperatively and associated with increase in interventions, time to feeding, and length of stay, it does not adequately describe the prolonged physical and mental suffering that these patients incur. The frequency with which an elective pancreas surgeon eventually cares for these patients is not insignificant. These "missed" injuries often mandate operative techniques such as cystgastrostomy, roux-en-y fistula-jejunostomy, or distal pancreatectomy and splenectomy for a disconnected left pancreatic remnant (DLPR). As a result, the optimal management of MPD injuries in the early setting remains crucial.

### For Patients with Distal Major Pancreatic Duct (MPD) Injury Undergoing Operative Management, Is Resection Preferred over Simple Drainage?

Further to the discussion, acceptance of drainage to convert a pancreatic leak into a controlled pancreatic fistula remains fraught with challenges for both the patient and surgeon. While temporary transampullary ERCP-placed stents are helpful in sealing off persistent side branch pancreatic fistulae, they are very rarely adequate for MPD leaks. Techniques such as cystgastrostomy, roux-en-y fistula-jejunostomy, or distal pancreatectomy and splenectomy for a DLPR remain the dominant options. Selection among these procedures in experienced hands is based upon anatomy of the gland, body habitus, interm generation of sinistral (left-sided) portal hypertension, endocrine and exocrine preoperative function, and patient age. It is also interesting to note the repeated discussion of pancreaticojejunostomy (i.e., akin to a central pancreatectomy). Given that most pancreatic gland injuries occur in young patients with soft glands and small MPDs, the technical requirement to adequately perform this anastamosis is substantial. More specifically, and as the authors insinuate, it should not be attempted by the occasional pancreatic surgeon.

### In Hemodynamically Stable Patients Undergoing Distal Pancreatectomy (DP) for Trauma, Is Splenic Preservation Associated with Better Outcomes Than Splenectomy?

Splenic preservation remains a commonly discussed and postulated technique. As summarized, the poor available evidence does not support one technique over another. Given the efficacy of vaccinations and rarity of overwhelming postsplenectomy infection (OPSI), most clinicians should not think twice about preserving the spleen in the context of a distal pancreatectomy if it is technically challenging or time consuming. More relevant technical discussions might include the benefits (less blood loss, fewer transfusions, faster operative times) associated with a medial to lateral approach, or the role of a Warshaw splenic preserving distal pancreatectomy (proximal division of the splenic artery and vein with maintenance of the left gastroepiploic and gastric vessels).

### Does Octreotide Reduce Postoperative Pancreatic-Related Complications after Trauma?

As described by this segment, the role of octreotide remains unclear, but is generally believed to be unhelpful in lowering clinically relevant (grade B—ISGPF) fistulas. A recent study in the *NEJM*, however, has indicated that perhaps, a longer-acting somatostatin analogue may significantly lower the fistula rate following pancreatic resections*. Use of this drug has not been described in injured patients to date.

* Allen PJ, Gonen M, Brennan MF et al. Pasireotide for postoperative pancreatic fistula. *N Engl J Med*. 2014;370(21):2014–2022.

### Should Pancreaticoduodenectomy (PDT) Be Done for Duodenal Injuries Involving the Ampulla or Distal Common Bile Duct or Massive Disruption of the Pancreaticoduodenal Complex (AAST Grade IV and V Injuries)?

Similar to comments on patients with missed grade III pancreatic injuries, those with chronic biliary and/or ampullary strictures can suffer significant disability. Although ERCP-based biliary balloon dilation and percutaneous transhepatic catheter-based dilation have improved dramatically, recurrent cholangitis and/or pancreatitis due to mechanical outflow obstructions is not infrequently encountered by an HPB surgeon. Similarly, massive disruptions to the pancreaticoduodenal complex can be treated in many ways, but are often best suited to a single intervention (i.e., Whipple operation) that eliminates chronic strictures, pain, and/or subsequent interventions. As indicated, in the critically ill patient, a pancreaticoduodenectomy is often a 2-stage procedure. It must be remembered, however, that an early return (<24 h) to the operating suite is optimal, because prolonged resuscitation and/or intervals lead to edematous intestines and leaky anastamoses.

# 26

## *Abdominal Vascular Trauma*

**Joseph E. Glaser and Alexandra A. MacLean**

**CONTENTS**



### 26.1 Introduction

The management of vascular trauma, and in particular injury to abdominal vessels, has changed dramatically in the United States over the last 15 years. Advances in interventional and endovascular techniques have brought a minimally invasive approach to some aspects of trauma management. In addition, advances in imaging studies techniques have increased the complexity of the decision tree that addresses questions of how to image, diagnose, treat, and follow such patients.

This chapter raises more questions than answers and highlights the need to continue to conduct quality studies so we can practice with confidence from evidence. It is challenging to answer each question without relying on dogma that is easily found in other textbooks and from surgical colleagues. With this in mind, we will pose questions and provide the best evidence currently available to answer them. And finally, at the end of the chapter, we will also delineate other questions without any evidenced answers to provide themes for further research.

### 26.2 Initial Evaluation and Diagnosis

The clinical indications for operative intervention on abdominal vessels are not always clear. The patient may be hemodynamically stable without obvious blood loss, but there may be a high index of suspicion of injury due to a minor decrease in femoral pulse examination or questionable findings on the initial trauma computed tomography (CT) exam that require further imaging. The armamentarium for examining abdominal vessels now includes duplex examination, computed tomography angiography (CTA), and magnetic resonance angiography (MRA). But which modality is most sensitive and specific for this vasculature?

### 26.2.1 When Comparing Duplex Ultrasonography, CTA, and MRA, What Is the Optimal Modality for Evaluation of Abdominal Vascular Trauma?

#### 26.2.1.1 Imaging Techniques: Background

Duplex ultrasound consists of several methods of vascular interrogation, including grayscale ("B mode"), spectral Doppler, and color Doppler ("angio-" or "power" Doppler may also be employed). It is classically a noninvasive, inexpensive way to assess the integrity and condition of vessels. The value of this technique in imaging peripheral vessels is well understood and established for many indications, including diagnosis and follow-up of chronic conditions (aortoiliac and peripheral arterial disease, post bypass graft surveillance, dialysis access assessment, cerebrovascular disease to name a few) as well as rapid and accurate diagnosis of more acute conditions (iatrogenic arteriovenous fistulas and pseudoaneurysms, acute arterial, and venous thromboembolism). Its advantages have typically included portability and low cost as well as lack of radiation or iodinated contrast exposure. Its portability confers an added advantage for intraoperative use or employment in the trauma bay or ICU for patients needing a rapid, focused vascular imaging study, but are too unstable for CT or MR imaging. Disadvantages have included a somewhat limited availability (many places may not employ an in-house ultrasound tech during off-hours) as well as greater interoperator variability.

CTA is the evaluation of the vascular tree using CT and iodinated contrast. It typically employs multidetector CT (MDCT) scanners. Contrast is rapidly injected using a power injector for rapid transit through and opacification of the arterial tree. Protocols can be timed and concentrations adjusted to evaluate different vessels and regions, with exams existing for a myriad of vascular beds. The most ubiquitously employed is probably familiar to most practitioners as CT pulmonary angiography for evaluation of pulmonary embolism. Its advantages include rapidity, both in acquisition, quick acquisition of a potentially large field of view (i.e., a lower extremity runoff exam), and lack of an arterial puncture. In some cases, delayed or multiphase imaging may be employed for additional perfusion, enhancement, or washout information. The classic example of this is a three-phase liver CT. Additionally, a good quality study will often provide much of the information provided by classical catheter angiography with additionally providing information about other tissues. For example, in the trauma setting it may be possible not only to see the arterial injury and extravasation but also the foreign object or fractured bone that caused it as well (if such exists). Disadvantages include lack of portability, exposure to ionizing radiation, and requirement for iodinated contrast. It may also require a higher dose of contrast than catheter angiography due to its need to traverse the venous system and the heart in order to reach the arterial tree, a requirement not entailed in invasive angiography.

MRA can also be an evaluation tool but, as will be discussed later, has markedly limited use in this setting. Other modalities have also been employed for evaluation of vascular injury. They are mentioned for the sake of completeness, but are not explored further in this discussion. This is for several reasons, including that they are typically employed in very specific situations (i.e., transcatheter embolization of bleeding vessels), or have been supplanted by other modalities in this arena (i.e., radionuclide scintiangiography).

#### 26.2.1.2 Imaging Techniques in Abdominal Vascular Trauma

Despite the widespread use of CTA, there are few studies examining the utility of this diagnostic tool for abdominal vascular trauma. A study by Maturen examined contrast-enhanced CT (CECT) and compared this with angiographic findings for the detection of torso hemorrhage in a retrospective study of 48 patients [1]. Of note, CECT was not specialized CTA. CECT findings were statistically associated with angiographic findings (active hemorrhage and need for intervention; $p < 0.0001$). The sensitivity of CECT was 94.1% and the negative predictive value (NPV) was 97.6% for active hemorrhage detection. The sensitivity and NPV for need for intervention were 92.6% and 91.2%, respectively.

There is also a study that examined 50 consecutive patients, where both CTA and MDCT were utilized to image all major arteries, veins, and parenchymatous organs [2]. Apart from the infrarenal venous cava, both modalities achieved high imaging quality.

It is fair to say that CTA is generally preferred for evaluation of abdominal vascular trauma. It should be noted that there is a relative abundance of literature regarding the use of CECT in the evaluation of trauma patients. Papers describing CTA, by contrast, are relatively few. Literature searches for this question included searching for papers specifically dealing with CTA, as well as reviewing papers describing standard CECT to see if they included CTA patients or in fact to see if the papers were referring to a CTA protocol as inferred by the description but were describing the use of CTA.

A 2012 systematic review published in the *British Journal of Surgery* evaluated radiologic diagnosis of vascular trauma over a 10-year period and included 58 articles. CTA showed "acceptable" sensitivity and specificity for blunt and penetrating vascular injuries in the neck and extremity and blunt aortic injury [3]. They suggest CTA as the first line study for patients with suspected vascular trauma without need for immediate operative intervention.

In some cases, invasive angiography is employed after CT [4]. A review from Taiwan showed of 182 patients who underwent such procedures included 26.4% negative findings at invasive angiography. About 31.7% of this group were due to renal findings and had the highest relative negative rate. For pelvic fractures and splenic injuries, nonselective proximal embolizations were often performed. Successful treatment without embolization after negative angiography was seen in liver, kidney, and pelvic fractures. Some rebleeding did occur with pelvic fractures even after embolization on negative angiography.

CTA may also be used for detection of late complications [5]. In a 2011 study evaluating 20 patients who underwent embolization for pseudoaneurysms after admission, MDCT scans were abnormal showing Grade III and IV splenic injuries. Seventy percent of these patients had pseudoaneurysms detected on MDCT. Seventy-five percent ($n$ = 15) of the vascular injuries were seen on the arterial phase of invasive angiograms, 66% ($n$ = 10) of which were seen on the CT. Of the remaining five patients with vascular injuries seen on delayed postcapillary phase of the CT, four had pseudoaneurysms. The authors recommended tailoring CT studies to mimic invasive angiography; this is essentially a CTA. Pseudoaneurysms may be seen at presentation or as a delayed complication (or iatrogenically) and CTA is helpful in their detection within the abdomen.

Although CTA is clearly superior, ultrasonography has been extensively described in the trauma literature. However, its ability to diagnose defects in abdominal vessels is not well demonstrated in the literature especially with respect to trauma. There are some case reports that detail experience in using duplex examination to diagnose postinjury pseudoaneurysms, arteriovenous fistulas, and dissections [6]. In a study of 68 patients, the three Doppler modalities (color duplex Doppler [CDD], power Doppler [PD], and B mode [BM]) were compared to assess injury to the iliac arteries and aorta among others. CDD had the lowest sensitivity versus PD and BM, 67%, 75%, and 98%, respectively, for iliac arteries and 85%, 85%, and 98% for the aorta [7]. Among the different Doppler modalities, BM Doppler was the best for the detection of intima flaps, fissures of membranes, and residual flow within the true and false lumen compared with CDD and PD. In addition, the laparoscopic color duplex ultrasound (LDCU) has been used to diagnose hepatic artery injury following laparoscopic injury in animals [8]. In this study, all injuries were correctly identified by LDCU. The applicability of this modality for humans is not well known.

Other aspects of ultrasonography deserve are mentioned here. One relatively new development is contrast-enhanced sonography (CES), which to date has found use in some specialized applications. It is analogous to bubble studies performed by echocardiographers. A 2013 study reviewed 63 stable patients with level II or greater splenic injuries without vascular involvement and use of CES to detect delayed posttraumatic splenic pseudoaneurysms. CES showed a "blush" consistent with a pseudoaneurysm in 6/63 patients that were all confirmed at subsequent control CT. Pooling of contrast was seen CT in two patients with negative contrast sonograms. No false-positive CES examinations were reported. When compared to CT, the study showed sensitivity, specificity, positive predictive value, and NPV of 75% (6/8), 100% (55/55), 100% (6/6), and 96% (55/57), respectively. The authors suggest it may be useful as a screening tool [9].

There is no literature pertaining to the use of MRA in abdominal vascular trauma. Its utility is mainly in the diagnosis of late complications, including dissections, pseudoaneurysms, and arteriovenous fistulas. It is used most commonly for preoperative mapping for intervention with angioplasty and stents and open procedures in patients with renal failure or other contraindications to intravenous contrast. The few references to trauma refer to these late complications, mostly in the extremities.

*Recommendation*: CTA is the imaging modality of choice in stable trauma patients. Duplex sonography may have roles in specific situations (intraoperative applications and patients who are difficult to move). MRA is not well described for these indications.

*Grade of recommendation*: B

## 26.3 Management

### 26.3.1 Is There a Role for Thoracotomy to Control of the Aorta in Abdominal Vascular Exsanguinations?

Laparotomy plays an important role in abdominal trauma especially vascular. But when is a thoracotomy the correct maneuver to gain control of the aorta? The purpose of cross-clamping the thoracic aorta is to obtain proximal control of exsanguinating abdominal hemorrhage and to redistribute intravascular volume to the heart and brain. This maneuver is also used when the infradiaphragmatic aorta is in a hostile environment or is injured.

In 2003, a retrospective review of 185 iliac vessel injuries revealed significant predictors of outcome: ED thoracotomy, associated aortic injury, inferior vena cava injurics, iliac artery and vein injury, intraoperative arrhythmia, and intraoperative coagulopathy. Logistic regression showed independent risk factors for survival: absence of thoracotomy in the emergency department, surgical management, and arrhythmia [10].

In a retrospective review of 470 patients with abdominal vascular injury, the mortality rate was 45% and patients where the aorta was injured proximal to the renal arteries, the mortality rate was 91%. Twenty-nine patients in their series had a good response to a prelaparotomy thoracotomy with aortic cross-clamping and this resulted in systolic blood pressure (SBP) >90 mmHg within 5 min and 38% of patients (11/29) survived [11].

In another retrospective review of 237 patients who underwent emergency department thoracotomy, 50 patients underwent this procedure prior to a laparotomy for abdominal exsanguination [12]. The authors' hypothesis was that Glasgow Coma Score, hemodynamic profile, and injury mechanism were more important than anatomic injury location in predicting which of these 50 patients would survive hospitalization. Sixteen percent of the 50 patients survived the hospitalization. The eight survivors were critical with multiple intra-abdominal injuries. Six of eight (75%) had major abdominal vascular injuries, including five iliac vessel injuries and one combined superior mesenteric artery and vein injury. Two of eight (25%) survivors had severe liver injuries. The authors concluded that prelaparotomy thoracotomy is not a futile procedure and can pass on survival benefit. Thoracotomy should remain as part of the arsenal for the approach to abdominal vascular trauma.

*Recommendation*: "Yes" for prelaparotomy thoracotomy for patients who are in critical status from abdominal vascular trauma.

*Grade of recommendation*: C

### 26.3.2 Regarding Optimal Control of the Aorta, Is There a Role for Resuscitative Endovascular Balloon Occlusion of the Aorta (REBOA)?

The guiding principle of vascular surgery is to obtain proximal and distal control of a vessel prior to repair or incision. This is typically performed with vessel loops, clamps, or Fogarty balloons. We now have an additional technique available: endovascular intra-aortic balloon. This can be inserted via the femoral or brachial artery and placed in the aorta to occlude the vessel from further blood flow. The literature detailing this experience is mainly in the clinical context of ruptured abdominal aortic aneurysms [13].

A case series from 2003 describes a novel technique of using CT guided balloon occlusion in polytrauma patients. The trauma CT scan showed active abdominal or pelvic bleeding, and patients subsequently became hypotensive with SBP <80. A 9 French sheath was introduced and a 20 × 40 mm balloon placed under CT guidance and subsequently evaluated with additional CT scans and CT fluoroscopy [14]. This innovative technique could be very useful in the case of bleeding seen on CT scan, as it could be followed immediately by placement of an occlusion balloon in the CT scanner without moving the patient to an angiography suite or operating room.

The teaching of REBOA has been studied at the R Adams Cowley *Shock Trauma* Center at the University of Maryland. The results show that REBOA is a teachable procedure for acute care surgeons when using the virtual reality simulation approach [15]. The implementation of REBOA was studied in six patients by Brenner et al. [16]; in this series "REBOA resulted in a mean (SD) increase in blood pressure of 55 (20) mmHg, and the mean (SD) aortic occlusion time was 18 (34) minutes. There were no REBOA-related complications, and there was no hemorrhage-related mortality."

*Recommendation*: Further studies are needed to elucidate the utility of this technology. Areas to address include developing and refining the techniques for use by trauma and endovascular personnel in these settings, and to establish standard, rapid algorithms for their use. The technique needs to be adequately compared to open aortic control and ultimately evaluated for incorporation into trauma algorithms and trauma training. It is a promising area but needs more experience before its use can become standard.

*Grade of recommendation*: There is not enough evidence to form a recommendation.

## 26.4 Intraoperative Management

### 26.4.1 Under What Circumstances Are Interventional Endovascular Techniques Superior to Open Vascular Repair?

Interventional techniques remain valuable in the treatment of bleeding vessels and solid organs. The main techniques involve angiographic embolization (AE) and stent placement. Velmahos et al. evaluated the role of AE to stop bleeding in 40 patients with penetrating wounds to the abdomen [17]. Embolization of both intraperitoneal and retroperitoneal vessels was performed for the following indications: angiographic findings in six patients (nonoperative), postsurgery with failure to control bleeding in 23 patients, and to treat late vascular complications in 11 patients. In 32 patients there was active bleeding and 29 underwent successful AE. In this retrospective series, AE proved to be a helpful technique to arrest bleeding from abdominal vessels.

The other important interventional technique with the widespread elective vascular use is the placement of stents (covered or uncovered). In the trauma literature, there are an increasing number of case reports that detail different experiences with stents. In 2006, results from a retrospective subgroup analysis of traumatic vascular injuries treated with a covered stent (data from a prospectively collected registry) were published in the *Journal of Trauma* [18]. The injuries included 33 iliac arteries, 18 subclavian, and 11 femoral arteries and indications were distributed among perforation/rupture, pseudoaneurysm, AV fistula, dissection. Imaging was performed postprocedure and at 12 months. In 93.5% of cases, exclusion was successful by the placement of the Wallgraft endoprosthesis. At 1 year follow-up, the exclusion rate was 91.3% and 90% for iliac and subclavian arteries, respectively, but was 62.3% for femoral arteries. Complications were 4.8% stenosis rate and 6.5% early and 1.6% late occlusion rates. The complication rates are less than open surgical repair at these follow-up points.

*Recommendation*: Whether one technique is superior to the other has not been specifically studied in abdominal vascular trauma. Angioembolization is a good method to arrest bleeding in hemodynamically stable patients with an active bleed. The indications for stent placement can be extrapolated from the vascular surgery literature especially in studies that examine the treatment of complications like pseudoaneurysms, fistulas, and dissections.

*Grade of recommendation*: C

### 26.4.2 Should Abdominal Vascular Injuries Be Ligated or Repaired?

There is a paucity of literature examining this subject so we can only gleam direction from looking at outcomes (retrospective) of different approaches. The approach for each vessel differs according to the presence of collateral supply, the degree of instability of the patient, the appearance of the bowel and other intra-abdominal organs.

For the direction on whether to repair or ligate the superior mesenteric vein (SMV), a retrospective study of all patients admitted at a level I trauma center with SMV injuries was published in 2007. In 59% of cases the vessels were ligated, 31% were primarily repaired, and 10% were exsanguinated prior to repair. The overall survival rate was 24/50 (47%). The study concluded that SMV injuries are highly lethal. Survival for patients apart from those with >3–4 associated injuries was 65%. Combined superior mesenteric artery (SMA) and SMV mortality was 55%, while SMV and portal vein was 40%. Multiple associated vessel injuries increase mortality further. Patients undergoing primary repair have higher survival rates (63%) and lesser numbers of associated vascular and nonvascular injuries, whereas those undergoing ligation have a smaller survival rate (40%) and a higher number of associated vascular and nonvascular injuries. Repair if possible should be performed, but hemodynamics, acid–base status, and temperature should dictate the approach. Ligation appears to be safe and should be selected for hemodynamically unstable patients with a large number of associated injuries [19].

For the other vessels we will detail the conventional surgical approach. The celiac artery can tolerate ligation as it has a good collateral network. In stable patients, a lateral arteriorrhaphy should be performed for a sharp partial superior mesenteric artery injury. If the injury is more substantial, but the patient is not critical then the surgical approach depends upon which zone the injury is in. In zone 1 and 2, ligation can result in severe bowel ischemia and therefore repair is recommended. In zone 3 and 4, ligation may lead to localized ischemia that may be tolerated depending on stability of the patient. If the SMA is injured proximally, then ligation can be performed only if the bowel is already necrotic; the consequences will be short bowel syndrome. In critical patients, an endoluminal shunt should be placed with reconstruction after stability is obtained and then a saphenous vein or polytetrafluoroethylene (PTFE) graft may be used.

Small iliac arterial injuries can be repaired, preferably with a venous or PTFE patch to avoid stenosis. Larger injuries should be approached with an end to end anastomosis with a PTFE graft. Spillage of bowel contents does not contraindicate reconstruction with a prosthetic graft. Iliac artery injuries should not be ligated and if the patient is critical, place an endoluminal shunt and delay repair. For the iliac vein the situation is quite different as a repair that results in stenosis can lead to thrombosis and pulmonary embolism. So, with an iliac vein, you should ligate instead of repair.

Renovasculature trauma in cases of penetrating to one kidney can be reconstructed or a nephrectomy performed depending on the stability of the patient and the presence of concomitant injuries. In blunt kidney vasculature injuries, the patient's kidney function should be followed carefully and endovascular approaches may be feasible. Renal vein injuries on the right that require ligation should lead to a nephrectomy, whereas on the left the vein can be ligated near the inferior vena cava (IVC) as drainage can occur through collateral paths (L gonadal vein, L adrenal vein, lumbar veins). With small renal artery trauma (intimal tears, fistulas, etc.) endovascular approaches can manage these.

Most IVC injuries should be repaired with ligation, only above the renal veins and in unstable patients. The portal venous system is delicate and supports important organs so many injuries in this system should be repaired by lateral venorrhaphy.

*Recommendation*: The decision to ligate or repair is dependent on collateral supply, bowel status, and patient criticality. There are some situations where ligation is preferred and others where repair is required. The use of endoluminal shunts can allow delay of repair. In addition, endovascular approaches for smaller injuries and complications seen later are very useful.

*Grade of recommendation*: C

### 26.4.3 In Difficult Vascular Repairs, Should Anticoagulation Be Used Postoperatively? And if So, for How Long?

There is no discernible level I, II, or III evidence on this subject. There were a plethora of papers on anticoagulation after repairs of difficult or traumatic related vascular conditions in the carotids, thoracic aorta, and extremities. The recommendation at this stage without appropriate abdominal vascular trauma literature would again refer us to extrapolated evidence from the general vascular literature.

**TABLE 26.1**

Abdominal Vascular Trauma

| Question | Answer | Levels of Evidence | Grade of Recommendation | References |
|---|---|---|---|---|
| When comparing Duplex ultrasonography, computed tomographic angiography (CTA), and magnetic resonance angiography (MRA), what is the optimal modality for evaluation of abdominal vascular trauma? | CTA is the imaging modality of choice in stable trauma patients. Duplex sonography may have roles in specific situations (intraoperative applications and patients who are difficult to move). MRA is not well described for these indications. | 4–5 | B | [1–9] |
| Is there a role for thoracotomy to control the aorta in abdominal vascular exsanguinations? | "Yes" for prelaparotomy thoracotomy for patients who are in critical status from abdominal vascular trauma. | 4–5 | C | [10–12] |
| Regarding optimal control of the aorta: is there a role for intraoperative placement of endovascular aortic occlusion balloon? | Further studies are needed to elucidate the utility of this technology. Areas to address include developing and refining the techniques for use by trauma and endovascular personnel in these settings and to establish standard, rapid algorithms for their use. The technique needs to be adequately compared to open aortic control and ultimately evaluated for incorporation into trauma algorithms and trauma training. It is a promising area but needs more experience before its use can become standard. | 4–5 | Not sufficient evidence | [13–16] |
| Under what circumstances are interventional endovascular techniques superior to open vascular repair? | Whether one technique is superior to the other has not been specifically studied in abdominal vascular trauma. Angioembolization is a good method to arrest bleeding in hemodynamically stable patients with an active bleed. The indications for stent placement can be extrapolated from the vascular surgery literature especially in studies that examine the treatment of complications like pseudoaneurysms, fistulas, and dissections. | 4–5 | C | [17,18] |
| Should abdominal vascular injuries be ligated or repaired? | The decision to ligate or repair is dependent on collateral supply, bowel status, and patient criticality. There are some situations where ligation is preferred and others where repair is required. The use of endoluminal shunts can allow delay of repair. In addition, endovascular approaches for smaller injuries and complications seen later are very useful. | 4–5 | C | [19] |
| In difficult vascular repairs, should anticoagulation be used postoperatively? And if so, for how long? | There is insufficient direct evidence for a recommendation. In the authors' opinion, the best available options are to extrapolate from the available data regarding difficult vascular repairs, even if nontraumatic. Examples provided in this chapter include abdominal aortic aneurysm repairs, spontaneous dissections, iatrogenic injuries, as well as highlights of concurrent injuries and comorbidities that must be considered. | 4–5 | Not sufficient evidence | [20,21] |

A small series reviewed 17 patients with spontaneous visceral artery dissections. Fifteen had no pain or ischemic changes. Treatment included observation without anticoagulation ($n$ = 3, 17.6%), anticoagulation ($n$ = 12, 70.6%), and endovascular stenting ($n$ = 2, 11.8%) with the disease stabilizing in all patients during follow-up. The authors concluded that if bowel perfusion is not compromised and patency is well compensated by collaterals then most cases can be managed conservatively with or without anticoagulation with close monitoring and regular follow-up [20]. Considerations in clinical decision-making include patient-specific factors, including comorbidities, type of injury (location in the abdomen, arterial versus venous, blunt versus penetrating) type of repair utilized (primary or patch arteriorrhaphy/venorrhaphy, ligation, vein or synthetic bypass, or endovascular methods), postoperative functional status and mobility, and overall risk of hemorrhage. If there is concern regarding the quality of the conduit or the patch, locations of nonrepaired intimal damage or if the patient has undergone extensive vascular operations for preexisting disease prior to the trauma and likely has poor runoff then it is reasonable to consider utilizing an antiplatelet agent and possibly heparin in the immediate postoperative period. Close clinical follow-up is obviously required to assess for durability of repairs although as aforementioned this is extrapolated from the general vascular literature. One observation to especially take into consideration is that the typical trauma patient may be younger and usually healthier than the generally older "vasculopaths" that undergo some of these procedures more often.

An additional concern is of concurrent injuries. In an extensive retrospective review of blunt abdominal aortic injury performed by the Western Trauma Association including 392,315 patients, reported concurrent injuries in such cases included spinal fractures (44%), pneumothorax/hemothorax (42%), solid organ (38%), small bowel (35%), and large bowel (28%). On CT, the injury itself presented as free aortic rupture (32%), pseudoaneurysm (16%), large intimal flaps (34%), or intimal tears (18%). Any of these concurrent injuries carry with them specific considerations that must be weighed in clinical decision-making, especially with regard to anticoagulation [21] (Table 26.1).

*Recommendation*: There is insufficient direct evidence for a recommendation. In the authors' opinion, the best available options are to extrapolate from the available data regarding difficult vascular repairs, even if nontraumatic. Examples provided here include abdominal aortic aneurysm repairs, spontaneous dissections, iatrogenic injuries as well as highlights of concurrent injuries and comorbidities that must be considered.

*Grade of recommendation*: Insufficient evidence for a recommendation with opinions noted as earlier.

## References

1. Maturen KE, Adusumilli S, Blane CE et al. Contrast-enhanced CT accurately detects hemorrhage in torso trauma: Direct comparison with angiography. *J Trauma.* 2007;62(3):740–745.
2. Loupatatzis C, Schindera S, Gralla J et al. Whole-body computed tomography for multiple traumas using a triphasic injection protocol. *Eur Radiol.* 2008;18(6):1206–1214.
3. Patterson BO, Holt PJ, Cleanthis M et al. Imaging vascular trauma. *Br J Surg.* Apr 2012;99(4):494–505.
4. Yuan KC, Wong YC, Lin B-C et al. Negative catheter angiography after vascular contrast extravasations on computed tomography in blunt torso trauma: An experience review of a clinical dilemma. *Scand J Trauma Resusc Emerg Med.* July 2012;20:46.
5. Atluri S, Richard HM III, Shanmuganathan K. Optimizing multidetector CT for visualization of splenic vascular injury. Validation by splenic arteriography in blunt abdominal trauma patients. *Emerg Radiol.* August 2011;18(4):307–312.
6. Al-Khayat H, Haider HH, Al-Haddad A et al. Endovascular repair of traumatic superior mesenteric artery to splenic vein fistula. *Vasc Endovascular Surg.* 2007;41(6):59–63.
7. Clevert DA, Rupp N, Reiser M et al. Improved diagnosis of vascular dissection by ultrasound B-flow: A comparison with color-coded Doppler and power Doppler sonography. *Eur Radiol.* 2005;15(2):342–347.
8. Birth M, Lossin P, Brugmans F et al. Vascular injuries within the hepatoduodenal ligament: Recognition by laparoscopic color Doppler ultrasound. *Surg Endosc.* 2000;14(3):246–249.
9. Poletti PA, Becker CD, Arditi D et al. Blunt splenic trauma: Can contrast enhanced sonography be used for the screening of delayed pseudoaneurysms? *Eur J Radiol.* November 2013;82(11):1846–1852.
10. Asensio JA, Petrone P, Roldan G et al. Analysis of 185 iliac vessel injuries: Risk factors and predictors of outcome. *Arch Surg.* 2003;138(11):1187–1193.
11. Tyburski, JG, Wilson RF, Dente C et al. Factors affecting mortality rates in patients with abdominal vascular injuries. *J Trauma Inj Infect Crit Care.* 2001;50(6):1020–1026.
12. Seamon, MJ, Pathak, AS, Bradley, KM et al. Emergency department thoracotomy: Still useful after abdominal exsanguination? *J Trauma Inj Infect Crit Care.* 2008;64:1–8.
13. Arthurs Z, Starnes B, See C et al. Clamp before you cut: Proximal control of ruptured abdominal aortic aneurysms using endovascular balloon occlusion—Case reports. *Vasc Endovascular Surg.* 2006;40(2):149–155.
14. Linsenmaier U, Kanz KG, Rieger J et al. CT-guided aortic balloon occlusion in traumatic abdominal and pelvic bleeding. *Rofo.* 2003;175(9):1259–1263.
15. Brenner M, Hoehn M, Pasley J et al. Basic endovascular skills for trauma course: Bridging the gap between endovascular techniques and the acute care surgeon. *J Trauma Acute Care Surg.* 2014;77(2):286–291.

16. Brenner ML, Moore LJ, DuBose JJ et al. A clinical series of resuscitative endovascular balloon occlusion of the aorta for hemorrhage control and resuscitation. *J Trauma Acute Care Surg*. 2013;75(3):506–511.
17. Velmahos GC, Demetriades D, Chahwan S et al. Angiographic embolization for arrest of bleeding after penetrating trauma to the abdomen. *Am J Surg*. 1999;178(5):367–373.
18. White R, Krajcer Z, Johnson M et al. Results of a multicenter trial for the treatment of traumatic vascular injury with a covered stent. *J Trauma*. 2006;60:1189–1195.
19. Asensio JA, Petrone P, Garcia-Nunez L et al. Superior mesenteric venous injuries: To ligate or to repair remains the question. *J Trauma Inj Infect Crit Care*. 2007;62(3):668–675.
20. Choi JY, Kwon OJ. Approaches to the management of spontaneous isolated visceral artery dissection. *Ann Vasc Surg*. August 2013;27(6):750–757.
21. Shalhub S, Starnes BW, Brenner ML et al. Blunt abdominal aortic injury: A Western Trauma Association multicenter study. *J Trauma Acute Care Surg*. December 2014;77(6):879–885.

## Commentary on Abdominal Vascular Trauma

*S.M. Cohn, M.O. Dolich, K. Inaba, and David V. Feliciano*

When all abdominal vascular injuries are considered, the etiology has been penetrating trauma in 88%–93% and blunt trauma in 7%–12% of patients in large civilian series over the past 25 years. For example, blunt injuries to the abdominal aorta and the iliac arteries have accounted for only 0.002% and 3.5% of all injuries reported in these vessels, respectively, in large reviews. The exceptions have been injuries to the superior mesenteric and renal arteries in which penetrating and blunt etiologies have been equal in recent series from centers with 70%–90% blunt trauma.

Patients with abdominal vascular injuries present with profound hypotension (especially an arterial injury), hypotension temporarily responsive to the infusion of crystalloids or blood (especially a venous injury), or are normotensive. With a penetrating injury to the abdomen and hypotension or peritonitis, an immediate laparotomy is indicated. The same is true with blunt trauma, hypotension, and a positive surgeon-performed FAST examination (free fluid present) using a 3.5 mHz probe. In a normotensive patient with blunt abdominal trauma and an equivocal or compromised physical examination or positive FAST examination, a CT scan with intravenous contrast is performed as noted by the authors.

In patients with emergent or urgent indications for a laparotomy, many trauma centers have specific indications to initiate a "massive transfusion protocol" once notified about the patient's status in the emergency room. Prior to laparotomy, perioperative prophylactic/therapeutic antibiotics are administered. The patient is prepped and draped from the chin (to allow for simultaneous thoracotomy or sternotomy) to the knees (to allow for retrieval of a greater saphenous vein).

Abdominal vascular injuries are actively bleeding, bleeding and partially tamponaded, or completely tamponaded at laparotomy. The sequence of operative management will depend on the presentation. Active bleeding from an abdominal vessel mandates vascular control, packing of solid organ injuries, and control of gastrointestinal perforations in sequence.

All intra-abdominal hematomas overlying abdominal vessels are explored after penetrating trauma. In contrast, only midline supramesocolic and inframesocolic hematomas are explored after blunt trauma; however, perirenal and pelvic hematomas are explored, as well, if ruptured, expanding, or pulsatile. A tamponaded injury mandates temporary packing of the hematoma if possible, packing of solid organ injuries, and control of gastrointestinal perforations in sequence.

Abdominal arterial injuries are controlled by direct compression, application of a side-biting clamp (Satinsky), the classical proximal and distal control, or balloon catheter tamponade. Repairs of solitary lacerations are performed in a transverse direction using a suture size appropriate to the vessel being repaired (3-0 or 4-0 polypropylene for aorta, 5-0 or 6-0 polypropylene for superior mesenteric, renal, or iliac arteries). Through-and-through wounds are connected, and the solitary wound is then closed in a transverse direction if at all possible. When the vessel injured is the abdominal aorta and narrowing will result from a primary repair, patch aortoplasty with thin-walled polytetrafluoroethylene (PTFE) is appropriate. A gaping wound (loss of substance) mandates segmental resection and an end-to-end anastomosis (impossible with wounds to the aorta) or insertion of an interposition graft. Even in the presence of gastrointestinal contamination, either a woven Dacron or PTFE graft is used to replace the abdominal aorta or the common or external iliac artery because of large luminal size. Saphenous vein interposition grafts may be used in other arteries with a smaller luminal size. No matter what type of graft is inserted, both anastomoses and the graft itself should be fully covered by mesentery, retroperitoneal tissue, or omentum at the completion of the procedure.

Abdominal venous injuries are controlled in the same fashion as arterial injuries, though proximal and distal compression with spongesticks can be used for vascular control. Because of the size mismatch with the saphenous vein retrieved from the groin, venous interposition often mandates the use of a ringed PTFE graft. Venous ligation is discussed in a later section.

### Optimal Imaging Modality

The precision and sensitivity of CT-arteriography continues to improve as the numbers of detectors increase. Much as with possible cervical, thoracic, or peripheral arterial injuries, CT-arteriography has rapidly become the imaging modality of choice in the highly selected group of patients where imaging is appropriate. This includes the patients who (1) have suffered blunt abdominal trauma with or without a pelvic fracture; (2) are hemodynamically stable or whose hemodynamic stability can be maintained by continuing blood transfusion; and (3) have perfusion abnormalities, intimal flaps, or pseudoaneurysms in the superior mesenteric, renal, or iliac arteries or branches of the iliac arteries in the pelvis as per the original CT.

When the results of CT-arteriography are equivocal or catheter-directed embolization is necessary, a standard digital subtraction abdominal aorta branch study is subsequently performed. Embolization for blunt bleeding from the spleen, liver, kidney, or a pelvic artery noted on an abdominal CT and subsequent aortogram is commonly performed. Obviously, the patient should have no other indication for a laparotomy. On occasion, the inability to attain hepatic hemostasis at laparotomy for a gunshot wound of the liver would mandates a standard selective hepatic arteriogram immediately after surgery with therapeutic embolization of bleeding branches.

### Role for Thoracotomy

A left anterolateral thoracotomy with cross-clamping of the descending thoracic aorta performed in the emergency room before an emergent laparotomy or before or simultaneously with the laparotomy in the operating room is occasionally indicated in patients with an abdominal vascular injury. The technique, however, will delay transfer to the operating room for 15–20 min, result in a rapid worsening of shock-induced hypothermia, and increase loss of blood in the coagulopathic patient. Highly selective indications for preceding or adding this operation to an emergency laparotomy include the following: (1) patient's systolic blood pressure is <70 mmHg and the operating room is geographically distant from the emergency room; (2) patient has prominent scars on the abdominal wall, suggesting the presence of extensive adhesions; and (3) the surgeon has limited operative experience with major abdominal vascular or hepatic trauma.

### Interventional Endovascular Techniques

As previously noted, therapeutic embolization of bleeding from pelvic arteries after blunt fractures has been a standard of care since first introduced at the Massachusetts General Hospital in 1971*. Embolization of intrahepatic bleeders following blunt trauma was introduced within 5 years and subsequently extended to splenic and renal parenchymal hemorrhage or pseudoaneurysms and to noncritical abdominal vessels.

The primary indications for use of endovascular stents or stent grafts in abdominal vascular injuries from blunt or penetrating trauma, but not catheter-associated injuries, are as follows: (1) delayed diagnosis of a pseudoaneurysm, arteriovenous fistula (aortocaval, renal, iliac), or intimal flap in a hemodynamically stable patient; and (2) acute or delayed diagnosis of a similar isolated vascular lesion in a hemodynamically stable patient with a hostile abdomen from previous laparotomies. Modest long-term data are available on the use of stent grafts in patients with noniatrogenic abdominal vascular injuries.

### Endovascular Aortic Occlusion Balloon

As technology has improved, this technique of retrograde passage of a collapsed balloon through the femoral artery and inflation of the balloon proximal to an intra-abdominal arterial bleeder has been revivified. With smaller introduced catheters now available, the technique has appeal in a patient with profound hypotension related to a pelvic fracture. As noted previously, it may prove to be of benefit in the following circumstances, as well: (1) inexperienced trauma surgeon and patient with bleeding from a presumed injury to a midline retroperitoneal or iliac vessel; and (2) presence of a hostile abdomen in a similar patient. There are no prospective data comparing operative control versus endovascular balloon occlusion of the abdominal aorta at this time.

### Ligation of Abdominal Vascular Injuries

Ligation of the proximal superior mesenteric artery (Fullen zones, 1, 2, 3), renal artery, common hepatic artery (beyond the gastroduodenal artery), and the common or external iliac artery should not be performed. If exsanguination is imminent and the surgeon is inexperienced, ligation may be used as a temporizing maneuver until an experienced surgeon is available with the exception of injuries to the superior mesenteric and iliac arteries. This author recommends the insertion of a temporary intraluminal shunt in patients with these injuries to avoid early loss of the midgut or ipsilateral lower extremity. The celiac axis may be ligated in all patients without a preoperative history of mesenteric angina.

All major named veins in the abdomen with the exception of the suprarenal or suprahepatic inferior vena cava may be ligated as long as the surgeon recognizes the likely sequelae. For example, ligation of the infrarenal inferior vena cava or common or external iliac vein is likely to lead to a below-knee compartment syndrome(s). Ligation of the right renal vein or the left renal vein lateral to the adrenal and ovarian veins will lead to renal infarction over time. And, ligation of the superior mesenteric or portal vein will cause splanchnic hypervolemia and systemic hypovolemia that can only be reversed by vigorous infusion of crystalloid solutions.

* Margolies MN, Ring EJ, Waltman AC et al. Arteriography in the management of hemorrhage from pelvic fractures. *N Engl J Med.* 1972;287(7): 317–321.

### Should Anticoagulation Be Used Postoperatively?

Patients with proximal dissections of the superior mesenteric or renal arteries that are not extensive enough to warrant operative repair or endovascular intervention should be considered for anticoagulation. The choice to do so or not will depend on whether a recent laparotomy has been performed and the presence of injuries to the brain or a solid abdominal organ. Should follow-up imaging demonstrate healing of the dissection or intimal flap, anticoagulation is discontinued.

Anticoagulation should also be considered after ligation or a narrowed operative repair of the inferior vena cava or common or external iliac artery. Pulmonary emboli have been reported after these forms of operative management. Therefore, in the absence of the contraindications listed earlier, anticoagulation for 3 months should be considered. With prospective data lacking, the surgeon may choose Coumadin, low molecular weight heparin, clopidogrel, or baby aspirin.

# 27

## *Evidence-Based Approach to Pregnant Trauma Patients*

**Igor Jeroukhimov**

**CONTENTS**



### 27.1 Introduction

Trauma is a leading cause for nonobstetric morbidity and mortality in pregnancy and complicates 6%–7% of all pregnancies [1]. Significant trauma occurs in 1 of 12 pregnant women. About two-thirds of these injures are the result of motor vehicle crash, while fall and physical abuse account for 10%–31% of injuries [2]. Maternal death from trauma ranges from 10% to 20% [3,4]. Fetal mortality of 9% has been reported [5] and increases to about two-thirds if maternal shock is present [6].

### 27.2 Anatomic and Physiologic Changes Unique to Pregnancy

The specific anatomic and physiologic changes that occur during pregnancy may alter the response to injury and, hence, necessitate a modified approach to management.

#### 27.2.1 Cardiovascular System

Plasma volume begins to expand at 10 weeks of gestation and increases to 45% of pregravid levels by full-term. Tubular resorption of sodium and water is significantly increased [7]. This hypervolemic state is protective for the mother because fewer red blood cells are lost during hemorrhage, and hence, the oxygen-carrying capacity of the blood is less affected [8]. Thus, volume expansion may cause a false sense of security for the resuscitating physician because as much as 35% of maternal blood may be lost before first signs of hemodynamic instability appear. Increases in plasma volume by 30%–40% are accompanied by a 15% increase in red blood cells cell mass, resulting in the physiological anemia of pregnancy.

A hypercoagulable state is common during the pregnancy. Factors VII, VIII, IX, X, and XII, and fibrinogen are increased, and fibrinolytic activity is reduced, putting the patient at increased risk for thromboembolic events.

Maternal heart rate increases by about 10–15 beats/min. As the diaphragm becomes progressively more elevated secondary to the enlarging uterus, the heart is displaced to the left and upward, resulting in a lateral displacement of the cardiac apex. Moreover, each pregnant woman has some degree of benign pericardial effusion. Both of these changes result in an enlarged cardiac silhouette and increased pulmonary vasculature on the chest radiograph [9].

Cardiac output increases to 25% above normal. In the healthy gravida, this increased workload on the heart is well-tolerated [7]. However, in supine position, gravid uterus partially obstructed the inferior vena cava, which decreases preload to the heart, resulting in a lower cardiac output, thereby causing the supine hypotensive syndrome. This syndrome is marked by dizziness, pallor, tachycardia, sweating, nausea, and hypotension. Turning the mother onto her left side restores the cardiac output.

### 27.2.2 Respiratory System

Secondary to uterus enlargement, the diaphragm rises about 4 cm and the diameter of the chest enlarges by 2 cm, increasing the substernal angle by 50% [7]. Care should be taken to consider these anatomical changes when thoracic procedures such as tube thoracostomies or thoracenteses are being performed.

The most prominent changes in respiratory physiology include progressive increase in tidal volume and minute ventilation. Functional residual capacity decreases because of a decline in expiratory reserve and residual volumes. Relative to these changes, the injured pregnant patient poorly tolerates hypoxia; hence, supplemental oxygen is always indicated.

Progesterone stimulates the medullary respiratory center, resulting in hyperventilation and respiratory alkalosis. $PCO_2$ decreases to level of 27–32 mmHg in pregnant woman. Therefore, pregnancy is a state of partially compensated respiratory alkalosis.

### 27.2.3 Gastrointestinal System

Increased levels of progesterone and estrogen inhibit gastrointestinal motility, intestinal secretion, and nutrient absorption. Additionally, the angle of the gastroesophageal junction is altered such that the lower esophageal sphincter is displaced into the thorax. This alteration decreases the competency of the lower gastroesophageal sphincter, which increases the potential for aspiration as early as 8–12 weeks [10]. It is, therefore, prudent to insert a nasogastric tube to decompress the stomach and prevent aspiration. Furthermore, as the uterus enlarges, it displaces the intestines upward and laterally, making physical examination unreliable.

### 27.2.4 Renal System

Renal blood flow increases by 30% during pregnancy. As pregnancy progresses, the ureters and bladder are compressed by the uterus, resulting in hydronephrosis and hydroureter; consequently, a dilated collecting system visualized on imaging studies is normal.

Increases in blood volume and cardiac output cause a rise in glomerular filtration rate and renal plasma flow. Therefore, more plasma is filtered, reducing the serum protein concentration and, hence, the plasma oncotic pressure [11]. This change also results in an increase in the renal clearance of many substances during pregnancy, and a review of the metabolism of pharmaceutical agents prior to their administration to pregnant patient is recommended [12].

### 27.2.5 Endocrine System

The placenta produces human chorionic gonadotropin and human placental lactogen (hPL), as well as progesterone, estrogen, thyroid-stimulating hormone, and adrenocorticotropic hormone [13].

Maternal utilization of glucose is decreased, whereas maternal lipolysis is enhanced, making nutrients available to the fetus. hPL is the physiologic antagonist of insulin and contributes to the diabetogenic effect of pregnancy by causing increased peripheral resistance to insulin. The pituitary gland enlarges during pregnancy by approximately 135%, and demands increased blood flow [13]. Shock may cause necrosis of the anterior pituitary gland, resulting in pituitary insufficiency or Sheehan syndrome.

### 27.2.6 Reproductive System

By the end of full-term gestation, the weight of the uterus increases to 20 times its prepregnancy weight. Intrapelvic location protects uterine from injury, but after the 12th week of pregnancy, it extends out of the pelvis and ascends into the abdominal cavity to displace the intestines laterally and superiorly. This makes the uterine more vulnerable for injury, but protects the intra-abdominal organs.

With progressive uterine enlargement, uterine blood flow increases, constituting up to 20% of the cardiac output at term. Uterine veins may dilate up to 60 times, increasing the risk of massive blood loss with pelvic injury.

### 27.2.7 Musculoskeletal System

The softening and relaxation of the interosseus ligaments during pregnancy cause increased mobility of the sacroiliac and sacrococcygeal joints and widening of the symphysis pubis. These changes, coupled with an enlarged uterus, disrupt the maternal center of gravity and gait stability, putting the gravida at increased risk for trauma, especially from falls.

## 27.3 Assessment of Pregnant Trauma Patients

A key management principle of injured pregnant patient is to treat the mother first because most medical measures which aid in the resuscitation of the mother will be helpful to the fetus. The pregnant patient is best cared for using team approach. The trauma surgeon and obstetrician should be involved early. All necessary tests and procedures should be performed if indicated. Because the most common cause of fetal death is maternal death, efforts to assess fetal well-being are secondary to resuscitation of the pregnant woman. However, fetal well-being may represent the most valuable measurement of maternal health. Fetal distress appears early and represents maternal hemorrhage even if the mother is hemodynamically stable. Waiting to maternal signs of instability will worsen the fetal compromise.

Assessment and establishment of the maternal airway are critical, and all pregnant patients should receive supplemental oxygen at a minimum. Late in gestation, the oropharynx is swollen from tissue edema and endotracheal intubation of the gravid patient can be difficult; therefore, use of a smaller than normal diameter endotracheal tube, such as a 6.5 mm or less, may be necessary [14]. During the pregnancy, the risk of aspiration increases and monitoring of oxygenation is necessary. Precaution must be taken when chest tube thoracostomy is required.

### 27.3.1 Should ß-Human Chorionic Gonadotropin Test Be Performed in Every Female Patient in Childbearing Age?

After the primary survey and stabilization of the patient, diagnostic modalities are used to determine extent of injuries to the mother and fetus. Laboratories pertinent to the trauma setting are obtained, and all female patients of childbearing age should have a ß-human chorionic gonadotropin test performed [15].

*Recommendation*: A rapid secondary survey must include evaluation of pregnancy. This consists of determination of fetal heart rate and movement, assessment of uterine size and tonus, and examination of vaginal bleeding, or leakage of amniotic fluid. Fetal monitoring is initiated. Fetal heart tones are discernable by Doppler by the 10th week of gestation, allowing a simple and non-invasive method of monitoring. After the 20th week of pregnancy, standard continuous fetal heart rate monitoring should be employed under the obstetrician guidance [2] (Grade B recommendation).

### 27.3.2 Should the Fetal Resuscitation Be Initiated in the Absence of Fetal Heart Tones?

If fetal heart tones are absent, resuscitation of the fetus should not be attempted. There were no fetal survivors in a series of 441 pregnant trauma patients with initially absent fetal heart tones [16].

*Recommendation*: If fetal heart tones are absent, resuscitation of the fetus should not be attempted. All female patients of childbearing age should have a ß-human chorionic gonadotropin test performed (Grade B recommendation).

### 27.3.3 What Is Appropriate Time for Fetal Monitoring after Trauma?

Controversies exist concerning the duration of fetal monitoring following trauma. Early studies indicating that placenta abruption can occur up to 48 h post-trauma recommend continues fetal monitoring during this period [17].

A widely used protocol is based on a prospective study of 60 patients at more than 20 weeks of gestation [18]. This protocol has a sensitivity of 100% for predicting adverse outcomes within 4 h. In the prospective study, 70% of patients required more than 4 h of fetal monitoring because of continued contractions (four or more per hour), abnormal laboratory values, or vaginal bleeding, but all of the patients discharged at the end of 4 or 24 h had similar outcomes compared with noninjured control patients. If fetal tachycardia is present or a non-stress test is nonreactive, monitoring usually is continued for 24 h, but no studies exist to support this practice.

Some experts recommend prolonged electronic fetal monitoring in patients with high-risk mechanisms of injury. These mechanisms include automobile versus pedestrian, and high-speed motor vehicle crashes [19]. No evidence supports the use of routine electronic fetal monitoring for more than 24 h after noncatastrophic trauma [20].

*Recommendation*: All pregnant trauma patients >20 weeks of gestation should have fetal monitoring for at least of 6 h (Grade B recommendations).

### 27.3.4 May Approach to Evaluation of Minor Trauma in Pregnancy Be Different?

Minor trauma during pregnancy requires only limited evaluation. In a prospective study of 317 patients with minor trauma, placental abruption appeared in only one case and was not predicted by conventional tests, including tocodynamometry, ultrasonography, and Kleihauer–Betke (KB) test. This led the authors to conclude that minor trauma can be appropriately evaluated with limited radiologic, laboratory, and fetal assessment [21].

*Recommendation*: Minor trauma during pregnancy requires only limited evaluation (Grade B recommendation). Five conditions are associated with signaling an acute status of the pregnancy. These include vaginal bleeding, rupture of the amniotic sac, presence of contractions, bulging perineum, and abnormal fetal heart rate and rhythm.

Vaginal bleeding before the onset of full-term labor is abnormal. It is potentially indicative of preterm labor, placental abruption, or placenta previa. Rupture of the amniotic sac can allow prolapse of the umbilical cord, resulting in compression of the cord and potential compromise of the fetal circulation. Suspected amniotic fluid can be tested using Nitrazine paper, which will turn deep blue if the test is positive. Rupture of the amniotic sac is an obstetrical emergency because of the risk of infection and umbilical cord prolapse. Bulging of the perineum represents pressure from a presenting part of the fetus, and delivery or spontaneous abortion may be in progress. The presence of strong contractions is associated with true labor.

### 27.3.5 Should KB Test Be Performed in Pregnant Trauma Patient?

Traumatic injury to the uterus can result in transplacental or fetomaternal hemorrhage. The KB test is used to detect the presence of fetal cells in the maternal circulation. Because of its high sensitivity, the KB test by itself does not necessarily indicate pathologic fetal-maternal hemorrhage [22]. The KB test is recommended for injured Rh-negative patients in the second or third trimester to detect impending fetal hemorrhage and determine the risk of Rh isosensitization.

As little as 0.001 mL of fetal blood can cause sensitization of an Rh-negative mother. Therefore, all Rh-negative pregnant trauma patients should receive immunoglobulin to suppress potential immune response [16]. Recent evidence suggests that the KB test accurately predicts the risk of preterm labor, and in a patient with a negative KB test, fetal monitoring duration can be terminated [23]. When used as a predictor of preterm labor, the KB test is beneficial to all maternal trauma patients, regardless of their Rh status.

*Recommendation*: KB test should be performed in all pregnant patients >12 weeks of gestation (Grade B recommendations).

## 27.4 Diagnostic Considerations

After maternal assessment, there is a need for rapid and accurate imaging. A pregnant patient with blunt abdominal injury or unconsciousness poses the greatest dilemma for imaging. Evaluation of the abdomen for hemoperitoneum can be performed by ultrasonography, diagnostic peritoneal lavage (DPL), computed tomography (CT) scan, or magnetic resonance imaging (MRI).

DPL can be performed safely in the pregnant patient and carries the same sensitivity as in the non-pregnant state [17]. In these cases, DPL is performed using an open technique in a supraumbilical location. DPL is rarely used with advent of focused abdominal sonography for trauma (FAST). It may be indicated when FAST is either unavailable or equivocal, particularly when the patient is hemodynamically unstable. The disadvantages of DPL include the relative invasiveness of the procedure and that, while hemoperitoneum is easily detected, the source of bleeding is not.

### 27.4.1 Should FAST Be Performed in Every Pregnant Patient with Suspected Abdominal Trauma?

FAST is an important tool performed for diagnosis of free intra-abdominal fluid. Sensitivity of this method ranges from 42% to 100% [24–26]. FAST is less sensitive in pregnant patients than in non-pregnant trauma patients, but this examination remains highly specific [24]. Some studies report false-negative ultrasound results and recommend further imaging or clinical follow-up [24,28]. However, a recent study showed that in patients with negative FAST results, 96% did not need additional testing that used ionizing radiation, and therefore, ultrasound was recommended as an accurate screening tool [27]. In that study, the patients who had false-negative findings were diagnosed within 24 h of the injury.

*Recommendation*: FAST should be performed in every pregnant trauma patient with suspected intra-abdominal injury (Grade C recommendations).

### 27.4.2 Should Diagnostic Radiologic Studies Be Withheld in Pregnant Trauma Patient?

During the period of major organogenesis (2–15 weeks), ionizing radiation has the highest potential for teratogenesis and neonatal neoplastic effect [2,28,29]. In the remainder of pregnancy, radiation may produce growth retardation, microcefaly, and mental retardation [30]. Exposure to a cumulative dose of less than 0.05 Gy (5 rad) equivalent to the radiation dose from approximately 500 chest radiographs or 100 abdominal CT scans has not been shown to affect pregnancy outcomes compared with control populations exposed to background radiation [31]. The American College of Obstetricians and Gynecologists stated that a 5-rad exposure to the fetus is not associated with increased risk of fetal loss or birth defects [32] (Grade C recommendation). Radiation dosage by study commonly used in trauma imaging is listed in Table 27.1. If multiple diagnostic studies are performed, particularly when radiation exposure approaches 5–10 rad, then consultation with radiologist or radiation specialist should be considered and alternative imaging methods, such as ultrasound or MRI should be performed when appropriate [32] (Grade C recommendation).

MRI is considered safe during pregnancy, as magnetic energy has been shown not to be harmful for fetus [33,34]. The most obvious advantage of it over CT is lack of ionizing radiation. On the other hand, most radiology providers recommend the use of gadolinium-based contrast agents, the safety of which for the fetus has never been proven. Although teratogenic effects have not been observed in a small number of human studies where gadolinium has been given in pregnancy, it is clear that gadolinium should not be administered during pregnancy unless there is an absolutely essential clinical indication, particularly during the period of organogenesis [34,35]. Moreover, MRI is a time-consuming examination, and gaining access to MRI scanners in an emergent fashion is generally impractical. Thus, MRI has no role in evaluation of acute trauma patient, and it is more useful in diagnosis of neurologic and musculoskeletal trauma, when most of life-threatening injuries were managed.

*Recommendation*: Radiologic studies requested for maternal evaluation should not be withheld on the basis of its potential danger to the fetus. Unnecessary duplication of studies should be avoided, and appropriate mandatory shielding should be used whenever possible (Grade and C recommendation).

**TABLE 27.1**

Fetal Radiation Exposure to Commonly Used Radiographic Studies

| Imaging Study | Fetal Radiation Exposure (rad) |
|---|---|
| Plain film | |
| Cervical spine | 0 |
| Chest AP | 0.0001 |
| Pelvis AP | 0.103 |
| Thoracic spine | 0.0001 |
| Lumbar spine | 0.090 |
| CT | |
| Head | <0.05 |
| Chest + abdomen | 1.6 |
| Abdomen + pelvis | 1.6 |
| Chest/abdomen/pelvis (angio)[a] | 4.5 |

[a] CT angiography protocol.

## 27.5 Emergent Cesarean Section for Trauma

### 27.5.1 What Is the Role of Perimortem Cesarean Section (CS) and When Should It Be Performed?

Performance of an emergency CS at more than 25 weeks' gestation for appropriate indications following trauma is associated with 45% fetal survival and 72% maternal survival [16]. The absence of fetal heart tones ordinarily predicts mortality from an emergency CS.

Perimortem CS should be performed in the traumatic maternal arrest with potential fetal viability, when resuscitative measures have failed. The best outcomes occur if the infant is delivered within 5 min of maternal cardiac arrest. This means that surgery should begin by 4 min into the arrest [16,36]. The latest reported survival was of an infant delivered 22 min after documented maternal cardiac arrest [37]. Several factors must be considered when deciding whether to undertake perimortem CS [36,38]. These include estimated gestational age of the fetus and the resources of the hospital. Before 23 weeks' gestational age, delivery of the fetus may not improve maternal venous return. Therefore, aggressive maternal resuscitation is the only indicated intervention [1].

*Recommendation*: Perimortem CS should be considered in moribund pregnant patient after 24 weeks of gestation. Delivery must occur in 20 min of maternal death, but should ideally begin within 4 min of maternal arrest (Grade C recommendations).

**TABLE 27.2**

Current Evidence and Recommendations

| Question | Answer | Level of Evidence | Grade of Recommendation | References |
|---|---|---|---|---|
| Should ß-human chorionic gonadotropin test be performed in every female patient in childbearing age? | All female patients of childbearing age should have a ß-human chorionic gonadotropin test performed. | II | B | [15] |
| Should resuscitation be initiated in case when fetal heart tones are absent? | If fetal heart tones are absent, resuscitation of the fetus should not be attempted. | II | B | [16] |
| What is appropriate time for fetal monitoring after trauma? | All pregnant trauma patients >20 weeks of gestation should have fetal monitoring for at least 6 h. | II | B | [17,18] |
| Should approach to evaluation of minor trauma in pregnancy be different? | Minor trauma during pregnancy requires only limited evaluation. | II | B | [21] |
| Should KB test be performed in pregnant trauma patient? | KB test should be performed in all pregnant patients >12 weeks of gestation. | II | B | [18,23] |
| Should FAST be performed in every pregnant patient with suspected abdominal trauma? | FAST should be performed in every pregnant trauma patient with suspected intra-abdominal injury. | III | C | [27] |
| Should diagnostic radiologic studies be withheld in pregnant trauma patient? | Radiologic studies necessary for maternal evaluation should not be withheld on the basis of its potential danger to the fetus. | III | C | [29–32] |
| What is the role of perimortem CS, and when it should be performed? | Perimortem CS should be considered in moribund pregnant patient after 24 weeks of gestation. Delivery must occur in 20 min of maternal death, but should ideally begin within 4 min of maternal arrest. | III | C | [16,36,38] |

## 27.6 Summary

Trauma is a leading cause of non-obstetrical maternal mortality. Knowledge of anatomic and physiologic alterations in pregnancy, correct evaluation of both mother and fetus, and careful considerations of conditions specific to pregnancy are essential to ensure the best outcome. Although the literature on trauma in pregnancy is quite extensive, it is characterized by several limitations. The majority of studies are retrospective, and even prospective works do not have a matching control group. Many studies relied on hospitalized patients rise a concern of ascertainment bias, as only severe trauma cases were identified (Table 27.2). Multi-institutional retrospective data collection following prospective phone follow-up may shed more light on the existing controversies.

## References


1. Muench MV, Canterio JC. Trauma in pregnancy. *Obstet Gynecol Clin N Am.* 2007;(34):555–583.
2. Tsuei BJ. Assessment of pregnant trauma patient. *Injury.* 2006;37:367–373.
3. Warner MW, Salfinger SG, Rao S et al. Management of trauma during pregnancy. *ANZ J. Surg.* 2004;74:125–128.
4. Hyde LK, Cook LJ, Olson LM et al. Effect of motor vehicle crashes on adverse fetal outcomes. *Obstet Gynecol.* 2003;102:279–286.
5. Rogers F, Rozycki G, Tuner O et al. A Multi-institutional study of factors associated with fetal death in injured pregnant patients. *Arch Surg.* 1999;134:1274–1277.
6. Scorpio RJ, Esposito TJ, Smith LG. Blunt trauma during pregnancy: Factors affecting fetal outcome. *J Trauma.* 1992;32(2):213–216.
7. Knudson MM, Rozycki GS, Paquin MM. 2004. Reproductive system trauma. In: Feliciano DV, Mattox KL, Moor EE (eds.), *Trauma,* 5th edn. McGraw-Hill: New York, pp. 609–643.
8. Smith CV, Phalen JP. 1991. Trauma in pregnancy. In: Clark SL, Cotton DB, Hankins GDV, Phelen JP (eds.), *Critical Care Obstetrics,* 2nd edn. Blackwell: Boston, MA, p. 498.
9. Lee W, Cotton DB. 1991. Cardiorespiratory changes during pregnancy. In: Clark SL, Cotton DB, Hankins GDV, Phelen JP (eds.), *Critical Care Obstetrics,* 2nd edn. Blackwell: Boston, MA, p. 2.
10. Bynum TE. Hepatic and gastrointestinal disorders in pregnancy. *Med Clin North Am.* 1977;61:129.
11. Dunlop W. Serial changes in renal hemodynamics during normal human pregnancy. *Br J Obstet Gynaecol.* 1981;88:1.
12. Briggs GC, Freeman RK, Yaffe SJ. 1990. *A Reference Guide to Fetal and Neonatal Risk: Drugs in Pregnancy and Lactation,* 3rd edn. Williams & Wilkins, Baltimore, MD.

13. Gonzalez JG, Elizondo G, Saldiver D et al. Pituitary gland growth during normal pregnancy: An in vivo study using magnetic resonance imaging. *Am J Med.* 1988;85:217.
14. Munnur U, de Boisblanc B, Suresh MS. Airway problems in pregnancy. *Crit Care Med.* 2005;33:S259–S268.
15. Bochicchio GV, Napolitano LM, Haan J et al. Incidental pregnancy in trauma patients. *J Am Coll Surg.* 2001;192: 566–569.
16. Morris JA, Jr., Rosenbower TJ, Jurkovich GJ et al. Infant survival after cesarean section for trauma. *Ann Surg.* 1996;223:481–491.
17. Esposito TJ. Evaluation of blunt abdominal trauma occurring during pregnancy. *J Trauma.* 1989;29:1621632.
18. Pearlman MD, Tintinalli JE, Lorenz RP. A prospective controlled study of outcome after trauma during pregnancy. *Am J Obstet Gynecol.* 1990;162:1502–1510.
19. Curet MJ, Schermer CR, Demarest GB, Bieneik EJ III, Curet LB. Predictors of outcome in trauma during pregnancy: Identification of patients who can be monitored for less than 6 hours. *J Trauma.* 2000;49:18–25.
20. Grossman NB. Blunt trauma in pregnancy. *Am Fam Physician.* 2004;70:1303–1313.
21. Cahill A, Bastek J, Stamilio D et al. Minor trauma in pregnancy—Is the evaluation unwarranted? *Am J Obstet Gynecol.* 2008;198:208.
22. Dhanraj D, Lambers D. The incidences of positive Kleihauer-Betke test in low-risk pregnancies and maternal trauma patients. *Am J Obstet Gynecol.* 2004;190:1461–1463.
23. Muench MV, Baschat AA, Reddy UM et al. Kleihauer-Betke testing is important in all cases of maternal trauma. *J Trauma.* 2004; 57:1094–1098.
24. Goodwin H, Holmes JF, Wisner DH. Abdominal ultrasound examination in pregnant blunt trauma patients. *J Trauma.* 2001;50(4):689–693.
25. Richards JR, Ormsby EL, Romo MV et al. Blunt abdominal injury in the pregnant patient: Detection with US. *Radiology.* 2004;233:463–470.
26. Brown MA, Sirlin SB, Farahmand N et al. Screening sonography in pregnant patients with blunt abdominal trauma. *J Ultrasound Med.* 2005;24:175–181.
27. Goldman SM, Wagner LK. Radiologic ABCs of maternal and fetal survival after trauma: When minutes may count. *RadioGraphics.* 1999;19:1349–1357.
28. Stalberg K, Haglund B, Axelsson O et al. Prenatal x-ray exposure and childhood brain tumours: A population-based case-control study on tumour subtypes. *Br J Canc.* 2007 3;97(11):1583–1587.
29. Harvey EB, Boice JD, Jr., Honeyman M et al. Prenatal x-ray exposure and childhood cancer in twins. *N Engl J Med.* 1985;312(9):541–545.
30. Otake M, Schull WJ. Radiation-related brain damage and growth retardation among the prenatally exposed atomic bomb survivors. *Int J Radiat Biol.* 1998;74(2): 159–171.
31. Brent RL. Saving lives and changing family histories: Appropriate counseling of pregnant women and men and women of reproductive age, concerning the risk of diagnostic radiation exposures during and before pregnancy. *Am J Obstet Gynecol.* 2009; 200(1):4–24.
32. American College of Obstetricians and Gynecologists Committee Opinion #299. 2004. Guidelines for diagnostic imaging during pregnancy. Washington, DC.
33. De Wilde JP, Rivers AW, Price DL. A review of the current use of magnetic resonance imaging in pregnancy and safety implications for the fetus. *Prog Biophys Mol Biol.* 2005;87:335–353.
34. Nagayama M, Watanabe Y, Okumura A et al. MR imaging in obstetrics. *Radiographics.* 2002;22:563–582.
35. Shellock FG, Kanal E. Safety of magnetic resonance imaging contrast agents *J Magn Reson Imaging.* 1999;10:477–484.
36. Katz VL, Dotters DJ, Droegemueller W. Perimortem cesarean delivery. *Obstet Gynecol.* 1986;68(4):571–576.
37. Lopez-Zeno JA, Carlo WA, O'Grady JP et al. Infant survival following delayed postmortem cesarean delivery. *Obstet Gynecol.* 1990;76(5):991–992.
38. Katz V, Balderston K, DeFreest M. Perimortem cesarean delivery: Were our assumptions correct? *Am J Obstet Gynecol.* 2005;192(6):1916–1920.

## Commentary on Evidence-Based Approach to Pregnant Trauma Patient

*Pieter J.S. Smit, Ronald Iverson, and Peter A. Burke*

Amongst the myriad high stakes situations that trauma surgeons face during their careers, none are as emotionally charged and require such a thorough understanding of specific physiology as the pregnant trauma patient. It is with this in mind that the tenets of ATLS should be applied to create a systematic, informed, approach to resuscitation and management of both mother and fetus. Developing this approach allows one to establish appropriate treatment priorities and mobilize the necessary resources to care for all involved patients, both living and unborn. While trauma resuscitations in general are dynamic situations that require the collection and interpretation of various data points in order to make treatment decisions, dealing with a pregnant patient adds another level of complexity to the equation. In this day and age, trauma is undoubtedly a team sport, with the trauma surgeon serving to orchestrate the multiple specialists involved in the care of the multitrauma patient. Being used to such multidisciplinary collaboration is of benefit when additional input is sought from our obstetrical colleagues, and ideally, their involvement begins prior to patient arrival in the trauma bay. It is with these multiple patient considerations in mind that a parallel processing approach should be applied. While initially used in computer science, parallel processing is more generally defined as simultaneously integrating multiple inputs to solve a problem. In this context, the inputs include not only the standard data points (physical exam, lab results, radiology findings, etc.) but also information regarding the fetus' health, namely, fetal heart rate. The parallel process aspect is further applicable, given the possibility of conflicting best interests of two separate but inexorably linked patients.

The initial resuscitation of the pregnant patient is not fundamentally different than any other adult resuscitation, except that there are two potential lives in the balance, which cannot help but add to an already tense situation. At times like these, it is important to fall back on first principles. A sequential primary survey aimed at identifying and intervening on any immediately life-threatening injuries is performed, with the added knowledge that shock may be related to supine hypotensive syndrome, and can be easily treated by off-loading the vena-cava being compressed by the gravid uterus. Our practice is to elevate the right side of all pregnant patients 10°–15° empirically in order to ameliorate the syndrome proactively. During the secondary survey, two crucial pieces of information specific to the pregnant patient need to be obtained: fetal heart rate and gestational age. The use of ultrasound either alone or at the conclusion of the FAST exam is a simple way of roughly evaluating this prior to formal fetal US. This information serves as the scaffolding on which the decision tree of care is built by establishing the fetal condition along with its extrauterine viability. While most literature supports 24 weeks as the cutoff for potential neonatal viability, we have adopted a lower threshold of 20 weeks in order to allow better treatment of possibly viable neonates if they are small for gestational age. While not as much of an issue for the alert and conversant patient, in the intubated or obtunded patient, the accuracy of fundal height and US estimation is not high enough to capture the small for date fetus that is potentially viable post delivery. If the fetus is truly less than 24 weeks gestation, then extrauterine viability is not likely and all efforts should be made to support the mother in order to optimize materno-placental perfusion. Furthermore, in the unfortunate event that the fetus is asystolic, there is no indication to emergently deliver the baby, as the fetus almost certainly will not be viable and delivery is unlikely to improve maternal hemodynamics. Moving to a different branch of the decision tree is the determination that the fetus is ≥24 weeks gestation, and therefore potentially viable. At this point, ongoing maternal resuscitation and monitoring of both mother and fetus is advised to aid in the early identification of instability of either the mother or fetus, which may push one toward exploratory laparotomy ± c-section. In this parallel processing framework, one has to realize that treatment priorities can quickly change, and that delivery of the child can benefit the mother by improving venous return, pulmonary mechanics, and by halting maternal to utero-placental blood flow. It is for this reason that delivery of a potentially viable fetus is performed in an unstable mother, in addition to removing the fetus from a suboptimally supportive environment. Regardless of the fetal age and viability, all Rh-negative women should receive an empiric dose of Rhogam 300 μg IM. The Kleihauer Betke test should then be obtained in the setting of abdominal trauma or any high-energy blunt mechanism to assess for the adequacy of the empiric dose, with additional immune globulin being given for estimated feto-maternal hemorrhage greater than 30mL of whole blood.

Surprisingly, it is not the scenario where the mother or fetus is in frank distress that creates the most challenging clinical situation, for these are the times when deranged physiology has declared itself and the need for decisive action becomes clear-cut. Rather it is the stable patient, or the transient responder, who wreaks havoc. The medico-legal hierarchy is that the mother's life takes primacy over that of the fetus, and that the goals of care ought to be focused on providing the adult patient appropriate care, despite potential harm to the fetus. While this sounds simple in practice, when faced with an alert, hemodynamically stable pregnant woman who has been involved in an MVC and is adamantly refusing all x-rays and CT scans, the question of what imaging is necessary and what can be omitted comes into play. At this point, a balance between identifying injuries that are likely to seriously injure the mother must be weighed against her wishes and the small, but real, risk of contributing to a radiation related disease in the fetus. Ultrasound, long used in the care of pregnant patients, has an important role to play, as it is safe for mother and fetus and can be performed serially. Shortcomings of US include its inability to identify the source of free fluid (liver, spleen, uterus?), and a lower threshold to explore a pregnant patient with transient hypotension and free intra-abdominal fluid should be entertained if CT has not been obtained. The role of MRI in pregnancy is unclear, and its use as a screening modality not well characterized in trauma. However, utilizing MRI for follow-up of imaging of known injuries is of potential use as it allows for a focused exam without additional radiation exposure. In the event that the radiologic evaluation is not completed in a manner consistent with the standard of care for a nonpregnant patient, we recommend that an extended period of observation of at least 24 h should be carried out prior to discharge, to allow the manifestations of occult injuries to present themselves. This is in contradistinction to the 6 h of fetal heart rate monitoring recommended for the identification of fetal distress or early labor. Obviously omitting portions of the work-up can only occur in a conscious and competent patient who is informed of the risks associated with delayed diagnosis.

Thankfully maternal and fetal well-being are not mutually exclusive, and in caring for the injured adult, optimization of materno-placental perfusion is attained. In general, the best place for the fetus to remain is in utero, and by optimally resuscitating the mother, this biologically perfect NICU can continue to function. This is why appropriate maternal care is generally the treatment of choice for the fetus. If, however, there is concern for fetal distress and the need for cesarean delivery in a fetus less than 34 weeks, consideration of antenatal steroids to assist in fetal lung development should be considered in consultation with Ob-Gyn. Maximal benefit is attained when the medication is given more than 24 h prior to delivery, a situation unlikely to occur in trauma. Additional interventions that can benefit the mother and/or fetus include the administration of antibiotics in the setting of premature or traumatic rupture of membranes and the consideration of magnesium sulfate infusion for neonatal neuroprotection. These treatments should be carried out in close consultation with obstetrics so that a discussion of risks and benefits can be had on a case-by-case basis.

No one wants to be in the trauma bay when a seriously injured woman with an obviously pregnant belly comes through the door, but by having a clear sense of priorities that focus first on maternal well-being, in addition to a secondary plan if things should deteriorate precipitously, then both mother and baby have the best chance of doing well. The importance of establishing a collaborative plan with obstetrical and neonatal specialists cannot be overemphasized, and the time to develop this framework is well before a pregnant trauma patient arrives on your door-step.

# 28

## *Pelvic Fractures*

**Panna A. Codner and Matthew O. Dolich**

**CONTENTS**



### 28.1 Introduction

Pelvic fractures are reported to account for 1%–3% of all skeletal injuries and are present in approximately 5% of trauma patients requiring hospitalization [1]. The fractures may occur through a variety of mechanisms, including motor vehicle collisions, pedestrian accidents, falls, and crush injuries. Pelvic fractures may present with a wide spectrum of severity ranging from relatively minor pubic ramus fractures to significant open-book or vertical shear-type injuries with exsanguinating hemorrhage or large soft tissue wounds. Associated extrapelvic injuries are common, and the clinician is frequently faced with a complex decision process in a multiple injured, unstable patient. This chapter will review the literature regarding diagnostic and therapeutic measures of particular interest to the trauma/acute care surgeon, and will provide recommendations based on the available evidence.

### 28.2 Which Patients with Pelvic Fractures Warrant Early Angiography with Arterial Angioembolization?

While most patients with pelvic fractures have an initial presentation of hemodynamic stability with relatively little blood loss, hemorrhage remains the leading cause of mortality with severe pelvic fractures. A number of arterial and venous branches course along the internal surfaces of the sacrum and ilium in the retroperitoneal space, and these structures may be disrupted following blunt fracture of the pelvis. In addition, patients with pelvic fractures have a high incidence of associated intra-abdominal injuries to organs, such as the liver and bladder. It can be difficult to diagnose the source of bleeding and prioritize treatment. Traditional methods for early detection of intracavitary hemorrhage, such as focused assessment with sonography in trauma (FAST) and diagnostic peritoneal lavage lack sensitivity for retroperitoneal pelvic hemorrhage. Clinical suspicion of pelvic fracture–associated retroperitoneal hemorrhage should increase in the hemodynamically unstable blunt trauma patient with an unremarkable chest x-ray, a negative FAST examination, and uninjured extremities. Although many authors report that more than 80% of pelvic fracture–associated hemorrhage is venous in origin, little scientific evidence exists to support this statement, and the exact role of pelvic arteriography continues to evolve.

Several studies have examined the role of contrast-enhanced computed tomography (CT) in the detection of arterial hemorrhage in blunt pelvic trauma and in predicting which patients might derive benefit from pelvic angiography and embolization. Cerva [2] retrospectively reviewed 30 patients with pelvic fractures who underwent both CT and pelvic angiography, and found that contrast extravasation or "blush" on CT had 84%

sensitivity, 85% specificity, and 90% accuracy for prediction of arterial injury or hemorrhage on angiography. A subsequent study by Stephen et al. [3] found contrast extravasation on CT to have 80% sensitivity and 98% specificity for arterial hemorrhage on subsequent angiography. Positive predictive value of a contrast blush was 80%, and negative predictive value was 98%. Pereira et al. [4] performed a retrospective study of 290 patients with pelvic fracture who underwent contrast-enhanced CT and noted contrast extravasation in 4.5%. More than two-thirds of the patients with contrast extravasation had evidence of hemodynamic instability, and all of these patients underwent therapeutic embolization. Overall sensitivity, specificity, and accuracy of CT for identifying patients requiring embolization were 90%, 98.6%, and 98.3%, respectively. In an endorsement of CT to identify pelvic fracture bleeding, the Eastern Association for the Surgery of Trauma group [5] reviewed radiologic findings predictive of hemorrhage. They found that patients with a pelvic hematoma >500 $cm^3$ in size had an increased likelihood of arterial injury and need for angiography. However, they also stated that lack of contrast extravasation on CT does not always exclude active hemorrhage. This was supported in a paper by Brasel et al. [6], who retrospectively reviewed their experience with 604 patients with pelvic fractures who underwent contrast-enhanced CT. Patients with contrast extravasation had a higher mean injury severity score (ISS) (24.5 vs. 18.3, $p < 0.001$) and higher mortality (24% vs. 6%, $p < 0.001$). However, therapeutic angioembolization was required in 33% of patients without contrast extravasation on CT. One possible explanation for this observation is a transient arterial hemorrhage that abated either during or shortly after the CT scan. ISS has been promoted as a better predictor of pelvic hemorrhage than the fracture pattern alone [5,7,8].

Miller et al. [9] examined the utility of clinical signs of ongoing hemorrhage for predicting the need for therapeutic angioembolization of arterial injuries. Thirty-five patients with hypotension attributable to pelvic fracture were retrospectively evaluated. One or more episodes of hypotension following resuscitation with ≤2 units of packed red blood cells (PRBCs) had 73% positive predictive value for arterial bleeding requiring embolization. The authors concluded that in the absence of other sources of hemorrhage, inadequate response to resuscitation should prompt early pelvic angiography.

*Recommendation*: Patients with evidence of extravasation on contrast-enhanced CT of the pelvis should undergo urgent pelvic angiography and embolization (Grade B). However, the absence of contrast extravasation should not preclude consideration of angiography, as bleeding may be transient in nature and ISS may be more predictive of the need for angiography. Patients with hemodynamic instability, pelvic fracture, and no obvious extrapelvic source of hemorrhage warrant consideration of pelvic angiography.

## 28.3 What Is the Role of Extraperitoneal Pelvic Packing in Hemodynamically Unstable Patients with Pelvic Fractures?

Current management of patients with hemodynamic instability related to hemorrhage from pelvic fracture has generally focused on mechanical stabilization of the pelvis, angiographic embolization of arterial hemorrhage, and prompt initiation of a balanced resuscitation. However, the belief that most pelvic hemorrhage is venous in origin coupled with the success of damage control packing techniques has generated renewed interest in pelvic packing as an adjunctive maneuver for control of pelvic hemorrhage. Extraperitoneal packing is accomplished via a lower midline incision, with division of the skin, subcutaneous tissue, and anterior rectus sheath. The preperitoneal space is entered, and blunt dissection is used to fully develop an extraperitoneal "pocket" that extends from the symphysis pubis to the sacroiliac joint. Three or four laparotomy pads are placed on each side, and the midline incision closed. The procedure may be followed by mechanical stabilization of the pelvis, laparotomy, or angiography as needed. Packs are generally removed after 24–48 h when hemodynamic stability has been achieved. Although the technique has achieved modest utilization in Europe [10], it did not generate much interest in North America until 2005, when a preliminary report by Smith et al. [11] described two blunt trauma patients with pelvic fracture–associated hemorrhage who underwent extraperitoneal packing and survived to hospital discharge.

In a larger, more recent study, Tötterman et al. [12] published a retrospective review of 18 pelvic trauma patients, who underwent extraperitoneal pelvic packing as part of an institutional protocol for control of massive pelvic hemorrhage. Thirty-day survival was 72%, and the authors reported a significant increase in systolic blood pressure (SBP) upon completion of pelvic packing ($p = 0.002$). Only one of the nonsurvivors was considered to have died of exsanguination rather than the associated injury. Interestingly, angiography performed after pelvic injury was positive for arterial injury in 80% of patients, suggesting that the presumed venous nature of pelvic hemorrhage is widely overstated.

Based largely on the aforementioned studies and their own clinical experience, Cothren et al. [13] adopted a clinical pathway for hemodynamically unstable patients with pelvic fracture that included aggressive use of extraperitoneal pelvic packing in addition to the mechanical stabilization and angiographic embolization. Twenty-eight patients underwent pelvic packing during a 1.5-year period and the mortality rate was 25%, which the authors felt was lower than expected for the injury severity in the group. Of note, no deaths were attributed to exsanguination from pelvic hemorrhage.

*Recommendation*: Although there are no prospective data, the technique of extraperitoneal pelvic packing appears to be a useful adjunct in hemodynamically unstable patients with suspected or actual pelvic fracture–associated hemorrhage. Limited retrospective studies support the concept of using extraperitoneal packing to achieve tamponade before or after mechanical stabilization (Grade C). This technique may be used as an adjunct to angiographic embolization of arterial hemorrhage.

## 28.4 What Is the Role of Intra-Aortic Balloon Occlusion to Salvage Patients with Uncontrolled Hemorrhagic Shock from Pelvic Fractures?

Although both venous and arterial bleeding may occur in pelvic fractures, hemorrhagic shock occurs primarily because of arterial hemorrhage [14,15]. Intra-aortic balloon occlusion (IABO) has been described for the treatment of hemorrhagic shock in cases of ruptured abdominal aortic aneurysms [16], abdominal trauma [17], and postpartum hemorrhage [18]. In the trauma setting, the procedure is more commonly referred to as resuscitative endovascular balloon occlusion of the aorta. In pelvic fractures with uncontrolled hemorrhage, balloon occlusion of the iliac artery has been proposed [19]. However, a blind technique for insertion of the balloon catheter into the infrarenal aorta has been described, eliminating the need for fluoroscopic guidance and permitting earlier control of bleeding in the emergency department. Martinelli et al. [20] evaluated 2064 patients with pelvic fractures, of which 13 underwent IABO to control massive pelvic bleeding. They performed the procedure in the emergency department with an intensive care unit physician, trauma surgeon, and interventional radiologist present. The procedure was performed by the senior interventional radiologist with access through the common femoral artery. A balloon was inserted through a 10F introducer sheath, inflated, and pulled back until wedged in the aortic bifurcation. The balloon was subsequently advanced 5 cm cephalad and inflated in the infrarenal aorta. Occlusion was confirmed by the bilateral absence of femoral pulses. All balloons were successfully placed and an immediate increase in SBP (70 mmHg, $p = 0.011$) was observed. Of the 13 patients, 12 were successfully transported to the angiographic suite after IABO; the 13th died prior to transport from the resuscitation area. Subsequent angiography was positive for arterial injury in 92% of patients, and nine underwent embolization. Overall survival was 46% (6 of 13) and was inversely related to length of inflation (survivors 46 min vs. nonsurvivors 91 min, $p = 0.026$) and mean ISS ($p = 0.011$). The authors concluded that IABO could be lifesaving in the management of uncontrolled hemorrhage in pelvic fractures by enabling transport to an angiography suite for definitive treatment.

Correct placement of the balloon has been described without fluoroscopic guidance. Brenner et al. successfully described fluoroscopy-free IABO of the descending aorta and infrarenal aorta by trauma and acute care surgeons following instruction and training in the procedure [21,22].

Although exciting as a potentially lifesaving procedure in hemorrhagic shock, the consequences of "delayed" multiple organ failure after aggressive fluid resuscitation for severe hemorrhage is well described [23]. As a result, investigators have studied the physiology of IABO in shock. Markov et al. induced shock in a swine model and showed that IABO improved mean central aortic pressures; however, lactate burdens increased [24]. Greater interleukin 6 release has also been shown in animals undergoing successful hemorrhage control with IABO [25].

*Recommendation*: Although there are no prospective data, the use of IABO for hemorrhage control in pelvic fractures appears to be a useful adjunct in hemodynamically unstable patients with suspected or actual pelvic fracture–associated hemorrhage. Limited retrospective and clinical case studies support the concept of using IABO to achieve tamponade before angioembolization (Grade C).

## 28.5 What Is the Role of Tranexamic Acid in Patients with Pelvic Fracture–Associated Hemorrhage?

Both major surgery and trauma resulting in severe blood loss can initiate similar hemostatic responses, particularly regarding coagulation. One part of that response is stimulation of clot breakdown (fibrinolysis), leading in some cases to hyperfibrinolysis. Antifibrinolytic agents have been shown to reduce blood loss in patients with both normal and deranged fibrinolytic responses to these stressors [26]. Tranexamic acid (TXA) is a synthetic derivative of the natural amino acid lysine, which inhibits fibrinolysis by blocking the lysine binding sites on plasminogen [27].

The use of antifibrinolytic agents, including TXA has been reported to reduce blood loss following major orthopedic surgery [28]. The blood loss occurred after staging, bilateral total hip arthroplasty with the TXA group experiencing significant (580 ± 237 mL vs. 869 ± 363 mL; $p < 0.001$) reductions in blood loss during the first 24 h of the postoperative period. Additional studies have demonstrated similar results in hip, knee, and pediatric and adult spine surgeries [28–30]. TXA has also been shown to be cost-effective compared with transfusion [31].

The collaborators of the CRASH-2 trial investigated the effects of TXA in trauma patients with significant hemorrhage [32] during a randomized controlled trial involving 274 hospitals in 40 countries. The study enrolled 20,211 adult trauma patients who had or were at risk for significant bleeding. The patients were assigned to receive TXA (loading dose 1 g over 10 min, followed by an infusion of 1 g over 8 h) or matching placebo. TXA was associated with a 1.5% reduction in 28-day all-cause mortality in adult trauma patients with signs of bleeding (SBP <90 mmHg, heart rate >100 beats/min, or both, within 8 h of injury). TXA had the greatest impact on reducing death caused by bleeding in the severe shock group (SBP ≤75 mmHg) (14.9% vs. 18.4%; RR, 0.81; 95% confidence interval [CI], 0.69–0.95). Early TXA (≤1 h from injury) was associated with the greatest reduction (32%) in deaths caused by bleeding (5.3% vs. 7.7%; RR, 0.68; 95% CI, 0.57–0.82; $p < 0.0001$). However, TXA given between 1 and 3 h also reduced the risk of death (4.8% vs. 6.1%; RR, 0.79; 95% CI, 0.64–0.97; $p = 0.03$). In addition, TXA treatment was not associated with an increased risk of vascular occlusive events.

Despite a subtle but significant outcome benefit, the clinical application of the CRASH-2 study results was challenged by several factors, including the inclusion criteria that diluted outpatients who were actually bleeding and the increase in risk of death due to bleeding if TXA was administered beyond 3 h. The MATTERS study [33] specifically addressed a cohort of patients who were actively bleeding. This retrospective observational study compared TXA with no TXA in patients receiving at least 1 unit of PRBCs. A subgroup of patients receiving massive transfusion (≥10 units of PRBCS) was also examined. Overall, the TXA group had lower mortality than the no-TXA group (17.4% vs. 23.9%, $p = 0.03$). This benefit was greatest in the massive transfusion group (14.4% vs. 28.1%, $p = 0.004$). The MATTERS study further supports the CRASH-2 trial in demonstrating an early mortality benefit and neutral risk profile.

There are still unanswered questions regarding use of TXA in the trauma population. Because the CRASH-2 trial did not assess fibrinolysis or coagulation testing, the mechanism by which TXA reduced mortality is unknown.

*Recommendation*: TXA use may be considered as a therapeutic adjunct in adult trauma patients with severe hemorrhagic shock (SBP ≤75 mmHg), those with known predictors of fibrinolysis, those with known fibrinolysis based on laboratory assessment, and those requiring massive blood transfusion. TXA should be administered less than 3 h from the time of injury, according to the following regimen: 1 g administered intravenously over 10 min and then 1 g administered intravenously over 8 h (Grade B).

## 28.6 What Is the Role of Fecal Diversion in Open Pelvic Fractures?

Open pelvic fracture is an uncommon clinical entity typically associated with high-energy blunt mechanisms and crush injuries. Historically, clinicians have voiced concern about communication of open perineal wounds with pelvic fractures generating an unacceptably high rate of osteomyelitis and pelvic sepsis. The practice of routine performance of a diverting colostomy in patients with open pelvic fractures arose largely based on this concern. However, few studies exist that provide scientific support for this practice, and the available data are further compromised by a lack of clearly accepted criteria for defining the anatomy and severity of open pelvic fractures. For example, most studies are of a heterogeneous patient population that includes full thickness rectal injuries, vaginal tears, perineal wounds, buttock lacerations, and groin wounds.

Raffa and Christensen [34] retrospectively reviewed 16 patients with open pelvic fracture and observed a high rate of sepsis and death in patients managed without colostomy, or in those who underwent delayed colostomy. This observation led the authors to strongly recommend fecal diversion in all patients with open fractures of the pelvis. One of the first large retrospective studies of open pelvic fracture was performed by Richardson in 1982 [35]. Thirty-seven patients were treated at a single center, of which 27 (73%) underwent diverting colostomy. The authors noted a correlation between wound location and infection. No patients with anterior wounds developed an infection, irrespective of fecal diversion, while infection was common with perineal wounds (43% in the colostomy group and 100% in patients in whom colostomy was not performed). Wounds of the buttock region fell into an intermediate category, with no infections in the colostomy group and 67% infection rate in those not receiving a colostomy. Infectious complications also increased when colostomy was delayed for more than 48 h, and all three patients who underwent fecal diversion more than 72 h after admission developed infections. No $p$ values were reported, making determinations of statistical significance difficult.

Apparently contradictory results were obtained by Faringer et al. [36], who retrospectively reviewed their experience with 33 open pelvic fracture patients. Although their overall mortality rate was relatively low (15%), wound infections occurred more commonly in the colostomy group than in those without fecal diversion (31% vs. 19%). This finding prompted the authors to suggest a more selective policy of fecal diversion in the setting of open pelvic fracture.

Jones et al. [37] performed a multicenter, retrospective analysis of 39 patients, who sustained open pelvic fractures. Overall mortality in the series was 25%, and associated extrapelvic injuries were present in 97% of patients. Of the eight patients who developed sepsis, seven had rectal injuries and one did not. Although the authors did not define the term "sepsis," the association with rectal injury was statistically significant ($p < 0.001$). The presence of a rectal tear ($p = 0.12$) and delay in performance of diverting colostomy ($p = 0.16$) showed nonsignificant trends toward correlation with mortality.

More recently, Pell et al. [38] performed a retrospective analysis of 14 patients with open pelvic fractures treated at a single center. Nine patients (64%) with nonperineal wounds did not undergo fecal diversion, and five (36%) with perineal wounds underwent colostomy. No patients with anterior wounds and an intact fecal stream developed pelvic sepsis. The authors concluded that colostomy might not be necessary in all patients with open pelvic fractures, particularly those with anterior wounds.

A systematic review of fecal diversion in preventing infection in the setting of open pelvic fracture was performed by Lunsjo and Abu-Zidan [39]. When the available data were pooled, no significant reduction in the rate of infectious complications was noted when colostomy was performed (38% infection rate in the colostomy group vs. 35% in the noncolostomy group, $p = 0.86$). Similarly, no significant benefit for sepsis-related mortality was noted in patients undergoing fecal diversion (15% for the colostomy group vs. 9% for the noncolostomy group, $p = 0.35$).

*Recommendation*: Diverting colostomy is not mandatory in all patients with open pelvic fractures. Selective application of fecal diversion in patients with rectal injuries or perineal wounds may be justified (Grade B).

## 28.7 Is Plain Radiography of the Pelvis Necessary in Stable Patients with Blunt Trauma to the Torso?

Current Advanced Trauma Life Support guidelines indicate that plain x-rays of the pelvis should be obtained in most patients sustaining blunt trauma to the torso [40]. This recommendation is intended to facilitate diagnosis of pelvic fracture early in the course of the evaluation of blunt trauma victims. However, the utility of this practice has recently been called into question, as CT of the abdomen and pelvis is obtained in the majority of hemodynamically stable patients with significant blunt torso trauma. Proponents of eliminating plain radiographs of the pelvis cite the superior sensitivity, specificity, and accuracy of CT for fractures of the pelvis, and find little clinical significance in the slight delay added by transportation to the CT scanner.

Guillamondequi et al. [41] performed a retrospective review of 686 patients with blunt trauma undergoing CT of the abdomen and pelvis. Of these, for 311 patients (45%), plain x-rays of the pelvis had been performed. The false-negative rate for pelvic radiography was 32%, and of the patients with a positive pelvic x-ray, 55% were noted to have additional fractures or a higher injury grade on CT scan.

In a more recent retrospective review of 129 stable blunt trauma patients, Kessel et al. [42] found that CT diagnosed 36% more pelvic fractures than plain radiography, with CT findings leading to pelvic angiography in 15% of these patients. In this study, the authors found that plain x-rays of the pelvis did not alter management.

Obaid et al. [43] performed a retrospective review of 174 trauma patients who underwent both CT and plain radiography of the pelvis. The false-negative rate for plain x-ray in this study was 22%, with 51% of patients underdiagnosed by plain x-ray. Additionally, they found that pelvic fracture patients with hypotension or transfusion requirements in the emergency department were more likely to require an angiogram (17% vs. 0%, $p < 0.0001$) and therapeutic embolization (9% vs. 0%, $p < 0.001$). The authors concluded that plain radiographs of the pelvis are of little value in hemodynamically stable patients, but that plain x-ray may have continued utility as a screening tool in unstable patients or those requiring blood transfusion.

*Recommendation*: In settings where multidetector CT is readily available, plain radiography of the pelvis adds little information and may be safely omitted in the majority of hemodynamically stable blunt trauma patients. Plain pelvic x-ray appears to have a continued role in triaging unstable patients or those requiring early blood transfusion (Grade B).

**TABLE 28.1**

Summary of Evidence and Recommendations

| Question | Answer | Level of Evidence | Grade of Recommendation | References |
|---|---|---|---|---|
| When is pelvic angiography and embolization indicated? | Contrast extravasation on CT. Hypotension with pelvic fracture and the absence of extrapelvic injury. | 2b | B | [2–9] |
| Does extraperitoneal pelvic packing aid in hemostasis? | Probably, in selected cases. | 4 | C | [10–13] |
| Does IABO aid in hemostasis? | Probably, in severe cases. | 4 | C | [20–22] |
| Should TXA be given routinely to facilitate hemostasis? | Probably, in cases of severe hemorrhage. | 2b | B | [28,31] |
| | Prophylactic use in the elective setting appears to diminish blood loss and is cost-effective. There is evidence to consider use in trauma. | 2c, 3 | B | [32,33] |
| Is fecal diversion mandatory in all patients with open pelvic fractures? | No. Fecal diversion should be considered in patients with rectal or perineal wounds. | 2a | B | [34–39] |
| Is plain radiography of the pelvis necessary in all blunt trauma patients? | No. In stable patients undergoing CT scanning, plain pelvic x-ray adds little information. | 3b | B | [40–43] |
| What is the optimal timing for operative pelvic fixation? | 3–7 days postinjury. | 2c | B | [44,45] |

## 28.8 What Is the Optimal Timing for Operative Pelvic Stabilization?

Controversy persists regarding the optimal timing of operative fixation of the pelvis. Proponents of an aggressive policy of early operative stabilization cite decreased blood loss, improved hemodynamics, decreased resuscitation requirements, earlier mobilization, and diminished pain. However, pelvic stabilization has been frequently a long, technically demanding procedure that may represent a "second hit" (after the initial trauma), which in turn increases the risk of multiple organ dysfunction syndrome (MODS). This concern, coupled with the relative success of "damage control" surgical techniques for abbreviating operations in unstable trauma patients, has generated increased interest in delaying definitive pelvic fixation until well after the initial resuscitation period.

Probst et al. [44] examined the relationship between timing and duration of operative pelvic stabilization on outcome. They retrospectively analyzed 290 patients with pelvic ring fractures undergoing operative stabilization. They observed that late operation (>3 days after admission) was associated with lower rates of MODS, renal failure, and death as compared with early (day 0) or intermediate (days 1–3) operation ($p < 0.025$). Long procedures (>3 h) were associated with a significantly higher incidence of hepatic dysfunction, but the length of the procedure did not correlate with MODS incidence or mortality. Additional delay of surgery does not appear to provide further benefit. In a retrospective review of 151 pelvic fracture patients, Connor [45] found that patients undergoing operative fixation within 1 week of injury had fewer pulmonary complications, reduced hospital length of stay, and reduced cost of care as compared with patients undergoing delayed surgery (Table 28.1).

*Recommendation*: Pelvic fractures should be repaired after the patient is fully resuscitated. Optimal timing of operative repair appears to be between 3 and 7 days postinjury (Grade B). Further delay may increase pulmonary complications and cost and therefore should be considered only when extrapelvic injuries or physiologic status preclude surgery within the first week.

## References

1. Mucha P, Farnell MB. Analysis of pelvic fracture management. *J Trauma*. 1984;24(5):379–386.
2. Cerva DS, Mirvis SE, Shanmuganathan K et al. Detection of bleeding in patients with major pelvic fractures: Value of contrast-enhanced CT. *Am J Roentgenol*. 1996;16(1):131–135.
3. Stephen DJ, Kreder HJ, Day AC et al. Early detection of arterial bleeding in acute pelvic trauma. *J Trauma*. 1999;47(4):638–642.
4. Pereira SJ, O'Brien DP, Luchette FA et al. Dynamic helical computed tomography scan accurately detects hemorrhage in patients with pelvic fracture. *Surgery*. 2000;128(4):678–685.
5. Cullinane DC, Schiller HJ, Zielinski MD et al. Eastern Association for the Surgery of Trauma practice management guidelines in pelvic fracture-update and systematic review. *J Trauma*. 2011;71(6):1850–1868.

6. Brasel KJ, Pham K, Yang H et al. Significance of contrast extravasation in patients with pelvic fracture. *J Trauma.* 2007;62(5):1149–1152.
7. Eastridge BJ, Starr A, Minei JP et al. The importance of fracture pattern in guiding therapeutic decision-making in patients with hemorrhagic shock and pelvic ring disruptions. *J Trauma.* 2002;53:446–450.
8. Lunsjo K, Tadros A, Hauggaard A et al. Associated injuries and not fracture instability predict mortality in pelvic fractures: A prospective study of 100 patients. *J Trauma.* 2007;62:687–691.
9. Miller PR, Moore PS, Mansell E et al. External fixation or arteriogram in bleeding pelvic fracture: Initial therapy guided by markers of arterial hemorrhage. *J Trauma.* 2003;54(3):437–443.
10. Ertel W, Keel M, Eid K et al. Control of hemorrhage using c-clamp and pelvic packing in multiply injured patients with pelvic ring disruption. *J Orthop Trauma.* 2001;15(7):468–474.
11. Smith WR, Moore EE, Osborn P et al. Retroperitoneal packing as a resuscitation technique for hemodynamically unstable patients with pelvic fractures: Report of two representative cases and a description of technique. *J Trauma.* 2005;59(6):1510–1514.
12. Tötterman A, Madsen JE, Skaga NO et al. Extraperitoneal pelvic packing: A salvage procedure to control massive traumatic pelvic hemorrhage. *J Trauma.* 2007;62(4):843–852.
13. Cothren CC, Osborn PM, Moore EE et al. Preperitoneal pelvic packing for hemodynamically unstable pelvic fractures: A paradigm shift. *J Trauma.* 2007;62(4):834–842.
14. Dondelinger RF, Trotteur G, Ghaye B et al. Traumatic injuries: Radiological hemostatic intervention at admission. *Eur Radiol.* 2002;12:979–993.
15. Ben-Menachem Y, Coldwell DM, Young JW et al. Hemorrhage associated with pelvic fractures: Causes, diagnosis, and emergent management. *AJR.* 1991;157:1005–1014.
16. Assar AN, Zarins CK. Ednovascular proximal control of ruptured abdominal aortic aneurysms: The internal aortic clamp. *J Cardiovasc Surg.* 2009;50:381–385.
17. Gupta BK, Khaneja SC, Flores L et al. The role of intra-aortic balloon occlusion in penetrating abdominal trauma. *J Trauma.* 1998;29:861–865.
18. Harma M, Harma M, Kunt AS et al. Balloon occlusion of the descending aorta in the treatment of severe post-partum haemorrhage. *Aust N Z J Obstet Gynaecol.* 2004;44:170–171.
19. Rieger J, Linsenmaier U, Euler E et al. Temporary balloon occlusion as therapy of uncontrollable arterial hemorrhage in multiple trauma patients. *Rofo.* 1999;70:80–83.
20. Martinelli T, Thony F, Declety P et al. Intra-aortic balloon occlusion to salvage patients with life-threatening hemorrhagic shocks from pelvic fractures. *J Trauma.* 2010;68(4):942–948.
21. Brenner ML, Moore LJ, DuBose JJ et al. A clinical series of resuscitative endovascular balloon occlusion of the aorta for hemorrhage control and resuscitation. *J Trauma Acute Care Surg.* 2013;75(3):506–511.
22. Scott DJ, Eliason JL, Villamaria C et al. A novel fluoroscopy-free, resuscitative endovascular aortic balloon occlusion system in a model of hemorrhagic shock. *J Trauma Acute Care Surg.* 2013;75(1):122–128.
23. Cotton BA, Guy JS, Morris JA, Jr. et al. The cellular, metabolic, and systemic consequences of aggressive fluid resuscitation strategies. *Shock.* 2006;26(2):115–121.
24. Markov NP, Percival TJ, Morrison JJ et al. Physiologic tolerance of descending thoracic aortic balloon occlusion in a swine model of hemorrhagic shock. *Surgery.* 2013;153(6):848–856.
25. Morrison JJ, Ross JD, Markov NP et al. The inflammatory sequelae of aortic balloon occlusion in hemorrhagic shock. *J Surg Res.* 2014;191(2):423–431.
26. Henry DA, Carless PA, Moxey AJ et al. Antifibrinolytic use for minimising perioperative allogeneic blood transfusion. *Cochrane Database Syst Rev.* 2007;4:CD001886.
27. Okamoto S, Hijikata-Okunomiya A, Wanaka K et al. Enzymes controlling medicines: Introduction. *Semin Thromb Hemost.* 1997;23:493–501.
28. Eubanks JD. Antifibrinolytics in major orthopedic surgery. *J Am Acad Orthop Surg.* 2010;18(3):132–138.
29. Yamasaki S, Masuhara K, Fuji T. Tranexamic acid reduces postoperative blood loss in cementless total hip arthroplasty. *Int Orthop.* 2004;28(2):69–73.
30. Imai N, Dohmae Y, Suda K et al. Tranexamic acid for reduction of blood loss during total hip arthroplasty. *J Arthroplasty.* 2012;27(10):1838–1843.
31. Sepah YJ, Umer M, Ahmad T et al. Use of tranexamic acid is a cost-effective method in preventing blood loss during and after total knee replacement. *J Orthop Surg Res.* 2011;6:22–26.
32. CRASH-2 Trial Collaborators. Effects of tranexamic acid on death, vascular occlusive events, and blood transfusion in trauma patients with significant haemorrhage (CRASH-2): A randomized, placebo-controlled trial. *Lancet.* 2010;376:23–32.
33. Morrison JJ, Dubose KK, Rasmussen TE et al. Military application of Tranexamic Acid in trauma emergency resuscitation (MATTERs) study. *Arch Surg.* 2012;147(2):113–119.
34. Raffa J, Christensen NM. Compound fractures of the pelvis. *Am J Surg.* 1976;132:282–286.
35. Richardson JD, Harty J, Amin M et al. Open pelvic fractures. *J Trauma.* 1982;22(7):533–538.
36. Faringer PD, Mullins RJ, Feliciano PD et al. Selective fecal diversion in complex open pelvic fractures from blunt trauma. *Arch Surg.* 1994;129(9):958–963.
37. Jones AL, Powell JN, Kellam JF et al. Open pelvic fractures: A multicenter retrospective analysis. *Orthop Clin North Am.* 1997;28(3):345–350.
38. Pell M, Flynn WJ, Seibel RW. Is colostomy always necessary in the treatment of open pelvic fractures? *J Trauma.* 1998;45(2):371–373.
39. Lunsjo K, Abu-Zidan FM. Does colostomy prevent infection in open blunt pelvic fractures? A systematic review. *J Trauma.* 2006;60(5):1145–1148.
40. American College of Surgeons. 2004. *Advanced Trauma Life Support for Doctors*, 7th edn. American College of Surgeons: Chicago, IL.

41. Guillamondequi OD, Pryor JP, Gracias VH et al. Pelvic radiography in blunt trauma resuscitation: A diminishing role. *J Trauma*. 2002;53(6):1043–1047.
42. Kessel B, Sevi R, Jeroukhimov I et al. Is routine portable pelvic x-ray in stable trauma patients always justified in a high technology era? *Injury*. 2007;38(5):559–563.
43. Obaid AK, Barleben A, Porral D et al. Utility of plain film pelvic radiographs in blunt trauma patients in the emergency department. *Am Surg*. 2006;72(10):951–954.
44. Probst C, Probst T, Gaensslen A et al. Timing and duration of initial pelvic stabilization after multiple trauma in patients from the German trauma registry: Is there an influence on outcome? *J Trauma*. 2007;62(2):370–377.
45. Connor GS, McGwin G, MacLennan PA et al. Early versus delayed fixation of pelvic ring fractures. *Am Surg*. 2003;69(12):1019–1023.

## Commentary on Pelvic Fractures

*Joseph P. Minei*

I often comment to my residents that trauma is a team sport, perhaps most evident in the treatment of complex pelvic fractures. Here the trauma surgeon, orthopedic surgeon, interventional radiologist, and other subspecialists often have to come together to devise a care plan in the setting of multiple competing priorities. Do I take the patient to the OR first or angiography? If we take the patient to the OR first, what procedure should be performed—external fixation of the pelvis, exploratory laparotomy, or extraperitoneal pelvic packing? These questions become very real when one is faced with an unstable patient with a complex pelvic fracture and concerns for an intra-abdominal bleeding source.

### Which Patients with Pelvic Fractures Warrant Early Angiography with Arterial Angioembolization?

The first question to be asked centers around hemodynamic status. Hemodynamically normal patients with pelvic fractures can undergo a series of tests to determine the likelihood of pelvic arterial bleeding and subsequent need for angioembolization. The fact that they have presented with normal vital signs already suggests they will not need invasive procedures to control bleeding. Those that are abnormal do not have the luxury of time and decisions must be made often with limited data. One of the first things I look at is the pelvic fracture type. I use the Young-Burgess classification* and will obtain an early pelvic plain film on these patients. If the patient has a low-grade LC or APC fracture, I am less concerned that they have substantial pelvic bleeding. If a patient has any of the high-grade fracture types, our next maneuver is to place a pelvic binder. The idea here is to stabilize fracture edges to prevent further damage to soft tissue and pelvic vessels as well as to reduce the pelvic volume of potential space that the patient can bleed into. Often, placing the pelvic binder results in substantial hemodynamic improvement.

At this point, I will pull together my known data. Is the FAST positive in multiple views and does the patient remain hemodynamically abnormal despite fluid and blood resuscitation? If yes, I am likely going to the OR for abdominal exploration. If no, I am heading to CT scan of the abdomen and pelvis. Factors that determine the need for subsequent angioembolization include free extravasation of contrast and size of the pelvic hematoma. All patients with free extravasation on CT scan will go to IR for angiography and embolization as needed. Patients without free extravasation, but who have (or had) abnormal vital signs will go to IR if they have a large pelvic hematoma and no source of cavitary bleeding elsewhere. Those with minimal pelvic hematomas will not go to IR.

### What Is the Role of Extraperitoneal Pelvic Packing in Hemodynamically Unstable Patients with Pelvic Fractures?

This issue comes back to the multidisciplinary nature of managing complex pelvic fractures. Our institutional protocol has IR ready for a patient within 30 min of request for pelvic angiography. Thus, our protocol is to consider angiography prior to any attempt at pelvic packing. The simple fact of the matter is that pelvic packing cannot control deep tissue arterial hemorrhage, particularly when it is from vessels that may be just outside the pelvis. Further, we have had excellent results controlling venous bleeding with mechanical stabilization from an externally placed pelvic binder. If IR consultants are not readily available, consideration for extraperitoneal pelvic packing might take on a higher priority.

In my opinion, there may be a role for pelvic packing in the setting of the patient who is being operated on for intra-abdominal bleeding. The potential use of pelvic packing has to be considered before the incision is made in order to separate the upper intra-abdominal incision from the lower extraperitoneal pelvic packing incision. If, during laparotomy, there is an expanding pelvic hematoma, a case can be made for extraperitoneal pelvic packing.

### What Is the Role of Intra-Aortic Balloon Occlusion (IABO) to Salvage Patients with Uncontrolled Hemorrhagic Shock from Pelvic Fractures?

In my opinion, while an exciting concept, the use of IABO or REBOA needs data before it can be recommended. The concept makes physiologic sense and the animal data is promising. However, there is very limited prospective data in humans and the procedure itself is not without potential peril. I agree with the authors that caution must be extended before recommendations can be made. A number of issues arise when discussing this procedure. How will trauma

* Young JW, Burgess AR, Brumback RJ, Poka A. Pelvic fractures: Value of plain radiography in early assessment and management. *Radiology.* 1986;160:445–451.

surgeons obtain the skills to perform this procedure and perhaps more importantly, how will they maintain those skills. The need for this procedure is rare. Even if one practices at the busiest of trauma centers, the likelihood of performing this procedure will also be infrequent. Perhaps with the use of hybrid ORs and duel trained trauma surgeons in vascular and endovascular techniques, expansion of this technique will be possible in the future.

### What Is the Role of Tranexamic Acid (TXA) in Patients with Pelvic Fracture–Associated Hemorrhage?

The use of TXA should not be limited to pelvic fracture–associated hemorrhage. The authors distill the data from the CRASH-2 and MATTERS trials and have made the appropriate recommendations. The use of TXA should be considered for all patients that have activation of a massive transfusion protocol as long as it is within the appropriate window of 3 h from the time of injury.

The use of viscoelastic analysis of coagulation either by TEG or TEM has gained significant interest in the trauma literature in recent years. The ability of viscoelastic analysis to complement traditional PT/PTT analysis by providing detail about specific phases of the clotting cascade as well as fibrinolysis activity gives the trauma surgeon the ability to target blood component therapy to address the specific defect. A small minority of severely injured patients have hyperfibrinolysis. These patients also have mortality rates approaching 100%. In the setting of hyperfibrinolysis, the role of TXA doses above the standard recommendation given in this chapter is being debated and investigated.

### What Is the Role of Fecal Diversion in Open Pelvic Fractures?

As the authors note, the quality of data evaluating the role of colostomy in patients with open pelvic fractures is wanting. The series are small and likely heterogeneous, including all patients with open pelvic fractures regardless where the wound is in relation to the fecal stream. Further, patients with and without rectal or vaginal tears are included in these studies. The author's recommendation seems appropriate and follows my own bias: divert those whose open wounds are in close proximity to the fecal stream. This would include all those with a rectal or vaginal laceration as well as those with perineal wounds not including the rectum/anus but in close proximity. The further the open wound is from the fecal stream, the less likely a colostomy is needed, particularly if the injury did not result in incontinence.

### Is Plain Radiography of the Pelvis Necessary in Stable Patients with Blunt Trauma to the Torso?

The author's recommendation follows my bias and was noted above in commentary to question 1. In unstable patients, the presence of a pelvic fracture seen by plain film taken in the ED will alter my decision tree and management scheme. The role of pelvic plain films in hemodynamically normal patients can probably be omitted if the patient is going to undergo abdominal and pelvic CT scan for other diagnostic purposes. Finally, in the ambulating trauma patient without complaints or findings on physical exam referable to the abdomen or torso, the pelvic plain film and CT scan can be omitted from the diagnostic work-up.

### What Is the Optimal Timing for Operative Pelvic Stabilization?

Orthopedic management of pelvic fractures has evolved significantly over the last decade. The use of percutaneous screw fixation techniques has significantly reduced the morbidity and blood loss associated with large incision, open fracture fixation. Further, recent publications from the Inflammation and Host Response to Injury consortium (Trauma Glue Grant) revealed no clinical or genetic basis for the second hit hypothesis and the development of multiple organ dysfunction, a hypothesis that has now fallen out of favor[*][†]. There appears to be no good reason to delay pelvic fracture fixation beyond the prerequisite need for a hemodynamically normal, resuscitated patient. Add to this modern techniques of percutaneous screw fixation of pelvic fractures and many patients can be fixed on postinjury day 1 or 2, allowing them to get out of bed earlier and start the rehabilitation process sooner, often leading to decreased pulmonary morbidity.

---

* Xiao W, Mindrinos MN, Seok J et al. A genomic storm in critically injured humans. *J Exp Med.* 2011;208:2581–2590.

† Minei JP, Cuschieri J, Sperry J et al. The changing pattern and implications of multiple organ failure after blunt injury with hemorrhagic shock. *Crit Care Med.* 2012;40:1129–1135.

# 29

# Evidence-Based Approach to Extremity Vascular Trauma

**Elizabeth Windell and Terence O'Keeffe**

**CONTENTS**



## 29.1 Introduction

Vascular injury caused by trauma remains a significant cause for mortality and morbidity in the injured patient, as it can be responsible for up to 20% of trauma deaths and is one of the highest hospital resource utilizers [1]. Vascular surgery has changed dramatically over the past decade, including the diagnosis and management of acute traumatic vascular injuries. There is a growing body of clinical trials and evidence on which to base both diagnostic and therapeutic decisions in the acutely injured trauma patient with extremity vascular injury.

In this chapter, recent data regarding the diagnosis and management of acute traumatic vascular injuries of the extremities are presented, divided into relevant clinical questions, with recommendations based on the most recent evidence.

## 29.2 Can a Diagnosis of Vascular Injury Be Adequately Made by Physical Exam Supplemented with the Ankle-Brachial Pressure Index?

Following the recognition that mandatory angiography was not required for penetrating wounds in close proximity to vessels, the role of physical examination in evaluating the presence or absence of vascular injury has been more closely scrutinized [2]. In 1998, Dennis et al. found that after adopting a policy of physical exam alone for asymptomatic penetrating extremity wounds, only 1.3% of patients presented following discharge with a need for vascular repair [3]. These patients all presented within a week and went on to have surgical repair without long-term sequelae. However, all patients were initially observed in the hospital for a full 24 h, and follow-up was only possible in 29% of patients.

There are considerably more data on the use of the ankle-brachial pressure index (ABI) as an adjunct to the physical diagnosis in the setting of vascular trauma. In a prospective study from 2004, the authors used an ABI cutoff value of 0.9 as a screening tool for angiography or immediate surgical exploration depending on the clinical condition [4]. An ABI of 0.9 was found to be 100% sensitive and specific for the diagnosis of arterial injury.

A retrospective review of 182 patients in 2009 by Sadjadi et al. examined whether or not patients could be safely discharged from the emergency department after sustaining penetrating trauma to their lower extremities if their ABI was >0.9. Their specificity was 100% with a negative predictive value of 98% [5]. This was then validated in a prospective study of 90 patients using the same evaluation criteria and again found a specificity of 100%. They felt that hemodynamically normal patients with lower-extremity gunshot wounds without fracture and an ABI of >0.9 were safe to discharge home without additional diagnostic imaging or evaluation.

One caveat to the aforementioned is with blast injuries. Physical exam, even with the adjunct of ABI measurement, is much less reliable. In 2007, a study performed by authors at Walter Reed Medical Center looked at using physical exam in predicting the presence of occult vascular injuries in solders injured during recent conflicts. They found a sensitivity of 38%, specificity of 90%, positive predictive value of 85%, and negative predictive value of 51% in using physical exam to diagnose vascular injury [6]. Therefore, they concluded that a normal physical exam did not reliably predict post-traumatic arterial lesions in complex trauma involving high amounts of energy, penetrating mechanism, or wounding patterns.

*Recommendation*: Physical exam alone can accurately detect "hard signs" of vascular injury. Patients with "soft signs" of vascular injury, but who have an ABI of >0.9 do not need additional work-up or imaging. Physical exam is not reliable in the presence of blast injuries and consideration should be given to additional imaging.

Physical examination with or without ABI as a screening tool for blunt or penetrating vascular injury:

*Level of evidence*: 2b

*Strength of recommendation*: B

## 29.3 Is CTA Adequate for the Diagnosis of Vascular Injury or Is Invasive Angiography Always Required?

As more and more facilities have access to multidetector computed tomography scanners, computed tomography angiography (CTA) as the initial diagnostic modality of choice for arterial injury has been increasingly promoted, with multiple retrospective reports regarding the use of CTA in vascular trauma being published.

In 2006, Inaba et al. retrospectively evaluated 63 examinations performed in 59 patients [7]. There was only one nondiagnostic study due to retained bullet fragments, although 19% of scans possessed some artifact from bullets, as 45% of these patients suffered penetrating injuries. Twenty-two lesions were diagnosed by CTA, with 19 being confirmed in the operating room and the other three were managed nonoperatively. Three patients underwent both CTA and conventional angiography with 100% concordance of findings. No missed injuries were found subsequently in patients with normal CTA, although follow-up was short at 48 days. These authors quoted a sensitivity and specificity of 100% for this modality.

Peng et al. [8] in 2008, reported their experience over a 5-year period, with 38 patients undergoing a CTA, with 17 abnormal scans. All findings were confirmed at surgery, and there were no false-negative findings or missed injuries. However, they did not specify a gold standard.

Another retrospective review by Wallin from 2011 looked specifically at penetrating trauma to the extremity and the use of CTA. Fifty-nine patients underwent CTA in their study, 34 studies were negative for vascular injury, and none of these patients required any operative intervention. Nineteen studies were positive and all underwent operative exploration. Six studies (10%) were indeterminate either due to bullet or bone artifacts or flawed timing of contrast injection [9].

Prospective studies evaluating the use of CTA where eventually conducted and confirmed the efficacy of CTA use for vascular trauma: by Seamon in 2009 and Inaba in 2011. In the first study, they evaluated the use of CTA in patients with extremity trauma and an ABI <0.9. Twenty-one patients were included and underwent CTA scan, which was then followed by either conventional angiography or operative exploration if the CTA suggested a limb-threatening injury. CTA had 100% sensitivity and specificity for clinically relevant vascular injury detection, and they concluded that CTA saves ~$13,000 in patient charges and $1,166 in hospital costs per extremity [10].

Inaba et al. tested CTA use against a composite gold standard of operative intervention, conventional angiography, or clinical follow-up. In their study, 89 CTAs were performed in 73 patients with "soft signs" of vascular trauma. Of these, 24 had positive studies and underwent operative exploration, 58 had negative studies, and all patients had clinical follow-up without any late findings of vascular compromise. Seven studies (9.6%) were inconclusive, five due to artifact from retained missile fragments and two due to reformatting errors. In the absence of artifact, multidetector CTA had 100% sensitivity and specificity in detecting clinically significant arterial injuries [11].

*Recommendation*: CTA is a highly useful screening tool for detecting vascular injury and may replace conventional angiography as the diagnostic modality of choice for injured extremities.

CTA as a screening tool for arterial injury:

*Level of evidence*: 2b

*Strength of recommendation*: B

## 29.4 Should Knee Dislocation Still Be Treated as a Special Circumstance, i.e., Is Routine Angiography Necessary?

Acute dislocation of the knee was previously thought to be a special circumstance due to a quoted injury prevalence rate of 20%–30% of the popliteal artery, with a concomitant high rate of amputation if restoration of flow takes longer than 8 h [12].

Multiple retrospective and prospective studies have been conducted over the past decade looking at mandatory imaging of the popliteal artery, with most concluding that physical exam and ABI were sufficient in diagnosing popliteal injury. The largest series ever reported was published in 2004 by Stannard et al., who reported on 138 knees treated by a protocol of selective angiography in a prospective, single-center study [13]. The prevalence of arterial injury was only 7% (9 patients) with a total of 17 patients undergoing angiography, despite a normal physical exam. Out of these 17 patients, 14 had normal findings, 2 had mild spasm, and there was one intimal tear, which was treated nonoperatively. Physical exam alone (without the use of ABI) had a sensitivity of 100% and specificity of 99% in this report.

A further report in 2004 on 57 knee dislocations in 55 patients again found no missed vascular injuries in the 32 patients who had a normal physical examination, although the gold standard was a composite of angiography and clinical follow-up (angiogram in 13 and follow-up in 19) [14]. The incidence of vascular injury in their study was higher at 21%. This study used physical exam with the addition of the ABI. One fasciotomy was performed for compartment syndrome without evidence of vascular injury. They quoted a lower sensitivity of 71% (as 13 patients with a normal exam had no injury on angiography) with a specificity of 100%.

A multicenter prospective study published in 2009 looked more specifically at bicruciate lesions of the knee with or without dislocation. Sixty-seven patients were included, and they found only nine vascular lesions (12%) in this group, all of which occurred in patients with true knee dislocation, not just ligamentous instability [15]. The absence of vascular injury was confirmed in 58 of the 59 patients with normal distal pulses. In one case, a vascular lesion was found on early imaging, but was not clinically significant. Of the remaining eight cases of abnormal exam, all patients had abnormal angiograms with no false-positive or false-negative findings. High-energy trauma was the cause in 68% of the cases and low energy in 32%.

*Recommendation*: Routine angiography in the setting of knee dislocation is unnecessary if a normal exam is present (including normal ABI).

Physical examination alone in knee dislocations:

*Level of evidence*: 2b

*Strength of recommendation*: B

## 29.5 Is There a Role for the Nonoperative Management of Vascular Injuries?

As diagnostic technologies have become more advanced, there has been an increase in our ability to detect minor vascular trauma. Originally, the surgical tenet was that all angiographic abnormalities must be surgically explored and repaired, which has been reexamined in recent years. One of the original studies for this approach came from Dennis et al., who compared a group of 43 patients who had angiographic abnormalities, but with patient distal vessels with no extraluminal extravasation >2 cm in size and without manifestations of "hard" signs of vascular injury [3]. They were observed in hospital for 24–48 h before discharge. Four of these patients (9%) represented with clinical deterioration within 1 month of injury and underwent immediate surgical repair without subsequent morbidity or problems during long-term follow-up. Mean follow-up was 9 years.

A study in the pediatric population by Shah et al. reported on 42 patients with peripheral vascular injuries. Most of these injuries (62%) involved the upper extremities. Of the total 42 patients, 67% underwent operative management of their vascular injuries, while 33% ($n = 14$) of patients were conservatively managed [16].

In 2011, Franz et al. published a 5-year review of patients who underwent management of lower-extremity arterial injuries. They had 65 patients included in their study with 75 lower-extremity arterial injuries. All patients presented with absent or diminished pulses and either were taken directly to OR for "hard signs" of vascular trauma or taken for CTA. The majority of patients in their study, 78.4%, underwent a surgical intervention, while 16 injuries (23.3%) were managed medically. Most of these patients had injuries to their tibial artery. Their criteria for nonoperative management were the following: patients with <5 mm intimal disruption, adherent intimal flaps, intact distal circulation, and no active hemorrhage. If patient's lesions persisted or worsened as seen by the change in ultrasound, ABI, CTA, or serial angiography, they were indicated for surgical exploration. None of their patients who were managed nonoperatively required subsequent surgery [17].

A study by Van Waes et al., published in 2013, looked specifically at nonoperative management after penetrating trauma to the extremities. In their study period of 10 years, 668 patients presented to the emergency department with penetrating trauma to the extremity. After initial assessment, 512 patients were discharged home, and none of these patients re-presented with complications. The other 156 patients were admitted for surgery or observation. Conservative observation was utilized in 134 patients (86%). Of this total, only two patients (1.5%) required a surgical intervention to treat late vascular complications. They concluded that a policy of selective nonoperative management for initial assessment and treatment of penetrating trauma to the extremities is both safe and feasible [18].

*Recommendation*: Minor vascular injuries (e.g., small intimal flaps or vasospasm) that do not compromise the distal blood supply may be safely treated nonoperatively, with close outpatient follow-up as a part of this algorithm.

Nonoperative management of vascular injuries:

*Level of evidence*: 2B

*Strength of recommendation*: C

## 29.6 What Is the Role of Endovascular Treatment, i.e., Stenting, in the Management of Acute Vascular Injuries?

With the increased expertise that has been gained in the use of vascular stent grafting in both aortic and extremity vessels, it was only a matter of time before these devices were used to repair vessels that had been acutely injured. One of the biggest debates about endovascular repair in trauma is whether or not this can be utilized for hemodynamically unstable patients. In 2008, Cohen et al. reported on six patients with penetrating subclavian artery injuries that were repaired by endovascular stent placement within 6 h of admission. They were successful with stent placement in all patients, and they had no procedural complications or acute stent thrombosis or infection. One patient developed arterial stenosis at 7 months, which was treated with angioplasty [19]. Another study by Tellopoulous et al. looked at 18 patients with peripheral arterial injuries and hemorrhagic shock who were treated with endovascular repair. Thirteen of these injuries were iatrogenic injuries, two spontaneous hemorrhages, and three from trauma (one penetrating, two blunt). They too had technical success with no procedural complications in all cases, and this series addressed injuries to the external carotid, vertebral, subclavian, common iliac, external iliac, internal iliac, profunda femoral, superficial femoral, and popliteal arteries. Thirteen patients had no complications in the postprocedure time period, but three patients died (17% mortality), one patient required a below knee amputation, and one developed hemiparesis [20].

In a larger study looking at subclavian artery injury, performed by du Toit et al., 57 patients who underwent endovascular repair were reviewed. During a 10-year period, 145 patients with subclavian artery injuries were seen, of which 88 underwent open repair and 57 endovascular [21]. Patients with active uncontrollable hemorrhage, critical limb ischemia, airway or brachial plexus compression, and infected wounds immediately went for open repair. They looked at both early and late complications associated with endovascular repair. Three patients had early stent thrombosis (none of which caused critical limb ischemia, but required catheter-directed thrombolysis and restenting), one femoral artery puncture site intimal flap, and one death due to multiorgan failure. Thirty-one patients were lost to follow-up, however, and late complications were identified with >50% graft stenosis in five patients (mean 11 months) and complete occlusion of graft in three patients (mean 26 months).

In 2007, a study analyzing the National Trauma Data Bank (NTDB) from 1994 to 2003 showed that only 281 of 12,732 patients with vascular trauma were treated with an endovascular procedure, with an overall utilization rate of endovascular repair of 3.7%. They did show a 27-fold increase in the number of endovascular procedures performed for arterial trauma from four procedures in 1997 to 37 in 2003, suggesting that this continues to be an evolving treatment [22]. This study found that there were no differences in the age or sex of patients or type of trauma (blunt vs. penetrating) in the groups evaluated, but more endovascular procedures were performed in public and university-based hospitals, which likely reflects the capability of these hospitals to perform interventional radiology (IR) procedures after hours and on weekends. Another key finding from this study was that patients undergoing endovascular repair had lower Injury Severity Score (ISS) and revised trauma score (RTS) values, suggesting that the endovascular patients were more stable on presentation than patients treated with open vascular repair. They did utilize a logistic regression to match for ISSs and showed that patients who underwent endovascular repair had a lower mortality and shorter length of stay.

In 2012 and 2014, two further papers were published utilizing data from the NTDB. The first study evaluated the predictors leading to endovascular repair for peripheral arterial injuries from 2007 to 2009. There were 8,977 patients in the NTDB with peripheral arterial injuries, and 5.9% (531 patients) underwent endovascular repair.

A risk adjustment analysis was then performed, and it was found that patients undergoing endovascular repair were older, more likely to have an injury to a lower-extremity vessel, had higher ISS, and had more comorbid illnesses than patients undergoing operative repair, suggesting some differences in the original analysis, which concluded that more stable patients were the ones undergoing endovascular repair. They also found no significant differences in postoperative mortality for those patients undergoing endovascular repair, again suggesting it is a safe alternative to open surgery [23]. The second study from the NTDB, published in 2014, looked at all cases of arterial trauma from 2002 to 2010, including patients with thoracic and abdominal aortic injuries. A total of 23,105 patients were found in the database. They found an increase in the number of endovascular procedures being performed per year, but this increase was highest for injuries to the internal iliac artery (from 8% in 2002 to 13.3% in 2010), the thoracic aorta (from 0.5% in 2002 to 21.9% in 2010), and common/external iliac arteries (0.4% in 2002 to 20.4% in 2010), along with a significant increase in those sustaining blunt trauma (0.4% in 2002 to 13.2% in 2010). After matching patients, the rate of in-hospital mortality was lower for those undergoing endovascular repair, 12.9% vs. 22.4%. These patients also had a higher ISS, had a lower rate of sepsis and surgical site infections, and required mechanical ventilation less frequently than the open procedure group [24].

*Recommendation*: Endovascular stenting for peripheral arterial trauma is often technically feasible with good short-term results, but little data exist on long-term safety and efficacy.

Endovascular treatment of vascular trauma:

*Level of evidence*: 4

*Strength of recommendation*: C

## 29.7 What Role Should Intravascular Shunting for Damage Control Vascular Surgery Play in the Management Scheme for Vascular Injuries?

Some of the most extensive experience with vascular shunting has been collected through the military experiences in Iraq and Afghanistan due to the special circumstances that prevent surgeons there from performing immediate vascular reconstructions. In 2008, prospective data were collected over a 7-month period, where they studied 23 proximal shunts placed in 16 patients, and found that 22 were patients (95.7%) at the time of reexploration. The mean time to presentation was 46 ± 15 min, whereas time to definitive repair at a higher-level facility was 5:48 ± 2:08 min [25]. The one failure was in a superficial femoral vein shunt and the vein was ultimately ligated without compromise to the extremity. All patients survived with limb salvage. The long-term follow-up for this study was only 2–30 days.

Additional military studies have looked more closely at the long-term complications with vascular shunting. In 2009, Gifford et al. looked at all American troops who sustained an extremity vascular injury from 2003 to 2007. They compared those treated with temporary vascular shunt to those with similar injuries and timing of injuries who did not have a vascular shunt placed. They had 64 vascular injuries with shunts and 61 vascular injuries without shunts included in their study. The overall amputation rate was 21% for all patients, with those sustaining a penetrating blast more likely to receive an amputation than those shot [26]. The groups were matched in regard to mechanism of injury, location of injury, rates of venous injury, and types of shunts used. They followed these patients on average 22 months after injury, and they found that those getting a shunt tended to be more injured (mean ISS 18 vs. 15), received more Level II care, and more fresh whole blood transfusion. Amputation-free survival for both groups was similar at 78%, suggesting that temporary vascular shunting can be used as a damage control option and will not lead to worse outcomes for a patient.

Another study by Borut et al. followed patients for 2 years who were treated with temporary vascular shunting. Eighty patients were included in their study, 46 who had temporary vascular shunts and 34 who underwent immediate surgical repair. Their overall amputation rate was 13%, with six in the shunt group and seven in the nonshunt group, and two of the shunt group amputations were performed late, whereas no late amputations occurred in the nonshunt group [27]. There were no differences between these groups in regard to ISS, age, mechanism of injury, or extremity injured.

In the civilian setting, studies still suggest that it is safe to perform temporary vascular shunting to reestablish perfusion to a threatened limb. In 2008, a study by Subramanian et al. looked at 786 patients with vascular injuries managed at a level 1 trauma center. Seventy-three patients (9%) had a total of 108 temporary vascular shunts placed, 76 in arteries and 32 in veins. In total, 53% of patients had the temporary shunt removed during the initial operation after orthopedic fixation was accomplished or their other injuries were managed appropriately. The remaining 31 patients went to the ICU with the shunt in place for an average placement time of 23.5 ± 15.7 h [28]. Of these patients with shunts in the ICU, three shunts occluded (9%). In total, 18% of patients despite shunting required secondary amputation. Reasons for a secondary amputation were thrombosis of the bypass graft, massive tissue loss, or associated infections.

*Recommendation*: Vascular shunts for damage control vascular surgery are useful and can allow for combined venous/arterial repair. Ischemia times are lower and patency rates are high without anticoagulation, but definitive repair should still be performed as soon as possible.

Use of vascular shunts in major vascular extremity trauma:

*Level of evidence*: 4

*Strength of recommendation*: C

## 29.8 What Role Do Tourniquets Play in the Management of Peripheral Vascular Injuries?

The use of tourniquets in civilian extremity trauma has generally been frowned upon in the past because of numerous complications reported with improper use in the civilian population. There has been increased interest in these devices, because of the nature of the injuries sustained by members of the armed forces in Iraq and Afghanistan, with some provisional reports suggesting that prehospital tourniquet use was associated with improved hemorrhage control.

Beekley et al. [29] reported on 166 patients with a major vascular extremity injury or traumatic amputation. In total, 65% of patients with tourniquets had hemorrhage control on arrival as opposed to 11% without tourniquets. The average time with tourniquet applied was 70 min. There were no differences in secondary amputation rates or mortality between groups. Analysis of the seven deaths estimated that four of these patients could have been saved with adequate tourniquet placement.

This study was followed up by Kragh et al. looking specifically at complications with tourniquet application. Over a 7-month period, patients were evaluated for tourniquet use, limb outcome, and morbidity. A total of 232 patients had 428 tourniquets applied on 309 injured limbs [30]. In total, 97% of the tourniquets were felt to be indicated, with 13 applied for reasons that were not indicated. Median tourniquet time was 1.0 h with an average of 1.3 h, and 91% of patients had the tourniquet on for less than 2 h. There were no associations between total tourniquet time and morbidity with regards to clots, myonecrosis, rigor, pain, palsies, or renal failure. Four patients (1.7%) sustained a transient nerve palsy at the level of the tourniquet, whereas six had palsies at the wound level. No amputations resulted from tourniquet use, and fasciotomy rates were not statistically significant. These studies certainly suggest that there is a role for tourniquets in treating hemorrhage from extremity trauma in the military setting.

There are much less data regarding their use in civilian trauma. A report by Kalish et al. from 2008 looked at tourniquet use in the management of civilian penetrating extremity injuries [31]. There were only 11 patients during their study period that had a prehospital tourniquet in place for a penetrating extremity injury. The mean tourniquet application time was 75 ± 38 min. One patient died with a tourniquet in place, but was pulseless at the scene initially. Of the remaining patients, two had motor and sensory nerve deficits, but this was due to the primary injury. No patients had neurologic deficits from the tourniquets, and only two patients underwent fasciotomy, both of which occurred at the primary operation.

*Recommendation*: The use of tourniquets for management of prehospital control of peripheral vascular trauma is supported by limited civilian and military data and has the potential to save lives with minimal morbidity, as long as first responders are trained to correctly apply them.

Tourniquet use for exsanguinating hemorrhage:

*Level of evidence*: 4

*Strength of recommendation*: C

## 29.9 Following Repair of an Acute Vascular Injury, Should Fasciotomies Be Performed Prophylactically or Should We Measure Compartment Pressures?

There has never been a randomized trial comparing routine prophylactic fasciotomy to a policy of careful clinical exam and/or measurement of compartment pressures. There is also continued lack of uniformity about how to measure compartment pressures.

O'Toole et al. looked specifically at the variation seen in the diagnosis of compartment syndrome by surgeons. They analyzed a consecutive cohort of patients with tibial shaft fractures. A total of 386 fractures were identified, and from this group, they looked at all patients who were diagnosed with "compartment syndrome" and, therefore, underwent fasciotomy. Forty patients with fracture underwent fasciotomy after physical examination by an orthopedic surgeon who deemed it was necessary. There was a range from 2% to 24% between surgeons in diagnosing compartment syndrome, which was statistically significant ($p < 0.005$) [32]. This study amply demonstrates the variability in the diagnosis and treatment seen between surgeons.

A study from 2008 tried to answer the question about the usefulness of continuous pressure monitoring versus intermittent clinical monitoring of compartment pressures, again after tibial fractures. In total, 109 consecutive patients in their study with a tibial fracture underwent 48 h of continuous pressure monitoring. This was compared to a group of historical controls that had been monitored by physical exam and intermittent pressure monitoring. In the continuous monitor group, 33 patients ultimately underwent fasciotomy. Compared to the historical controls, the rate of fasciotomy was not different (15.6% for continuous monitoring vs. 14.7% for intermittent exams), suggesting that continuous pressure monitoring did not change outcomes or unnecessary fasciotomies [33].

*Recommendation*: There are very little quality data on which to base recommendations. Clinical experience and frequent reexaminations (with/without pressure monitoring) remain the only way to detect this syndrome.

Prophylactic fasciotomy following vascular repair:

*Level of evidence*: 2b

*Strength of recommendation*: C

## 29.10 Conclusions

Although certain questions regarding vascular trauma appear to have been definitively answered, the majority of the vascular literature is limited by small patient numbers, varying definitions of injuries and complications, questionable gold standards, and limited follow-up. Accurate evidence-based guidelines are therefore difficult to formulate. Multicenter prospective cooperative trials may be the only way to definitively answer many of the remaining questions.

Until such data are available, we have attempted to synthesize and summarize the recent accumulated evidence relating to the management of acute vascular injuries. We hope that a similar review in another 10 years' time will be able to draw on studies of higher quality and make more definitive recommendations.

## References

1. Perkins ZB, De'Ath HD, Aylwin C et al. Epidemiology and outcome of vascular trauma at a British Major Trauma Centre. *Eur J Vasc Endovasc Surg*. 2012;44(2):203–209.
2. Britt LD, Weireter LJ, Cole FJ. Newer diagnostic modalities for vascular injuries; the way we were, the way we are. *Surg Clin North Am*. 2001;81(6):1263–1279.
3. Dennis JW, Frykberg ER, Veldenz HC et al. Validation of nonoperative management of occult vascular injuries and accuracy of physical examination alone in penetrating extremity trauma: 5- to 10-year follow up. *J Trauma*. 1998;44(2):243–252; discussion 242–243.
4. Mills WJ, Barei DP, McNair P. The value of the ankle-brachial index for diagnosing arterial injury after knee dislocation: A prospective study. *J Trauma*. 2004;56(6):1261–1265.
5. Sadjadi J, Cureton EL, Dozier KC, Kwan RO, Victorino GP. Expedited treatment of lower extremity gunshot wounds. *J Am Coll Surg*. 2009;209:740–745.
6. Johnson ON, Fox CJ, White P et al. Physical exam and occult post-traumatic vascular lesions: Implications for the evaluation and management of arterial injuries in modern warfare in the endovascular era. *J Cardiovasc Surg*. 2007;48:581–586.
7. Inaba K, Potzman J, Munera F et al. Multi-slice CT angiography for arterial evaluation in the injured lower extremity. *J Trauma*. 2006;60(3):502–506; discussion 506–507.
8. Peng PD, Spain DA, Tataria M et al. CT angiography effectively evaluates extremity vascular trauma. *Am Surg*. 2008;74(2):103–107.
9. Wallin D, Yaghoubian A, Rosing D et al. CT angiography as the primary diagnostic modality in penetrating lower extremity vascular injuries: A level 1 trauma experience. *Ann Vasc Surg*. 2011;25(5):620–623.
10. Seamon MJ, Smoger D, Torres D et al. A prospective validation of a current practice: The detection of extremity vascular injury with CT angiography. *J Trauma*. 2009;67:238–244.
11. Inaba K, Branco BC, Reddy S et al. Prospective evaluation of multidetector computed tomography for extremity vascular trauma. *J Trauma*. 2011;70(4):808–815.
12. Perron AD, Brady WJ, Sing RF. Orthopedic pitfalls in the ED: Vascular injury associated with knee dislocation. *Am J Emerg Med*. 2001;19(7):583–588.
13. Stannard JP, Sheils TM, Lopez-Ben RR et al. Vascular injuries with knee dislocations: The role of physical examination in determining the need for angiography. *J Bone Joint Surg Am*. 2004;86-A(5):910–915.
14. Klineberg EO, Crites BM, Flinn WR et al. The role of arteriography in assessing popliteal artery injury in knee dislocations. *J Trauma*. 2004;56(4):786–790.
15. Boisrenoult P, Lustig S, Bonneviale P et al. Vascular lesions associated with bicruciate and knee dislocation ligamentous injury. *Ortho Trauma Surg Res*. 2009;95:621–626.
16. Shah SR, Wearden PD, Gaines BA. Pediatric peripheral vascular injuries: A review of our experience. *J Surg Res*. 2009;153:162–166.
17. Franz RW, Shah KJ, Halaharvi D et al. A 5-year review of management of lower extremity arterial injuries at an urban level 1 trauma center. *J Vasc Surg*. 2011;53:1604–1610.
18. Van Waes OJF, Van Lieshout EM, Hogendoorn W et al. Treatment of penetrating trauma of the extremities: Ten years' experience at a Dutch level 1 trauma center. *Scand J Trauma*. 2013;21:2.
19. Cohen JE, Rajz G, Gomori JM et al. Urgent endovascular stent-graft placement for traumatic penetrating subclavian artery injuries. *J Neuro Sci*. 2008;272:151–157.
20. Trellopoulous G, Georgiadis GS, Aslanidou EA et al. Endovascular management of peripheral arterial trauma in patients presenting in hemorrhagic shock. *J Cardiovasc Surg*. 2012;53:495–506.

21. Du Toit DF, Lambrechts AV, Stark H, Warren BL. Long-term results of stent graft treatment of subclavian artery injuries: Management of choice for stable patients? *J Vasc Surg*. 2008;47:739–743.
22. Reuben BC, Whitten MG, Sarfati M, Kraiss LW. Increasing use of endovascular therapy in acute arterial injuries: Analysis of the National Trauma Data Bank. *J Vasc Surg*. 2007;46:1222–1226.
23. Worni M, Scarborough JE, Gandhi M et al. Use of endovascular therapy for peripheral arterial lesions: An analysis of the national trauma data band from 2007 to 2009. *Ann Vasc Surg*. 2013;27(3):299–305.
24. Branco BC, DuBose JJ, Zhan LX et al. Trends and outcomes of endovascular therapy in the management of civilian vascular injuries. *J Vasc Surg*. November 2014;60(5):1297–1307.
25. Taller J, Kamdar JP, Greene JA et al. Temporary vascular shunts as initial treatment of proximal extremity vascular injuries during combat operations: The new standard of care at Echelon II facilities? *J Trauma*. 2008;65:595–603.
26. Gifford SM, Aidinian G, Clouse WD et al. Effect of temporary shunting on extremity vascular injury: An outcome analysis from the global war on terror vascular surgery initiative. *J Vasc Surg*. 2009;50:549–556.
27. Borut J, Acosta JA, Tadlock M et al. The use of temporary vascular shunts in military extremity wounds: A preliminary outcome analysis with 2-year follow up. *J Trauma*. 2010;69:174–178.
28. Subramanian A, Vercruysse G, Dente C et al. A decade's experience with temporary intravascular shunts at a civilian level 1 trauma center. *J Trauma*. 2008;65:316–326.
29. Beekley A, Sebestra J, Blackborne L, Holcomb J. Prehospital tourniquet use in operation Iraqi freedom: Effect on hemorrhage control and outcomes. *J Trauma*. February 2008;64(2 Suppl):S28–S37; discussion S37.
30. Kragh JF, Walters TJ, Baer DG et al. Practical use of emergency tourniquets to stop bleeding in major limb trauma. *J Trauma*. 2008;64(2):S38–S50.
31. Kalish J, Burke P, Felman J et al. The return of tourniquets. *JEMS*. 2008;33(8):44–54.
32. O'Toole RV, Whitney A, Merchant N et al. Variation in diagnosis of compartment syndrome by surgeons treating tibial shaft fractures. *J Trauma*. 2009;67(4):735–741.
33. Al-Dadah OQ, Darrah C, Cooper A, Donell ST, Patel AD. Continuous compartment pressure monitoring vs clinical monitoring in tibial diaphyseal fractures. *Injury*. 2008;39:1204–1209.

## Commentary on Evidence-Based Approach to Extremity Vascular Trauma

*Rao R. Ivatury*

No other area in trauma management arguably has more controversial topics than extremity vascular trauma. The different approaches and opinions exist, absent high-grade evidence from randomized, controlled trials (RCTs). Excellent practice management guidelines, such as those formulated by WEST*†, based on collective evidence from large multicenter trials, albeit nonrandomized, form the spring-board for our constantly evolving principles. And, as the current chapter very nicely and succinctly summarizes, many of these concepts are undergoing frequent transformation.

The author(s) have taken common clinical questions and summarized the evidence favoring the current management. I agree with them that many of these recommendations are based on a level of evidence of 2B and deserve a grade B recommendation at best. The trauma surgeon, nevertheless, is likely to be enthralled at the refined concepts in many of these areas: the avoidance of "routine" angiographic evaluation of all "proximity" penetrating injuries (we can rely to a large extent on physical examination and Doppler pressure measurements: huge benefit in cost and morbidity); CTA is rapidly gaining superiority over catheter angiography in the evaluation of extremity vascular trauma, in the absence of artifacts and reformatting errors (benefits in speed, cost, and personnel); we need not routinely perform angiography for knee dislocation *if* the patient is not morbidly obese and the physical examination and ABI are normal (benefits in cost and morbidity).

The newer concepts do not stop at just diagnostics. Significant therapeutic strategies are evolving, with a similar strength of evidence (2b) and level of recommendation (B): nonoperative management of *selected* vascular injuries with careful, long-term follow-up (benefits in cost and morbidity), endovascular management of *selected* vascular lesions (benefits in cost and minimally invasive procedures).

Other impressive and highly exciting developments are in the area of vascular trauma with hemodynamic instability: rapid hemorrhage control in austere conditions (battlefield, on the street) with appropriate application of tourniquets; injuries with difficult access (subclavian vessel, head, and neck major vessel injuries) with endovascular interventions. I believe damage-control vascular surgery with intravascular shunting is one of the greatest advances in civilian and military injury management. Carefully and appropriately performed, these temporary shunts can provide immense benefit with minimal disadvantages. None of these concepts are likely to be subjected to very rigid testing by RCT but are supported by multiple series with similar results.

The last topic addressed by the authors, the role of fasciotomy in extremity trauma, in my opinion, is the most vexed issue in acute care surgery. As reviewed recently‡, the diagnosis of compartment syndromes and the indications for fasciotomy and are, at best, imprecise. Measurement of compartmental pressure is a worthy endeavor. Their interpretation, however, is highly capricious. The only certain fact is the poor outcome if the diagnosis is late or missed and fasciotomy is late or incomplete. I agree with the authors' recommendation that clinical experience and frequent re-examinations (with/without pressure monitoring) are absolutely necessary. It is also an area where we need more research and more evidence-based management guidelines.

* Feliciano DV, Moore FA, Moore EE et al. Western trauma association critical decisions in trauma: Evaluation and management of peripheral vascular injury, Part I. *J Trauma*. 2011;70:1551–1556.

† Feliciano DV, Moore EE, West M et al. Western Trauma Association critical decisions in trauma: Evaluation and management of peripheral vascular injury, Part II. *J Trauma Acute Care Surg*. 2013;75(3):391–397.

‡ Ivatury RR. Pressure, perfusion and compartments: Challenges for the acute care surgeon. *J Trauma Acute Care Surg*. 2014;June;76(6):1341–1348.

# 30

# *Surgery of Upper Extremity*

**Wendie Grunberg, Shari Lawson, and Howard T. Wang**

**CONTENTS**



## 30.1 How Are Common Soft Tissue Infections Such as Human or Animal Bites, Flexor Tenosynovitis, and Hand Abscess Treated, and Are the Current Empiric Antibiotic Used Based on Clinical Evidence?

Infections of the hand can occur because of bites from humans or animals. A "fight bite" is when a closed fist punch results in breaking of the skin by a tooth. This violates the extensor tendon and joint capsule and may injure the metacarpal head, inoculating the metacarpophalangeal (MCP) joint [1]. Because of the limited soft tissue envelope that covers the deeper structures and numerous tight compartments, bite wounds to the hand have a higher infection rate [2].

Although most bites are polymicrobial, antibiotic selection initially is empiric and based on the most common organisms found in the mouth. This includes *Staphylococcus* species and *Eikenella corrodens* for humans and *Pasteurella* species for animals. Unusual microbial contamination can often complicate human and animal bites, as these are often associated with plant, water, and soil exposure [3]. A broad-spectrum antibiotic such as Unasyn or Augmentin is usually the first line of therapy. Tetanus prophylaxis and rabies prevention should also be considered. Transmission of viruses is less common, especially after human bites, but hepatitis B and C, human immunodeficiency virus (HIV), syphilis, herpes simplex virus, and human T-lymphotropic virus-1 have been documented [4–9].

If the wound is relatively superficial, generous cleansing of the wound may be all that is needed. Deeper and more complex bites may require operative intervention and debridement of necrotic tissue. Patients should be placed on antibiotics and the hand splinted and elevated for comfort.

Hand infections can be more severe in those who are immunocompromised, including diabetics and smokers [10,11]. Flexor tenosynovitis can occur when infection affects the flexor tendon sheath. Purulent fluid in the synovial space surrounding the tendon denies the tendon vital nutrition, and increased pressure in the infected sheath can inhibit blood flow to the tendon, causing necrosis [12].

The classic sign of flexor tenosynovitis is Kanavel's sign: pain on extension of digit, semiflexed position of digit, fusiform swelling of digit, and tenderness along the flexor sheath with frequent extension into the palm [13]. Early infection, less than 24 h since onset, can be successfully managed medically with antibiotics, elevation, and splinting. For infections with subcutaneous purulence or necrotic tendon, open exposure of the sheath and irrigation through windows sparing the A2 and A4 pulleys is necessary. In all but the most severe infections, drainage can be accomplished through the placement of an irrigation catheter at the A1 pulley (distal palmar crease) with a counter incision and drain left at the A5 pulley (volar distal interphalangeal [DIP] joint). Irrigation of the sheath is then accomplished using normal saline. The catheter may be left and irrigation attempted on the floor for the next 24–48 h without the need to return to the OR [14].

Other forms of hand infections like an abscess or felon needs to be drained as any other abscess in the body. A longitudinal incision from the distal flexion crease to the pulp apex avoids the neurovascular bundles and permits disruption of the septal compartments [1].

Current guidelines show that penicillin-based antibiotics are useful in soft tissue infections. Augmentin is suitable for its broad-spectrum therapy and is commonly used in the management of open fractures [15]. The ineffectiveness of flucloxacillin, erythromycin, and cephalosporins in *Pasteurella* infections suggests that Augmentin should be used routinely in animal bites and scratches [16]. Clindamycin is a good alternative in penicillin-allergic patients, unless *Pasteurella* species is identified [17]. Oral antibiotic therapy should continue between 10 and 14 days for cellulitis and at least 3 weeks if deeper tissue is involved.

*Recommendation*: Bacteriology of animals and humans are studied and general guidance is given regarding antibiotic coverage. Thorough cleansing of the wound for shallow wounds and excisional debridements for deeper wounds may be necessary.

*Recommendation grade*: B

## 30.2 When Is It Appropriate to Operate on Scaphoid Fractures, and What Are the Diagnostic Techniques Employed?

Scaphoid fractures of the wrist are one of the most common fractures clinicians will manage. Unfortunately, it is also relatively difficult to manage, as imaging studies can often miss the fracture. Failure to immobilize scaphoid fractures risks nonunion, functional morbidity, and eventual arthritic degeneration [18].

The presenting symptom of these fractures is "snuff box" tenderness along the radial side of the wrist. Alternatively, pain with digital pressure over the scaphoid tubercle may indicate scaphoid fracture [19]. History and physical examination alone are inadequate to rule out scaphoid fractures [20]. Imaging studies generally start with plain wrist views.

Computed tomography (CT), magnetic resonance imaging (MRI), and bone scanning are other modalities of imaging. Advanced imaging in patients with signs of a scaphoid injury within days of the injury reduces unnecessary immobilization that limits activity in patients who ultimately do not have a scaphoid fracture [20]. MRI is diagnostically superior to CT, bone scan, ultrasound, or physical examination [20].

The traditional treatment for nondisplaced scaphoid fractures is nonoperative. The blood supply of the scaphoid bone travels from a distal to proximal direction; thus, fractures at the waist are much more likely to develop a nonunion. A clear overall benefit of early fixation has not been demonstrated [21,22]. Instead, an aggressive conservative management should remain the mainstay for scaphoid fractures. Fracture healing can be assessed with plain radiographs or CT after 6–8 weeks of cast immobilization. Surgical fixation with or without bone grafting can be performed if a gap is identified at the fracture site [21]. Studies have shown that cast immobilization of the thumb appears to be unnecessary for CT or MRI image confirmed nondisplaced or minimally displaced fractures of the waist [23].

Displaced fractures of the scaphoid have four times higher risk of nonunion than nondisplaced fractures when treated with cast only [24]. These fractures can be reduced surgically with traction, placement of Kirschner wires (K-wires), or open realignment, followed by internal fixation of the screw.

*Recommendation*: Fracture healing can be assessed with plain radiographs or CT after 6–8 weeks of cast immobilization. Surgical fixation with or without bone grafting can be performed if a gap is identified at the fracture site. MRI is useful to diagnose scaphoid fractures.

*Recommendation grade*: B

## 30.3 What Are the Indications for Replantation of Digits and Extremities?

### 30.3.1 Indications

- Thumb
- Multiple digits
- Single digit distal to FDP insertion
- Upper extremity and palm/wrist/forearm
- Proximal to elbow if a sharp amputation
- Almost any amputation in a child

### 30.3.2 Contraindications

- Crushed/mangled parts
- Multilevel amputation
- Prolonged ischemia time
- Medical comorbidities
- Life-threatening injuries

### 30.3.3 Relative Contraindications

- Single digit in an adult
- Heavy contamination
- Self-mutilation
- Avulsion

The goals of replantation are to restore circulation and regain sufficient function and sensation of the amputated part as well as to allow patients to return to their previous employment [25]. Not all amputees will benefit from replantation. Strict selection criteria should be defined to optimize the result.

Amputations are characterized into two main categories: complete and incomplete [26]. Incomplete segments are connected to the proximal stump with a bridge of tissue. Incomplete amputations are further subdivided based on the viability of the remaining stump, whether the distal tissue segment maintains sufficient blood circulation and if it needs major additional microvascular reconstruction.

The type of injury is the single most important factor in determining the survival rate and overall functional outcome [27]. Clean-cut amputations are a good indication for replant, whereas crush injuries and avulsion amputations generally have poorer outcomes [28].

The level of functional disability should be determined. For instance, the thumb should be given first priority for replantation, as it is responsible for about 40% of hand function [29]. Patients with multiple digit amputations should be given first priority for replant in order to preserve function of the hand [25].

Amputation at the midpalm is also an absolute indication for replant and is seen to have high functional outcome when at the level of the superficial or deep palmar arch [25]. Replantation following amputation at the wrist has excellent potential for functional recovery and should be attempted.

The amount of ischemia time tolerated is directly proportional to the amount of muscle present in the amputated segment. Because digits lack muscle, the duration of warm ischemia is up to 12 h, while only 6 h for a major limb. Cooling an amputated digit allows for extended ischemia time up to 30 h. One must be cognizant that life-threatening complications may follow major replantation because of free radical production at the time of vascular reperfusion [30].

The presence of life-threatening injuries or general conditions that prohibit a long surgical procedure is a contraindication to replantation attempts. Patients who smoke should be advised to quit smoking, as the vasoconstrictive properties of nicotine correlate with a decreased survival rate as compared to nonsmokers [31]. Diseases that deteriorate peripheral circulation, like atherosclerosis, autoimmune disease, and diabetes mellitus, can reduce survival rate and functional outcome, thus constituting a relative contraindication for replantation [32].

*Recommendation*: Indications replantation include thumb, multiple digits, upper extremity amputated at the wrist, midpalm, forearm, and almost any amputation in a child.

*Recommendation grade*: B

## 30.4 What Are the Indications for Release of Forearm Compartment Syndrome, Hand Compartment Syndrome, and Acute Carpal Tunnel Syndrome?

Compartment syndrome is a surgical emergency. Compartment syndrome exists when fascial compartment pressures exceed perfusion pressure leading to tissue ischemia [33]. Delaying diagnosis can lead to functional, cosmetic, and legal ramifications.

The diagnosis of compartment syndrome is often clinical with the main symptom being pain out of proportion to the injury. Paresthesias may occur early; this represents a potentially reversible state because peripheral nerves are more sensitive to ischemia than muscle [34]. Irreversible ischemia begins about 8 h after the onset of ischemia [35]. By the time pallor, pulselessness, and poikilothermia are observed, and ischemic changes may be irreversible.

When physical diagnosis is inconclusive, compartmental pressures can be measured. Some believe that absolute ischemia occurs at pressures of 30–50 mmHg [36]. The use of pulse pressure (diastolic blood pressure, intramuscular pressure) better represents the quantitative diagnosis. A value below 30 mmHg is the cutoff for inadequate perfusion to the extremity [37].

The forearm contains five interconnected compartments with significant amount of musculature. The hand contains 10 compartments that have much less muscle mass. Even though the digits lack muscle, they can undergo increased pressures because of restriction caused by Cleland's and Grayson's ligaments and also because of the adherence at the flexor creases [38,39].

The median nerve is the most frequently damaged nerve in the forearm because of its course deep in the volar forearm. Some authors advocate routine decompression of the carpal tunnel in conjunction with the forearm fasciotomies [40].

Although compartment syndrome has the potential for devastating consequences, if intervention is provided on a prompt basis, patients can recover fully with minimal residual dysfunction of the forearm or hand [39].

*Recommendation*: Intramuscular pressure within 20 mmHg of the diastolic blood pressure causes ischemic muscle necrosis, and success of treatment is both time and pressure dependent.

*Recommendation grade*: B

## 30.5 What Are the Current Options to Treat Flexor and Extensor Tendon Injuries?

The treatment options to restore tendon integrity include primary repair, secondary repair, immediate reconstruction with tendon graft, staged reconstruction, and tendon transfer. If direct repair of tendon is possible, it should be performed. More complex tendon injuries that occur in the presence of compromised overlying soft tissues will require staged reconstruction [41].

Injury patterns are differentiated into open or closed, sharp or blunt, traumatic or degenerative lesions [42]. Open tendon injuries are common findings in trauma and orthopedic patients. A differentiation between partial rupture and complete rupture needs to be determined. Lacerations less than 60% can be treated conservatively [43].

### 30.5.1 Extensor Tendon Injuries

The ideal suture technique for primary extensor repair should ensure high tensile strength, low rupture, and minimal tendon shortening. Extensor tendon injuries are divided into eight zones.

The most common closed tendon injury is the mallet finger (Zone 1). Soft tissue mallet finger injury is generally caused by direct trauma that forces the extended finger into flexion at the DIP joint, or by laceration of the extensor tendon at the level of the middle phalanx [44]. These can be treated conservatively with extension splinting of the DIP joint with the proximal interphalangeal (PIP) joint left free for 4–6 weeks [45]. An osseous disruption of the extensor tendon is called a mallet fracture [44]. These fractures are treated by using osteosynthesis techniques, like screws, tension band, and K wiring.

Zone II injuries are related to direct trauma. Surgical repair is recommended for complete tendon lacerations. If there is partial extensor laceration with a loss of active extension, repair is recommended [46].

The boutonniere deformity (Zone III) is an interruption of the central slip of the extensor tendons, leading to flexion at the PIP joint with hyperextension at the DIP joint. Management of the injury is treated with splinting the PIP joint in extension while leaving the DIP joint free, thus allowing dorsal translation of the lateral bands that occur with DIP flexion [46]. Surgical repair is recommended for open injuries, volar dislocations, or fracture dislocations of the PIP joint, lacerations over the central slip, failed splinting, and large displaced avulsion fractures [47].

Zone IV injuries are typically lacerated tendons. The management is identical to Zone II injuries.

Zone V (sagittal band rupture and fight bites) are located over the MCP joint. Treatment can involve splinting the injured and adjacent digit in a hand-based splint for 3–4 weeks with the MCP joint flexed 30° and the interphalangeal joints free [46]. If the immobilization is unsuccessful, repair is performed through a dorsal longitudinal approach. The two leaflets of the sagittal band are elevated off the dorsal capsule, and repair is performed with a braided non-absorbable suture.

Zone VI injuries occur with a laceration. These are typically managed with direct surgical repair of the tendon using a core stitch and epitendinous stitch. A flexion blocking splint is placed.

Zone VII injuries are located over the extensor retinaculum and result from penetrating trauma. Direct repair of the tendon is followed by repair of the retinaculum. Repair of the retinaculum will prevent bowstringing and subluxation of the tendons [45].

Zone VIII injuries are found at the musculotendinous junction of the extensor compartment of the forearm. They occur after traumatic lacerations or forceful flexion with or without pronation of the forearm. After repair of the tendons, 3–4 weeks of immobilization should occur.

### 30.5.2 Flexor Tendon Injuries

The surgical method of tendon repair depends on the level of injury. These injuries are classified into five anatomic zones. The goal of flexor tendon injury is to achieve normal range of motion while allowing the repair to be strong enough to permit early movement though the first 5 weeks with a dorsal splint [48].

Repair should occur within 1 week of injury [49]. If experienced hand surgeons are not available, primary wound closure should be performed. Delayed primary repair can then be performed days to weeks after the tendon trauma [49].

Incisions can be made using Bruner's incisions in the area of the palmar digit. Alternatively, a midlateral incision can be used. In an end-to-end repair, a multistrand core suture (4-0) is placed to avoid gapping. In a retrospective clinical study comparing six-strand repair to a two-strand Kessler repair, the six-strand repair had a better result in total active movement and grip strength [50]. Epitendinous suture with a 6-0 monofilament can increase the strength of the repair [51].

Zone 1 tendon disruption is due to either a laceration of the FDP tendon distal to the insertion of the FDS, or to an avulsion at the proximal aspect of the distal phalanx. If the distal stump is longer than 1 cm, primary end-to-end repair is indicated. If the distal stump is less than 1 cm long, a tendon to bone repair is indicated.

Zone II injuries are between the A1 pulley and the insertion of the FDS tendon. The proper relationship of the FDS tendon and the FDP need to be determined with appropriate repair.

Zone III, IV, and V injuries are located proximal to the A1 pulley. The tendon repair is similar to injuries described earlier. These injuries tend to have a better prognosis because the repaired tendons move through a more spacious area [52].

Patients are splinted postoperatively, with the wrist in neutral or slightly flexed position, the MCP joint at 70°, and the interphalangeal (IP) joints should be straight [53]. Aftercare of flexor tendon injuries requires early mobilization, which allows passive flexion carried out by a rubber string and active extension for 6 weeks [54]. The next 6 weeks, rehabilitation will continue with active flexion.

*Recommendation*: Most hand surgeons would operate when laceration is >50% of flexor tendon. Early mobilization recommended for flexor tendon injury repairs. Extensor tendons should be primarily repaired with core sutures followed by 3–4 weeks of immobilization.

*Recommendation grade*: B

## 30.6 How Are Common Fractures of the Hand Such a Phalanx, Boxer's, Bennett's, and Rolando Fractures Treated?

### 30.6.1 Phalanx Fracture

Indications for conservative treatment include fractures with adequate reduction; fracture with suboptimal reduction, good longitudinal alignment that does not involve the joint, and no rotational deformity; and noncompliant patients [55]. Indications for surgical treatment include persistently unstable fractures after reduction; inability to obtain satisfactory reduction with shortening rotation, angulation, or articular step-off (>1 mm); open fractures with severe soft tissue injuries; displaced articular surface; or multiple fragments that cannot be reduced adequately [55].

Nonoperative treatment is managed with a cast or splint immobilization for 4 weeks. For nondisplaced fractures, buddy taping is an accepted method. This will allow for finger motion that will decrease joint stiffness.

Operative treatment for displaced and unstable fractures can be reduced via closed reduction and percutaneous fixation with two crossing K-wires. If adequate reduction is achieved, gentle range of motion can start within a week of surgery. K-wire removal and progression of therapy can commence within 4 weeks. Open reduction is warranted in fractures with nerve or tendon injuries and fractures with significant bone loss. Methods of fixation include K-wires, low-profile titanium plates, lag screw, cerclage wires, or dynamic external fixators [55].

Tuft fractures require only a short period of immobilization of 2–4 weeks. Displaced, unstable, or painful tuft fractures with delayed union may require reduction and internal splinting with K-wires. A concomitant nail bed injury should be repaired.

### 30.6.2 Boxer's Fracture

A boxer's fracture is a common name for a fracture of the distal fifth metacarpal commonly caused by punching an object with a closed fist. If the forces are severe, the fractures can be comminuted and displaced and may result in an obvious deformity. The angulation of the metacarpal head may be accompanied by impaction or rotation of the metacarpal head.

Treatment of the fracture can be accomplished with closed or open reduction and limiting joint fixation. This will often depend on the degree of angulation and the rotation of the metacarpal head. If the angulation is greater than 45° with little or no rotation and slight displacement, minimal immobilization is an option [56]. The little finger can be strapped to the ring finger. If the angulation is greater than 45°, or if rotation is greater than 20°, external reduction is required. Once again, the little finger is taped to the ring finger. If the rotation of the metacarpal head is great, 80°–90°, the fracture site may require open reduction and internal fixation with the use of K-wires.

### 30.6.3 Bennett's Fracture

Bennett's fracture is an intra-articular fracture separating the volar ulnar aspect of the metacarpal base from the remaining thumb metacarpal [57]. Treatment for this type of fracture with closed reduction and percutaneous K-wire fixation of the metacarpal shaft to the trapezium in the reduced position [58]. For fractures that are deemed irreducible with an intra-articular step-off greater than 1 mm, open reduction should be performed [57].

### 30.6.4 Rolando Fracture

Rolando fracture refers to comminuted fractures of the base of the first metacarpal that are in a Y or T shape including the volar ulnar Bennett fragment in addition to a dorsal radial fragment. This type of fracture has a worse prognosis than a Bennett fracture. If there are two large fragments, open reduction and internal fixation through a Wagner approach is performed [59]. Various methods of fixation can be used such as K-wires, tension banding, and plate and screw fixation [60].

*Recommendation*: Closed reduction or open reduction of fractures may be attempted; however, technique must be adjusted for the individual fracture with the goal of preservation of function through stabilizing an adequate reduction.

*Recommendation grade*: C

**TABLE 30.1**

Levels of Evidence

| No. | Subject | Year | References | Level | Strength | Findings |
|---|---|---|---|---|---|---|
| 1 | Bacteriology of animal bites | 1993 | [3] | IIB | B | Complex mix of bacteria including *Pasteurella*. |
| 2 | Compare cast immobilization with internal fixation in nondisplaced scaphoid fractures and MRI to CT | 2008, 2012, 2014 | [22–24] | IA, IIB IIC | B | Percutaneous screws allow faster return to work; no long-term benefit of internal fixation. |
| 3 | Upper limb replantation success | 2000, 2001, 2010, 2012, 2014 | [25–30] | IIC | C | Large retrospective reviews confirming successful outcomes in 70%–87% of patients. |
| 4 | Compartment syndrome | 1979, 1994, 2014 | [33,34,36] | IIC | C | Pressure within 20 of diastolic cause ischemic muscle necrosis and success of treatment is both time- and pressure-dependent. |
| 5 | When lacerations should be repaired, compare dynamic with static splinting for extensor tendon injury | 2013, 2014 | [41,45] | III, IIB | C | Most hand surgeons would operate when laceration is >50% of flexor tendon; early improved function with dynamic splinting up to 6 months, then no difference. |
| 6 | How are common fractures of the hand such as phalanx, boxer's, Bennett's, and Rolando fractures treated? | 2006, 2009 | [56,59] | IIC IIC | C | Closed reduction or open reduction of fractures may be attempted; the technique must be adjusted for the individual fracture with the goal of preservation of function through stabilizing an adequate reduction. |
| 7 | What do you do with a fingertip amputation that is too distal for replantation? | 1998, 2003 | [60,61] | IIC IIC | C | Defects smaller than 1 cm$^2$ can be allowed to heal by secondary intent; otherwise, a composite graft or local flap can be used instead. |

## 30.7 What Do You Do with a Fingertip Amputation That Is Too Distal for Replantation?

The goal of treatment for fingertip amputations too distal for microvascular replantation is to restore a painless, minimally shortened digit and durable sensate skin on the tip [60]. Therapeutic options range from allowing the wound to heal by secondary intention to primary closure with or without bone shortening, skin grafts, composite grafts, and local, regional, or distant flaps [61]. Composite grafts may allow for the patient to maintain digital length and function while retaining a cosmetically pleasing finger. If it does not survive, then finger shortening and closure can then be performed [61] (Table 30.1).

*Recommendation*: Defects smaller than 1 cm$^2$ can be allowed to heal by secondary intent; otherwise, a composite graft or local flap can be used instead.

*Recommendation grade*: C

## References


1. Osterman M, Draeger R, Stern P. Acute hand infections. *J Hand Surg*. 2014;39(8):1628–1635.
2. Wiggins ME, Akelman E, Weiss AP. The management of dog bites and dog bite infection to the hand. *Orthopedics*. 1994;17(7):617–623.
3. Moran GJ, Talan DA. Hand infections. *Emerg Med Clin North Am*. 1993;11(3):601–619.
4. Figueiredo JF, Borges AS, Martinez R et al. Transmission of hepatitis C virus but not human immunodeficiency virus type 1 by a human bite. *Clin Infect Dis*. 1994;19:546–547.
5. Bartholomew CF, Jones AM. Human bites: A rare risk factor for HIV transmission. *AIDS*. 2006;20:631–632.
6. Shapiro CN. Transmission of hepatitis viruses. *Ann Intern Med*. 1994;120(1):82–84.
7. Vidmar L, Poljak M, Tomazic J, Seme K, Klavs I. Transmission of HIV-1 by human bite. *Lancet*. 1996;347(9017):1762.
8. Dusheiko GM, Smith M, Scheuer PJ. Hepatitis C virus transmitted by human bite. *Lancet*. 1990;336:503–504.
9. Davis LG, Weber DJ, Lemon SM. Horizontal transmission of hepatitis B virus. *Lancet*. 1989;1:889–893.
10. Robinson RA, Pugh RN. Dogs, zoonoses and immunosuppression. *J R Soc Promot Health*. 2002;122(2):95–98.
11. Oya J, Hanai K, Miura J et al. Diabetic gangrene in multiple fingers and toes after a dog bite in an elderly patient with type 2 diabetes. *Intern Med*. 2011;50(12):1303–1307.
12. Schnall SB, Vu-Rose T, Holtom PD, Doyle B, Stevanovic M. Tissue pressures in pyogenic flexor tenosynovitis of the finger: Compartment syndrome and its management. *J Bone Joint Surg Br*. 1996;78(5):792–795.
13. Pang HN, Teoh LC, Yam AK et al. Factors affecting the prognosis of pyogenic flexor tenosynovitis. *J Bone Joint Surg Am*. 2007;89(8):1742–1748.
14. Draeger RW, Bynum DK. Flexor tendon sheath infections of the hand. *Jam Acad Orthop Surg*. 2012;20(6):373–382.
15. Talan DA, Abrahamian FM, Moran GJ et al. Clinical presentation and bacteriologic analysis of infected human bites in patients presenting to emergency departments. *Clin Infect Dis*. 2003;37(11):1481–1489.
16. Holm M, Tarnvik A. Hospitalization due to Pasteurella multocida infected animal bite wounds: Correlation with inadequate primary antibiotic medication. *Scand J Infect Dis*. 2000;32(2)181–183.
17. Malahias M, Jordan D, Hughes O et al. Bite injuries to the hand: Microbiology, virology and management. *Open Orthop J*. 2014;8:157–161.
18. Barton NJ. Twenty questions about scaphoid fractures. *J Bone Joint Surg Br*. 1992;17:289–310.
19. Freeland P. Scaphoid tubercle tenderness: A better indicator of scaphoid fractures? *Arch Emerg Med*. 1989;6:46–50.
20. Carpenter C, Pines JM, Schuur JD et al. Adult scaphoid fracture. *Acad Emerg Med*. 2014;21(2):101–121.
21. Dias JJ, Wildin CJ, Bhowal B, Thompson JR. Should acute scaphoid fractures be fixed? A randomized controlled trial. *J Bone Joint Surg Am*. 2005;87(10):2160–2168.
22. Vinnars B, Pietreanu M, Bodestedt A et al. Nonoperative compared with operative treatment of acute scaphoid fractures. A randomized clinical trial. *J Bone Joint Surg Am*. 2008;90(6):1176–1185.
23. Buijze GA, Goslings JC, Rhemrev SJ et al. Cast immobilization with and without immobilization of the thumb for nondisplaced and minimally displaced scaphoid waist fractures: A multicenter, randomized controlled trial. *J Hand Surg Am*. 2014;39(4):621–627.
24. Singh HP, Taub N, Dias JJ. Management of displaced fractures of the waist of the scaphoid: Meta analyses of comparative studies. *Injury*. 2012;43(6):933–939.
25. Beris AE, Lykissas MG, Korompilias AV et al. Digit and hand replantation. *Trauma Surg*. September 2010;130(9):1141–1147.
26. Soucacos PN. Indications and selection for digital amputation and replantation. *J Hand Surg*. 2001;26:572–581.
27. Dec W. A meta-analysis of success rates for digit replantation. *Tech Hand Up Extrem Surg*. 2006;10(3):124–129.
28. Waikakul S, Sakkarnkosal S, Vanadurongwan V et al. Results of 1018 digital replantations in 522 patients. *Injury*. 2000;31:33–40.
29. Soucacos PN, Beris AE, Malizos KN, Touliatos AS. Bilateral thumb amputation. *Microsurgery*. 1994;15:454–458.
30. Lloyd MS, Teo TC, Pickford MA, Arnstein PM. Preoperative management of the amputated limb. *Emerg Med J*. 2005;22:478–480.
31. Wei DH, Strauch RJ. Smoking and hand surgery. *J Hand Surg*. 2013;38(1):176–179.

32. Heistein JB, Cook PA. Factors affecting composite graft survival in digital tip amputations. *Ann Plas Surg.* 2003;50:299–303.
33. Garner MR, Taylor SA, Gausden E, Lyden JP. Compartment syndrome: Diagnosis, management, unique concerns in the twenty-first century. *HSS J.* 2014;10(2):143–152.
34. Matava MJ, Whitesides TE, Seiler JG, Hewan-Lowe K, Hutton WC. Determination of the compartment pressure threshold of muscle ischemia in a canine model. *J Traumu.* 1994;37(1):50–58.
35. Heckman MM, Whitesides TE, Grewe SR, Rooks MD. Compartment pressure in association with closed tibial fractures. The relationship between tissue pressure, compartment, and the distance from the site of the fracture. *J Bone Joint Surg Am.* 1994;76(9):1285–1292.
36. Halpern AA, Nagel DA. Compartment syndromes of the forearm: Early recognition using tissue pressure measurement. *J Hand Surg Am.* 1979;4(3):258–263.
37. Whitesides TE, Haney TC, Morimoto K, Harada H. Tissue pressure measurements as a determinant for the need of fasciotomy. *Clin Orthop Relat Res.* 1975;113:43–51.
38. Cha J, York B, Tawfik J. Forearm compartment syndrome. *Eplasty.* 2014;14:ic10.
39. Friedrich JB, Shin AY. Management of forearm compartment syndrome. *Hand Clin.* 2007;23(2):245–254.
40. Gelberman RH, Garfin SR, Hergenroeder PT, Mubarak SJ, Menon J. Compartment syndromes of the forearm: Diagnosis and treatment. *Slin Orthop Relat Res.* 1981;161:252–261.
41. Carty MJ, Blazar PE. Complex flexor and extensor tendon injuries. *Hand Clin.* 2013;29(2):283–293.
42. Schoffl V, Heid A, Kupper T. Tendon injuries of the hand. *World J Orthop.* 2012;3(6):62–69.
43. Kondratko J, Duenwald-Kuehl S, Lakes R, Vanderby R. Mechanical compromise of partially lacerated flexor tendons. *J Biomech Eng.* 2013;135(1):011001.
44. Altan E, Bulent N, Basser R, Yalcin L. Soft-tissue mallet injuries: A comparison of early and delayed treatment. *J Hand Surg.* 2014;39(10):1982–1985.
45. Baratz ME, Schmidt CC, Hughes TB et al. 2005. Extensor tendon injuries. In: Green D et al. (eds.), *Green's Operative Hand Surgery*, 5th edn. Elsevier Churchill Livingstone: Philadelphia, PA, pp. 187–217.
46. Chauhan A, Jacobs B, Andoga A, Baratz M. Extensor tendon injuries in athletes. *Sports Med Arthroscopy Rev.* 2014;22(1):45–55.
47. Stern PJ. Extensor tenotomy: A technique for correction of posttraumatic distal interphalangeal joint hyperextension deformity. *J Hand Surg Am.* 1989;14:546–549.
48. Elliot D. Primary flexor tendon repair-operative repair, pulley management and rehabilitation. *J Hand Surg Br.* 2002;27:507–513.
49. Lalonde DH. An evidence based approach to flexor tendon laceration repair. *Plast Reconstr Surg.* 2011;127:885–890.
50. Hoffman GL, Buchler U, Vogelin E. Clinical results of flexor tendon repair in zone II using a six stand double loop technique compared with a two strand technique. *J Hand Surg Eur.* 2008;33:418–423.
51. Diao E, Hariharan JS, Soejima O et al. Effect of peripheral suture depth on strength of tendon repairs. *J Hand Surg Am.* 1996;21:234–239.
52. Mehling IM, Arsalan-Wener A, Sauerbier M. Evidence-based flexor tendon repair. *Clin Plast Surg.* 2014;41(3):513–523.
53. Lehfeldt M, Ray E, Sherman R. MOC-PS (SM) CME article: Treatment of flexor tendon laceration. *Plast Reconstr Surg.* 2008;121:1–12.
54. Hernandez J, Stern PJ. Complex injuries including flexor tendon disruption. *Hand Clinics.* 2005;21(2):187–197.
55. Bhatt RA, Schmidt S, Stang F. Methods and pitfalls in treatment of fractures in the digits. *Clin Plast Surg.* 2014;41(3):429–450.
56. Altizer L. Boxer's fracture. *Orthopaedic Nurs.* 2006;25(4):271–273.
57. Edmunds JO. Traumatic dislocations and instability of the trapeziometacarpal joint of the thumb. *Hand Clin.* 2006;22:365–392.
58. Demi C, Smekal V, Kastenberger T et al. Pressure distribution in carpometacarpal joint, due to step off in operatively treated Bennett's fractures. *Injury.* 2014;45(10):1574–1578.
59. Carlsen BT, Moran SL. Thumb trauma: Bennett fractures, Rolando fractures, and Ulnar collateral ligament injuries. *J Hand Surg.* 2009;34(5):945–952.
60. Martin C, Gonzalez del Pino J. Controversies in the treatment of fingertip amputations. Conservative versus surgical reconstruction. *Clin Orthop Relat Res.* 1998;353:63–73.
61. Heistein J, Cook P. Factors affecting composite graft survival in digital tip amputation. *Ann Plas Surg.* 2003;50(3):299–303.

# 31

# *Lower Extremity Injury*

**Hany Bahouth and Yoram Kluger**

**CONTENTS**



## 31.1 Introduction

Acute lower extremity trauma is a very common health problem. In 2012, 278,100 lower extremity injuries were entered into the civilian National Trauma Data Bank [1]. According to the Health Care Cost and Utilization Project, more than 746,000 people in 2003 were hospitalized for lower limb fractures [1]. Because of the increasing use of the safety devices in vehicles, trauma caregivers are managing more severely injured survivors with catastrophic lower extremity injuries. This chapter will discuss several highly important issues in several lower extremity injuries.

## 31.2 Do Clinical Findings Aid in the Diagnosis of Compartment Syndrome of the Lower Extremity?

Compartment syndrome (CS) is defined as an increase in pressure within confined anatomic space resulting in ischemic changes to the encompassed tissues [2]. Vascular impairment leads to decreased tissue oxygenation, and if persistent, cellular death will follow. Nervous and muscular tissues appear to be the most sensitive to ischemia. The incidence of CS is 7.3 per 100,000 in men and 0.7 per 100,000 in women [3]. Fractures are the most common etiology and the most common location for CS is the lower leg, which is reported to occur in 1%–10% of all tibial fractures [4]. Clinical findings (pain, paresthesia, pain with passive stretch, and paresis) have a low sensitivity (13%–19%) and low positive predictive value (11%–15%) [5] for the diagnosis of the lower extremity CS in alert patients. In unconscious patients, compartment pressure measurements may facilitate diagnosis of CS.

*Recommendation*: Clinical findings are poor predictors of compartmental syndrome of the lower extremity, particularly in patients with altered mental status (Grade C recommendation).

## 31.3 Which Compartment Pressure Measurement Method Is Optimal for the Diagnosis of Acute Lower Leg CS?

The utility of compartment pressure in the diagnosis of CS and the subsequent need for fasciotomy is controversial. Various methods of measuring compartment pressures have been described [5–9]. In a prospective observational study over 6 months, Koiser et al. [10] evaluated 45 patients who were admitted to a trauma intensive care unit (ICU) and met one or more of the risk factors for CS, which included pulmonary artery catheter–directed shock resuscitation, open or closed tibial shaft fracture, major vascular injury below the aortic bifurcation, abdominal CS, or pelvic or lower extremity crush injury. Initial screening included a comprehensive physical examination and compartment pressure measurements (anterior and deep posterior compartments) when physical examination was suspicious or unreliable. Subsequent examination was performed every 4 h for 48 h. A difference of less than 30 mmHg between the diastolic blood pressure and the measured compartment pressure mandated four-compartment fasciotomy. During this time period, the incidence of acute lower leg CS in the screened patients was 20%. No limb loss was subsequently reported in this group of patients. The authors concluded that aggressive screening in high-risk patients may provide some diagnostic insights. Compartment pressure should be measured by devices designed for this purpose. If this specific equipment is unavailable, compartmental pressures may be measured by a standard 16-gauge cannula connected to a pressure transducer and monitor [10]. No other screening protocols for the diagnosis of the acute lower extremity CS were found in the English literature.

*Recommendation*: It is unclear what the value or optimal method of measuring compartmental pressure is (Grade C recommendation).

## 31.4 Is It Safe to Use Tourniquets in Major Lower Extremity Trauma?

Since the first description of tourniquets in the seventeenth century, their use has remained of uncertain benefit. The controversy exists on a number of tourniquet-related issues; the indications for tourniquet use, the optimal type of tourniquet, site (prehospital and emergency room) and timing of application and removal; and finally, who should apply the device [12]. Experiments in World War I revealed that tourniquet use was not without potential risks. Observations in World War II suggested that misuse or inadequate assessment was dangerous and, therefore, the standard of care was to limit tourniquet use in patients with obvious arterial bleeding [13]. In the modern military trauma management, the approach to tourniquet use has been changed owing to the recognition that external hemorrhage is a major cause of potentially preventable death following severe lower extremity injury in the battlefield [14–17]. Lessons learned from the recent conflicts in Iraq and Afghanistan have resulted in a more liberal use of tourniquets [18,19].

Five recent studies regarding the use of military tourniquets have given us a greater understanding of potential utility. The Norwegian military in Iraq in 1991 [20] reported on 68 patients who suffered traumatic amputations. Patients were compared during two different time spans. During the first time period, tourniquets were liberally used. In the second time period, wounds were managed by removing the tourniquet early and replacing with a tight elastic bandage. The mortality in the first group was 17% (3/18) but decreased in the second group to 2% (1/50). The transfusion requirements in the first group were 56% versus 27% in the second. The conclusion of the authors was that the use of tourniquet for traumatic amputations was ineffective and potentially dangerous. However, we feel the difference may be exclusively related to the severity of injury. The second study is from the Israeli Defense Force Medical Services [21], where 110 tourniquets were applied to 91 casualties; 53% were judged to have been applied properly, 78% (71% for the lower limbs) were felt to be effective, and 53% were thought to have been clinically indicated. They concluded that the use of field tourniquet was justified. The next study conducted by the 31st U.S. Combat Support Hospital in Iraq [22] studied 166 matched patients with significant extremity injuries. Sixty-seven patients who received prehospital tourniquets were compared with 99 who did not. Twenty-three percent of tourniquets were ineffective at controlling bleeding. The amputation rate was 42% in the tourniquet group and 26% in the nontourniquet group ($p < 0.04$). Tourniquet use was felt to have resulted in the unnecessary loss of 2% of limbs.

Kragh et al. [23] performed a prospective observational study at the U.S. combat support hospital in Baghdad, Iraq. Among 2838 injured and admitted civilian and military casualties with major limb trauma, 232 (8%) had 428 tourniquets applied on 309 injured limbs. Tourniquet use when shock was absent was strongly associated with survival (90% vs. 10%; $p = 0.001$). Prehospital applied tourniquet was 11%, whereas 38 patients had emergency department (ED) application of which nine died (24% mortality; $p = 0.05$). The five casualties indicated for tourniquets but had none used had a survival rate of 0% versus 87% for those casualties with tourniquets used ($p = 0.001$); patients (1.7%) sustained transient nerve palsy at the level of the tourniquet.

The same author [24] in a continuation of the previous study added 267 new patients to have a total population of 499 patients (232 in the previous study and 267 in the current study). In all, 862 tourniquets were applied on 651 limbs. Survival was 87% for both study periods. Morbidity rates for palsies at the level of the tourniquet were 1.5% for this study. Survival was associated with prehospital application (89% vs. 78% hospital, $p < 0.01$) and application before the onset of shock (97% vs. 4% after).

The authors of these two studies concluded that tourniquet use when shock was absent was strongly associated with saved lives, and prehospital use was also strongly associated with lifesaving. No limbs were lost due to tourniquet use.

The use of tourniquet in civilian trauma is much less clear and is not well studied. The Advanced Trauma Life Support (ATLS) manual [25] recommends judicious use of tourniquets to help save a life in potentially life-threatening extremity injury with major arterial bleeding. Even as recently as 2011, the Guidelines for Field Triage of Injured Patients does not include a recommendation for tourniquet use as a trauma triage criteria [26]. Lessons learned from the military management of these injuries are beginning to be adopted in the civilian community and the recent Boston marathon bombing event highlighted this issue [27].

The American College of Surgeons Committee on Trauma, in their evidence-based prehospital guideline for external hemorrhage control, recommends the use of tourniquets in the prehospital setting for the control of significant extremity hemorrhage if direct pressure is ineffective or impractical [28]. In a recent retrospective study of trauma patients at two large Canadian trauma centers with arterial injury after isolated extremity trauma, 190 patients were included in the study and only four patients had a prehospital tourniquet applied and four patients had a tourniquet applied in the emergency room within 1 h of injury. Of these eight patients, none died. Six patients died without tourniquet, all from hemorrhage. The authors concluded that tourniquets may prevent exsanguination in the civilian setting for patients with blunt or penetrating trauma to the extremity [29].

*Recommendation*: Tourniquet use appears indicated on the battlefield when required for hemorrhage control for limited time intervals (Grade B recommendation). Civilian use of tourniquets is justified in exsanguinating patients due to extremity injury with uncontrolled hemorrhage (Grade C recommendation).

## 31.5 Is a "Damage Control" Approach Justified for the Orthopedic Care of Multiple Trauma Patients?

Rotondo et al. [30] found a remarkable salvage rate of over 70% in a limited number of patients treated with damage control for abdominal vascular injury and massive shock, hypothermia, and acidosis. Since then, the damage control approach to unstable trauma patients has gained widespread use in other trauma fields (chest, vascular, urology) along with orthopedic injuries. Damage control orthopedic intervention appears to be a suitable alternative to definitive orthopedic surgery (i.e., open reduction, internal fixation) for patients at high risk of developing posttraumatic systemic complications such as acute respiratory distress syndrome (ARDS), fat embolism syndrome, and multiple organ failure. The orthopedic damage control approach in lower extremity trauma includes the following:

1. External fixation (EF) and temporary soft tissue coverage at open fracture sites
2. Distal perfusion of the injured extremity with temporary intraluminal shunting
3. Liberal use of fasciotomy in the setting of ischemia

Early stabilization of major skeletal injuries was the mainstay of treatment in trauma surgery in the 1980s and early 1990s. The early total care (ETC) involves definitive surgical stabilization of all long bone fractures during the early phase of treatment (24–48 h) [31]. The ETC concept was not suitable for all multiple trauma patients since in an unstable patient, it was associated with a high rate of pulmonary complications. The shift from ETC to damage control orthopedics (DCO) came after significant advances in the understanding of pathophysiological and immunological mechanisms regulating the host responses to injuries. EF has become the DCO workhorse. For most upper extremity injuries, simple stabilization with splints or slings will suffice, and for closed fractures below the knee, splinting is the best option [32].

EF is a viable alternative to attain temporary rigid stabilization in patients with multiple injuries. It is rapid, with negligible blood loss, and can be followed by intramedullary nailing (IMN) when the patient has normalized hemodynamically [33]. In one retrospective study, investigators tracked the clinical course of adult trauma patients admitted with femur fractures who were treated with EF versus IMN. The patients treated with EF were more seriously injured and less physiologically stable than those treated with standard IMN. The authors' conclusion was that immediate EF followed by early closed medullary nailing is a safe method for treating femoral shaft fractures in badly injured patients [33].

Pape et al. [34] assessed the impact of time on femur shaft fracture repair in 514 multiple blunt trauma patients. They demonstrated a significant increased incidence of ARDS in patients during the damage control era when they were submitted to primary intramedullary stabilization of the femur shaft when compared with EF. They also noted a decrease in the relative percentage of patients who developed ARDS, 54.6% (ETC) to 26.4% (DCO) when primary IMN was performed, which decreased from 97.4% (ETC) to 22.1% when primary EF was performed.

Importantly, in a systematic literature review conducted by the German Trauma Society, controlled trials were tested and failed to support a "generalized management strategy" [35,36]. A total of 1465 femur shaft fracture treatments in 8057 trauma registry patients (age 19–35 years; Injury Severity Score [ISS] 14.9–23.5; 17.3% mortality) were treated initially (<24 h) by EF, nail, or plate in 47.0%, 41.1%, and 11.9%, respectively. Despite large interhospital variability, EF was more likely with increasing severity of ISS, Glasgow Coma Score (GCS), thoracic trauma, base deficit, coagulation abnormalities, and initial probability of death. Although decision making is currently based on poorly validated criteria, anatomic and physiologic injury severity appears to influence the choice of management concept.

A prospective cohort-controlled trial [37], in 409 patients with multitrauma, 75 (mean ISS = 37.3) required DCO surgery for 135 fractures, whereas 334 patients (ISS of 30.4) did not require immediate fracture fixation. Mean surgical time was short and ranged 30–62 min for DCO. Duration of EF averaged 13.7 days (range, 3–46 days). Overall mortality in DCO patients was significantly lower than predicted by Trauma and Injury Severity Score (TRISS) (20% vs. 39.3%), as it was in the 334 patients without immediate fracture fixation (29.5% vs. 24.3%). In this study, DCO appears to reduce operation time and blood loss in the primary treatment period among severely injured patients compared with historical data. In addition, the authors found that DCO did not appear to be associated with an increased rate of procedure-related complications. They concluded that DCO with early and one-stage conversion seems to be a safe strategy of primary fracture treatment in patients with multiple injuries.

DCO is the preferred approach in unstable in extremis patients and the ETC approach is the gold standard in stable patients [38]. Pape coined the term "borderline" patient to describe a patient who is stable before surgery but deteriorates unexpectedly and develops organ dysfunction postoperatively [38].

In a retrospective cohort study by Doussoux et al. [39], 41 multitrauma patients with femur fracture were treated with EF following damage control orthopedic surgery. The mortality rates, TRISS analysis, incidence of ARDS, and multiorgan failure (MOF) were analyzed. Five patients with EF died. The difference between predicted mortality by TRISS and actual mortality showed a reduction of 15.9% in favor of damage control orthopedic surgery.

The European Polytrauma Study Group on the Management of Femur Fractures performed a randomized multicenter study, comparing ETC and DCO. Among "borderline" patients, the incidence of ARDS was 16.7% in the ETC group and 11.1% in the DCO group ($p$ = 0.618) [40] A lower incidence of ARDS is usually reported in North American studies. In the recent North American retrospective series, the incidence of ARDS was 1.5% in the ETC group and 0.0% in the DCO group ($p$ = 1.000) [41]. From these data, we may conclude that an adequate resuscitation before surgery is essential.

In a prospective randomized controlled study by Nicholas et al. [42] of 66 patients with femoral shaft fracture, 68% were stable and 32% were borderline. ETC was utilized in 98% of the stable patients and in 86% of the borderline group. The patients in this study were compared with similar groups from another randomized control study [39]. The studied approach resulted in shorter ICU and ventilator days, fewer septic complications, and a potentially lower incidence of organ failure than in the compared RCT study.

Finally, bilateral femoral fractures represent a separate entity with different prognosis and therapeutic options. This injury pattern is associated with a higher mortality and ARDS rates [43] and increased number of associated injuries (up to 80%). Although there is a paucity of literature data on this subset of patients, DCO seems to be the ideal strategy.

*Recommendation*: Damage control orthopedic is recommended in severely unstable and underresuscitated injured multiple trauma patients (Grade B recommendation). ETC is recommended in stable injured patients with femoral fracture (Grade B recommendation).

## 31.6 When Should Antibiotics Be Utilized in the Setting of Open Lower Extremity Fracture?

Open fractures require urgent surgical treatment to reduce the risk of infection. Failure to utilize prophylactic antibiotics and increased time from injury to initiation of antimicrobial agent and operative debridement are among the primary factors that increase the risk of infection [44].

Prophylactic antibiotics for open fracture frequently exceeds guideline recommendations in the duration and spectrum of coverage. This noncompliance with guidelines may cause increase in hospital morbidity [46].

Gustilo et al. [52] were first to recognize that fracture location, mechanism, grade, and operative management all influence the development of infection. In a double-blind prospective trial, Dellinger et al. randomized 248 patients with open fractures to receive 1 or 5 days of cefonicid sodium therapy or 5 days of cefamandole nafate therapy as part of the initial treatment. Rates of fracture-associated infections in the three groups were 10 of 79 (13%), 10 of 85 (12%), and 11 of 84 (13%), respectively. The 95% confidence limit for the difference in infection rates between the 1-day group and the combined 5-day groups was 0%–8.3%. The actual difference was 0.2%. They concluded that a brief course of antibiotic administration was not inferior to a prolonged course of antibiotics for prevention of postoperative fracture site infections [45,46].

In a retrospective case–control study by Dunkel et al. [47], 1492 open fractures were retrieved; these were Gustilo and Anderson Grade I (44.4%), Grade II (24.8%), Grade III (20.8%), and unclassifiable (10.0%). The study did not show any significant differences in the infection between 1 day to more than 5 days of antibiotic treatment.

In their prospective clinical trial, Saveli et al. [48] studied 130 patients with open fractures. The patients were randomized to receive cefazolin as control arm and the experimental arm to receive vancomycin and cefazolin from presentation to the emergency department until 24 h after surgery. The authors prospectively assessed the patients for surgical site infection for no less than 30 days and up to 12 months, they found no significant difference between the regimens.

Rodriguez et al. [49] examined an evidence-based protocol for prophylactic antibiotics in open fractures and implemented a new protocol for antibiotic prophylaxis based on grade of open fracture. Grade II fractures received cefazolin (clindamycin if allergy), and Grade III received ceftriaxone (clindamycin and aztreonam if allergy) for 48 h. One hundred seventy-four femur and tibia/fibula open fractures were analyzed. Aminoglycoside, vancomycin, and penicillin were removed from the protocol. The authors found no increase in skin and soft tissue infection rates before and after the protocol implementation.

*Recommendation*: In the setting of open extremity fractures, no more than 24 h are required postoperatively. First- and second-generation cephalosporins are recommended for Gustilo I, II, and III, respectively (Grade C recommendation).

## 31.7 What Is the Optimal Timing of Long Bone Fracture Stabilization in the Multiple Trauma Patient?

The potential advantages of the early surgery for the long bone fracture stabilization (defined as <48 h from injury) include increased patient mobilization and decreased pulmonary morbidity (fat emboli syndrome, pneumonia, ARDS), late septic sequelae, mortality, hospital length of stay (LOS), ICU LOS, and ventilator days. The known disadvantages of the early stabilization in polytrauma patients include increased blood loss, fluid administration, and surgical stress; fat embolism and possibly a greater likelihood of pulmonary complication risks; and mortality [50].

There have been concerns regarding the timing of long bone stabilization in patients with brain or chest injury. Problems with early fixation of long bones in patients with brain injury include secondary brain injury as a result of hypoxemia, hypotension, and/or complexity of controlling intracranial hypertension, as well as increased fluid administration, which might exacerbate cerebral edema.

This question was addressed by a subcommittee of the Practice Management Guideline Committee of the Eastern Association for the Surgery of Trauma that conducted a systematic review and meta-analysis regarding the optimal timing (early <24 h vs. late >24 h) for internal fixation of open or closed femur fractures. No significant reduction in mortality, infection, or venous thromboembolic events (VTE) was associated with early stabilization. There was only a trend toward a lower risk of mortality, infection, and VTE in early open reduction and internal fixation [51].

*Recommendation*: There is no difference in survival of polytrauma patients who undergo early or late long bone fracture stabilization. It is unclear whether timing of bone fracture stabilization impacts outcome in the setting of chest or brain injury (Grade C recommendation).

## 31.8 What Is the Best Method for Prediction of Amputation after Severe Lower Extremity Injuries?

Several limb salvage scoring systems have been devised to help clinicians determine when to attempt limb salvage or whether to perform early amputation [54,55]. The level of the vascular injury, degree of bony injury, degree of muscular injury, and the warm ischemia time have been utilized to predict the outcome after lower extremity injury [31].

The Predictive Salvage Index (PSI) [32] calculated score by dividing dermal, muscular, and bony damage into slight, moderate, or severe and counted one to three points, respectively. This score showed a sensitivity of 78% and specificity of 100%. In 1985, Lange et al. showed [56] that in patients with similar local injuries, the age, comorbidities, and the social environment of the patients also play an important role in the outcome. In 1990, Helfet et al. [57] found Lange's absolute indications for amputation difficult to determine in certain patients. From the retrospective analysis of 26 severe injuries to the lower extremity with vascular injuries (Gustilo Grade IIIC), four parameters were found to be significant: extent of the bone and soft tissue damage, time of ischemia, initial shock, and age of the patient. In 1994, McNamara et al. [58] published the Nerve Injury, Ischemia, Soft Tissue Injury, Skeletal Injury, Shock, and Age (NISSSA) Score by retrospective evaluation of 24 patients with Grade IIIc injury. Boss et al. [59], in a prospective study of 556 limbs, found that all the lower extremity injury scoring systems have limited usefulness and cannot be used as the sole criterion by which amputation decisions are made (Tables 31.1 and 31.2).

*Recommendation*: At present, there is no predictive scale that can be used with confidence to determine

**TABLE 31.1**
Grade Recommendation

| Subject | Findings | Grade of Recommendation |
|---|---|---|
| How well do clinical findings aid in the diagnosis of CS of the lower extremity? | Clinical findings are poor predictors for the diagnosis of CS of the lower extremity. | C |
| Which compartmental pressure measurement method is optimal for the diagnosis of acute lower leg CS? | It is unclear what the value of optimal method of measuring compartmental pressure is. | C |
| What is the optimal method for screening and diagnosing CS? | No recommendation on this subject. | C |
| Is it safe to use tourniquets in major lower extremity trauma? | Tourniquet use appears indicated on the battlefield when required for hemorrhage control for limited time intervals. | B |
| | Tourniquet use in civilian trauma needs to be addressed with more prospective studies. | C |
| Is damage control justified for the orthopedic care of multiple trauma patients? | Damage control orthopedic is recommended in unstable severely injured multiple trauma patients. | B |
| When should antibiotics be utilized in the setting of open lower extremity fracture? | Prophylactic antibiotics are required for open fractures. | C |
| What is the optimal time from injury to long bone fracture stabilization in the multiple trauma patient? | There is no difference in survival in polytrauma patients who undergo early or late long bone fracture stabilization. It is unclear whether timing of bone fracture stabilization impacts mortality infectious rare and VTE. | C |
| What is the best method for prediction of amputation after severe lower extremity injuries? | There is no predictive scale that can be used with confidence to determine whether to amputate or attempt to salvage a mangled lower extremity. Scoring systems should be used only as guides to supplement the surgeon's clinical judgment and experience. | C |

**TABLE 31.2**
Levels of Evidence

| Subject | Level of Evidence | Grade of Recommendation | Findings |
|---|---|---|---|
| Clinical findings for the diagnosis of CS | IIb | B | The predictive value of the clinical findings for the diagnosis of CS of the lower extremity has to be defined. |
| The optimal method for the measurement of the compartment pressure | III | C | No recommendation for one of the screened methods. |
| The optimal method for screening and diagnosing CS | IIb | C | No recommendation on this subject. |
| The safety of tourniquet use | IIb | B | Appropriate use of tourniquets in the battlefield for a short time can be safe. |
| Justification for the damage control orthopedic | IIb | B | Damage control orthopedic is recommended in severely injured patients. |
| Antibiotic prophylaxis in open fractures | Ia | B | 24 h of first-generation cephalosporin agent is sufficient in Grade I open fracture. |
| The optimal time for long bone fracture stabilization | III | C | No deference in outcome between early and late stabilization. |
| The best scoring system for the clinical decision in mangled extremity | IIb | B | The scores are adjuncts tools to aid the clinician but are not a sole criterion. |

whether to amputate or attempt to salvage a mangled lower extremity. Scoring systems should be used only as guides to supplement the surgeon's clinical judgment and experience (Grade C recommendation).

## References


1. Nance ML. National Trauma Data Bank Annual Report. 2012. http://www.facs.org/trauma/ntdb/pdf/ntdb-annual-report-2012.pdf (Accessed on October 22, 2013).
2. Konstantakos EK, Dalstrom DJ, Nelles ME et al. Diagnosis and management of extremity compartment syndromes: An orthopaedic perspective. *Am Surg.* December 2007;73(12):1199–1209.
3. McQueen MM, Gaston P, Court-Brown CM. Acute compartment syndrome: Who is at risk? *J Bone Joint Surg Br.* 2000;82:200–203.
4. Elliot KGB, Johnstone AJ. Diagnosing acute compartment syndrome. *J Bone Joint Surg Br.* 2003;85:625–632.
5. Ulmer T. The clinical diagnosis of compartment syndrome of the lower leg: Are clinical findings predictive of the disorder? *J Orthop Trauma.* 2002;16(8):572–577.
6. Ktz LM, Nauriyal V, Nagarj S et al. Infrared imaging of trauma patients for detection of acute compartment syndrome of the leg. *Crit Care Med.* 2008;36(6):1756–1761.
7. Wilson SC, Varhas MS, Berson L, Paul EM. A simple method to measure compartment pressures using an intravenous catheter. *Orthopedics.* 1997;20:403–406.
8. Gianotti G, Cohn SM, Brown M et al. Utility of near infrared spectroscopy in the diagnosis of lower extremity compartment syndrome. *J Trauma.* 2000;48(3):396–401.
9. Arbabi S, Brundage SI, Gentilello LM. Near infrared spectroscopy: A potential method for continuous, transcutaneous monitoring for compartment syndrome in critically injured patients. *J Trauma.* 1999;47:829–833.
10. Koiser R, Moore F, Selby JH, Coucanour C, Kozar R, Gonzalez E, Todd R. Acute lower extremity compartment syndrome screening protocol in critically ill trauma patients. *J Trauma.* 2007;63(3):268–275.
11. Wilson SC, Varahas MS, Berson L et al. A single method to measure pressures using an intravenous catheter. *Orthopedics.* 1997;20:403–406.
12. Thomas JW, Robert LM. Issues related to the use of tourniquet on the battlefield. *Mil Med.* 2005;270:770–775.
13. Welling DR, Burris DG, Hutton JE et al. A balanced approach to tourniquet use: Lessons learned and relearned. *J Am Coll Surg.* 2006;203(1):107–115.
14. Kragh JF Jr, Walters TJ, Baer DG et al. Practical use of emergency tourniquets to stop bleeding in major limb trauma. *J Trauma.* 2008;64(Suppl):S38–S49.
15. Beekly AC, Sebesta JA, Blackbourne LH et al. Prehospital tourniquet use in Operation Iraqi Freedom: Effect on hemorrhage control and outcomes. *J Trauma.* 2008;64(Suppl):S28–S37.
16. Bellamy RF. The causes of death in conventional land warfare: Implications for combat casualty care research. *Mil Med.* 1984;149:55–62.
17. Holocomb JB, McMullin NR, Pearse L et al. Causes of death in U.S, special operation forces in the global war on terrorism: 2001–2004. *Ann Surg.* 2007;245:986–991.
18. Kam PC. Uses and precautions of tourniquets. *Surgery.* 2005;23(2):76–77.
19. Thomas JW, Robert LM. Issues related to the use of tourniquet on the battlefield. *Mil Med.* 2005;270:770–775.
20. Pillgram-Larsen J, Mellesmo S. Not a tourniquet but compressive dressing: Experience from 68 traumatic amputations after injuries from mines. *Tidsskr Nor Laegeforen.* 1992;112(17):2188–2190.
21. Lakstein D, Blumenfield A, Sokolow T et al. Tourniquet for hemorrhage control in battlefield: A four year accumulated experience. *J Trauma.* 2003;54:S221–S225.
22. Beekley AC, Sebesta JA, Mullinex P et al. Pre-hospital tourniquet use in operation iraqi freedom: Effect on hemorrhage control and outcomes. 31st Combat Support Hospital Research Group. *J Trauma.* February 2008;64(2 Suppl):S28–S37.
23. Kragh JF, Walters TJ, Baer DG et al. Survival with emergency tourniquet use to stop bleeding in major limb trauma. *Ann Surg.* 2009;249(1):1–7.
24. Kragh JF, Littrel ML, Jones JA et al. Battle casualty survival with emergency tourniquet use to stop limb bleeding. *J Emerg Med.* 2011;41(6):590–597.
25. Advanced Trauma Life Support (ATLS), Student Course Manual, 9th Edition, American College of Surgeons, Committee on Trauma, 2012.
26. Sasser SM, Hunt RC, Faul M, Sugarman D et al. Guidelines for field triage of injured patients: Recommendations of the national expert panel on field triage, 2011. *Morb Mort Wkly Rep.* 2012;61(RR-1):1–20.
27. Walls RM, Zinner MJ. The Boston Marathon response: Why it did it work so well? *JAMA.* 2013; 309(23):2441–2442.
28. Bulger EM, Snyder D, Schoelles K et al. An evidence based prehospital guideline for external hemorrhage control. *Prehospital Emerg Care.* 2014;18:163–173.
29. Passos E, Dingley B, Smith A et al. Tourniquet use for peripheral vascular injuries in the civilian setting. *Injury.* 2014;45:573–577.
30. Rotondo MF, Schwab CW, McGonial MD et al. Damage control: An approach for improved survival in exsanguinating penetrating abdominal injury. *J Trauma.* 1993;35:375–382.
31. Riska EB, Bonsdroff HV, Hakkinen S. Primary operative fixation of long bone fractures in patients with multiple injuries. *J Trauma.* 1977;17(2):111–121.
32. Carson JH. Damage control orthopedics-when and why. *J Lancaster General Hosp.* 2007;2(3):103–105.
33. Scalea TM, Boswell SA, Scott JD et al. External fixation as a bridge to intramedullary nailing for patients with multiple injuries and with femur fractures: Damage control orthopedics. *J Trauma.* 2002;48:613–662.
34. Pape HC, Hildebrand F, Pertschy S et al. Changes in the management of femoral shaft fractures in polytrauma patients: From early total care to damage control orthopedic surgery. *J Trauma.* September 2006;53(3):452–461.

35. Rixen D, Grass G, Sauerland S, Lefering R, Raum MR, Yücel N, Bouillon B, Neugebauer EA; Polytrauma Study Group of the German Trauma Society. Evaluation of criteria for temporary external fixation in risk-adapted damage control orthopedic surgery of femur shaft fractures in multiple trauma patients: "evidence-based medicine" versus "reality" in the trauma registry of the German Trauma Society. *J Trauma*. 2005;59:1375–1395.
36. Taeger G, Ruchholtz S, Waydhas C et al. Damage control orthopedics in patients with multiple injuries is effective, time saving, and safe. *J Trauma*. 2005;59:408–415.
37. Pape HC. Damage control orthopedic surgery in polytrauma: Influence on the clinical course and its pathologic background. *Eur Instruct Lect*. 2009;9:67–74.
38. Pape HC, Giannoudis PV, Krettek C et al. Timing of fixation of major fractures in blunt polytrauma: Role of conventional indicators in clinical decision making. *J Orthop Trauma*. 2005;19(8):551–562.
39. Doussoux PC, Baltasar JL, Fuentes CG et al. Damage control in severe polytrauma with femur fracture. *Injury*. 2012;43:S42–S46.
40. Pape HC, Rixen D, Morley J et al. Impact of the method of initial stabilization for femoral shaft fractures in patients with multiple injuries at risk for complication (borderline patients). *Ann Surg*. 2007;246(3):491–499.
41. O'Tool RV, O'Brien M, Scalea TM et al. Resuscitation before stabilization of femoral fractures limits acute respiratory distress syndrome in patients with multiple traumatic injuries despite low use of damage control orthopedics. *J Trauma*. 2009;67(5):1013–1020.
42. Nicholas B, Toth L, Wessem KV et al. Border line femur fracture patients: Early total care or damage control orthopedics?. *AZN J Surg*. 2011;81(3):148–153.
43. Copeland CF, Mitchell KA, Brumback RJ et al. Mortality in patients with bilateral femoral fractures. *J Orthop Trauma*. 1998;12(5):315–319.
44. Dellinger EP, Caplan ES, Weaver LD et al. Duration of preventive antibiotic administration for open extremity fractures. *Arch Surg*. March 1988;123(3):333–339.
45. Dellinger EP, Caplan ES, Weaver LD. Duration of preventative antibiotic administration for open extremity fractures. *Arch Surg*. 1988;123:333–339.
46. Barton CA, Mackmillian WD, Crookes B et al. compliance with EAST guidelines for prophylactic antibiotics after open extremity fracture. *Inter J Crit Illness Inj Sci*. 2012;2(2):57–62.
47. Dunkel N, Pettet D, Tovmirzaeva L et al. Short duration of antibiotic prophylaxis in open fractures does not enhance risk of subsequent infection. *Bone Joint J*. 2013;95(6):831–837.
48. Saveli CC, Morgan SJ, Belknap RW et al. Prophylactic antibiotics in open fractures: A pilot randomized clinical safety study. *J Orthop Trauma*. 2013;27(10):552–557.
49. Rodriguez L, Jung SJ, Goulet J et al. Evidence based protocol for prophylactic antibiotics in open fractures: Improved antibiotic stewardship with no increase in infection rates. *J Trauma Acute Care Surg*. 2014;77(3):400–408.
50. Hoff WS1, Bonadies JA, Cachecho R et al. East practice management guidelines work group: Practice management guidelines for prophylactic antibiotics use in open fractures. *J Trauma*. March 2011;70(3):751–754.
51. Gandhi R, Overton TL, Haut ER et al. Optimal timing of femur fracture stabilization in polytrauma patients: A practice management guideline from the eastern association for the surgery of trauma. *J Trauma Acute Care Surg*. 2014;77(5):787–795.
52. Gustilo RB, Anderson JT. Prevention of infection in the treatment of one thousand and twenty-five open fractures of long bones: Retrospective and prospective analyses. *J Bone Joint Surg*. 1976;58A:453–458.
53. Dunham CM, Bosse MJ, Clancy TV et al. Practice management guidelines for the optimal timing of long bone fracture stabilization in polytrauma patients: The EAST practice management guidelines work group. *J Trauma*. May 2001;50(5):958–967.
54. Gregory RT, Gould RJ, Peclet M et al. The mangled extremity syndrome (M.E.S.): A severity grading system for multisystem injury of the extremity. *J Trauma*. 1985;25:1147–1150.
55. Howe HR, Jr, Poole GV, Jr, Hansen KJ et al. Salvage of lower extremities following combined orthopedic and vascular trauma. A predictive salvage index. *Am Surg*. 1987;53:205–208.
56. Lange RH, Bach AW, Hansen ST, Jr. et al. Open tibial fractures with associated vascular injuries: Prognosis for limb salvage. *J Trauma*. 1985;25:203–208.
57. Helfet DL, Howey T, Sanders R et al. Limb salvage versus amputation. Preliminary results of the Mangled Extremity Severity Score. *Clin Orthop Rel Res*. 1990;256:80–86.
58. McNamara MG, Heckman JD, Corley FG. Severe open fractures of the lower extremity: A retrospective evaluation of the Mangled Extremity Severity Score (MESS). *J Orthop Trauma*. 1994;8:81–87.
59. Boss MJ, Mackenzie EJ, Kellam JF et al. A prospective evaluation of the clinical utility of the lower extremity injury severity scores. *J Bone Joint Surg Am*. 2001;83:3–14.

## Commentary on Lower Extremity Injury

*Hasan B. Alam*

Management of complex lower extremity injuries, especially in the presence of vascular trauma, fractures, soft tissue loss, and nerve damage, is extremely challenging. To be successful, you must set the appropriate priorities and design a logical plan of interventions, which often involves close coordination between numerous subspecialty services. A good understanding of the contemporary literature is also essential due to the rapidly changing data. The information that has emerged from the battlefields of Iraq and Afghanistan has redefined the roles of emergency tourniquet application, damage control surgery with the use of temporary vascular shunts, and innovative limb salvage strategies*. There has also been a revolution in the technology behind the design and manufacturing of limb prosthesis†. All of these advancements have resulted in some of the best outcomes after lower extremity injuries that have been recorded in the history of modern warfare.

Although revolutionary, almost none of these new developments have been tested through large multi-institutional randomized clinical trials, and thus, strictly speaking, they would command a rather low level of recommendation. However, in reality, some of these strategies have now become standard of care, and it may be considered unethical to not use them in severely injured patients:

1. *Use of tourniquets and advanced hemostatic dressings for hemorrhage control*: Early and effective hemorrhage control is the leading priority in bleeding patients. A review of 10 years of data from a military registry showed that of 4297 casualties with extremity trauma, 30% underwent application of tourniquets‡. Over this period, tourniquet use increased by tenfold, and survival rates improved markedly for casualties that had injuries amenable for tourniquets. Recently, special tourniquets have also been designed for really proximal/junctional injuries that are not suitable for conventional tourniquets§. In addition, a number of advanced hemostatic dressings are now available that can be used to pack the wound to help with hemorrhage control¶. In my opinion, emergency medical personnel and trauma surgeons should be trained in the proper use of tourniquets and advanced hemostatic dressings.
2. *Strategies to minimize ischemia time*: Rapid restoration of distal flow is a priority that is secondary only to rapid hemorrhage control. Our goal should be to restore blood flow as soon as possible (definitely within 6 h) to minimize the chances of limb loss. One strategy that has recently gained favor in the military and civilian settings is the placement of temporary intravascular shunts (TIVSs) to control the injury, to restore distal flow (arterial), and enhance drainage if needed (venous shunts)**††. Typical indications for the use of shunts are to: (1) control exsanguination ("damage control"), or to (2) maintain distal flow in the setting of combined orthopedic and vascular injuries (Gustillo IIIc fractures where skeletal stabilization is required before vascular repair). When dealing with combined vascular and orthopedic injuries, my preference is to start by placing the TIVS to restore distal flow, which converts a rushed operation into a much more controlled situation. At this stage, the orthopedic team can focus on stabilizing the fractures while I use this time to harvest the vein graft. Once the fracture has been reduced and stabilized, the definitive vascular repair can be performed without rush. TIVSs are also a reasonable bailout option for surgeons who do not have the expertise to perform the definitive repair, as it can maintain limb viability during the transfer of patient to higher levels of care (without need for systemic anticoagulation). For example, even in complex battlefield injuries, patency rates of 86% for proximal shunts have been reported with >90% viability

* Alam HB, DiMusto PD. Management of lower extremity vascular trauma. Current trauma reports 2015 (accepted for publication). Electronically published ahead of print. Available at http://link.springer.com/article/10.1007/s40719-014-0007-2.

† Hoyt BW, Pavey GJ, Pasquina PF, Potter BK. Rehabilitation of lower extremity trauma: A review of principles and military perspective on future directions. Current trauma reports 2015 (accepted for publication). Electronically published ahead of print. Available at http://link.springer.com/article/10.1007/s40719-014-0004-5.

‡ Kragh JF Jr., Dubick MA, Aden JK, McKeague AL, Rasmussen TE, Baer DG, Blackbourne LH. U.S. Military use of tourniquets from 2001 to 2010. *Prehosp Emerg Care*. 2015 April–June;19(2):184–190.

§ Kragh JF Jr., Parsons DL, Kotwal RS et al. Testing of junctional tourniquets by military medics to control simulated groin hemorrhage. *J Spec Oper Med*. 2014;14(3):58–63.

¶ Bennett BL, Littlejohn LF, Kheirabadi BS et al. Management of external hemorrhage in tactical combat casualty care: Chitosan-based hemostatic gauze dressings—TCCC guidelines-change 13-05. *J Spec Oper Med*. 2014;14(3):40–57.

** Subramanian A, Vercruysse G, Dente C, Wyrzykowski A, King E, Feliciano DV. A decade's experience with temporary intravascular shunts at a civilian level I trauma center. *J Trauma*. 2008;65(2):316–324.

†† Gifford SM, Aidinian G, Clouse WD et al. Effect of temporary shunting on extremity vascular injury: An outcome analysis from the Global War on Terror vascular injury initiative. *J Vasc Surg*. 2009;50(3):549–555.

after eventual reconstruction*. Almost any tubing can be placed through the proximal and distal ends of a torn vessel and secured in place, but Javid, Argyle, and Pruitt-Inahara shuts are the most commonly used. We should place the largest diameter shunt that can be accommodated by the injured vessel, and return the patient to the operating room as soon as possible (preferably within 24 h) for definitive repair of the injury.

3. *Compartment syndrome and fasciotomies*: Compartment syndrome is often the silent enemy that can cause limb loss, even in patients that have received excellent early care. Diagnosis of compartment syndrome can be difficult in patients that are sedated and on mechanical ventilation. Pain, which is an early symptom, is often masked by drugs and other associated injuries. In addition, the injured limb is typically covered in dressings and casts that further obscures the clinical exam. Thus, an extremely high index of suspicion is needed for early detection. A prophylactic four-compartment lower leg fasciotomy should be considered when the total ischemia time is more than 4 h or if there are associated injuries (especially combined arterial and venous injuries)†. As fasciotomy is not without complications, this decision must be made judiciously based on the nature of injuries, ischemia time, and the ability to monitor the patient closely. If a decision is made to not perform prophylactic fasciotomy, then it is prudent to serially measure the compartment pressures to facilitate early detection. Due to logistical and ethical issues, it is highly unlikely that a prospective randomized trial will ever be performed to compare serial pressure measurements to simple observation (without measurement) in high-risk patients. I personally think that compartment pressure measurement, although not infallible, is an invaluable adjunct to the clinical exam in patients that are sedated or have traumatic brain injuries (TBIs).

4. *Early fixation of long bone fractures in patients with TBIs or severe respiratory failure*: Early fixation of bony injuries is highly desirable in the vast majority of patients, with the possible exception of these two categories. In patients with TBI, secondary brain injury can significantly worsen the neurological outcomes. Patients with severe TBI are unlikely to derive the benefits of early fixation (quicker ambulation and rapid rehabilitation) and are especially susceptible to the adverse consequences of hypotension, bleeding, hypoxia, hyperventilation, etc. during the orthopedic repair. Similarly, patients with severe respiratory failure may not survive additional insults such as fat emboli syndrome, intraoperative bleeding, or excessive fluid administration. The risk–benefit ratio in these patients is not the same as in the general trauma population. A practical approach, in my opinion, is to allow these critically ill patients to stabilize for 48 h or so before proceeding with an orthopedic repair. Even at this time, a quick procedure to achieve stabilization (damage control approach) is preferable compared to a definitive (but longer) operation.

Often the literature provides no clear recommendations for the most complicated situations. As the clinicians at the bedside, we must not only evaluate the literature, but also apply this knowledge in a thoughtful fashion to develop plans that are customized to the unique needs of our patients. These difficult decisions require thoughtful discussions between the different teams: trauma, ICU, orthopedics, neurosurgery, plastics, etc, that often have conflicting priorities. Development of clear, logical, and evidence-based practice recommendations is likely to result in a more uniform approach and enhance the quality of care.

* Rasmussen TE, Clouse WD, Jenkins DH, Peck MA, Eliason JL, Smith DL. The use of temporary vascular shunts as a damage control adjunct in the management of wartime vascular injury. *J Trauma*. 2006;61(1):8–12.

† Branco BC, Inaba K, Barmparas G et al. Incidence and predictors for the need for fasciotomy after extremity trauma: A 10-year review in a mature level I trauma centre. *Injury*. 2011;42(10):1157–1163.

# 32

# *Limb Salvage for the Mangled Extremity*

**Charles J. Fox and Todd E. Rasmussen**

**CONTENTS**



## 32.1 Introduction

The patient exposed to limb-threatening trauma presents the surgeon with a complex array of early and critical challenges that persist well beyond the time of injury. Although the multifaceted and emergent nature of this injury pattern has precluded the highest levels of clinical study, evidence-based guidelines can be discerned from available clinical reviews, case series, and general clinical consensus. From the multitude of published literature on this topic, several strategies have been advocated in order to simplify the process and minimize the morbidity and mortality from extremity trauma. The objective of this chapter is to identify and expand on evidence-based strategies that influence treatment decisions aimed at maximizing functional recovery following traumatic extremity injury.

Across the spectrum of extremity injury, the mangled lower extremity requires the greatest attention. The term *mangled extremity* describes a limb in which at least three of the four components (soft tissue, nerve, bone, vessel) are severely injured [1]. While *limb salvage* is defined as an attempt to restore structure and neurovascular function to a mangled extremity, often, the decision whether to repair or to perform an amputation hinges not only on the feasibility but also on the anticipated functional outcome. These decisions are often made in the context of additional associated life-threatening injuries. While substantial advances have been made in reconstructive techniques that have created opportunities to address both life- and limb-threatening injuries, heroic measures for limb salvage do not necessarily provide superior quality of life and limb outcomes even if reconstructive efforts produce a viable limb [2–5].

*Primary amputation* is defined as an extremity amputation that is performed at the original operation for injury (i.e., in which limb salvage efforts were not pursued). In some cases, a primary amputation may offer the patient an expedited and superior functional outcome [6,7]. A *secondary amputation* is defined as an extremity amputation that takes place following any attempt for limb salvage (i.e., following intent to treat or intent to salvage). Secondary amputation is further divided into *early* (an amputation within 30 days following the initial intent to salvage) and *late* (an amputation performed greater than 30 days following the initial intent to salvage). Whether early or late, a secondary amputation is performed at a subsequent operation when the measures to salvage a limb are deemed unsuccessful, futile, or detrimental to the patient.

Beyond initial stabilization of critically ill patients with injured extremities, and in addition to the complexity that operative intervention entails, an overarching factor that guides early decision making is selecting the course that will optimize functional recovery. An intricate limb repair that does not enable the patient to perform activities at a level comparable to a similar patient with a primary or secondary amputation does a disservice to the patient and poses an economic burden on health care resources [3,8,9]. While there is a paucity of high-level data that guide strategies in the treatment of the mangled extremity, this chapter poses eight relevant questions and recommendations to highlight the strongest clinical evidence on this challenging topic.

## 32.2 Which Management Strategies Reduce the Impact of Ischemia and Reperfusion Injury on Limb Salvage Following Trauma?

In the setting of extremity vascular injury, the ability to save an injured limb is based in large part on the ability to restore adequate perfusion. Over 50% of patients with severe extremity injuries will have additional injuries, many of which are life threatening [10,11]. Treatment of a life-threatening torso, head, or neck injury takes priority over definitive repair of an extremity vascular injury, leaving the limb at high risk of amputation as the negative impact of ischemic time is increased [5,12].

While placement of an autologous vein interposition graft is the most common and often ideal form of repair, it is a time-consuming endeavor that is not feasible in the setting of progressive coagulopathy, acidosis, and hypothermia. In the setting of life-threatening polytrauma, successful application of damage control techniques is based upon early recognition of pending patient demise with adjustment of the operative plan. Damage control strategies for extremity arterial and venous injuries include abbreviated lateral vessel repair, placement of a temporary vascular shunt (TVS), and vessel ligation with or without performance of a primary amputation.

Many consider vessel ligation as a technique of last resort, but as demonstrated over 50 years ago by DeBakey and Simeone in a series of 2471 vascular injuries treated during World War II, ligation of a major extremity vessel does not uniformly lead to amputation [13]. The introduction of *selective vessel ligation* in the setting of extremity vessel injuries reduced the amputation rate from nearly 100% to 49%. Another example of the concept of selective vessel ligation rests in an analysis of patients with brachial artery injury, which demonstrated a twofold difference in amputation rates depending upon whether the artery was ligated above (55%) or below (26%) the profunda brachii artery. A similar relationship in the rates of lower extremity amputation has been reported for femoral artery injuries: 81% lower extremity amputation rate if the ligation is above the profunda femoris artery versus 55% if ligation occurs below the profunda femoris artery.

Venous ligation is generally better tolerated than arterial ligation. While the direct impact of venous ligation on amputation rates has been reported to be low, ligation of large lower extremity veins has been found to result in thrombosis, significant venous hypertension and postphlebitic syndrome [14,15]. Injuries resulting from high-energy mechanisms, particularly those resulting from explosive devices or high-velocity gunshot wounds, strip collateral venous drainage from the extremity-potentiating lifestyle-limiting venous hypertension [16]. In the largest post-Vietnam review of venous injuries, Quan and associates from Walter Reed reported a retrospective analysis of 82 patients with 103 extremity venous injuries due to combat injuries [15]. In this 2008 study, 63% of extremity venous injuries were treated by ligation, while the remaining 37% were repaired. Importantly, this study reported an 84% midterm patency of venous repair and showed that patients with extremity vein repair did not experience a higher incidence of pulmonary embolus than patients treated with venous ligation. All patients in this landmark report developed postinjury edema of the extremity, and there was a trend toward increased deep venous thrombosis (DVT) rate (14% vs. 7%) and phlegmasia (2% vs. 0%) in the group treated by venous ligation [16].

Another tool that can be used in the setting of vascular injury is the TVS. These devices are used routinely during the performance of carotid endarterectomy but have also been utilized as a damage control adjunct as a means of quickly restoring perfusion to an extremity in the setting of vascular injury. Large animal studies by Dawson et al. at Lackland Air Force Base demonstrated the safety and efficacy of TVS in restoring distal perfusion during hemorrhagic shock [17]. In this model, TVS remained patent and functioning for nearly 24 h without systemic heparinization. Several retrospective clinical series have also reported the short-term efficacy of TVS in the setting of extremity vascular injury, the largest being a report from the Air Force Theater Hospital on Balad AB, Iraq [18–21]. This series demonstrated that although shunts placed in smaller, more distal arteries and veins are more likely to thrombose, there is no adverse impact on limb salvage [20]. Gifford et al. have recently reported the impact of TVS on long-term limb salvage in a case–control study of 125 patients with severe extremity injuries [22]. In this sentinel report, there were more early amputations performed in the control than the TVS group (13% vs. 3%; $p = 0.04$);

however, after nearly 2 years of follow-up, there was no significant difference in the amputation rate (17% vs. 23%; $p = 0.42$). After adjusting for a Mangled Extremity Severity Score (MESS) greater than 8, the TVS group had a significantly lower risk of amputation (HR = 0.43; $p = 0.04$). Outcomes data such as these suggest that TVS does not cause harm in the setting of extremity vascular injury, and likely extends the window of opportunity for limb salvage.

*Recommendations*:

1. Arterial ligation may be used as a damage control maneuver understanding that there is an increased incidence of extremity amputation.
2. Large vessel venous injuries should be repaired when feasible.
3. TVSs are an effective damage control adjunct, and the long-term impact on amputation is most beneficial in the subset of patients with mangled extremities (MESS ≥8).

   *Level of evidence*: 3b

   *Grade of recommendation*: C

## 32.3 Is There a Difference in Limb Salvage Strategies in the Setting of Upper versus Lower Extremity Injury?

While severe extremity injuries are less common in the upper extremity, the complex and important function of the hand presents unique considerations that require modification in management strategies. Because of the relative smaller size and increased collateralization, ligation of upper extremity vascular injuries is better tolerated than those of the lower extremity [13,14]. Conversely, interwoven tendons and nerves of the upper extremity play an integral role in arm, hand, and digit function and require more meticulous debridement and repair. Finally, the relative paucity of soft tissue in the upper compared to the lower extremity makes coverage of nerve and vascular repairs more challenging in many cases.

Civilian literature, consisting of smaller case series describing blunt and penetrating injuries, reports a very high rate of upper limb salvage (95%) [23,24]. Even in the setting of combined neural and vascular trauma, after repair and nearly 4 years of rehabilitation, 87% of patients showed improvement as assessed by the American Medical Association's standardized disability impairment scale [24].

In contrast, wartime injuries to the upper extremity are high-energy wounds often with penetrating, blast, and burn components. In this setting, upper extremity injuries are associated with more extensive soft tissue, nerve, and bone destruction. Data in two separate reports from the Global War on Terrorism demonstrated that upper extremity amputation rates in wartime may be as high as 10%, perhaps reflecting attempts to salvage more severely injured upper extremities than those in the civilian setting [25,26]. Despite high upper extremity limb salvage rates reported by Rich et al. from the Vietnam Vascular Registry, nearly 75% of patients with mangled upper extremities report significant long-term disability [16]. This is especially the case for proximal upper extremity injuries that frequently involve the axillary structures including the brachial plexus.

*Recommendations*:

1. Limb salvage rates are higher for upper extremities than lower extremities in setting of civilian trauma.
2. The rate of upper extremity amputation is higher in the setting of complex wartime injury.

   *Level of evidence*: 4

   *Grade of recommendation*: D
3. Three-quarters of patients with upper extremity injury report significant functional disability in the long term.

   *Level of evidence*: 3b

   *Grade of recommendation*: C

## 32.4 What Prehospital Adjuncts Are Available That Impact Limb Salvage Following Traumatic Extremity Injury?

Tourniquets have been utilized as an adjunct for extremity hemorrhage control for over 100 years and have been reintroduced during military conflicts as a lifesaving measure while preparing for transport from the battlefield [27,28,29]. Uncontrolled hemorrhage remains a leading cause of preventable battlefield death, and the second most common cause of death for civilian trauma [11]. During each recent major conflict, attention has been directed to the proper design, application, and utility of tourniquets [30]. A recent randomized control trial evaluating the effectiveness of seven different self-applied tourniquets suggests that only the Combat Application Tourniquet (North American Rescue Products, Greenville, SC), the Emergency Medical Tourniquet (Delfi Medical, Vancouver, Canada), and the Special Operations Forces Tactical Tourniquet (Tactical Medical Solutions,

Anderson, SC) were effective in eliminating Doppler evidence of distal arterial signal after self application to the thigh and proximal arm [31]. Subsequently hundreds of thousands of these commercially designed tourniquets have been issued for use on the battlefields of Iraq and Afghanistan [32].

A prospective review of tourniquet usage at a combat support hospital in Baghdad was conducted to evaluate potential adverse events associated with tourniquet usage [33]. Of 232 patients with 428 tourniquets in place; none of the 309 limbs were lost as a result of tourniquet use. There were many secondary outcomes investigated, including fasciotomy, DVT, pain, and nerve palsy. However, the only complications reported were transient nerve palsies in <2%. Nonetheless, improperly applied tourniquets may cause increased hemorrhage when placed above a venous injury, and properly placed tourniquets cause significant pain if left in place for extended periods of time. In 2009, Kragh and colleagues also prospectively reported an observed survival benefit with emergency tourniquet use to stop bleeding in major limb trauma. The authors concluded that both prehospital tourniquet use and tourniquet use when shock was absent was strongly associated with survival (90% vs. 10%; $p < 0.001$) [64]. It is a current consensus that the efficacy of tourniquet use on the battlefield is inversely related to the time in which it takes for the tourniquet to be evaluated, loosened, or removed by a surgical team.

An additional prehospital adjunct that has gained attention is the topical hemostatic agent designed to stop bleeding from large proximal arterial and venous injuries. In addition to standard pressure dressings, there are two component agents (zeolite and chitosan) Food and Drug Administration (FDA) approved for military use [34]. Studies supporting the safety and efficacy of these agents have been based on large animal work that suggest that zeolite dressings significantly reduce blood loss after large vessel laceration and uncontrolled hemorrhagic shock. Alam et al. compared the mortality and blood loss after the application of five hemostatic agents to an iliac injury in a swine model of uncontrolled hemorrhage [35]. Animals in the zeolite group demonstrate a statistically significant mortality benefit; no animals died in the zeolite group, while mortality rates in the remaining treatment groups ranged from 28% in the chitosan group to 100% in the untreated group. While the hemostatic properties of the zeolite dressing appears promising, the associated exothermic reaction cause tissue damage that may complicate wound healing or cause thrombosis. Despite concern and anecdotal reports that topical hemostatic agents may compromise the ability to perform vascular reconstruction and limb salvage there are no studies that support this line of thinking.

*Recommendations*:

1. Tourniquets should be placed early and above arterial extremity injuries and remain in place until further resuscitation and evaluation by qualified teams.

   *Level of evidence*: 2b

   *Grade of recommendation*: B
2. Chemical hemostatic agents limit life-threatening blood loss in select extremity injury patterns at the expense of thermal tissue injury. (* based on animal studies)

## 32.5 What Strategies in Skeletal Reconstruction Impact Limb Salvage Following Traumatic Injury?

Like vascular injuries, patients with skeletal injuries will benefit most from primary definitive stabilization. Similarly, definitive stabilization is often time consuming and represents an additional physiologic burden for the patient. Principles of damage control for orthopedic injuries include external fixation with delayed intramedullary nailing (IMN) of long bone fractures [36,37]. Initial small, randomized multicenter trials conducted by the European Polytrauma Study on the Management of Femur Fractures demonstrated that patients with severe polytrauma (Injury Severity Score [ISS] 22) and femur fractures exhibited a significantly greater cytokine response following early IMN versus external fixation followed by delayed IMN [38]. These findings were not corroborated when the same group randomized 165 patients across 10 European centers to receive either early IMN or external fixation followed by delayed IMN [39]. Regression analysis of the most severely injured patients (ISS 32 vs. 24) with thorax injuries (Abbreviated Injury Scale [AIS] 2.8) suggests a lower risk of pulmonary complications and sepsis if treated with early external fixation (EF) rather than early IMN. Conversely, stable patients did not benefit from a two-staged repair (e.g., EF followed by delayed IMN). In fact, in this less severely injured group, EF followed by delayed IMN was associated with nearly double the ICU hours (212 vs. 133) and ventilator hours nearly tripled (142 vs. 66), although neither was statistically significant.

Open fractures carry a significantly higher incidence of infection than closed fractures (52% vs. 4%, respectively) and gram-negative bacterial infections are over three times more common in the setting of an open extremity fracture [39]. Gustilo classified open lower extremity fracture patterns based on wound size, presence of contamination, degree of soft tissue injury, and associated vascular injuries [40]. In his series of 511 patients, those with open fractures and associated vascular injuries (Gustilo Class IIIc) had a 41% chance of developing either an infection or requiring a secondary amputation [40].

*Recommendations*:

1. Severely injured patients with long bone fracture benefit from early external fixation followed by IMN.
2. Less severely injured patients are best served with definitive stabilization in the form of IMN within the first 24 h of injury.

   *Level of evidence*: 1b

   *Grade of recommendation*: A
3. Due to increased incidence of wound-related sepsis after open fractures, gram-negative coverage should be provided in addition to a first generation cephalosporin for 3 days from the time of initial evaluation.

   *Level of evidence*: 1b

   *Grade of recommendation*: A

## 32.6 How Do Advances in Soft Tissue Wound Management Strategies Impact Limb Salvage?

Severe lower extremity trauma is often associated with extensive soft tissue loss. Large soft tissue wounds create an independent physiologic burden on the patient in the form of insensible fluid loss, infection, and metabolic demands during healing. Among the most commonly employed tools used to manage extremity soft tissue wounds are the negative pressure vacuum–assisted closure device (V.A.C.® KCI, San Antonio, TX), tissue flaps, free tissue transfers, and skin grafts.

V.A.C. therapy (using reticulated open cell foam) acts to remove interstitial fluids that contain inflammatory cytokines that suppress the proliferative phase of wound healing and bacteria. Negative pressure wound therapy also reduces capillary afterload that increases local circulation and a properly sealed system decreases the burden of external contamination [41–43]. The applications of V.A.C. therapy are extensive and the techniques especially effective when placed over properly debrided, well vascularized tissues such as muscle and subcutaneous fat. Several case series have demonstrated that the use of the V.A.C. device decreases the time to wound closure or coverage with a skin graft without the aid of tissue flaps [43–45].

Use of V.A.C. therapy has been extensive in the management of wartime extremity injury and has become standard in some phase of nearly all soft tissue wounds. Leininger et al. reported in 2006 on a series of local patients injured in Iraq with large soft tissue wounds [46]. In this study, a strict wound management strategy that included repeat debridement, irrigation, initiation of delayed primary closure, and V.A.C. changes in the operating room resulted in no wound complications or skin graft failures. Each patient in this series received definitive wound treatment at a level III surgical hospital from one group of surgeons using one uniform wound management strategy. Leininger's results were confirmed and extended by Peck et al. a year later in a report describing the utility of V.A.C. therapy in the complete management of soft tissue wounds associated with extremity vascular injury [63].

For those extremity wounds with extensive devitalized tissues, a rotational flap or free tissue transfer may be delivered in to a clean wound bed to aid in definitive wound closure. An analysis of the timing of tissue transfer after extremity trauma was completed by Markus Godina in 1986 [47]. This multicenter retrospective series included 532 patients receiving early (within 72 h of injury), delayed (between 72 h and 3 months of injury), or late (between 3 months and 12 years of injury) free-flap transfer. Those patients undergoing delayed free tissue transfer had significantly higher rate of wound infections (delayed 18% vs. early 2%), and the average hospitalization was over four times as long (130 days vs. 27 days). The author also highlights the steep learning curve associated with the microsurgical reconstruction of free tissue transfers as failures occurred in 26% of the first 100 flaps and only 4% of the last 100.

The value of surgical expertise in tissue reconstruction is particularly relevant in light of the decreasing use of free tissue transfers for complex extremity injuries. A retrospective review of 290 Gustilo Grade III injuries collected from 1992 to 2003 reports a decrease in free tissue transfers from 20% in the first 4 years of the study, 11% in the second 4 years, and 5% in the most current 4 years [48]. A reciprocal increase in the use of skin grafts and delayed primary closure was noted over the same interval (22% in the first 4 years of the study and 49% in the last 4 years of the study). No significant difference was noted in secondary amputation or wound infection rates in this study.

*Recommendations*:

1. Frequent and adequate surgical debridement of soft tissue wounds is paramount in the preparation of extremity soft tissue wounds.
2. Negative pressure wound therapy (V.A.C.) as a standard surgical adjunct that aids in the management of extremity injury is associated with low infection rates and decreased time to closure or coverage with skin graft.

   *Level of evidence*: 2b

   *Grade of recommendation*: B

3. When necessary, reconstruction of wounds using free tissue transfers should occur early and be performed by experienced subspecialists.

   *Level of evidence*: 3b

   *Grade of recommendation*: C

## 32.7 How Do Patient and Injury Characteristics Impact Decision Making regarding Extremity Salvage?

Six factors that influence the initial decision to amputate or attempt limb salvage are as follows:

1. Physiologic reserve of the patient
2. Extent and severity of associated injuries
3. Nature of the extremity injury
4. Preinjury functional status
5. The presence of significant comorbidities
6. Access to adequate resources during rehabilitation

Authors of the Lower Extremity Assessment Project (LEAP) assessed the relationships among these factors and the functional outcome after extremity reconstruction and limb salvage or amputation [2,49–52]. The LEAP project is a multicenter prospective study of 600 patients with severe lower extremity injury who underwent either amputation or reconstruction. Results from this important study have shown that factors associated with the injury itself are the most significant in influencing the decision to amputate [51]. Specifically, muscle injury, arterial and/or deep venous injury, and absence of plantar sensation are three factors shown to be associated with a fivefold risk of amputation [2,49,51].

To address the absence of plantar sensation as an indication for extremity amputation, three groups of patients were selected based on the absence of plantar sensation on initial evaluation and successful limb salvage (Group 1), the absence of plantar sensation and amputation (Group 2), and the presence of plantar sensation and limb salvage (Group 3) [62]. There was no difference in functional outcomes between the groups, and approximately half (55%) of the entire cohort had normal plantar sensation after 2 years.

These studies found no difference in functional outcome from either group based on injury characteristics or presence of a limb. In fact, subset analysis suggests that the factors most likely to influence functional outcome are related to preinjury social characteristics such as level of education, income level, and access to health care [2,49,61].

Similar findings are reported by Sohn and associates for a cohort of 153 patients wounded during Operation Iraqi Freedom [10]. In contrast to participants in the LEAP project, who were 16–69-year-old civilians, the injured Troops Sohn's study were young (mean 23 years), otherwise healthy, and had sustained greater percentages of high-energy complex wounds. Upon initial presentation, one quarter was hypotensive and 80% had a base deficit ≥6. The median military Injury Severity Score of the cohort was 13, all of which suggest a significant physiologic derangement as a result of their injuries. Despite the extent of their injuries, the authors report an 80% early limb salvage rate, which is comparable to that observed in the LEAP project (83%) [2,10].

*Recommendations*:

1. Patient factors most highly correlated with extremity amputation are severe soft tissue injury, nerve injury, and vascular injury in descending order.

   *Level of evidence*: 1b

   *Grade of recommendation*: A

2. Limb salvage rates associated with complex wartime extremity injuries are similar than those reported in the civilian trauma literature.

   *Level of evidence*: 3b

   *Grade of recommendation*: C

## 32.8 What Is the Role of Mangled Extremity Scores and Indices on Decision Making in Limb Salvage?

Based on data from the previously mentioned studies and others, factors have been identified that influence functional outcome after limb salvage. In order to guide the decision-making process during initial and early management of patients with severe extremity trauma, scoring systems have been developed that incorporate several of these factors. An ideal mangled extremity scoring system needs to be simple to implement during the initial evaluation, based upon readily available information and able to predict limb salvage and functional outcome. Unfortunately no single scoring system has been designated as ideal and as a result, several options are now available. Among the most common are the MESS; the Predictive Salvage Index (PSI); the Limb Salvage Index (LSI); the Nerve Injury, Ischemia, Soft Tissue Injury, Skeletal Injury, Shock, and Age of Patient (NISSSA) Score; and the Hannover Fracture Scale-98 (HFA-98).

The most commonly reported scoring system, the MESS, was derived by Johansen and associates from the initial retrospective and subsequent prospective outcomes of 52 patients, 21 of whom underwent an amputation [53]. Factors considered in the calculation of a score include the following:

1. Presence or absence of skeletal/soft tissue injury (graded 1–4)
2. Presence or absence of limb ischemia (graded 1–3)
3. Presence or absence of shock (graded 0–2)
4. Patient age (graded 0–2)

Each variable is graded and the individual scores added to provide a score from 2 to 11. The authors of the MESS recognize limb ischemia as time dependent and suggest limb ischemia scores be doubled if perfusion has not been restored within 6 h of injury. The authors of the MESS found that a score ≥7 predicted amputation with 100% accuracy and scores <6 also predicted limb salvage in all cases [53]. Interestingly, patients with significant peripheral nerve deficits were excluded from the study because they were assumed to require amputation. Larger prospective trials with long-term follow-up have not successfully duplicated the results of the MESS report [10,54,55]. The MESS and scoring systems like it tend to have high specificities with low scores accurately able to predict limb salvage. However, the sensitivity of these metrics lacks as their ability to predict amputation in the setting of high scores is variable (i.e., low positive predictive values).

Less commonly utilized scoring systems are available, each more complex than the MESS. Examples include the PSI developed by Howe et al. that includes the level of arterial injury, the degree of bone injury, the degree of muscle injury, and the time to surgery [56]. A score greater than or equal to 8 should be predictive of need for amputation. The LSI designed by Russell et al. measures seven components including artery, deep vein, nerve, bone, skin, muscle, and warm ischemia time [57]. Again variables are graded and an additive score ≥6 predicts the need for amputation. The NISSSA, developed by McNamara et al. in 1994, contains six variables including nerve injury, ischemia, soft tissue injury, skeletal injury, shock, and patient age [58]. Amputations are recommended with scores ≥11. The HFS-98 proposed in revised form by Krettek et al. is the most complex and involves the determination of: fracture type, the degrees of bone loss, periosteal stripping, skin injury, muscle injury, wound contamination, local circulation, systemic circulation, and neurologic function [59]. The scoring system is designed to be employed during the initial operation by the operating surgeon and ranges from 0 to 22 with a score ≥11 being predictive of amputation.

In the most comprehensive evaluation of extremity injury scoring metrics to date, the designers of the LEAP applied the criteria for each of the previously listed scoring systems to the 407 patients in their study group with the intent to evaluate long-term *functional outcomes* after attempted limb salvage [55]. In this important part of the LEAP report there was found to be no correlation between any of the injury severity scores and reported *functional outcome* at either 6 or 24 months.

*Recommendations*:

1. Mangled extremity severity scoring systems have limited predictive value in terms of the need for amputation.
2. No scoring system is able to reliably predict functional outcome.

   *Level of evidence*: 1b

   *Grade of recommendation*: A

## 32.9 What Is the Financial Cost of Extremity Reconstruction versus Early Amputation and the Impact on Quality of Life?

Extremity injury presents a significant physical and emotional burden for the patient as well as an economic challenge for the health care system, acute and long term. Several groups have evaluated the costs associated with pursuit of limb salvage as opposed to early amputation and placed these in relation to functional outcomes [5,17,20,31,48,60]. There are significant differences in the length of hospital stay, need for rehospitalization, number of operations, and length of time to return to work in patients receiving primary amputation versus those with limb salvage. In nearly every report, these variables are significantly greater for groups after limb salvage [5,17,31]. As an example, Boundurant reported that patients who required a secondary amputation remained in the hospital more than twice as long as those who underwent primary amputation (53 vs. 22 days) [5]. Patients in limb salvage groups also require a significantly greater number of operations than patient receiving primary amputation (19% vs. 5%) [49]. Nearly half of patients in both groups (limb salvage and primary amputation) failed to return to work within 24 months following injury, illustrating the persistent morbidity associated with severe extremity injury [5,17,31,49]. Finally, Boundurant, documented the fiscal cost of secondary versus early primary amputation by showing a fivefold increase in the number of operations (2 vs. 7) and doubling of hospital costs ($28,964 vs. $53,462—1988 dollars) in the secondary amputation group [5].

**TABLE 32.1**

Grading of Clinical Strategies to Improve Limb Salvage for the Mangled Extremity

| Question | Answer | Level of Evidence | Grade | References |
|---|---|---|---|---|
| Which management strategies improve ischemia and reperfusion injury following traumatic extremity injury? | Damage control techniques aid in limb salvage after life-threatening trauma. | 3b | C | [5,10–22] |
| | Large vessel venous injuries should be repaired when feasible. | 3b | C | |
| | Temporary vascular shunts are safe and fewer amputations are performed in patients with severely mangled extremities. | 2b | B | |
| Is there a difference in limb salvage strategies in the setting of upper versus lower extremity injury? | Limb salvage rate exceeds 90% in upper extremities, but with poor functional outcomes. | 4 | D | [16,23–26] |
| | The rate of upper extremity amputation is higher in the setting of complex wartime injury. | 4 | D | |
| What prehospital adjuncts are available that impact limb salvage following traumatic extremity injury? | Tourniquets are lifesaving when placed before shock is present and do not adversely impact limb salvage. | 2b | B | [27–35,64] |
| | Hemostatic agents effectively control hemorrhage. | * | * | |
| What contemporary strategies in skeletal reconstruction impact limb salvage following traumatic injury? | Definitive stabilization (intramedullary nail) within 24 h of injury in stable patients. | 1b | A | [36–40] |
| | Early external fixation followed by intramedullary nail in unstable patients. | 1b | A | |
| | Early antibiotic coverage continued for 3 days from time of injury. | 1b | A | |
| How do advances in soft tissue wound management strategies impact limb salvage following traumatic injury? | Frequent and adequate debridement is a critical component of soft tissue wound closure. | 2b | B | [41–48,63] |
| | Negative pressure wound therapy (V.A.C.) decreases infection rates and hastens time to wound closure. | 3b | C | |
| | Complex reconstruction of soft tissue defects should occur within 72 h of injury and by experienced subspecialists. | | | |
| How do injury patterns impact decision-making regarding extremity salvage? | Severe soft tissue injuries, nerve injuries, and vascular injuries influence decision to amputate but no difference in functional outcome. | 1b | A | [2,10,49–52,61,62] |
| | Limb salvage rates associated with wartime extremity injuries are comparable to that reported in civilian literature. | 3b | C | |
| Which extremity severity scores predict limb salvage and functional outcome? | No scoring system accurately predicts limb salvage or functional outcome. | 1b | A | [10,53–59] |
| What are the costs of reconstruction and quality of life? | There is no significant difference in functional outcome between limb salvage and amputation. | 1b | A | [5,7,17,20,31,48,49,60] |
| | Limb salvage is associated with more operations, longer recovery time, and more than 2× the cost than amputation. | 1b | A | |

In a notable finding, the LEAP demonstrated no difference in quality of life between patients with primary amputation and those with successful limb salvage at 2 years [49]. Using the validated, self-reporting questionnaire called the Sickness Impact Profile that assesses 12 categories of function including ambulation, mobility, body care, social interaction, and ability to work, the LEAP failed to show improved quality of life in those with successful limb salvage following severe extremity injury at 24 months [7]. These findings may be attributable to the increasing quality of prosthetics as well as the social and financial support required for optimal care and rehabilitation following limb salvage attempts (Table 32.1).

*Recommendations*:

1. There is no significant difference in functional outcome after limb salvage versus amputation following severe extremity injury.
2. There is a significant economic, health care, and rehabilitation cost associated with limb salvage.

*Level of evidence*: 1b

*Grade of recommendation*: A

## References


1. Gregory RT, Gould RJ, Peclet M, Wagner JS, Gilbert DA, Wheeler JR, Snyder SO, Gayle RG, Schwab CW. The mangled extremity syndrome (M.E.S.): A severity grading system for multisystem injury of the extremity. *J Trauma.* 1985;25(12):1147–1150.
2. Bosse MJ, MacKenzie EJ, Kellam JF et al. An analysis of outcomes of reconstruction or amputation after leg-threatening injuries. *N Engl J Med.* 2002;347(24):1924–1931.
3. Fern KT, Smith JT, Zee B et al. Trauma patients with multiple extremity injuries: Resource utilization and long-term outcome in relation to injury severity scores. *J Trauma.* 1998;45(3):489–494.
4. Holbrook TL, Anderson JP, Sieber WJ et al. Outcome after major trauma: 12-month and 18-month follow up results from the Trauma Recovery Project. *J Trauma.* 1999;46(5):765–771.
5. Katzman SS, Dickson K. Determining the prognosis for limb salvage in major vascular injuries with associated open tibial fractures. *Orthop Rev.* 1992;21(2):195–199.
6. Purry NA, Hannon MA. How successful is below-knee amputation for injury? *Injury.* 1989;20(1):32–36.
7. Quirke TE, Sharma PK, Boss WK, Jr., Oppenheim WC, Rauscher GE. Are type IIIC lower extremity injuries an indication for primary amputation. *J Trauma.* 1996;40(6):992–996.
8. Bondurant FJ. Cotler HB, Buckle R et al. The medical and economic impact of severely injured lower extremities. *J Trauma.* 1988;28(8):1270–1273.
9. Dischinger PC, Read KM, Kufera JA et al. Consequences and costs of lower extremity injuries. *Annu Proc Assoc Adv Automot Med.* 2004;48:339–353.
10. Sohn VY, Arthurs ZM, Herbert GS, Beekley AC, Sebesta JA. Demographics, treatment, and early outcomes in penetrating vascular combat trauma. *Arch Surg.* 2008;143(8):783–787.
11. Starnes BW, Beekley AC, Sebesta JA et al. Extremity vascular injuries on the battlefield: Tips for surgeons deploying to war. *J Trauma.* 2006;60(2):432–442.
12. Clarke P, Mollan RA. The criteria for amputation in severe lower limb injury. *Injury.* 1994;25(3):139–143.
13. Debakey ME, Simeone FA. Battle injuries of the arteries in World War II: An analysis of 2471 cases. *Ann Surg.* 1946;123(4):534–537.
14. Timberlake GA, Kerstein MD. Venous injury: To repair or ligate, the dilemma revisited. *Am Surg.* 1995;61:139.
15. Quan RW, Gillespie DL, Stuart RP et al. The effect of vein repair on the risk of venous thromboembolic events: A review of more than 100 traumatic military venous injuries. *J Vasc Surg.* 2008;47(3):571–577.
16. Rich NM, Mattox KL, Hirschberg A. 2004. *Vascular Trauma*, 2nd edn. Elsevier Saunders: Philadelphia, PA, pp. 3–73, 353–392.
17. Dawson DL, Putnam AT, Light JT et al. Temporary vascular shunts to maintain limb perfusion after arterial injury: An animal study. *Trauma.* 1999;47(1):64–71.
18. Clouse WD, Rasmussen TE, Peck MA et al. In-Theater Management of Vascular Injury: 2 Years of the Balad Vascular Registry. *J. Am Coll Surg.* 2007;204(4):625–632.
19. Chambers LW, Green DJ, Sample K et al. Tactical Surgical Intervention with temporary shunting of peripheral vascular trauma sustained during Operation Iraqi Freedom: One units experience. *J Trauma.* 2006;61:824–830.
20. Rasmussen TE, Clouse WD, Jenkins DH et al. The use of temporary vascular shunts as a damage control adjunct in the management of wartime vascular injury. *Trauma.* 2006;61:8–12.
21. Taller J, Kamdar JP, Greene JA et al. Temporary vascular shunts as initial treatment of proximal extremity vascular injuries during combat operations: The new standard of care at echelon II facilities? *J Trauma.* 2008;65:595–603.
22. Gifford S, Aidinian G, Clouse WD et al. 2008. Improved long-term outcomes following temporary vascular shunting for wartime vascular injury: A case control analysis from the GWOT vascular initiative. *Presented at the American Association of Surgery for Trauma*, Maui, HI.
23. Joshi V, Harding GE, Bottoni DA, Lovell MB, Forbes TL. Determination of functional outcome following upper extremity arterial trauma. *Vasc Endovascular Surg.* 2007;41(2):111–114.
24. Manford JD, Garard CL, Kline DG, Sternberg WC, Money SR. Management of severe vascular and neural injury of the upper extremity. *J Vasc Surg.* 1998;27(1):43–49.
25. Clouse WD, Rasmussen TE, Perlstein J et al. Upper extremity vascular injury: A current in-theater wartime report from Operation Iraqi Freedom. *Ann Vasc Surg.* 2006;20(4):431–434.
26. Weber MA, Fox CJ, Adams E et al. Upper extremity arterial combat injury management. *Perspect Vasc Surg Endovasc Ther.* 2006;18(2):141–145.
27. Fox CJ, Starnes BW. Vascular surgery on the modern battlefield. *Surg Clin North Am.* 2007;87:1193–1211.
28. Fox CJ, Gillespie DL, O'Donnell SD et al. Contemporary management of wartime vascular trauma. *J Vasc Surg.* 2005;41(4):638–644.
29. Lakstein D, Blumenfeld A, Sokolov T et al. Tourniquets for hemorrhage control on the battlefield: A 4-year accumulated experience. *J Trauma.* 2003;54:S221–S225.
30. Welling DR, Burris DG, Hutton JE et al. A balanced approach to tourniquet use: Lessons learned and relearned. *J Am Coll Surg.* 2006;203(1):106–115.
31. Walters TJ, Wenke JC, Kauvar DS, McManus JG, Holcomb JB, Baer DG. Effectiveness of self-applied tourniquets in human volunteers. *Prehosp Emerg Care.* 2005;9(4):416–422.
32. Rasmussen TE, Clouse WD, Jenkins DH, Peck MA, Eliason JL, Smith DL. Echelons of care and the management of wartime vascular injury: A report from the 332nd EMDG/Air Force Theater Hospital, Balad Air Base, Iraq. *Perspec Vasc Surg Endovascular Ther.* 2006;18(2):91–99.
33. Kragh JF, Walters TJ, Baer DG, Fox CJ, Wade CE, Salinas J, Holcomb JB. Practical use of emergency tourniquets to stop bleeding in major limb trauma. *J Trauma.* 2008;64(2):S38–S50.
34. Pusateri AE, Holcomb JB, Kheirabadi BS, Alam HB, Wade CE, Ryan KL. Making sense of the preclinical literature on advanced hemostatic products. *J Trauma.* 2006;60:674–682.

35. Alam HB, Uy GB, Miller D et al. Comparative analysis of hemostatic agents in a swine model of lethal groin injury. *J Trauma*. 2003;54:1077–1082.
36. Rixen D, Grass G, Sauerland S et al. Evaluation of criteria for temporary external fixation in risk-adapted damage control orthopedic surgery of femur shaft fractures in multiple trauma patients: "evidence-based medicine" versus "reality" in the trauma registry of the German Trauma Society. *J Trauma*. 2005;59:1375–1395.
37. Scalea TM, Boswell SA, Scott JD et al. External fixation as a bridge to intramedullary nailing for patients with multiple injuries and with femur fractures: Damage control orthopedics. *J Trauma*. 2000;48(4):613–621.
38. Pape HC, Grimme K, Van Griensven M et al. Impact of intramedullary instrumentation versus damage control for femoral fractures on immunoinflammatory parameters: Prospective randomized analysis by the EPOFF Study Group. *J Trauma*. 2003;55:7–13.
39. Pape HC, Rixen D, Morley J et al. Impact of the method of initial stabilization for femoral shaft fractures in patients with multiple injuries at risk for complications (borderline patients). *Ann Surg*. 2007;246(3):149–157.
40. Gustilo RB, Mendoza RM, Willimas DN. Problems in the management of type III severe open fractures: A new classification of type III open fractures. *J Trauma*. 1984;24(8):742–746.
41. Georgiadis GM, Behrens FF, Joyce MJ, Earle AS, Simmons AL. Open tibial fractures with severe soft-tissue loss. Limb salvage compared with below-the-knee amputation. *J Bone Joint Surg Am*. 1993;75(10):1431–1441.
42. Pirela-Cruz MA, Machen MS, Esquivel D. Management of large soft-tissue wounds with negative pressure therapy-lessons learned from the war zone. *J Hand Ther*. 2008;21(2):196–202.
43. DeFranzo AJ, Argenta LC, Marks MW, Molnar JA, David LR, Webb LX, Ward WG, Teasdall RG. The use of vacuum-assisted closure therapy for the treatment of lower-extremity wounds with exposed bone. *Plastic Reconstr Surg*. 2001;108(5):1184–1191.
44. Herscovici D, Sanders RW, Scaduto JM et al. Vacuum-assisted wound closure (VAC therapy) for the management of patients with high-energy soft tissue injuries. *J Orthop Trauma*. 2003;17(10):683–688.
45. Geiger S, McCormick F, Chou R, Wandel AG. War wounds: Lessons learned from Operation Iraqi Freedom. *Plast Reconstr Surg*. 2008;122(1):146–153.
46. Leininger BE, Rasmussen TE, Smith DL, Jenkins DH, Coppola C. Experience with wound VAC and delayed primary closure of contaminated soft tissue injuries in Iraq. *J Trauma*. 2006;61(5):1207–1211.
47. Godina M. Early microsurgical reconstruction of complex trauma of the extremities. *Plast Reconstr Surg*. 1986;78:285–292.
48. Parrett BM, Matros E, Pribaz JJ, Orgill DP. Lower extremity trauma: Trends in the management of soft-tissue reconstruction of open tibia-fibula fractures. *Plast Reconstr Surg*. 2006;117(4):1315–1322.
49. Bosse MJ, MacKenzie EJ, Kellam JF et al. A prospective evaluation of the clinical utility of the lower-extremity injury-severity scores. *J Bone Joint Surg Am*. 2001;83-A(1):3–14.
50. Bosse MJ, McCarthy ML, Jones AL, Webb LX, Sims SH, Sanders RW, MacKenzie EJ. The insensate foot following severe lower extremity trauma: An indication for amputation? *J Bone Joint Surg Am*. 2005;87(12):2601–2608.
51. MacKenzie EJ, Bosse MJ, Kellam JF et al. Factors influencing the decision to amputate or reconstruct after high-energy lower extremity trauma. *J Trauma*. 2002;52(4):641–649.
52. Treiman RL, Doty D, Gaspar MR. Acute vascular trauma: A fifteen year study. *J Surg*. 1966;111:469–473.
53. Johansen K, Daines M, Howey T, Helfet D, Hansen ST, Jr. Objective criteria accurately predict amputation following lower extremity trauma. *J Trauma*. 1990;30(5):568–572; discussion 572–573.
54. Jurkovich G, Mock C, MacKenzie E, Burgess A, Cushing B, deLateur B, McAndrew M, Morris J, Swiontkowski M. The sickness impact profile as a tool to evaluate functional outcome in trauma patients. *J Trauma*. 1995;39(4):625–631.
55. Ly TV, Travison TG, Castillo RC, Bosse MJ, MacKenzie EJ, LEAP Study Group. Ability of lower-extremity injury severity scores to predict functional outcome after limb salvage. *J Bone Joint Surg Am*. 2008;90:1738–1743.
56. Howe HR, Jr., Poole GV, Jr., Hansen KJ, Clark T, Plonk GW, Koman LA, Pennell TC. Salvage of lower extremities following combined orthopedic and vascular trauma. A predictive salvage index. *Am Surg*. 1987;53(4):205–208.
57. Russell WL, Sailors DM, Whittle TB, Fisher DF, Jr., Burns RP. Limb salvage versus traumatic amputation. A decision based on a seven-part predictive index. *Ann Surg*. 1991;213(5):473–480; discussion 480–481.
58. McNamara MG, Heckman JD, Corley FG. Severe open fractures of the lower extremity: A retrospective evaluation of the Mangled Extremity Severity Score (MESS). *J Orthop Trauma*. 1994;8(2):81–87.
59. Krettek C, Seekamp A, Kontopp H, Tscherne H. Hannover Fracture Scale '98-re-evaluation and new perspectives of an established extremity salvage score. *Injury Int J Care Injured*. 2001;32:317–328.
60. Hierner R, Betz AM, Comtet JJ, Berger AC. Decision making and results in subtotal and total lower leg amputations: Reconstruction versus amputation. *Microsurgery*. 1995;16(12):830–839.
61. MacKenzie EJ, Bosse MJ, Pollak AN et al. Long-term persistence of disability following severe lower-limb trauma. Results of a seven-year follow-up. *J Bone Joint Surg Am*. 2005;87(8):1801–1809.
62. MacKenzie EJ, Bosse MJ, Kellam JF et al. Factors influencing the decision to amputate or reconstruct after high-energy lower extremity trauma. *J Trauma*. 2002;52(4):641–649.
62. Bosse MJ, McCarthy ML, Jones AL et al. The insensate foot following severe lower extremity trauma: An indication for amputation. *J Bone Joint Surg Am*. 2005;87(12):2601–2608.
63. Peck MA, Clouse WD, Cox MW et al. The complete management of extremity vascular injury in a local population: A wartime report from the 332nd Expeditionary Medical Group/Air Force Theater Hospital, Balad Air Base, Iraq. *J Vasc Surg*. 2007;45:1197–1205.
64. Kragh JF, Jr., Walters TJ, Baer DG, Fox CJ, Wade CE, Salinas J, Holcomb JB. Survival with emergency tourniquet use to stop bleeding in major limb trauma. *Ann Surg*. January 2009;249(1):1–7.

## Commentary on Limb Salvage for the Mangled Extremity

*William Schecter*

The mangled extremity is a common problem after blunt and high-velocity penetrating trauma. After attention to the primary survey (including control of extremity hemorrhage by local pressure and/or tourniquets), attention is focused on the extremity during the secondary survey. In the presence of active hemorrhage, the patient should be transported immediately to the operating room for exploration, hemostasis, and restoration of perfusion without preoperative vascular imaging. On-table angiography to assess the injury or the results of reconstruction can be done in the OR.

The primary goal of reconstruction is achievement of a stable skeleton, free of infection, covered by well-vascularized soft tissue. All secondary reconstruction and rehabilitation aims depend on achievement of this primary goal. The ultimate objective is a mobile functional patient.

The extremity is composed of a skin envelope containing fascia, muscle-tendon units, arteries, veins, nerves, and bone. The priorities of management are: (1) assessment and restoration of arterial perfusion, (2) restoration of venous drainage, (3) prevention or treatment of compartment syndrome, (4) skeletal stabilization, (5) debridement of nonviable or infected soft tissue, (6) assessment and treatment of nerve injury, (7) repair of muscle-tendon units, and (8) coverage of exposed bone with well vascularized soft tissue and skin. A multidisciplinary approach is frequently necessary depending upon the complexity of the injury and the skill set of the responsible surgeon.

### Which Management Strategies Reduce the Impact of Ischemia, and Reperfusion Injury on Limb Salvage Following Trauma?

If the patient presents with an ischemic limb, the clock is ticking. If transport time is very short, a rapid CT angiogram of the extremity can provide useful information regarding the vascular and skeletal anatomy in the hemodynamically stable patient. This should be a 15 min experience if the surgeon is in constant attendance. If the patient is unstable, ischemia time is prolonged, or a CT scanner is unavailable, the patient should go directly to the OR. There are few relevant questions that cannot be answered by a combination of exploration, on-table angiography and intra-operative radiography. Occasionally an unstable patient has life-threatening intra-abdominal, intrathoracic or intracranial injuries demanding immediate attention prior to definitive management of the extremity injury. In this situation, a two-team approach should be considered. The extremity team should focus their initial attention on restoration of perfusion.

Vascular shunts to rapidly restore arterial flow and venous drainage prior to skeletal stabilization have changed our approach to this complex problem. Definitive vascular repair should be avoided in the presence of cardiovascular instability and/or adverse local wound conditions. Hemodynamic instability, coagulopathy, acidosis, and hypothermia are all contraindications to complex vascular reconstruction. Skeletal instability, gross contamination, or major soft tissue loss are relative contraindications to definitive repair. The skill set of the surgeon and the available equipment may also affect the decision regarding primary vascular repair. Inexperienced vascular surgeons or surgeons working in austere environments should consider temporary vascular shunts to restore limb perfusion prior to transfer for definitive care.

A variety of commercial vascular shunts are available. However, any plastic tube irrigated with heparin saline can function as a temporary shunt. Intravenous tubing, tubes in closed system suction sets, pediatric endotracheal tubes, or even small chest tubes cut to size may be used depending upon the size of the injured vessel. The shunt should be secured with heavy ligatures. The vessel should be debrided and irrigated with heparin saline solution after distal thrombectomy prior to shunt insertion. Shunt patency should be monitored by direct observation or Doppler examination of the distal pulses. Definitive vascular repair should be delayed until achievement of cardiovascular stability and improvement in local wound conditions. Intravascular shunts have been left in place for up to 10 days*, but as a general rule, definitive vascular reconstruction should be performed as soon as the patient is stable. All truly mangled extremities with vascular compromise require four-compartment fasciotomy at the initial procedure. One final point: it is imperative to cover all exposed vessels with soft tissue (preferably local muscle flaps if available) to prevent desiccation and anastomotic disruption.

### Is There a Difference in Limb Salvage Strategies in the Setting of Upper versus Lower Extremity Injury?

There are several points regarding the upper extremity that deserve emphasis. Denervation of the upper extremity is not an indication for amputation. The results of neurorrhaphy and nerve grafting in the upper extremity are reasonable (depending on the level and the nature of the nerve injury). Even replantation can result in a useful assistive extremity.

It is critical to manage the upper extremity in the "position of function." The wrist should be extended,

* Feliciano DV. Heroic procedures in vascular injury management: The role of extra-anatomic bypass. *Surg Clin North Am.* 2002 February;82(1):115–124.

the metacarpophalangeal joints flexed, and the thumb abducted. This permits initiation of grasp and power finger flexion.

The elbow should be extended in the postoperative period. It is much easier to achieve elbow flexion with physical therapy than to extend an elbow frozen in the flexed position. Range of motion of all joints should be initiated as soon as possible.

### What Prehospital Adjuncts Are Available That Impact Limb Salvage Following Traumatic Extremity Injury?

When I was a young surgeon, the use of tourniquets was discouraged in the management of vascular injuries. In fact, if a tourniquet is left in place for a prolonged period of time, severe iatrogenic injury can result. Nevertheless, as the authors eloquently describe, the reintroduction of this useful prehospital tool to control extremity hemorrhage has saved countless lives. It should be part of every combat soldier's kit and every emergency medical service rig.

### What Strategies in Skeletal Reconstruction Impact Limb Salvage Following Traumatic Injury?

The introduction of external fixation in the management of Gustillo Grade 111 c injuries has greatly improved management by providing rapid stabilization and access to the wound with minimal physiologic insult. I prefer to place shunts, stabilize the skeleton, and only then do a definitive vascular repair even in stable patients to avoid anastomotic disruption during fracture reduction. Intramedullary fixation is the preferred definitive stabilization technique when possible. Osteotomy, bone lengthening, and bone grafting with the Ilizarov technique have extended the boundaries of limb salvage in selected patients*.

### How Do Advances in Soft Tissue Wound Management Strategies Impact Limb Salvage?

Several principles deserve emphasis. The initial debridement should be conservative. It is often difficult to determine tissue viability at the initial exploration. Conservative debridement allows the subsequent use of well-vascularized soft tissue for bone coverage.

Frequent repeated soft tissue debridement is essential to achieve a clean wound bed. There are numerous lower and upper extremity pedicle muscle flaps that can be used effectively to cover exposed bone. These flaps should be in the armamentarium of surgeons responsible for the definitive management of these wounds†.

Free flaps are another option for wound coverage as described by the authors. However, recent Israeli experience suggests that luxuriant granulation tissue will usually cover even exposed bone after negative pressure wound management (Alexander Lerner, personal communication). This permits definitive wound closure with split-thickness skin grafts instead of more complex procedures. Negative pressure sponges should never be applied to a fresh vascular anastomosis without protective overlying soft tissue.

### How Do Patient, and Injury Characteristics Impact Decision Making Regarding Extremity Salvage?

### What Is the Role of Mangled Extremity Scores and Indices on Decision Making in Limb Salvage?

Both sections "How Do Patient, and Injury Characteristics Impact Decision Making Regarding Extremity Salvage?" and "What Is the Role of Mangled Extremity Scores and Indices on Decision Making in Limb Salvage?" deal with amputation. In spite of the truly remarkable progress in reconstructive surgery, the authors point out that "heroic measures for limb salvage do not necessarily provide superior quality of life and limb outcomes." Furthermore, advances in prosthetics and rehabilitation have produced remarkable functional results. Unfortunately, the decision to amputate rather than reconstruct a mangled lower extremity cannot be made on the basis of any known scoring system. Mature clinical judgment taking into account variables such as ischemia time, muscle necrosis, nerve injury, comorbidities, and wound contamination is the best guide for treatment. Lower extremity prostheses are generally more functional than upper extremity prostheses at the present time. An assistive upper extremity is better than a prosthesis in most cases. Aggressive efforts to salvage an upper extremity are usually justified.

It takes more courage to do a primary amputation than attempt limb salvage. I usually consult one or two colleagues prior to primary amputation unless the indications are obvious. Undue delay in amputation complicates the ultimate decision. I find that patients "get attached" to their infected, functionless, and occasionally necrotic limbs, delaying consent often to the detriment of their health and rehabilitation.

---

* Sen C, Kocaoglu M, Eralp L et al. Bifocal compression-distraction in the acute treatment of grade 111 open tibia fractures with bone and soft-tissue loss: A report of 24 cases. *J Orthop Trauma*. 2004;18:150–157.

† Reddy V, Stevenson TR. MOC-PS CME article: Lower extremity reconstruction. *Plast Reconstr Surg*. 2008;121(4 Suppl.):1–7.

# 33

## *Critical Questions in Support of the Burned Patient*

**Eileen Bernal and Steven E. Wolf**

**CONTENTS**



### 33.1 Introduction

Burn care has advanced dramatically in the last 50 years to the point that almost any injury in a young person might be expected to survive. Most of these advances were reached through both observational and prospective research done at the bench and bedside. The days of conservative wound management and wait-and-see critical care have given way to goal-directed fluid management, early excision and grafting of burn wounds for wound closure, aggressive organ support, and directed rehabilitation strategies. Primary advances have been in the areas of resuscitation, wound care, prevention of infection, and critical care; some nascent work in the assessment of rehabilitation outcomes and scar management is underway with no current definitive answers.

Even with these advances, important questions still arise about what exactly the advances have been and how these should be considered in decision for patient treatment, particularly in those with severe burns. Most define burns of greater than 20% of the total body surface area (TBSA) to be severe, with real risk of mortality and other poor outcomes. In this chapter, we will consider the following relevant questions in the severely burned: exactly how much fluid to give and when in the first 24 h after injury, when to go to the operating theatre and how to manage the patient when there, the best treatment for those treated without operation, how to reduce infectious complications, and how to manage a relevant pulmonary complication peculiar to this population. Each of these questions is vitally important in outcomes.

### 33.2 What Is the Optimal Resuscitation Method Following Severe Burn?

Current guidelines outlining the resuscitation of severely burned patients were developed over 30 years ago, and the most commonly used are the Parkland formula [1] and Modified Brooke formula [2]. Each of these was developed in preclinical studies and then was trialed in patients without contemporaneous controls (class V evidence); evidence to support their use was simply success of the formulae. Both of these formulae make recommendations for the first 24 h after injury and are crystalloid based with no provision for colloid during this time period. This notion is based on the finding that fluid given in the first 24 h escapes from the intravascular space into the interstitium regardless of its molecular size; thus the purported advantage of colloid to expand the intravascular space is lost during this time period [2], although early administration seems to have a volume-sparing pulmonary benefit [3]. This led Dr. Pruitt to state that "in early burn resuscitation, colloid is no more than expensive salt water" [4]. Any more fluid than that required for normovolemia will increase tissue turgor and necrosis, increasing burn depth [5]. Many studies exist that examine alterations or adjustments in resuscitation protocols that may lead to improved outcomes; however, none are definitive nor have replaced the tried and true standards.

In the last several years, many adjuncts to resuscitation of the severely burned have been suggested, some with supporting data. These include the use of fluids other than isotonic crystalloid such as hypertonic saline (class V) [6] and the colloids albumin (class V) [7], pentastarch (class II) [8], and plasma (class II) [9]. In the case of hypertonic saline, one class III study showed increased mortality and renal failure with the use of this modality, and thus, it is not in common use [10]. A class I study found hydroxyethyl starch-supplemented burns resuscitation allowed smaller fluid volume requirements and less tissue edema in the first 24 h and was associated with a dampened inflammatory response at 48 h after injury [11]. Of these agents, perhaps plasma shows the most promise with the findings of improved base deficit and abdominal pressures in a class II study, but recommendations from the national blood transfusion councils do not justify its use for volume expansion, where synthetic and/or natural colloids are to be preferred [3,12,13]. Other proposed adjuncts include infusion of high-dose antioxidants such as vitamin C [14] (class II) and use of plasma exchange [15] (class III) or continuous hemofiltration [16] (class IV). Although each of these studies provides compelling evidence that perhaps these treatments may improve resuscitation in the severely burned, none of these is in the worldwide standard of care; common use remains only in specific centers. Large-scale trials are indicated to provide findings generalizable to broad practice.

In the future, we expect a shift from the Parkland and Brooke formulae as the recognition of better and more frequent monitoring is better established. Perhaps the best way to resuscitate the severely burned will be to define a starting dose of a defined fluid, then adjust therapy based on response with the use of decision support technology with allocations for expected biologic responses over time [17]. This method has been tested (class II) and was shown to significantly decrease fluid volumes with improved clinical outcomes [18]. Currently, the outcome measured to define response is urine output, but this also may change in the future.

*Recommendation*: The available data and established expert opinion favor crystalloid resuscitation with lactated Ringers' solution infused at 2–4 mL/kg/% TBSA burned with one-half given in the first 8 h after injury and the second in the subsequent 16 h (Grade B recommendation). Adjuncts such as the use of plasma in resuscitation (Grade B), high-dose vitamin C (Grade B), and guidance of volumes through decision support methodology (Grade B) hold the most promise for advances in the field, but are not established standards of care. Further, decision support technology (Grade B) is likely to play a role in guiding resuscitation in the future.

## 33.3 How Is Burn Depth Best Determined?

Wound depth determination is critical to the decision to operate in burned patients. This is based on the notion that deep partial- and full-thickness burns will not heal in a timely fashion and therefore are best treated with prompt excision and grafting. Central to this idea is the ability to properly discern wound depth such that the decision to operate is made only in those who receive benefit, i.e., those with partial thickness burns that will heal with conservative therapies are not subjected to skin grafting. Typically, this is done through clinical assessment by an expert examiner; however, this method has only 60%–80% accuracy in well-done descriptive studies using histologic analysis from biopsy of the wound as the standard [19]. This method is therefore insufficient.

Many alternative methods have been tested to evaluate wound depth [20], the most promising of which is the laser Doppler. This technology images blood flow using laser Doppler assessment of moving red blood cells to detect vascularity and thus viability. Images are collected of normal and burned skin; normal skin has a moderate level of blood flow, while superficial burns have significantly increased blood flow associated with increased local inflammation. Deep partial- and full-thickness burns have significantly decreased blood flow. Images can be obtained at any time after injury with reasonable accuracy (>90% sensitivity and specificity with wound biopsies and requirement for surgery) [21]. Several trials testing this modality have been performed, all of which confirm the superiority of laser Doppler imaging to clinical assessment (class II). The greatest usefulness is in those wounds where clinical assessment is least accurate (class II) [22], in burns that neither clearly superficial nor clearly full thickness. Even with this evidence, most will still rely on clinical assessment until the technology is more widespread.

*Recommendation*: The preponderance of the evidence suggests that burn depth is best determined by laser Doppler imaging to the exclusion of clinical assessment (Grade B recommendation). For wounds in doubt, this technology should be considered.

## 33.4 When Is the Optimal Time for Burn Wound Excision?

Deep partial- and full-thickness burns benefit from excision and grafting for timely closure. Dr. Cope and others first espoused early excision and grafting for treatment of the acutely burned in the 1940s [23], initially as a means of accelerating time to healing [24]. These initial efforts led to the practice followed by most burn centers, which is to excise the majority of the wound within the first week after injury. The question that arises is precisely when in this time frame should these procedures be performed? Is there some benefit to performing these procedures in the first day after injury compared to a week or more later? Unfortunately, the answer to these questions has not been addressed in a prospective randomized controlled trial, so we are left with lesser evidence to make a determination.

Herndon and Parks in 1986 compared two groups of patients with massive burns (mean >70% TBSA) treated in their center over a 4-year period; some underwent complete excision and grafting within 48 h of admission, and others underwent serial excision and grafting over a several-week period. They found that mortality was not different; however, wound closure was 33% more rapid in the early excision group, which was associated with a similar decrease in the length of hospital stay (class III) [25]. The group in Seattle had similar findings in a related study with a significant decrease in burn wound sepsis (class III) [26]. These data indicate that early excision and grafting decreases burn wound infections and length of stay without effects on mortality. To further refine whether excision and grafting done within the first 48 h compared to sometime in the first week was beneficial, the group in Galveston compared patients who were admitted to the hospital within the first day of injury and thus, at their center, underwent excision and grafting within 48 h of injury compared to those who were admitted later, associated with long-distance transport, with excision and grafting over 48 h after injury. They found that excision greater than 48 h after injury was associated with a higher incidence of invasive wound infection and sepsis and longer total length of hospital stay [27], which is in agreement with the earlier studies (class III). A recent meta-analysis of all studies in this regard showed a significant reduction in mortality for early excision in those *without* inhalation injury (class II) [28].

*Recommendation*: The optimal time for burn wound excision is within 48 h of injury to minimize infectious wound complications and expedite length of hospital stay (Grade B recommendation).

## 33.5 How Is Blood Loss Best Minimized during Burn Excision Procedures?

It is well known that blood loss is common during burn wound excision and grafting procedures. Reported blood loss is from 0.3 to 1.0 cc/cm$^2$ excised, and in one study, was best predicted by larger body size, higher wound bacterial counts, wound area excised, and operative time [29]. Given then that approximately 0.5 cc will be lost per 1 cm$^2$ excised, a normal-sized man with a 50% TBSA burn excision will be predicted to lose 5000 cc of blood, or 10 units. Therefore, the issue at hand is obvious.

Blood loss can be reliably measured in the burned patient by calculating the change in hemoglobin concentration during the operation and the amount of blood that was replaced during and after the operation. To determine whether a technique to decrease blood loss was effective, this number should proportionally decrease in relation to the surface area excised. Reported techniques to decrease blood loss during burn surgery include the use of tourniquets for extremity injuries (class II in favor) [30], subcutaneous clysis of donor sites with vasoconstrictors (class III showing no benefit) [31], thrombin spray to excised areas and donor sites (class II in favor) [32], or fibrin spray to excised areas and donor sites (class II in favor) [33]. In practice, burn surgeons use a combination of these techniques to attempt to minimize transfused blood products. Other considerations such as timing of surgery (less blood loss early in the course) also have merit (class III in favor) [34].

*Recommendation*: Burn wound excision is a bloody business. Efforts to decrease bleeding should include the use of tourniquets on the extremities (class B recommendation) and topical thrombin and/or fibrin sealant (class B recommendation). No particular fibrin or thrombin product has been found to be definitively superior to another.

## 33.6 How Should Partial Thickness Burns Be Treated?

Determining the best treatment for partial thickness wounds with sufficient remaining cellular elements to produce timely wound closure is complex. This is related to trade-offs between minimizing wound complications, allowing for rapid healing, and maximizing patient comfort while minimizing provider effort. Topical treatment of the burn wound is most often the only indicated treatment, and it is optimally a dressing that is antimicrobial, has minimal inhibition of wound healing, does not interfere with wound assessment, and minimizes pain and provider effort through decreasing dressing changes. The tried and true method of burn wound care was twice daily dressing changes with a topical antibiotic salve such as silver sulfadiazine, but this is labor intensive with significant daily patient pain associated with the change. This can be reduced safely to once a day (class III) [35], but it is still suboptimal. Further, silver sulfadiazine inhibits wound healing (class IV) [36] and obscures the wound for evaluation for healing because of the development of pseudoeschar. In fact, this can lead to inappropriate decisions for operative care regarding "conversion" of the wound to what appears to have "become full thickness."

Alternative approaches include use of a skin substitute such as Biobrane (class III) [37] or xenograft (class III) [38] that allows for rapid healing, maximizes patient comfort, and minimizes provider effort and allows for wound assessment; however, the trade-off is potential wound colonization and infection. Another alternative is the use of longer-term silver cloth dressings (e.g., Aquacel Ag, Silverlon, Therabond) that are changed every 3–7 days (class II) [39], some with some effort to keep them moist, and thus diminish pain and provider effort while maintaining antimicrobial activity. The drawbacks are some inhibition of wound healing and loss of ability of daily evaluation of the wound.

*Recommendation*: The best treatment is one that controls antimicrobial growth and allows for frequent wound assessment while minimizing dressing changes. All potential treatments have at least one drawback in this regard, but treatment with a skin substitute or a long-term silver cloth dressing appears to be the best alternative with the current technology (Grade B recommendation).

## 33.7 How Is Burn Wound Infection Effectively Minimized?

Burn wound infection is common in the severely burned due to loss of innate defense associated with the skin, the rich pabulum of the denatured protein comprising eschar, and relative burn-induced immune suppression making burn patients particularly susceptible to sepsis. These three conditions combine to result in the occurrence of invasion of microorganisms into remaining viable tissue as the established criterion for this diagnosis. Organisms typically causing burn wound infection are of a wide spectrum, from gram positives and gram negatives to opportunistic fungi and viruses.

Burn wound infection, therefore, can be minimized in two ways. The first is early excision and grafting for wound closure to re-establish the skin barrier and remove the culture medium of the eschar. We have already seen that early excision of the wound in deep partial- and full-thickness burns is associated with decreased incidence of wound infection (class III evidence), and another study showed that wounds excised greater than 6 days from injury had increased bacterial counts, which was associated with an increased rate of graft loss (class III evidence) [40]. The second is to provide topical antimicrobial therapy directly to the wound, which was shown with class III evidence to be beneficial in burn wounds between 40% and 80% TBSA [41], or systemic antibiotics, which has almost no supportive evidence in the literature yet is a common practice. Antimicrobial selection should be for a broad spectrum agent effective against gram-positive and gram-negative bacteria, and fungi. This is typically achieved topically with the use of a silver-containing agent such as silver sulfadiazine, silver ion-containing dressings, or through alternating use of highly effective soaks and salves such as 5% sulfamylon and/or Dakins' and Domboro's solutions.

*Recommendation*: Infection remains a leading cause of death in burn patients. Burn wound infection is most effectively minimized through the aggressive early use of excision and grafting for wound closure (Grade B recommendation) and judicious use of topical antimicrobials (Grade B recommendation). Systemic antibiotics are commonly used with no supporting evidence in the literature.

## 33.8 What Is the Best Method of Ventilation after Smoke Inhalation Injury to Minimize Lung Complications?

The diagnosis of inhalation injury is generally made by a history of being in an enclosed space with smoke, physical findings of soot in the airway or perioral/perinasal burns, high concentrations of carbon monoxide in the blood, and evidence on bronchoscopy of erythema, edema, loss of epithelium, and/or carbonaceous secretions. Prudent medical practice dictates early intubation to secure the airway of patients with significant inhalation injury, particularly in those with coexistent significant cutaneous burns, before significant edema of the airway develops during resuscitation. With the diagnosis of inhalation injury, the actual damage to the airway and lung is variable ranging from some mild irritation of the upper airways to full-thickness burns of the upper and lower airways.

**TABLE 33.1**
Clinical Questions and Recommendations

| Question | Answer | Level of Evidence | Recommendation Grade | References |
|---|---|---|---|---|
| What is the optimal resuscitation method following severe burn? | Parkland or modified Brooke formula with isotonic crystalloid | II | B | [1–18] |
| How is burn depth best determined? | Laser Doppler imaging | II | B | [19–22] |
| When is the optimal time for burn wound excision? | First 48 h after injury | II | B | [23–28] |
| How is blood loss best minimized during burn excision procedures? | Tourniquets, topical thrombin, and fibrin sealant | III | B | [29–34] |
| How should partial thickness burns be treated? | Skin substitute, silver-containing cloths | III | C | [35–39] |
| How is burn wound infection effectively minimized? | Early excision and grafting, topical antimicrobials | II | B | [40,41] |
| What is the best method of ventilation after smoke inhalation injury to minimize lung complications? | High-frequency percussive ventilation | II | B | [42–50] |

Many modes of ventilation are available for patients intubated with inhalation injury from standard methods used daily in all patient groups to very specialized modes used primarily in this population. These include conventional volume-controlled mechanical ventilation, high-frequency percussive ventilation (HFPV), high-frequency oscillatory ventilation (HFOV), or permissive hypercapnia in association with conventional ventilation. The best studied of these modes is HFPV [42], which was first shown to improve rates of pneumonia and improve survival compared to historic controls [43] (class IV). The survival data were confirmed by another study with contemporaneous nonrandomized controls in burns >40% TBSA (class III) [44]. One randomized controlled study in this population showed only early improvements in oxygenation, but no demonstrable improvement in survival or other clinical outcomes (class II) [45]. Another single-center randomized controlled trial found that low tidal volume (LTV) conventional ventilation was inadequate to meet oxygenation and ventilation goals, especially in patients with inhalational injury, and no significant different between HFPV and LTV with respect to lung protection (class II) [46]. These investigators did find that episodes of rescue ventilation were lower with HFPV. That said, while some of the early data are compelling, no firm clinical evidence with properly controlled trials exists for the superiority of HPRV over conventional ventilation.

Other modes reported in the literature for inhalation injury include HFOV and permissive hypercapnia with conventional ventilation. HFOV was found to improve oxygenation as a salvage technique, with the conclusion that it can be effective for this use in this population (class V) [47]. A similar report was made for the use of permissive hypercapnia, with no controls and the conclusion that this mode can be used safely [48].

Other newer modes of ventilatory support have been reported recently in other populations, most particularly airway pressure release ventilation (APRV) [49]. No reports of its effectiveness in humans in those with inhalation injury are extant. However, one study found that in swine with inhalational injury, APRV-treated animals developed acute respiratory distress syndrome faster than conventional mechanical ventilation-treated animals [50] (Table 33.1).

*Recommendation*: No ventilator strategy has been found to be definitively superior to another in the condition of inhalation injury. HFPV has shown the most promise, however, with some class II, III, and IV studies showing benefit. At the current time, this is the recommended mode of ventilation until more definitive trials are completed (Grade B recommendation).

## 33.9 Conclusion

Data exist in the literature to support the use of many therapies to improve the lot of the severely burned; however, most of these methods have not been rigorously tested. The highest grade of recommendation for these central questions for burn care is only at the class II level for the quality of evidence, and thus, only Grade B recommendations can be made. Well-defined and conducted trials are required to provide further answers to these questions, in particular the method of resuscitation, timing of burn excision and grafting, and optimal method of ventilation in those with smoke-induced lung injury.

## References


1. Baxter CR. Physiological response to crystalloid resuscitation of severe burns. *Ann N Y Acad Sci*. 1968;150(3):874–883.
2. Pruitt BA, Mason AD, Moncrief JA. Hemodynamic changes in the early post-burn patient: The influence of fluid administration and of a vasodilator (hydralazine). *J Trauma*. 1971;11:36–46.
3. Holm C. Resuscitation in shock associated with burns: Tradition or evidence-based medicine? *Resuscitation*. 2000;44(3):157–164.
4. Pruitt BA. Protection from excessive resuscitation: "pushing the pendulum back". *J Trauma*. 2000;49:567–568.
5. Diver AJ. The evolution of burn fluid resuscitation. *Int J Surg*. 2008;6(4):345–350.
6. Monafo WW. The treatment of burn shock by the intravenous and oral administration of hypertonic lactated saline solution. *J Trauma*. 1970;10(7):575–586.
7. Cochran A, Morris SE, Edelman LS, Saffle JR. Burn patient characteristics and outcomes following resuscitation with albumin. *Burns*. 2007;33(1):25–30.
8. Waxman K. Hemodynamic and oxygen transport effects of pentastarch in burn resuscitation. *Ann Surg*. 1989;209(3):341–345.
9. O'Mara MS, Slater H, Goldfarb IW, Caushaj PF. A prospective, randomized evaluation of intra-abdominal pressures with crystalloid and colloid resuscitation in burn patients. *J Trauma*. 2005;58(5):1011–1018.
10. Huang PP, Stucky FS, Dimick AR, Treat RC, Bessey PQ, Rue LW. Hypertonic sodium resuscitation is associated with renal failure and death. *Ann Surg*. 1995;221(5):543–554; discussion 54–57.
11. Contreras M, Ala FA, Greaves M et al. Guidelines for the use of fresh frozen plasma. British Committee for Standards in Haematology, Working Party of the Blood Transfusion Task Force. *Transfus Med*. 1992;2(1):57–63.
12. Contreras M, Ala FA, Greaves M et al. Guidelines for the use of fresh-frozen plasma. *Transfus Med*. 1992;2(1):57–63.
13. Guideline for the use of fresh-frozen plasma. Medical Directors Advisory Committee, National Blood Transfusion Council. *S Afr Med J*. 1998;88(10):1344–1347.
14. Tanaka H. Reduction of resuscitation fluid volumes in severely burned patients using ascorbic acid administration: A randomized, prospective study. *Arch Surg*. 2000;135(3):326–331.
15. Kravitz M, Warden GD, Sullivan JJ, Saffle JR. A randomized trial of plasma exchange in the treatment of burn shock. *J Burn Care Rehabil*. 1989;10(1):17–26.
16. Chung KK, Juncos LA, Wolf SE et al. Continuous renal replacement therapy improves survival in severely burned military casualties with acute kidney injury. *J Trauma*. 2008;64(2 Suppl):S179–S185; discussion S85–S87.
17. Alvarado R, Chung KK, Cancio LC, Wolf SE. Burn resuscitation. *Burns*. 2009;35:4–14.
18. Salinas J, Chung KK, Mann EA et al. Computerized decision support system improves fluid resuscitation following severe burns: An original study. *Crit Care Med*. 2011;39(9):2031–2038.
19. Pape SA, Skouras CA, Byrne PO. An audit of the use of laser Doppler imaging (LDI) in the assessment of burns of intermediate depth. *Burns*. 2001;27(3):233–239.
20. Hemington-Gorse SJ. A comparison of laser Doppler imaging with other measurement techniques to assess burn depth. *J Wound Care*. 2005;14(4):151–153.
21. Jeng JC, Bridgeman A, Shivnan L et al. Laser Doppler imaging determines need for excision and grafting in advance of clinical judgment: A prospective blinded trial. *Burns*. 2003;29(7):665–670.
22. Khatib M, Jabir S, Fitzgerald O'Connor E, Philp B. A systematic review of the evolution of laser Doppler techniques in burn depth assessment. *Plast Surg Int*. 2014;2014:621792.
23. Cope O, Langohr JL, Moore FD, Webster RC. Expeditious care of full thickness burn wounds by surgical excision and grafting. *Ann Surg*. 1947;125:1–22.
24. Burke JF, Bondoc CC, Quinby WC. Primary burn excision and immediate grafting: A method shortening illness. *J Trauma*. 1974;14(5):389–395.
25. Herndon DN, Parks DH. Comparison of serial debridement and autografting and early massive excision with cadaver skin overlay in the treatment of large burns in children. *J Trauma*. 1986;26(2):149–152.
26. Gray DT, Pine RW, Harnar TJ, Marvin JA, Engrav LH, Heimbach DM. Early surgical excision versus conventional therapy in patients with 20 to 40 percent burns. A comparative study. *Am J Surg*. 1982;144(1):76–80.
27. Xiao-Wu W, Herndon DN, Spies M, Sanford AP, Wolf SE. Effects of delayed wound excision and grafting in severely burned children. *Arch Surg*. 2002;137(9):1049–1054.
28. Ong YS, Samuel M, Song C Meta-analysis of early excision of burns. *Burns*. 2006;32(2):145–150.
29. Hart DW, Wolf SE, Beauford RB, Lal SO, Chinkes DL, Herndon DN. Determinants of blood loss during primary burn excision. *Surgery*. 2001;130(2):396–402.
30. O'Mara MS, Goel A, Recio P et al. The use of tourniquets in the excision of unexsanguinated extremity burn wounds. *Burns*. 2002;28(7):684–687.
31. Barret JP, Dziewulski P, Wolf SE, Desai MH, Nichols RJ, Herndon DN. Effect of topical and subcutaneous epinephrine in combination with topical thrombin in blood loss during immediate near-total burn wound excision in pediatric burned patients. *Burns*. 1999;25(6):509–513.
32. Prasad JK, Taddonio TE, Thomson PD. Prospective comparison of a bovine collagen dressing to bovine spray thrombin for control of haemorrhage of skin graft donor sites. *Burns*. 1991;17(1):70–71.
33. Nervi C, Gamelli RL, Greenhalgh DG et al. A multicenter clinical trial to evaluate the topical hemostatic efficacy of fibrin sealant in burn patients. *J Burn Care Rehabil*. 2001;22(2):99–103.
34. Desai MH, Herndon DN, Broemeling L, Barrow RE, Nichols RJ, Rutan RL. Early burn wound excision significantly reduces blood loss. *Ann Surg*. 1990;211(6):753–759; discussion 9–62.
35. Sheridan RL, Petras L, Lydon M, Salvo PM. Once-daily wound cleansing and dressing change: Efficacy and cost. *J Burn Care Rehabil*. 1997;18(2):139–140.

36. Muller MJ, Hollyoak MA, Moaveni Z, Brown TL, Herndon DN, Heggers JP. Retardation of wound healing by silver sulfadiazine is reversed by Aloe vera and nystatin. *Burns.* 2003;29(8):834–836.
37. Lal S, Barrow RE, Wolf SE et al. Biobrane improves wound healing in burned children without increased risk of infection. *Shock.* 2000;14(3):314–318; discussion 8–9.
38. Bukovcan P, Koller J. Treatment of partial-thickness scalds by skin xenografts—A retrospective study of 109 cases in a three-year period. *Acta Chir Plast.* 2010;52(1):7–12.
39. Verbelen J, Hoeksema H, Heyneman A, Pirayesh A, Monstrey S. Aquacel((R)) Ag dressing versus Acticoat dressing in partial thickness burns: A prospective, randomized, controlled study in 100 patients. Part 1: Burn wound healing. *Burns.* 2014;40(3):416–427.
40. Barret JP, Herndon DN. Effects of burn wound excision on bacterial colonization and invasion. *Plast Reconstr Surg.* 2003;111(2):744–750; discussion 51–52.
41. Brown TP, Cancio LC, McManus AT, Mason AD. Survival benefit conferred by topical antimicrobial preparations in burn patients: An historical perspective. *J Trauma.* 2004;56(4):863–866.
42. Cioffi WG, Graves TA, McManus WF, Pruitt BA. High-frequency percussive ventilation in patients with inhalation injury. *J Trauma.* 1989;29(3):350–354.
43. Cioffi WG, Rue LW, Graves TA, McManus WF, Mason AD, Pruitt BA. Prophylactic use of high-frequency percussive ventilation in patients with inhalation injury. *Ann Surg.* 1991;213(6):575–580; discussion 80–82.
44. Hall JJ, Hunt JL, Arnoldo BD, Purdue GF. Use of high-frequency percussive ventilation in inhalation injuries. *J Burn Care Res.* 2007;28(3):396–400.
45. Reper P, Wibaux O, Van Laeke P, Vandeenen D, Duinslaeger L, Vanderkelen A. High frequency percussive ventilation and conventional ventilation after smoke inhalation: A randomised study. *Burns.* 2002;28(5):503–508.
46. Chung KK, Wolf SE, Renz EM et al. High-frequency percussive ventilation and low tidal volume ventilation in burns: A randomized controlled trial. *Crit Care Med.* 2010;38(10):1970–1977.
47. Cartotto RC, Ellis S, Gomez M, Cooper AB, Smith T. High frequency oscillatory ventilation in burn patients with the acute respiratory distress syndrome. *Burns.* 2004;30(5):453–463.
48. Sheridan RL, Kacmarek RM, McEttrick MM et al. Permissive hypercapnia as a ventilatory strategy in burned children: Effect on barotrauma, pneumonia, and mortality. *J Trauma.* 1995;39(5):854–859.
49. Varpula T, Valta P, Niemi R, Takkunen O, Hynynen M, Pettila VV. Airway pressure release ventilation as a primary ventilatory mode in acute respiratory distress syndrome. *Acta Anaesthesiol Scand.* 2004;48(6):722–731.
50. Batchinsky AI, Burkett SE, Zanders TB et al. Comparison of airway pressure release ventilation to conventional mechanical ventilation in the early management of smoke inhalation injury in swine. *Crit Care Med.* 2011;39(10):2314–2321.

## Commentary on Critical Questions in Support of the Burned Patient

*Basil A. Pruitt, Jr.*

Comment: The authors have identified important questions that the surgeon taking care of a burn patient must address to provide optimum management of fluid resuscitation, burn wound care, and ventilator support for those with inhalation injury. In large part, they have provided answers that define best-evidence standards of care.

The authors note the recent emphasis on lesser-volume fluid resuscitation focused on maintaining organ function with the least infused volume of crystalloid fluid in the first 24 h post burn to minimize edema formation. Consequently, their unqualified recommendation to estimate first 24 h fluid needs as being 2–4 milliliters of lactated Ringer's solution per kilogram body weight per % TBSA burn is surprising. Consensus, as expressed in the current Advanced Burn Life Support Provider Manual, recommends use of only 2 mL/kg body weight/% TBSA burned and 3 mL/kg body weight/% TBSA burned as the initial estimate of lactated Ringer's solution needed in the first 24 h by adults and children, respectively. An initial 24 h estimate of 4 mL of lactated Ringer's solution/kg body weight/% TBSA burned is reserved for adults with high-voltage electric injuries*. The initial infusion rate is increased or decreased depending upon the individual patient's response in terms of timed urinary output. Also surprising is the author's implication that the two most commonly used formulae to guide fluid therapy are only useful for predicting fluid needs for the first 24 h when each formula clearly encompasses the first 48 h and recommends the use of colloid containing fluid (albumin diluted to physiologic concentration in normal saline) in the second 24 h and even in the latter half of the first 24 h after injury if the infusion rate needed to maintain the urinary output goal exceeds the formula estimate by twofold or more. Additionally, the reader should be warned that there are patients who typically require more fluid than that predicted by formulae, i.e., those patients with inhalation injury, those in whom resuscitation has been delayed, those with high-voltage electric injury, those with associated mechanical injuries, those who are drunk when burned, and nursing home patients who are typically dehydrated when burned.

As indicated by the authors, the most promising means of minimizing resuscitation fluid volume appears to be the use of a computer-based closed loop decision support system such as the one developed by investigators at the US Army Burn Center. In that system, the fluid infusion rate is adjusted on the basis of frequently monitored urinary output. In initial studies using an animal model in which the infusion rate was adjusted in response to urinary volume on an hourly basis, a significant reduction in resuscitation volume was observed†. As noted by these authors, the early clinical experience has confirmed a reduction in the volume of fluid required for resuscitation when that system was employed and the investigators speculated that further reduction in volume could be achieved with more frequent adjustment of the infusion rate based on 10 min urinary volume collections.

In answer to the question about the best way to determine burn depth, the authors recommend use of laser Doppler imaging on the basis of what they consider to be class II data but properly point out that such diagnostic assistance is needed only in those burns of equivocal depth, i.e., those that are between clearly superficial and clearly full thickness by clinical assessment. The determination of depth in those burns has been used to support excision of deep partial thickness burns to prevent the hypertrophic scarring that commonly occurred with their prolonged spontaneous healing. The current use of laser therapy to remodel or "re-engineer" postburn scars to reduce or eliminate their complications and limiting features may make the identification and excision of such wounds unnecessary‡.

The authors pose a question about the optimal time for burn wound excision and supply "within 48 h" as the answer. They note that the supporting data for that statement is based on a study involving only 64 patients, all of whom had extensive burns and were treated at a pediatric burn center. In that study, no significant difference in mortality could be attributed to early excision as opposed to serial excision and grafting extending over a several week period. There was a significant reduction in hospital stay in the survivors, but blood loss was 10-fold greater in the early excision patients who did not survive. With topical antimicrobial chemotherapy, there is a predictable and generally slow increase in the microbial density within unexcised eschar such that bacteremia induced by excision is rare within the first 10 days post burn. Consequently, there is no absolute necessity to excise the burn wound within 48 h and fluid resuscitation can be completed and the wound excised and

* American Burn Association. 2011. Shock and fluid resuscitation. *ABLS Provider Manual*. American Burn Association: Chicago, IL, pp. 41–51.

† Salinas J, Drew G, Gallagher J et al. Closed-loop and decision-assist resuscitation of burn patients. *J Trauma*. 2008;64:S321–S332.

‡ Hultman CS, Friedstat JS, Edkins RE et al. Laser resurfacing and remodeling of hypertropic burn scars: The results of a large prospective, before-after cohort study, with long-term follow-up. *Ann Surg*. 2014;260:519–532.

grafted, prior to the 10th postburn day, when the patient has been stabilized without compromising survival*.

As the authors state, "burn wound excision is a bloody business." And in response to the question how best to minimize blood loss during burn wound excision procedures and presumably to reduce the risk of transfusion-related acute lung injury, they note the documented benefits of the use of tourniquets during the excision of extremity burns and the use of topical thrombin and/or fibrin sealant on the excised wound bed and donor sites during the excision and grafting procedure. Even though transfusion to increase hemoglobin concentration can decrease cardiac stress in hyperdynamic septic burn patients, of greatest potential benefit in the elderly, the increased risk of infection associated with transfusion recommends caution in such use of blood[†‡].

In answer to the question about how partial-thickness burns should be treated, the authors nicely balance control of microbial proliferation, acceleration of healing, and the conservation of medical resources to minimize expenditures. The possible treatment regimens are reviewed with the benefits of silver-impregnated dressings emphasized. As noted earlier, laser therapy to re-engineer scars has decreased the use of excision for even some deep partial-thickness burns, which some clinicians now allow to heal spontaneously with any scarring treated by the use of a variety of lasers.

Burn wound infection represents a persistent problem with continuous change in the predominance of causative organisms. As the authors note, the use of topical antimicrobial chemotherapy and prompt burn wound excision are the principal agents of microbial control. To ensure the adequacy of infection control, the burn wound should be examined frequently and if signs of microbial invasion are present, a biopsy of that area of the burn wound including the underlying unburned subcutaneous tissue should be performed[§]. The microbial status of the wound can be determined by histologic examination of the biopsy specimen. If invasive infection is confirmed, i.e., microorganisms present in the underlying unburned tissue, prompt excision of the infected tissue is mandated. The authors state "systemic antibiotics are commonly used with no supporting evidence in the literature," but it should be further emphasized that systemic antibiotics should never be used prophylactically in the burn patient and only as therapeutic agents for confirmed infections. The recent emergence of fungi as the predominant causative agent of invasive burn wound infection and the significant comorbid effect of fungal infections in burn patients speak for close control of antibiotic therapy and meticulous surveillance of burn wounds that have not healed or been excised within 14 days[¶].

Lastly, the authors address the question of the best method of ventilation after smoke inhalation injury to minimize lung complications and recommend the use of high-frequency positive pressure interrupted flow ventilation (HFPV). That recommendation is strengthened by a study at the US Army Burn Center indicating that high-frequency percussive ventilation improved both oxygen and carbon dioxide tensions, attenuated lung inflammation and histologic lung injury, improved static compliance and other selected indices of pulmonary function, and was associated with decreased ventilator associated pneumonia and improved survival of inhalation injury patients. Those investigators concluded that HFPV had the unique capacity to "exploit both high- and low-frequency ventilation to favorably influence gas exchange while still adhering to a lung protective low tidal volume ventilation strategy"[**]. Other studies at the Army Burn Center have indicated that prone positioning markedly improved oxygenation (increased $FIO_2$ ratio) in 12 of the 14 survivors out of a group of 18 burn patients with severe ARDS[††].

The questions posed by these authors and their answers provide a secure road map, which will enable surgeons caring for burn patients to deliver best evidence-based care including physiologically attuned fluid resuscitation, sound burn wound management including infection control, and optimum ventilatory support for those patients with inhalation injury. These comments are meant in no way to impugn the recommendations of the authors but merely to supplement and refine what they have presented to the reader.

* Mozingo DW, McManus AT, Kim SH, Pruitt BA Jr. Incidence of bacteremia after wound manipulation in the early postburn period. *J Trauma.* 1997;42:1006–1011.

† Farrell KJ, McManus WF, Mason AD Jr., Pruitt BA Jr. Interrelationship of cardiac index and hemoglobin concentration in a subset of hyperdynamic septic burn patients. *Surg Forum.* 1986;371:75–78.

‡ Graves TA, Cioffi WG, Mason AD Jr., Pruitt BA Jr. Relationship of transfusion and infection in burn population. *J Trauma.* 1989;29:948–954.

§ Pruitt BA Jr., McManus AT, Kim SH et al. Burn wound infections: Current status. *World J Surg.* 1998;22:135–145.

¶ Horvath EE, Murray CK, Vaughan GM et al. Fungal wound infection (not colonization) is independently associated with mortality in burn patients. *Ann Surg.* 2007;246:978–985.

** Allan PF, Osborn EC, Chung KK et al. High frequency percussive ventilation revisited. *J Burn Care Res.* 2010;31:510–520.

†† Hale DF, Cannon JW, Batchinsky AI et al. Prone positioning improves oxygenation in adult burn patients with severe acute respiratory distress syndrome. *J Trauma Acute Care Surg.* 2012;72:1634–1639.

# 34

## *Inhalation Injury*

**Leopoldo C. Cancio***

CONTENTS



### 34.1 Introduction

Smoke inhalation injury (II) occurs in about 10% of patients admitted to burn centers and greatly increases postburn pneumonia and mortality risk, especially at the mid-range of age and burn size [1,2]. II is also an independent risk factor for acute respiratory distress syndrome (ARDS) in burn patients, which, in turn, predicts increased mortality [3]. Acute care surgeons frequently provide initial care to patients with II. This chapter will review the evidence for current standards of care in the treatment of these patients, summarized in Tables 34.1 and 34.2. The acute care surgeon, faced with a patient with severe II, must address the following questions:

- What are the indications for endotracheal intubation and for tracheostomy in patients with II?
- What diagnostic procedures should be performed in patients with suspected II?
- What mode of mechanical ventilation is most effective for these patients?
- What drugs and fluid management strategies, if any, improve outcomes?

* The opinions or assertions contained herein are the private views of the author and are not to be construed as official or as reflecting the views of the Department of the Army or Department of Defense.

**TABLE 34.1**

Clinical Questions: Inhalation Injury

| Question | Answer | Recommendation Grade | References |
|---|---|---|---|
| What are the indications for endotracheal intubation? | Early prophylactic airway control is indicated for most symptomatic patients with II and for patients with extensive burns during initial resuscitation. | C | [4] |
| What are the indications for tracheostomy? | Tracheostomy is an option for long-term airway management and may facilitate pulmonary toilet. | C | [9–11] |
| What diagnostic procedures should be performed? | A presumptive diagnosis can be made on clinical grounds, supplemented by FOL. Definitive diagnosis requires bronchoscopy. | B | [14,81] |
| What mode of mechanical ventilation is most effective? | High-frequency percussive ventilation improves ventilation and oxygenation and may reduce pneumonia and mortality. | B | [25,29,82] |
| What IV fluid strategies improve outcome? | Avoid under- or over-resuscitation. II patients frequently require larger volumes for burn shock resuscitation, but no evidence supports initiation of resuscitation at higher infusion rates. | C | [31,32] |
| What drugs improve outcome? | Inhaled heparin may prevent obstructing clots and casts. | C | [37,38] |
| How is CO poisoning diagnosed? | CO-oximetry (measurement of COHb and MetHb levels) should be performed in patients with II. | D | [57] |
| What treatment is safe and effective for CO poisoning? | One hundred percent oxygen should be given to all patients with CO poisoning until the COHb is normal (<5%). | D | [59] |
| What is the role of HBOT? | HBOT is an option for patients with CO poisoning to prevent the delayed neurocognitive syndrome. | C | [64] |
| What treatments are safe and effective for cyanide? | Hydroxocobalamin should be considered for patients with known or suspected cyanide poisoning. | C | [73] |
| Should II patients be transferred to a burn center? | Consultation with the regional burn center should be performed upon admission. | D | [76] |

*Notes:* The reader is cautioned that, e.g., recommendations concerning airway management, 100% oxygen for treatment of CO poisoning, and burn center referral are considered standard of care in the United States despite the cited levels of evidence.

**TABLE 34.2**

Levels of Evidence

| Subject | Year | References | Level of Evidence | Strength of Recommendation | Findings |
|---|---|---|---|---|---|
| Long-term airway management | 2002, 2004 | [9–11] | 4 | C | Both endotracheal intubation and tracheostomy may be equally safe for long-term airway management. |
| Diagnosis of II | 2004, 2007 | [14,81] | 2b | B | FOB permits diagnosis of II and grading of severity. |
| Best mode of mechanical ventilation | 1991, 2007 | [25,29,82] | 2b | B | High-frequency percussive ventilation may reduce pneumonia and mortality in II and improves oxygenation and ventilation. |
| Pharmacologic therapy | 1998, 2008 | [37,38] | 3b | C | Inhaled heparin may improve outcome in II. |
| HBOT for CO | 2005 | [64] | 2a(-) | C | HBOT may reduce incidence of delayed neurocognitive syndrome. Its role in burn patients is undefined. |
| Antidote for cyanide | 2007 | [73] | 4 | C | Hydroxocobalamin is safe and may be effective for CN poisoning in II. |

- What immediate treatments are safe and effective for metabolic asphyxiation, e.g., by carbon monoxide (CO) or cyanide?
- Should patients with II be transferred to a burn center?

Inhalation injury can be classified into three types based on the anatomic location of the lesion: (1) Upper airway injuries are those caused primarily by thermal injury to the mouth, oropharynx, and larynx. (2) Lower airway and parenchymal injuries are those tracheal, bronchial, and alveolar injuries caused by the passage of the chemical and particulate constituents of smoke past the glottis. (3) Metabolic asphyxiation is the process by which smoke constituents (CO, cyanide) or their by-products (methemoglobinemia due to oxidation of hemoglobin by, e.g. nitrogen dioxide) impair oxygen delivery to, and/or consumption by, the tissues. All three types of II may coexist in a given patient, whose care may be further complicated by cutaneous thermal injury or mechanical trauma. However, unless otherwise specified, the term "inhalation injury" usually means "lower airway and parenchymal injury."

In conducting this review, the primary methodology was a PubMed search for all English language publications for 1966–2008 with the keywords "smoke inhalation injury" or "burns, inhalation," limited to clinical trial, randomized controlled trial (RCT), meta-analysis, or practice guideline. The entirety of the literature was then searched for the period 2009–2014. *The reader is cautioned that, although the level of evidence is low for some recommendations, many of these are considered the current standard of care in the United States. These include prophylactic intubation of symptomatic II patients, provision of 100% oxygen to patients with CO poisoning, and burn center consultation for II patients.*

## 34.2 Airway Management

### 34.2.1 What Are the Indications for Endotracheal Intubation and for Tracheostomy in Patients with II?

The indications for intubation include decreased mental status from inhalation of toxic gases (see the following) or from other injuries; airway obstruction caused by II or generalized postburn edema; and pulmonary failure from subglottic II. The evidence in favor of early intubation of patients with II is primarily that gained by hard experience, rather than that derived from RCTs. Direct thermal injury to the upper airway (to include the larynx, oropharynx, mouth, and tongue) causes edema, which may progress within minutes or hours to complete airway obstruction. Orotracheal intubation of such patients after the onset of obstruction is often impossible, and immediate cricothyroidotomy should then be considered. To avoid that scenario, prophylactic intubation is appropriate.

Premedication for direct laryngoscopy should be performed with an appreciation for the fact that many patients with burns and II are hypovolemic and may become profoundly hypotensive upon induction of anesthesia. The primary risk associated with prophylactic intubation in these patients is catastrophic loss of the airway, especially during transport. Thus, cotton ties (1/2 inch umbilical "tape"), rather than adhesive tape, is used to secure the endotracheal tube circumferentially around the patient's neck. Second, the tube may become obstructed in patients with copious mucus production. This may be prevented by frequent (hourly or more) suctioning.

Concomitant skin burns compound airway swelling and increase the risk of airway obstruction. While II directly damages the airway, cutaneous thermal injury causes generalized edema throughout the body, to include the airway. Zak et al. showed that some children with scald injuries and no II whatsoever required endotracheal intubation, in particular when age <2.8 years and burn size >19% of the total body surface area (TBSA) [4]. In adults, we recommend prophylactic endotracheal intubation for burn patients with greater than 40% TBSA burns until the resuscitation period is complete (first 48 h)—even when II is absent.

Not all patients with smoke exposure require endotracheal intubation. Of the 96 patients with isolated II (no skin burns) from a Korean subway fire, only seven (7%) were intubated [5]. In another retrospective study, of 41 patients who underwent fiberoptic laryngoscopy (FOL), eight (20%) were intubated. Soot in the mouth, facial burns, body burns, edema of the true vocal cords, and edema of the false vocal cords were associated with the decision to intubate [6]. FOL can be used as a screening tool in a multiple-casualty incident [7]. In questionable cases, we recommend awake transnasal FOL as a quick way of assessing laryngeal patency. We use a bronchoscope for this purpose, as it also permits evaluation of the subglottic airway, discussed in the next section.

#### *34.2.1.1 Tracheostomy*

Should patients with II undergo a tracheostomy? If so, when? These questions continue to be debated. In a 1989 report, there were 74 deaths among 99 burn patients who underwent tracheostomy—including 7% due to lost airway and 4% due to massive hemorrhage [8]. In a recent retrospective review of 38 burned children, tracheostomy was performed at a mean of 4 days after admission. Indications included expectation of prolonged ventilation (63%), ARDS (13%), or partial occlusion of endotracheal tube (24%). The operation led to improvements in compliance and in oxygenation ($PaO_2$-to-$FiO_2$ ratio). Twenty-three were performed through neck burns. There were no surgical site infections, tracheostomy-related deaths, or tracheal stenoses [9]. In another retrospective study, 98 burned children underwent mechanical ventilation for at least 7 days (mean 20 ventilator days). Two of these required tracheostomy. At a mean follow-up time of 3 years, subglottic stenosis was noted in only one patient [10]. In a prospective trial in adult burn patients, an early predictor of ventilator dependence was used to select patients for study. Then, patients were randomized to early tracheostomy (Day 4, $n = 21$) or tracheostomy if still intubated at 2 weeks (Day 15, $n = 23$). There was no difference in length of stay, ventilator days, survival, or pneumonia [11].

In brief, in both adults and children, the route of intubation seems less important than avoidance of high peak inspiratory pressures and high cuff pressures. Our practice is to perform tracheostomy at 14 days for those patients who remain ventilator-dependent. But earlier tracheostomy may be necessary for pulmonary toilet. By facilitating pulmonary toilet, tracheostomy may be lifesaving in patients with severe II when they begin to slough the airway mucosa, bleed into the airway, and form obstructing clots and casts. This may begin within a few days of injury.

We, and others, frequently perform bedside percutaneous tracheostomy in these patients [12]. However, caution should be employed when considering the percutaneous route for patients with copious purulent or bloody secretions, as may be the case in severe II. For these patients, open tracheostomy may be safer.

*Recommendation*: Early prophylactic intubation is indicated for most symptomatic patients with II and for patients with extensive burns during initial resuscitation (Grade C recommendation). Tracheostomy is an option for long-term airway management and may facilitate pulmonary toilet (Grade C recommendation).

## 34.3 Diagnosis of Inhalation Injury

### 34.3.1 What diagnostic procedures should be performed in patients with suspected II?

Definitive diagnosis of II before transferring a patient to a burn center is not necessary; it is sufficient to identify the patient at risk for airway and breathing problems and to protect the airway. For this purpose, FOL (see Section 3.2), history and physical exam, and carboxyhemoglobin (COHb) levels (if available) suffice. Mechanism of injury, signs, symptoms, and physical examination provide clues to the presence of II but not diagnostic certainty. Shirani et al. in a retrospective study of 1058 burn patients, 373 (35%) of whom had II by fiberoptic bronchoscopy (FOB) and/or xenon$^{133}$ lung scans, generated the following equation to predict the presence of II:

$P(II) = e^k/(1 - e^k)$, where $k = -4.4165 + 1.61$ (closed space) + 1.77 (facial burn) + 0.0237 (TBSA; %) + 0.0268 (age; years). P ranges from 0 to 1; values for closed space and facial burn are 0 (absent) or 1 (present).

In other words, patients with a history of injury in a closed space, facial burns, large burn sizes, and/or advanced age are more likely to have II [1]. Other historical clues to diagnosis include loss of consciousness at the fire scene and the presence of noxious fumes at the fire. In a retrospective review of the presenting symptoms of 805 patients with burns and II, classic signs of airway obstruction (stridor, voice change, dyspnea) were frequently absent [13].

#### 34.3.1.1 Fiberoptic Bronchoscopy

FOB has been called a "gold standard" for the diagnosis of II. Several authors have developed grading schemes for severity of injury based on FOB that may correlate with outcome [14–16]. FOB may disclose hyperemia, edema, necrosis, pallor, varying amounts of carbonaceous material (soot) in the airways, copious or no secretions, and/or progressive sloughing of the mucosa. Finally, FOB may be falsely negative if performed immediately after injury in patients with burn shock (due to decreased blood flow, thus decreased erythema, during shock). A repeat FOB 24–48 h later may be more revealing.

#### 34.3.1.2 Imaging

Aside from FOB, radiographic and nuclear medicine techniques have been used to diagnose II. Most patients with II have a normal chest radiograph upon initial presentation. The percentage of abnormal initial radiographs in patients with II ranges from 8% to 73% in various retrospective series. Thus, a normal chest radiograph cannot be used to rule out II. Bronchial thickening, perivascular fuzziness or cuffing, alveolar or interstitial pulmonary edema, consolidation, and atelectasis have been reported.

Other imaging technologies used to diagnose II include xenon$^{133}$ ventilation scans, computed tomography (CT) scans (including virtual bronchoscopy) [17–19], and bronchoscopic optical coherence tomography (OCT) scans [15,20]. CT and OCT are mainly used for research, but are evolving into clinically useful tools.

*Recommendation*: A presumptive diagnosis of II and a decision to transfer to a burn center can be made on clinical grounds, but definitive diagnosis requires FOB and/or advanced imaging techniques (Grade B recommendation).

## 34.4 Mechanical Ventilation

### 34.4.1 What Mode of Mechanical Ventilation is Most Effective for Patients with II?

Despite the ARMA trial conducted by the ARDSNet, which showed that lower tidal volumes are associated with improved survival, the best ventilation mode for burn and II patients is still debated; ARMA excluded patients with burns in excess of 30% TBSA [21]. There is reason to believe that the ARMA results may not be fully applicable to patients with II. The principal cause of hypoxemia in ARDS induced by pulmonary contusion, systemic injury, or sepsis is alveolar flooding and

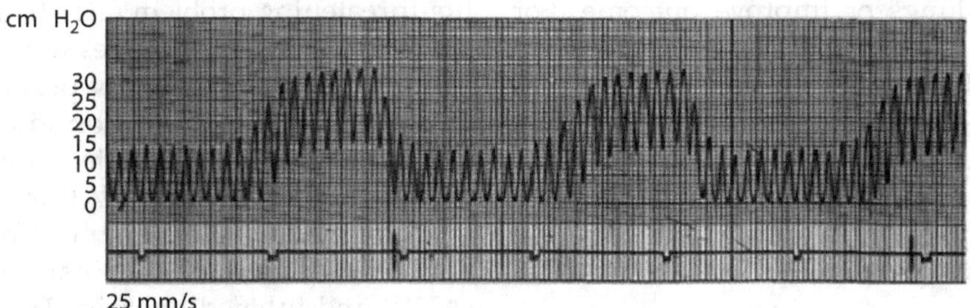


**FIGURE 34.1**
High-frequency percussive ventilation: pressure-time waveform for the VDR-4® ventilator. High-frequency subtidal breaths are combined with low-frequency tidal breaths. The "percussive" action of the high-frequency breaths improves gas exchange, recruits collapsed alveoli, and affects pulmonary toilet. (Reproduced with permission from Percussionaire, Inc., Sandpoint, ID.)

an increase in true shunt. In II, chemical damage to the small airways predominates, causing an increase in blood flow to poorly ventilated lung segments, and ventilation-perfusion (V/Q) mismatch [22]. As small airway obstruction progresses, atelectasis followed by consolidation and pneumonia ensue. Thus, ventilation of II patients, in contrast to other forms of ARDS, should focus not only on avoiding ventilator-induced lung injury but also on actively providing pulmonary toilet and recruiting and stabilizing collapsed alveoli.

This is the rationale for the use of high-frequency percussive ventilation by means of the volumetric diffusive respiration (VDR-4®) ventilator (Percussionaire, Sandpoint, ID). This device is different from high-frequency jet or oscillation ventilators. It combines both subtidal, high-frequency (e.g., 400–1000 breaths per min) and tidal, low-frequency (e.g., 0–20 breaths per min) ventilations (Figure 34.1). With the VDR-4, gas exchange at lower peak and mean airway pressures occurs as a result of a variety of mechanisms, to include more turbulent flow and enhanced molecular diffusion [23,24]. Unique to the VDR-4, the high-frequency, flow-interrupted breaths effect dislodgement of debris and cause its retrograde expulsion out of the airways. For this reason, we partially deflate the endotracheal tube cuff (to a minimal leak level) and frequently suction the oropharynx, as plugs and secretions in II patients can be copious. Finally, VDR-4, like airway-pressure release ventilation (APRV, also known as bi-level ventilation) enables spontaneous ventilation throughout the inspiratory and expiratory phases. In most cases, this improves patient–ventilator synchrony, and as in APRV may have other beneficial effects on gas distribution and respiratory muscle strength. The main disadvantage of the VDR-4 is the extra training required of nurses and respiratory therapists in its operation.

Cioffi described 54 II patients treated with VDR-4 during 1987–1990 and compared observed mortality and pneumonia rates to those predicted by data from the recent past, in which conventional ventilation was employed (12–15 mL/kg tidal volumes). The VDR-4 was associated with a reduction in mortality from 43% (predicted) to 19% (observed), and with a reduction in pneumonia from 46% (predicted) to 26% (observed) [25]. Others showed an improvement in gas exchange at lower airway pressures [26–28]. In a recent RCT performed at the U.S. Army Burn Center, Chung et al. randomized burn patients (with or without II) requiring mechanical ventilation to VDR-4 versus low-tidal-volume ventilation. They found that the VDR-4 group achieved ventilation and oxygenation goals more frequently and required a lower rate of rescue to other forms of mechanical ventilation [29].

Other advanced ventilation techniques have not fared as well as the VDR-4. For example, in an animal model, APRV ventilation was no better than low-tidal-volume ventilation with respect to survival [30].

*Recommendation*: In comparison to conventional mechanical ventilation, high-frequency percussive ventilation improves ventilation and oxygenation in patients with II and may reduce pneumonia and mortality (Grade B recommendation).

## 34.5 Fluid and Pharmacologic Therapy

### 34.5.1 What Drugs and Fluid Management Strategies, If Any, Improve Outcomes in Patients with II?

Patients with isolated II rarely have prodigious fluid resuscitation requirements. But addition of II to cutaneous burns greatly increases fluid resuscitation requirements during the first 48 hours postburn [31]. In one study, patients resuscitated with the modified Brooke formula (which predicts 2 mL/kg/TBSA burned as the lactated Ringer's dose for the first 24 h) actually received over 5 mL/kg/TBSA burned [32]. Efforts to anticipate this response by starting patients out on higher infusion rates are likely to result in increased complications of volume overload [33]. On the other hand, fluid restriction does not protect the lungs or improve outcome. For example, Herndon et al. demonstrated an increase in lung lymph flow (indicating increased microvascular permeability) in fluid-restricted sheep with combined II and burns [34]. Thus, resuscitation of patients with combined II and burns should be conducted with close attention to providing neither too much nor too little fluid by hourly attention to endpoints such as the urine output.

#### 34.5.1.1 Inhaled Heparin

II causes a hypercoagulable state in the lungs [35,36], one manifestation of which is the formation of obstructing clots and casts (Figure 34.2). Inhaled heparin is one way in which we routinely address this. Desai reported a reduction in reintubation rates and in mortality (from 19% to 4%) in those burned children treated with inhaled heparin and *N*-acetylcystine, in comparison with recent historical controls [37]. On the other hand, Holt et al. reviewed their experience with inhaled heparin and *N*-acetylcystine in adults with II. There were no differences in ventilator days or in mortality between those who received it and those who did not [38]. The divergent results of the two studies may be due to the fact that children, with smaller airways and endotracheal tubes, are more vulnerable to airway obstruction [4]. Because obstructing clots and casts are a common life-threatening problem after II, and because this therapy is inexpensive and does not cause systemic anticoagulation [39], we routinely provide nebulized heparin to all II patients, beginning on admission and continuing as long as they are intubated, and the airways remain friable. Traber's group took this concept a step further in the ovine model of combined burn and II, providing both intravenous recombinant human antithrombin (ATIII) and inhaled heparin. This resulted not only in improved lung function and reduced airway obstruction but also in decreased edema and inflammation. These data suggest that ATIII, in addition to enhancing airway patency in combination with heparin, also exerts anti-inflammatory effects, to include inhibition of neutrophil activation [40].

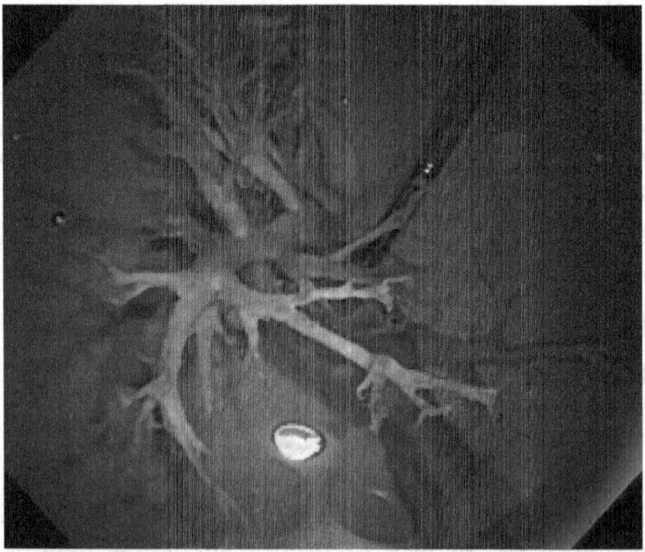

**FIGURE 34.2**
Obstructing airway cast following severe inhalation injury in sheep: an extreme example of a common problem. This tree-like cast of the airways was removed with bronchoscopic forceps (and placed in a bowl of saline for the photograph). Airway obstruction may present at any time in patients with inhalation injury, requiring immediate intervention to remove the casts. Inhaled heparin, high-frequency percussive ventilation, and scheduled pulmonary toilet help prevent it.

#### 34.5.1.2 Other Therapies

Inhaled nitric oxide (NO), by improving blood flow to well-ventilated lung segments, modestly improves oxygenation following II [41]. Although RCTs of inhaled NO in this patient population are not available, we deliver it, if necessary, via the VDR-4 ventilator, to patients with severe oxygenation failure [42]. We also use prone positioning in selected patients who respond to that maneuver with improved oxygenation [43].

II causes a variety of immunologic changes which, in combination with the physical damage to the airways and the need for prolonged intubation, place patients at high risk of pneumonia [44]. Pneumonia is the most common cause of death in patients with burns and II [1,45]. Previously, intravenous corticosteroids were often used to treat patients with II. However, corticosteroids are to be avoided because of their immunosuppressive effects, except in those patients who are adrenally insufficient or who (rarely) have refractory bronchospasm.

Bronchodilators such as albuterol, with or without *N*-acetylcystine, are routinely given to intubated II patients, in order to improve ventilation. But there likely is an advantage to using a less selective adrenergic agonist: nebulized epinephrine improved oxygenation in the ovine II model, along with a reduction in excessive levels of blood flow to the trachea and bronchi (a cause of V/Q mismatch) [46].

Prophylactic antibiotics have not been shown to prevent infection in II or burn patients. Especially, when hospitalized for weeks to months, these patients are at risk of colonization and infection with multiple-drug-resistant organisms; this risk increases with indiscriminant antibiotic exposure. On the other hand, they are also at high risk for pneumonia, which greatly increases postburn mortality [1,47]. Compounding the problem is the fact that burn injury alone causes a hyperdynamic systemic inflammatory response syndrome, characterized by many of the same signs and symptoms of sepsis.

Thus, elevated temperature or white blood cell count do not correlate well with systemic infection [48]. Therefore, other clinical indicators (e.g., insulin resistance, tachycardia, tube-feeding intolerance) are frequently considered [49]. Early institution of broad-spectrum antibiotics, an aggressive diagnostic approach to include bronchoalveolar lavage, and rapid tailoring of the regimen to match organism sensitivities are crucial.

Oxidative and nitrosative stress are major mechanisms implicated in II pathophysiology [50]. Several experimental therapies have been used to address these mechanisms. For example, nebulized γ-tocopherol (one of the vitamin E compounds) improved lung function in the ovine model [51]. A clinical study of high-dose ascorbic acid (vitamin C, 66 mg/kg/h IV) during burn shock resuscitation included many patients with both burns and inhalation injury and demonstrated an improvement in lung function in the treatment arm [52].

*Recommendation*: Fluid resuscitation of patients with II should be carefully titrated to physiologic endpoints such as adequacy of urine output (range 30–50 mL/h in adults), avoiding both fluid excess and fluid restriction (Grade C recommendation). Inhaled heparin may prevent obstructing clots and casts in patients with II at low risk and cost (Grade C recommendation).

## 34.6 Metabolic Asphyxiants

### 34.6.1 What Immediate Treatments Are Safe and Effective for Metabolic Asphyxiation by Systemic Toxins (CO or Cyanide)?

Along with smoke, patients may inhale compounds which impair oxygen delivery to or utilization by the tissues. Chief among these is CO. CO is produced by the partial combustion of carbon-containing compounds such as cellulosics (e.g., wood, paper, coal, charcoal), natural gases (methane, butane, propane), and petroleum products. CO poisoning is a common cause of death at fire scenes [53,54], and is a leading cause of nonfire-related fire deaths in the United States [55]. In addition to combining with hemoglobin to form COHb with an affinity 200 times that of oxygen, CO also impairs mitochondrial function and causes brain injury by pathways involving oxidative stress, inflammation, and excitatory amino acids [56]. The organs most vulnerable to CO poisoning are those most affected by oxygen deprivation, namely, the cardiovascular system and the brain. The diagnosis requires measurement of arterial COHb levels using a CO-oximeter; the $PaO_2$ in these patients is frequently normal or high. A standard two-wavelength pulse oximeter will falsely provide a high $SpO_2$ reading even with COHb levels in the lethal range (≥50%) because it cannot discriminate between COHb and oxygenated hemoglobin [57]. The half-life of COHb is a function not of the $FiO_2$ but of the $PaO_2$, which in II patients may be quite variable even at an $FiO_2$ of 100%. In one retrospective study of 240 patients, the COHb half-life of patients treated with 100% oxygen was 74 min ± 25 SD (range = 26–148 min) [58].

The mainstay of treatment is 100% oxygen by non-rebreather mask or endotracheal tube until the COHb level is less than 5% [59] or for 6 h [60]. Hyperbaric oxygen therapy (HBOT) has been used to treat these patients. Although HBOT accelerates the clearance of CO beyond that achieved by 100% oxygen at one atmosphere, the main rationale is prevention of a delayed neurocognitive syndrome. This features memory loss and other cognitive defects with onset 2–28 days after exposure and is thought to be caused by binding of CO to brain mitochondrial cytochromes and by other mechanisms [60,61]. In an important RCT, Weaver et al. provided HBOT to symptomatic patients with COHb exposure, consisting of three treatments over 24 h, beginning less than 24 h after exposure. There was a decrease in the neurocognitive syndrome from 46% to 25% at 6 weeks. Of note, COHb levels were normal by the time of HBOT in these patients [62]. Loss of consciousness and higher COHb levels (≥25%) were factors associated with successful HBOT, i.e., prevention of the syndrome [63]. The Cochrane group reviewed six RCTs of HBOT for prevention of neurological sequelae. Four studies showed no benefit, two studies did show benefit, and the pooled analysis showed no benefit. Because of design flaws, etc., they concluded that the efficacy of HBOT in this setting is uncertain [64]. The American College of Emergency Physicians published a clinical policy in 2008 stating that Level C data support HBOT as an option in CO poisoning, and that its use is not mandated [65].

#### *34.6.1.1 Cyanide*

Hydrogen cyanide (CN) is produced by the combustion of nitrogen-containing materials such as plastics, foam, paints, wool, and silk. It impairs cellular utilization of oxygen by binding to the terminal cytochrome (cytochrome a, $a_3$) of the electron transport chain, causing lactic acidosis and, potentially, elevated mixed venous oxygen saturation. The half-life in the human body is about 1 h.

The role of CN in fire deaths and the prevalence of CN poisoning in patients with II is less clear than that of CO. In their review of 364 fire deaths in New Jersey, Barillo et al. found that only eight casualties (2%) had high CN and low COHb levels [53]. On the other hand, Baud et al. obtained CN and COHb levels at the scene of residential fires in Paris. The mean CN level in 66 II patients who lived was 21.6 μmol/L (0.6 mg/L) and in 43 who died it was 116 μmol/L (3 mg/L). CN was linearly correlated with COHb and with plasma lactate. Plasma lactate levels above 10 mmol/L were a sensitive indicator of a toxic CN level >40 μmol/L (1 mg/L) [66]. Other studies have found a poor correlation between CO and CN levels [67]. Thus, CN may be a significant factor in a variable percentage of II patients.

Diagnosis of CN poisoning is difficult because a rapid assay is not available; CN and CO poisoning share many features to include signs and symptoms related to the central nervous and cardiovascular systems [68]. Three types of antidote are available for CN. The Cyanide Antidote Kit in the United States contains amyl nitrite for inhalation, and sodium nitrite and sodium thiosulfate for IV injection. The nitrites oxidize hemoglobin to methemoglobin (MetHb), which chelates CN. Sodium thiosulfate combines with CN to form thiocyanate, which is excreted in the urine. We do not recommend the use of nitrites in patients with II and suspected CN poisoning. They can cause severe hypotension, and the MetHb does not transport oxygen [69]. This is problematic, particularly in patients with burn shock and impaired oxygen transport and utilization from CO and CN. Certainly, nitrites should not be used in II victims without knowledge of the COHb and MetHb levels [70]. Sodium thiosulfate has slower onset [71] and lacks efficacy compared to hydroxocobalamin [72].

Hydroxocobalamin (a form of vitamin $B_{12}$) is now available in the United States as the Cyanokit for IV injection. This drug is well-tolerated and rapidly chelates CN. A prospective uncontrolled observational trial in Paris documented a 67% survival rate in 69 II patients with decreased mental status and CN ≥39 μmol/L who received hydroxocobalamin at the fire scene [73]. It would be reasonable to administer hydroxocobalamin IV to II patients with signs and symptoms suggestive of CN poisoning, such as persistent lactic acidosis (despite fluid resuscitation) and unexplained decreased level of consciousness (Glasgow Coma Scale [GCS] score ≤13) [68]. The dose is 5 g (70 mg/kg), which can be repeated once after 2 h in the absence of an improvement [67].

#### *34.6.1.2 Methemoglobinemia*

Methemoglobinemia is another life-threatening syndrome of metabolic asphyxiation which is rarely seen in II patients. Certain smoke constituents such as NO and nitrogen dioxide oxidize hemoglobin to MetHb, a species which is incapable of carrying oxygen. This problem may also be caused by several drugs, to include nitrites (see earlier) or topical anesthetics such as benzocaine. As with COHb, a two-wavelength pulse oximeter cannot distinguish MetHb, and falsely gives $SpO_2$ readings in the 80s. Patients with high levels of MetHb may have chocolate-brown-colored blood and, if light-skinned, central cyanosis. Diagnosis is by CO-oximetry, and treatment consists of IV methylene blue, preferably in consultation with a poison control center or similar [74].

It is likely that COHb, CN, and/or MetHb act additively such that toxicity occurs at lower individual levels when more than one toxin is present. However, there are limited data on such combined effects [75].

*Recommendation*: CO-oximetry (measurement of COHb and MetHb levels) should be performed in patients with II (Grade D recommendation). One hundred percent oxygen should be given to all patients with known or suspected COHb poisoning until the COHb is normal (less than 5%) (Grade D recommendation). HBOT is an option for patients with COHb poisoning for prevention of the delayed neurocognitive syndrome (Grade C recommendation). Hydroxocobalamin treatment should be given to patients with known or suspected cyanide poisoning (Grade C recommendation).

## 34.7 Burn Center Referral

### 34.7.1 Should Patients with II Be Transferred to a Burn Center?

II is one of the American Burn Association criteria for burn center referral [76]. Although we are not aware of prospective data comparing the outcomes of II patients treated in burn centers versus those treated elsewhere, many of the modalities mentioned in this paper are not routinely available outside of burn centers—to include, most importantly, the expertise of respiratory therapists and other health-care professionals with the experience to provide optimal care to patients with this highly lethal injury. Certainly, smoke-exposed patients with an unremarkable physical examination, alert mental status, and normal blood gases and COHb levels may safely be discharged home [77]. For all those II patients requiring admission, we recommend at a minimum prompt consultation with the regional burn center.

*Recommendation*: Consultation with the regional burn center should be performed upon admission of a patient with II (Grade D recommendation).

## 34.8 Conclusion

The advances described in this review, along with general improvements in the care of burn patients, have resulted in a significant reduction in mortality following

II over the past 70 years [78]. Still, II remains a significant independent predictor of postburn death [79]. A recent American Burn Association State of the Science symposium identified four priorities for II research: diagnosis and grading of severity of injury, therapeutics (mechanical ventilation, extracorporeal life support, drugs, role of tracheostomy), long-term outcomes, and basic science mechanisms [80]. Randomized controlled multicenter trials, in particular, are needed in order to address these unsolved issues.

## Acknowledgment

The author gratefully acknowledges the assistance of Annette Collins in conducting this review. Conflict of interest statement: The author received reimbursement from Percussionaire, Inc., for travel expenses to speak at the Bird Institute in 2013.

## References

1. Shirani KZ, Pruitt BA, Jr., Mason AD, Jr. The influence of inhalation injury and pneumonia on burn mortality. *Ann Surg.* 1987;205:82–87.
2. Tredget EE, Shankowsky HA, Taerum TV, Moysa GL, Alton JD. The role of inhalation injury in burn trauma. A Canadian experience. *Ann Surg.* 1990;212:720–727.
3. Belenkiy SM, Buel AR, Cannon JW et al. Acute respiratory distress syndrome in wartime military burns: Application of the Berlin criteria. *J Trauma Acute Care Surg.* 2014;76:821–827.
4. Zak AL, Harrington DT, Barillo DJ, Lawlor DF, Shirani KZ, Goodwin CW. Acute respiratory failure that complicates the resuscitation of pediatric patients with scald injuries. *J Burn Care Rehabil.* 1999;20:391–399.
5. Cha SI, Kim CH, Lee JH et al. Isolated smoke inhalation injuries: Acute respiratory dysfunction, clinical outcomes, and short-term evolution of pulmonary functions with the effects of steroids. *Burns.* 2007;33:200–208.
6. Madnani DD, Steele NP, de Vries E. Factors that predict the need for intubation in patients with smoke inhalation injury. *Ear Nose Throat J.* 2006;85:278–280.
7. Goh SH, Tiah L, Lim HC, Ng EK. Disaster preparedness: Experience from a smoke inhalation mass casualty incident. *Eur J Emerg Med.* 2006;13:330–334.
8. Jones WG, Madden M, Finkelstein J, Yurt RW, Goodwin CW. Tracheostomies in burn patients. *Ann Surg.* 1989;209:471–474.
9. Palmieri TL, Jackson W, Greenhalgh DG. Benefits of early tracheostomy in severely burned children. *Crit Care Med.* 2002;30:922–924.
10. Kadilak PR, Vanasse S, Sheridan RL. Favorable short- and long-term outcomes of prolonged translaryngeal intubation in critically ill children. *J Burn Care Rehabil.* 2004;25:262–265.
11. Saffle JR, Morris SE, Edelman L. Early tracheostomy does not improve outcome in burn patients. *J Burn Care Rehabil.* 2002;23:431–438.
12. Gravvanis AI, Tsoutsos DA, Iconomou TG, Papadopoulos SG. Percutaneous versus conventional tracheostomy in burned patients with inhalation injury. World *J Surg.* 2005;29:1571–1575.
13. Clark WR, Bonaventura M, Myers W. Smoke inhalation and airway management at a regional burn unit: 1974–1983. Part I: Diagnosis and consequences of smoke inhalation. *J Burn Care Rehabil.* 1989;10:52–62.
14. Endorf FW, Gamelli RL. Inhalation injury, pulmonary perturbations, and fluid resuscitation. *J Burn Care Res.* 2007;28:80–83.
15. Chou L, Batchinsky A, Belenkiy S et al. In vivo detection of inhalation injury in large airway using three-dimensional long-range swept-source optical coherence tomography. *J Biomed Opt.* 2014;19:36018.
16. Albright JM, Davis CS, Bird MD et al. The acute pulmonary inflammatory response to the graded severity of smoke inhalation injury. *Crit Care Med.* 2012;40:1113–1121.
17. Park MS, Cancio LC, Batchinsky AI et al. Assessment of severity of ovine smoke inhalation injury by analysis of computed tomographic scans. *J Trauma.* 2003;55:417–427.
18. Oh JS, Chung KK, Allen A et al. Admission chest CT complements fiberoptic bronchoscopy in prediction of adverse outcomes in thermally injured patients. *J Burn Care Res.* 2012;33:532–538.
19. Kwon HP, Zanders TB, Regn DD et al. Comparison of virtual bronchoscopy to fiber-optic bronchoscopy for assessment of inhalation injury severity. *Burns.* 2014;40:1308–1315.
20. Brenner M, Kreuter K, Ju J et al. In vivo optical coherence tomography detection of differences in regional large airway smoke inhalation induced injury in a rabbit model. *J Biomed Opt.* 2008;13:034001.
21. Anonymous. Ventilation with lower tidal volumes as compared with traditional tidal volumes for acute lung injury and the acute respiratory distress syndrome. The Acute Respiratory Distress Syndrome Network. *N Engl J Med.* 2000;342:1301–1308.
22. Shimazu T, Yukioka T, Ikeuchi H, Mason AD, Jr., Wagner PD, Pruitt BA, Jr. Ventilation-perfusion alterations after smoke inhalation injury in an ovine model. *J Appl Physiol.* 1996;81:2250–2259.
23. Krishnan JA, Brower RG. High-frequency ventilation for acute lung injury and ARDS. *Chest.* 2000;118:795–807.
24. Salim A, Martin M. High-frequency percussive ventilation. *Crit Care Med.* 2005;33:S241–S245.
25. Cioffi WG, Jr., Rue LW III, Graves TA, McManus WF, Mason AD, Jr., Pruitt BA, Jr. Prophylactic use of high-frequency percussive ventilation in patients with inhalation injury. *Ann Surg.* 1991;213:575–582.
26. Rodeberg DA, Housinger TA, Greenhalgh DG, Maschinot NE, Warden GD. Improved ventilatory function in burn patients using volumetric diffusive respiration. *J Am Coll Surg.* 1994;179:518–522.

27. Reper P, Wibaux O, Van Laeke P, Vandeenen D, Duinslaeger L, Vanderkelen A. High frequency percussive ventilation and conventional ventilation after smoke inhalation: A randomised study. *Burns.* 2002;28:503–508.
28. Carman B, Cahill T, Warden G, McCall J. A prospective, randomized comparison of the Volume Diffusive Respirator vs conventional ventilation for ventilation of burned children. 2001 ABA paper. *J Burn Care Rehabil.* 2002;23:444–448.
29. Chung KK, Wolf SE, Renz EM et al. High-frequency percussive ventilation and low tidal volume ventilation in burns: A randomized controlled trial. *Crit Care Med.* 2010;38:1970–1977.
30. Batchinsky AI, Burkett SE, Zanders TB et al. Comparison of airway pressure release ventilation to conventional mechanical ventilation in the early management of smoke inhalation injury in swine. *Crit Care Med.* 2011;39:2314–2321.
31. Navar PD, Saffle JR, Warden GD. Effect of inhalation injury on fluid resuscitation requirements after thermal injury. *Am J Surg.* 1985;150:716–720.
32. Lund T, Goodwin CW, McManus WF et al. Upper airway sequelae in burn patients requiring endotracheal intubation or tracheostomy. *Ann Surg.* 1985;201:374–382.
33. Pruitt BA, Jr. Protection from excessive resuscitation: Pushing the pendulum back. *J Trauma.* 2000;49:567–568.
34. Herndon DN, Traber DL, Traber LD. The effect of resuscitation on inhalation injury. *Surgery.* 1986;100:248–251.
35. Midde KK, Batchinsky AI, Cancio LC et al. Wood bark smoke induces lung and pleural plasminogen activator inhibitor 1 and stabilizes its mRNA in porcine lung cells. *Shock.* 2011;36:128–137.
36. Hofstra JJ, Vlaar AP, Knape P et al. Pulmonary activation of coagulation and inhibition of fibrinolysis after burn injuries and inhalation trauma. *J Trauma.* 2011;70:1389–1397.
37. Desai MH, Mlcak R, Richardson J, Nichols R, Herndon DN. Reduction in mortality in pediatric patients with inhalation injury with aerosolized heparin/N-acetylcystine therapy. *J Burn Care Rehabil.* 1998;19:210–212.
38. Holt J, Saffle JR, Morris SE, Cochran A. Use of inhaled heparin/N-acetylcystine in inhalation injury: Does it help? *J Burn Care Res.* 2008;29:192–195.
39. Yip LY, Lim YF, Chan HN. Safety and potential anticoagulant effects of nebulised heparin in burns patients with inhalational injury at Singapore General Hospital Burns Centre. *Burns.* 2011;37:1154–1160.
40. Rehberg S, Yamamoto Y, Sousse LE et al. Antithrombin attenuates vascular leakage via inhibiting neutrophil activation in acute lung injury. *Crit Care Med.* 2013;41:e439–e446.
41. Ogura H, Saitoh D, Johnson AA, Mason AD, Jr., Pruitt BA, Jr., Cioffi WG, Jr. The effect of inhaled nitric oxide on pulmonary ventilation-perfusion matching following smoke inhalation injury. *J Trauma.* 1994;37:893–898.
42. Cancio LC, Galvez E, Jr., Jordan BS, Allies WE. Delivery of nitric oxide by high-frequency percussive ventilation: System design and evaluation. *Clin Intensive Care.* 2006;17:41–48.
43. Hale DF, Cannon JW, Batchinsky AI et al. Prone positioning improves oxygenation in adult burn patients with severe acute respiratory distress syndrome. *J Trauma Acute Care Surg.* 2012;72:1634–1639.
44. Davis CS, Janus SE, Mosier MJ et al. Inhalation injury severity and systemic immune perturbations in burned adults. *Ann Surg.* 2013;257:1137–1146.
45. Cioffi WG, Kim SH, Pruitt BA, Jr. 1993. Cause of mortality in thermally injured patients. In: Lorenz S, Zellner P-R (eds.), *Die Infektion beim Brandverletzten: Proceedings of the "Infektionsprophylaxe und Infektionshekampfung beim Brandverletzten" International Symposium.* Steinkopff Verlag: Darmstadt, Germany, pp. 7–11.
46. Lange M, Hamahata A, Traber DL et al. Preclinical evaluation of epinephrine nebulization to reduce airway hyperemia and improve oxygenation after smoke inhalation injury. *Crit Care Med.* 2011;39:718–724.
47. Edelman DA, Khan N, Kempf K, White MT. Pneumonia after inhalation injury. *J Burn Care Res.* 2007;28:241–246.
48. Murray CK, Hoffmaster RM, Schmit DR et al. Evaluation of white blood cell count, neutrophil percentage, and elevated temperature as predictors of bloodstream infection in burn patients. *Arch Surg.* 2007;142:639–642.
49. Hogan BK, Wolf SE, Hospenthal DR et al. Correlation of American Burn Association sepsis criteria with the presence of bacteremia in burned patients admitted to the intensive care unit. *J Burn Care Res.* 2012;33:371–378.
50. Park MS, Cancio LC, Jordan BS, Brinkley WW, Rivera VR, Dubick MA. Assessment of oxidative stress in lungs from sheep after inhalation of wood smoke. *Toxicology.* 2004;195:97–112.
51. Yamamoto Y, Enkhbaatar P, Sousse LE et al. Nebulization with gamma-tocopherol ameliorates acute lung injury after burn and smoke inhalation in the ovine model. *Shock.* 2012;37:408–414.
52. Wolf SE. Vitamin C and smoke inhalation injury. *J Burn Care Res.* 2009;30:184–186.
53. Barillo DJ, Goode R, Esch V. Cyanide poisoning in victims of fire: Analysis of 364 cases and review of the literature. *J Burn Care Rehabil.* 1994;15:46–57.
54. McGwin G, Jr., Chapman V, Rousculp M, Robison J, Fine P. The epidemiology of fire-related deaths in Alabama, 1992–1997. *J Burn Care Rehabil.* 2000;21:75–3; discussion 4.
55. Centers for Disease Control Prevention. Carbon monoxide-related deaths—United States, 1999–2004. *Morb Mortal Wkly Rep.* 2007;56:1309–1312.
56. Thom SR. Hyperbaric-oxygen therapy for acute carbon monoxide poisoning. *N Engl J Med.* 2002;347:1105–1106.
57. Hampson NB. Pulse oximetry in severe carbon monoxide poisoning. *Chest.* 1998;114:1036–1041.
58. Weaver LK, Howe S, Hopkins R, Chan KJ. Carboxyhemoglobin half-life in carbon monoxide-poisoned patients treated with 100% oxygen at atmospheric pressure. *Chest.* 2000;117:801–808.
59. Ilano AL, Raffin TA. Management of carbon monoxide poisoning. *Chest.* 1990;97:165–169.
60. Piantadosi CA. Carbon monoxide poisoning. *N Engl J Med.* 2002;347:1054–1055.

61. Piantadosi CA, Sylvia AL, Jobsis-Vandervliet FF. Differences in brain cytochrome responses to carbon monoxide and cyanide in vivo. *J Appl Physiol.* 1987;62:1277–1284.
62. Weaver LK, Hopkins RO, Chan KJ et al. Hyperbaric oxygen for acute carbon monoxide poisoning. *N Engl J Med.* 2002;347:1057–1067.
63. Weaver LK, Valentine KJ, Hopkins RO. Carbon monoxide poisoning: Risk factors for cognitive sequelae and the role of hyperbaric oxygen. *Am J Respir Crit Care Med.* 2007;176:491–497.
64. Juurlink DN, Buckley NA, Stanbrook MB, Isbister GK, Bennett M, McGuigan MA. Hyperbaric oxygen for carbon monoxide poisoning. *Cochrane Database Syst Rev.* 2005;Issue 1, Art. No. CD002041.
65. Wolf SJ, Lavonas EJ, Sloan EP, Jagoda AS, American College of Emergency Physicians. Clinical policy: Critical issues in the management of adult patients presenting to the emergency department with acute carbon monoxide poisoning. *Ann Emerg Med.* 2008;51:138–152.
66. Baud FJ, Barriot P, Toffis V et al. Elevated blood cyanide concentrations in victims of smoke inhalation. *N Engl J Med.* 1991;325:1761–1766.
67. Anseeuw K, Delvau N, Burillo-Putze G et al. Cyanide poisoning by fire smoke inhalation: A European expert consensus. *Eur J Emerg Med.* 2013;20:2–9.
68. Baud FJ. Cyanide: Critical issues in diagnosis and treatment. *Hum Exp Toxicol.* 2007;26:191–201.
69. Hall AH, Kulig KW, Rumack BH. Suspected cyanide poisoning in smoke inhalation: Complications of sodium nitrite therapy. *J Toxicol Clin Exp.* 1989;9:3–9.
70. Kirk MA, Gerace R, Kulig KW. Cyanide and methemoglobin kinetics in smoke inhalation victims treated with the cyanide antidote kit. *Ann Emerg Med.* 1993;22:1413–1418.
71. Dart RC. Hydroxocobalamin for acute cyanide poisoning: New data from preclinical and clinical studies; new results from the prehospital emergency setting. *Clin Toxicol.* 2006;44(Suppl 1):1–3.
72. Bebarta VS, Pitotti RL, Dixon P, Lairet JR, Bush A, Tanen DA. Hydroxocobalamin versus sodium thiosulfate for the treatment of acute cyanide toxicity in a swine (Sus scrofa) model. *Ann Emerg Med.* 2012;59:532–539.
73. Borron SW, Baud FJ, Barriot P, Imbert M, Bismuth C. Prospective study of hydroxocobalamin for acute cyanide poisoning in smoke inhalation. *Ann Emerg Med.* 2007;49:794–801, e1–e2.
74. Hoffman RS, Sauter D. Methemoglobinemia resulting from smoke inhalation. *Vet Hum Toxicol.* 1989;31:168–170.
75. Levin BC, Rechani PR, Gurman JL et al. Analysis of carboxyhemoglobin and cyanide in blood from victims of the Dupont Plaza Hotel fire in Puerto Rico. *J Forensic Sci.* 1990;35:151–168.
76. Anonymous. Guidelines for the operation of burn centers. 2006. *Resources for Optimal Care of the Injured Patient.* Committee on Trauma, American College of Surgeons: Chicago, IL, pp. 79–86.
77. Mushtaq F, Graham CA. Discharge from the accident and emergency department after smoke inhalation: Influence of clinical factors and emergency investigations. *Eur J Emerg Med.* 2004;11:141–144.
78. Rue LW, 3d, Cioffi WG, Mason AD, McManus WF, Pruitt BA, Jr. Improved survival of burned patients with inhalation injury. *Arch Surg.* 1993;128:772–780.
79. Cancio LC, Galvez E, Jr., Turner CE, Kypreos NG, Parker A, Holcomb JB. Base deficit and alveolar-arterial gradient during resuscitation contribute independently but modestly to the prediction of mortality after burn injury. *J Burn Care Res.* 2006;27:289–296.
80. Palmieri TL. Inhalation injury: Research progress and needs. *J Burn Care Res.* 2007;28:549–554.
81. Chou SH, Lin SD, Chuang HY, Cheng YJ, Kao EL, Huang MF. Fiber-optic bronchoscopic classification of inhalation injury: Prediction of acute lung injury. *Surg Endosc.* 2004;18:1377–1379.
82. Hall JJ, Hunt JL, Arnoldo BD, Purdue GF. Use of high-frequency percussive ventilation in inhalation injuries. *J Burn Care Res.* 2007;28:396–400.

## Commentary on Inhalation Injury

*Nicholas Namias*

Inhalation injury continues to be a significant contributor to burn mortality. Dr. Cancio has presented an excellent overview of inhalation injury (II) for the acute care surgeon. I have always worked in the world of both the acute care surgeon and the burn surgeon, and I have frequently had to view II from both perspectives, and provide "translational" services for my acute care surgery colleagues.

Dr. Cancio provided a section on indications for endotracheal intubation and for tracheostomy in patients with II. I have no disagreement with anything in this section, but would like to provide the translation for the acute care surgeon. First, the indications for intubation that apply to any other patient also apply to the burn and inhalation injury patient. To explain, in any disease where there is obstruction or impending obstruction of the airway, inability to protect the airway, or impaired gas exchange, intubation is indicated. This is true in burns and II as well. One special situation worth noting is that of the large burn. Large burns (>40%) will require large volume resuscitation, and are at risk of losing the airway from swelling. I agree with Dr. Cancio that it is best to avoid the "hard experience" of losing the airway to swelling a few hours into the resuscitation. Since these patients may have a good mental status at presentation, and the intubation is not a stat emergency, take the opportunity to explore issues surrounding code status and end of life wishes of the patient. Finally, Dr. Cancio mentions securing the tube with umbilical ties instead of adhesive tape. Alternatives to adhesive tape also include commercial tube holders and fastening the tube to an incisor tooth with wire.

Dr. Cancio devotes a large section to tracheostomy. Respiratory benefits of tracheostomy remain controversial; however, there is one incontrovertible fact about the tracheostomy. The use of double cannula tracheostomies allows for easy cleaning or exchange of the inner cannula as needed. The sheer quantity of secretions with the likely addition of soot leads to a tenacious film adherent to the inner surface of the artificial airway. In the University of Miami/Jackson Memorial experience, if the patient is not clearly on a trajectory to extubation by day 7, tracheostomy with a double cannula tracheostomy is performed to facilitate airway hygiene.

The diagnostic section is very complete, and explains the role of fiber-optic bronchoscopy (FOB) and imaging studies for the diagnosis of II. We have not embraced the use of routine FOB for diagnosis. We have performed it sporadically for diagnosis, and have found soot-coated airways that never displayed any degree of respiratory compromise, and alternatively, have found pristine airways that have gone on to severe respiratory failure. Therefore, we rely almost exclusively on history and physical examination for the diagnosis of II. Significant II is very unlikely in the absence of a history of entrapment in an enclosed, smoke-filled space. We agree that chest radiograph is neither sensitive nor specific, and that the nuclear medicine and tomographic examinations are mostly of research interest.

The role of the VDR ventilator is given an expanded focus in the chapter. This mode of ventilation has been championed by the U.S. Army Institute for Surgical Research (ISR) and the generations of trainees counted in its educational progeny, Dr. Cancio included. Many outside this academic genealogy have not so enthusiastically embraced the VDR. While I have no doubt that it is effective in the hands of those well trained in its use, all of the evidence supporting its use as an alternative to other modes is significantly flawed. In fact, in the prospective trial comparing VDR to low tidal volume ventilation referenced in the chapter*, there were no outcome differences except in the frequency of needing to switch to a salvage mode of ventilation. In the absence of universal availability and widespread training in VDR ventilation, I would have to agree with the accompanying editorial that concluded "the mode of ventilation that is best in a given clinical situation is the mode that the user is most familiar with and most comfortable using"†.

Other adjuncts in the treatment of II mentioned in the chapter do not require as much of an investment in money and training as does the VDR, and these can easily be adopted by any hospital. We agree with Dr. Cancio on the use of nebulized heparin, and combine it with inhaled n-acetylcysteine. Prone positioning can be a short-term life-saving intervention, and we have occasionally used it. Inhaled nitric oxide can help oxygenation in the short term, and we have used it as well. None have convincing evidence of survival benefit; however, we have accepted what little evidence there exists, since these interventions are easily implemented and have little potential for harm when used properly. Vitamin C is mentioned briefly as an adjunct, and is unlikely to ever be studied again, since there is limited commercial benefit in marketing a nutrient. However,

* Chung KK, Wolf SE, Renz EM et al. High-frequency percussive ventilation and low tidal volume ventilation in burns: A randomized controlled trial. *Crit Care Med.* 2010;38:1970–1977.

† Kacmarek RM, Villar J. Clinical repercussions of high-frequency percussive ventilation: A burning issue. *Crit Care Med.* 2010;38:2069–2070.

we were convinced early on from a published trial on parenteral ascorbic acid* and have been using it in major burns since the early 2000s.

Hyperbaric oxygen remains controversial, and although Dr. Cancio presents some evidence on improved neuropsychological outcome improvement with hyperbaric oxygen, there are significant barriers to instituting this modality (paucity of specialized centers that can provide this 24 h/day, with ability to monitor and care for critically ill patients while under therapy). As Dr. Cancio also mentions, the Cochrane group deemed the use of hyperbaric oxygen therapy for this indication uncertain†.

Finally, the issue of metabolic asphyxiants is an underrecognized cause of mortality in burn patients, and is covered well in this chapter. Early recognition, primarily by co-oximetry in the laboratory, point-of-care testing with specialized pulsoximeters that can report co-oximetry values, and persistent refractory acidosis should prompt the use of one of the antidotes. Early recognition and involvement of poison control experts may help improve survival.

* Matsuda T, Tanaka H, Williams S, Hanumadass M, Abcarian H, Reyes H. Reduced fluid volume requirement for resuscitation of third-degree burns with high-dose vitamin C. *J Burn Care Rehabil.* 1991;12:525–532.

† Juurlink DN, Buckley NA, Stanbrook MB, Isbister GK, Bennett M, McGuigan MA. Hyperbaric oxygen for carbon monoxide poisoning. *Cochrane Database of Syst Rev.* 2005;1:CD002041.

# 35

## *Electrical, Cold, and Chemical Injuries*

**Stephanie A. Savage**

**CONTENTS**



### 35.1 Introduction

Traumatic injury to tissues is a common occurrence and sequelae may range from the relatively benign to major functional alterations or even death. The most common mechanisms include interpersonal violence and motor vehicular crashes. The less common causes of injury may often be more difficult to treat due to the lack of familiarity with the disease process, potential complications, and long-term derangements. Injuries resulting from electrical, cold, and chemical exposures fall into this latter category. In cases such as these, evidence-based medicine is a sound foundation upon which to base practice decisions (Table 35.1).

### 35.2 Electrical Injuries

Electrical injuries account for 3%–5% of burn unit admissions annually, with a mortality rate approaching 40% (approximately 1000 deaths annually) [1–3]. Age distribution tends to be bimodal with the majority of injuries occurring in young children, from accidental contact with power sources, and in adults [3]. In adult patients, electrocutions occur preferentially as a work-related injury, with electricians, line men, and construction workers displaying the most frequent occurrence. Due to gender distribution in these trades, occurrence favors males in their fourth and fifth decade of life [4,5].

Lightning strikes are an uncommon source of electrical injury as well, with approximately 400 lightning injuries occurring annually in the United States. Though the current in a lightning bolt is between 30,000 and 110,000 A, time of contact ranges only from 10 to 100 ms, which limits transference of energy [6]. Therefore, overall mortality is only 10%–30% [7]. Simultaneous cardiac and respiratory arrest are most likely to lead to mortality and are managed with standard Adult Cardiac Life Support measures. Long-term cardiac sequelae following lightning strike are uncommon. Long-term neurologic sequelae may occur secondary to hypoxic injury or intracranial hemorrhage due to primary strike or secondary falls. Keraunoparalysis is a transient neurologic effect specific to lightning strikes. This transient paralysis more commonly affects lower limbs over upper and is attributed to parasympathetic overstimulation with secondary vascular spasm [6].

Burns related to lightning strikes tend to be linear, from evaporation of sweat from the skin ("flashover") or punctate from current egress. Lichtenburg's figures are fern-like patterns seen under the skin, which are pathognomonic for lightning strike but do not represent a true burn. They typically resolve within 24 hours [6,7].

Finally, cataracts and tympanic membrane rupture are also common following these injuries. Care for victims of lightning strikes is supportive.

Electrical injuries may be especially challenging for the trauma or burn surgeon to treat, as external evidence of injury (entrance and exit wounds) frequently grossly under-represent the true extent of tissue damage. The severity of injury is determined by the magnitude of energy delivered, the resistance to current flow, duration of contact with the electric source, and the pathway through which the current travels [8,9]. Mechanisms of tissue injury are varied and contribute to the difficulty of caring for these patients. The direct effect of the electric current on the tissue, especially cardiac, may result in asystole, ventricular fibrillation, or apnea in cases of respiratory muscle spasm. Electrical current may be converted to thermal energy, resulting in burns. Arcing, the transition of current across a charged space, may throw a patient, resulting in blunt injuries from falls. Tetanic contractions of muscles may also lead to fractures and the blunt disruption of soft tissues [1,10].

At a cellular level, three major mechanisms can result in cellular death. Joule heating literally results in "frying" of tissues and disrupts the lipid bilayer. Electroporation, a process used in laboratories to introduce DNA into cells, causes the formation of temporary pores in the lipid bilayer. The influx of charged particles, especially calcium, can alter membrane gradients and lead to cellular apoptosis. Electroconformational denaturation results in a change in orientation of proteins that result in denaturation [3]. All of these processes occur with electrical injury, contributing to tissue injury and death at the macroscopic and microscopic level.

### 35.2.1 Which Patients Suffering Electrical Injury Require More Comprehensive Monitoring, Including Urine Myoglobin Levels?

With potential injury to such varied systems as cardiac, respiratory, nervous, renal, ocular, and skeletal systems, many management conundrums arise. The pool of evidence-based data in the case of electrical injuries is primarily Levels II and III data. Owing to the uneven distribution of cardiac injury from current, with necrotic cells next to viable ones, cardiac manifestations of electrical injury may include arrhythmias and conduction abnormalities [1,11,12]. Low-voltage injuries have a lesser rate of serious injury. If patients exposed to a low-voltage electric source have no evidence of injury, discharge from the emergency room is a reasonable option [13]. Purdue and Hunt proposed a series of criteria to determine whether patients require admission following electrical injury. These criteria include loss of consciousness at the scene or cardiac arrest in the field, a documented cardiac arrhythmia in the field, an abnormal electrocardiogram (ECG) (with broad criteria extending as far as bradycardia or tachycardia), or a separate indication for admission [13]. Blackwell and Hayllar looked at 212 consecutive patients presenting to an Australian hospital with low-voltage electrical injury. They detected no late rhythm abnormalities in patients who originally had normal ECGs. Much like other studies, this group recommended continuous cardiac monitoring of patients with a history of loss of consciousness, documented arrhythmia, or abnormal ECG at presentation [14].

Creatine kinase (CK) levels are frequently elevated in electrical injury due to diffuse muscle damage. The average CK level following an electrical burn is 18,900 IU. Associated with this is the release of myoglobin from damaged muscle. Myoglobin may lead to renal constriction with associated ischemia and cast formation in the distal convoluted tubule. Grossly pigmented urine is highly suspicious for significant muscle damage, and urine myoglobin levels should be evaluated [15]. Some authors have even advocated using myoglobin levels as a marker for severity of injury, as there is an association between myoglobinuria and morbidity [16]. The presence of myoglobin in the urine following electrical injury should prompt continued close monitoring. Urine output should be maintained at a higher level, often greater than 100 cc/h, until myoglobinuria clears. There is no Level 1 evidence to support the use of urine alkalization in this process or of osmotic diuresis with mannitol [15]. Persistent myoglobinuria or elevations in CK levels should prompt evaluation for necrotic tissue requiring debridement.

*Recommendation*: Low-voltage injuries without signs of injury do not require further monitoring. Patients with sequelae of electrical injury, including recent history of cardiac arrest, arrhythmias, and myoglobinuria, should be monitored closely (Grade C recommendation).

Based on the current evidence, the majority comprising Level III data, recommendations for the management of electrical injuries include the following points. Low-voltage (<1000 V) electrocutions with no history of arrhythmia and a normal ECG at presentation may be discharged without further evaluation. High-voltage injuries and/or those with abnormal ECG, a history of arrhythmia, or other indications for admission should be monitored with telemetry. Patients with myoglobinuria should be monitored closely as well, with maintenance of elevated urine output. Persistent myoglobin abnormalities are suspicious for necrotic tissue.

### 35.2.2 Is There Any Role for Advanced Imaging to Evaluate Muscle Damage?

Electrical injuries may be misleading, as the external evidence of injury may be a poor reflection of actual tissue damage. Identification of necrotic tissue is important to allow proper debridement. Although monitoring of serum CK levels and urine myoglobin may provide important information, they are not very specific. Conversely, the aggressive use of early fasciotomy has been associated with increased rates of amputation, as high as 35%–40% [13]. Therefore, some research have focused on the use of magnetic resonance imaging (MRI) or nuclear scanning to pinpoint damaged muscle.

Overall, MRI has demonstrated poor sensitivity in detecting damaged tissue in nonperfused regions, as there is a lack of local edema [17]. Xenon[133] and Technetium-99 pyrophosphate radionuclide imaging are accurate predictors of tissue damage [17–20]. However, use of these imaging modalities neither shortened duration of hospital stay nor contributed to clinical decision-making in multiple studies [15,19]. Therefore, there is little practical application for these diagnostic adjuncts in managing patients with electrical injury.

*Recommendation*: There is little role for MRI or nuclear imaging in the management of electrical injury (Grade C recommendation).

Patients with significant electrical injury should be admitted to a monitored setting with telemetry and serial evaluation of laboratory values, including urine myoglobin. There is little practical utility in the use of MRI or radionuclide imaging in identifying damaged muscle or influencing clinical care.

## 35.3 Cold Injuries

Frostbite remains a significant problem. While often associated with eras in which adequate heating and protection from the elements was not the norm, in modern times at-risk groups include the homeless, outdoor enthusiasts, and patients with altered mental status. Vretenar et al. identified risk factors for cold injury to include alcohol use, a history of psychiatric illness, vehicular trauma or failure, and drug abuse [21,22]. Additionally, patient factors that may exacerbate injury include atherosclerotic disease, smoking, diabetes mellitus, and a history of prior cold-related tissue injury [23]. Cold-related injuries are more common in males, with incidence approaching 10:1 and with a mean age of 30–49 years. Injuries preferentially affect regions distant from the core, isolated by heat conservation reflexes. Areas of frequent injury include the digits and hands, feet, and the nose and ears [23].

Frostbite represents the most severe degree of tissue injury that may lead to necrosis and the potential for tissue loss. As freezing of the tissues occurs, ice crystals form in extracellular fluids. These crystals damage cell membranes, resulting in altered concentration gradients with abnormal cellular electrolyte concentrations. Further temperature decreases result in intracellular ice crystal formation and cell death. Direct tissue freezing is not the only source of cell death, however. Endothelial injury and local tissue edema from the release of inflammatory mediators lead to occlusion of small vessels and sludging within vessels. Interruption of oxygen delivery also clearly results in tissue ischemia [23].

The degree of tissue loss is often hard to delineate at the time of the injury. Traditionally, frostbite has been described on a scale of first through fourth degree, similar to descriptive methods used to describe burn injuries. However, it is not possible to classify the degree of injury before rewarming occurs and complete delineation of necrotic tissue is not apparent until days to weeks later. A less specific but more accurate grading system is simply classifying frostbite wounds as superficial (encompassing first and second degree) or deep (third and fourth degree). Murphy et al. note this system to be more accurate at predicting clinical outcome than the degree system [23].

Hypothermia is the most life-threatening of the cold injury disorders, despite the lack of obvious external injury as seen in frostbite. As patients progress from mild hypothermia (32°C–35°C) to severe hypothermia (<28°C), systemic sequelae increase. Hypothermia causes decreased cardiac contractility. Combined with relative volume depletion due to fluid sequestration and cellular crystallization, patients with hypothermia experience decreased cardiac output and shock, which easily transitions to cardiac arrest. Additionally, hypothermia contributes to cardiac irritability often resulting in intractable arrhythmias during attempts to resuscitate patients. Hypothermia leads to vasoconstriction and endothelial injury with sludging and vessel thrombosis. Cold diuresis results from inhibition of antidiuretic hormone and cold-induced glycosuria, further contributing to volume depletion [24].

Clearly, hypothermia is a component of the "deadly triad," which includes acidosis and coagulopathy and frequently results in mortality in trauma patients. Reports of the impact of hypothermia on trauma patients from Operation Iraqi Freedom also emerged from military hospitals. In the report by Arthurs et al., they noted that no patient presenting to the 31st Combat Support Hospital with a temperature <32°C survived [25].

### 35.3.1 What Is the Most Appropriate Method of Rewarming the Severely Hypothermic Patient?

Rewarming the hypothermic patient may be life saving. However, there are conflicting descriptions of the most appropriate methods to restore normothermia. The majority of evidence regarding rewarming following cold injury is Level III or IV. The most important aspect of rewarming, as noted in multiple citations, however, is that rewarming should not occur until there is no further potential of refreezing [26]. Refreezing may convert damaged but viable tissue to frankly ischemic tissue [23,24,27–30]. Rapid and repeated freeze-thaw cycles promote the inflammatory response, resulting in increased production of arachidonic acid and thromboxane [31]. Limiting freeze-thaw cycles will limit production of these inflammatory mediators.

Severe hypothermia, with temperatures less than 28°C, mandates rapid rewarming as the primary modality of therapy. As inappropriate rewarming can lead to reperfusion injury, it is important to minimize this risk while avoiding the pitfalls that accompany a hypothermic state—namely, cardiac irritability, respiratory depression, acidosis, and coagulopathy. Class 2b data using a swine model investigated the optimal rate of rewarming to improve outcome. In this uncontrolled hemorrhage model, optimal rewarming (defined as survival without significant neurological deficit) was achieved at 0.5°C/min [27].

Multiple consensus statements confirm that extracorporeal rewarming with cardiopulmonary bypass is the gold standard for rewarming, especially in instances of hypothermic cardiac arrest [32]. Cardiopulmonary bypass has demonstrated less instances of ventricular fibrillation, better overall survival, and higher Glasgow Outcome Scores in affected patients. A further benefit of active rewarming is decreased time required for cardiopulmonary resuscitation, in which the patient risks the sequelae of possibly inadequate resuscitation (i.e., chest compressions) or thoracic trauma [33]. Active rewarming should continue until the patient's core temperature reaches 33°C–35°C. Some evidence has demonstrated that rapidly warming patients above this threshold may contribute to cerebral edema [32].

*Recommendation*: Rewarming should wait until there is no further risk of freezing. Active rewarming is favored in patients suffering severe hypothermia (Grade C recommendation).

Rewarming should not occur until there is no further risk of refreezing. For hypothermic patients, active rewarming to achieve a rate of 0.5°C/min is ideal. Cardiopulmonary bypass should be reserved for the profoundly hypothermic or in patients with cardiac irritability/instability. When used promptly, however, patients may achieve good neurologic outcomes.

### 35.3.2 What Is the Role of Amputation in the Management of Significant Frostbite?

Blood-thinning agents and thrombolytics are the areas of most vigorous research in cold injury. Hypothermia contributes to intravascular sludging, which impairs delivery of oxygen and nutrients. During thaw cycles, endothelial damage may also contribute to thrombosis of small vessels, resulting in tissue ischemia and necrosis [24]. Delineation of nonviable tissue may take weeks to months, however, and surgical debridement should be left for as late as possible [26].

Multiple studies have demonstrated the utility of Technetium-99 scans in delineating areas of significant tissue injury from frostbite. In studies by Twomey et al. and Bruen et al., at-risk areas were identified and directed infusion of tissue plasminogen activator (tPA) were administered intravascularly. Both studies demonstrated preservation of at-risk tissue. The latter study demonstrated significantly lower amputation rates when compared to patients not receiving tPA [28,30]. Early institution of this therapy seemed to be a key component of its success.

*Recommendation*: Surgical debridement should be conservative, as it may take weeks to months to determine viability of tissues. Early use of thrombolytic therapy may assist with tissue perfusion and preservation (Grade C recommendation).

Rewarming is the mainstay of therapy for frostbite. In those with a poor response to rewarming who have evidence of diminished perfusion, the use of thrombolytics (in the form of tPA) with heparin should be considered, if there is no known bleeding risk. Surgical debridement should be conservative.

## 35.4 Chemical Injuries

Injuries from chemical exposures are not common in the United States. The group at most routine risk for a caustic burn includes laborers. In examining work-related burn injuries from 1995 to 2004, only 5.8% of burns were found to be chemical in nature as opposed to 45.8% electrical burns and 39.6% thermal burns [24]. Despite the very serious nature of work-related chemical burns, with morbidity and loss of productivity, caustic ingestions are a far more common source of chemical burn seen by the emergency room and surgeons. Included in the category of accidental caustic burns seen routinely would be burns to the pulmonary system due to aspiration pneumonitis. Caustic ingestion occurs in a bimodal age distribution, and the severity of injury is often linked to the reason behind the ingestion. Caustic ingestions in young children are accidental and attributed to mistaking household cleaning items for beverages. Conversely, in adults, the most common cause of caustic ingestion is purposeful during a suicide attempt.

Overall, caustic ingestions in adults tend to be more severe due to the purposeful nature [34]. These patients may typically ingest larger volumes and not seek evaluation for prolonged periods. The extent of tissue damage depends on multiple factors including the type of agent (alkali or acid), the physical properties of the agent, agent concentration, duration of the contact, and volume of substance ingested [35–38]. Solutions with a pH <2 or >12 tend to be highly corrosive, and solid or powdered forms may be more damaging due to the tendency to adhere to the mucosal surface [34]. Alkali ingestion results in liquefactive necrosis, with thrombosis of small vessels and local heat production compounding the injury. In a similar fashion, acids cause liquefactive necrosis with eschar formation. By 4–7 days following the injury, mucosal sloughing begins. This allows the potential for bacterial invasion with a robust inflammatory response and deposition of granulation tissue. Tensile strength of tissue is low for the first 3 weeks and the inflammatory response and tissue sloughing renders tissues weakened starting at 48 h. This increases the likelihood of perforation. Scar formation, which may begin as early as the second week following surgery, may result in esophageal shortening and stricture formation. A shortened esophagus has altered pressures at the lower esophageal sphincter, allowing increased acid reflux to exacerbate injuries [34].

Caustic ingestions in children are quite variable in degree of severity. Accidental ingestions are seen more commonly in developing countries, where household cleaners and other chemicals may be stored in reused containers, thereby leading children to think the contents are potable. Twenty-six percent of children with accidental ingestions are ultimately found to have severe lesions, and 1%–5% of children with accidental ingestions ultimately develop a stenosis [38].

While topical chemical burns are not common, white phosphorus has been a source of significant morbidity and mortality in military, industrial, and rural settings. White phosphorus is highly toxic in this regard and has been used in munitions, in fertilizers, and in production of semiconductors. White phosphorus spontaneously ignites at 30°C and may cause severe burns when in contact with skin. Further, if the burn allows deep invasion, white phosphorus is very lipophilic and may spread rapidly beneath the dermis. This chemical is easily absorbed via the skin, lungs, and gut and may ignite at body temperature, if it dries. Further, it may cause profound electrolyte imbalances (hyperphosphatemia and hypocalcemia), which may result in fatal arrhythmias. Treatment is thorough decontamination with cold water lavage and monitoring of electrolytes, if absorption is suspected [39].

### 35.4.1 What Is the Optimal Role of Endoscopy in Evaluating and Treating Patients with Caustic Ingestions?

The degree of esophageal injury is assessed with endoscopy and graded on a scale of 0-IIIb [35,38]. The primary concern during endoscopy is not in detecting perforation, which may be diagnosed with other modalities, but in differentiating minimal injury from severe injury, which then influences management. In a retrospective cohort study of 50 patients with caustic ingestions from 1988 to 2003 in Israel, the overall rate of stricture formation was 10%. However, patients with third-degree esophageal injuries had a 71% rate of stricture formation [35]. In a series of 48 pediatric patients reported in Level IIb evidence from France, 26% of the patients with accidental ingestions had severe lesions. However, this study found that all patients at risk of stenosis with severe lesions presented with symptoms, such as hematemesis and respiratory distress [38]. No particular symptom is predictive of increased severity of esophageal lesion and, thus, risk of stenosis.

In light of these findings, children with accidental caustic ingestions who are asymptomatic at presentation do not require endoscopy. Owing to intent to harm, all suicidal ingestions, and patients presenting with symptoms, should receive endoscopy. Endoscopy should occur within the first 48 h, as after this time point, tensile strength is decreased and the risk of iatrogenic perforation increases [34]. Additionally, endoscopy should not proceed past circumferential burns due to the increased risk of perforations at these points. Further evaluation of the gastrointestinal tract may occur with a barium study, if necessary.

Subsequent management of patients with injury will depend on patient condition, injury severity, and physician practice. Although the use of nasogastric tubes to stent the esophagus and injury sites has been promulgated, some evidence indicates that this may actually promote stricture formation. Zargar et al., in a prospective endoscopic evaluation of 81 patients with corrosive esophageal burns, determined that all patients with Grades 0-IIa burns recovered without sequelae. Further, approximately three quarters of patients with 2b burns and all those with Grades 3a and 3b injuries ultimately developed esophageal stricture. These authors postulated that early resection of the most severe injuries (Grade IIIb) may improve outcome as defined by morbidity and mortality [40].

*Recommendation*: Endoscopy should be reserved for symptomatic patients or for ingestions secondary to suicidal intent (Grade C recommendation).

The majority of the evidence in caustic injuries falls somewhere within the realm of Grade C data. Endoscopy clearly has a role in the management of patients with caustic ingestions and should be used routinely for symptomatic patients or patients with ingestion due to suicide attempt. Results of endoscopy can then be used to determine prognosis and to formulate a management plan.

### 35.4.2 Is There Any Role for Exogenous Agents to Limit Damage after Chemical Ingestion or Aspiration Pneumonitis?

In light of the potentially serious effects of caustic damage to the esophagus, research has focused on interventions that may mitigate or prevent negative long-term outcomes. The most commonly used modality to prevent stricture formation is steroids [41]. While some animal models have indicated a potential benefit, evidence in human subjects is mixed. A meta-analysis retrospective review of 361 patients with corrosive esophageal injury found a stricture rate of 19% in patients treated with steroids (40–60 mg/day intravenous) and antibiotics versus 40% stricture rate in those not receiving steroids [42]. However, a randomized control trial of 60 children suffering caustic ingestions and treated with steroids (2 mg/kg/day intravenous) versus no steroids found no decrease in stricture rate [43]. The only firm recommendation regarding the use of steroids in caustic ingestion patients is that antibiotics and antireflux medications should be given concurrently with steroids to mitigate the immunosuppressive effect [34,41].

Considerable research effort continues to look at unusual adjuncts to decrease stricture formation, although most of these efforts are small studies. Halofuginone, an alkaloid plant derivative, suppresses collagen synthesis and has been shown to improve esophageal patency in rats following caustic ingestion [44]. Topical application of dilute hyaluronic acid has suppressed local inflammation and decreased stricture formation in another rat study [41]. Human study has looked at the use of biodegradable esophageal stents for patients with existing esophageal strictures. This study demonstrated temporary improvement in symptoms but little long-term benefit [45].

Finally, caustic injury secondary to aspiration pneumonitis is an intensive care unit (ICU) challenge that continues to plague clinicians. Following aspiration, one-third of patients will develop severe pulmonary symptoms and up to 22% are at risk of acute respiratory distress syndrome (ARDS) with the associated morbidity and mortality. Aspiration may result in a profound inflammatory response, with activation of cytokines including TNFα, IL-1, and IL-8. Attempts to modulate the development of ARDS increasingly focus on anti-inflammatory agents and immunomodulators. Pawlik et al. examined the role of pentoxifylline, which inhibits the release of TNFα, in limiting the development of ARDS following aspiration. In this animal model ($n$ = 24), animals receiving pentoxifylline had significantly improved oxygenation, less atelectasis, and less evidence of inflammation on CT than animals in the untreated group. Mortality was also significantly less in the treated group. These results are directly opposite to findings in the ARDSNet trial using lisofylline, a pentoxifylline derivative. However, method of drug administration and ventilatory methods were quite different between the studies, making direct comparison between the two studies difficult [46].

*Recommendation*: Supportive care with the use of antibiotics and antireflux medications is the mainstay of therapy. Steroids may have some benefits as well. Evidence supporting other agents is very limited (Grade C recommendation).

Adjuncts minimizing the formation of esophageal stricture are poorly defined. The strongest evidence

**TABLE 35.1**

Management Questions and Evidence-Based Recommendations for Electrical, Cold, and Caustic Injuries

| Question | Answer | Grade of Recommendation | References |
|---|---|---|---|
| Which patients suffering electrical injury require more comprehensive monitoring, including urine myoglobin levels? | Low-voltage injuries without signs of injury do not require further monitoring. Patients with sequelae of electrical injury should be monitored closely. | C | [1,9–14] |
| Is there any role for advanced imaging to evaluate muscle damage after electrical injury? | There is little role for MRI or nuclear imaging in the management of electrical injury. | C | [11,14–18] |
| What is the most appropriate method of rewarming the severely hypothermic patient? | Rewarming should wait until there is no further risk of freezing. Active rewarming is favored in patients suffering severe hypothermia. | C | [21,22,24–31] |
| What is the role of amputation in the management of significant frostbite? | Surgical debridement should be conservative, as it may take weeks to months to determine tissue viability. Early use of thrombolytic therapy may assist with tissue perfusion and preservation. | C | [22,24,26,28] |
| What is the optimal role of endoscopy in evaluating and treating patients with caustic ingestions? | Endoscopy should be reserved for symptomatic patients or for ingestions secondary to suicidal intent. | C | [32,33,36,37] |
| Is there any role for exogenous agents to limit damage after chemical ingestion or aspiration pneumonitis? | Supportive care with antibiotics and antireflux medications is the mainstay of therapy. Steroids may have some benefits. Evidence supporting other agents is very limited. | B | [32,38–43] |

involves the use of steroids, though significant morbidities may occur. Nevertheless, if steroids are incorporated, they should be used in conjunction with antibiotics and antireflux agents. Additional agents are promising in animal studies but require more analysis in human trials.

## 35.5 Conclusion

Injuries secondary to electricity, cold exposure, and caustic ingestions are uncommon. Subsequently, the library of evidence-based data is limited. As with all injuries, the most effective management is prevention. However, as discussed in this chapter, these injuries remain areas of active scientific investigation. The results should be used to guide decision-making and management when these injuries are encountered. Further study is warranted.

## References


1. Spies C, Trohman RG. Narrative review: Electrocution and life-threatening electrical injuries. *Ann Intern Med.* 2006;145:531–537.
2. Maghsoudi H, Adyani Y, Ahmadian N. Electrical and lightning injuries. *J Burn Care Res.* 2007;28(2):255–261.
3. Tuttnauer A, Mordzynski SC, Weiss YG. Electrical and lightning injuries. *Contemp Crit Care.* 2006;4(7):1–10.
4. Laupland KB, Kortbeek JB, Findlay C et al. Population-based study of severe trauma due to electrocution in the Calgary Health Region, 1996–2002. *Can J Surg.* 2005;48(4):289–292.
5. Fordyce TA, Kelsh M, Lu ET et al. Thermal burns and electrical injuries among electric utility workers, 1995–2004. *Burns.* 2007;33:209–220.
6. Davis C, Engeln A, Johnson E et al. Wilderness medical society practice guidelines for the prevention and treatment of lightning injuries. *Wilderness Environ Med.* 2012;23:260–269.
7. Forster SA, Silva IM, Ramos MLC et al. Lightning burn—Review and case report. *Burns.* 2013;29:e8–e12.
8. Bailey B, Gaudreault P, Thivierge R. Cardiac monitoring of high-risk patients after an electrical injury: A prospective multicentre study. *Emerg Med J.* 2007;24(5):348–352.
9. 2005 American Heart Association Guidelines for Cardiopulmonary Resuscitation and Emergency Cardiovascular Care. Part 10.9: Electric shock and lightning strikes. *Circulation.* 2005;112(Suppl IV):154–155.
10. Li M, Hamilton W. Review of autopsy findings in judicial electrocutions. *Am J Forensic Med Pathol.* 2005;26(3):261–267.
11. Pham TN, Gibran NS. Thermal and electrical injuries. *Surg Clin North Am.* 2007;87:185–206.
12. Purdue GF, Hunt JL. Electrocardiographic monitoring after electrical injury: Necessity of luxury. *J Trauma.* 1986;26:166.
13. Arnoldo B, Klein M, Gibran NS. Practice guidelines for the management of electrical injuries. *J Burn Care Res.* 2006;27(4):439–447.
14. Blackwell N, Hayllar J. A three year prospective audit of 212 presentations to the emergency department after electrical injury with a management protocol. *Postgrad Med J.* 2002;78:283–285.
15. Arnoldo BD, Purdue GF. The diagnosis and management of electrical injuries. *Hand Clinics.* 2009;25:469–479.
16. Rosen CL, Adler JN, Rabban JT et al. Early predictors of myoglobinuria and acute renal failure following electrical injury. *J Emerg Med.* 1999;17:783–789.
17. Fleckenstein JL, Chasson DP, Bonte FJ et al. High-voltage electric injury: Assessment of muscle viability with MR imaging and Tc-99m pyrophosphate scintigraphy. *Radiology.* 1993;195:205–210.
18. Hunt JL, Lewis S, Parkey R et al. The use of technetium 99 stannous pyrophosphate scintigraphy to identify muscle damage in acute electric burns. *J Trauma.* 1979;19:409–413.
19. Hammond J, Ward CG. The use of technetium-99 pyrophosphate scanning in management of high voltage electrical injuries. *Am Surg.* 1994;68:886–888.
20. Clayton JM, Hayes AC, Hammond J et al. Xenon-133 determination of muscle blood flow in electric injury. *J Trauma.* 1977;17:293–298.
21. Koljonen V, Andersson K, Mikkonen K et al. Frostbite injuries treated in the Helsinki area from 1995 to 2002. *J Trauma.* 2004;57(6):1315–1320.
22. Vretenar DF, Urschel JD, Parott JC et al. Cardiopulmonary bypass resuscitation for accidental hypothermia [review]. *Ann Thorac Surg.* 1994;58:895–898.
23. Murphy JV, Banwell PE, Roberts AHN et al. Frostbite: Pathogenesis and treatment. *J Trauma.* 2000;48(1):171–178.
24. Biem J, Koehncke N, Classen D et al. Out of the cold: Management of hypothermia and frostbite. *CMAJ.* 2003;168(3):305–311.
25. Arthurs Z, Cuadrado D, Beekley A et al. The impact of hypothermia on trauma care at the 31st combat support hospital. *Am J Surg.* 2006;191:610–614.
26. Roche-Nagle G, Murphy G, Collins A et al. Frostbite: Management options. *Eur J Emerg Med.* 2008;15(3):173–175.
27. Alam HB, Rhee P, Honma K et al. Does the rate of rewarming from profound hypothermic arrest influence the outcome in a swine model of lethal hemorrhage? *J Trauma.* 2006;60(1):134–146.
28. Bruen KJ, Ballard JR, Morris SE et al. Reduction of the incidence of amputation in frostbite injury with thrombolytic therapy. *Arch Surg.* 2007;142:546–553.
29. McGillion R. Frostbite: Case report, practical summary of ED treatment. *J Emerg Nurs.* 2005;31(5):500–502.
30. Twomey JA, Peltier GL, Zera RT. An open-label study to evaluate the safety and efficacy of tissue plasminogen activator in treatment of severe frostbite. *J Trauma.* 2005;59(6):1350–1355.

31. Robson MC, Heggers JP. Evaluation of hand frostbite blister fluid as a clue to pathogenesis. *J Hand Surg [Am]*. 1981;6:43–47.
32. Monika BM, Martin D, Balthasar E et al. The Bernese Hypothermia Algorithm: A consensus paper on in-hospital decision-making and treatment of patients in hypothermic cardiac arrest at an alpine level 1 trauma centre. *Injury*. 2011;42:539–543.
33. Morita S, Inokuchi S, Yamagiwa T et al. Efficacy of portable and percutaneous cardiopulmonary bypass rewarming versus that of conventional internal rewarming for patients with accidental deep hypothermia. *Crit Care Med*. 2011;39(5):1064–1068.
34. Ramasamy K, Gumaste VV. Corrosive ingestion in adults. *J Clin Gastroenterol*. 2003;37(2):119–124.
35. Arevalo-Silva C, Eliashar R, Wohlgelernter J et al. Ingestion of caustic substances: A 15 year experience. *The Laryngoscope*. 2006;116:1422–1426.
36. Wedler V, Guggenheim M, Moron M et al. Extensive hydrofluoric acid injuries: A serious problem. *J Trauma*. 2005;58(4):852–857.
37. Mattos GM, Lopes DD, Mamede RCM et al. Effect of time of contact and concentration of caustic agent on generation of injuries. *The Laryngoscope*. 2006;116:456–460.
38. Lamireau T, Rebouissoux L, Denis D et al. Accidental caustic ingestion in children: Is endoscopy always mandatory? *J Pediatr Gastroenterol Nutr*. 2001;33:81–84.
39. Berndtson AE, Fagin A, Sen S et al. White phosphorus burns and arsenic inhalation: A toxic combination. *J Burn Care Res*. 2013;35(2):e128–e131.
40. Zargar SA, Kuchhar R, Mehta S et al. The role of fiberoptic endoscopy in the management of corrosive ingestion and modified endoscopic classification of burns. *Gastroint Endos*. 1991;37:165–169.
41. Cevik M, Demir T, Karadag CA et al. Preliminary study of efficacy of hyaluronic acid on caustic esophageal burns in an experimental rat model. *J Pediatr Surg*. 2013;48:716–723.
42. Howell JM, Dalsey WC, Hartsell FW et al. Steroids for the treatment of corrosive esophageal injury: A statistical analysis of past studies. *Am J Emerg Med*. 1992;10:421–425.
43. Anderson KD, Rouse TM, Randolph JG. A controlled trial of corticosteroids in children with corrosive injury of the esophagus. *N Engl J Med*. 1990;323:637–640.
44. Arbell D, Udassin R, Koplewitz BZ et al. Prevention of esophageal strictures in a caustic burn model using halofuginone, an inhibitor of collagen type I synthesis. *The Laryngoscope*. 2005;115:1632–1635.
45. Karakan T, Utku OG, Dorukoz O et al. Biodegradable stents for caustic esophageal strictures: A new therapeutic approach. *Dis Esophagus*. 2013;26:319–322.
46. Pawlik MT, Schreyer AG, Ittner KP et al. Early treatment with pentoxifylline reduces lung injury induced by acid aspiration in rats. *Chest*. 2005;127(2):613–621.

# 36

# *Evidence-Based Wound Care Management*

**Shari Lawson, Wendie Grunberg, and Howard T. Wang**

**CONTENTS**



## 36.1 Principles of Wound Healing

The management of chronic, complicated, and slow-healing wounds is a significant challenge in medicine today. Knowledge of wound management is imperative to providing adequate patient care. In the trauma setting, a wound usually begins with an acute injury. The healing process begins immediately after the inciting injury through four integrated and overlapping phases: hemostasis, inflammation, proliferation, and maturation. This process is followed by orchestrated molecular and cellular events, leading to either a complete healing of the injury or the development of a chronic wound. Many factors can interact with this process, impairing the body's natural ability for wound healing.

Despite the clinician's optimization of local and systemic factors affecting healing, it is still difficult to treat some chronic wounds. In this case, further wound care is attempted with more advanced modalities such as negative pressure, hyperbaric oxygen (HBO2), and topical products before reconstruction with flap coverage is considered. Below are evidence-based recommendations to be used for treating these more complex wounds.

## 36.2 What Are the Common Factors Adversely Affecting Wound Healing?

There are many different factors that negatively affect wound healing, and these can generally be divided into two groups: local factors and systemic factors [1]. Local factors are described as those that affect the wound directly, and systemic factors are those that impact the innate ability to heal. All of these factors interact with each other to impact a patient's wound healing potential.

### 36.2.1 Local Factors

*Infection*: Wound infection is defined as colonization of bacteria beyond $10^5$ per gram of tissue or the presence of beta-hemolytic streptococcus. These replicating bacteria induce continued inflammation secondary to host defenses, which, if prolonged, will result in delayed wound healing [2].

*Oxygenation*: Cells require oxygen for metabolic activity and adenosine triphosphate production. Wound hypoxemia, caused by atherosclerosis, wound tension, anemia, or cardiac failure can impair fibroblast activity when tissue oxygen level is below 35 mmHg. Several systemic factors decrease wound oxygenation as well, including smoking, diabetes, and peripheral vascular disease [3].

### 36.2.2 Systemic Factors

*Diabetes mellitus*: The disease process thickens capillary basement membranes and decreases wound perfusion microenvironment [4]. It also impairs phagocytic function and prolongs inflammation, leading to delayed healing.

*Nutritional status*: As macronutrients such as amino acids, carbohydrates, and fatty acids are the building blocks of the human cellular makeup, it follows that adequate nutrition is essential for wound healing. Albumin levels of <2 g/dL are associated with delayed healing and wound dehiscence. Improving nutrition alone has significant effect on closure of chronic wounds [5].

*Smoking*: Smoking reduces tissue perfusion and oxygenation, impairs normal inflammatory cells and processes, as well as attenuates of reparative processes and collagen deposition [6].

*Age, stress, and medications*: Increased age, as well as stress, causes a decrease in the inflammatory process and results in delayed wound healing. Medications such as steroids, hormones, and chemotherapy drugs also can inhibit the healing process by altering collagen synthesis and cell reproduction [1].

*Recommendation*: Both local and systemic factors affect wound healing, including infection, oxygenation, foreign bodies, nutritional status, smoking, diabetes, age, medications, and obesity. Optimization or elimination of any negative factors will improve the individual's capacity to heal (Grade B recommendation).

## 36.3 How Much Does Preoperative Smoking Cessation Affect Postoperative Wound Healing?

Mosely and Finseth first demonstrated the detrimental effect of smoking on healing of hand wounds in 1977, and since that time, surgical patients have been routinely advised against smoking perioperatively [7]. One such study by Goldminz and Bennett [7] demonstrated a threefold increase in the risk of flap or graft necrosis in current smokers. In this study, former smokers and low-level smokers (less than one pack per day) had no significant increase in necrosis compared to nonsmokers.

A randomized clinical trial by Sorensen et al. [8] studied the effects of smoking in patients with lateral sacral incisional biopsy sites. After 2 weeks of observation, there was a higher rate of wound infection in smokers as opposed to never-smokers (12% vs. 2%, $p < 0.05$). Another prospective study by Bartsch et al. [9] showed the effect of nicotine on breast reduction. Impaired wound healing was noted in 40% of smokers, compared with 16% of nonsmokers. Chan et al. [10] studied the effect of smoking abstinence during perioperative period in breast reduction in 173 patients. As expected, smokers were more likely to develop wound healing problems compared with nonsmokers (55.4% vs. 33.7%, $p < 0.05$). More importantly, when they stopped smoking 4 weeks prior to operation, wound healing impairment dropped from 55.4% to 33.3%.

*Recommendation*: Smoking may delay, complicate, or cause failure of wound healing, and preoperative and/or postoperative smoking cessation may improve an individual's ability to heal (Grade B recommendation).

## 36.4 What Is the Mechanism of Accelerated Wound Healing Using Negative Pressure Therapy?

Negative pressure wound therapy (NPWT) has increased in popularity over the past 15 years, becoming ubiquitous in most health-care settings [11]. The NPWT commercial devices consist of a polyurethane or polyvinyl alcohol porous open-cell sponge which is applied directly to the wound and covered with an occlusive dressing to sustain negative pressure in the local wound environment. A tube connecting the sponge with a vacuum pump maintains subatmospheric pressure in continuous or intermittent fashion. The sponge dressing is changed approximately every 2–3 days until the desired effect is obtained.

A variety of mechanisms have been proposed for the clinical effects seen through the use of NPWT. One major mechanism is reduction of tissue edema and, thus, improved oxygenation and nourishment of cells [12]. This is not the only mechanism, however, as wounds with minimal fluid excretion have been known to improve with NPWT [13]. Studies also show increased vascularity of the wound with NPWT, which may explain increased rate of granulation tissue formation [14]. Given that stretched cells in the presence of growth factors are prone to proliferation and induction of angiogenesis, micro-mechanical forces on individual wound cells are another possible mechanism of improved wound healing [14–16]. Wound effluent (including neutrophil degradation products) can inhibit wound healing, and removal of this fluid from the wound bed by NPWT can aid in the wound healing process [16]. Drawing soft tissues together may minimize retraction of wound edges and promotion of wound closure [17]. Although reducing infectious load has been advocated based on animal studies, retrospective human studies are less convincing [17].

*Recommendation*: The mechanism of action of NPWT is multifactorial, including edema reduction, increase in blood flow, mechanical stimulation of cells, reduction of inhibitory wound exudates, and potential reduction of bacterial load (Grade B recommendation).

## 36.5 Does NPWT Affect Healing Time? Is It Cost-effective?

In 2001, Evans and Land [18] reviewed Cochrane randomized controlled clinical studies comparing NPWT with standard of care dressing changes in an attempt to determine the efficacy of NPWT. This review found significant reduction in wound volume; however, no significant decreases in wound healing time were observed. Joseph et al. found a reduction in wound volume while observing 24 patients with chronic wounds treated with either NPWT or standard normal saline dressing changes [19]. McCallon et al. assessed 10 patients with diabetic foot ulcers and found that satisfactory healing was obtained sooner with NPWT (22.8 vs. 42.8 days) [20]. A randomized clinical trial by Armstrong et al. [21] found an increase in rate of wound healing as well as granulation tissue formation with NPWT as opposed to standard saline dressings in diabetic foot ulcer patients (56% vs. 39% over 16 weeks). Although differences were statistically significant, concerns over this study include low power and funding by manufacturer of the NPWT device [21].

Apelqvist et al. [22] compared resource utilization and direct economical cost of healing diabetic foot wound between NPWT and moist wound therapy. A total of 162 patients were enrolled into a 16-week, multicenter randomized clinical trial. Although the study found no difference between NPWT and moist wound therapy in inpatient hospital stays, the NPWT group underwent fewer surgical procedures (120 vs. 43; $p < 0.001$), had fewer outpatient visits (4 vs. 11; $p = 0.044$), and ultimately cost significantly less money (27K vs. 36K) than standard treatment.

These and other NPWT studies have historically suffered from poor reporting of statistical analysis, low power and selection, attrition, and performance bias. Reviewers of the earlier studies have concluded that the data at hand are weak evidence in favor of NPWT [23]. There is further need for additional multicenter randomized controlled trials with adequate power to evaluate the contribution of NPWT to the healing of chronic wounds and the cost-effectiveness of the treatment.

*Recommendation*: There is currently weak evidence for decreased healing time with NPWT wound compared to wet to dry dressing. Very few studies currently address the cost-effectiveness of the modality (Grade B recommendation).

## 36.6 How Does Acellular Replacement Dermis Affect Final Wound Healing in Burn and Reconstructive Surgery?

Although acellular replacement dermis was initially developed in the 1970s for coverage of burn wounds, its clinical application has widened dramatically in reconstructive surgery. Acellular dermal matrix has many advantages, especially in burn and reconstructive surgery, as it forms a barrier that reduces moisture loss, guards against bacterial infection, and promotes epithelial migration [24]. More importantly, however, the acellular dermal matrix also reduces donor site morbidity in that it functions as a skin graft during the early stages of healing [25]. The first use of acellular replacement dermis was reported by Burke et al. in 1981 on 10 burn patients [26]. After the Food and Drug Administration granted the license to the manufacturer in 1996, the first multicenter trial published in 2003 showed favorable outcomes in function and patient satisfaction [27].

There are many acellular dermal matrix products on the market today, differing according to composition and source of tissue. The tissue can be obtained from a human cadaver (allograft) or from an animal donor (xenograft). Regardless of the tissue source, the dermis undergoes multiple processes to destroy any pathogens and remove the donor cells before packaging. As it lacks these donor cells, the matrix does not elicit an immune response in the host [28].

In the original case series by Burke et al. in 1981, 10 patients with artificially grafted dermis were described as closely resembling normal skin in palpation, elasticity, softness, and pliability. The conventionally meshed autograft was described to have hypertrophic scars in areas of interstices and feels stiff and thick to palpation without normal skin resilience.

Although histologic biopsies of artificially grafted skins were shown to resemble normal skin with a "neodermis" and the paper describes in detail the technique involved in placing the artificial dermis, the clinical evidence was weak [30].

In Heimbach et al.'s 11-center prospective randomized trial in patients with major burns [29], acellular replacement dermis was compared with autograft, allograft, xenograft, or a synthetic dressing. Median take of the acellular dermis was reported to be 80%, compared with median take of all controls of 95%. At the conclusion of the study, there was less hypertrophic scarring of artificial dermis and more patients and surgeons preferred the final result of the artificial dermis to the control graft. Another multicenter study involving 216 burn injury patients by the same group confirmed safe and effective treatment modality in the hands of properly trained clinicians in burn centers [30].

In addition to its utility in acute burn setting, acellular replacement dermis has been increasingly used in contracture release and reconstruction. Given the scarcity of full thickness skin grafts for large areas of deep skin defects, the dermal regeneration template has been advocated as a substitute for full thickness skin graft, skin expansion, and even skin flaps in reconstructive surgery. Unfortunately, no randomized clinical trials have been reported to date in reconstructive application of acellular replacement dermis, although several studies have examined its utility in this setting.

Dantzer and Braye [31] reported their experience with artificial dermis in general plastic surgery as one of the first series. In their series of 31 patients, scar tissues or skin tumor were excised and replaced immediately with the acellular replacement dermis. An ultra-thin autograft was placed over the neodermis 3 weeks later. In every case, the coverage was described as flexible and nonadherent to deep tissue. Furthermore, the skin was uniform in color and texture.

Given the benefits of dermal regeneration template in reconstructive surgery and acceleration of wound healing by NPWT, the methods can be combined to optimize therapy. A retrospective case series presented by Molnar et al. [32] showed that NPWT applied over acellular replacement dermis would improve take as well as expedite tissue infiltration of the dermal template. In this series of eight patients, the authors used NPWT for an average of 7.25 days (almost 2 weeks less than the standard therapy) over the acellular replacement dermis followed by split thickness graft and re-application of NPWT for another 4 days. Acellular replacement dermis take was reported 95%, and the take of autograft over neodermis was 93%, similar to original reports of Burke et al. Furthermore, splinting was not necessary due to the structure provided by NPWT sponges. Jeschke et al. improved artificial dermis take to 98% from 78% ($p$ = 0.003) by adding fibrin glue prior to application of the dermal matrix and NPWT [33]. This study also confirmed reduction of time for graft take (10 vs. 24 days). Thus, NPWT combined with acellular replacement dermis appears to decrease healing time, simplify wound care, and potentially conserve significant resources.

*Recommendation*: Acellular replacement dermis appears to decrease hypertrophic scarring and improve contractures, which benefit both burn surgery as well as reconstructive surgery. Furthermore, acellular replacement dermis allows the use of ultra-thin skin grafts, which improves donor site morbidity (Grade B recommendation).

## 36.7 Is Hyperbaric Oxygen Therapy Beneficial to Ischemic or Irradiated Flaps?

The clinical efficacy of HBO2 therapy has been demonstrated in a variety of clinical problems, including diabetic foot ulcers [34], carbon monoxide toxicity [35], gas gangrene [36], and osteoradionecrosis of the mandible [37]. However, there are currently little concrete data demonstrating the superiority of HBO2 for improving ischemic and irradiated tissues when compared to traditional wound care modalities.

Several studies have attempted to study the effect of HBO2 on ischemic tissue.

One of the earliest attempts was by Perrins [38] in 1975. In this nonrandomized prospective study, ischemic flaps were treated with HBO2 between 2.0 and 3.0 atmospheres absolute. Of the 150 flaps per year performed in his institution, there was 4.5% failure rate. This was a decrease from his previous (retrospective) failure rate of 8.5%–1.8%. Bowersox et al. [39] reviewed HBO2 therapy for threatened failure of skin flaps between 1976 and 1983. Fifty-five percent of the patients were reported to heal completely and an additional 34% showed marked improvement.

A Cochrane review was published in 2012 that studied randomized controlled trials comparing the effects of therapeutic regimens on chronic wound healing, including HBO2 therapy [40]. The study found that HBO2 therapy significantly improved wound healing in people with diabetic foot ulcers in short-term follow-up. Further studies with adequate power are needed to properly evaluate HBO2 therapy in patients with a spectrum of chronic wounds.

*Recommendation*: Although HBO2 therapy has been shown to be effective in a number of settings, there is little convincing evidence for the use of HBO2 therapy in trauma or reconstructive surgery (Grade C recommendation).

## 36.8 What Are the Current Effective Treatments against Formation of Keloid and Hypertrophic Scar?

Keloid formation results from excessive fibroblast activity and abnormally high collagen deposition. Normally after full thickness dermal injury, matrix accumulates and scar forms. Initially, the wound enters evolutional phase marked by increase in height, firmness, and redness. This is followed by stability and finally the involutional stage, which is marked by flattening, softness, and pallor. A keloid does not follow this normal pattern of wound healing. Hypertrophic scars are different both clinically and histologically from keloids, as they exhibit similarities to normal wound healing but with prolonged time course and excessive deposition of collagen within the borders of the scar.

Although a variety of treatments are available for keloid and hypertrophic scar management, the standard of care remains surgical excision, steroid injection, and pressure therapy with occasional use of silicone gel and radiation therapy. Druit [41] documented the first description of surgical excision as a mode of therapy for keloid formation in 1844; however, the futility of surgical excision alone soon became apparent, as initially noted by DaCosta [42] in 1903. Surgical excision alone simply replays the cascade of healing biology that previously led to keloid formation, and potentially results in larger keloid. Recurrence rate of 40%–100% [43] is expected when simple surgical excision is employed.

Intralesional steroid injection remains first line of therapy for keloid and the most common treatment used [44]. Although the use of steroids for treatment of keloid was first reported by Conway and Stark [45] in 1951, their systemic route of injection, photographs, and end results obtained did not impress the contemporary surgical community. Intralesional injection of triamcinolone for "dermatoses" was first described by Hollander [46]. In the frequently cited 1963 paper by Murray [47], 87 patients with hypertrophic and keloid scars were treated with triamcinolone. Overall, in the group treated with triamcinolone injection with excision and triamcinolone ointment massage postoperatively, 82% were reported as good or fair with better outcome in Caucasian population. He achieved similar results by addition of 800 roentgen units of x-ray therapy. In 1966, Griffith reported his results of intralesional injection of 37 keloids in 29 patients. Fifty-one percent of keloids completely flattened out, and an additional 40% became much softer. All had relief of symptoms. Lesions that were not completely flattened had 15% recurrence rate on an average follow-up of 10.3 months. Of the 19 keloids that were excised in addition to injected with triamcinolone, he had only one recurrence in a 10–16-month average follow-up. Intralesional injection of triamcinolone was further confirmed by subsequent studies to have greater than 80% efficacy, typically 10 mg per centimeter of incision wound monthly [48].

The efficacy of radiation in treatment of keloid has been documented, but its use is limited owing to the risk of inducing malignancy. Radiation is contraindicated in

**TABLE 36.1**
Levels of Evidence

| No. | Subject | Year | References | Level | Strength | Findings |
|---|---|---|---|---|---|---|
| 1 | Factors affecting wound healing | 1969, 1979, 2008, 2010, 2013 | [1–5] | IIB | B | Infection, smoking, diabetes, and poor nutrition negatively affect wound healing. |
| 2 | Effects of preoperative smoking on wound healing | 1991, 2003, 2006, 2007, 2012 | [6–10] | IIB | B | Smoking may delay, complicate, and cause failure of wound healing. |
| 3 | Mechanism of accelerated wound healing in NPWT | 1997, 2004, 2014 | [11–23] | IIB | B | Multifactorial: edema reduction, increase blood flow, mechanical stimuli, reduce exudates, decrease bacterial load |
| 4 | Effect of NPWT on healing time or cost | 1997, 2004, 2014 | [11–23] | IIB | B | NPWT may decrease healing time and potentially cost. |
| 5 | Effects of acellular dermal replacement on wounds in burn and reconstructive surgery | 1994, 1998, 2001, 2003, 2004, 2008, 2011, 2014 | [23–33] | IIB | B | Acellular dermis decreases hypertrophic scars, lessens contracture in burn scars, and reduces donor site morbidity. |
| 6 | Effects of HBO2 therapy on ischemic or irradiated flaps | 1975, 1986, 1993, 1996, 2000, 2002, 2012 | [34–40] | IIIB | C | There is no convincing evidence that HBO2 helps ischemic or irradiate flaps. |
| 7 | Effective treatments against keloid and hypertrophic scar | 1844, 1903, 1942, 1951, 1961, 1963, 1966, 1992, 1994, 1996, 2002, 2006 | [41–53] | IIB | B | Excision, intralesional triamcinolone injection, silicone gel/pressure therapy, and radiation |

pediatric population and pregnant women as well as sites with underlying visceral structures. In addition to excision, radiation has been shown to have 65%–99% efficacy and consistently better than excision alone [49].

Other common methods of treatment for keloid include silicone gel and pressure therapy. Silicone gel, a cross-linked polymer of ethylsiloxane, has been shown to be efficacious in treatment of hypertrophic scars [50]. Silicone gel is placed as a covering layer over wounds for 12–24 h a day. Results are appreciated after 4–6 months of application. One study shows superiority of silicone gel over triamcinolone injection in treatment of hypertrophic scars [51]. However, this has not been established in keloid treatment. Pressure therapy is a simple and cost-effective method of reducing keloid recurrence to less than 20% [52]. This effect was shown as early as 1942 by Nason et al. in a controlled trial where recurrence of keloid was reduced from 67% to 18% (Table 36.1) [53].

*Recommendation*: Triamcinolone injection with or without excision as the first line of therapy for keloid scars. Hypertrophic scars may be managed with silicone gel and pressure therapy initially, although eventual excision and triamcinolone injection may be needed. Radiation is reserved for selected patient populations with lesions that are refractory to conventional therapy (Grade B recommendation).

## References

1. Guo S, DiPietro LA. Factors affecting wound healing. *J Dent Res.* March 2010;89(3):219–229.
2. Robson MC, Heggers JP. Surgical infection. II. The beta-hemolytic streptococcus. *J Surg Res.* 1969;9:289–292.
3. Rodriguez PG, Felix FN, Woodley DT, Shim EK. The role of oxygen in wound healing: A review of the literature. *Dermatol Surg.* September 2008;34(9):1159–1169.
4. Goodson WHD, Hunt TK. Deficient collagen formation by obese mice in a standard wound model. *Am J Surg.* 1979;138:692–694.
5. Dryden SV1, Shoemaker WG, Kim JH. Wound management and nutrition for optimal wound healing. *Atlas Oral Maxillofac Surg Clin North Am.* March 2013;21(1):37–47.
6. Sørensen LT. Wound healing and infection in surgery: The pathophysiological impact of smoking, smoking cessation, and nicotine replacement therapy: A systematic review. *Ann Surg.* June 2012;255(6):1069–1079.
7. Goldminz D, Bennett RG. Cigarette smoking and flap and full-thickness graft necrosis. *Arch Dermatol.* 1991;127(7):1012–1015.
8. Sorensen LT, Karlsmark T, Gottrup F et al. Abstinence from smoking reduces incisional wound infection: A randomized controlled trial. *Ann Surg.* 2003;238(1):1–5.
9. Bartsch RH, Weiss G, Kästenbauer T et al. Crucial aspects of smoking in wound healing after breast reduction surgery. *J Plast Reconstr Aesthet Surg.* 2007;60(9):1045–1049.
10. Chan LK, Withey S, Butler PE. Smoking and wound healing problems in reduction mammaplasty: Is the introduction of urine nicotine testing justified? *Ann Plast Surg.* 2006;56(4):358.
11. Huang C, Leavitt T, Bayer LR, Orgill DP. Effect of negative pressure wound therapy on wound healing. *Curr Probl Surg.* July 2014;51:301–331.
12. Argenta LC, Morykwas MJ. Vacuum-assisted closure: A new method for wound control and treatment: Clinical experience. *Ann Plast Surg.* 1997;38:563.
13. Saxena V, Hwang C, Huang S, Eichbaum Q, Ingber D, Orgill DP. Vacuum-assisted closure: Microdeformations of wounds and cell proliferation. *Plast Reconstr Surg.* 2004;114:1086.
14. Morykwas MJ, Argenta LC, Shelton-Brown EI, McGuirt W. Vacuum-assisted closure: A new method for wound control and treatment: Animal studies and basic foundation. *Ann Plast Surg.* 1997;38(6):553–562.
15. Iwasaki H, Eguchi S, Ueno H, Marumo F, Hirata Y. Mechanical stretch stimulates growth of vascular smooth muscle cells via epidermal growth factor receptor. *Am J Physiol Heart Circ Physiol.* 2000;278(2):H521–H529.
16. Yager Dorne R, Zhang LY, Liang HX et al. Wound fluids from human pressure ulcers contain elevated matrix metalloproteinase levels and activity compared to surgical wound fluids. *J Invest Derm.* 1996;107(5):743–748.
17. Fenn CH, Butler PE. Abdominoplasty wound-healing complications: Assisted closure using foam suction dressing. *Br J Plast Surg.* 2001;54(4):348–351.
18. Evans D, Land L. Topical negative pressure for treating chronic wounds. *Brit J Plast Surg.* 2001;54(3):238–242.
19. Joseph E, Hamori CA, Bergman S, Roaf E, Swann NF, Anastasi GW. A prospective randomized trial of vacuum assisted closure versus standard therapy of chronic nonhealing wounds. *Wounds.* 2000;12:60–67.
20. McCallon SK, Knight CA, Valiulus JP, Cunningham MW, McCulloch JM, Farinas LP. The effectiveness of vacuum assisted closure vs. saline moistened gauze in the healing of post-operative diabetic foot wounds. *Ost Wound Manage.* 2000;46(8):28–32, 34.
21. Armstrong DG, Lavery LA; Diabetic Foot Study Consortium. Negative pressure wound therapy after partial diabetic foot amputation: A multicentre, randomised controlled trial. *Lancet.* 2005;366(9498):1704–1710.
22. Apelqvist J, Armstrong DG, Lavery LA et al Resource utilization and economic costs of care based on a randomized trial of vacuum-assisted closure therapy in the treatment of diabetic foot wounds. *Am J Surg.* June 2008;195(6):782–788.
23. Ubbink DT, Westerbos SJ, Evans D, Land L, Vermeulen H. Topical negative pressure for treating chronic wounds. *Cochrane Database Syst Rev.* 2008;(3):CD001898.
24. Zhang Z, Lv L, Mamat M, Chen Z, Liu L, Wang Z. Xenogenic (porcine) acellular dermal matrix is useful for the wound healing of severely damaged extremities. *Exp Ther Med.* March 2014;7(3):621–624.
25. Wainwright DJ, Bury SB. Acellular dermal matrix in the management of the burn patient. *Aesthet Surg J.* September 2011;31(7 Suppl):13S–23S.

26. Burke JF, Yannas IV, Quinby WC, Jr., Bondoc CC, Jung WK. Successful use of a physiologically acceptable artificial skin in the treatment of extensive burn injury. *Ann Surg.* 1994;413:1981.
27. Heimbach DM, Warden GD, Luterman A et al. Multicenter postapproval clinical trial of Integra dermal regeneration template for burn patients. *J. Burn Care Rehabil.* 2003;24:42.
28. Sclafani AP, Romo T III, Jacono AA, McCormick SA, Cocker R, Parker A. Evaluation of acellular dermal graft (AlloDerm) sheet for soft tissue augmentation: A 1-year follow-up of clinical observations and histological findings. *Arch Facial Plast Surg.* April–June 2001;3(2):101–103.
29. Heimbach D, Luterman A, Burke J et al. Artificial dermis for major burns: A multi-center randomized clinical trial. *Ann Surg.* 1988;208:313–320.
30. Heimbach DM, Warden GD, Luterman A et al. Multicenter postapproval clinical trial of integra® dermal regeneration template for burn treatment. *J Burn Care Rehabil.* 2003;24:42–48.
31. Dantzer E, Braye EM. Reconstructive surgery using an artificial dermis (Integra): Results with 39 grafts. *Br J Plast Surg.* December 2001;54(8):659–664.
32. Molnar, JA DeFranzo AJ, Hadaegh A et al. Acceleration of integra incorporation in complex tissue defects with subatmospheric pressure. *Plast Reconstr Surg.* April 2004;113(5):1339–1346.
33. Kopp J, Jeschke MG, Bach AD, Kneser U, Horch RE. Applied tissue engineering in the closure of severe burns and chronic wounds using cultured human autologous keratinocytes in a natural fibrin matrix. *Cell Tissue Bank.* 2004;5(2):89–96.
34. Faglia E, Favales F, Aldehgi A et al. Adjunctive systemic hyperbaric oxygen therapy in treatment of severe prevalently ischemic diabetic foot ulcer: A randomized study. *Diabetes Care.* 1996;19:1338.
35. Weaver LK, Hopkins RO, Chan K et al. Hyperbaric oxygen for acute carbon monoxide poisoning. *N Engl J Med.* 2002;347:1057.
36. Hirn M. Hyperbaric oxygen in the treatment of gas gangrene and perineal necrotizing fasciitis. *Eur J Surg.* 1993;570(Suppl):1.
37. Curi MM, Dib LL, Kowalski LP. Management of refractory osteoradionecrosis of the jaws with surgery and adjunctive hyperbaric oxygen. *Int J Oral Maxillofac Surg.* 2000;29:430.
38. Perrins DJD. 1975. The effect of hyperbaric oxygen on ischemic skin flaps. In: Grabb WC, Myers MB (eds.), *Skin Flaps.* Little, Brown: Boston, MA, p. 53.
39. Bowersox JC, Strauss MB, Hart GB. Clinical experience with hyperbaric oxygen therapy in the salvage of ischemic skin flaps and grafts. *J Hyperbaric Med.* 1986;1:141.
40. Kranke P, Bennett MH, Martyn-St James M, Schnabel A, Debus SE. Hyperbaric oxygen therapy for chronic wounds. *Cochrane Database Syst Rev.* April 2012;4:CD004123.
41. Druit R. 1844. *Modern Surgery.* Lea and Blanchard: Philadelphia, PA.
42. DaCosta JC. 1903. *Modern Surgery.* Saunders: Philadelphia, PA.
43. Al-Attar, AMD, Mess S, Thomassen JM, Kauffman, CL, Davison SP. Keloid pathogenesis and treatment. *Plast Reconstr Surg.* January 2006;117(1):286–300.
44. Mustoe TA, Cooter RD, Gold M et al. International clinical recommendations on scar management. *Plast Reconstr Surg.* 2002;110:560.
45. Conway H, Stark RB. ACTH in plastic surgery. *Plast Reconstr Surg.* 1951;8:354.
46. Hollander A. Intralesional injections of triamcinolone acetonide: A therapy for dermatoses. *Antibiotic Med Clin Ther.* 1961;8:78–81.
47. Murray RD. Kenalog and the treatment of hypertrophied scars and keloids in Negroes and whites. *Plast Reconstr Surg.* March 1963;31:275–280.
48. Ketchum LD, Smith J, Robinson DW, Masters FW. The treatment of hypertrophic scar, keloid and scar contracture by triamcinolone acetonide. *Plast Reconstr Surg.* 1966;38:209.
49. Darzi MA, Chowdri NA, Kaul SK, Khan M. Evaluation of various methods of treating keloids and hypertrophic scars: A 10-year follow-up study. *Br J Plast Surg.* 1992;45:374.
50. Gold MH. A controlled clinical trial of topical silicone gel sheeting in the treatment of hypertrophic scars and keloids. *J Am Acad Dermatol.* 1994;30:506.
51. Sproat JE, Dalcin A, Weitauer N, Roberts RS. Hypertrophic sternal scars: Silicone gel sheet versus Kenalog injection treatment. *Plast Reconstr Surg.* 1992;90:988.
52. Lawrence WT. Treatment of earlobe keloids with surgery plus adjuvant intralesional verapamil and pressure earrings. *Ann Plast Surg.* 1996;37:167.
53. Nason KH. Keloids and their treatment. *N Engl J Med.* 1942;226:883.

## Commentary on Evidence-Based Wound Care Management

*Victor C. Joe*

Chronic nonhealing wounds not only pose a tremendous clinical challenge, they are an increasing problem in healthcare. The estimated prevalence is 2% of the general U.S. population (over 6 million) at an annual cost of over $50 billion per year*. The prevalence of these complex and difficult wounds is expected to increase with the aging of the population. While chronic wound care is becoming more specialized from a both provider (certified wound specialist nurses, therapists, and physicians) and institutional (advanced wound healing centers) standpoint, not all patients have access to such care. In these situations, it has been my experience that we, as acute care surgeons, are consulted due to our experience in treating acute traumatic wounds as well as skin and soft tissue infections. It is vital, therefore, that we maintain the requisite knowledge and competency.

A chapter on evidence-based wound care management is highly appropriate as the Office of the Inspector General has voiced concern over the years in regard to growing healthcare expenditures related to chronic wound care. In 2011, the Agency for Healthcare Research and Quality (AHRQ) awarded the Johns Hopkins Evidence-based Practice Center a $475,000 grant to perform a comprehensive systematic review of the wound care literature. In one sobering example, of 10,066 citations specific to the topic of chronic venous leg ulcers, only 66 (0.06%) met inclusion criteria for review†. A common theme in this chapter is that there is a need for more rigorously performed studies in wound care in order to generate higher level practice recommendations. As the field of comparative effectiveness research grows and payor sources insist upon evidence-based justifications for resource utilization, it will become even more incumbent upon us to produce such data.

### What Are Common Factors Adversely Affecting Wound Healing?

The local and systemic factors enumerated in this chapter have potentially significant roles in derailing the normal pattern (i.e., phases) of wound healing. What results is a local milieu that is no longer conducive to healing. There are increased levels of inflammatory mediators, cytokines, and matrix metalloproteinases (MMPs), causing a destruction of both structural (extracellular matrix) and cellular (through impairment of growth factors and receptors) components of the wound environment. Most of us can recount scenarios where these issues helped turn relatively straightforward acute traumatic or surgical wounds into difficult nonhealing wounds. Many of these factors are clearly at play in the three most common types of chronic wounds encountered in practice: venous leg ulcers, diabetic foot ulcers, and pressure ulcers. In addition, there are several rheumatologic (e.g., scleroderma) and dermatologic (e.g., pyoderma gangrenosum, hidradenitis suppurativa) diseases that may result in recalcitrant nonhealing wounds. Successful care of chronic wounds necessitates a multidisciplinary approach in order to identify and address each of the complex, intertwined elements that comprise the causative and/or exacerbating factors for the existence of the chronic wound.

### How Much Does Preoperative Smoking Cessation Affect Postoperative Wound Healing?

The negative effects of smoking on overall health and healthcare expenditure are well known. The studies reviewed in this section demonstrate the negative impact smoking has on wound healing outcomes in a postoperative setting. However, there are several questions that remain in terms of the dose-related and time-related effects of smoking on the wound healing process. These issues are important in determining the recommendations or requirements for cessation of smoking prior to surgery/therapy. The extent to which we can quantify the impact of smoking will help determine how much we ascribe it an absolute or relative contraindication to offering patients therapies that carry increased risk and/or cost. Nevertheless, it is clear that we must continue to advocate for and offer access to smoking cessation programs.

### What Is the Mechanism of Accelerated Wound Healing Using Negative Pressure Therapy?

The cellular, biochemical, physiologic, and structural discoveries highlighted in this section provide the basis for the ongoing enthusiasm shown for the use of negative pressure wound therapy (NPWT). It addresses a majority of the adverse circumstances mentioned previously in wound healing. Thus, it can have a direct effect in altering the local wound environment and make it more favorable to achieving wound closure.

### Does NPWT Affect Healing Time? Is It Cost-Effective?

The attractiveness of NPWT rests not only on the potential mechanistic effects of the therapy on the local wound environment, but with the versatility and convenience of the modality on the wound itself for both the patient

* Fife CE, Carter MJ. Wound care outcomes and associated cost among patients treated in US outpatient wound centers: Data from the US Wound Registry. Wounds. 2012;24(1):10–17.

† Lazarus G, Valle F, Malas M et al. Chronic venous leg ulcer treatment: Future research needs. *Wound Repair Regen.* 2014;22:34–42.

and the practitioner. Many practical advantages to traditional wound dressings exist including frequency, hygiene, and labor. These then may have implications for pain control and psychosocial well-being. Whether these mechanisms and advantages translate into meaningful outcomes, defined by the goal of complete wound closure in a cost-effective manner, is the key question. The literature thus far is not conclusive in the matter. As ongoing fervor and widespread use of NPWT is likely to continue, high-quality data with carefully delineated patient groups, adequate power, and clearly delineated outcome measures must be generated. Until then, providers endeavoring to employ best practices must be judicious in their use of NPWT and balance considerations of efficiency (time and resources) and effectiveness (local wound environment and eventual outcome) to each clinical circumstance.

## How Does Acellular Replacement Dermis Affect Final Wound Healing in Burn and Reconstructive Surgery?

The growing experience with the use of acellular dermal matrices has altered the traditional reconstructive ladder and provides an attractive alternative step to traditional flap coverage of difficult wounds. It has also provided more flexibility to burn surgeons for the coverage of extensive deep full-thickness burns in the acute setting, particularly over areas of important cosmesis and function and for scar contracture release in the reconstructive phase. There are numerous products available and more in development. There are differences among the products in the origin of the matrix (human, porcine, bovine) and biochemical properties (type of collagen, glycosaminoglycans, proteoglycans, growth factors). Randomized, controlled trials to provide direct comparisons between products and to standard wound care are difficult due to the number of permutations that would need to be studied. As these products are often cost-prohibitive, patient selection is of the utmost importance and the choice of product must match the characteristics of the matrix to the type of patient and wound being addressed.

## Is Hyperbaric Oxygen (HBO) Therapy Beneficial to Ischemic or Irradiated Flaps?

Both the American College of Hyperbaric Medicine (ACHM) and the Undersea and Hyperbaric Medicine Society (UHMS) have approved 13–14 indications for the use of HBO, including compromised skin grafts and tissue flaps. These indications are reimbursable through the Centers for Medicare & Medicaid Services (CMS). Nevertheless, HBO has been described as "a therapy in search of an indication" and viewed with skepticism by many medical professionals. This is due in large part to the proliferation of stand-alone hyperbaric centers catering to patients with difficult disease processes and utilizing HBO for nonapproved indications. Much of the literature regarding HBO is flawed at best, but must be evaluated thoughtfully. Patient selection is important; there are patients who may benefit from this therapy as an adjunct to standard best practices in wound care.

## What Are the Current Effective Treatments against Formation of Keloid and Hypertrophic Scar?

The treatment of keloids and hypertrophic scars (HTSs) is often difficult and frustrating. The use of silicone gel sheeting and pressure therapy are relatively simple, depending on location and size of the scar. They are also noninvasive, though at times considered uncomfortable. Steroid injection is generally repeated at 6 week intervals until the desired result or a plateau is reached. One caution is that there have been reports of the development of Cushing's syndrome after intralesional steroid injection. While this has not been seen when recommended doses are not exceeded in adults, children appear to be at more risk. It has been suggested that monthly dosage not exceed 30 mg in this population*. A modality that has gained much attention in the media and increasing interest in the burn and wound community is the use of laser therapy, particularly the fractional $CO_2$ laser. This body of literature is growing and being generated by a few higher volume research centers around the United States. Some encouraging results and therapeutic approaches are being developed. As more studies are published in the peer-reviewed literature, systematic review will be eagerly anticipated. A more effective tool against HTS has been identified as a priority by burn survivors in particular.

* Fredman R, Tenenhaus M. Cushing's syndrome after intralesional triamcinolone acetonide: A systematic review of the literature and multinational survey. *Burns*. 2013;39(4):549–557.

# 37

# *Viperidae Snakebite Envenomation*

**Steven Granger and Ronald Stewart**

**CONTENTS**



## 37.1 Introduction

This chapter addresses common questions surrounding pit viper (Viperidae) envenomations common in North America. As envenomations are not reportable, and few maintain registries, the exact incidence is uncertain. Approximately 45,000 snakebites occur per year in the United States with 8,000 from venomous snakes and with 5–15 associated deaths [1–4]. To place this in perspective, Chippaux estimated 5,000 deaths in Central and South America and up to 125,000 worldwide [5].

The two clinically important families of venomous snakes in the North America include the Viperidae and Elapidae. A majority of these bites are from one of the three relevant Viperidae (subfamily crotalines or pit vipers) including the rattlesnake (genera Crotalus and Sistrurus), copperhead (*Agkistrodon contortrix*), and the cottonmouth water moccasin (*Agkistrodon piscivorus*). There are also three relevant elapids in the United States, including the eastern coral snake (*Micrurus fulvius*), the Texas coral snake (*Micrurus tener*), and the Sonoran coral snake (*Micruroides euryxanthus*) [1,6].

Envenomations from the Viperidae and Elapidae are clinically different in terms of presentation and treatment. These differences include the significant local findings and consequences of Viperidae envenomation compared to the systemic consequences of Elapidae envenomation. Most envenomations evaluated by physicians in North America are caused by Viperidae. Bites from these pit vipers are a rare but a challenging problem, occurring more commonly in the Southern United States and Mexico than elsewhere in North America. Like most other traumatic illnesses, men are more common victims. Roughly half of patients are bitten during recreational activity or while working outdoors, whereas the remaining half are bitten by those intentionally handling snakes as a hobby or for some other reason. Although they are typically the most severe of the Crotalinae envenomations, rattlesnake bites are responsible for a very small number of deaths in the United States. These snakes are characterized by broad triangular heads and facial pits (Figures 37.1 through 37.4). All but one species of rattlesnakes have a terminal namesake rattle (Figure 37.5). Most major medical centers where these bites occur have on-hand stocks of antivenin, whereas the antivenom for Elapidae is usually available at regional repositories where these snakes are indigenous.

Clinically relevant questions surrounding pit viper bites include the following:

1. What is the initial type of first aid?
2. When (if ever) should an antivenom therapy be administered?
3. What is the initial dose of antivenin and whether redosing is indicated?
4. What are the indications for surgical intervention, including when (if ever) to employ fasciotomies?
5. Should antibiotics be administered?

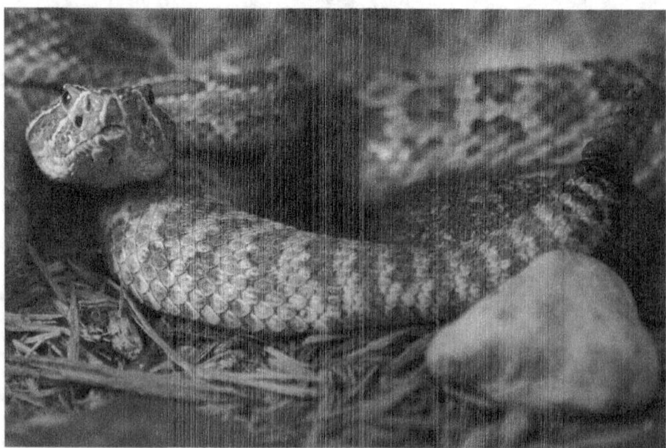

**FIGURE 37.1**
*Crotalus viridis* (prairie rattlesnake) with the characteristic facial pits, elliptical pupils, and the rattle.

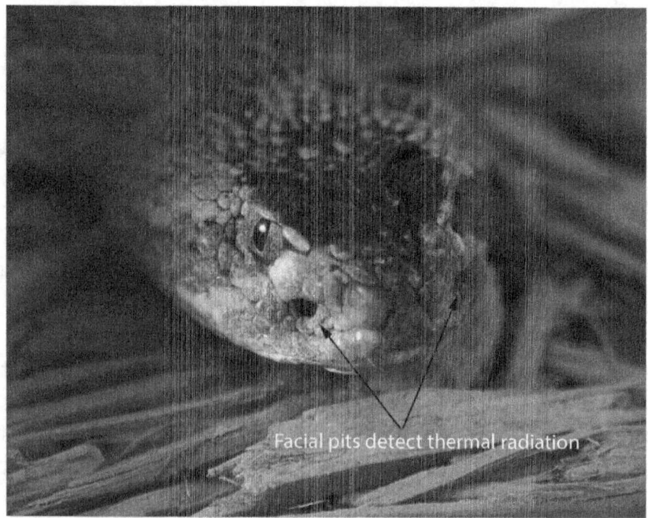


**FIGURE 37.2**
Pit vipers are named for their prominent infrared sensing facial pits (*Crotalus scutulatus*, Mojave rattlesnake).

## 37.2 What Initial First Aid Should Be Administered after a Venomous Snakebite?

Not all pit viper bites lead to envenomation. Most experts believe there is no envenomation in approximately 20% of bites. Severe envenomations are infrequent, depending on the type of snake and the volume of venom injected. Initial first aid for snakebite has changed over the last 100 years. Historic treatments, based on anecdotal experience, included application of ice (cryotherapy), incision and suction on the wound by laypersons, tourniquets, and even electric-shock therapy [1,7–10]. Each of these therapies has the potential to create harm independently of the snakebite itself.

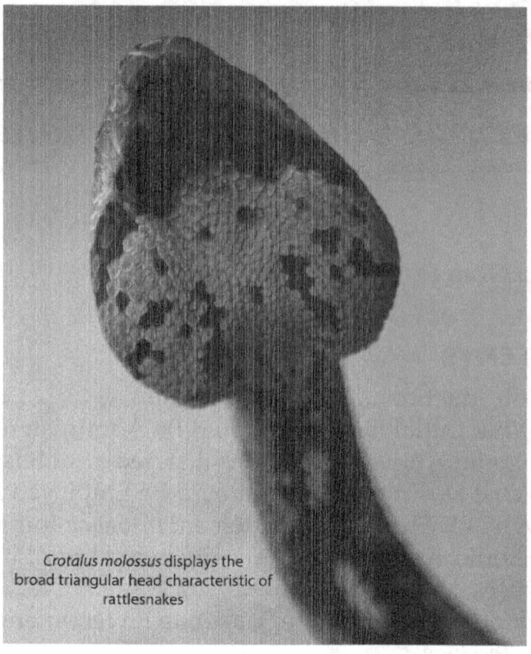


**FIGURE 37.3**
Rattlesnakes and other vipers have a broad, somewhat triangular-shaped, head.

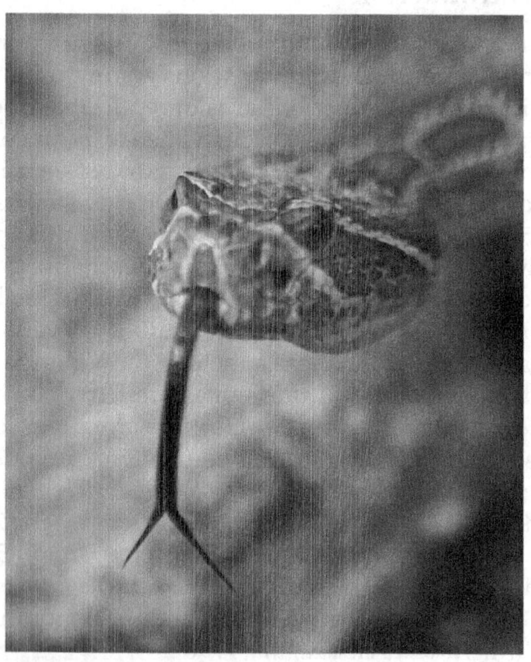

**FIGURE 37.4**
Pit vipers use their tongue to sample the environment which is sensed by their vomeronasal organ (Jacobson's organ).

Current treatment efforts emphasize supportive measures including removal of the victim and caregivers from danger/proximity to the snake, establishment of airway, breathing and circulation as indicated, cleansing of the wound, removal of any restrictive jewelry or clothing, and rapid transport to the nearest

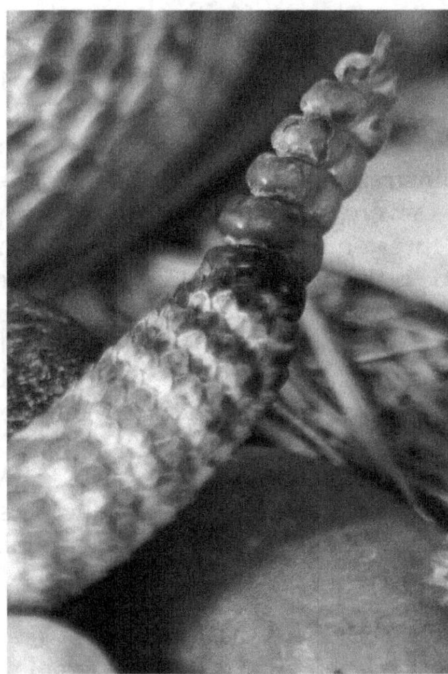

**FIGURE 37.5**
The namesake of rattlesnakes is their terminal rattle. All but one species of rattlesnakes have this characteristic morphologic feature.

medical facility. Additional proposed initial treatments after snakebite include immobilization of the affected extremity at or below the level of the heart, placement of a compression dressing, application of suction on the wound by a bystander or with a commercially available venom extraction device within 5 min of envenomation, and proximal placement of a lymphatic constriction band.

Data regarding the use of an extraction device are sparse. Two recent studies have shown that no clinically significant venom was extracted. Alberts et al. performed a prospective human trial where radioactively labeled mock venom was injected at a depth of 1 cm into the leg of human volunteers—followed in 3 min by application of a popular commercially available suction device. Only 2% of the mock venom was extracted, despite extracting a larger amount of "bloody fluid" [11]. Bush et al. performed a controlled animal trial using real rattlesnake venom. Clinical endpoints were measured including swelling and local effects. These authors concluded that the extractor did not reduce swelling but caused further injury in some subjects [12]. Several small studies dating back to the 1960s had previously suggested benefit from these devices [13–15]. Based on the lack of data showing efficacy and the potential for harm, suction device use for snakebites cannot be recommended (Level IIIb evidence; Grade C recommendation) [8,16–18].

Local and/or circumferential compression therapy is aimed at slowing the systemic absorption of crotaline venom. The theoretic advantage would be to delay serious systemic toxicity until arrival at a health-care facility. Arterial tourniquets are not supported by any data or academic body because of the risk for limb ischemia [17,19]. Insufficient data and concerns regarding uniform application of venous tourniquets and compression devices have similarly led to a lack of universal acceptance. However, some experimental data suggest that these measures slow systemic absorption of venom or—in most cases—mock venom. The theoretic disadvantage to these methods is the trapping of venom locally. The pit viper venom, in particular, has significant local hemolytic/tissue effects. In an animal study injecting rattlesnake venom into the legs of a porcine model, Burgess et al. demonstrated how a constriction band use delayed venom absorption without causing increased swelling [20]. A slightly different technique, pressure-immobilization, has been demonstrated as effective in slowing the systemic absorption of a mock venom. This method employs pressure wrapping the extremity between 40 and 70 mmHg and splinting of the entire affected extremity [21,22]. Conflicting animal data have suggested worsened local effects from these constriction devices as well as a possible bolus effect from venom upon releasing the device [17,20,21,23,24]. There are insufficient data and potential harm to these devices, so routine use of constriction bands and pressure-immobilizing techniques cannot be recommended for pit viper envenomations (Level IIIb evidence; Grade C recommendation). In individual cases where a patient is suffering from systemic decompensation secondary to neurotoxic venom, use of a constriction device or compressive bandage may decrease the systemic effects of venom until a medical facility can be reached [17,24].

Simple extremity immobilization has been shown in several animal models to decrease lymphatic and subsequent systemic absorption of venom, which leads to an increase in the lethal dose of venom tolerated. Early work by Leopold et al. showed that simple immobilization of all four limbs in a rabbit model allowed an increase in the lethal dose of Cadamanteus venom that could be tolerated [15]. Similarly, Snyder et al. showed an increase in the lethal dose of venom after immobilization, and Anker et al. showed slowed transit of radiolabeled isotope with extremity immobilization (Level IIIb evidence) [17,25–27]. Patient and affected extremity immobilization may decrease the rate of systemic absorption of venom and has minimal associated risk (Grade C recommendation).

Although no specific studies have been performed, common sense suggests that rapid transport to a medical facility will likely provide improved care after snake envenomation—allowing more skilled supportive therapy, access to antivenom, and access to specialists when needed.

*Recommendation*: "Do no harm" first aid consisting of immobilization and rapid transport to a medical facility are recommended (Level IIIb evidence; Grade C recommendation). Suction devices, application of constrictive dressings, or tourniquets are not recommended (Level IIIb; Grade C recommendation).

## 37.3 Should Antivenin Be Administered after Suspected Pit Viper Snakebite?

Multiple historic animal studies have shown that pretreatment or early postbite treatment with antivenom is effective at reducing morbidity and mortality. These same studies have mixed results when treatment is delayed past 4 h from the envenomation [14,27–29]. Data regarding the translation of these results to clinically relevant scenarios are lacking. One prospective randomized clinical trial has been performed in the United States. In 1963, Reid randomized patients admitted with pit viper envenomation to antivenom, steroids, and untreated controls. Patients with severe symptoms were excluded. The three groups differed only in less hemorrhagic complications in the antivenom treated group but did not differ in local swelling or tissue necrosis [30]. Rojnuckarin et al., in 2006, published a randomized double-blind placebo-controlled trial of antivenom for green pit viper bites in Thailand. Twenty-eight patients with marked limb swelling but without coagulopathy were randomized to receive placebo versus antivenom. Plasma venom levels and affected extremity swelling were reduced in the antivenom group versus placebo. No difference in pain scores or outcomes was noted, leading these authors to conclude that general use of antivenom, in the absence of coagulopathy, was not warranted after green pit viper envenomation [31].

Determining the need for antivenom administration is complicated by the unpredictability of whether snakebite has occurred, whether it is from a venomous snake, if yes, whether the strike was envenoming, and whether the consequences/clinical course will be minor or severe, warranting antivenom. Definitive diagnosis requires experienced identification of the snake and clinical manifestations of envenomation. In the absence of snake identification, clinical signs and symptoms become the focus.

In the United States, absolute indications for antivenom administration have not been rigorously studied or established. Envenomation severity scores have been published that attempt to classify the severity of pit viper envenomation as a guide to directing therapy. These are often based on local, systemic, laboratory, and organ system involvement with some authors advocating no treatment in asymptomatic patients, as up to 25% of confirmed bites may be avenomous [1,6]. Most cases of pit viper envenomation are associated with minimal morbidity, which ultimately may not warrant antivenom administration [32]. Approximately 7%–13% are classified as severe, including those with early presentation of life-threatening symptoms [33]. The venom from copperheads is the least potent U.S. pit viper venom relative to rattlesnake and water moccasin venom. Several authors have published their experiences with conservative management of select pit viper snakebites and specifically mildly symptomatic copperhead envenomations (Level IV evidence) [6,30–32,34–36]. Crotalidae polyvalent immune Fab (ovine) (CroFab; FabAV) is the antivenin of choice [37–43]. This product is safer and very likely more effective than the older equine-based polyvalent antivenin.

*Recommendation*: Early administration of antivenom appears most effective and should be employed when symptomatic snakebite victims present (Level 2b evidence; Grade C recommendation). Asymptomatic patients and those with mild symptoms after confirmed copperhead snakebites may be initially managed without antivenom when serial examinations and close observation can be rigorously performed (Grade C recommendation).

## 37.4 What Dosing Regimen Should Be Employed for Pit Viper Envenomation?

The timing for administration and exact dosing has not been rigorously elucidated. Several prospective studies have demonstrated a rebound phenomenon after FabAV administration, which suggests that redosing is often necessary [39,44]. The exact initial dose and redosing interval is not known. Most authors who recommend antivenom after pit viper snakebite suggest initial immediate dosing of enough vials of FabAV to gain control of the effects of the envenomation, followed by regularly scheduled redosing. Dart et al. showed, in two prospective studies, that an initial dose of six vials was sufficient in 65% of patients with redosing of two vials every 6 h for maintenance or redosing of four to six vials at any time that progression was apparent (Level IIIb evidence) [1,39]. Lavonas et al. reviewed their experience with FabAV retrospectively for copperhead envenomations. Seventy-two percent of their treated patients required an initial dose of four vials to halt progression of swelling, and 18% suffered recurrent swelling. They report that during this same time period after release of FabAV, they treated 92% of copperhead snakebite victims without antivenom [43].

*Recommendation*: Initial dosing of six vials with repeated dosing until control of progression is witnessed, followed by redosing of two vials for maintenance at 6, 12, and 18 h or six vials at any point that worsening of signs or symptoms is appreciated (Grade C recommendations). Symptomatic copperhead snakebite victims may require less antivenom than other crotalid envenomations (Grade D recommendation).

## 37.5 When Is Surgical Debridement or Fasciotomies Indicated after Pit Viper Snake Envenomation?

Historically, early surgical debridement was thought to be effective in removing venom from the wound and was employed as a preferred treatment over (or adjunct treatment with) antivenom [27,45–47]. Medical and surgical treatments both have been shown to be efficacious and are associated with potentially significant morbidity. Treatment for envenomation has evolved, with many authors suggesting that surgical debridement is rarely needed and with the improved safety profile of FabAV. Burch et al. published a series of 81 pit viper snakebite (mostly copperhead) patients that were managed without medical or surgical therapy [32]. Numerous authors have noted that the vast majority of envenomations are superficial to the fascia, with the possible exception of the fingers, hand, and anterolateral lower leg, making compartment syndrome extremely rare. Nonetheless, clinical judgment cannot be eliminated, as some patients still suffer from severe envenomations and will develop necrosis and compartment syndromes, requiring surgical debridement and fasciotomy [8]. In a controlled animal study, Stewart et al. showed antivenom alone to provide the best control of local muscle necrosis over the surgical arm alone and the combined medical and surgical arm [47]. In this animal model, it was very clear that fasciotomy and debridement led to the removal of viable muscle in those animals treated with antivenom. Authors of large series advocate antivenom, observation, and delayed minimal debridement of obviously necrotic tissue (Level IIb evidence) [18].

As with early aggressive surgical debridement, early fasciotomy was once recommended and employed after pit viper snakebite [46]. Compartment syndrome has since been found to be a rare but morbid complication after envenomation [8,48–50]. In a controlled animal study with intramuscular injections of venom leading to elevated compartment pressures clearly demonstrated that fasciotomy and debridement were associated with worse outcomes than antivenom (Level IIIb evidence) [47]. In Hall et al.'s review of 1,257 snakebite cases, fasciotomy was performed in only two cases [8].

*Recommendation*: Antivenom alone is sufficient in almost all envenomations. Surgical debridement has no role in acute treatment of envenomation. Compartment fasciotomy is indicated for the very rare patient with documented elevations in compartment pressures despite medical therapy (Grade C recommendation).

**TABLE 37.1**

Clinical Questions

| Question | Answer | Grade of Recommendation | References |
|---|---|---|---|
| First aid after pit viper snakebite? | Extremity/patient immobilization and immediate transport to a medical facility | C | [11,12,25–27] |
| Should snake antivenom be administered? | Early/immediate administration of antivenom for symptomatic snakebite victims.<br>Asymptomatic patients may undergo a trial of initial observation.<br>Minimally symptomatic patients who suffered a confirmed copperhead envenomation may not require antivenom. | B | [14,28,30–32,34] |
| What is the dosing regimen for FabAV? | Initial dosing of six vials, repeated until control of venom effects, then maintenance with two vials at 6, 12, and 18 h. Redosing with six vials if worsening occurs during this 24 h observation period. | C | [39,43,44] |
| When is surgical debridement indicated and are fasciotomies still needed after pit viper snake envenomation? | Early surgical debridement has no role in the treatment of envenomation. Debridement of necrotic tissue may be required after medical therapy. Fasciotomy should be performed for documented elevations in compartment pressures refractory to antivenom and conservative therapy. | C | [8,32,47,50] |
| Should antibiotics be administered after pit viper snake envenomation? | No | A | [51,53] |

## 37.6 Should Antibiotics Be Administered after Pit Viper Snake Envenomation?

Each animal's mouth has a unique resident flora, which may lead to infection following a bite. Prophylaxis after a bite from an animal is routine in some circumstances. Historically, this was true after snakebite, which includes the proteolytic factors from venom causing local tissue destruction as well as bacterial flora from the snake's mouth. When infections do occur, they can be associated with significant morbidity. Kerrigan et al. performed a prospective randomized controlled trial to evaluate the need for antibiotics after pit viper snakebite. One hundred and fourteen patients with local and/or laboratory evidence of pit viper envenomation were randomized over a 3-year period. No difference in abscess rate was found between the two groups with an overall abscess rate of 7.8% (Level 1b evidence) [51]. While thoroughly cleansing the wound should be employed, prophylactic antibiotics have not been shown to decrease wound infection rates which have been reported at 3%–8% after snakebite (Grade A recommendation) [51–53] (Table 37.1).

*Recommendation*: Prophylactic antibiotics after pit viper snakebite is not warranted (Grade A recommendation).

## References


1. Gold BS, Dart RC, Barish RA. Bites of venomous snakes. *N Engl J Med*. 2002;347(5):347–356.
2. Watson WA, Litovitz TL, Rodgers GC, Jr. et al. 2002 Annual report of the American Association of Poison Control Centers Toxic Exposure Surveillance System. *Am J Emerg Med*. 2003;21(5):353–421.
3. Watson WA, Litovitz TL, Klein-Schwartz W et al. 2003 Annual report of the American Association of Poison Control Centers Toxic Exposure Surveillance System. *Am J Emerg Med*. 2004;22(5):335–404.
4. O'Neil ME, Mack KA, Gilchrist J et al. Snakebite injuries treated in United States emergency departments, 2001–2004. *Wilderness Environ Med*. 2007;18(4):281–287.
5. Chippaux JP. Snake-bites: Appraisal of the global situation. *Bull World Health Organ*. 1998;76(5):515–524.
6. Juckett G, Hancox JG. Venomous snakebites in the United States: Management review and update. *Am Fam Physician*. 2002;65(7):1367–1374.
7. McCollough N. Evaluation of venomous snake bite in the southern United States from parallel clinical and laboratory investigations: Development of treatment. *J Fla Med Assoc*. 1963;49:959–967.
8. Hall EL. Role of surgical intervention in the management of crotaline snake envenomation. *Ann Emerg Med*. 2001;37(2):175–180.
9. Meier J. 1995. *Handbook of Clinical Toxicology of Animal Venoms and Poisons*. CRC Press: Boca Raton, FL, p. 477.
10. Dart RC, Gustafson RA. Failure of electric shock treatment for rattlesnake envenomation. *Ann Emerg Med*. 1991;20(6):659–661.
11. Alberts MB, Shalit M, LoGalbo F. Suction for venomous snakebite: A study of "mock venom" extraction in a human model. *Ann Emerg Med*. 2004;43(2):181–186.
12. Bush SP. Hegewald KG, Green SM et al. Effects of a negative pressure venom extraction device (Extractor) on local tissue injury after artificial rattlesnake envenomation in a porcine model. *Wilderness Environ Med*. 2000;11(3):180–188.
13. Reitz CJ, Willemse GT, Odendaal MW et al. Evaluation of the Venom Ex apparatus in the initial treatment of puff adder envenomation. A study in rabbits. *S Afr Med J*. 1986;69(11):684–686.
14. Ya P. Experimental evaluation of methods for the early treatment of snakebite. *Surgery*. 1960;47:975–981.
15. Leopold R. An evaluation of the mechanical treatment of snakebite. *Mil Med*. 1957;120:414–416.
16. Bush SP. Snakebite suction devices don't remove venom: They just suck. *Ann Emerg Med*. 2004;43(2):187–188.
17. McKinney PE. Out-of-hospital and interhospital management of crotaline snakebite. *Ann Emerg Med*. 2001;37(2):168–174.
18. Wingert WA, Chan L. Rattlesnake bites in southern California and rationale for recommended treatment. *West J Med*. 1988;148(1):37–44.
19. Gold BS, Wingert WA. Snake venom poisoning in the United States: A review of therapeutic practice. *South Med J*. 1994;87(6):579–589.
20. Burgess JL, Dart RC, Egen NB et al. Effects of constriction bands on rattlesnake venom absorption: A pharmacokinetic study. *Ann Emerg Med*. 1992;21(9): 1086–1093.
21. Sutherland SK, Coulter AR. Early management of bites by the eastern diamondback rattlesnake (*Crotalus adamanteus*): Studies in monkeys (*Macaca fascicularis*). *Am J Trop Med Hyg*. 1981;30(2):497–500.
22. Sutherland SK, Coulter AR, Harris RD. Rationalisation of first-aid measures for elapid snakebite. *Lancet*. 1979;1(8109):183–185.
23. Pearn J, Morrison J, Charles N et al. First-aid for snakebite: Efficacy of a constrictive bandage with limb immobilization in the management of human envenomation. *Med J Aust*. 1981;2(6):293–295.
24. Watt G, Padre L, Tuazon ML et al. Tourniquet application after cobra bite: Delay in the onset of neurotoxicity and the dangers of sudden release. *Am J Trop Med Hyg*. 1988;38(3):618–622.
25. Anker RL, Straffon WG, Loiselle DS et al. Retarding the uptake of "mock venom" in humans: Comparison of three first-aid treatments. *Med J Aust*. 1982;1(5):212–214.
26. Anker RL, Straffon WG, Loiselle DS et al. Snakebite. Comparison of three methods designed to delay uptake of 'mock venom'. *Aust Fam Physician*. 1983;12(5):365–368.

27. Snyder CC, Pickins JE, Knowles RP et al. A definitive study of snakebite. *J Fla Med Assoc.* 1968;55(4):330–337.
28. Fischer F. Antivenin and antitoxin in the treatment of experimental rattlesnake venom intoxication (Crotalus adamanteus). *Am J Trop Med Hyg.* 1962;102:75–79.
29. Brubacher JR, Lachmanen D, Hoffman RS. Efficacy of Wyeth polyvalent antivenin used in the pretreatment of copperhead envenomation in mice. *Wilderness Environ Med.* 1999;10(3):142–145.
30. Reid H. Specific antivenin and prednisone in viper-bite poisoning: Controlled trial. *Br Med J.* 1963;2:1378–1380.
31. Rojnuckarin P, Chanthawibun W, Noiphrom J et al. A randomized, double-blind, placebo-controlled trial of antivenom for local effects of green pit viper bites. *Trans R Soc Trop Med Hyg.* 2006;100(9):879–884.
32. Burch JM, Agarwal R, Mattox KL et al. The treatment of crotalid envenomation without antivenin. *J Trauma.* 1988;28(1):35–43.
33. Litovitz TL, Klein-Schwartz W, Dyer KS et al. 1997 Annual report of the American Association of Poison Control Centers Toxic Exposure Surveillance System. *Am J Emerg Med.* 1998;16(5):443–497.
34. Whitley RE. Conservative treatment of copperhead snakebites without antivenin. *J Trauma.* 1996;41(2):219–221.
35. Patrick Walker J, Morrision R, Stewart R, Gore D, Stewart RM. Venomous bites and stings. *Curr Probl Surg.* January 2013;50(1):9–44.
36. Walker JP, Morrison RL. Current management of copperhead snakebite. *J Am Coll Surg.* April 2011;212(4):470–474.
37. Minton SA, Jr. Polyvalent antivenin in treatment of experimental snake venom poisoning. *Am J Trop Med Hyg.* 1954;3(6):1077–1082.
38. Jurkovich GJ, Luterman A, McCullar K et al. Complications of Crotalidae antivenin therapy. *J Trauma.* 1988;28(7):1032–1037.
39. Dart RC, Seifert SA, Boyer LV et al. A randomized multicenter trial of crotalinae polyvalent immune Fab (ovine) antivenom for the treatment for crotaline snakebite in the United States. *Arch Intern Med.* 2001;161(16):2030–2036.
40. Corneille MG, Larson S, Stewart RM et al. A large single-center experience with treatment of patients with crotalid envenomations: Outcomes with and evolution of antivenin therapy. *Am J Surg.* 2006;192(6):848–852.
41. Clark RF, McKinney PE, Chase PB et al. Immediate and delayed allergic reactions to Crotalidae polyvalent immune Fab (ovine) antivenom. *Ann Emerg Med.* 2002;39(6):671–676.
42. Consroe P, Egen NB, Russell FE et al. Comparison of a new ovine antigen binding fragment (Fab) antivenin for United States Crotalidae with the commercial antivenin for protection against venom-induced lethality in mice. *Am J Trop Med Hyg.* 1995;53(5):507–510.
43. Lavonas EJ, Gerardo CJ, O'Malley G et al. Initial experience with Crotalidae polyvalent immune Fab (ovine) antivenom in the treatment of copperhead snakebite. *Ann Emerg Med.* 2004;43(2):200–206.
44. Dart RC, Seifert SA, Carroll L et al. Affinity-purified, mixed monospecific crotalid antivenom ovine Fab for the treatment of crotalid venom poisoning. *Ann Emerg Med.* 1997;30(1):33–39.
45. Huang TT, Lynch JB, Larson DL et al. The use of excisional therapy in the management of snakebite. *Ann Surg.* 1974;179(5):598–607.
46. Glass TG, Jr. Early debridement in pit viper bites. *JAMA.* 1976;235(23k0):2513–2516.
47. Stewart RM, Page CP, Schwesinger WH et al. Antivenin and fasciotomy/debridement in the treatment of the severe rattlesnake bite. *Am J Surg.* 1989;158(6):543–547.
48. Grace TG, Omer GE. The management of upper extremity pit viper wounds. *J Hand Surg [Am].* 1980;5(2):168–177.
49. Curry SC, Kraner JC, Kunkel DB et al. Noninvasive vascular studies in management of rattlesnake envenomations to extremities. *Ann Emerg Med.* 1985;14(11):1081–1084.
50. Garfin SR, Mubarak SJ, Davidson TM. Rattlesnake bites: Current concepts. *Clin Orthop Relat Res.* 1979;140:50–57.
51. Kerrigan KR, Mertz BL, Nelson SJ et al. Antibiotic prophylaxis for pit viper envenomation: Prospective, controlled trial. *World J Surg.* 1997;21(4):369–372; discussion 372–373.
52. Clark RF, Selden BS, Furbee B. The incidence of wound infection following crotalid envenomation. *J Emerg Med.* 1993;11(5):583–586.
53. Kularatne SA, Kumarasiri PV, Pushpakumara SK et al. Routine antibiotic therapy in the management of the local inflammatory swelling in venomous snakebites: Results of a placebo-controlled study. *Ceylon Med J.* 2005;50(4):151–155.

## Commentary on Viperidae Snakebite Envenomation

*Eric A. Toschlog*

The human obsession with snakes and serpents is primordial, and perhaps, no event engenders more trepidation, fascination, and lore than snake envenomation. As an avid outdoorsman and naturalist, I have had a long-standing passion for wilderness medicine. Over the past 15 years in Eastern North Carolina, I have had the privilege of being permitted by my wary but gracious trauma and acute care surgery partners to convert hobby into practice, caring for all manner of bites and stings, from black widow spider envenomation to shark attack. I find it interesting that the response to snake envenomation is analogous to that of shark attack. The event provokes a fear and fascination that are disproportionate to the statistical reality; both are rare events with extremely rare mortality. Snake envenomation is unique in that there does seem to be a relationship between the degree of fascination and the number and complexity of treatments proposed. Unfortunately, the vast majority of historical treatment options, many still perpetuated today, not only lacks an evidence basis but also can be overtly harmful. The goal of a chapter on snake envenomation would be to present an evidence basis for care while dispelling treatment myth, which Drs. Granger and Stewart have very effectively accomplished.

### What Initial First Aid Should Be Administered after a Venomous Snakebite?

The answer to this question, presented well by the authors, is *primum non nocere*: first, do no harm. As I have traveled the Southeast lecturing on snakebite, I have been astounded at the number and complexity of suggestions regarding first aid, many remedies well-intended but frankly dangerous. I agree with the authors that very little should be done to the wound, and most attempts to control venom spread have the potential to produce ischemia as a unifying detrimental complication. Therefore, venom extraction through suction, particularly oral, and tourniquets or constrictive bands are not advised. First aid should consist of pain control and reassurance, immobilization of the extremity, and rapid transfer to an appropriate medical facility. I like to preach in our very rural region that the most valuable first aid tool after snakebite is a cell phone.

### Should Antivenin Be Administered after Suspected Pit Viper Snakebite?

In the prior era of equine-based polyvalent antivenin, it was often stated that the antivenin was worse than the snakebite. That statement is not an indictment of the older product, but it is fortunate for our patients that our current ovine-based Fab antivenin has less associated side effects. It is true that indications for antivenin have not been rigorously studied, and the improved safety profile of the current antivenin has likely led to an increase in utilization. There is reasonable evidence to treat envenomation by pit vipers other than copperheads with antivenin, given early, for systemic and progressive local symptoms. Copperhead envenomation presents a conundrum. *Agkistrodon contortrix* venom is not used in the creation of the current antivenin, but cottonmouth venom (*Agkistrodon piscivorus*) is included, and venom homology likely produces cross-reactivity. A prospective multi-institutional trial is underway focusing specifically on antivenin use in copperhead envenomation, so an evidence basis may be forthcoming. I currently treat copperhead envenomation similar to other pit vipers, definitely administering for the rare systemic symptoms and for truly progressive local symptoms, most commonly extremity edema with neurologic symptoms.

### What Dosing Regimen Should Be Employed for Pit Viper Envenomation?

Dosing regimens for antivenin have also not been well studied, although there is evidence that 4–6 vials as an initial dose are effective in most cases, and should be repeated within 1–2 h if symptoms do not abate. It is unclear how many times the initial dose should be repeated, and to what clinical end point. Again, the need for antivenin and amount administered in copperhead envenomation remain to be determined.

### When Is Surgical Debridement or Fasciotomy Indicated after Pit Viper Envenomation?

The answer to this question is both important and well presented. Again, *primum non nocere* should rule the day. We published an extensive review of the literature on the surgical treatment of snake envenomation recently, and concur with the authors' recommendations*. First, necrosis is relatively rare, and wounds should be provided time to demarcate if the patient's physiology is amenable. Second, true compartment syndrome is rare, and a course of antivenin should be first-line treatment unless definitive indications for urgent fasciotomy exist. Snake envenomation is a great mimicker of compartment syndrome, but most often represents subcutaneous edema rather than true compartment syndrome. Compartment pressure measurement is strongly encouraged to guide need for fasciotomy.

* Toschlog EA, Bauer CR, Hall EL, Dart RC, Khatri V, Lavonas EJ. Surgical considerations in the management of pit viper snake envenomation. *J Am Coll Surg*. 2013;217(4):726–735.

### Should Antibiotics Be Administered after Pit Viper Snake Envenomation?

I spend a significant amount of time educating our region on this topic, as antibiotics are commonly and inappropriately utilized for snakebite. As with many animal bites, the incidence of infection is rare, and the use of antibiotics is not only not indicated, but may lead to resistant organisms.

# 38

# *Evidence-Based Surgery: War Wounds*

**Thomas A. Mitchell, Michael S. Clemens, and Lorne H. Blackbourne**

**CONTENTS**



## 38.1 Introduction

*War Wounds* offer unique challenges to evidence-based surgical practice secondary to the absence of prospective studies within austere environments. This chapter offers insight into wartime casualty management using the most recent medical literature from Operations Enduring Freedom and Iraqi Freedom.

Penetrating injurious mechanisms from gunshots and explosive device weaponry are responsible for 75% of all war wounds [1]. Specifically, these explosive devices result in fragmentation wounds and large soft tissue injuries [2]. Improvised explosive devices induce blast injuries independently and synergistically through four distinct phases: primary, secondary, tertiary, and quaternary. Primary blast injuries describe the initial effect of the blast wave on the patient. Secondary blast injuries involve projectiles that strike the patient. If the patient is thrown by the blast, this causes tertiary injuries. Quaternary injuries include other effects such as burns, crush injuries, and infections. Military literature addressing explosive injuries may include any or all of these phases.

After sustaining injuries on the battlefield, the combat wounded are evacuated over several continents through multiple surgical facilities in route to the continental United States. Initially at the point of injury, immediate life-saving measures are implemented by combat medics or corpsmen trained in tactical combat casualty care (TCCC). The patient is immediately transferred to a North American Treaty Organization

(NATO) Role 1 medical treatment facility (MTF) that may include a physician, physician assistant, or medic who will triage, implement life-saving treatment, and activate emergency evacuation as needed. Aeromedical evacuation then proceeds to a NATO Role II MTF with capabilities approaching a 20-person team including several surgeons with the capabilities of two operating rooms. After stabilization, patients continue to a Role III MTF that is a fixed medical facility with up to 248 beds, six operating rooms, and subspecialty support. Patients are then aeromedically evacuated to Landstuhl Regional Medical Center in Germany, which is equivalent to a United States Medical Center. Finally, patients are transported to the Continental United States (CONUS) at facilities, such as San Antonio Military Medical Center (SAMMC), which is an American College of Surgeons (ACS) verified level I trauma facility. Throughout these extensive geographical movements, injured service members encounter different physicians and undergo multiple operations at several geographic sites; the logistical coordination of the service members' movement creates ample opportunities for unique challenges not encountered in civilian trauma. Importantly, the survivability on the battlefields of Iraq and Afghanistan has reached 90%, compared to 84% in Vietnam, and 80% in World War II [2].

Soldiers are considered a potential "vulnerable" population and are often unable to give consent by the nature of their trauma physiology. By default, all combat-related research is based on "waiver of consent" retrospective or prospective medical chart data collections. The confluence of unique wounding patterns with global patient evacuation and the constraints of ethical research in the combat wounded result in all "evidence-based" combat casualty information as—at best—level II data [3].

## 38.2 Prehospital Combat Casualty Care

From 2001 to 2011, 4596 battlefield casualties from Iraq and Afghanistan were retrospectively reviewed, demonstrating that lethality was induced by explosives (73.7%), gunshots (22.1%), and other mechanisms (4.2%) [2]. Importantly, 87.3% of mortalities occurred in a pre-MTF environment. Of battlefield deaths, 35.2% were instantaneous, 52.1% were acute (minutes to hours) pre-MTF, and 12.7% died of wounds after reaching the MTF. Of 976 service members deemed potentially survivable retrospectively, 90.9% were related to hemorrhage. Specifically, the hemorrhagic origin was noted to be truncal (67.3%), junctional (19.2%), and peripheral extremity (13.5%).

Eastridge et al. in a retrospective evaluation between 2001 and 2009, noted that 4.6% of patients died of wounds, with over half presenting to the MTF in extremis [4]. Overall, 51.4% of MTF fatalities were deemed to be potentially survivable with predominantly acute hemorrhage (80%) from a penetrating mechanism. Holcomb et al. reviewed soldiers' autopsies and revealed that compressible extremity hemorrhage was the most common potentially preventable cause of death [5]. Other potentially preventable causes of death included loss of airway, compressible nonextremity hemorrhage, and tension pneumothorax.

The back-and-forth of counterinsurgency warfare prompted evolution of medical and protective equipment; this resulted in changing the dynamics of injuries. The advances in body armor have provided augmented protection to the head, thorax, and abdomen; however, this may explain the increased prevalence of extremity injuries [6].

### 38.2.1 Tension Pneumothorax

Early in the Global War on Terror, anecdotal evidence identified treatment of tension pneumothorax with needle decompression as inadequate using standard 14-gauge angiocatheters in the combat wounded. A review of autopsy and computed tomography (CT) imaging demonstrated that many men and women have a chest wall thickness surpassing the length of standard 14-gauge angiocatheters [7]. As a result, 14-gauge decompression catheters of >3.25 in. are now carried by combat medics and many first responders (Class V, Grade D).

### 38.2.2 Hemorrhage

#### *38.2.2.1 What Battlefield Techniques Are Available to Combat Medics to Treat Potentially Preventable Deaths?*

##### *38.2.2.1.1 Extremity Hemorrhage: Tourniquets*

After 2005, military medical experts recommended issuing tourniquets to all deploying forces. Eastridge et al. estimated that this decreased mortality from peripheral-extremity hemorrhage from 23.3 deaths per year prior to 3.5 deaths per year after 2007 [3]. Furthermore, tourniquet implementation is attributed to saving one to two thousand lives throughout the current conflicts in Iraq and Afghanistan [8].

Despite concerns regarding ischemic injuries, several retrospective reviews have documented the prehospital use of tourniquets to be both safe and effective [9]. Several tourniquets have been tested on the battlefield and deemed suitable for both medical and nonmedical personnel [10].

The ACS Committee on Trauma (COT) extrapolated combat data to strongly recommend the use of tourniquets by civilians to control extremity hemorrhage if direct pressure was ineffective or impractical [11].

*Recommendations*: Tourniquet use for prehospital prevention of exsanguination from significant extremity hemorrhage (Class III, Grade B).

*38.2.2.1.2 Junctional Hemorrhage*

*38.2.2.1.2.1 Junctional Tourniquets* Eastridge et al. demonstrated that 21% of potentially survivable injuries in patients who died of wounds in Iraq and Afghanistan involved junctional hemorrhage from the neck, groin, or axilla [2]. Junctional tourniquets provide a unique solution to these proximal extremity injuries. There are currently four U.S. Food and Drug Administration approved devices for junctional hemorrhage: Combat Ready Clamp (CRoC; Combat Medical Systems, Fayetteville, NC), Junctional Emergency Treatment Tool (JETT; North American Rescue Products, Greer, SC), SAM Junctional Tourniquet (SJT; SAM Medical Products, Wilsonville, OR), and the Abdominal Aortic Tourniquet (AAT; Compression Works, Hoover, AL).

The Defense Health Board approved the use of junctional tourniquets for TCCC in 2011 and this was expanded to include the CRoC, JETT, and SJT devices in 2013 [12]. As the majority of medical knowledge regarding these devices is conducted through personal communication and case reports, the ACS COT did not find sufficient evidence to make recommendations regarding controlling junctional hemorrhage [11].

*Recommendations*: A junctional tourniquet should be applied as early as possible in circumstances of appropriate hemorrhage. Digital compression and Combat Gauze application can mitigate hemorrhage while preparing the junctional tourniquet (Class IV, Grade D).

*38.2.2.1.3 Truncal Tourniquet*

Early studies in human volunteers and large porcine models suggest the possibility of using an AAT to control junctional hemorrhage [13,14]. This device utilizes an abdominal strap placed at the level of the umbilicus with an inward-facing, inflatable bladder and windlass style mechanism. There have been a handful of case reports of in-theater use by Special Operations Forces for control of groin hemorrhage [15,16]. However, due to its relative contraindication in the setting of penetrating abdominal trauma, concerns regarding device reliability, and patient discomfort with placement, the 2013 Committee on TCCC recommended against its use [12]. Large porcine models and sporadic human reports of AAT are ongoing and it remains a potential tool in life-threatening circumstances.

*38.2.2.1.4 Hemostatic Wound Dressings*

In 2005, the U.S. Army advanced the ubiquitous fabric gauze and manual pressure by deploying a hemostatic chitosan-based dressing to every soldier. The positively charged chitin interacts with negatively charged red blood cells to facilitate coagulation and is efficacious in several animal models [17]. Retrospective analysis of chitosan-based dressings document a 97% success rate for hemostasis in combat injured [18]. Practical application demonstrated a superiority of impregnated gauze over granular hemostatic agents in austere environments.

In 2008, the TCCC committee recommended the use of Combat Gauze, a kaolin-based gauze (Z-Medica Corporation, Wallingford, Connecticut) for compressible extremity and junctional hemorrhage. Newer chitosan-based hemostatic agents were added in 2014: Celox Gauze (Medtrade Products Ltd., Crewe, United Kingdom) and ChitoGauze (HemCon Medical Technologies, Portland, Oregon) [19].

The ACS COT weakly recommended topical hemostatic agents, in the prehospital setting where tourniquets cannot be applied and where sustained direct pressure is impractical or ineffective [11]. Furthermore, they recommended that these topical hemostatic agents be delivered in a gauze format with wound packing.

*Recommendation*: Hemostatic dressings should be considered by pre-hospital personnel if gauze dressing fails to stop bleeding from an injury that is not amenable to tourniquet placement (Class III, Grade C).

### 38.2.3 Tranexamic Acid

The CRASH-2 trial suggested that tranexamic acid (TXA) could reduce mortality in patients suffering from hemorrhagic shock [20]. Utilization of TXA in a NATO Role III MTF in Afghanistan was identified as having a lower unadjusted mortality than the no-TXA group (17.4% vs. 23.9%, respectively; $p$ = 0.03). Specifically, in patients who received a massive transfusion, the mortality benefit was improved from 14.4% to 28.1% with and without TXA utilization, respectively ($p$ = 0.04, and independently associated with survival (odds ratio = 7.228; 95% CI: 3.016–17.322) [21]. Because the CRASH-2 study [20] was performed primarily in the third world and half the patients did not require transfusion, and the MATTERS study [21] involved historical controls, the use of TXA remains a Grade B recommendation.

*Recommendation*: TXA may be considered as an adjunct to active resuscitation in patients who require a massive transfusion (Grade B).

## 38.3 Combat Damage Control Resuscitation

### 38.3.1 How Should Combat-Injured Patients Undergoing Massive Blood Transfusion Be Resuscitated?

Combat damage control surgery requires integration of multiple surgical facilities and surgeons, as well as en-route care through a multistage global transit while resuscitating patients to prevent the "lethal triad" of coagulopathy, hypothermia, and acidosis [22]. The U.S. military has adopted a minimal resuscitation policy (aka "hypotensive resuscitation") with the goal of achieving a systolic blood pressure of approximately 90 mmHg based on civilian trauma data and animal research data documenting a rebleeding threshold [23,24]. Predictive factors for combat-related massive transfusion requirements include heart rate >105 beats/min, pH <7.25, systolic blood pressure <110 mmHg, hematocrit <25%, and an international normalization ratio (INR) >1.5 on admission [25,26]. Crystalloid administration is minimized during active damage control resuscitation (DCR) with the goal of restoring the coagulation system and oxygen-carrying capacity [27]. Further, Borgman et al. retrospectively found that the increased use of fresh frozen plasma (FFP) in a packed red blood cells (PRBCs)-to-FFP ratio of 1.4 was associated with a lower mortality rate when compared to patients receiving a higher ratio of PRBCs [28].

This decreased mortality with a lower ratio of blood products became the tenant for the DCR CPG in 2006 that recommended transfusion of component blood products in a 1:1:1 ratio of FFP to platelets (PLTs) to PRBC. A 10-year review of transfusion in Iraq and Afghanistan noted that increased FFP-to-RBC and PLT-to-RBC ratios reduced mortality despite increased injury severity scores (ISS) [29].

INR and PLT count measurements are the standard method for assessing coagulopathy in trauma patients; however, thrombelastography (TEG) has been shown to be a more accurate indicator of the need for blood products in the combat wounded [30]. TEG may play a significant role in DCR in the near future within an austere environment.

Since World War I, Western physicians have intermittently utilized whole blood transfusions to supplement the limited availability of component blood products in combat environments. Currently, Role III MTFs have a limited quantity of PRBCs and very limited access to FFP, PLTs, or cryoprecipitate. Therefore, warm fresh whole blood (FWB) transfusions that comprise all necessary component factors may be utilized for injuries that require any blood product that is not immediately available. Six thousand units of FWB were given from 2003 to 2007 in Iraq and Afghanistan, or approximately 4% of all blood products transfused [31]. The FWB utilized in austere environments derives from hospital and military personnel who were prescreened for eligibility. Acquisition optimally takes 20–30 min, as the units are transfused without leukoreduction or irradiation [31]. Larger MTFs may send selected blood for infectious disease testing back in the United States. Importantly, all U.S. soldiers are immunized against Hepatitis B and screened for HIV every 2 years. Finally, any soldier receiving FWB is screened upon return to the United States for transfusion-related diseases. The Oraquick advance test (Orasure, Bethlehem, Palestine) has been utilized to rapidly screen for HIV [31].

*Recommendations*: A Grade B recommendation supports the use of "hypotensive resuscitation," titrating intravenous fluid to a palpable radial pulse or normal mental status (in nonhead injured patients). Patients requiring a massive transfusion should receive PRBCs: FFP: PLTs in a 1:1:1 ratio with minimal intravenous crystalloid. In austere environments, the use of warmed FWB is effective for massive transfusion and correction of coagulopathy (Class II, Grade B).

### 38.3.2 Hematological Resuscitation (Prehospital)

#### *38.3.2.1 What Is the Role of Freeze-Dried Plasma in the Prehospital Environment?*

Freeze-dried plasma (FDP) was initially created and utilized in World War II. This concept was revisited with the onset of dilutional coagulopathy and abdominal compartment syndromes in Somalia, Afghanistan, and Iraq. FDP offers the advantage of portability and ambient storage compared to FFP that must be stored at −18°C with a post-thaw shelf life of 4 days. French studies suggest that FDP has a 2-year shelf life and can be reconstituted in 6 min [32]. The Israeli Defense Forces have instituted widespread usage of FDP from point of injury to fixed medical facilities with preliminary data suggesting a relative speed of reconstitution and minimal difficulty with usage or patient tolerance [33].

*Recommendation*: FDP may be used for patients in shock where whole blood or a balanced resuscitation of plasma, RBC, and PLTs is unavailable (Class IV, Grade C).

### 38.3.3 Hypothermia Prevention

#### *38.3.3.1 How Can Hypothermia Be Avoided during Transportation of Combat-Injured Patients?*

Hypothermia (<35°C) has been associated with increased resuscitation requirements, prolonged clotting times, and dysfunction of the coagulation cascade [8].

Six percent of U.S. combat injuries present with hypothermia and this population is associated with an increased mortality [8]. Wade et al. demonstrated in military populations that hypothermia (<36°C) had a sixfold increased mortality, 12% vs. 2% [34]. Hypothermia prevention strategies include utilization of the Hypothermia Prevention and Management Kit (HPMK) to provide warmth for several hours during transport [6]. This includes a reflective, hooded blanket with four built-in chemical heating elements [6]. An educational curriculum change in TCCC and the HPMK implementation have effectively reduced the number of wounded soldiers experiencing hypothermia.

*Recommendation*: HPMKs may reduce mortality by preventing hypothermia during extended transport of combat patients. (Class III, Grade B).

## 38.4 Combat Burn Care

### 38.4.1 What Are the Advances in Combat Burn Care?

Approximately 5%–10% of combat wounded patients suffer burn injury. Large burns (>20% total body surface area [TBSA]) require a carefully balanced fluid resuscitation to avoid complications associated with either under- or over-resuscitation [35,36]. Specifically, over-resuscitation can result in abdominal compartment syndrome or acute respiratory distress syndrome and is associated with a higher mortality rate.

This systemic concern led to implementation of a burn flow sheet that tracked the hourly urine output and intravenous fluid administration throughout transportation. In a retrospective review, Ennis et al. demonstrated a dramatically lower incidence of over-resuscitation compared to the preimplementation period [37]. Furthermore, the "rule of ten" was implemented to simplify fluid resuscitation where the patient's TBSA was multiplied by 10 cc/h in order to set a starting fluid rate of resuscitation [38].

In the critical care environment, Chung et al. performed a retrospective review of combat burn patients with greater than 40% TBSA, acute kidney injury (RIFLE I or RIFLE F criteria), and the need for vasopressors and found that early administration of CRRT was associated with a decrease in mortality when compared to a historically matched control non-CRRT group [39].

Current wound therapy for burn care relies upon topical antimicrobial agents including silver sulfadiazines and sulfamylon cream. Newer modalities include items like Silver Nylon that allows wounds to be wrapped for several days, increasing portability and reducing dressing changes during transport.

*Recommendations*: Burn patients treated with multiple facilities should be resuscitated with the benefit of a burn resuscitation flow sheet to ensure appropriate volume resuscitations. During the critical care portion of burn care, CRRT should be considered in the patient with renal failure from sepsis (Class II, Grade B).

#### 38.4.1.1 Transportation of Wounded Soldiers

Major advances in combat casualty care included implementation of the Critical Care Air Transport Team (CCATT) and the Army's Burn Flight Team (BFT). The CCATT is composed of a critical care physician, a respiratory therapist, and a critical care nurse. These teams are equipped to optimize patient care for flights ranging from 1 h (intratheater) to 18 h (trans-Atlantic). In comparison to Vietnam where patients would be evacuated from the theater to a remote hospital in 21 days, the average time of movement with CCATT is 28 h [22]. Similarly, the BFT consists of a critical care surgeon, a registered nurse, a licensed vocational nurse, and a respiratory therapist. These severely injured patients can be transported from the theater to the United States in 3–4 days providing state-of-the-art critical care support [22,40]. A recent review of the first 10 years of CCATT operations in Iraq and Afghanistan suggested an overall efficacy with low en-route mortality (0.02%) [41].

Intratheater transport largely relies on helicopter emergency medical services based on the large distances from the point of injury to fixed medical facilities. However, there remains significant variability in composition and capabilities of these services, ranging from a single emergency medical technician (EMT) basic to a critical care team with physicians, nurses, and paramedics. A 2012 review suggested that services with critical care trained paramedics alone had an overall 66% lower estimated risk of 48 h mortality compared to basic EMTs [42]. Further studies have suggested that the use of physician-led critical care teams for medical evacuation increases the rate of unexpected survivors over three times that of less skilled services [43].

## 38.5 Workup of Patients with Fragmentation Wounds

### 38.5.1 How Are Fragmentation War Wounds to the Abdomen, Flank, and Back Evaluated?

Explosion injuries account for the majority of combat wounds, often resulting in multiple fragmentation wounds [44]. Although classically penetrating abdominal wounds mandate exploratory laparotomy, this is difficult to implement practically in the combat setting secondary to the possibility of mass casualties, limited operating room availability that renders mandatory exploration untenable. Furthermore, the rapid evacuation of patients through multiple facilities makes observation by the same surgeon impossible. In response to these limitations, CT has revolutionized the care of the hemodynamically normal patient with multiple fragmentation wounds.

CT triage of stable patients with multiple abdominal, flank, and/or back fragmentation wounds has allowed successful nonoperative management of these patients. Physical exam is unreliable with a sensitivity of 30.2% for predicting a therapeutic laparotomy [45]. Ultrasound was also found to have a low sensitivity of 11.7%, but with 100% specificity ($n$ = 4) [45]. CT has a high sensitivity of 97.8% for documenting intraperitoneal fragments and predicting the need for therapeutic laparotomy. Beekley et al. demonstrated the successful nonoperative treatment of up to 60% of stable patients with penetrating fragments to the abdomen in the absence of frank peritoneal signs or evidence of intra or retroperitoneal violation by fragments [45]. Future intentions include diagnostic laparoscopy in the armamentarium of deployed surgeons to avoid the complications of nontherapeutic laparotomies.

*Recommendation*: Patients with multiple fragmentation wounds to the abdomen, flank, and/or back with normal hemodynamics should undergo a CT scan for the evaluation of intraperitoneal fragments. Intraperitoneal fragments mandate surgical exploration, and their absence can safely allow observation. A negative ultrasound cannot safely rule out intraperitoneal injury, and if hemodynamically normal, patients should undergo a CT scan (Class III, Grade C).

## 38.6 Soft Tissue War Wound Management

### 38.6.1 How Can Large Soft Tissue Injuries from Explosions Be Treated?

The majority of combat wounds are due to fragments from explosives (secondary blast injury). These wounds are grossly contaminated, often carrying clothing and other foreign bodies into the underlying subcutaneous tissues and muscles. Classic war teaching involves debridement, irrigation, and packing all wounds to remain open, requiring multiple painful packing changes and environmental exposure to sand or dust [2]. Leininger et al. [46] in a retrospective review of 77 consecutive patients in Iraq with soft tissue wounds demonstrated that negative-pressure wound therapy (NPWT) had an excellent wound infection and complication rate (0% and 0%) [26]. The wounds were initially irrigated and debrided to remove all gross contamination and subsequently placed in a NPWT (Wound VAC, San Antonio, Texas) with suction set at −125 mmHg. Furthermore, NPWT has also been utilized to facilitate damage control laparotomy as a means to keep the fascia open during resuscitation or aeromedical evacuation.

*Recommendations*: Wound VAC negative-pressure dressings can be used after the initial debridement and irrigation in patients with soft tissue injuries from explosions (Class IV, Grade C).

## 38.7 Combat Vascular Surgery

### 38.7.1 How Is a Major Vessel Injury Treated in an Austere Surgical Environment?

Approximately 60% of combat traumas have major extremity injuries with vascular injury occurring in about 5% [47]. The combat wounded seen at far forward facilities undergo placement of a temporary vascular shunt (TVS) until transfer to a more robust surgical facility. On retrospective reviews, extremity vascular shunts placed in the combat wounded had a patency rate of 78%–95% with no documented amputation due to shunt thrombosis [48]. A review of 125 patients from 2003 to 2007 noted an overall 79% amputation-free survival at 3 years, without significant difference between TVS patients compared to controls. Venous ligation, associated fracture, and penetrating blast mechanisms were associated with higher rates of amputation [49]. Patients with prolonged extremity ischemia should undergo a prophylactic extremity compartment fasciotomy, as delayed fasciotomy is also retrospectively associated with increased mortality and amputation rates [50].

Selective tibial artery revascularization was assessed by Burkhardt et al. noting that the majority of patients (83%) can be successfully managed without formal reconstruction [51]. However, patients with a persistent absence of a Doppler signal and a tolerable ISS are candidates for reconstruction, leading to an overall 79% limb salvage rate. They also noted that a mangled extremity severity score (MESS) greater than five was independently associated with amputation [51].

**TABLE 38.1**

Summary of Evidenced-Based Recommendations

| No. | Question | Answer | Grade | References |
|---|---|---|---|---|
| 1 | What battlefield techniques are available to combat medics to treat potentially preventable deaths? | Tourniquet use for prehospital prevention of exsanguination from significant extremity hemorrhage. | Class III, Grade B | [3,8,10,11] |
| 2 | | A junctional tourniquet should be applied as early as possible in circumstances of appropriate hemorrhage Digital compression and Combat Gauze application can mitigate hemorrhage while preparing the junctional tourniquet. | Class IV, Grade D | [2,11,12] |
| 3 | | Hemostatic dressings should be considered by prehospital personnel if gauze dressing fails to stop bleeding from an injury that is not amenable to tourniquet placement | Class III, Grade C | [11,17–19] |
| 4 | | TXA may be considered as an adjunct to active resuscitation in patients who require a massive transfusion | Class I, Grade B | [20,21] |
| 5 | How should combat-injured patients undergoing a massive blood transfusion be resuscitated? | A Grade B recommendation supports the use of "hypotensive resuscitation," titrating intravenous fluid to a palpable radial pulse or normal mental status (in non-head injured patients). Patients requiring a massive transfusion should receive PRBCs: FFP: PLTs in a 1:1:1 ratio with minimal intravenous crystalloid. In austere environments, the use of warmed FWB is effective for massive transfusion and correction of coagulopathy. | Class II, Grade B | [22–31] |
| 6 | What is the role of FDP in the prehospital environment? | FDP may be used for patients in shock where whole blood or a balanced resuscitation of plasma, RBC, and PLTs is unavailable | Class IV, Grade C | [32,33] |
| 7 | How can hypothermia be avoided during transportation of combat-injured patients? | HPMKs may reduce mortality by preventing hypothermia during extended transport of combat patients. | Class III, Grade B | [6,8,34] |
| 8 | What are the advances in combat burn care? | Burn patients treated at multiple facilities should be resuscitated with the benefit of a burn resuscitation flowsheet. During the critical care portion of burn care, CRRT should be considered in the patient with renal failure from sepsis | Class II, Grade B | [35–39] |
| 9 | How are fragmentation war wounds to the abdomen, flank, and back evaluated? | Patients with multiple fragmentation wounds to the abdomen, flank, and/or back with normal hemodynamics should undergo a CT scan for the evaluation of intraperitoneal fragments. Intraperitoneal fragments mandate surgical exploration, and their absence can safely allow observation. A negative ultrasound cannot safely rule out intra-peritoneal injury, and if hemodynamically normal, patients should undergo a CT scan | Class III, Grade C | [44,45] |
| 10 | How can large soft tissue injuries from explosions be treated? | Wound VAC negative-pressure dressings can be used after the initial debridement and irrigation in patients with soft tissue injuries from explosions | Class IV, Grade C | [2,26] |
| 11 | How is a major vessel injury treated in an austere surgical environment? | Patients with large vessel injury in an austere environment with access to rapid evacuation should have a temporary shunt placed and undergo definitive repair with saphenous vein at the receiving facility. Adequate and timely prophylactic fasciotomies should be performed in patients with prolonged extremity ischemia. Tibial artery injuries should undergo selective repair based on persistent lack of a distal pulse and associated injury factors | Class II, Grade B | [46–50] |

*Recommendation*: Patients with large vessel injury in an austere environment with access to rapid evacuation should have a temporary shunt placed and undergo definitive repair with saphenous vein at the receiving facility. Adequate and timely prophylactic fasciotomies should be performed in patients with prolonged extremity ischemia. Tibial artery injuries should undergo selective repair based on persistent lack of a distal pulse and associated injury factors (Class III, Grade C). A summary of final recommendations is included in Table 38.1.

The opinions or assertions contained herein are the private views of the authors and are not to be construed as official or as reflecting the views of the Department of the Army or the Department of Defense.

## References

1. Champion HR, Bellamy RF, Roberts CP, Leppaniemi A. A profile of combat injury. *J Trauma*. May 2003 [cited 2014 Nov 8]; 54(5 Suppl):S13–S19.
2. Eastridge BJ, Mabry RL, Seguin P et al. Death on the battlefield (2001–2011): Implications for the future of combat casualty care. *J Trauma Acute Care Surg*. December 2012 [cited September 29, 2014];73(6 Suppl 5):S431–S437.
3. Brosch LR, Holcomb JB, Thompson JC, Cordts PR. Establishing a human research protection program in a combatant command. *J Trauma*. Feb 2008 [cited November 8, 2014];64(2 Suppl):S9–S12; discussion S12–S13.
4. Eastridge BJ, Hardin M, Cantrell J et al. Died of wounds on the battlefield: Causation and implications for improving combat casualty care. *J Trauma*. 2011;71:S4–S8.
5. Holcomb JB, McMullin NR, Pearse L et al. Causes of death in U.S. Special Operations Forces in the global war on terrorism: 2001–2004. *Ann Surg*. Jun 2007 [cited November 8, 2014];245(6):986–991.
6. Belmont PJ, McCriskin BJ, Sieg RN, Burks R, Schoenfeld AJ. Combat wounds in Iraq and Afghanistan from 2005 to 2009. *J Trauma Acute Care Surg*. Jul 2012 [cited November 6, 2014];73(1):3–12.
7. Cordts PR, Brosch LA, Holcomb JB. Now and then: Combat casualty care policies for Operation Iraqi Freedom and Operation Enduring Freedom compared with those of Vietnam. *J Trauma*. 2008;64:S14–S20; discussion S20.
8. Blackbourne LH, Baer DG, Eastridge BJ et al. Military medical revolution: Prehospital combat casualty care. *J Trauma Acute Care Surg*. Dec 2012 [cited October 10, 2014];73(6 Suppl 5):S372–S377.
9. Beekley AC, Sebesta JA, Blackbourne LH et al. Prehospital tourniquet use in Operation Iraqi Freedom: Effect on hemorrhage control and outcomes. *J Trauma*. February 2008 [cited November 8, 2014];64(2 Suppl):S28–S37; discussion S37.
10. Walters TJ, Wenke JC, Kauvar DS, McManus JG, Holcomb JB, Baer DG. Effectiveness of self-applied tourniquets in human volunteers. *Prehosp Emerg Care*. October–December 2005 [cited November 8, 2014];9(4):416–422.
11. Bulger EM, Snyder D, Schoelles K et al. An evidence-based prehospital guideline for external hemorrhage control: American College of Surgeons Committee on Trauma. *Prehosp Emerg Care*. 2014 [cited November 8, 2014];18(2):163–173.
12. Kotwal RS, Butler FK, Gross KR et al. Management of Junctional Hemorrhage in Tactical Combat Casualty Care : TCCC Guidelines—Proposed Change 13-03. *J Spec Oper Med*. 2013 Winter;13(4):85–93.
13. Taylor DM, Coleman M, Parker PJ. The evaluation of an abdominal aortic tourniquet for the control of pelvic and lower limb hemorrhage. *Mil Med*. January 2013 [cited November 8, 2014];178(11):1196–201.
14. Lyon M, Shiver S, Greenfield EM et al. Use of a novel abdominal aortic tourniquet to reduce or eliminate flow in the common femoral artery in human subjects. *J Trauma Acute Care Surg*. August 2012 [cited November 8, 2014];73(2 Suppl 1):S103–S105.
15. Croushorn J. Abdominal aortic and junctional tourniquet controls hemorrhage from a gunshot wound of the left groin. *J Spec Oper Med*. January 2014 [cited November 8, 2014];14(2):6–8.
16. Anonymous. Abdominal aortic tourniquet? Use in afghanistan. *J Spec Oper Med*. January 2013 [cited November 8, 2014];13(2):1–2.
17. Pusateri AE, McCarthy SJ, Gregory KW et al. Effect of a chitosan-based hemostatic dressing on blood loss and survival in a model of severe venous hemorrhage and hepatic injury in swine. *J Trauma*. January 2003 [cited November 7, 2014];54(1):177–182.
18. Wedmore I, McManus JG, Pusateri AE, Holcomb JB. A special report on the chitosan-based hemostatic dressing: Experience in current combat operations. *J Trauma*. March 2006 [cited November 7, 2014];60(3):655–658.
19. Bennett B, Littlejohn L. Management of External Hemorrhage in Tactical Combat Casualty Care: Chitosan-Based Hemostatic Gauze Dressings—TCCC Guidelines-Change 13-05. *J Spec Oper Med*. 2014 [cited November 8, 2014];14(3):12–29.
20. Roberts I, Shakur H, Afolabi A et al. The importance of early treatment with tranexamic acid in bleeding trauma patients: An exploratory analysis of the CRASH-2 randomised controlled trial. *Lancet*. 2011;377:1096–1101, 1101, e1–e2.
21. Morrison JJ, Dubose JJ, Rasmussen TE, Midwinter MJ. Military Application of Tranexamic Acid in Trauma Emergency Resuscitation (MATTERs) Study. *Arch Surg*. February 2012 [cited October 13, 2014];147(2):113–119.
22. Blackbourne LH, Baer DG, Eastridge BJ et al. Military medical revolution: Deployed hospital and en route care. *J Trauma Acute Care Surg*. December 2012 [cited October 13, 2014];73(6 Suppl 5):S378–S387.
23. Bickell WH, Wall MJ, Pepe PE et al. Immediate versus delayed fluid resuscitation for hypotensive patients with penetrating torso injuries. *N Engl J Med*. October 1994 [cited November 8, 2014];331(17):1105–1109.
24. Sondeen JL, Coppes VG, Holcomb JB. Blood pressure at which rebleeding occurs after resuscitation in swine with aortic injury. *J Trauma*. May 2003 [cited November 8, 2014];54(5 Suppl):S110–S117.
25. McLaughlin DF, Niles SE, Salinas J et al. A predictive model for massive transfusion in combat casualty patients. *J Trauma*. February 2008 [cited November 8, 2014];64(2 Suppl):S57–S63; discussion S63.
26. Schreiber MA, Perkins J, Kiraly L, Underwood S, Wade C, Holcomb JB. Early predictors of massive transfusion in combat casualties. *J Am Coll Surg*. October 2007 [cited November 8, 2014];205(4):541–545.
27. Holcomb JB, Jenkins D, Rhee P et al. Damage control resuscitation: Directly addressing the early coagulopathy of trauma. *J Trauma*. February 2007 [cited October 7, 2014];62(2):307–310.

28. Borgman MA, Spinella PC, Perkins JG et al. The ratio of blood products transfused affects mortality in patients receiving massive transfusions at a combat support hospital. *J Trauma*. October 2007 [cited October 20, 2014];63(4):805–813.
29. Pidcoke HF, Aden JK, Mora AG et al. Ten-year analysis of transfusion in Operation Iraqi Freedom and Operation Enduring Freedom: Increased plasma and platelet use correlates with improved survival. *J Trauma Acute Care Surg*. December 2012 [cited November 8, 2014];73(6 Suppl 5):S445–S452.
30. Plotkin AJ, Wade CE, Jenkins DH et al. A reduction in clot formation rate and strength assessed by thrombelastography is indicative of transfusion requirements in patients with penetrating injuries. *J Trauma*. February 2008 [cited November 8, 2014];64(2 Suppl):S64–S68.
31. Spinella PC. Warm fresh whole blood transfusion for severe hemorrhage: U.S. military and potential civilian applications. *Crit Care Med*. July 2008 [cited November 8, 2014];36(7 Suppl):S340–S345.
32. Sailliol A, Martinaud C, Cap AP et al. The evolving role of lyophilized plasma in remote damage control resuscitation in the French Armed Forces Health Service. *Transfusion*. January 2013 [cited October 23, 2014];53(Suppl 1):65S–71S.
33. Glassberg E, Nadler R, Gendler S et al. Freeze-dried plasma at the point of injury: From concept to doctrine. *Shock*. December 2013 [cited November 8, 2014];40(6):444–450.
34. Wade CE, Salinas J, Eastridge BJ, McManus JG, Holcomb JB. Admission hypo- or hyperthermia and survival after trauma in civilian and military environments. *Int J Emerg Med*. January 2011 [cited November 30, 2014]; 4(1):35.
35. Ivy ME, Atweh NA, Palmer J, Possenti PP, Pineau M, D'Aiuto M. Intra-abdominal hypertension and abdominal compartment syndrome in burn patients. *J Trauma*. September 2000 [cited November 8, 2014]; 49(3):387–391.
36. Chung KK, Wolf SE, Cancio LC et al. Resuscitation of severely burned military casualties: Fluid begets more fluid. *J Trauma*. August 2009 [cited November 8, 2014];67(2):231–237; discussion 237.
37. Ennis JL, Chung KK, Renz EM et al. Joint Theater Trauma System implementation of burn resuscitation guidelines improves outcomes in severely burned military casualties. *J Trauma*. February 2008 [cited November 4, 2014];64(2 Suppl):S146–S151; discussion S151–S152.
38. Chung KK, Salinas J, Renz EM et al. Simple derivation of the initial fluid rate for the resuscitation of severely burned adult combat casualties: In silico validation of the rule of 10. *J Trauma*. July 2010 [cited October 21, 2014]; 69(Suppl 1):S49–S54.
39. Chung KK, Juncos LA, Wolf SE et al. Continuous renal replacement therapy improves survival in severely burned military casualties with acute kidney injury. *J Trauma*. February 2008 [cited November 8, 2014];64(2 Suppl):S179–S185; discussion S185–S187.
40. Renz EM, Cancio LC, Barillo DJ et al. Long range transport of war-related burn casualties. *J Trauma*. February 2008 [cited November 8, 2014];64(2 Suppl):S136–S144; discussion S144–S145.
41. Ingalls N, Zonies D, Bailey JA et al. A review of the first 10 years of critical care aeromedical transport during operation iraqi freedom and operation enduring freedom: The importance of evacuation timing. *JAMA Surg*. August 2014 [cited November 3, 2014];149(8):807–813.
42. Mabry RL, Apodaca A, Penrod J, Orman JA, Gerhardt RT, Dorlac WC. Impact of critical care-trained flight paramedics on casualty survival during helicopter evacuation in the current war in Afghanistan. *J Trauma Acute Care Surg*. August 2012 [cited November 3, 2014];73(2 Suppl 1):S32–S37.
43. Clarke JE, Davis PR. Medical evacuation and triage of combat casualties in Helmand Province, Afghanistan: October 2010–April 2011. *Mil Med*. November 2012 [cited November 8, 2014];177(11):1261–1266.
44. Kelly JF, Ritenour AE, McLaughlin DF et al. Injury severity and causes of death from Operation Iraqi Freedom and Operation Enduring Freedom: 2003–2004 versus 2006. *J Trauma*. March 2008 [cited September 29, 2014];64(2 Suppl):S21–S26; discussion S26–S27.
45. Beekley AC, Blackbourne LH, Sebesta JA, McMullin N, Mullenix PS, Holcomb JB. Selective nonoperative management of penetrating torso injury from combat fragmentation wounds. *J Trauma*. February 2008 [cited November 8, 2014];64(2 Suppl):S108–S116; discussion S116–S117.
46. Leininger BE, Rasmussen TE, Smith DL et al. Experience with wound VAC and delayed primary closure of contaminated soft tissue injuries in Iraq. *J Trauma*. November 2006;61(5):1207–1211.
47. Clouse WD, Rasmussen TE, Peck MA et al. In-theater management of vascular injury: 2 years of the Balad Vascular Registry. *J Am Coll Surg*. April 2007 [cited November 8, 2014];204(4):625–632.
48. Taller J, Kamdar JP, Greene J et al. Temporary vascular shunts as initial treatment of proximal extremity vascular injuries during combat operations: The new standard of care at Echelon II facilities? *J Trauma*. September 2008 [cited November 8, 2014];65(3):595–603.
49. Gifford SM, Aidinian G, Clouse WD et al. Effect of temporary shunting on extremity vascular injury: An outcome analysis from the Global War on Terror vascular injury initiative. *J Vasc Surg*. September 2009 [cited November 8, 2014];50(3):549–555; discussion 555–556.
50. Ritenour AE, Dorlac WC, Fang R et al. Complications after fasciotomy revision and delayed compartment release in combat patients. *J Trauma*. February 2008 [cited November 7, 2014];64(2 Suppl):S153–S161; discussion S161–S162.
51. Burkhardt GE, Cox M, Clouse WD et al. Outcomes of selective tibial artery repair following combat-related extremity injury. *J Vasc Surg*. July 2010 [cited November 8, 2014];52(1):91–96.

## Commentary on Evidence-Based Surgery: War Wounds

*Donald H. Jenkins*

Management of war wounds is perhaps one of the longest documented surgical management techniques described by humanity dating to 490 BC in artwork in which Achilles applies a battlefield tourniquet to the arm wounds of Patroclus during the Trojan war. It suggests overall that there is nothing new under the sun, but perhaps rediscovered or repurposed techniques/devices or the development of a better mousetrap (not the idea to create a mousetrap, merely improve upon it) is at the core of recent success in military medicine. The authors have done an excellent job in outlining the evidence supporting the care rendered to injured combatants in the latest conflict in southwest Asia and along the continuum of care. This includes tourniquets, fresh whole blood, far forward damage control surgery, hypothermia prevention, negative pressure wound therapy, vascular shunts, and movement of the critically injured combatant with critical care teams out of the theater of operations while still undergoing resuscitation.

### What Battlefield Techniques Are Available to Combat Medics to Treat Potentially Preventable Deaths?

Direct pressure on hemorrhaging wounds is the natural first maneuver undertaken by bystanders or even the patient themselves. The days of cries by the wounded for "medic! medic!" as famously depicted in numerous Hollywood war movies are long gone. The military has invested heavily in training and equipping all of its combatants to achieve self-aid and buddy care at the earliest possible moment following injury.

Tourniquets, reinvented and brought into the inventory during this conflict, were controversial early in the war and, surprisingly, fielded with essentially no evidence to support their efficacy. The evidence came later. This was the first in a series of decisions and actions employing a strategy of "focused empiricism"; a problem with no deployed/accepted solution was investigated and solutions brought to bear based on expert opinion of experienced senior medics. Extremity wound care was transformed by the use of tourniquets. As IEDs became more powerful, extremity wounds gave way to high amputations at the junction with the trunk and new tourniquets were fielded based upon need alone. In both examples, the experts reasoned that extremity tourniquets used in orthopedic operating rooms thousands of time per year without significant morbidity while cardiac catheterization and vascular/radiology suites make use of junctional tourniquets with great success following vascular access in the groin could be adopted/adapted to the battlefield. They were right.

Early versions of hemostatic dressings, some embedded into gauze, others directly applied to the wound were successful but were quickly replaced by a second (and now third) generation of products, which are more conformable to the wound space and more effective.

TXA use is not, today, routinely employed by the combat medic but is employed with increasing frequency by specially trained medics during evacuation from the point of wounding to initial surgical care. This was the only prehospital hemorrhage control technique with Class I evidence to support its use.

Increasingly, the success achieved and evidence gathered with these techniques is resulting in more widespread use in the civilian sector.

### How Should Combat Injured Patients Undergoing a Massive Transfusion Be Resuscitated?

The history of resuscitation, similar to the use of tourniquets, has come full circle. Whole blood was first used to treat injured combatants during WWI and remained the fluid of choice until the end of the Vietnam war. Faced, for the first time in over 40 years, with large combat forces in remote locations days distant from resupply, physicians and surgeons resurrected fresh whole blood transfusion as the standard as it was the only source of plasma in most outposts and the only source of platelets at even the largest combat hospitals for several years. It was a comparative study of components versus whole blood and improved survival that allowed scientists to determine that to replace blood loss in injured combatants in order to achieve the best survival, one should use whole blood or a rough reconstitution of it in a 1:1:1 fashion. This too is being adopted across the civilian trauma community.

### What Is the Role of Freeze-Dried Plasma in the Prehospital Environment?

History repeats itself again. FDP was a standard resuscitation in WWII but fell out of favor during Korea due to the rise of transfusion transmissible disease (hepatitis B). Thankfully, the Germans and French kept this technology in their inventory, improved upon it, and have deployed this, albeit somewhat quietly, since the earliest days of the invasion in Afghanistan and thousands injured in north and central Afghanistan benefitted from this product. Every critical access hospital and long-distance transfer organizations in the United States would change their practices when an FDA-approved product comes to the market.

### How Can Hypothermia Be Avoided during Transportation of Combat Injured Patients?

The very first system-wide trauma management guideline published was on hypothermia prevention and resulted in development of the hypothermia prevention management kit successfully deployed across both theatres in the combat zone. This initiative was a direct result of one of the very first studies done in theater and subsequently published by the 31st Combat Support Hospital, arguably the single medical unit ever deployed in combat zone with the most influence on changing practice (negative pressure wound dressings, hypothermia prevention, whole blood, 1:1 transfusion, damage control resuscitation, study of tourniquets, massive transfusion triggers, practice guideline development, etc.) for the entire theater and conflict. Rightfully proud. This was also the focus of the very first performance improvement effort of the newly formed Joint Theater Trauma System in January 2005.

### What Are the Advances in Combat Burn Care?

The resuscitation of the burned combatant was one of the first DoD wide system guidelines implemented and resulted in one of the largest and most successful injury prevention initiatives ever undertaken during combat operations. Fire retardant flight suits were issued to patrols, vehicles resistant to burning were developed, fuel reconfigured to limit fire risk (the fuel can even be used to put out a fire), fire retardant undergarments manufactured and fielded, and eventually all uniforms manufactured using better fire retardant materials.

### How Are Fragmentation War Wounds to the Abdomen, Flank, and Back Evaluated?

The advent of CT imaging in theater has revolutionized combat casualty care effectively taking the term "austere" right out of the combat casualty care lexicon. Early generations of field deployable scanners were reminiscent of early 1990s technology but have quickly been upgraded and the modern combat hospital resembles a robust urban trauma center. Too numerous to count, unnecessary explorations of the abdomen were avoided by the use of this technology.

### How Can Large Soft Tissue Injuries from Explosions Be Treated?

Repeated wound debridements along echelons of care with application of negative pressure wound therapy in theater and eventually for transcontinental and trans oceanic flights has replaced high amputations and excessive initial debridement with definitive closure after 7 days as described up through the Vietnam war. No longer satisfied with wound salvage, DoD is focusing on long-term quality of injured extremity outcomes. Early use of antibiotics (as early as at the point of injury by the casualty themselves taking their "combat pill pack" of pain killers and antibiotics pioneered by the Tactical Combat Casualty Care group) appears to result in lower wound infection rates; long-term morbidity related to osteomyelitis and nonunion are being evaluated.

### How Is Major Vessel Injury Treated in an Austere Surgical Environment?

Following the principles of civilian damage control surgery developed during the 1980s and 1990s, hemorrhage control while maintaining distal perfusion when possible is the guiding doctrine in vascular injury in theater. Shunts are used at initial operation, including venous shunts where needed and possible, as well as liberal use of prophylactic fasciotomies in extremity wounds. Definitive vascular repair, including venous reconstruction where indicated and possible, in theater with coverage of the graft with healthy tissue is at the core of the practice guideline covering vascular injury management. Torso major vascular injury management today includes a full array of endovascular techniques with a newly designed and deployed endovascular suite that would be the envy of any county trauma center in the country.

In every instance of care addressed in this chapter, movement of the critically injured casualty to the next echelon of care by individuals trained in critical care in an unfriendly (aircraft) and resource limited (if it is not in your pack, there is no way to get it or improvise) environment has likely been the number one reason for the overall success of the system of care. This is an area of military medicine untested prior to this conflict during actual combat operations, especially as it relates to rotary wing transport from far forward locations to combat support hospitals. It is also, to date, one of the most poorly studied and reported upon areas in modern military medicine. As with nearly every other topic discussed, the civilian sector stands to gain benefit from the experience gained in this arena during the recent conflicts.

# 39

# *Evidence-Based Surgery: Pediatric Trauma*

**Erin E. Perrone and Gerald Gollin**

**CONTENTS**



## 39.1 Introduction

Injuries in children are frequently managed in a similar manner as in adults. However, the unique anatomy, physiology, and psychology of children mandate care in the application of evidence obtained from studies of adults to the pediatric population. The following chapter focuses upon five questions in pediatric trauma that are relevant to the daily practice of those who care for injured children.

## 39.2 When Is a CT Scan of the Head Indicated in Pediatric Head Trauma?

There are over 600,000 emergency department visits a year in the United States for head injuries in children 18 years old and younger [1,2]. Among these, 60,000 are hospitalized and about 7,400 die. CT scanning has become an indispensable tool in the identification of significant intracranial injuries in children.

A study of 400 children with a Glasgow Coma Score (GCS) of greater than 12 and a negative CT scan of the head found that only four patients were readmitted with a neurological diagnosis and only one, who was on Coumadin, required craniotomy [3]. Based upon this and similar findings in adults, most clinicians confidently discharge head-injured children with unremarkable CT scan findings. However, a protocol of CT scanning for all pediatric head injuries is neither cost-effective nor safe, considering that one in a thousand CT scans in children may result in a malignancy [4].

Some had believed that a patient with normal mental status and no history of a loss of consciousness is at such a low risk for intracranial injury that a CT scan need not be performed. Simon et al. cast significant doubt on this in a retrospective review of 429 children with head trauma and GCS of 14 or 15 [5]. Among 219 with a GCS of 15 and a reliable history of no loss of consciousness there were 35 intracranial injuries (16%), of which four required operative intervention and one needed intubation. Based upon these findings the authors recommended a policy of "liberal" CT scanning.

Subsequent studies have aimed to more precisely define the population at risk for intracranial injury by expanding the criteria examined beyond mental status and loss of consciousness. Haydel and Shembekar reviewed 175 children between 5 and 17 years of age who had a loss of consciousness but a GCS of 15 and a normal neurological exam [6]. If CT scans had been obtained only in children with at least one of these six conditions: headache, vomiting, intoxication, short-term memory loss, seizure, or physical evidence of trauma above the clavicles, intracranial injuries would have been identified with a sensitivity of 100% (95% CI 73%–100%) and the use of CT scanning would have been reduced by 23%. Generalization of these criteria is limited by a very low confidence limit and the exclusion of children under 5 years of age.

In 2003, a prospective evaluation of 2,043 children with nontrivial head trauma, including 327 under 2 years of age, was published [7]. Head CT scans were done for 1,271 children. Of the 98 who had evidences of brain injury on CT scan, 96 had at least one of the following: abnormal mental status (GCS <15), clinical signs of skull fracture, scalp hematoma (when <2 years old), or a history of vomiting. The sensitivity of an algorithm using these variables to identify patients who require CT scanning was 98% (95% CI = 92.8%–99.8%). In an effort to derive a decision tool to identify those at risk for the more worrisome occurrence of a head injury that requires an intervention, another set of variables (GCS <15, signs of skull fracture, vomiting, and headache) was identified for which the presence of at least one identified these more serious injuries with a sensitivity of 100% (95% CI = 97.2%–100%). Finally, the finding of a focal neurological deficit, GCS <15 and/or vomiting predicted all 29 cases in which a neurosurgical procedure was required, yielding a sensitivity of 100% (95% CI = 90.2%–100%).

The National Emergency X-Radiography Utilization Study II (NEXUS II) was a prospective, multicenter study of adults and children with blunt head trauma that sought to derive a decision tool that could be used to identify patients at risk for intracranial injury who should undergo CT scanning [8]. An algorithm was developed that identified intracranial injuries with a sensitivity of 98.3% (95% CI = 97.2%–99%). Oman et al. evaluated this decision instrument in the subset of 1,666 children in the original study [9]. The NEXUS II decision tool for children included seven variables: clinical evidence of skull fracture, altered alertness, neurological deficit, persistent vomiting, scalp hematoma, abnormal behavior, and coagulopathy. The occurrence of one or more of these variables identified 136 of 138 significant injuries for a sensitivity of 98.6% (95% CI = 94.9%–99.8%). All of the 25 clinically important injuries in children under 3 years were identified, although the confidence interval for this subset was large due to the small population.

The importance of using precision in applying the two decision tools described here was highlighted by Sun et al. [10], who assessed a subtle modification of the criteria described by Palchak et al. [7] with the pediatric subset of the NEXUS II database. By substituting the criteria "severe headache" for "headache" and "high-risk vomiting" for "vomiting," 13 (9%) of patients with clinically important intracranial injuries would not be identified as needing head CT scanning.

In 2006 and 2008, two other large studies developed decision-making algorithms in children with blunt head trauma. Dunning et al. prospectively evaluated 766 children who underwent head CT scan and found that if at least 1 of the 13 conditions were present (including loss of consciousness, seizure, and evidence of basilar skull fracture) patients with an intracranial injury could be identified with a sensitivity of 98% (95% CI = 96%–100%) [11]. The four missed injuries included two depressed skull fractures and one case that required craniotomy.

Atabaki et al. evaluated an eight-component decision tool (including evidence of basilar skull fracture, age under 2 years, and dizziness) in 1,000 children with GCS >13 [12]. The sensitivity of this algorithm was 95.4% (95% CI = 86.2%–98.8%). None of the potentially missed injuries required neurosurgical intervention.

To add further support to limiting routine head CT scan in children, a 2009 multi-institutional prospective cohort study of over 40,000 children enrolled with GCS 14–15 was done [2]. The authors identified prediction rules for children with low risk of clinically significant traumatic brain injuries in which CT scans could be avoided. For children less than 2 years of age, a head CT scan is not indicated if they have normal mental status, no scalp hematoma except frontal, no loss of consciousness or loss of consciousness for less than 5 s, nonsevere injury mechanism, no palpable skull fracture, and acting normally according to parents. These criteria had 100% sensitivity and no child with a clinically significant head injury was missed. For children aged 2 years and older, a head CT scan was not needed if they had normal mental status, no loss of consciousness, no vomiting, nonsevere injury mechanism, no signs of basilar skull fracture, and no severe headache. These criteria had a 96.8% sensitivity in predicting clinically significant head injuries. Two children in this group were classified as low risk but did have clinically significant head injury (subdural hematoma and occipital lobe contusion); neither child required neurosurgical intervention.

*Recommendation*: A Grade B recommendation can be made for using the decision tools described in the NEXUS II study, by Palchak et al., or prediction rules, as described by Kuppermann et al., in determining which children with head trauma require a head CT scan. No protocol of selective CT scanning will ever identify every intracranial injury. Ultimately, decision making must weigh how many and what missed injuries are justified by the prevention of a radiation-induced malignancy or the saving of several million dollars.

## 39.3 Is There a Role for Hypertonic Saline in Pediatric Head Injuries?

Head injuries result in direct and indirect costs of 56 billion dollars [13]. Apart from prevention, the devastating impact of childhood injury can only be reduced by advancements in treatment.

Intracranial hypertension accompanies serious brain injury and is contributed to by multiple factors. The initial injury may result in hemorrhage in the subdural, epidural, and/or subarachnoid space thereby increasing the volume within the rigid cranial vault.

The secondary response to injury is characterized by the development of edema due to alterations in cerebral blood flow, ischemia, and ultimately cellular necrosis. The resultant inflammatory response, while beneficial for healing, leads to further edema and a continuing cycle of ischemia, necrosis, and inflammation. If this scenario is not controlled, herniation and global cerebral ischemia ensue.

The cornerstone of management of brain injury in children and adults is the prevention of intracranial hypertension and the maintenance of cerebral perfusion pressure (CPP) through medical and operative interventions. Depending upon the neurological examination and the intracranial pressure (ICP) and CPP, interventions such as elevation of the head of the bed, prevention of hyperthermia, and sedation may progress to mechanical ventilation with mild hyperventilation, chemical paralysis, administration of a hyperosmolar solution, barbiturate coma, and decompressive craniotomy.

The role of hyperosmolar agents in reducing experimental cerebral edema has been known for almost a century [14]. In the early 1960s mannitol began to be used in patients with head injury [15], but its efficacy in adults and children remains unclear [16,17]. In that context, this discussion focuses on the question of whether the administration of hypertonic saline is a safe and effective adjunct to other, more traditional, means of controlling ICP dynamics in children.

Each of the studies that have been performed assessing hypertonic saline in pediatric head trauma have limited numbers of subjects and unique protocols and none have directly compared hypertonic saline to mannitol.

In 1992, Fisher performed a double-blind, crossover study in 18 children with traumatic brain injury that assessed the short-term efficacy of 3% saline in reducing ICP as compared to normal (0.9%) saline (NS) [18]. Each child received a bolus of each fluid after which ICP was followed for 2 h. On average, after administration of NS, ICP changed minimally from 19.3 to 20.0 mmHg. In contrast, after a bolus of 3% saline ICP decreased from 19.9 to 15.8 mmHg ($p = 0.003$). After hypertonic saline infusion there was a reduced requirement for additional interventions to control ICP.

A randomized controlled trial that compared the efficacy of hypertonic saline to lactated Ringer's solution (LR) was carried out in 35 children with GCS <8 [19]. Subjects received either 1.75% saline, with an aim of increasing serum sodium to 145–150 meq/L, or LR for 72 h. The group treated with hypertonic saline required fewer interventions to maintain an ICP less than 15 mmHg ($p < 0.02$), had shorter ICU stays ($p = 0.04$), and a lower incidence of acute respiratory distress syndrome (ARDS) ($p = 0.01$) and other complications than the group that received LR.

Khanna et al. reported a prospective trial of 3% saline in 10 children with traumatic brain injury in 2000 [20]. In this study hypertonic saline was continuously infused and titrated to maintain ICP less than 20 mmHg when other measures failed. More patients were not enrolled because standard measures, including mannitol, sedation, and hyperventilation, were usually successful in lowering ICP. The elevation in serum sodium concentration was limited to 15 meq/L/day. At the start of therapy the mean ICP of the subjects was 26 mmHg. A statistically significant inverse correlation between serum sodium and ICP was demonstrated. Beyond 72 h, the frequency of ICP spikes decreased ($p < 0.01$) and CPP increased ($p < 0.01$). Reversible renal failure developed in two of the subjects. One patient, who presented 2 days after nonaccidental trauma, died.

A retrospective study of 68 children with intracranial hypertension treated with hypertonic saline was published in 2000 [21]. In this series 3% saline was used as rescue therapy in a similar manner as in Khanna's study when mannitol, hyperventilation, and other measures failed to maintain ICP less than 20 mmHg. The mean serum sodium in these cases was 160 meq/L. Mortality was 15% and was less than what would be expected based upon injury severity. Two deaths were due to cerebral edema, five were as a consequence of sepsis and multisystem organ failure, and one was from ARDS. Seventy-four percent of patients had complete recovery or only moderate neurological deficits and 11% had severe deficits. When serum sodium exceeded 180 meq/L only one of four patients survived and that subject had severe neurological deficits. Two theoretical complications of hypertonic saline administration, central pontine myelinolysis, and subarachnoid hemorrhage due to rapid brain shrinkage, did not occur in any subjects.

Guidelines for use of hyperosmolar therapy were published in 2003 and again in 2012 [16,22]. A weak recommendation based on the studies listed here is given for hypertonic saline therapy in pediatric traumatic brain injury. The recommended dosing for 3% saline ranges between 0.1 and 1.0 mL/kg/h administered on a sliding scale to maintain ICP <20 mmHg. Further recommendation was given to maintain serum osmolarity <360 mOsm/L.

The use of hypertonic saline has expanded to patients with mild traumatic brain injury. In 2014, Lumba-Brown et al. reported a randomized controlled trial that compared the use of a 3% saline bolus to a normal saline bolus for concussive pain [23]. This study enrolled 44 pediatric patients and used a self-reported pain score at pretreatment, 1 h posttreatment, and after 2–3 days with a follow-up phone call. Subjects given 3% saline had a greater degree of improvement in their pain scale scores at 1 h posttreatment (mean improvement 3.5 with 3% saline vs. 1.1 in the NS group, $p < 0.001$). This improvement in pain scores was also seen after 2–3 days with the 3% saline group having a mean improvement of 4.61 and the NS group having a mean improvement of 3 ($p = 0.01$).

*Recommendation*: Only a Grade C recommendation can be made for the use of hypertonic saline to reduce ICP in children. Although it is listed as one of the recommended acute therapies of severe traumatic brain injury, its efficacy in lowering the incidence of mortality or severe neurological morbidity is not well supported. Expanded use of hypertonic saline for reducing pain in mild traumatic brain injury has promise but requires further evaluation.

## 39.4 When Is Clinical Clearance of the Cervical Spine Appropriate in Children?

Cervical spine injuries are diagnosed in 1%–2% of cases of pediatric trauma [24,25]. As compared to adult trauma patients, the incidence of cervical spine injury in the pediatric trauma population is much lower. In children with pain and tenderness of the cervical spine or neurological deficits it is imperative that imaging studies be obtained and interpreted carefully by a radiologist with pediatric expertise. The unique bony anatomy of the developing spine can lead to overdiagnosis of injuries and ligamentous laxity can result in a spinal cord injury without radiological abnormality (SCIWORA), in which plain films and even CT scans may show no evidence of a dangerous spinal instability. In pediatric trauma victims with no obvious signs or symptoms of injury to the cervical spine clinicians must balance the risk of a potentially disastrous missed injury against the cost and radiation exposure of universal imaging.

The concept of "clinical clearance" of the cervical spine has evolved over the last 20 years. In an effort to reduce the time and expense of cervical spine imaging in trauma patients investigators have worked to define the circumstances under which imaging may be omitted without resultant missed injuries. Early studies in adults [26] suggested that as many as 20% of cervical spine injuries would be missed with protocols of selective imaging based on a lack of neck pain and mechanism of injury.

Velmahos et al. [27] refined the selection criteria used to determine eligibility for a clinical clearance protocol in a prospective study of trauma victims without neck pain by eliminating cases in which patients were intoxicated and had otherwise an altered level of consciousness, a subset that accounted for most of the missed injuries in previous reports. They identified 549 cases in which there was no neck tenderness with palpation or active motion. Patients with distracting injuries and head/facial injuries were included in subgroup analysis. Of these 549 cases there were no cervical spine injuries identified by imaging studies. However, this cohort included only 18 patients less than 10 years of age.

A large, prospective, multicenter study evaluated the efficacy of the NEXUS decision instrument for cervical spine imaging in 31,000 trauma victims without neck pain or neurological deficit [28]. A substudy by Vicello et al. [29] focused on 3,065 patients younger than 18 years of age. There were 2,160 patients between age 9 and 17, 817 between age 2 and 8 and 88 less than 2 years of age. About 20% of the 3,065 cases evaluated were deemed "low risk," based upon a lack of pain or midline tenderness, alertness, no neurological deficit, and no "painful distracting injury." In none of these cases was there a cervical spine injury. Thirty patients (0.98%) who did not satisfy low risk criteria had cervical spine injuries. However, even this large study is not definitive evidence for the safety of clinical cervical spine clearance in children. This study found no cases of SCIWORA, only four injuries in children under 9 years of age, and none in those under two, making interpretation particularly difficult in the younger child. While the sensitivity of the NEXUS instrument for the identification of cervical spine injury in children was 100%, due to the low incidence of injury in this population, the lower limit of the 95% confidence interval for sensitivity was only 88%. In order to achieve a confidence interval for sensitivity of only 0.5%, a study of 80,000 children would be required.

Garton and Hammer [30] retrospectively reviewed the 20-year experience with cervical spine injury in children at a single institution. This study included 190 children with cervical spine injury, many more than in the study of Vicello. The sensitivity of the NEXUS criteria for injury was 100% in those 8 years of age and older, but 2 of the 33 patients under 8 years of age (6 and 18 months old) were found to have cervical spine injuries despite fulfilling "low risk" NEXUS criteria.

Pieretti-Vanmarcke et al. [31] retrospectively reviewed 12,537 patients younger than 3 years of age at 22 trauma centers. The incidence of cervical spine injury was 0.66%. They identified four simple clinical predictors of cervical spine injury, giving a weighted score to each: GCS <14 (3 points), $GCS_{EYE} = 1$ (2 points), MVC (2 points), and age ≥2 years (1 point). This was labeled PEDSPINE and a score of 0–1 had a negative predictive value of 99.9% for cervical spine injury with a sensitivity of 92.9% and specificity of 69.9%. They identified 8707 patients who had scores of 0–1 and suggested that cervical spine clearance could be achieved without further imaging based upon clinical exam. Five patients were reported as outliers, with scores <2 and with a clinically important cervical spine injury. These patients all presented with physical findings of head and neck injury and underwent CT scanning with timely identification of cervical spine injury.

*Recommendation*: A Grade B recommendation may be made for clinical clearance of the cervical spine in teens and preteens using the NEXUS criteria, based upon the available pediatric studies and more abundant adult data. In all children under 8 years of age who fulfill the NEXUS criteria, due to the infrequency of injury, the relative paucity of data, and the variability in patients' ability to focus during a neck examination, more clinical judgment is necessary. A clinical scoring system (PEDSPINE) for children under 3 years of age has been done but requires further validation.

## 39.5 How Should Femur Fractures Be Managed in Children?

Femur fractures occur relatively frequently in the multiply injured pediatric patient [32] and it is in that context that most trauma surgeons encounter this condition. Expedient and effective treatment is imperative for a good long-term outcome. The options for management of femur fractures depend mostly on the age of the patient, the type of fracture and fractures, or the presence of other relevant injuries.

Most pediatric orthopedic surgeons agree that for the majority of fractures in children under 5 years of age the most appropriate management is traction and spica cast placement [33]. For the mature adolescent, intramedullary nailing is usually best [34] except in the case of very proximal or distal fractures, extensive soft tissue injury, gross comminution, or significant contamination [33,35]. The optimal management of children between 5 years and 16 years is more controversial [36] and is the subject of this section.

Multiple case series have documented successful experience with traction and spica cast application, external fixation, compression plating, and internal fixation with either rigid or flexible intramedullary nails. However, due to a paucity of randomized controlled trials and a tremendous heterogeneity of clinical material in the available studies, a 2001 evidence-based working group of pediatric orthopedic surgeons was unable to reach consensus as to the optimal care for children with femur fracture [36].

Comparative assessment of the management options for femur fracture must address the short- and long-term anatomical and psychosocial outcomes as well as the potential complications inherent to specific treatment methods, such as pressure ulceration with spica casting, pin infections with external fixation, and migration of intramedullary nails and the necessity for their removal. Differences in the definitions used by authors to determine adequate initial reduction or malunion can make the comparison of results difficult. Interpretation of even the most well-powered, randomized studies requires weighing of the significance of these "apples and oranges" of outcomes.

One of the largest reports of a consecutive series of external fixation of femur fractures studied 96 children between 3 and 15 [37]. In this population, there was an average hospital stay of 8.7 days and fixators were removed at an average of 61 days. There were 2 refractures (6%) and 36 pin tract infections (37%). Although external fixation comes with increased complications over internal fixation or spica casting, it remains an option for femoral shaft fracture fixation when the patient presents with length-unstable fractures, metadiaphyseal fracture location, pathologic fractures, or refractures [38].

Hip spica application was compared to external fixation for the treatment of femur fracture in a multicenter, randomized, controlled trial published in 2005 [39]. In this study of children between 4 and 10 years of age, 60 were randomized to hip spica and 48 to external fixation. In the hip spica group, the mean duration of initial hospitalization (3.4 vs. 5.3 days, $p = 0.01$), total hospitalization (4.1 vs. 5.9 days, $p = 0.02$) and overall treatment (58 vs. 77 days, $p = 0.01$) was significantly less than for those treated with external fixation. Malunions, including leg length discrepancies and excessive angulations occurred in 45% of the patients managed with hip spica but in only 16% of the external fixator group ($p = 0.002$) The clinical significance of this difference is unclear as assessment concluded at 2 years and the potential to remodel in this age group is significant. However, permanent gait abnormalities can result from substantial malunions. Pin site infections occurred in 45% of those treated with external fixation. No pressure ulcers or other direct complications of spica casting were reported. Psychosocial assessment outcomes were similar in the two groups.

Despite similar rates of patient and child satisfaction with the two treatments, these results suggest a trade-off between a shorter treatment duration with hip spica versus a lower rate of malunion with external fixation.

A large, consecutive series of 52 children between 5 and 14 years of age who were treated with intramedullary nailing demonstrated excellent outcomes [40]. The average hospital stay for those with isolated injuries was 3 days and full weight bearing was achieved within 30 days. There were good functional results and only minor complications.

A prospective, nonrandomized, cohort study published in 2004 compared traction followed by hip spica application to treatment with elastic, titanium nails in children between 6 and 16 years of age with diaphyseal femur fractures [35]. Skeletal traction and spica cast application was used in 35 patients and titanium nails in 49. All fractures healed and only three (8.5%) of those treated with traction and spica casting had malunions at the time of healing. The group treated with titanium elastic nails had significantly shorter times to discharge (5 vs. 24 days, $p < 0.0001$), walking unaided (14 vs. 70 days, $p < 0.0001$), and returning to school (48 vs. 103 days, $p < 0.0001$). Although operative costs for the traction/spica were less, they were made up for by the cost of longer hospitalization yielding similar total costs for the two groups. An outcome questionnaire showed a trend toward better functional outcome at 6 months in the group managed with the titanium elastic nail but this was equivalent after a year. Complications among the patients treated with traction and spica casting occurred in 34% that included malunion (3), loss of reduction (2), refracture (2), and pressure ulceration (4). In the titanium nail group, 21% of the patients sustained complications, including irritation at the nail entry site (8), refracture after early nail removal (1), and bending of the nail after a fall (1). There were no malunions with titanium nailing.

Though this study was limited by a lack of randomization, long-term follow-up, and insufficient functional assessment, it demonstrated a faster recovery with the use of titanium elastic nails compared to traction and spica cast application. Overall costs were comparable and the incident rate of complications was similar.

In 2013, Prata do Nascimento et al. retrospectively reviewed 30 children treated with titanium elastic nails and 30 children treated with plaster casts [41]. In the surgical patients, they reported a decreased length of hospital stay (9.4 vs. 20.5 days) and decreased time to return to activities (3.7 vs. 9.5 weeks). Patients in the surgical group also had significantly less shortening (6.7% vs. 63.3%) with mean shortening 0.25 vs. 1.14 cm. In the same year, a subsequent study by Sela et al. reviewed 212 children treated with different modalities (spica cast, skin traction, titanium elastic nail, external fixator, intramedullary nail, or plating) [42]. They reported more complications (contact dermatitis and loss of reduction requiring remanipulation) and greater limb length discrepancy in the spica casting group when compared to all other treatment modalities.

In 2014, Crosby et al. reported their experience with 241 patients in a 12-year period treated with intramedullary nailing of femoral shaft fractures in children aged 8–17 years [43]. The complication rate was 9.8% (24 patients) that included 11 patients with heterotopic ossification, 3 delayed unions, 3 malunions, 3 interlocking screw migrations, 2 asymptomatic coxa valga, 1 deep tissue infection, and 1 malrotation. There were no reports of femoral head osteonecrosis.

*Recommendation*: Based upon the available evidence, a Grade B recommendation may be made for intramedullary nailing in most children with femur fractures between 5 and 15 years of age who lack the exclusion criteria discussed previously. If performed by an experienced surgeon, this treatment would reduce hospital stay and time to return to school, minimize early complications and psychosocial impact and optimize long-term anatomical and functional outcome at a cost comparable to other methods.

## 39.6 How Should Blunt Pancreatic Injury Be Managed in Children?

Pancreatic injuries are rare in children, occurring in only 0.3%–0.7% of trauma admissions [44–46]; however, they are present in 3%–12% of children sustaining blunt abdominal trauma [47,48]. As with other solid organs, the severity of pancreatic trauma is based upon the extent and location of injury [49]. Grade I and II injuries are minor and major contusions, respectively. Distal transections and duct injuries are classified as Grade III, proximal transactions are Grade IV, and massive disruptions of the pancreatic head are Grade V. It is generally accepted that most Grade I and II injuries are initially best managed nonoperatively [44,46,50]. Grade V injuries are often devastating due to duodenal and biliary involvement and frequently necessitate laparotomy.

Diagnosis of pancreatic injuries requires a high index of suspicion in patients sustaining blunt abdominal trauma. Serum amylase and lipase elevations are seen in pancreatic injuries, however the values do not correlate with the grade of injury, LOS, or mortality [51]. The values can be used as a screening tool and confirm pancreatic injury on CT, magnetic resonance cholangiopancreatography, and/or endoscopic retrograde cholangiopancreatography (ERCP). There is limited value in repeated amylase and lipase levels.

For children with pancreatic transections that do not involve the duodenum or bile duct (Grade II and III injuries) there are several initial management strategies that have been advocated and used with success including

(1) expectant management, (2) early ERCP and ductal stenting, and (3) distal pancreatectomy [52,53]. Due to the infrequent occurrence of pancreatic transection there are no level 1 and limited level 2 data on which to base management. Determinations of what constitutes best practice for pediatric pancreatic transection must be made from consecutive case series and multi-institutional reviews.

In 1998, The Hospital for Sick Children in Toronto reported the outcome of nonoperative management of 35 children who sustained pancreatic injuries, including 11 cases of transection [47]. Only 5 of these 11 patients with transections developed pseudocysts. No operative intervention was required in any, although percutaneous drainage was performed in four children. The average length of stay (LOS) was 25 days and less for those that did not develop a pseudocyst. A subsequent study from the same institution focused on nine cases managed nonoperatively [54]. Long-term follow up (47 months) revealed complete healing of the gland in 25% of patients and body/tail atrophy in 75% of patients. None of the patients suffered endocrine or exocrine dysfunction.

Initial experiences with ductal stenting in children was in the form of case reports [52, 55] in which three cases with good outcomes were presented. In the largest series of ductal stenting, 12 children with presumed pancreatic transection underwent ERCP [56]. In 11 cases, a ductal injury was identified and an attempt was made to place a stent. Stents were technically feasible in nine cases. Three of these stents were advanced beyond the site of injury and six were placed via the pancreatic duct into a pseudocyst. In two cases an endoscopic cyst-gastrostomy was subsequently performed and in another, percutaneous cyst drainage was required. The remaining stented patients required no further interventions. Average LOS for the children who received stents was 27 days (3–51 days). If the cases in which a percutaneous or cyst-enteric drainage was not required, the LOS was 18 days.

Multiple studies support the use of early operative intervention (less than 48–72 h) when operative intervention is chosen [44,57]. In 1999, the Children's Hospital of Pittsburgh documented early operative management of pancreatic injury, usually a distal pancreatectomy, resulted in a median LOS of 11.5 days [58]. LOS was substantially longer after delayed diagnosis or failed nonoperative management.

In 2009, Wood et al. compared nonoperative vs. operative management of pancreatic injuries in children admitted to a single institution [59]. Although median LOS increased with worsening pancreatic injury grade, there was no significant difference in LOS or readmission rates in patients with Grade II–IV injuries. Nonoperative management, however, was associated with an increased incidence of pancreatic complications (pancreatic pseudocyst, leak, or fistula). These complications were identified in 73% of patients treated nonoperatively as opposed to 21% of the patients treated with pancreatic resection.

Recently multi-institutional collaborations have led to better evaluation of treatment choice. In 2011, Paul and Mooney collected data on 131 children with rade II or III injuries from nine different level 1 pediatric trauma centers [60]. Nonoperative management was associated with a higher rate of pseudocyst formation and an increased use of total parenteral nutrition (TPN) although LOS was similar. In 2013, Beres et al. reviewed 39 patients with Grade III or IV pancreatic injuries from two level 1 pediatric trauma centers [61]. Nonoperative management was associated with increased LOS (mean 27.5 vs. 15 days), increased days on TPN (21.8 vs. 7.9), and more complications, most commonly pseudocyst formation.

The largest multi-institutional collaboration to date is on behalf of the Pancreatic Trauma in Children (PATCH) Study Group and included 14 pediatric trauma centers with evaluation of 167 patients with Grade II and III blunt pancreatic injuries [48]. Patients treated nonoperatively had a higher rate of pseudocyst formation (18% vs. 0%) and increased requirement for endoscopic or interventional radiologic procedures to manage them. Patients treated with operative resection had shorter times to initial (4.5 vs. 8.9 days) and goal (7.8 vs. 15.1 days) feedings with a corresponding decreased use of parenteral nutrition. Subset analysis was performed in patients with evidence of main pancreatic duct injury (Grade III) and the results were even more compelling. For patients with Grade III injuries, 44% developed a pseudocyst with an even longer delay of initial (12.7 days) and goal (26.1 days) enteral feedings. These patients also had a significantly increased LOS when compared to those undergoing operative resection (17.5 vs. 12.6 days) (Table 39.1).

*Recommendation*: A Grade B recommendation can be made regarding pancreatic blunt trauma in children. (1) If a distal pancreatectomy is performed in the first 48–72 h after injury, a LOS of 11–16 days, on average, could be predicted. (2) When there is a delay in diagnosis and pancreatectomy is undertaken after 3 days, the LOS and morbidity may be substantially greater. (3) LOS with initial nonoperative management and selective, percutaneous or cyst-enteric drainage of resultant pseudocysts may result in an average LOS as low as 14 days, although hospitalizations of many months and TPN-related complications will occur in some cases. (4) Blunt pancreatic injury with main duct involvement (Grade III) is best managed with operative resection.

**TABLE 39.1**

Summary of References Including Study Design, Findings, and Level of Evidence

| Author | Reference | Year | Level of Evidence | Groups | Design | Median Follow-up | End-Point |
|---|---|---|---|---|---|---|---|
| Palchak | [7] | 2003 | 2b | Brain injury on CT scan, no brain injury on CT scan | PCS | NR | Prediction of brain injury by CT decision tool |
| Oman | [9] | 2006 | 2b | Brain injury on CT scan, no brain injury on CT scan | PCS | NR | Prediction of brain injury by CT decision tool |
| Dunning | [11] | 2006 | 2b | Brain injury on CT scan, no brain injury on CT scan | PCS | NR | Prediction of brain injury by CT decision tool |
| Kuppermann | [2] | 2009 | 2b | Brain injury on CT scan, no brain injury on CT scan | PCS | 1 week–3 months | Prediction of brain injury by CT decision tool |
| Fisher | [18] | 1992 | 2b | 3% saline, normal saline | RCT | 2 h | ICP change |
| Simma | [19] | 1998 | 2b | Lactated Ringer's, normal saline | RCT | NR | ICP, CPP, hospital and ICU stay, survival |
| Khanna | [20] | 2000 | 4 | 3% saline | CS | 72 h | ICP spike frequency, serum sodium, renal failure |
| Peterson | [21] | 2000 | 4 | 3% saline | CS | NR | ICP, renal failure |
| Lumba-Brown | [23] | 2014 | 2b | 3% saline | RCT | 3 days | Self-reported pain improvement |
| Vicello | [29] | 2001 | 2b | Low risk for cervical spine injury, high risk for injury | PCS | NR | Cervical spine injury |
| Garton | [30] | 2008 | 2b | Low risk for cervical spine injury, high risk for injury | RCS | NR | Cervical spine injury |
| Pieretti-Vanmarcke | [31] | 2009 | 2b | Low risk for cervical spine injury, high risk for injury | RCS | NR | Cervical spine injury |
| Cramer | [40] | 2000 | 4 | Intramedullary rod | CS | NR | Malunion, rotation, leg length discrepancy, hospital stay, time to weight bearing |
| Flynn | [35] | 2004 | 2b | Traction/hip spica, intramedullary rod | PCS | 1 year | Malunion, refracture, pressure ulcer, hospital stay, return to school |
| Prata do Nascimento | [41] | 2013 | 2b | Intramedullary rod vs. nonoperative management | RCS | 24–59 months | Time to weight bearing, LOS, shortening |
| Sela | [42] | 2013 | 2b | Surgical treatment vs. nonoperative management | RCS | 12 months | Overall complications, leg length discrepency |
| Keller | [46] | 1997 | 4 | Early diagnosis and operation, late diagnosis | RCS | 12 months–12 years | Hospital stay, pseudocyst development |
| Shilyansky | [47] | 1998 | 4 | Nonoperative management | CS | 10 months | Time to enteral feeding, hospital stay, pseudocyst development |
| Nadler | [58] | 1999 | 4 | Early diagnosis and operation, late diagnosis | RCS | NR | Hospital stay, morbidity |
| Meier | [44] | 2001 | 4 | Distal pancreatectomy, observation | CS | NR | Hospital stay, pseudocyst development |
| Wales | [54] | 2001 | 4 | Nonoperative management | CS | 47 months | Time to enteral feeding, hospital stay, pseudocyst development, endocrine/exocrine dysfunction |
| Houben | [56] | 2007 | 4 | Pancreatic ductal stenting | CS | 2 years | Time to enteral feeding, hospital stay, requirement for cyst-enterostomy |
| Wood | [59] | 2010 | 2b | Nonoperative and operative management | RCS | NR | Hospital stay, readmission rates, pancreatic complications |
| Paul | [60] | 2011 | 2b | Nonoperative and operative management | RCS | NR | Time to enteral feeding, hospital stay, pseudocyst development |
| Beres | [61] | 2013 | 2b | Nonoperative and operative management | RCS | NR | Time to enteral feeding, hospital stay, pancreatic complications |
| Iqbal | [48] | 2013 | 2b | Nonoperative and operative management | RCS | NR | Time to enteral feeding, hospital stay, pancreatic complications |

*Abbreviations:* CS, case series; RCT, randomized controlled trial; PCS, prospective cohort study; RCS, retrospective cohort study; NR, not reported.

## References

### CT Scan in Head Injury


1. Langlois JA, Rutland-Brown W, Thomas KE. 2006. Traumatic brain injury in the United States: Emergency department visits, hospitalizations, and deaths. Centers for Disease Control and Prevention, Nation Center for Injury Prevention and Control: Atlanta, GA.
2. Kuppermann N, Holmes JF, Dayan PS et al. Identification of children at very low risk of clinically important brain injuries after head trauma: A prospective cohort study. *Lancet*. 2009;374:1160–1170.
3. Davis RL, Hughes M, Gubler KD et al. The use of cranial CT scans in the triage of pediatric patients with mild head injury. *Pediatrics*. 1995;95:345–349.
4. Brenner DJ, Elliston CD, Hall EJ et al. Estimated risks of radiation induced fatal cancer from pediatric CT. *AJR*. 2001;176:289–296.
5. Simon B, Letorunean P, Vitorino E et al. Pediatric minor head trauma: Indications for computed tomographic scanning revisited. *J Trauma*. 2001;51:231–238.
6. Haydel MJ, Shembekar AD. Prediction of intracranial injury in children aged five years and older with loss of consciousness after minor head injury due to nontrivial mechanisms. *Ann Emerg Med*. 2003;42:507–514.
7. Palchak MJ, Holmes JF, Vance CW et al. A decision rule for identifying children at low risk for brain injuries after blunt head trauma. *Ann Emerg Med*. 2003;42:492–506.
8. Mower WR, Hoffman JR, Herbert M et al. for the NEXUS II Investigators: National Emergency X-Radiology Utilization Study. Developing a clinical decision instrument to rule out intracranial injuries in patients with minor head trauma: Methodology of the NEXUS II investigation. *Ann Emerg Med*. 2002;40:505–514.
9. Oman JA, Cooper RJ, Holmes JF et al. for the NEXUS II investigators: Performance of a decision rule to predict need for computed tomography among children with blunt head trauma. *Pediatrics*. 2006;117:e238–e246.
10. Sun BC, Hoffman JR, Mower WR. Evaluation of a modified prediction instrument to identify significant pediatric intracranial injury after blunt head trauma. *Ann Emerg Med*. 2007;49:325–332.
11. Dunning J, Daly JP, Lomas J-P et al. Derivation of the children's head injury algorithm for the prediction of important clinical events decision rule for head injury in children. *Arch Dis Child*. 2006;91:885–891.
12. Atabaki, SM, Stiell IG, Bazarian JJ et al. A clinical decision rule for cranial computed tomography in minor pediatric head trauma. *Arch Pediatr Adolesc Med*. 2008;162:439–445.


### Hypertonic Saline in Head Injury


13. Thurman D. 2001. The epidemiology and economics of head trauma. In: Miller L, Hayes R (eds.), *Head Trauma Basic, Preclinical and Clinical Directions*. Wiley & Sons: New York.
14. Weed LH, Mc Kibben PS. Pressure changes in the cerebro-spinal fluid following intravenous injection of solutions of various concentrations. *Am J Physiol*. 1919;48:512–530.
15. Wise BL, Chater N. Use of hyperosmolar mannitol solutions to lower cerebrospinal fluid pressure and decrease brain bulk in man. *Surg Forum*. 1961;12:398–399.
16. Adelson PD, Bratton SL, Carney NA et al. Guidelines for the acute medical management of severe traumatic brain injury in infants, children, and adolescents. Chapter 11. Use of hyperosmolar therapy in the management of severe pediatric traumatic brain injury. *Pediatr Crit Care Med*. 2003;4(3 Suppl):S40–S44.
17. Wakai A, Roberts I, Schierhout G. Mannitol for acute traumatic brain injury. *Cochrane Database Syst Rev*. 2005;(4):CD001049.
18. Fisher B, Thomas D, Peterson B. Hypertonic saline lowers raised intracranial pressure in children after head trauma. *J Neurosurg Anesth*. 1992;4:4–10.
19. Simma B, Burger R, Falk M et al. A prospective, randomized, and controlled study of fluid management in children with severe head injury: Lactated Ringer's solution versus hypertonic saline. *Crit Care Med*. 1998;26:1265–1270.
20. Khanna S, Davis D, Petersoon B et al. Use of hypertonic saline in the treatment of severe refractory posttraumatic intracranial hypertension in pediatric traumatic brain injury. *Crit Care Med*. 2000;28:1144–1151.
21. Peterson B, Khanna S, Fisher B et al. Prolonged hypernatremia controls elevated intracranial pressure in head-injured pediatric patients. *Crit Care Med*. 2000;28:1136–1143.
22. Kochanek PM, Carney N, Adelson PD et al. Guidelines for the acute medical management of severe traumatic brain injury in infants, children, and adolescents—Second Edition. *Pediatr Crit Care Med*. 2012;13(1):S36–S41.
23. Lumba-Brown A, Harley J, Lucio S et al. Hypertonic saline as a therapy for pediatric concussive pain: A randomized controlled trial of symptom treatment in the emergency department. *Pediatr Emerg Care*. 2014;30:139–145.


### Clinical Clearance of the Cervical Spine


24. Brown RL, Brunn MA, Garcia VF. Cervical spine injuries in children: A review of 103 patients treated consecutively at a level 1 pediatric trauma center. *J Pediatr Surg*. 2001;36:1107–1114.
25. Leonard JR, Jaffe DM, Kuppermann N et al. Cervical spine injury patterns in children. *Pediatrics*. 2014;133(5):e1179–e1188.
26. Jacobs LM, Schwartz R. Prospective analysis of acute cervical spine injury: A methodology to predict injury. *Ann Emerg Med*. 1986;15:44–49.
27. Velmahos GC, Theodorou D, Tatevossion R et al. Radiographic cervical spine evaluation in the alert asymptomatic blunt trauma victim: Much ado about nothing? *J Trauma*. 1996;40:768–774.

28. Hoffman JR, Mower WR, Wolfson AB et al. Validity of a set of clinical criteria to rule out injury to the cervical spine in patients with blunt trauma. National Emergency X-Radiography Utilization Study Group. *N Engl J Med.* 2000;343:94–99.
29. Vicello P, Simon H, Pressman BD et al. A prospective multicenter study of cervical spine injury in children. *Pediatrics.* 2001;108:e20.
30. Garton HJ, Hammer MR. Detection of pediatric cervical spine injury. *Neurosurgery.* 2008;62:700–708.
31. Pieretti-Vanmarcke R, Velmahos GC, Nance ML et al. Clinical clearance of the cervical spine in blunt trauma patients younger than 3 years: A multi-center study of the American Association for the Surgery of Trauma. *J Trauma.* 2009;67(3):543–550.


## Femur Fracture Management


32. Jawandi AH, Letta M. Injuries associated with fracture of the femur secondary to motor vehicle accidents in children. *Am J Orthop.* 2003;32:459–462.
33. Kuremsky MA, Frick SL. Advances in surgical management of pediatric femoral shaft fractures. *Curr Opin Pediatr.* 2007;19(1):51–57.
34. Reeves RB, Ballard RI, Hughes JL. Internal fixation versus traction and casting of adolescent femoral shaft fractures. *J Pediatr Orthop.* 1995;15:457–460.
35. Flynn JM, Luedtke LM, Canley TJ et al. Comparison of titanium elastic nails with traction and a spica cast to treat femoral fractures in children. *J Bone Joint Surg Am.* 2004;86:770–777.
36. Saunders JO, Browne RH, Mooney JF et al. Treatment of femoral fractures in children by pediatric orthopedists: Results of a 1998 survey. *J Pediatr Orthop.* 2001;21:436–441.
37. Hedin H, Hjorth K, Rehnberg L et al. External fixation of displaced femoral shaft fractures in children: A consecutive study of 98 fractures. *J Orthoped Trauma.* 2003;17:250–256.
38. Kong H, Sabharwal S. External fixation for closed pediatric femoral shaft fractures: Where are we now? *Clin Orthop Relat Res.* 2014;472(12):3814–3822.
39. Wright JG, Wang EEL, Owen JL et al. Treatments for paediatric femoral fractures: A randomized trial. *Lancet.* 2005;365:1153–1158.
40. Cramer KE, Tornetta P, Spero CR et al. Ender rod fixation of femoral shaft fractures in children. *Clin Ortho.* 2000;376:119–123.
41. Prata do Nascimento F, Santili C, Akkari M et al. Flexible intramedullary nails with traction versus plaster cast for treating femoral shaft fractures in children: Comparative retrospective study. *Sao Paulo Med J.* 2013;131(1):5–12.
42. Sela Y, Hershkovich O, Sher-Lurie N et al. Pediatric femoral shaft fractures: Treatment strategies according to age—13 years of experience in one medical center. *J Orthop Surg Res.* 2013;8:23.
43. Crosby SN, Kim EJ, Koehler DM et al. Twenty-year experience with rigid intramedullary nailing of femoral shaft fractures in skeletally immature patients. *J Bone Joint Surg Am.* 2014;96:1080–1090.


## Pancreatic Transection


44. Meier DE, Coln CD, Hicks BA et al. Early operation in children with pancreas transection. *J Pediatr Surg.* 2001;36:341–344.
45. Jobst MA, Canty TG, Lynch FP. Management of pancreatic injury in pediatric blunt abdominal trauma. *J Pediatr Surg.* 1999;34:818–823.
46. Keller MS, Stafford PW, Vand DW. Conservative management of pancreatic trauma in children. *J Trauma.* 1997;42:1097–1100.
47. Shilyansky J, Sena LM, Kreller M et al. Nonoperative management of pancreatic injuries in children. *J Pediatr Surg.* 1998;33:343–349.
48. Iqbal CW, St Peter SD, Tsao K et al. Operative vs nonoperative management for blunt pancreatic transection in children: Multi-institutional outcomes. *J Am Coll Surg.* 2014;218(2):157–162.
49. Moore EE, Cogbill TH, Malangoni MA et al. Organ injury scaling II: Pancreas, duodenum, small bowel, colon and rectum. *J Trauma* 1990;30:1427–1429.
50. Graham CA, O'Tolle SJ, Watson AJ et al. Pancreatic trauma in Scottish children. *JR Coll Surg Edinb.* 2000;45:223–226.
51. Herman R, Guire KE, Burd RS et al. Utility of amylase and lipase as predictors of grade of injury or outcomes in pediatric patients with pancreatic trauma. *J Pediatr Surg.* 2011;46:923–926.
52. Canty TG, Weinman D. Treatment of pancreatic duct disruption in children by an endoscopically placed stent. *J Pediatr Surg.* 2001;36:345–348.
53. Rescorla FJ, Plumley DA, Sherman S et al. The efficacy of early ERCP in pediatric pancreatic trauma. *J Pediatr Surg.* 1995;30:336–240.
54. Wales PW, Shuckett B, Kim PCW. Long-term outcome after nonoperative management of complete traumatic pancreatic transection in children. *J Pediatr Surg.* 2001;36:823–827.
55. Cay A, Mustafa I, Bektas O et al. Nonoperative treatment of traumatic pancreatic duct disruption in children with an endoscopically placed stent. *J Pediatr Surg.* 2005;40:e9–e12.
56. Houben CH, Niyi AA, Patel S et al. Traumatic pancreatic duct injury in children: Minimally invasive approach to management. *J Pediatr Surg.* 2007;42:629–635.
57. Snajdauf J, Rygl M, Kalousova J et al. Surgical management of major pancreatic injury in children. *Eur J Pediatr Surg.* 2007;17:317–321.
58. Nadler EP, Gardner M, Schall LC et al. Management of blunt pancreatic injury in children. *J Trauma.* 1999;47:1098–1103.
59. Wood JH, Partrick DA, Bruny JL et al. Operative vs nonoperative management of blunt pancreatic trauma in children. *J Pediatr Surg.* 2010;45:401–406.
60. Paul MD, Mooney DP. The management of pancreatic injuries in children: Operate or observe. *J Pediatr Surg.* 2011;46:1140–1143.
61. Beres AL, Wales PW, Christison-Lagay ER et al. Nonoperative management of high-grade pancreatic trauma: Is it worth the wait? *J Pediatr Surg.* 2013;48:1060–1064.

## Commentary on Evidence-Based Surgery: Pediatric Trauma

*Michael P. Hirsh and Jonathan Green*

In my 30 years of pediatric surgery practice, I have witnessed the evolution of pediatric traumatology as a branch of both trauma care and pediatric surgical practice. Under the influence of giants in pediatric surgical care, such as Drs. Izant, Haller, Ramenofsky, Eichelberger, Koop, Templeton, O'Neill, and Barlow, it was recognized that pediatric trauma victims were not just smaller versions of their adult counterparts. Their unique anatomy and physiology dictated alternative approaches to the "trauma ABC's." It was also recognized that above 95% of pediatric trauma was predictable, hence preventable. We began to discard the term accidents from the pediatric trauma vernacular[*,†,‡,§,¶,**,††].

Initially, our pediatric trauma education efforts attempted to highlight the differences between kids and adults, and this inevitably led to trauma providers unfamiliar with pediatrics to lose their comfort level with their care and to regard pediatric trauma victims as "of another species." Pediatric traumatologists needed to swing the pendulum back to encourage adult trauma care providers both in the prehospital arena and in trauma centers that the priorities of airway, breathing, and circulation were still the same, just the ways of securing them slightly altered by the size, anatomy, and physiology of the kids.

Now there is robust regionalization of pediatric trauma care with rigorous accreditation of pediatric trauma centers by the American College of Surgeons and various state trauma accrediting bodies. The truth remains that only about 40% of pediatric trauma patients nationwide are cared for in pediatric hospitals. Thus, the wide dissemination of basic pediatric trauma resuscitation and care techniques is vitally important to optimize excellent outcomes. Additionally, the continuum of trauma care for children, from prehospital to rehabilitation hospitals, has been recognized as an important element for these improved outcomes. Though the national pediatric trauma mortality rate is less than 2%, for every pediatric trauma death, there are scores admitted to pediatric trauma centers, hundreds seen in the emergency rooms and thousands of children injured yearly overall. No pediatric trauma program can now be fully accredited without efforts with its own injury prevention program, as prevention education is the vaccination for this scourge of epidemic proportions.

This chapter and its reviewers summarize five of the key areas of pediatric trauma that have a unique care algorithm in the pediatric population.

### When Is a CT Scan of the Head Indicated in Pediatric Head Trauma?

I feel that the NEXUS criteria are good identifiers. If any are present and their mechanism of injury fits with concern for severe head trauma, these patients are more inclined to receive a head CT scan. However, the value of admission, with observation and serial neurologic exams, cannot be overlooked. This allows time for us to reassess the patient and put together the sequence of events of the injury. It also gives us the opportunity to investigate the social issues and family dynamics of our pediatric (especially nonverbal) patients to make sure that the mechanism of injury correlates with the patient's actual injuries. Sometimes however, we do not have the luxury of admitting all of these patients due to hospital geography or need for timely disposition of these patients, which will lead to a CT scan of the head in case of some problem. We must keep in mind that a lot of the radiation burden of CT scanning has made it into the lay literature and informed parents are driving whether or not a CT scan is done[‡‡]. We need to be prepared for both why we would proceed or not with CT scanning. It is important to note that even with the most inclusive criteria, we will still miss pediatric head injuries and that we must rely on our clinical judgment to make the ultimate determination for radiographic evaluation of our patients.

*Additional empirical criteria are the CATCH Criteria that I find helpful:

High risk: failure to reach score of 15 on the Glasgow coma scale within 2 h, suspicion of open skull fracture, worsening headache, and irritability

* Izant RJ, Hubay CA. The annual injury of 15,000,000 children: A limited study of childhood accidental injury and death. *J Trauma.* 1966;6:65–74.

† Haller JA Jr. Newer concepts in emergency care of children with major injuries. *Pediatrics.* 1973 October;52(4):485–487.

‡ Ramenofsky ML, Ramenofsky MB, Jurkovich GJ, Threadgill D, Dierking BH, Powell RW. The predictive validity of the Pediatric Trauma Score. *J Trauma.* 1988 July;28(7):1038–1042.

§ Eichelberger MR, Randolph JG. Progress in pediatric trauma. *World J Surg.* 1985 April;9(2):222–235.

¶ Garcia V, Eichelberger M, Ziegler M, Templeton JM, Koop CE. Use of military antishock trouser in a child. *J Pediatr Surg.* 1981 August;16(4 Suppl. 1):544–546.

** Barlow B, Niemirska M, Gandhi RP. Ten years' experience with pediatric gunshot wounds. *J Pediatr Surg.* 1982 December;17(6):927–932.

†† O'Neill JA. Advances in the management of pediatric trauma. *Am J Surg.* 2000 November;180(5):365–369.

‡‡ Wall, B. European Community Radiation Protection Report 118. National Radiological Protection Board, Chilton, U.K.

Low risk: Boggy hematoma of the scalp; signs of basal skull fracture; dangerous mechanism of injury*

### Is There a Role for Hypertonic Saline in Pediatric Head Injuries?

I would agree with the chapter's assessment that the data referring to hypertonic saline administration in children has been less than compelling. There have been recent studies (in publication Falman et al. of Cincinnati Children's) that have shown that overexuberant use of hypertonic saline in traumatic brain injury patients has resulted in increased ventilatory days, prolonged ICU stays,and complications including DVTs. With these factors in mind, the use of hypertonic saline in TBI patients has not demonstrated significant benefit in our pediatric patients unlike their adult counterparts. We must also take into account the inability of immature kidneys to clear sodium effectively, which can result in large serum sodium shifts, predisposing pediatric patients to seizures. Perhaps, the efficacy of hypertonic saline might benefit adolescent patients whose physiology is closer to that of an adult.

### When Is Clinical Clearance of the Cervical Spine Appropriate in Children?

In children with verbal skills, the incidence of cervical spine injury without complaints of neck pain, neurological deficit, distracting injury, or unreliable mental status exam is exceedingly low. This is consistent with the NEXUS guidelines. My concern is elevated in patients who are less than 3 years of age. Their large head mass, weak neck musculature, and developing spine predispose them to increased risk of cervical spine injury. Patients in this age group are more predisposed to spinal cord injury without radiographic abnormality (SCIWORA), although the risk is still quite low. Because the radiation burden in the neck is even higher than the head, the concern of subsequent development of thyroid neoplasia is a real one. In a cooperative child, the standard 3 view C-spine plain film evaluation is a very effective tool. In the head-injured child, who is already going to receive a CT scan of the brain, we have found that extending the scan to the level of C-2, coupled with a lateral C-spine down to C7-T1, allows us to examine the odontoid process and clear up to 95% of our patients. This eliminates the excess radiation from a traditional formal CT C-Spine.

### How Should Femur Fractures Be Managed in Children?

In patients who are not mobile or under 5 years of age, a spica cast can be effective in treating femoral fractures. Significantly, this reduces the risk of anesthesia complications and possible surgical infection. However, with concern for combined intra-abdominal/pelvic trauma, coordination needs to be obtained to allow for an intra-abdominal window for on-going abdominal evaluation. Patients, who are aged 5–15 years and more mobile, benefit from intramedullary nail fixation of femoral fractures. The use of a flexible intramedullary nail allows for growth of the child with great fixation of the fracture. In multitrauma, having a patient undergo anesthesia and a intramedullary nail fixation of the femur can cloud further neurologic or abdominal examinations. This must be taken into account with pediatric patients who have combined neurologic and musculoskeletal injuries.

### How Should Blunt Pancreatic Injury Be Managed in Children?

There is an overarching trend of less invasive treatment and management. Only documentation of a total ductal disruption, location of pancreatic injury, or a duodenal injury leads to surgical intervention (pancreatic injuries class III–V). Advancements of ERCP and interventional radiology have limited operative intervention in patients with minor pancreatic duct leaks or pancreatic pseudocysts. Also of note are complications of parenteral nutrition. The data in this chapter support the concept that distal pancreatic ductal injury should be managed with distal pancreatectomy instead of allowing them to fester with pseudocyst or other necrotizing complications. These procedures should be performed earlier rather than later to prevent prolonged hospitalizations and necrotizing pancreatitis.

* Osmand, M. et al. CATCH: A clinical decision rule for the use of computed tomography in children with minor head injury. *Can Med Assoc J*. February 2010;182(4):341–348.

# 40

## *Evidence-Based Approach to Geriatric Trauma*

**Juliet J. Ray and Carl I. Schulman**

**CONTENTS**



### 40.1 Introduction

Geriatric trauma is becoming an increasingly important facet of trauma care. The projected population in 2050 of those aged 65 years and over is 83.7 million, which is almost double that in 2012 [1]. As of 2010, trauma is the fifth leading cause of death in all age groups and the ninth leading cause for those 65 years and older (2.3% of deaths in this cohort) [2]. Perhaps even more important is the added influence of comorbid conditions in this age group. Aging data from 2010 reflect the high percentage of people 65 and over with selected chronic health conditions, such as heart disease (30.4%), hypertension (55.9%), stroke (8.6%), cancer (24.0%), and diabetes (20.%)[3]. Apart from specific health concerns, the elderly are plagued by unique social and economic challenges. For example, elder abuse has become a recognized health threat and screening for abuse should be considered in the aging trauma population.

The definition of "geriatric" is the subject of much controversy, as the absolute age of the patient may not be the most important factor in defining the population of older adults who require specialized care. Rather, a combination of factors including chronological age, physiological age, and the presence of preexisting conditions play a role. The most commonly used age cutoff for elderly or geriatric patients is 65 years. There are, however, some data to suggest that those even as young as 45 years old may have poorer outcomes than their younger counterparts, and that those greater than 75 years old may be at especially high risk [4,5]. It is important to be able to identify those at increased risk, while recognizing that the studies used to make clinical decisions are based on various definitions of the "geriatric" trauma patient.

### 40.2 Are There Any Patient Characteristics, Circumstances, or Premorbid Conditions Known to Increase Morbidity/Mortality or Require Specialized Care?

There is a preponderance of evidence to suggest that elderly trauma patients have a higher level of injury-related mortality than their younger counterparts. The presence of preexisting conditions (PEC) contributes to this increased risk of death and is greatest in patients with the least severe injuries, with a lesser effect on those with moderate injuries [6,7]. In addition, this increased risk of death varies according to the type and number of preexisting conditions. The concept of "physiologic age" is often used as a surrogate for the presence of preexisting conditions. Examination of hospital discharge data for trauma patients in the state of California found that preexisting conditions were important predictive factors of mortality, independent of age [5,7]. A similar study of 8000 trauma patients demonstrated a threefold increase in mortality in patients with preexisting conditions, compared to those without preexisting conditions [8].

A review of a state trauma database with over 30,000 records over a 13-year period showed an overall mortality of 7.6% with an increase of 6.8% for each year over age 65. The presence of preexisting conditions was found to have an independent effect on mortality after controlling for initial vital signs, Glasgow Coma Scale (GCS) score and Injury Severity Score (ISS). The strongest effects were seen for hepatic disease (odds ratio 5:1), renal disease (odds ratio 3:1), and cancer (odds ratio 1:8). In this study, warfarin therapy was not an independent predictor of mortality [9].

Preinjury functional status has also been shown to be predictive of postinjury mortality. A study of elderly patients with lateral compression pelvic type 1 fractures showed that patients who were nonfunctional ambulators were five times more likely to die within 1 year of injury [10]. Due to the complex interplay between the geriatric patient's preexisting conditions and often poor preinjury functional status, trauma outcomes may be negatively affected.

*Effect of preexisting conditions on outcome in geriatric trauma patients*

*Level of evidence*: 3

*Strength of recommendation*: C

*Recommendation*: The current evidence, although all retrospective, points to worse outcomes for geriatric patients with preexisting chronic disease. Preinjury functional status is an important consideration. There are no recommendations, however, for how this information can be used to improve outcomes.

## 40.3 What Is the Impact on Treatment and Outcome for Patients with Medication-Induced Coagulopathy?

The use of anticoagulation in the elderly is increasing and is an important consideration in the trauma population, especially in the setting of traumatic brain injury. A survey of 75 trauma surgeons shows that variability exists in the practice patterns of coagulopathy correction, indicating that physician preference plays a role in treatment thresholds [11]. Pieracci found that in patients with a therapeutic INR (≥2), there was an increased odds of intracranial hemorrhage (OR = 2.59, 95% CI 0.92–7.32, $p = 0.07$) and overall mortality (OR = 4.48, 95% CI 1.60–12.50, $p = 0.004$) [12]. Warfarin use in the absence of a therapeutic INR was not associated with adverse outcomes. Another retrospective review confirmed increased mortality in those >70 years old if on oral anticoagulants and that both mortality and ICH were increased with increasing INR (INR over 4.0 had mortality 50%, risk of ICH 75%) [13]. A small series found those >55 years with warfarin use had more severe injuries and a higher mortality [14]. A prospective study of 159 patients with a mean age of 75 ± 13 years compared to age-matched historical controls demonstrated no increased risk of fatal hemorrhagic complications in the absence of head trauma. When intracranial injury was present, those taking warfarin had a statistically higher mortality rate [15]. This is contrasted by two older retrospective reviews of large registries suggesting no adverse impact on mortality or length of stay [16,17].

Less is known regarding management of patients on aspirin or plavix in geriatric trauma. Small retrospective studies show that preinjury use of antiplatelet agents is associated with increased mortality after traumatic intracranial hemorrhage [18,19]. A study of geriatric patients requiring surgical repair for hip fractures showed that patients on clopidogrel were at increased risk of requiring blood transfusions [20]. A review of 350 patients on anticoagulants and prescription antiplatelets (ACAP) showed that anticoagulant users were more likely to have progression of intracranial hemorrhage (aRRR = 3.23; 95% CI, 1.21–8.62; $p = 0.02$) and that antiplatelet users were more likely to die in the hospital (HR = 3.09; 95% CI, 1.03–9.23; $p = 0.04$) compared with non-ACAP patients [21]. There is limited data, however, regarding the impact of correcting iatrogenic platelet dysfunction.

The new anticoagulants, dabigatran (a direct thrombin inhibitor), rivaroxaban, and apixaban (both factor Xa inhibitors), present additional challenges for the trauma surgeon. Coagulopathy due to these agents cannot be fully assessed with the coagulation assays that are routinely used. Specialized tests such as thrombin clotting time or ecarin clotting time for dabigatran and anti-Xa assays for the factor Xa inhibitors may not be readily available, and practitioner's knowledge of how to interpret these results may be limited. Importantly, there are no direct reversal agents. At this time there are no evidence-based guidelines for the management of trauma patients taking these medications although delay of nonemergent surgeries for minor trauma is recommended when feasible [22].

*Impact on treatment and outcome for geriatric trauma patients with medication-induced coagulopathy*

*Level of evidence*: 3

*Strength of recommendation*: C

*Recommendation*: Geriatric patients with warfarin use, elevated INR, or antiplatelet use and intracranial hemorrhage have worse outcomes. Patients receiving warfarin with post-traumatic intracranial hemorrhage should receive therapy to correct INR within 2 h of admission [23]. There are no distinct recommendations for correcting platelet dysfunction in injured patients. As there are no reversal agents for the new anticoagulants, nonemergent surgery should be delayed when possible.

## 40.4 What Is the Impact on Treatment and Outcome for Patients on Beta-Blockers, and When Should They Be Used?

This issue is certainly not limited to the geriatric trauma patient, but surprisingly there are few studies on beta-blocker use in trauma patients. A retrospective review of adult trauma victims found that the odds ratio for fatal outcome was 0.3 ($p < 0.001$) for the cohort using beta-blockers compared to controls and was more pronounced in patients with a significant head injury. They concluded beta-blocker therapy is safe and may be beneficial in selected trauma patients with or without head injury [24]. However, a study of geriatric patients in particular found that preinjury beta-blockade had a significant association with mortality (OR 2.1, 95% CI 1.1–4.3) [25].

Bone marrow dysfunction is a known phenomenon after severe trauma that can lead to persistent anemia. Beta-blockers have been considered as an adjunctive treatment modality during the resuscitation stage of management to help mediate this response. A prospective randomized pilot trial of 45 patients was performed to evaluate the effect of propranolol treatment to decrease heart rate by 10%–20% postinjury. They found that treatment safely mediated surrogate measures of bone marrow function by reducing hematopoietic progenitor cell mobilization and resulted in a faster return to baseline of the peak in granulocyte colony-stimulating factor [26]. Larger clinical trials regarding the role of beta-blockers for therapeutic hematologic benefit are needed.

*Impact on treatment and outcome for patients on beta-blockers*

*Level of evidence*: 3

*Strength of recommendation*: C

*Recommendation*: No specific recommendation can be made as to the effect of pre-hospital use of beta-blockers on physiologic response or outcomes in the geriatric trauma patient. Beta-blockade may show promise as an adjunctive treatment strategy in the severely injured patient to reduce bone marrow dysfunction post injury.

## 40.5 What Are the Risk Factors for Elder Abuse and the Common Patterns of Injury to Be Recognized by the Trauma Provider?

Elder abuse can be divided into five subtypes, of which physical abuse is one. A review evaluating 838 injuries showed the most common anatomic distribution of injuries as follows: upper extremity, 43.98%; maxillofacial, dental, and neck, 22.88%; skull and brain, 12.28%; lower extremity, 10.61%; and torso, 10.25% [27]. One case–control study showed that victims of elder abuse, which resulted in traumatic injury, were more likely to have more severe injuries than controls with higher mean ISS and case fatality [28]. They also were more likely to require ICU admission and mechanical ventilation. In this study, the perpetrator was most often the spouse/partner or child, and the most common types of injuries were open wounds. To our knowledge, no studies have evaluated screening techniques for abuse in the geriatric trauma population.

*Impact on treatment and outcome for patients on elder abuse*

*Level of evidence*: 3

*Strength of recommendation*: D

*Recommendation*: Elder abuse is a significant cause of trauma in the geriatric population resulting most often in injury to the upper extremities and maxillofacial regions.

## 40.6 What Are the Optimal Triage Guidelines for the Geriatric Trauma Patient?

Triage is the process of sorting patients based on their need for immediate medical treatment as compared to their chance of benefiting from such care. Triage attempts to maximize patient benefit based on available resources. "Resources for Optimal Care of the Injured Patient 2014" from the American College of Surgeons Committee on Trauma recommends patients greater than 55 years old be considered for transport to a trauma center [29]. The reality, however, is that elderly trauma patients are less likely to be triaged to a trauma center. Several studies have documented that undertriage is much more common in patients over the age of 55 and even worse for those over 65 [30,31].

A retrospective cohort study looked at the implementation of a specific geriatric triage criteria compared to adult triage criteria. Modifications to the standard criteria included "consideration of systolic blood pressure less than 100 mmHg, any abnormality in GCS, fracture of any long bone in a motor vehicle crash, injury to two or more body regions, pedestrian struck by motor vehicle, and any fall with evidence of traumatic brain injury" [32]. The use of geriatric specific trauma criteria significantly improved sensitivity in identifying ISS and other surrogate markers of the need for trauma center care [32]. Nevertheless, no specific geriatric trauma criteria have been widely adopted. Only with better recognition of the importance of identifying severe injury in elderly patients can triage be improved by prehospital and hospital providers.

The most common scoring systems (RTS, GCS, APACHE, etc.), along with more basic measures, such as initial blood pressure, respiratory rate, and base deficit, have been shown to correlate with outcome in the geriatric population. The Trauma Score (TS) may be the most useful in the prehospital and early hospital setting as a triage tool. It varies from 0 to 16 and contains blood pressure, respiratory rate, respiratory effort, GCS, and capillary refill. Several studies have documented the correlation between the TS (or Revised Trauma Score) and mortality in the geriatric population. A case-matched review of 100 elderly patients showed that no patient hospitalized with severe injuries survived with a TS <9 and no elderly patients with a TS <7 survived to reach the hospital [33]. Another study confirmed this 100% mortality with a TS <7 [34]. These population-based studies may provide some guidance when counseling families about the expected outcomes and making end-of-life decisions, but they cannot be directly translated to individual patients.

ISS is a good predictor of survival in most trauma populations, including the elderly cohort. A systematic review with a pooled sample size of 65,897 patients showed a higher rate of mortality in geriatric patients with ISS of >16. In fact, their likelihood of death was 10 times that of those with a score <16. Furthermore, geriatric patients with a score >24 had a 50 times higher likelihood of death [35]. Unfortunately, the delay in obtaining the data required to calculate the ISS makes it not useful as a triage tool. The basic physiologic variables contained in the TS are the only available alternatives. None of these markers, however, is specific enough to make decisions on definitive care, although they may provide some guidance for direction of future research efforts in this area.

*Optimal triage guidelines for the geriatric trauma patient*
*Level of evidence*: 3
*Strength of recommendation*: C

*Recommendation*: There is insufficient evidence to make any conclusions on the optimal triage guidelines for the geriatric trauma patient. The current recommendations from the American College of Surgeons Committee on Trauma will remain the standard until further studies are performed.

## 40.7 What Are the Optimal Strategies for Resuscitation and Monitoring of the Geriatric Trauma Patient?

Geriatric trauma patients are more likely to present in shock than younger patients matched for trauma and ISS [36]. It is unclear, however, which geriatric patients will benefit from more aggressive resuscitation and invasive monitoring. This decision may be more difficult due to the coexistence of underlying disease in the geriatric population.

A prospective study of elderly patients (>65 years of age) who presented with predefined criteria attempted to help answer these questions. The criteria were a pedestrian-motor vehicle mechanism, initial BP less than 150 mmHg, acidosis, multiple fractures, and head injuries. Patients meeting these criteria were treated with invasive hemodynamic monitoring including a pulmonary artery catheter and moved to the intensive care unit as soon as possible to optimize hemodynamic parameters including cardiac index and oxygen consumption. The ability to optimize cardiac output and systemic vascular resistance was greater in survivors compared to nonsurvivors. Occult shock was found in 13 of 30 (43%) of patients, despite being hemodynamically stable upon initial presentation. Mortality was high in these patients (54%) [37]. This underscores the fact that geriatric trauma patients with significant underlying physiologic abnormalities may be difficult to identify early in the course of treatment and may be at greater risk for mortality.

A prospective cohort study sought to determine whether implementing a geriatric resuscitation protocol using lactate-guided therapy was associated with lower mortality through the early recognition of occult hypoperfusion [38]. All individuals 65 and older with admission venous lactate >2.5 had ATLS resuscitation initiated. Occult hypoperfusion was seen in 20.5% of the participants based on lactate level and a significant decrease in mortality was observed over time in this group [38].

A prospective study compared the responses of old (≥65 years old) and young (<65 years old) trauma patients resuscitated using a standardized protocol to attain and maintain an oxygen delivery index of 600 mL/min/m$^2$ or greater ($DO_2I \pm 600$) for the first 24 h in the intensive care unit. Inclusion criteria were designed to select patients at high risk of postinjury multiple organ failure and included major organ or vascular injury and/or skeletal fractures, initial base deficit of 6 mEq/L or greater, need for 6 units or more of packed red blood cells in the first 12 h, or age of 65 years or older with any two previous criteria. The clinical endpoint was a $DO_2I \geq 600$ using a pulmonary artery catheter, infusion of crystalloid solutions, transfusion of packed red blood cells, and moderate inotropic support as needed in that sequence. A total of 12 old patients and 54 young patients were resuscitated according to the protocol. For old patients, 9 (75%) attained $DO_2I \geq 600$, and 11 (92%) survived 7 or more days and 5 (42%) 30 or more days. For young patients, 45 (83%) attained the $DO_2I$ goal, and 48 (89%) survived 30 or more days. Outcomes were worse for the elderly cohort but they concluded resuscitation is not futile [39]. This study is limited by the lack of a control group of elderly patients who were not resuscitated with the study protocol.

A retrospective review by Mitra et al. revealed that of 311 patients who received a massive transfusion, 51 (16.4%) were over the age of 65. In this group there were 20 (39.2%) deaths, which was significantly higher than the 21.1% of deaths among the younger cohort. However, the volume of red cells transfused was not associated with increased mortality. The authors conclude, therefore, that a restrictive transfusion practice based on age alone is not supported [40].

The only randomized trial of resuscitation in geriatric trauma patients was in hip fracture patients. They compared monitoring with the use of a pulmonary artery catheter to a standard central venous catheter. A significant increase in mortality was noted in the non-monitored group (29% vs. 2.9%) [41]. Unfortunately, the study did not include the polytrauma patient, and the exact protocol by which patients were optimized with the use of the PA catheter is not clear. Additionally, this study was performed in 1995, before the current era of more modern critical care, with less reliance on invasive monitoring and the more recent literature showing no benefit to the use of a PA catheter in most situations.

The precise cohort of patients in need of aggressive resuscitation and monitoring has yet to be determined. A trauma score <15, a base deficit of −6 or worse, or the presence of shock (SBP <90) have all been associated with worse outcomes and may help identify patients who would benefit from aggressive resuscitation [34,42–44]. The Eastern Association for the Surgery of Trauma practice management guidelines support the use of base deficit of −6 mEq/L or less for consideration of ICU admission [23]. The geriatric trauma patient may exhibit subtle or no signs of shock so that a heightened level of suspicion is required at all times while assessing and treating these patient.

*Optimal strategies for resuscitation and monitoring of the geriatric trauma patient*

*Level of evidence*: 2

*Strength of recommendation*: B

*Recommendation*: It appears that aggressive therapy and monitoring improves outcomes in a very select subset of geriatric trauma patients. Identifying these patients and the exact intervention remains in need of further high quality studies. Lactate levels provide better insight into the perfusion status of geriatric trauma patients. Geriatric resuscitation protocols that use lactate are in use at various institutions and should be considered. Restrictive resuscitation in the elderly is not supported.

## 40.8 Are There Any Injury-Prevention Programs That Have Been Shown to Work for Geriatric Patients?

The ultimate ability to influence outcome lies in the reduction of injuries. Injury prevention has proven to be successful for a wide variety of traumatic injuries. Since the majority of elderly injuries result from falls, this has been the most studied area. Many methods and programs already exist and have been proven effective in elderly populations. Some examples include regular exercise, supplementation of vitamin D and calcium, withdrawal of psychotropic medication, cataract surgery, professional assessment and modification of environmental hazards, hip protectors, and multifactorial prevention programs [45]. Walking devices in theory are used to maintain balance and decrease falls; however, they may actually contribute to this risk. One study showed that the injury risk was 3.1 per 100 users of four-wheeled walkers in all those >65. This number increased to 6.2 per 100 users in the subset of women >85 [46]. It is worthwhile for the trauma surgeon to be aware of elderly injury prevention programs and serve as a source of information, referral, and perhaps even program implementation in high-need, underserved areas.

As there are many studies that have shown a decrease in the rate of falls, few have focused on the actual decrease of fractures. A prospective study with a 10-year follow-up showed that a program of back-strengthening exercises for 2 years reduced the risk of spine fractures by more than 60% [47]. A larger randomized trial showed that impact exercise in 72–74 year old women reduced fracture risk by over 60% [48]. This is coupled with numerous other population-based studies confirming these effects [45].

An interesting approach worth mentioning is the use of hip protectors. Many studies of their use, including a recent review of randomized trials, suggested a benefit and a cost savings for those at high risk, such as nursing home or institutionalized patients [49].

*Injury-prevention programs that have been shown to work for geriatric patients*

*Level of evidence*: 1

*Strength of recommendation*: A

*Recommendation*: Based on an overwhelming amount of population-based data (not all presented here), regular strength and balance exercises are effective at preventing falls and injuries in elderly people. Hip protectors can be considered in high-risk groups. Walkers, although often used in those with balance deficits, may actually contribute to fall risk in the elderly.

## 40.9 Are There Any Circumstances Where Withholding/Withdrawing Care Is Appropriate?

The combination of age, injury severity, and underlying disease makes even the most advanced modern medical care futile for certain patients. This, however, is a very individualized decision. Some patients and families might consider a 1% chance of any type of survival (i.e., even a poor functional outcome) acceptable and desire all possible medical efforts. Patients who cannot reasonably be expected to maintain their quality of life as the result of severe injuries may not wish to continue with possible life-saving treatment. While no prospective trial will ever be done to definitively identify the criteria by which care should be withheld, there are several studies attempting to provide some insight.

Arterial base deficit has been correlated with mortality in the geriatric population and provides some insight into prognosis. In a study of elderly (>55) trauma patients those with a severe base deficit (−10 or worse) had an 80% mortality, those with a moderate (−6 to −9) base deficit had a 60% mortality, and those with a mild base deficit (−3 to −5) had a 23% mortality. Highlighting the difficulty in identifying severe injuries in this population is the fact that even those patients with a normal base deficit (2 to −2) had an 18% mortality [42].

A review of the National Trauma Data Bank attempts to provide criteria for the futility of care in elderly trauma patients. They stratified the patients into "young" old (65–74 years) and "old" old (75–84 years). A multiple regression analysis of over 76,000 records was performed to identify predictors of a 95% probability of death. This cutoff to determine a futile effort is subject to controversy and individual interpretation. Injuries to the brain, chest, and abdomen were the strongest anatomic injury predictors of mortality ($p < 0.001$ for all), while worsening base deficit and systolic blood pressure less than 90 were the strongest physiologic predictors of mortality. In the 65–74 year old age group, only hypotensive patients admitted with a severe thoracic and/or abdominal injury who also had severe injuries to the brain (AIS ≥4) or profound shock (BD ≤−12) had a less than 5% chance of survival. For those aged 75–84, even moderate injury to the brain (AIS ≤3) and moderate shock (BD ≤−6) were associated with a less than 5% chance of survival. Finally, for those aged 85 or older, profound shock or the combination of moderate shock and moderate injury to the head was associated with a less than 5% chance of survival [50]. Unfortunately, none of these criteria are specific enough to make decisions on withdrawal of care for any individual patient, but they may aid in decisions at the end-of-life.

*Circumstances where withholding/withdrawing care is appropriate*

*Level of evidence*: 3

*Strength of recommendation*: C

*Recommendation*: Based on poor quality trials and the inability to apply population-based data to individual patients, current recommendations cannot be made at this time. The existing data, however, can be used to aid physicians in their conversations with patients and families about end-of-life decisions.

## 40.10 Conclusion

Geriatric trauma remains a significant cause of morbidity and mortality. Practitioners need to be aware of the anatomic, physiologic, and mechanistic differences encountered in this population. The effects of preexisting medical conditions and preinjury functional status place the elderly patient at increased risk and make it difficult for them to compensate in the face of injury. In addition, geriatric trauma patients may present atypically and a heightened level of suspicion, starting with appropriate triage to a trauma center and continuing throughout the spectrum of care, is the only way to reduce the risk of poor outcomes (Table 40.1).

High quality trials are sparse relating to the care of the elderly trauma patient, but the prevention literature shows that strength and balance programs are effective at reducing injury. The ultimate decision, to withhold or withdraw care, is also a difficult question that remains to be answered, and may never reach the level of evidence required for any firm recommendation.

**TABLE 40.1**

Literature Supporting Evidence-Based Recommendations for Geriatric Trauma

| | | | | | | | | |
|---|---|---|---|---|---|---|---|---|
| Morris | 1 | 5 | 1990 | IIIb | Adult trauma patients | RCS/CC | N/A | In-hospital mortality |
| McGwin | 1 | 6 | 2004 | IIIb | 50–65 and >65 | RCS | N/A | In-hospital mortality |
| Morris | 1 | 7 | 1990 | IIIb | Adult trauma deaths and injured survivors | CC | N/A | In-hospital mortality |
| Milzman | 1 | 8 | 1992 | IIIb | 8,000 adult trauma patients 1986–1990 | RCS | N/A | Mortality |
| Grossman | 1 | 9 | 2002 | IIIb | >65 Statewide trauma database | RCS | N/A | 30 day in-hospital mortality |
| Ting | 1 | 10 | 2014 | IV | >80 with isolated lateral compression Type 1 fractures | CS | N/A | 1-year mortality |
| Coimbra | 1a | 11 | 2005 | N/A | Survey on clinical practice regarding reversal of anticoagulation | E | N/A | N/A |
| Pieracci | 1a | 12 | 2007 | IIIb | >65 suspected head injury single Level 1 center | RCS | N/A | ICH and mortality |
| Franko | 1a | 13 | 2006 | IIIb | Adult TBI patients, young vs. >70 | RCS | N/A | ICH and mortality |
| Lavoie | 1a | 14 | 2004 | IIIb | >55 with TBI and warfarin use | RCS | N/A | Severity of injury and mortality |
| Mina | 1a | 15 | 2003 | IIb | All trauma patients taking warfarin | PCS | Hospital Discharge | Hemorrhagic complications and mortality |
| Kennedy | 1a | 16 | 2000 | IIIb | All trauma patients taking warfarin | RCS | N/A | Mortality |
| Wojcik | 1a | 17 | 2001 | IIIb | All trauma patients taking warfarin | RCS | N/A | LOS and mortality |
| Ohm | 1a | 18 | 2005 | IIIb | >50 with ICH on or off antiplatelets | CC | N/A | Mortality |
| Ivascu | 1a | 19 | 2008 | IIIb | >50 with ICH on or off antiplatelets | CC | N/A | Mortality, hemorrhage progression |
| Wallace | 1a | 20 | 2012 | IV | Geriatric hip fracture patients on or off antiplatelets | CC | N/A | Need for transfusion |
| Peck | 1a | 21 | 2014 | IV | >55 with blunt force TBI on or off antiplatelets | CC | N/A | In-hospital mortality, hemorrhage progression |
| Moorman | 1a | 22 | 2014 | N/A | N/A | G | N/A | Review of new anticoagulants |
| Calland | 1a, 3 | 23 | 2012 | N/A | Geriatric trauma patients—EAST guidelines | G | N/A | Trauma management guidelines |
| Arbabi | 1b | 24 | 2007 | IIIb | All trauma patients receiving beta-blockers | RCS | N/A | Mortality |
| Neideen | 1b | 25 | 2008 | IV | >65 on or off beta-blockers | CC | N/A | In-hospital mortality |
| Bible | 1b | 26 | 2014 | IIIb | Trauma patients 18–79 with "severe" injury | RCT | N/A | Bone marrow dysfunction |
| Murphy | 1c | 27 | 2013 | IIIa | Geriatric elder abuse patients | SR | N/A | Anatomic distribution of injuries |
| Friedman | 1c | 28 | 2011 | IIIb | Geriatric elder abuse patients | CC | N/A | Risk factors for elder abuse |
| ACS-COT | 2 | 29 | 2014 | N/A | Resources for optimal care of injured patients | G | N/A | Trauma management guidelines |
| Ma | 2 | 30 | 1999 | IIIb | 1995 Maryland Statewide prehospital data | RCS | N/A | Transfer to trauma center |
| Phillips | 2 | 31 | 1996 | IIIb | Florida triage records | RCS | N/A | Appropriate triage |
| Ischwan | 2 | 32 | 2014 | IIb | Trauma patient age >16 | RCS | Hospital Discharge | Triage criteria, ISS |
| Osler | 2 | 33 | 1988 | IIIb | Geriatric trauma patients | RCS | N/A | Mortality |
| Knudson | 2, 3 | 34 | 1994 | IIIb | >65 Blunt trauma—3 registries | RCS | N/A | Mortality |
| Hashmi | 2 | 35 | 2014 | IV | Geriatric trauma patients | SR | N/A | Mortality and severity of injury |
| Clancy | 3 | 36 | 1997 | IIIb | >17 with splenic injury | CC | N/A | Resource utilization and mortality |

(*Continued*)

**TABLE 40.1 (*Continued*)**

Literature Supporting Evidence-Based Recommendations for Geriatric Trauma

| | | | | | | | | |
|---|---|---|---|---|---|---|---|---|
| Scalea | 3 | 37 | 1990 | IIb | >65 PHBC, BP <150, acidosis, fx, and TBI | PCS | Hospital Discharge | Hemodynamic parameters and mortality |
| Bar-Or | 3 | 38 | 2013 | IIb | >65 with blunt trauma and hemodynamically stable | PCS | Hospital Discharge | Mortality |
| McKinley | 3 | 39 | 2000 | IIb | > and <65 yo, high risk, BD <−6, >6u PRBC | PCS | Hospital Discharge | LOS and mortality |
| Mitra | 3 | 40 | 2014 | IIb | Trauma patients receiving massive transfusion | RCS | Hospital Discharge | Mortality |
| Schultz | 3 | 41 | 1985 | IIb | Elderly hip fractures | PCS | Hospital Discharge | Mortality |
| Davis | 3, 5 | 42 | 1998 | IIIb | >55 yo Trauma Registry Level 1 Center | RCS | N/A | ISS and mortality |
| Pellicane | 3 | 43 | 1992 | IIIb | >65 trauma patients | RCS | N/A | Trauma Score, complications and mortality |
| Van Aalst | 3 | 44 | 1991 | IIb | >65 years, blunt trauma, ISS >16 | PCS | 2.8 years | 20 measures of functional ability |
| Kannus | 4 | 45 | 2006 | I | Elderly people | SR | N/A | Prevention of falls |
| Van Riel | 4 | 46 | 2014 | N/A | >65 four-wheeled walker use | E | N/A | Falls |
| Sinaki | 4 | 47 | 2002 | I | Postmenopausal women | RCT | 10 years | Vertebral fracture |
| Korpelainen | 4 | 48 | 2006 | I | >70 yo women | RCT | 30 months | Fall-related fractures |
| Parker | 4 | 49 | 2004 | I | Multiple trials | RCT | Variable | Hip fracture |
| Nirula | 5 | 50 | 2004 | IIIb | >65, NTBD 1994–2001 | RCS | N/A | Mortality |

*Abbreviations:* RCT, randomized controlled trial; PCS, prospective cohort study; RCS, retrospective cohort study; CS, case series; CC, case control; SR, systematic review; E, epidemiologic study; G, guidelines.

## Disclaimer

There were no sources of funding or conflicts of interest in the writing of this chapter.

## References


1. Ortman JM, Velkoff VA. May, 2014. *An Aging Nation: The Older Population in the United States.* U.S. Department of Commerce, Economics and Statistics Administration: Washington, DC.
2. CDC. National Vital Statistics Report; Death: Leading causes for 2010, Vol. 62, No. 6, 2013.
3. Shirts BH, Burt RW, Mulvihill SJ, Cannon-Albright LA. A population-based description of familial clustering of pancreatic cancer. *Clin Gastroenterol Hepatol.* September 2010;8(9):812–816.
4. Champion HR, Copes WS, Buyer D, Flanagan ME, Bain L, Sacco WJ. Major trauma in geriatric patients. *Am J Public Health.* September 1989;79(9):1278–1282.
5. Morris JA Jr., MacKenzie EJ, Damiano AM, Bass SM. Mortality in trauma patients: The interaction between host factors and severity. *J Trauma.* December 1990;30(12):1476–1482.
6. McGwin G, Jr., MacLennan PA, Fife JB, Davis GG, Rue LW III. Preexisting conditions and mortality in older trauma patients. *J Trauma.* June 2004;56(6):1291–1296.
7. Morris JA, Jr., MacKenzie EJ, Edelstein SL. The effect of preexisting conditions on mortality in trauma patients. *JAMA.* April 1990;263(14):1942–1946.
8. Milzman DP, Boulanger BR, Rodriguez A, Soderstrom CA, Mitchell KA, Magnant CM. Pre-existing disease in trauma patients: A predictor of fate independent of age and injury severity score. *J Trauma.* February 1992;32(2): 236–243; discussion 243–244.
9. Grossman MD, Miller D, Scaff DW, Arcona S. When is an elder old? Effect of preexisting conditions on mortality in geriatric trauma. *J Trauma.* February 2002;52(2): 242–246.
10. Ting B, Zurakowski D, Herder L, Wagner K, Appleton P, Rodriguez EK. Preinjury ambulatory status is associated with 1-year mortality following lateral compression Type I fractures in the geriatric population older than 80 years. *J Trauma Acute Care Sur.* May 2014;76(5):1306–1309.
11. Coimbra R, Hoyt DB, Anjaria DJ, Potenza BM, Fortlage D, Hollingsworth-Fridlund P. Reversal of anticoagulation in trauma: A North-American survey on clinical practices among trauma surgeons. *J Trauma.* August 2005;59(2):375–382.
12. Pieracci FM, Eachempati SR, Shou J, Hydo LJ, Barie PS. Degree of anticoagulation, but not warfarin use itself, predicts adverse outcomes after traumatic brain injury in elderly trauma patients. *J Trauma.* September 2007;63(3):525–530.
13. Franko J, Kish KJ, O'Connell BG, Subramanian S, Yuschak JV. Advanced age and preinjury warfarin anticoagulation increase the risk of mortality after head trauma. *J Trauma.* July 2006;61(1):107–110.

14. Lavoie A, Ratte S, Clas D et al. Preinjury warfarin use among elderly patients with closed head injuries in a trauma center. *J Trauma*. April 2004;56(4):802–807.
15. Mina AA, Bair HA, Howells GA, Bendick PJ. Complications of preinjury warfarin use in the trauma patient. *J Trauma*. May 2003;54(5):842–847.
16. Kennedy DM, Cipolle MD, Pasquale MD, Wasser T. Impact of preinjury warfarin use in elderly trauma patients. *J Trauma*. March 2000;48(3):451–453.
17. Wojcik R, Cipolle MD, Seislove E, Wasser TE, Pasquale MD. Preinjury warfarin does not impact outcome in trauma patients. *J Trauma*. December 2001;51(6):1147–1151; discussion 1151–1152.
18. Ohm C, Mina A, Howells G, Bair H, Bendick P. Effects of antiplatelet agents on outcomes for elderly patients with traumatic intracranial hemorrhage. *J Trauma*. March 2005;58(3):518–522.
19. Ivascu FA, Howells GA, Junn FS, Bair HA, Bendick PJ, Janczyk RJ. Predictors of mortality in trauma patients with intracranial hemorrhage on preinjury aspirin or clopidogrel. *J Trauma*. October 2008;65(4):785–788.
20. Wallace HC, Probe RA, Chaput CD, Patel KV. Operative treatment of hip fractures in patients on clopidogrel: A case-control study. *Iowa Orthop J*. 2012;32:95–99.
21. Peck KA, Calvo RY, Schechter MS et al. The impact of preinjury anticoagulants and prescription antiplatelet agents on outcomes in older patients with traumatic brain injury. *J Trauma Acute Care Surg*. February 2014;76(2):431–436.
22. Moorman ML, Nash JE, Stabi KL. Emergency surgery and trauma in patients treated with the new oral anticoagulants: Dabigatran, rivaroxaban, and apixaban. *J Trauma Acute Care Surg*. September 2014;77(3):486–494; quiz 486–494.
23. Calland JF, Ingraham AM, Martin N et al. Evaluation and management of geriatric trauma: An Eastern Association for the Surgery of Trauma practice management guideline. *J Trauma Acute Care Surg*. November 2012;73(5 Suppl 4):S345–S350.
24. Arbabi S, Campion EM, Hemmila MR et al. Beta-blocker use is associated with improved outcomes in adult trauma patients. *J Trauma*. January 2007;62(1):56–61; discussion 61–62.
25. Neideen T, Lam M, Brasel KJ. Preinjury beta blockers are associated with increased mortality in geriatric trauma patients. *J Trauma*. November 2008;65(5):1016–1020.
26. Bible LE, Pasupuleti LV, Alzate WD et al. Early propranolol administration to severely injured patients can improve bone marrow dysfunction. *J Trauma Acute Care Surg*. July 2014;77(1):54–60; discussion 59–60.
27. Murphy K, Waa S, Jaffer H, Sauter A, Chan A. A literature review of findings in physical elder abuse. *Can Assoc Radiol J*. February 2013;64(1):10–14.
28. Friedman LS, Avila S, Tanouye K, Joseph K. A case-control study of severe physical abuse of older adults. *J Am Geriatr Soc*. March 2011;59(3):417–422.
29. Committee on Trauma ACoS. 2014. *Resources for the Optimal Care of the Injured Patient*, 6th edn. American College of Surgeons: Chicago, IL.
30. Ma MH, MacKenzie EJ, Alcorta R, Kelen GD. Compliance with prehospital triage protocols for major trauma patients. *J Trauma*. January 1999;46(1):168–175.
31. Phillips S, Rond PC, 3rd, Kelly SM, Swartz PD. The failure of triage criteria to identify geriatric patients with trauma: Results from the Florida Trauma Triage Study. *J Trauma*. February 1996;40(2):278–283.
32. Ichwan B, Darbha S, Shah MN et al. Geriatric-specific triage criteria are more sensitive than standard adult criteria in identifying need for trauma center care in injured older adults. *Ann Emerg Med*. January 2015;65(1):92–100.
33. Osler T, Hales K, Baack B et al. Trauma in the elderly. *Am J Surg*. December 1988;156(6):537–543.
34. Knudson MM, Lieberman J, Morris JA, Jr., Cushing BM, Stubbs HA. Mortality factors in geriatric blunt trauma patients. *Arch Surg*. April 1994;129(4):448–453.
35. Hashmi A, Ibrahim-Zada I, Rhee P et al. Predictors of mortality in geriatric trauma patients: A systematic review and meta-analysis. *J Trauma Acute Care Surg*. March 2014;76(3):894–901.
36. Clancy TV, Ramshaw DG, Maxwell JG et al. Management outcomes in splenic injury: A statewide trauma center review. *Ann Surg*. July 1997;226(1):17–24.
37. Scalea TM, Simon HM, Duncan AO et al. Geriatric blunt multiple trauma: Improved survival with early invasive monitoring. *J Trauma*. February 1990;30(2):129–134; discussion 134–136.
38. Bar-Or D, Salottolo KM, Orlando A, Mains CW, Bourg P, Offner PJ. Association between a geriatric trauma resuscitation protocol using venous lactate measurements and early trauma surgeon involvement and mortality risk. *J Am Geriatr Soc*. August 2013;61(8):1358–1364.
39. McKinley BA, Marvin RG, Cocanour CS, Marquez A, Ware DN, Moore FA. Blunt trauma resuscitation: The old can respond. *Arch Surg*. June 2000;135(6):688–693; discussion 694–695.
40. Mitra B, Olaussen A, Cameron PA, O'Donohoe T, Fitzgerald M. Massive blood transfusions post trauma in the elderly compared to younger patients. *Injury*. September 2014;45(9):1296–1300.
41. Schultz RJ, Whitfield GF, LaMura JJ, Raciti A, Krishnamurthy S. The role of physiologic monitoring in patients with fractures of the hip. *J Trauma*. April 1985;25(4):309–316.
42. Davis JW, Kaups KL. Base deficit in the elderly: A marker of severe injury and death. *J Trauma*. November 1998;45(5):873–877.
43. Pellicane JV, Byrne K, DeMaria EJ. Preventable complications and death from multiple organ failure among geriatric trauma victims. *J Trauma*. September 1992;33(3):440–444.
44. van Aalst JA, Morris JA, Jr., Yates HK, Miller RS, Bass SM. Severely injured geriatric patients return to independent living: A study of factors influencing function and independence. *J Trauma*. August 1991;31(8):1096–1101; discussion 1101–1192.
45. Kannus P, Sievanen H, Palvanen M, Jarvinen T, Parkkari J. Prevention of falls and consequent injuries in elderly people. *Lancet*. November 26, 2005;366(9500):1885–1893.
46. van Riel KM, Hartholt KA, Panneman MJ, Patka P, van Beeck EF, van der Cammen TJ. Four-wheeled walker related injuries in older adults in the Netherlands. *Inj Prev*. February 2014;20(1):11–15.

47. Sinaki M, Itoi E, Wahner HW et al. Stronger back muscles reduce the incidence of vertebral fractures: A prospective 10 year follow-up of postmenopausal women. *Bone.* June 2002;30(6):836–841.
48. Korpelainen R, Keinanen-Kiukaanniemi S, Heikkinen J, Vaananen K, Korpelainen J. Effect of impact exercise on bone mineral density in elderly women with low BMD: A population-based randomized controlled 30-month intervention. *Osteoporos Int.* January 2006;17(1):109–118.
49. Parker MJ, Gillespie LD, Gillespie WJ. Hip protectors for preventing hip fractures in the elderly. *Cochrane Database Syst Rev.* 2004;(3):CD001255.
50. Nirula R, Gentilello LM. Futility of resuscitation criteria for the "young" old and the "old" old trauma patient: A national trauma data bank analysis. *J Trauma.* July 2004;57(1):37–41.

## Commentary on Evidence-Based Approach to Geriatric Trauma

*Carlos V.R. Brown*

Geriatric trauma patients are here to stay. Trauma and acute care surgeons will be increasingly responsible for caring for the ever-increasing population of geriatric trauma patients. Unfortunately, despite a growing number of elderly trauma patients, very few studies have been published regarding the optimal approach to caring for the geriatric trauma patient. Dr. Ray and Dr. Schulman use this chapter to review the existing evidence surrounding geriatric trauma and provide some insight as to what areas need further investigation. The authors evaluate the literature surrounding pre-existing conditions, medications, elderly abuse, triage guidelines, resuscitation, injury prevention, and end-of-life care, shedding light on the current state of an evidenced-based approach to geriatric trauma.

Elderly patients, almost by definition, will present with an abundance of comorbidities and preinjury medical conditions that appear to negatively contribute to their ultimate outcome. The physiology of aging affects almost every organ system and in particular can profoundly impact the cardiovascular, pulmonary, and renal systems. In addition to the physiology of aging, elderly trauma patients may have an impaired functional status before sustaining an injury. Elderly patients should be screened for current functional status using one for the existing tools such as the short simple screening test for functional assessment. While it appears from the existing literature (retrospective in nature) that elderly trauma patients have worse outcomes due to chronic conditions and poor preinjury functional status, there is a gap in knowledge and literature to guide the trauma surgeon in improving outcomes in this population of patients.

Hand-in-hand with chronic medical conditions in elderly trauma patients come medications to treat those disease processes. In particular, anticoagulation is the bane of trauma surgeons' existence, as we are in the business of stopping bleeding. Geriatric trauma patients may present taking warfarin, antiplatelet agents, or any of a number of the new anticoagulants, all of which appear to be associated with worse outcomes. While warfarin can be monitored with INR, and elevated INR should be corrected in elderly trauma patients, there is almost no evidence to guide reversal of either antiplatelet agents or any of the new oral anticoagulants. Optimal management of geriatric trauma patients taking anticoagulants (new and old) and antiplatelet agents should be a primary focus of future investigations to improve the care of geriatric trauma patients. Once admitted to the hospital, geriatric trauma patients should have their medications catered to their specific needs and the Beers Criteria for Potentially Inappropriate Medication Use in Older Adults are an excellent guide for the clinician tasked with caring for these patients.

Elderly abuse appears to be a significant source of trauma in geriatric patients, putting them at risk for injuries to the face and upper extremities. Elderly abuse may be perpetrated by family members or caregivers at an assisted living or nursing facility. Any elderly patients suspected of sustaining elderly abuse should be screened for abuse by one of the many existing tools: the American Medical Association (AMA) screening tool, the conflict tactics scale (CTS), the brief abuse screen for the elderly (BASE), the elder assessment instrument (EAI), or the comprehensive geriatric assessment (CGA).

Triage can be a complex issue with any trauma patient, and the issue becomes even more challenging for geriatric trauma patients. Undertriage of geriatric trauma patients will lead them to be taken to nontrauma centers or have unnecessary mobilization of resources upon arrival to a trauma center, while overtriage will lead to excess cost and waste of resources. Unfortunately, the current literature is not robust enough to draw any conclusions regarding the optimal triage system for elderly trauma patients and trauma surgeons and trauma centers will need to depend on the current guidelines provided by the American College of Surgeons. Future studies will need to focus on altering triage criteria for elderly trauma patients to make sure they are prioritized appropriately. In addition, prehospital criteria are needed to determine which geriatric trauma patients need to be transferred to a trauma center and which subset might be appropriately cared for at nontrauma centers.

Similar to younger trauma patients, geriatric trauma patients may require resuscitation early after injury. This may be an area of confusion for the clinician as geriatric patients may not manifest typical clinical signs of shock (tachycardia, hypotension) due to their inability to mount a physiologic response. The lack of physiologic response is due to a blunted alpha-adrenergic stimulation that limits vasoconstriction and beta-adrenergic stimulation that limits the ability to mount a tachycardic response. In addition, geriatric patients may be taking medications such as beta-blockers that limit their ability to mount a tachycardic response. Geriatric trauma patients should be resuscitated in a manner similar to their younger counterparts, and resuscitation should not be withheld or limited solely based on advanced age.

Thankfully, some of the best geriatric trauma literature that exists is in the important realm of injury prevention in elderly individuals. Falls are the most common mechanism in geriatric trauma patients, and fall prevention can be accomplished through a variety of mechanisms. In addition to exercises targeted at improving balance and strength, elderly trauma patients and their caregivers should be educated regarding home and lifestyle modifications that may prevent future falls. The Centers for Disease Control (CDC) has an informative website dedicated to preventing falls in older adults (http://www.cdc.gov/Features/OlderAmericans/).

A large percentage of in-hospital deaths among geriatric trauma patients will involve decisions to withdraw or withhold potentially life-savings interventions. While the literature is limited regarding which specific circumstances were withholding care in geriatric trauma patients is appropriate, it is critically important for the health care team to determine if advanced directives are in place to help guide decisions. Unfortunately, many geriatric patients will not have advanced directives at time of injury to the care team and there is a need to have early discussions with the patient or their family to determine the best course of action for a specific patient in a specific situation. If the elderly trauma patient cannot speak for themselves, it will be important to identify as health care proxy or medical power of attorney to assist in providing the appropriate, individualized care for each patient. In situations where care is being withdrawn or withheld, the physician in charge and care team will also need to ensure that the geriatric trauma patient and their family are provided a comfortable and dignified death experience.

The current chapter delves into the existing literature available to help us take care of geriatric trauma patients. More importantly, it makes it very clear that a tremendous amount of work is needed to determine the optimal way to care for this complex and challenging patient population.

# 41

# *Rural Trauma*

**Burke Thompson**

**CONTENTS**



## 41.1 Introduction

Trauma system development has evolved over the past 30 years. Prior to this time, the delivery of trauma care by physicians was quite inconsistent [1]. The implementation of Advanced Trauma Life Support (ATLS) both revolutionized and helped standardize the care of injured patients. What has yet to be standardized is the best system to get the injured to a location where the teachings of ATLS can be applied.

The care of patients injured in a rural setting has not been studied extensively. The literature that exists often shows that patients injured in a rural setting do not do as well as those injured in urban areas. The improvement in rural trauma patient outcomes is an important avenue of current research.

Some literature does exist regarding the epidemiology of trauma care related to patients in rural settings. MacKenzie et al. studied the differences in mortality between level 1 trauma centers and non-trauma centers [2]. This study was designed to see if the added cost related to organized trauma systems led to added benefit to the patients. The sample of level 1 centers included 18 hospitals. The sample of non-trauma centers included 51 small, medium, and large hospitals with many in rural areas across 14 states. Mortality outcomes were compared for over 5000 patients. Adjustments were made for differences in case mix. In-hospital mortality was significantly lower at trauma centers than at nontrauma centers (7.6% vs. 9.5%). One year mortality was also significantly lower at the trauma centers (10.4% vs. 13.8%). Analysis revealed the differences were primarily in patients with multiple injuries.

Nathens et al. looked at the relationship between trauma center volume and outcomes [3]. This was a retrospective cohort study that focused on 31 academic trauma centers, both level 1 and level 2. They measured inpatient mortality and hospital length of stay comparing high volume (>650 trauma admissions per year) with low volume (≤650 trauma admissions per year). Patients with penetrating abdominal injury and shock had significantly improved survival at the high volume centers. No benefit was seen in the penetrating abdominal injury patients without shock. Blunt multisystem injury patients also had significantly better survival if they had severe traumatic brain injury. Those without severe traumatic brain injury did not have lower mortality at the high volume centers. The blunt multisystem injury patients overall did have significantly shorter hospital length of stay at the higher volume centers. Rural hospitals as a whole have low volumes of trauma patients and may be expected to perform as low volume centers.

Nathens et al. also looked at the effectiveness of an integrated approach to trauma care. They did a cross-sectional time series analysis of crash mortality from 1979 to 1995 [4]. Rates of death due to motor vehicle crashes were compared before and after implementation of an organized trauma care system. They found that 10 years after initial trauma system implementation, mortality after motor vehicle crashes began to decline. Enforcement of restraint laws and laws deterring drunk driving were seen to decrease mortality by 13%. Relaxed speeding laws increased mortality by 7%. They concluded an organized trauma system can lead to decreased mortality after motor vehicle crashes, but the effect may take 10 or more years to realize.

In this chapter, we will review the available literature addressing several important clinical questions regarding rural trauma and discuss the varied levels of evidence presented.

## 41.2 Does the Mode of Transportation of Rural Trauma Patients Impact Mortality?

Patients who are injured in rural or remote areas are usually transported by emergency helicopter or ground transportation. Much of the literature that exists compares these modes. Often, cost analysis is the goal but outcome analysis has been measured [5–7]. Mann and colleagues found an increase in mortality following the loss of an air medical program. Nicholl et al. compared cost and performance of air versus ground transport of injured patients in the rural setting.

In order to investigate this further, Mitchell et al. devised a study to compare the mortality of blunt trauma patients transported by air versus ground in a rural trauma system in Nova Scotia [8]. Their trauma center serves a predominately rural province. Communications and dispatch are centralized. This study used the trauma registry and included all trauma activations over a 4-year period from March 27, 1998, to March 28, 2002. Penetrating trauma was not included. 791 patients were evaluated using the trauma and injury severity score (TRISS) to determine whether there was a difference in outcomes between patients transported by air and those transported by ground ambulance. This included transportation both from the scene and from small regional hospitals.

The air transport patients fared better with 6.4 more survivors than expected per 100 patients. The ground transport cohort showed outcomes that were worse than expected. There were 2.4 unexpected deaths per 100 patients taken by ground. There was a 25% reduction in mortality with the use of air medical services. This difference was statistically significant.

*Recommendation*: Air transport systems are costly. There is a lack of level-1 evidence to support universal application of these systems. The data that exist do not suggest a common pattern. Geographical limitations do come into play in different regions and this must be considered. Further investigation is warranted.

*Grade of recommendation*: D

## 41.3 Are Mortality Rates Higher for Trauma Patients Injured in Rural Areas?

National Center for Health Statistics (NCHS) data has shown that death rates for unintentional injury in 2001 were higher in rural counties compared with large metropolitan counties [9]. This is also reflected in Centers for Disease Control (CDC) data for 2004 [10]. More recent data is included in a report by Singh and Siahpush regarding widening rural-urban disparities in mortality from major causes of death, 1969–2009 [11]. Residents in metropolitan areas have experienced larger mortality reductions during the past four decades compared to nonmetropolitan residents. U.S. victims of unintentional injury from 2005 to 2009 had mortality rates in metropolitan areas of 36.08 per 100,000 and in nonmetropolitan areas of 54.20 per 100,000. This is after population adjustment for age.

According to Esposito et al., among patients who survive long enough to reach a hospital, there is a threefold increase in risk of emergency department death among those injured in a region with limited access to trauma center care [12].

The leading cause of unintentional injury death in the United States is motor vehicle crash (MVC) [13]. There has been a disparity noted comparing rural to urban death rates after MVC [14,15]. The mortality is inversely proportional to population density. This disparity may be increasing.

Muelleman et al. designed a study to investigate this concept further [16]. The purpose was to analyze if there is a regional variation in the risk of death after MVC controlling for injury severity. All fatal and injury-related crashes in Nebraska from 1996 through 1999 were evaluated using the Crash Outcome Data Evaluation System data set. Injury Severity Scores (ISS) were calculated. The odds ratio for death was calculated for three rural county groupings compared with urban locations. This study included a large volume of patients. About one half of patient records had adequate information to calculate ISS and this amounted to 28,859 patients. Adjusting for ISS, the odds of death were 1.98 higher in small rural counties compared with urban counties. When speed limit (higher in rural areas), age, and alcohol use were controlled-for, odds of death in rural crashes were still significantly higher. The authors postulated that variations in medical care might account for some of this difference.

Another outcomes study was done by McCowan et al. at the University of Utah [17]. This was a retrospective review of all adult helicopter emergency transports in 2001 and it compared rural versus urban trauma patients. It included the registry data for three level 1 trauma centers. This study examined in-hospital mortality, length of stay, and discharge status of victims of blunt trauma. Included were 271 urban and 141 rural transports. After controlling for age, gender, and ISS, there were no significant mortality differences between the two groups, despite longer transport times.

Gerhardt et al. analyzed trauma transfers in South Central Texas and compared outcomes with current U.S. combat operations in the RemTORN-1 study [18]. Prolonged evacuation and its consequences are seen both in rural trauma and in armed conflict. In this study, a retrospective cohort was collected including demographics, epidemiology, and time data. Clinical data was included. The civilian patients in this geographic area were older, spent longer times en route to level 1 trauma centers, and had higher ISS than the military comparison group. Blood transfusion rates and survival to discharge were similar. The authors plan to use this model to compare data to other regional trauma systems and to the contemporary operational environment encountered by deployed military personnel. They found civilian-military collaboration in prehospital trauma care research was feasible. This was felt to demonstrate a capacity for the military to continue such efforts in interwar periods.

*Recommendation*: While there are federal statistics supporting the existence of a higher mortality rate associated with rural versus urban trauma, there is no level 1 data. The data that does exist in the literature is inconsistent.

*Grade of recommendation*: C

## 41.4 What Are the Roles of Rural Physicians?

In studies showing a disparity in outcomes between rural and urban trauma patients, the inexperience of rural physicians is often listed as a possible cause. A rural trauma course is being piloted in North Carolina in order to address this issue. Results have not been published as of yet. Investigation into the role of rural physicians in trauma management has been undertaken in Australia due to its particular population distribution.

Lopez et al. investigated early trauma management skills in Australian general practitioners [19]. A course is taught in Australia called the Early Management of Severe Trauma (EMST). This is similar to ATLS. Lopez et al. sought to evaluate the skill and comfort levels of general practitioners in managing trauma patients. All general practitioners who completed the EMST course between 1989 and 2004 and resided in rural Western Australia were surveyed. Background and open-ended questions were included. Results showed the physicians were confident with IV access and fluid resuscitation. They felt least comfortable doing procedures such as diagnostic peritoneal lavage and surgical airway insertion. Low confidence was also seen in interpretation of cervical spine radiographs and in the management of penetrating torso injuries and severe head injuries. Most felt able to intubate and insert chest tubes. Those with more recent trauma experience were more confident of their abilities.

The surveyed physicians also listed ways to improve the EMST course. Popular suggestions were making refresher courses more accessible, increasing procedure instruction, and teaching from a rural perspective.

Cheffins et al. looked specifically at rural general practitioner management of vehicle related trauma patients [20]. Australian data have shown morbidity and mortality resulting from rural MVC's to be twice that resulting from urban crashes [21]. The study by Cheffins et al. looked specifically at management challenges facing rural physicians via an interview process. The physicians were selected from areas having high road crash numbers. Still, about half of those surveyed reported treating vehicle-related injury less than monthly. Less than 6% reported weekly experience. Lack of frequent exposure limited comfort level with severely injured patients. The physicians also often saw patients with delayed presentation of injuries, such as soft tissue injuries, whiplash, and chronic pain syndromes. Access to specialty services was a big concern. The specialties felt to be most in need were orthopedics, acute care surgery, and rehabilitation. Chronic pain and mental health services were also felt to be lacking. Whether or not the patients had private insurance was often seen to determine the level of care. In general, there was also a perceived need for better injury prevention efforts in the rural setting.

*Recommendation*: The lack of high volume experience for rural physicians in managing injured patients may impact the care they provide. Structured educational programs that focus on initial stabilization followed by transfer to a definitive care center are critical to address this world-wide problem.

*Grade of recommendation*: B

## 41.5 Has Rural Trauma System Development Impacted Care?

A wealth of literature exists regarding the benefits of trauma center care. Most articles, though, describe urban trauma centers with large patient volumes. Much less in known about the performance of rural trauma centers and how they perform as part of a larger trauma system.

Lipsky et al. compared the survival of trauma patients in urban versus rural settings after the implementation of a novel rural nontrauma center alternative care model called the Model Rural Trauma Project [22]. They compared the outcomes at two urban level 1 trauma centers to the outcomes at eight rural hospitals. The Model Rural Trauma Project included three key elements to attempt to improve care. They created a warning system for the arrival of major trauma patients using trauma triage criteria. They began early activation of a trauma team in the emergency department. Finally, periodic systems review was employed to evaluate the system and make modifications. These are key elements found in designated trauma centers across the country. After implementation of this project, they found overall survival indistinguishable between urban and rural hospitals once they corrected for differences in patient populations. It was clearly acknowledged that rural trauma populations are predominately blunt by mechanism and had extended transport times.

A retrospective study by Helling at the University of Missouri investigated the performance of rural trauma centers and how the experience of their trauma surgeons might shape future educational efforts to optimize rural trauma care [23]. Missouri has three levels of trauma centers. Level I centers are large, urban, tertiary referral facilities with full subspecialty support. Level III centers are rural and do not require orthopedic or neurosurgical coverage. The state trauma registry was reviewed over a 2-year period from 2002 and 2003. Admissions to level III centers were examined for acuity, severity, and type of injury. Experiences with chest, abdominal, and neurologic trauma were examined in detail. Dr. Helling found acuity and severity of injuries to be greater at level I and level II centers. Mortality at level III centers was significantly lower than at the other centers but the rate of death within 24 h of admission was no different. Only 1% of patients admitted to level III centers needed emergent chest or abdominal surgery. The level III centers were seen to perform as expected as part of the integrated state trauma system. The relative paucity of severe head, chest, and abdominal injuries seen at such centers presents a challenge to the rural trauma surgeon to maintain the skills required in caring for these patients.

System development and improvement is the key to successful rural trauma management. McDermott et al. in Victoria, Australia looked specifically at motor vehicle crash mortality before and after implementing a new trauma care system [24]. This system included a division of rural trauma services. Prior to the new system, patients injured in a rural setting were usually transported to the nearest public hospital and were treated by junior emergency department staff. A few severely injured patients were flown to the single level I trauma center from the scene. Many errors and potentially preventable deaths were noted. Despite reporting these, outcomes did not improve. A new system was then devised [25].

This new system was based on a tiered designation of trauma centers. Rural locations were served by "regional trauma services" and "urgent care services." Triage criteria determined the destination of patients transported from the scene. Later, transfer to a higher level of care was done as appropriate. A trauma registry was started to allow evaluation of results. The study compared patients treated from 1997 to 1998 with those from 2002 to 2004. Demographics and Injury Severity Scores (ISS) were not significantly different. The mean time from crash to hospital increased in the later group. The rural ambulance service also had longer on-scene times. TRISS analysis showed the two patient populations to be similar. The preventable death rate dropped from 5% to 3% after the new system was implemented. Combined preventable and potentially preventable death rates decreased significantly as well. Management deficiencies were also reduced. Some of these improvements were attributed to quicker triage and transfer of severely injured patients to a level I trauma center. All in all, this was seen as a successful system.

Shafi et al. in the United States hypothesized that state wide trauma systems independently reduce injury mortality [26]. This was a nationwide cross-sectional study that used data from the CDC, the National Highway Traffic Safety Administration, the United States Department of Transportation, and the United States Census Bureau. Motor vehicle death rates per 100,000 population were compared between states with and without trauma systems. Management of rural population distribution was analyzed. Death rates have declined over time as new state-wide trauma systems came on line. Rural population distribution, however, remained an independent predictor of mortality. The explanation of this was felt to be multifactorial.

Tiesman et al. investigated the effects of a rural trauma system on traumatic brain injuries [27]. Timely arrival at definitive care is especially important in traumatic brain injury (TBI). The Iowa System Trauma Registry Dataset was analyzed before (1997–1998) and after (2002–2003) implementation of a rural trauma system. There was a significant reduction in 72-h mortality for TBI after system implementation. More severely injured patients were triaged or transported to a higher level of care. Inhospital mortality was reduced.

More recent work has been done by the American College of Surgeons. The ad hoc Rural Trauma Committee of the American College of Surgeons, Committee on Trauma developed the Rural Trauma Team Development Course. This is a training and education program focused on providing quality care despite geographic, demographic, and limited resource challenges that can be a hindrance [28]. Delays in care are present both in transport times and after arrival at rural medical centers. This education process serves to reduce the "authority gradient" and standardize the patient information through the system to expedite transfer of critically injured patients to a trauma center. The course includes a module on team building and emphasizes the decision to transfer should be made within the first 15 min after patient arrival.

The Rural Trauma Team Development Course was found to be an effective educational tool and team building exercise. It is inclusive knowing team members at a small, rural facility may include untrained volunteers. They found the segment on communication increased efficiency specifically by reducing delays in the transfer process.

*Recommendation*: The literature that is available suggests that rural trauma care is significantly improved if it is part of a regional trauma system. There is also evidence that education and training can help expedite transfer of patients to appropriate facilities.

*Grade of recommendation*: B

## 41.6 Does the Availability of Surgeons Impact Mortality in Rural Trauma?

The availability of surgeons varies widely based on geography. The American College of Surgeons Health Policy Research Institute publishes these data based on counties in the United States [29]. In 2011, 1144 rural counties had no general surgeons. 386 counties had only 0.1–4.6 general surgeons per 100,000 population. Most large metropolitan areas have 6–25 general surgeons per 100,000 population. This disparity can affect access to care for all patients with general surgery needs, including trauma patients.

Chang et al. found the density of surgeons (all types) to be significantly associated with risk of death from motor vehicle collisions [30]. They did a retrospective analysis of the 3-year average of MVC deaths per one million population for each county studied from 2001 to 2003. That average was their primary outcome variable. Their independent variable was the density of surgeons per 1 million population in 2003. They analyzed 3225 counties. The median number of surgeons per one million of population was 55. On interval analysis, each increase of one surgeon per million was associated with 0.16 fewer deaths per million population. Rural location was associated with a significant increase in mortality.

*Recommendation*: The availability of surgeons does impact mortality from motor vehicle crashes.

*Grade of recommendation*: C

## 41.7 Has ATLS Training Affected Trauma Outcomes in Rural Communities?

The advanced Trauma Life Support program, (ATLS), by the American College of Surgeons serves to educate physicians who care for injured patients in emergency rooms—often not at trauma centers. Hedges et al. tried to determine if the practices taught in the course affect survival at rural level 3 trauma centers in the Oregon trauma system [31]. This was a retrospective observational analysis of rural injured patient survival. They identified high-risk groups of patients. There was considerable variation in measured care interventions among the 21 level 3 centers. There was a strong association of transfer to a higher level of care with survival in patients presenting with GCS <9 and in patients with ISS >20 but no hypotension. Transfer to a higher level of care is a key tenant of ATLS. They found the contribution of surgeon presence upon initial resuscitation, ED intubation, and blood product administration warranted further study.

*Recommendation*: McCrum et al. specifically looked at ATLS guideline adherence in the management of adult trauma patients transferred from rural hospitals to level 1 trauma centers [32]. They did a retrospective analysis of all adult major trauma patients transferred ≥50 km from a rural hospital to a level 1 trauma center from 2007 to 2009 in Alberta. They found that key aspects of ATLS were often missed. Common deficiencies were patient warming, chest tube insertion, adequate IV access, and motor/sensory exam. Patients with higher ISS scores and those transported by air were more likely to receive ATLS recommended interventions. Comprehensive quality improvement initiatives with targeted training and education were recommended to improve the quality of care (Table 41.1).

*Grade of recommendation*: C

**TABLE 41.1**

Rural Trauma: Question Summary

| Question | Answer | Grade of Support | References |
|---|---|---|---|
| Does mode of transportation impact mortality? | Unclear | D | [5–8] |
| Are mortality rates higher for patients injured in rural areas? | Yes | C—there is inconsistency | [15–17] |
| What are the roles of rural physicians? | Assess, resuscitate, perform initial stabilizing procedures | B | [16,17] |
| Has rural trauma system development impacted care? | Yes | B | [19,20,28] |
| Does the availability of surgeons impact mortality in rural trauma | Yes | C | [30] |
| Has ATLS training affected trauma outcomes in rural communities? | Yes | C | [31,32] |

## References


1. The American College of Surgeons. 1997. *Advanced Trauma Life Support for Doctors*, 6th edn. Chicago, IL, p. 11.
2. MacKenzie EJ, Rivara FP, Jurkovich GJ et al. A national evaluation of the effect of trauma-center care on mortality. *N Engl J Med.* 2006;354:366–378.
3. Nathens AB, Jurkovich GJ, Maier RV et al. Relationship between trauma center volume and outcomes. *JAMA.* 2001;285:1164–1171.
4. Nathens AB, Jurkovich GJ, Cummings P et al. The effect of organized systems of trauma care on motor vehicle crash mortality. *JAMA.* 2000;283:1990–1994.
5. Mann NC, Pinkney KA, Price DD, et al. Injury mortality following the loss of air medical support for rural interhospital transport. *Acad Emerg Med.* 2002;9: 694–698.
6. Cummings G, O'Keefe g. Scene disposition and mode of transport following rural trauma: A prospective cohort study comparing patient costs. *J Emerg Med.* 2000;18: 349–354.
7. Nicholl JP, Beeby NR, Brazier JE. A comparison of the costs and performance of an emergency helicopter and land ambulances in a rural area. *Injury.* 1994;25: 145–153.
8. Mitchell AD, Tallon JM, Sealy B. Air versus ground transport of major trauma patients to a tertiary trauma centre: A province-wide comparison using TRISS analysis. *Can J Surg.* 2007;50:129–133.
9. Eberhardt MS, Ingram DD, Makuc DM et al. 2001. *Urban and Rural Chartbook, Health United States 2001.* National Center for Health Statistics: Hyattsville, MD.
10. National Center for Health Statistics, Centers for Disease Control and Prevention. 2004. NCHS data on injuries. http://cdc.gov/nchs/data/factsheets/injury.pdf (accessed February 13, 2007).
11. Sing GK, Siahpush M. Widening rural-urban disparities in all-cause mortality and mortality from major causes of death in the USA, 1969–2009. *J Urban Health.* 2013;91(2):272–292.
12. Esposito TJ, Maier RV, Rivara FP et al. The impact of variation in trauma care times: Urban versus rural. *Prehosp Disaster Med.* 1995;10:161–166.
13. Vyrostek SB, Annest JL, Ryan GW. Surveillance for fatal and non-fatal injuries- United States. 2001. *MMWR.* 2004;53:1–57.
14. Baker SP, Whitfield RA, O'Neill B. Geographic variations in mortality from motor vehicle crashes. *N Engl J Med.* 1987;316:1384–1387.
15. Muelleman RL, Mueller K. Fatal motor vehicle crashes: Variations of crash characteristics within rural regions of different population densities. *J Trauma.* 1996;11: 316–320.
16. Muelleman RL, Wadman MC, Paul Tran T et al. Rural motor vehicle crash risk of death is higher after controlling for injury severity. *J Trauma.* 2007;62: 221–226.
17. McCowan CL, Swanson, ER, Thomas F et al. Outcomes of blunt trauma victims transported by HEMS from rural and urban scenes. *Prehosp Emerg Care.* 2007;11:383–388.
18. Gerhardt RT, Koller AR, Rasmussen TE et al. Analysis of remote trauma transfers in South Central Texas with comparison with current US combat operations: Results of the RemTORN-1 study. *J Trauma Acute Care Surg.* 2013;75(2):164–168.
19. Lopez DG, Hamdorf JM, Ward AM et al. Early trauma management skills in Australian general practitioners. *ANZ J Surg.* 2006;76:894–897.
20. Cheffins TE, Blackman R, Veitch C. Rural GPs' management of vehicle related trauma. *Aust Fam Physician.* 2007;36:782–784.
21. Strong K, Trickett P, Titulaer I, Bhatia K. 1998. Health in rural and remote Australia. Australian Institute of Health and Welfare: Canberra, Australian Capital Territory, Australia.
22. Lipsky AM, Karsteadt LL, Gausche-Hill M et al. A comparison of rural versus urban trauma care. *J Emerg Trauma Shock.* 2014;7:1:41–46.
23. Helling TS. Trauma care at rural level III trauma centers in a state trauma system. *J Trauma.* 2007;62: 498–503.
24. McDermott FT, Cordner SM, Cooper DJ et al. Management deficiencies and death preventability of road traffic fatalities before and after a new trauma care system in Victoria, Australia. *J Trauma.* 2007;63:331–338.
25. Review of Trauma and Emergency Services: Victoria. 1999. Final Report of the Ministerial Task Force on Trauma and Emergency Services and the Department Working Party on Emergency and Trauma Services. Melbourne, Victoria, Australia: Human Services.
26. Shafi S, Nathens AB, Elliott AC et al. Effect of trauma systems on motor vehicle occupant mortality: A comparison between states with and without a formal system. *J Trauma.* 2006;61:1374–1379.
27. Tiesman H, Young T, Torner JC et al. Effects of a rural trauma system on traumatic brain injuries. *J Neurotrauma.* 2007;24:1189–1197.
28. Kappel DA, Rossi DC, Polack EP et al. Does the rural trauma team development course shorten the interval from trauma patient arrival to decision to transfer? *J Trauma.* 2011;70:2:315–319.
29. American College of Surgeons Health Policy Research Institute, Cecil G. Sheps Center for Health Services Research, University of North Carolina at Chapel Hill, Chapel Hill, NC, 2011.
30. Chang DC, Eastman B, Talamini MA et al. Density of surgeons is significantly associated with reduced risk of deaths from motor vehicle crashes in US counties. *J Am Coll Surg.* 2011;1:862–866.
31. Hedges JR, Adams AL, Gunnels MD. ATLS practices and survival at rural level 3 trauma hospitals. *Prehosp Emerg Care.* 2002;6:299–305.
32. McCrum ML, McKee J, Lai M et al. ATLS adherence in the transfer of rural trauma patients to a level 1 facility. *Injury.* 2013;44:1241–1245.

## Commentary on Rural Trauma

*Michael F. Rotondo*

In the first 10 years of my career at the University of Pennsylvania, a Level I university–based urban trauma center, I became well versed with the nuances of managing an injury demographic that was characteristic of a densely populated city in America. I had only "brushed up" against rural injury in the time spent working at an affiliated Level II center 44 miles away from center city, Philadelphia, in the middle of Chester County, Pennsylvania, during that same time frame. It did not take long to understand that there were some fundamental differences in the patients and the system of care surrounding them. When I began to think seriously about next steps after my career at Penn, the call to eastern North Carolina was too compelling to ignore. The move to East Carolina University was fueled by a personal agenda to help create an organized trauma system in a region that was otherwise underserved. The eastern third of the state of North Carolina area is a relatively sparsely populated region with 1.4 million people spread out over an area a little larger than the state of New Hampshire. At the time, injury mortality rates were extraordinarily high in that region compared to the rest of the country and in many ways, rural trauma appeared to be a totally different disease than urban trauma. It was in this decision, made with clear intentionality, that I became familiar with the challenges of providing injury care to a rural population and in this case, a people that lived in the shadow of the White House, only 4 h driving time south of Washington DC.

The differences between the urban and rural population populations in injury care were striking. A high percentage of penetrating injury, a young healthy patient population, short prehospital transport, a sophisticated EMS response system, and transport directly to the trauma center characterized the urban population of injured patients. In contrast, the rural population was characterized by high percentage of blunt injury, an older patient population with attendant multiple comorbidities, long pretrauma center times frequently featuring a stop at a small rural hospital, and a primarily volunteer prehospital response with oftentimes only basic life support training. Air medical transport was limited to what we could provide at the time with our one hospital-based helicopter—often down for maintenance or the unstable weather patterns of the eastern coastal plain of North Carolina. As you can imagine these factors presented a whole different set of challenges from what I had encountered in the 10 years that I spent surrounded by the sophisticated resource-rich environment of University of Pennsylvania.

When the rural trauma outcome facts are examined related to these stark differences in the characteristics of the patient population, what is identified is not surprising:

- There are a disproportionate high number of deaths relative to the total population.
- There is a high preventable death rate.
- There is an increased death rate at an equivalent or even lower injury severity.
- There is an increased death rate with decreasing population density.
- The elderly and the young have higher mortality rates.
- There is clear susceptibility in poverty-stricken, illiteracy-rich, high unemployment, and under-resourced areas.

Now one would think that in a country as prolific as America we would have this problem solved by now. We are, after all, the richest country in the world—are not we? How is it that we have evolved to a system of care that yields these results?

The work of Branas and Mackenzie in 2006 helps us understand the nature of the challenge. Their data demonstrate that we while have a reasonable coverage in the suburban and urban areas, there are nearly 50 million rural Americans that do not have access within 1 h.

While 85% of U.S. residents access within 1 h, only about 25% of the land in the United States is located within 1 h of a Level I or Level II trauma center. That means that 75% of our land mass in the United States does not have adequate access to trauma care resources and as you would expect, the northeast has the highest land coverage, and the intermountain west has the least land coverage, hence, long discover, extrication, and transport times. This may explain why nearly 60% of all trauma deaths occur in rural areas despite the fact that only 20% of the nation's population lives in these areas. This is not a small number of deaths—it translates to about 60,000 lives lost each year in rural America.

There are other factors that must be considered as well. In rural areas, there is a higher prevalence of alcohol use while driving, a higher prevalence of loaded unlocked firearms at home, and an increase in life-threatening/serious farm related-injuries due to exposure to agricultural machinery. As compared to trauma patients sustaining the same types of injuries treated in an urban or larger metropolitan hospital, rural hospitals have fewer resources.

The problem while complex and vexing is not insurmountable, there are some things that can be done. The first is to realize and confront who we are as a country. At 3000 miles across with a general populace of nearly 350 million with an "all healthcare is local" culture—we must first acknowledge that a one size, all approach is unlikely to work. At its broadest—the solution lays in local activism state-by-state and region-by-region: the solution focusing on improving the general health and well-being of our population and a population health management approach rooted in public health principles. Creative collaborations between state departments of health, state offices of rural health, the Office of Rural Health Policy, the National Rural Health Association, state offices of emergency medical services, state committees on trauma and regional trauma councils, trauma centers, critical access hospitals must pursue the issue as a central health issue.

Perhaps most importantly, the things than can be done should be done including

- Injury prevention education
- Prehospital resuscitation and triage management
- Development of triage, destination, and activation protocols
- Improved utilization and development of critical access hospitals
- Dissemination of the rural trauma team development course
- Exploration and utilization of telemedicine along with creative payment vehicles
- Development of objective methods to measure regional trauma systems efficacy
- Commitment to need-based trauma system resource

While the development of statewide regional trauma systems has demonstrated improvement in injury-related mortality as compared to states will less developed trauma systems. We should also confront the fact that while we might believe in the importance of this, our investment pattern belies this notion. Currently, only 24 of the 42 states with trauma systems are state funded, 8 states have no system at all which means that over half the country has systems that are either unfunded or nonexistent. For us to make serious headway—we will have to invest time, creative energy, thoughtful consideration, and money.

The authors of this chapter have done an exemplary job in addressing five important questions related to injury care in rural America and to my way of thinking, they have reached the proper conclusions. It is our job now to get to work and endeavor to address the problem—region-by-region and state-by-state and extinguish this considerable health problem in our country today.

# 42

# *Evidence-Based Management of Genitourinary Trauma*

**Patrick C. Samson and Jay A. Motola**

**CONTENTS**



## 42.1 Evidence-Based Management of Genitourinary Trauma

The field of genitourinary trauma has evolved over the past few decades. With the advent of better imaging technology and improvements in hemodynamic monitoring, management has become less surgically aggressive. Trauma-related injuries remain as the leading cause of death for the younger population in the United States [1], with about 10% of abdominal traumas involving the genitourinary tract, and frequently occurring concomitantly with injuries to other abdominal organs. Urologists must be involved in the management of these patients to maximize outcomes. Hematuria, a hallmark of injury to the urinary tract, is not specific to the location or severity of the injury. The clinician must take into account the mechanism of injury, the patient's hemodynamic stability, and those resuscitative efforts required to stabilize the patient, in order to decide the best management route. This chapter provides an evidence-based approach in tackling well-established management practices as well as controversial ones for traumatic injuries to the genitourinary (GU) tract. The studies cited are mostly retrospective, due to the logistics and ethics of executing prospective, randomized studies in the trauma setting.

## 42.2 Renal Trauma

### 42.2.1 When Does Renal Trauma Require Immediate Surgical Exploration?

The kidney is the most commonly injured organ in the genitourinary system. A population-based observational study has shown that 1.2% of all trauma patients suffered renal injuries, with blunt trauma being the major cause of injury [2]. The injury severity score (assessment of the patient's global status), penetrating injury, and the renal injury severity were independent predictors for the need for nephrectomy. Other studies have also assessed the usefulness of the American Association for the Surgery of Trauma (AAST) injury scale and found retrospective and prospective data, suggesting that the scale correlates with clinical outcome and need for nephrectomy [3,4]. Grade of injury must be determined with a CT of the abdomen and pelvis, with intravenous contrast in stable patients who have suffered blunt trauma with gross or microscopic hematuria and systolic blood pressure <90 mmHg [5]. The scan should be obtained with intravenous contrast when the mechanism of injury or findings on physical examination are concerning for renal injury. The degree of hematuria does not necessarily correlate with the grade of injury, and should not preclude imaging studies [6]. Immediate and delayed imaging should be obtained to show the location of renal lacerations and the presence of extravasation from the urinary collecting system.

Most renal injuries can be managed conservatively, depending on the severity of injury and the patient's stability. Limited prospective, randomized data exist to support the concept that conservative management is superior to initial operative management, however, there are data showing that trauma centers that adopt a conservative approach to renal trauma have decreased rates of renal exploration and nephrectomy without any increase in complications. A study comparing outcomes between patients in different time periods, whereas in the earlier time period surgical management was primarily involved, and during the later time period, conservative management prevailed [7]. Those treated conservatively had decreased operative, but similar complication rates. A 2005 literature review demonstrates that hemodynamically stable and patients with grade I–IV renal injuries can be managed nonoperatively with close hemodynamic monitoring, bed rest, and blood transfusions if necessary [8]. Grade IV injuries can also be treated with close observation, with the understanding that delayed complications such as bleeding or renovascular hypertension may necessitate nephrectomy. Patients with blunt Grade IV renal injury treated conservatively required delayed surgical intervention 0%–40% of the time, and up to 20% requiring nephrectomy [8]. McGuire et al. demonstrated a 9.3% complication rate with high-grade blunt injuries that were treated conservatively [9]. Some blunt Grade V injuries have been shown to be amenable to nonoperative management [10]. Patients managed conservatively were younger, had less comorbidity, and did not have imaging findings suspicious of renal pedicle injury. Although this study was limited by a small population size, nonoperative management resulted in fewer ICU days, significantly lower transfusion rates ($p = 0.124$), and fewer complications. The clinician must take into account many factors in deciding which patients can be managed conservatively.

Selective nonoperative management in penetrating renal injuries has also been associated with low complication rates. Bjurlin et al. [11] found that the selective nonoperative management of penetrating renal injuries resulted in lower transfusion rates, shorter ICU and hospital length of stay, and decreased mortality when compared with nephrectomy, but results were similar when compared to renorrhapy. Patients undergoing nonoperative management were hemodynamically stable, had an absence of the following CT findings: gross urinary extravasation, contrast blush indicative of arterial hemorrhage, and hilar disruption. The absence of these radiographic findings was indicative of a potentially viable, salvageable kidney.

There is Grade B evidence to support immediate intervention with surgery or angioembolization in hemodynamically unstable patients with no or minimal response to resuscitation. Again, the need for emergent intervention is not only based on the grade of the injury, but the patient's clinical status. A retrospective study of high-grade blunt renal injuries revealed that the ongoing need for fluid, blood, and blood products predicted the need for emergent intervention [9]. A higher proportion of Grade V injuries required immediate intervention, however 50% of patients with Grade V injuries were managed nonoperatively. Others have advised that grade V vascular injuries should be treated with immediate surgical intervention, usually requiring nephrectomy [12].

When experienced interventional radiologists are available, some patients requiring immediate intervention because of bleeding may benefit from angioembolization. In a retrospective series of 26 patients, angioembolization was found to be an effective option for patients with Grade IV renal trauma that have failed conservative management [13]. However, patients with Grade V injuries did not respond well to embolization and either immediate nephrectomy or death occurred. In a recent study, nine hemodynamically unstable patients with Grade V renal injuries secondary to blunt trauma were all successfully treated with angioembolization and none required any further intervention [14]. It is unclear why there is such discrepancy in outcomes between the two studies, however it is most likely attributable to either differences in techniques used by the interventional radiologists or the mechanism of injury. Regardless, there is insufficient evidence to support or reject angioembolization as a treatment option for Grade V renal injuries.

The American Urological Association (AUA) Urotrauma guidelines state that urinary extravasation and renal parenchymal injuries can be managed nonoperatively, however there is not enough evidence to make this formal recommendation. Patients with isolated urinary extravasation from parenchymal injury, who were treated nonoperatively had >90% rate of resolution of urinary leakage [15], and those taken to the operating room had a 19% nephrectomy rate. None of the patients initially treated nonoperatively required nephrectomies, but 9% required ureteral stent placement due for persistent leakage.

*Recommendation*: Hemodynamically stable patients with renal injury may initially be treated nonoperatively, while hemodynamically unstable patients who do not respond to resuscitation must undergo immediate intervention, with either surgery or angioembolization (Grade B).

## 42.3 Ureteral Injury

### 42.3.1 How Should Traumatic Ureteral Injuries Be Repaired?

Injuries to the ureter are relatively rare and are usually iatrogenic, accounting for only about 1% of all GU traumatic injuries and usually occurring in either the operating room during gynecologic, urologic, or colorectal surgery, or as a result of penetrating trauma [16]. Iatrogenic ureteral injuries usually occur in the distal 1/3 and pelvic ureter while ureteral injuries from external trauma usually occur in the upper 1/3 of the ureter [17,18]. Diagnosis may be missed or delayed since ureteral injuries may not manifest with obvious signs and symptoms. A high index of suspicion is necessary for prompt diagnosis and management.

As with renal injuries, the management of ureteral injuries depends on the hemodynamic stability of the patient, as well as the timing and location of injury. Stable patients with suspected ureteral injuries should be evaluated with a CT of the abdomen and pelvis with delayed imaging. Ureteral injuries are suggested by contrast extravasation, delayed pyelogram, hydronephrosis, or lack of contrast in the ureter distal to the injury [19–21]. Many ureteral injuries occur in the operating room, and visual inspection of the ureters at the time of laparotomy without imaging is recommended [1]. The efficacy of this approach is demonstrated in a study that revealed no missed ureteral injuries during surgical exploration for patients who had a penetrating mechanism of injury [22]. A meta-analysis of ureteral injuries showed that delayed diagnosis of ureteral injuries is associated with a prolonged length of stay and increased rate of nephrectomy [23]. If there is clinical suspicion of a ureteral injury, every effort should be made to identify it. Primary repair is the treatment of choice, unless the patient is hemodynamically unstable and complex repair is not technically feasible within a reasonable amount of time [1]. A retrospective review showed favorable results when ureteral injuries were repaired primarily [24]. The majority of patients underwent complex repairs with nearly a 100% renal salvage rate. Deferred management with percutaneous nephrostomy tube with or without ureteral ligation almost always resulted in significant strictures and eventual loss of ureteral length. Primary repair is the main goal, if diagnosed early and if technically feasible.

If the patient is unstable, primary repair is not a practical option. These patients should undergo temporary diversion with a nephrostomy tube, ureteral ligation, and planned delayed repair, which prevents urinary extravasation and urinoma formation, however this is mostly based on anecdotal accounts [1]. Placing a ureteral stent will ensure patency of the ureter in incomplete ureteral injuries if the injury was initially missed or presented in a delayed manner [25]. Ku et al. showed that patients who underwent urinary diversion alone without a stent had a higher rate of ureteral stenosis [26] however, if stent placement is not possible, the patient should be treated in the same manner as unstable patients.

The method of choice for ureteric repair depends on the location, extent, and mechanism of injury. Ureteral injuries distal to the iliac vessels should be repaired either primarily or with ureteral reimplant (ureteroneocystostomy) over a ureteral stent [17,18]. Long defects >2 cm will likely require a psoas hitch or Boari flap to provide a tension-free anastomosis [18]. Injuries above the iliac vessels should be repaired primarily with a spatulated, tension-free primary repair (ureteroureterostomy) over a ureteral stent after all nonviable tissue has been debrided [17]. If the anastomosis is not tension-free, mobilization of the ureter needs to be performed. If mobilization does not permit for tension-free anastomosis, then ureteral reimplantation can be attempted with other maneuvers such as a psoas hitch and/or Boari flap to bring the ureter closer to the bladder. Complex reconstruction such as autotransplant and bowel interposition should not be attempted in the acute setting [17,18]. Autotransplant can be used with large length ureteral loss and involves placing the affected kidney into the iliac fossa with vascular anastomoses of the renal to iliac vessels and a ureterovesicostomy. Bowel interposition, usually performed with ileum requires a standard mechanical and antibiotic bowel preparation. Success rates can be as high as 81%, but there are associated complications such as mucus formation, stones, recurrent infections, and metabolic acidosis [7]. These procedures are too complex and time-consuming to be appropriately performed in the trauma setting.

*Recommendations*: Hemodynamically stable patients with ureteral injuries should undergo primary repair or ureteral reimplant if time permits. Delayed management almost always results in significant stricture (Grade C).

## 42.4 Bladder Trauma

### 42.4.1 What Types of Bladder Injuries Need to Be Surgically Repaired?

The bladder is a hollow organ located deep in the pelvis, usually protected from external trauma. Bladder injuries only occur in 1.6% of blunt abdominal trauma cases since such high forces are required to disrupt the integrity of the bony pelvis [28]. Other causes include a direct blow to a distended bladder, penetrating injuries, and other various iatrogenic causes.

Bladder injuries (60%–90%) are associated with pelvic fractures, while only a 2%–11% of patients with pelvic fractures have bladder injuries [28], thus not all patients with pelvic fracture require imaging to rule out bladder injury. When combined with the presence of gross hematuria, pelvic fractures are highly indicative of a bladder injury. A retrospective review of 53 patients with bladder rupture secondary to blunt trauma revealed that all 85% with gross hematuria also sustained a pelvic fracture [29]. Stable patients with gross hematuria and pelvic fracture must have retrograde cystography (RC) to rule out bladder perforation or rupture. RC may be performed with either plain radiographs or CT; both have high specificity and sensitivity for bladder injury [30]. Associated injuries, the hemodynamic stability of the patient, and the availability of the test need to be considered when choosing between the two.

Stable patients with gross hematuria and mechanisms concerning for bladder injury, or in those with pelvic ring fractures and clinical suspicion for bladder rupture should also undergo RC, although the evidence is not as strong as with gross hematuria in the setting of a pelvic fracture. Some patients with pelvic fractures with bladder injuries will present with microscopic hematuria. Patients who suffered pelvic fractures with hematuria >30 RBC/HPF had an increased risk for bladder injury, while none of the patients with <30 RBC/HPF had bladder injuries [31]. Additionally, patients with wide diastasis of the symphysis pubis or sacroiliac joints, and displaced fractures of the obturator ring were at increased risk for bladder injury.

The standard of care for intraperitoneal (IP) bladder rupture in the setting of blunt or penetrating external trauma is immediate surgical repair [29,32,33]. These injuries are located at the dome of the bladder and rarely heal with catheter drainage alone. Failure to repair or recognize IP bladder injuries can lead to urinary ascites, ileus, abdominal distention, peritonitis, localized abscesses, or sepsis [28]. Patients who require complex repairs, those involving the trigone or ureteral reimplantation, should undergo a postoperative cystogram to ensure complete healing of the bladder, while patients who undergo simple repairs may not necessarily need any follow-up imaging at all. All simple IP injuries had negative post-operative cystograms while one of three of the complex IP injuries had a cystogram positive for a leak [34], with the postoperative cystogram being performed between 1 and 4 weeks. There are no prospective data to determine the optimal timing of the postoperative cystogram and catheter removal in these patients, but current practice involves obtaining the cystogram at 2 weeks.

Extraperitoneal bladder ruptures (EP) account for about 55% of all bladder injuries and are seen almost exclusively with pelvic fractures [28]. As opposed to patients with IP bladder injuries, patients with uncomplicated EP bladder injury can be managed conservatively with Foley catheter drainage [22]. No statistical differences in outcomes were identified between patients whose EP bladder injuries were explored surgically or treated with Foley drainage [28,35]. As with IP bladder injuries, cystography should be performed after 2 weeks to ensure complete healing of the bladder injury [34].

Patients with complicated EP bladder injuries, such as those with exposed bone spicules in the bladder lumen, concurrent rectal or vaginal lacerations, or bladder neck injuries should undergo surgical repair as patients in these circumstances will likely develop long-term sequelae if the injuries were not primarily repaired [21]. Patients undergoing open reduction internal fixation or repair of abdominal injuries may benefit from concurrent repair of EP bladder injuries as the typical bladder repair can be executed with little morbidity [28,33].

Patients who undergo IP or EP bladder repair should have urethral catheter drainage without the need for a suprapubic cystotomy. Several studies have shown that the use of suprapubic tubes with urethral catheterization vs. catheterization alone does not offer any advantage in terms of altering catheter related complications [16,36,37]. Alli et al. showed that the use of urethral catheters alone is associated with shorter hospital stays and lower morbidity including a decreased incidence of UTIs, fistula formation, and the development of urinary retention than drainage with both suprapubic and urethral catheters [36].

*Recommendations*: IP bladder ruptures in the setting of blunt or penetrating external trauma should undergo prompt surgery and be primarily repaired (Grade B). Uncomplicated EP bladder injuries should be treated conservatively with Foley catheter drainage, while complicated EP bladder injuries should be primarily repaired (Grade C).

## 42.5 Urethral Trauma

### 42.5.1 How Should Urethral Trauma Be Managed in the Acute Setting?

Urethral injury can occur to the anterior urethra (penile or bulbar) or posterior urethra (proximal to the membranous urethra). The mechanism of injury tends to differ with straddle injuries (a crushing of the immobile portion of the urethra between the undersurface of the pubis) and penetrating trauma affecting the anterior urethra. Posterior urethral injuries tend to be associated with pelvic fracture. Of paramount importance to the successful management of urethral trauma is the degree of suspicion of injury. Any blood at the urethral meatus in the setting of pelvic trauma needs to be considered a significant finding and be evaluated with retrograde urethrography (RUG), which will help establish the diagnosis of urethral injury [38], however, establishing the full extent of injury may be prevented by external sphincter, pelvic floor, and periurethral spasm.

*Recommendation*: Acute management of suspected urethral injury must include RUG (Grade C).

### 42.5.2 Should Straddle (Anterior) Injuries Be Treated Acutely or Should Management Be Delayed?

The timing of the repair of these injuries has been debated and several series have satisfactorily provided evidence-based outcomes. RUG is required to determine a complete or incomplete injury. The most common complication related to these injuries is the subsequent development of a urethral stricture, with a statistically greater likelihood of stricture formation in those who had a complete bulbar urethral rupture [38].

The incidence of stricture formation is greater in those who underwent primary urethral realignment (82% vs. 35%; $p < 0.001$) [38], supporting the use of an initial suprapubic cystotomy (SP). In patients with partial urethral disruption, stricture formation occurred in 11% of patients with SP and 87% in patients who underwent realignment. Patients with complete disruption who underwent realignment demonstrated a 100% incidence of stricture formation compared to 75% treated with SP. The San Francisco General experience included only 19% of patients having primary realignment, and patients who underwent primary realignment required complex flaps or graft urethroplasty at a greater rate compared to men who underwent SP [39].

In patients with complete bulbar disruption that occurred as a result of blunt trauma, statistically higher rates of urethral stricture formation were noted in patients who underwent delayed repair than in those who underwent immediate urethral realignment (69% vs. 31%; $p = 0.014$) [40].

Gong et al. assessed additional endpoints in another study comparing immediate and primary repair after initial suprapubic cystotomy insertion, and did not find any statistical difference in stricture formation related to the time of the repair, however, a significantly shorter return to spontaneous voiding and the length of time needed for suprapubic diversion with immediate repair were noted [41]. No differences were noted in erectile dysfunction, or continence rates between the two groups, and without any outcome advantages, it does not appear that immediate primary repair is indicated in a trauma patient who likely has more serious concomitant injuries.

*Recommendation*: In bulbar urethral injuries, urinary drainage should occur with a suprapubic cystostomy tube. Primary realignment can be considered in patients with complete bulbar disruption (Grade C).

### 42.5.3 What Is the Ideal Management of Posterior Urethral Injuries Associated with Pelvic Fractures?

Posterior urethral disruption has been reported in 5%–25% of patients sustaining pelvic fractures. Immediate urinary drainage must be established with the placement of a suprapubic tube and controversy exists regarding the subsequent management of the urinary drainage. Traditionally, delayed repairs have been advocated, especially in those patients who may be hemodynamically unstable. The early endoscopic realignment of posterior urethral disruptions has been advocated with long-term follow-up revealing no increased incidence of impotence, stricture formation or incontinence compared to delayed repair [42,43], providing that the realignment is done in a fairly expeditious manner [1].

The most common complication seen in these patients is the subsequent development of a urethral stricture, and long-term surveillance needs to be pursued. Stricture formation in this group of severely ill patients who have sustained significant concomitant injuries resulting in 51% mortality rates, is extremely high regardless of early versus delayed reconstruction, but clearly favors the early realignment group (49% vs. 100%) [43,44]. Delayed repair was also associated with a greater degree of complexity of the resultant stricture, further supporting early realignment.

Urethral trauma that requires a suprapubic tube raises concerns amongst orthopedic surgeons who worry about the proximity of a foreign body to a site of hardware insertion. On occasion, this has led on occasion to the conservative management of orthopedic injuries and possible suboptimal outcomes [44]. However, there has not been any proven increased incidence of hardware infection despite these concerns [44,45], and orthopedic repair should occur irrespective of the need for suprapubic cystostomy. To allay some of these fears, the urologist can place the tube as high as possible in the bladder and use a subcutaneous tunnel.

*Recommendation*: Endoscopic early realignment of posterior urethral injuries should be attempted if possible. (Grade C).

## 42.6 Penile and Scrotal Trauma

### 42.6.1 Does Penetrating Penile or Scrotal Trauma Need to Be Explored?

Penetrating penile or scrotal trauma in the civilian population usually occurs as a result of low velocity projectiles. They are rather rare occurrences and there is a paucity of studies in the literature, most which come from the larger trauma centers in the country [46–48]. Exploration of penetrating scrotal trauma occurring from either gunshot wounds (GSWs) or stab wounds (SWs) has been shown to result in testicular salvage, and exploration is indicated. Salvage rates of GSWs have been reported between 52% and 75% [47,48], with GSWs showing statistically significant higher salvage rates than SWs ($p < 0.001$) [48]. Studies such as these are consistent with the European Association of Urology (EAU) 2005 guidelines [49], which recommend scrotal exploration for all penetrating scrotal injuries. Only injuries that were superficial, nonpenetrating, and had a low clinical suspicion of injury deep to the dartos layer were managed without surgery.

Given the high rate of testicular loss despite exploration, these outcomes may help influence preoperative counseling with regard to patient's expectations. This center advocates surgical exploration in lieu of ultrasound evaluation in all injuries that have penetrated or are suspected to have penetrated the dartos fascia, and to perform conservative debridement. The vascularity of the scrotal contents helps to contribute to the low rate of infectious complications seen postoperatively.

GSWs to the external genitalia result in a lower incidence of urethral injury compared to SWs (6% vs. 17%) [48]. GSWs may be associated with urethral injury (15%–29%) and blood at the urethral meatus is indication to perform a RUG which has been shown to have a sensitivity of 92%, specificity of 100%, a positive predictive value of 100% and a negative predictive value of 97% [50]. Spatulated primary repair of the injury should be undertaken when injury in the anterior urethra is identified. Conservative treatment can be undertaken for superficial injuries, however an injury to the cavernosal bodies should be repaired [46].

*Recommendation*: Penile, urethral, or testicular injury should be explored and repaired in the hemodynamically stable patient (Grade C).

### 42.6.2 Does Penile Fracture Need to Be Treated Emergently?

A penile fracture refers to a tear of the corpus cavernosum in an erect penis. Patients commonly complain of a snapping or popping sensation that occurs during sexual activity followed by pain, detumescence, discoloration, and penile swelling. Koifman et al. categorized patients into either low or high suspicion of injury and managed only the highly suspicious group with surgical intervention [51]. None of the nonoperative group experienced complications related to subsequent erectile dysfunction (ED), and similarly in the 88% of patients in the surgical group who followed up, ED did not occur. Penile curvature was noted in 5.6% [51]. The history, physical findings, and mechanism of injury help determine treatment.

Satisfactory and painless erectile function was reported in 95% of surgical patients who underwent immediate repair, with a few long-term complications (4.7%), and erectile dysfunction rates similar to a control population [52]. Urethral injury may also occur in these patients and blood at the meatus must be evaluated either with urethrography or cystoscopy at the time of intervention. Up to 50% of patients treated conservatively have been shown to have complications of erectile dysfunction and penile curvature [53].

In a series of 300 patients, all undergoing repair within 48 h of injury, complications reported including erectile dysfunction (0.6%), penile pain with erection or intercourse (3.3%), and mild penile curvature in 14 patients (4.6%) that did not hinder intercourse in 10 of them [54]. Older series had advocated conservative management of this problem using ice, pressure dressings, and anti-inflammatories; however, complication rates in these earlier series are reported up to 53% [55].

Whether the repair of the defect in the corpora cavernosum must be treated emergently has been debated. There are no studies that show any adverse effects related to the immediate repair of the injury, and clearly emergent repair can be undertaken. A retrospective study of 180 patients with long-term follow-up (mean 8 years) demonstrated that regardless of early repair (within 24 h) or delayed repair (within 7 days), no statistically significant differences in outcomes were noted (Table 42.1) [56].

*Recommendation*: Penile fracture should be surgically corrected either immediately or delayed (within 7 days) to maximize outcomes such as erectile function and lack of penile deviation (Grade B).

**TABLE 42.1**
Evidence-Based Management of Urotrauma

| Question | Answer | Grade of Recommendation | Level of Evidence | References |
|---|---|---|---|---|
| When does renal trauma require immediate surgical exploration? | Hemodynamically stable patients with renal injury may initially be treated nonoperatively, while hemodynamically unstable patients who do not respond to resuscitation must undergo immediate intervention, whether via surgery or angioembolization. | B | III, IV | [1–15] |
| How should traumatic ureteral injuries be repaired? | Hemodynamically stable patients with ureteral injuries should undergo primary repair or ureteral reimplant if time permits. Delayed management almost always results in significant stricture. | C | III, IV | [1,16–27] |
| What types of bladder injuries need to be surgically repaired? | IP bladder ruptures in the setting of blunt or penetrating external trauma should be primarily repaired.<br>Uncomplicated EP bladder injuries should be treated conservatively with Foley catheter drainage, while complicated EP bladder injuries should be primarily repaired. | B<br>C | III<br>III | [21,22, 28–37] |
| How should urethral trauma be managed in the acute setting? | Acute management of suspected urethral injury must include RUG. | C | III | [38] |
| Should straddle injuries be treated acutely or should management be delayed? | In bulbar urethral injuries, urinary drainage should occur with a suprapubic tube. Primary realignment can be considered in patients with complete bulbar disruption. | C | III | [39–42] |
| What is the ideal management of posterior urethral injuries associated with pelvic fractures? | Endoscopic early realignment should be attempted if possible. | C | III, IV | [1,42–45] |
| Does penetrating penile or scrotal trauma need to be explored? | Penile, urethral or testicular injury should be explored and repaired in the hemodynamically stable patient. | C | IV | [46–50] |
| Does penile fracture need to be treated emergently? | Penile fracture should be corrected either immediately or delayed to maximize outcomes such as erectile function and lack of penile deviation. | B | III | [50–54] |

## References


1. Morey A, Brandes S, Dugi D et al. Urotrauma: AUA guidelines. *J Urol.* 2014;192:327–335.
2. Wessells H, Suh D, Porter JR et al. Renal injury and operative management in the United States: Results of a population-based study. *J Trauma.* 2003;54:423–430.
3. Santucci RA, McAninch JW, Safir M et al. Validation of the American Association for the Surgery of Trauma organ injury severity scale for the kidney. *J Trauma.* 2001;50:195–200.
4. Shariat SF, Roehrborn CG, Karakiewicz PI et al. Evidence-based validation of the predictive value of the American Association for the Surgery of Trauma kidney injury scale. *J Trauma.* 2007;62:933–939.
5. Miller KS, McAninch JW. Radiographic assessment of renal trauma: Our 15-year experience. *J Urol.* 1995;154:352–355.
6. Brandes SB, McAninch JW. Urban free falls and patterns of renal injury: A 20-year experience with 396 cases. *J Trauma.* 1999;47:643–649.
7. Danuser H, Wille S, Zöscher G, Studer U. How to treat blunt kidney ruptures: Primary open surgery or conservative treatment with deferred surgery when necessary? *Eur Urol.* 2001;39:9–14.
8. Santucci RA, Fisher MB. The literature increasingly supports expectant (conservative) management of renal trauma—A systematic review. *J Trauma.* 2005;59:493–501.
9. McGuire J, Bultitude MF, Davis P et al. Predictors of outcome for blunt high grade renal injury treated with conservative intent. *J Urol.* 2011;185:187–191.
10. Altman AL, Haas C, Dinchman KH, Spirnak JP. Selective non-operative management of blunt grade 5 renal injury. *J Urol.* 2000;164:27–30.
11. Bjurlin MA, Jeng EI, Goble SM et al. Comparison of non-operative management with renorrhaphy and nephrectomy in penetrating renal injuries. *J Trauma.* 2011;71:554–558.
12. Knudson MM, Harrison PB, Hoyt DB et al. Outcome after major renovascular injuries: A Western Trauma Association multicenter report. *J Trauma.* 2000;49: 1116–1122.
13. Breyer BN, McAninch JW, Elliott SP et al. Minimally invasive endovascular techniques to treat acute renal hemorrhage. *J Urol.* 2008;179:2248–2253.
14. Brewer ME, Strnad BT, Daley BJ et al. Percutaneous embolization for the management of grade 5 renal trauma in hemodynamically unstable patients: Initial experience. *J Urol.* 2009;181:1737–1741.

15. Alsikafi NF, McAninch JW, Elliott SP, Garcia M. Nonoperative management outcomes of isolated urinary extravasation following renal lacerations due to external trauma. *J Urol.* December 2006;176(6 Pt 1):2494–2497.
16. Al-Awadi K, Kehinde EO, Al-Hunayan A et al. Iatrogenic ureteric injuries: Incidence, aetiological factors and the effect of early management on subsequent outcome. *Int Urol Nephrol.* 2005;37:2235–2241.
17. Elliott SP, McAninch JW. Ureteral injuries from external violence: The 25-year experience at San Francisco General Hospital. *J Urol.* 2003;170:1213–1216.
18. Brandes S, Coburn M, Armenakas N et al. Diagnosis and management of ureteric injury: An evidence-based analysis. *BJU Int.* 2004;94:277–289.
19. Carver BS, Bozeman CB, Venable DD. Ureteral injury due to penetrating trauma. *South Med J.* 2004;97:462–464.
20. Gayer G, Zissin R, Apter S et al. Urinomas caused by ureteral injuries: CT appearance. *Abdom Imag.* 2002;27:88–92.
21. Ortega SJ, Netto FS, Hamilton P et al. CT scanning for diagnosing blunt ureteral and ureteropelvic junction injuries. *BMC Urol.* 2008;8:1–5.
22. Digiacomo JC, Frankel H, Rotondo MF et al. Preoperative radiographic staging for ureteral injuries is not warranted in patients undergoing celiotomy for trauma. *Am Surg.* 2001;67:969–973.
23. Kunkle DA, Kansas BT, Pathak A et al. Delayed diagnosis of traumatic ureteral injuries. *J Urol.* 2006;176(Pt 1): 2503–2507.
24. Best CD, Petrone P, Buscarini M et al. Traumatic ureteral injuries: A single institution experience validating the American Association for the Surgery of Trauma-Organ Injury Scale grading scale. *J Urol.* 2005;173: 1202–1205.
25. Koukouras D, Petsas T, Liatsikos E et al. Percutaneous minimally invasive management of iatrogenic ureteral injuries. *J Endourol.* 2010;24:1921–1927.
26. Ku JH, Kim ME, Jeon YS et al. Minimally invasive management of ureteral injuries Recognized later after obstetric and gynaecologic surgery. *Injury.* 2003;34: 480–483.
27. Kochakarn W, Tirapanich W, Kositchaiwat S. Ileal interposition for the treatment of a long gap ureteral loss. *J Med Assoc Thai.* 2000;83:37–41.
28. Gomez RG, Ceballos L, Coburn M et al. Consensus statement on bladder injuries. *BJU Int.* 2004;94:2732.
29. Morey AF, Iverson AJ, Swan A et al. Bladder rupture after blunt trauma: Guidelines for diagnostic imaging. *J Trauma.* 2001;51:683–686.
30. Quagliano PV, Delair SM, Malhotra AK. Diagnosis of blunt bladder injury: A prospective comparative study of computed tomography cystography and conventional retrograde cystography. *J Trauma.* 2006;61:410–421.
31. Avey G, Blackmore CC, Wessells H et al. Radiographic and clinical predictors of bladder rupture in blunt trauma patients with pelvic fracture. *Acad Radiol.* 2006;13:573–579.
32. Wirth GJ, Peter R, Poletti PA et al. Advances in the management of blunt traumatic bladder rupture: Experience with 36 cases. *BJU Int.* 2010;106:1344–1349.
33. Pereira BM, de Campos CC, Calderan TR et al. Bladder injuries after external trauma: 20 years' experience report in a population-based cross-sectional view. *World J Urol.* 2013;31:913–917.
34. Inaba K, McKenney M, Munera F et al. Cystogram follow-up in the management of traumatic bladder disruption. *J Trauma.* 2006;60:23–28.
35. Corriere JN, Sandler CM. Management of the ruptured bladder: Seven years of experience with 111 cases. *J Trauma.* 1986;26:830–833.
36. Alli MO, Singh B, Moodley J et al. Prospective evaluation of combined suprapubic and urethral catheterization to urethral drainage alone for intraperitoneal bladder injuries. *J Trauma.* 2003;55:1152–1154.
37. Volpe MA, Pachter EM, Scalea TM et al. Is there a difference in outcome when treating traumatic intraperitoneal bladder rupture with or without a suprapubic tube? *J Urol.* 1999;161:1103–1105.
38. Elgammal MA. Straddle injuries to the bulbar urethra: Management and outcome in 53 patients. *Int Braz J Urol.* 2009;34:450–458.
39. Park S, McAnnich JW. Straddle injuries to the bulbar urethra: Management and outcomes in 78 patients. *J Urol.* 2004;171:722–725.
40. Ku JH, Kim ME, Jeon YS et al. Management of bulbous urethral disruption by blunt external trauma: The sooner, the better? *Urology.* 2002;60:579–583.
41. Gong IH, Oh JJ, Choi DK et al. Comparison of immediate primary repair and delayed urethroplasty in men with bulbous urethral disruption after blunt straddle injury. *Kor J Urol.* 2012;53:569–572.
42. Moudouni SM, Parard JJ, Manunta A et al. Early endoscopic realignment of post-traumatic posterior urethral disruption. *Urology.* 2001;57:628–632.
43. Mouraview V, Coburn M, Santucci R. The treatment of posterior urethral disruption associated with pelvic fractures: Comparative experience of early realignment versus delayed urethroplasy. *J Urol.* 2005;173:873–876.
44. Mayher BE, Guyton JL, Gingrich JR. Impact of urethral management on the treatment and outcome of concurrent pelvic fractures. *Urology.* 2001;57:439–442.
45. Bepple JL, Virasoro R, Williams MB et al. Incidence of infection in patients with orthopedic interventions for pelvic fracture and a suprapubic catheter placed secondary to posterior urethral distraction. *J Urol.* 2007;77:115.
46. Cerwinka W, Block NL. Civilian gunshot injuries of the penis: The Miami experience. *Urology.* 2009;73:877–880.
47. Simhan JH, Rothman J, Canter D et al. Gunshot wounds to the scrotum: A large single-institutional 20-year experience. *BJU Int.* 2012;190:1704–1708.
48. Phonsombat S, Master VA, McAninch JW. Penetrating external genital trauma: A 30-year single institution experience. *J Urol.* 2008;180:192–196.
49. Lynch TH, Marinez-Pineiro L, Plas E et al. EAU guidelines on urological trauma. *Eur Urol.* 2005;47:1–15.
50. Kunkle DA, Leed BD, Mydlo JH et al. Evaluation and management of gunshot wounds of the penis: 20-year experience at an urban trauma center. *J Trauma.* 2008;64:1038–1042.

51. Koifman L, Barros R, Junior R et al. Penile fracture: Diagnosis, treatment and outcomes of 150 patients. *Urology*. 2010;76:1488–1492.
52. Zargooshi J. Penile fracture in Kermanshah, Iran: The long-term results of surgical treatment. *BJU Int*. 2002;89:890–894.
53. Gamal WM, Osman MM, Hammady AH et al. Penile fracture: Long-term results of surgical and conservative management. *J Trauma*. 2011;71:491–493.
54. El Atat R, Sfaxi M, Benslama MR et al. Fracture of the penis: Management and long-term results of surgical treatment. Experience in 300 cases. *J Trauma*. 2008;64: 121–125.
55. Mydlo JH. Surgeon experience with penile fracture. *J Urol*. 2001;166:526–529.
56. El-Assmy A, El-Tholoth HJ, Mohsen T et al. Does timing of presentation of penile fracture affect outcome of surgical intervention? *Urology*. 2011;77:1388–1392.

## Commentary on Evidence-Based Management of Genitourinary Trauma

*Steven B. Brandes*

### When Does Renal Trauma Require Immediate Surgical Exploration?

The short answer is that in patients who are unstable from bleeding that is sourced to be coming from the kidney, exploration is mandatory to prevent exsanguination and/or death. Everything else is a relative indication for kidney exploration. As to blunt renal trauma, the only absolute indication for exploration is a Grade 5 injury. Grade 5 injuries are by definition life threatening. Shattered kidney is under the category Grade 5, but the definition of a "shattered" kidney is vague—and thus spawns papers that conclude that select Grade 5 injuries can be managed conservatively. I think such papers are deceptive and their cohorts are just severe Grade 4 injuries, and not true grade 5 injuries.

If a blunt trauma patient undergoes abdominal exploration and a pulsatile, expanding or uncontained retroperitoneal hematoma (Zone 2) is noted—this suggests that there is a major arterial injury—and thus requires opening the hematoma—with the knowledge that opening the hematoma and releasing the tamponade effect will often result in a nephrectomy. A Zone 1 hematoma, which by definition overlies the great vessels, demands exploration because of its potential for exsanguination. It is wise to get proximal vascular control for a Zone 1 hematoma, but for a Zone 2 hematoma, it is controversial. We feel that vascular control of the kidney parenchyma can be achieved by just manual compression. If the injury is so severe that bleeding cannot be controlled manually, then place a hilar pedicle clamp. The key here is to bring the kidney to the midline and scoop the kidney out of the retroperitoneal space. If there is a large perinephric hematoma, then the blood has done the dissection for you. When mobilizing the kidney, be careful not to iatrogenically strip the kidney capsule off, because the renorrhaphy bolster sutures then will easily pull through.

All other injuries, irrespective of the degree of urine extravasation, renal parenchymal infarct, and hilar vessel thrombosis, are relative indications for operative intervention. Contrast extravasation that is medial to the kidney, and no contrast seen in the ureter on CT imaging, suggests an ureteropelvic junction (UPJ) injury. This warrants further evaluation by retrograde urogram. If the injury is partial, place a ureteral stent. The textbook answer for an UPJ avulsion is immediate repair, but the tissue is usually very friable and the anatomy distorted. We prefer instead to place a nephrostomy tube followed by a definitive repair weeks later.

For gunshot wounds (GSWs) to the kidney, the *best* management is debatable. Civilian injuries are typically low-velocity injuries, so the degree of blast injury and delayed tissue damage are limited. This said, we feel that isolated penetrating injuries to kidneys that do not violate the peritoneal cavity should be managed grade for grade, the same as a blunt injury. The proviso is that Grade 3 and 4 penetrating injuries have a 20%–25% chance for a delayed bleed when managed conservatively. Delayed bleeds can be managed by angiography and selective embolization. For GSWs that violate the retroperitoneum and there is a stable hematoma, by definition the hematoma is uncontained, as it has a hole in it, and thus demands exploration. Once explored, if the kidney just has a thru and thru hole and is not bleeding, then we typically just cover the hole with an absorbable hemostat such as Surgicel™ and place a closed suction drain in proximity. However, if the kidney injury had been properly staged by CT preoperatively, and the hematoma is stable and the Gerota's bullet hole is not bleeding, it is reasonable to manage the hematoma expectantly—and not open it.

### How Should Traumatic Ureteral Injuries Be Repaired?

Nearly all ureteral injuries (except for UPJ) are from a penetrating mechanism. Blunt injuries are typical to the UPJ, classically seen in adolescents with flexion-extension injuries. I agree with the statement that hemodynamically stable patients should have the ureteral injury repaired, while unstable patients should be damaged controlled—and the definitive repair delayed until the patient fully resuscitated. For the unstable patient, good options are to ligate the ureter with a long silk and come back for a planned and delayed repair, or place a single J ureteral stent up the cut end of the ureter. Do not mobilize the ureter and just bring the stent out of a stab incision in the skin (like a JP drain) and place a urostomy bag over it.

For the stable patient with a pelvic ureteral injury—reimplant the ureter into the dome of the bladder or perform a Psoas hitch and reimplant. Fancy repairs like a Boari flap or trans-ureteroureterostomy or Ileal ureter or auto transplant have no place in the acute setting and should be delayed till resuscitation is performed and in a delayed fashion.

### What Types of Bladder Injuries Need to Be Surgically Repaired?

#### *Blunt Injuries*

Intraperitoneal bladder ruptures to the dome of the bladder from blunt trauma to a full bladder should be surgically repaired, because the dome injury is on average 6 cm long. Urine leaking into the abdomen can result in severe morbidity (metabolic acidosis, AKI and ascites). Extraperitoneal bladder injuries almost always can be managed conservatively. Concomitant rectal or vaginal injuries are very rare—yet demand repair, to prevent a fistula. Interposing omentum between the repairs is wise. The textbook answer for a bladder injury that also involves the bladder neck (BN) is to open the bladder and fix the BN injury from within—the reason is that the rates of BN contracture or severe incontinence are high if not repaired. Extraperitoneal bladder injuries that require repair are ones where the pelvic hematoma is evacuating out the Foley, and thus does not drain well from clots. Extraperitoneal bladder injuries are nearly always from shearing forces. When repairing extraperitoneal bladder injuries acutely, it is important not to disturb the pelvic hematoma and to enter the bladder from the dome and to explore the bladder and repair all injuries from within. Two narrow handheld Deaver retractors are helpful to expose the inside of the bladder, the ureteral orifices for clear efflux, and the bladder neck.

For patients with an open book pelvic fracture and an extraperitoneal bladder injury, who undergo internal fixation of the pubic diastasis—this is an ideal time to also fix the bladder. Orthopedics will make a Pfannenstiel incision, open up the space of Retzius and suck out the pelvic hematoma, and, in so doing, expose the whole anterior bladder.

#### *Penetrating Injuries*

GSWs to the bladder from a low velocity bullet demand bladder exploration so as to look at the trigone and to see if the GSW is in proximity to the ureteral orifice (UO) or bladder neck. Injuries in proximity to the UO demand ureteral stent placement. Injuries through the UO or intramural tunnel demand ureteral reimplantation. All GSWs to the trigone demand evaluation of the rectum or vagina for possible injury. This is very different from a 5 mm trocar injury to the bladder dome. Such injuries to the dome are small and do not involve the trigone, and thus can typically be managed by prolonged Foley drainage.

### How Should Urethral Trauma Be Managed in the Acute Setting?

Urethral injuries from pelvic fracture are caused by shearing forces. Gentle placement of a Foley catheter is safe and reasonable to try. If the patient is young and awake, inability to place a Foley is usually because he is in pain and clamping down the external sphincter. Moreover, a gentle attempt at a Foley catheter does not convert a partial urethral injury to a complete injury, unless the Foley balloon is inflated at the injury site. Foley placement should not be relegated to the nurse or medical student.

If the bladder is full and there is a urethral injury on imaging, a percutaneous suprapubic tube can be placed in the emergency room. If there is an associated bladder injury and the bladder is decompressed, then an SP needs to be placed in the OR.

### What Is the Ideal Management of Posterior Urethral Injuries Associated with Pelvic Fractures?

I agree with the authors that the ideal time for primary realignment is at the same time that orthopedics performs their ORIF surgery—usually 2–5 days after acute injury. Primary realignment with fluoroscopy guidance and two cystoscopes is a good method to help reduce long-term urethral stricture formation—without negatively affecting eventual potency or urine control. Primary realignment, however, entails a high degree of selection bias. So the actual benefit from primary realignment is less than the historical 50% reduction in stricture rate. Regardless, there is little downside.

### Should Straddle Injuries Be Treated Acutely or Should Management Be Delayed?

Urethral injuries from pelvic fracture and those from a straddle injury are very different, and should not be treated the same. A urethral injury from pelvic fracture is typically a distraction injury, either at the prostatomembranous or bulbo-membranous junction. The urethral ends are pulled apart, and the interposing space fills with scar. Straddle injuries are a crush injury to the corpus spongiosum and urethra between the object and the pubic bone. The urethra remains in continuity and is not distracted at all. From the limited literature, it is best to manage straddle injuries just by SP tube and avoid attempts at urethral realignment.

### Does Penetrating Penile or Scrotal Trauma Need to Be Explored?

All penetrating scrotal wounds should be explored, in the stable patient. Wounds that result in blood at the meatus, hematuria (microscopic or gross), perineal swelling, or ecchymosis appear to be in the trajectory of the urethra, and hence demand urethral evaluation. If the patient is unstable and has other pressing issues, the penis or scrotum can be explored safely within 48–72 h. Penetrating wounds to the scrotum with associated swelling and/or ecchymosis demand exploration, because physical exam is unreliable and a normal feeling testis can still be severely injured.

As to GSWs to the penis—if the wounds are in proximity to or in the path of the urethra—when the penis is degloved and explored—the urethra can be directly examined for injury. The reason for closing the holes in the corpora and Buck's fascia is to prevent venous leak impotence.

**Does Penile Fracture Need to Be Treated Emergently?**

Do not believe the hype—penile fracture is not a true urologic emergency. Fractures can safely be scheduled for surgical repair, in an elective fashion. All penile fractures should eventually undergo repair, in order to prevent penile curvature, penile fibrosis, and organic impotence. We prefer to explore within 48hrs of injury, but many patients are embarrassed and avoid early presentation. In such cases, we have safely and successfully explored patients even up to 7–10 days post injury. The injury to the corpora is typically transverse at the mid penis on the ventrum. The exception to a delayed repair is an associated urethral injury—which demands immediate repair, as the patient either cannot urinate or will void urine into the penile tissue.

# Section II

# Surgical Emergencies

# 43

# *Small Bowel Surgery*

**Rafael M. Bustamante and John J. Hong**

**CONTENTS**



## 43.1 Postoperative Ileus

### 43.1.1 Introduction

Ileus is defined as bowel dysmotility in the absence of a mechanical obstruction. It is usually a self-limiting process, but can produce significant morbidity and increase hospital length of stay and hospital cost. Ileus fall into two categories: expected postoperative ileus or paralytic ileus. Postoperative ileus (POI) is the uncomplicated ileus occurring following surgery, generally resolving spontaneously in about 2–3 days, while paralytic POI lasts longer than 3 days [1]. Risk factors for paralytic ileus include overuse of narcotics, retroperitoneal inflammation, sepsis, and spinal cord injury.

Artinyan and colleagues examined the extent and duration of POI in 88 patients who underwent elective abdominal surgery. The duration of POI was 10 days or less in 96.6% of patients and the median duration was 5 days. The mean number of days to initiation of unrestricted clear liquids were 1.6% and 22.7% of patients were tolerating a solid diet by postoperative day (POD) 6. Variables within the patient population such as age, body mass index (BMI), anesthesia time, surgery time, estimated blood loss (EBL), and total opioid dose were examined to determine whether correlation exists to the duration of POI. Statistically, only EBL and total opioid dose were independently and significantly associated with duration of POI [2].

Symptoms of POI include increasing abdominal pain, distention, nausea and vomiting, and obstipation. POI affects all portions of the gastrointestinal (GI) tract and the recovery of each occurs at different rates. The function of the small intestine returns first, within 4–24 h after surgery, followed by the stomach in 24–48 h, and large intestine function returns last within 48–72 h [3].

There is no diagnostic test that can exclude or confirm the diagnosis of POI. Radiographs of the abdomen may show diffused dilated loops of small bowel, with air fluid levels resembling small bowel obstruction (SBO). Additional findings may include colonic dilatation. Upper GI series and abdominal computerized axial tomography (CAT) scans may be utilized when it is required to differentiate an ileus from bowel obstruction. The recognition of POI is based on the usual signs and symptoms in the proper postoperative setting.

The resolution of POI is marked with the passage of flatus or defecation, as colonic motility is the last portion of the GI tract to recover from ileus. Other criteria that can demonstrate the resolution of POI include the return of bowel sounds, a decrease in nasogastric tube (NGT) drainage, a change in the consistency of NGT drainage with decreasing amounts of bile, and the tolerance of oral intake.

#### 43.1.1.1 Does Chewing Gum Shorten the Duration of Postoperative Ileus?

Based on the evidence that early enteral feedings lessened the extent of POI, Asao and colleagues examined the effect of gum chewing as an alternative approach to stimulate bowel function in the postoperative period. Gum is theorized to increase vagal tone, normally provided by food, and to stimulate the release of GI hormones associated with bowel motility. Their data showed an earlier return of bowel function in a small series of 19 patients who underwent laparoscopic colon resection for cancer that were prospectively randomized to either a gum chewing or a control group. The first passage of flatus was about 24 h sooner and the first defecation was approximately 2.7 days sooner in the gum chewing group than in controls [4]. Another prospective study, published by Schuster and colleagues, randomized 34 patients scheduled for elective open sigmoidectomy for diverticular disease or cancer into a gum chewing or control group. The first passage of flatus occurred on postoperative hour 65.4 in the gum chewing group versus 80.2 in the control group. The first bowel movement occurred on postoperative hour 63.2 and 89.4 in the gum chewing and control groups, respectively [5]. A meta-analysis of 17 randomized controlled trials conducted by Li and Liu in 2013 identified trials studying the use of chewing gum in patients undergoing abdominal surgery. Days' reduction of return to flatus, bowel movement, and length of stay (LOS) were 0.31, 0.51, and 0.72 days, respectively [6].

*Recommendation*: According to prospective studies, gum chewing has shortened the duration of POI and hospital LOS and should be employed in postoperative patients.

*Grade of recommendation*: B

#### 43.1.1.2 Does the Use of Selective Opiate Receptor Inhibitors Decrease the Duration of Postoperative Ileus?

With the high cost of increased LOS and the increased morbidity associated with prolonged postoperative ileus, a novel approach has been the development of a selective opioid receptor antagonist. There are three opioid receptor subtypes, μ, κ, and δ, involved in regulation of GI tract function [7]. The μ receptor is the important subtype involved in GI motility, transit time, and central pain management [8]. Alvimopan is a synthetic, peripherally acting μ opioid antagonist that has limited GI absorption and does not cross the blood–brain barrier [9]. Clinical trials have supported the use of alvimopan as an agent to accelerate GI recovery and reduce time to patient discharge. In the first published study of 78 patients undergoing partial colectomy of total abdominal hysterectomy, 6 mg of alvimopan shortened the POI, measured by the median time to first flatus that decreased from 70 to 49 h, median time to first bowel movement that decreased from 111 to 70 h, and median time until readiness to hospital discharge that decreased from 91 to 68 h compared to placebo [10]. Wolff and colleagues prospectively randomized 500 patients undergoing bowel resection or radical hysterectomy to receive either alvimopan or placebo and demonstrated that the time to GI recovery was improved by 15–20 h following doses of 6 mg and 22–28 h following doses of 12 mg of alvimopan. The mean time to hospital discharge was 13 and 20 h sooner for patients treated with the 6 or 12 mg doses, respectively [11]. Vaughan performed a meta-analysis to determine the role of alvimopan in accelerating GI recovery and hospital discharge. Three trials were involved 1388 patients, in which 685 patients received 12 mg of alvimopan. The analysis showed a reduced time to hospital discharge that was reduced between 15.2 and 24 h, but the recovery for bowel function was reduced between 12.7 and 28 h with alvimopan. In these trials, alvimopan reduced time to GI recovery and hospital discharge in patients undergoing abdominal surgery [12]. Harbaugh et al. hypothesized that alvimopan significantly decreases the incidence of prolonged ileus and reduces LOS in patients who had undergone colectomy. Approximately 528 patients received pre- and postoperative alvimopan and compared to control group and they showed a lower incidence of prolonged ileus (2.3% vs. 7.9%) and significantly shorter LOS (4.84 vs. 6.40) than control patients [13]. These trials observed no differences between placebo and alvimopan-treated patients for postoperative opioid consumption and POI-related morbidity as shown by a lower postoperative NGT insertion, increased LOS, or readmission. Using pooled data from alvimopan trials, Wolff and colleagues [11] showed that overall POI morbidity in the placebo groups ranged from 14.1% to 19.7%, while those groups treated with alvimopan had ranged from 6.6% to 11.2%. With the reduction in POI and LOS, there was the added benefit of cost reduction. In a retrospective matched cohort study performed by Poston et al., 480 patients received alvimopan compared to 960 matched controls. Mean hospital cost was $12,865 for alvimopan patients, compared with $13,905 for controls [14]. Kauf et al. examined the effect of alvimopan treatment versus placebo on health care costs related to GI recovery in patients treated with radical cystectomy. They showed that mean hospital stay was 2.63 days shorter for alvimopan than placebo. POI-related health care cost was $2340 lower for alvimopan versus placebo and mean total combined costs were decreased by $2640 per patient [15].

*Recommendation*: Alvimopan has improved the duration of POI, hospital LOS, and cost in several prospective randomized studies.

*Grade of recommendation*: B

## 43.2 Intra-Abdominal Adhesions

### 43.2.1 Introduction

Intra-abdominal adhesions are one of the most frequent complications of abdominal surgery. They arise from the abdominal cavity's ability to form scar tissue after peritoneal violation.

The peritoneal cavity is the space between the visceral and parietal peritoneum making up a closed sac in the male and an open sac in the female through the gynecological tract. The peritoneum consists of a connective tissue layer covered by a mesothelium, which under normal conditions contains approximately 10 cc of serous fluid. This fluid circulates within the abdominal cavity through well-defined routes and is in continuity with the vascular system via lymphatics.

Intra-abdominal adhesions are formed after surgical trauma or inflammation of the peritoneum resulting in a denuded surface, submesothelial damage, and injury to blood vessels provoking an inflammatory response. This inflammatory response results in a simultaneous activation of the coagulation cascade and fibrin deposition, as well as the release of histamine and $PGE_2$ caused by increased vessel permeability [16]. Inactive fibrinogen at the site of peritoneal injury then becomes activated to a fibrin gel that connects the two damaged layers of peritoneum. There is a fibrinolytic process that attempts to control fibrin formation by hydrolyzing this to fibrin split products that is initiated by plasmin, an active protease formed by the action of plasminogen activators on its precursor, plasminogen. Surgery dramatically diminishes fibrinolytic activity, by increasing levels of plasminogen activator inhibitors and reducing tissue oxygenation. Eventually, in the absence of an effective fibrinolytic response, there exists a fibrin gel matrix that may serve as the scaffolding for the development of mature adhesions [16]. Adhesions contain inflammatory cells that include fibroblasts, macrophages, mast cells, eosinophils, red blood cells, and tissue debris. Over time the numbers of cells decrease, and adhesions mature into fibrous bands composed of collagen and covered by mesothelium.

The causes of SBO include internal hernias, intra-abdominal malignancy, and abdominal adhesions with over 70% resulting from previous surgery. Patients presenting with high-grade obstruction necessitating open laparotomies have an increased morbidity secondary to a higher risk of bowel injury. Reviews of hospital admissions for adhesional SBO have identified a mortality rate of almost 10% [17], increasing to approximately 15% in patients undergoing small bowel resection [18]. Adhesional SBO requiring surgical treatment has a 33% risk of inadvertent enterotomy and the presence of adhesions have a 19% risk of inadvertent enterotomy during a reoperative laparotomy [19]. There is a 20%–50% mortality rate in those patients who have an undetected bowel injury when undergoing operation for adhesional SBO [17].

#### *43.2.1.1 Which Is More Advantageous: Open or Laparoscopic Adhesiolysis?*

Small bowel obstruction requiring adhesiolysis is a frequent problem in the United States resulting with increased morbidity, complication, and LOS. Open adhesiolysis has long been the established operation of choice. With the advent of laparoscopy, there has been a debate as to whether it provides a benefit when compared to open adhesiolysis. In a comparison analysis performed by Kelly, 9619 patients with SBO were analyzed in which 14.9% of patients were performed laparoscopically. Patients undergoing laparoscopic procedures had shorter mean operative times (77.2 vs. 94.2 min) and decreased postoperative length of stay (4.7 vs. 9.9 days). After controlling for comorbidities and surgical factors, patients undergoing laparoscopic adhesiolysis were less likely to develop major complications. Therefore, laparoscopic adhesiolysis demonstrated a benefit in 30-day morbidity and mortality [20]. More recent studies suggest that laparoscopic adhesiolysis carries a lower rate of postoperative morbidity compared with laparotomy as well as a shorter hospital stay. Lombardo compared outcomes of over 6762 who underwent adhesiolysis and stratified patients into laparoscopically versus open laparotomy. They showed that laparoscopy was associated with significantly lower rates of any complications with odds ratio of 0.41, including surgical sites infections (OR 1.15), and shorter hospital stay (4 vs. 10 days) [21]. Adhesiolysis remains the treatment for adhesions, although adhesions reform in approximately 85% of patients [22]. These findings have been repeated multiple times by Li et al. who showed through a meta-analysis analyzing 334 patients enrolled into four retrospective comparative studies that laparoscopic adhesiolysis was associated with a reduced overall complication rate, prolonged ileus rate, and pulmonary complication rate [23].

*Recommendation*: Performing laparoscopic adhesiolysis in the hands of an experienced surgeon provides improved outcomes compared to those of conventional open adhesiolysis.

*Grade of recommendation*: B

#### 43.2.1.2 Should the Sun Set on an SBO?

Much controversy exists on the timing of operative interventions for SBO. The question of proper timing of operative planning depends on the patient's clinical presentation. Patient symptoms, radiological finding, and presence of metabolic derangements influence the management of SBO. It is important to identify those patients who would fail nonoperative management. O'Leary et al. performed a retrospective review in which 219 consecutive patients were studied and revealed four readily evaluable clinical parameters that may be used to predict the need for surgery that included persistent abdominal pain, abdominal distention, fever at 48 h, and CT findings of high-grade obstruction as factors that were predictive of nonoperative failure [24]. How many days should a surgeon wait until considering operation? Schraufnagel et al. attempted to answer this question with a large retrospective study in 2013. A total of 27,046 patients were identified with SBO in which 4826 required adhesiolysis. The study showed that complications, prolonged postoperative LOS, and death were more likely in patients for whom surgery was delayed 4 days or more. Patients on the fourth day or later had a 26% greater risk of staying more than 7 days postoperatively [25].

*Recommendation*: In the absence of hard signs such as intra-abdominal sepsis, peritoneal examination findings, strangulation, it is safe to say that there is an increased risk of complications, LOS, and death in patients who are delayed by 4 or more days.

*Grade of recommendation*: A

#### 43.2.1.3 Should Patients with SBO in the Setting of a Virgin Abdomen Undergo Early Intervention?

The majority of SBOs are the result of adhesions caused by previous abdominal surgeries. Other causes of SBO include congenital bands, internal hernias, and malignancies. The thought of missing a malignant disease resulting in SBO prompted surgeons to approach SBO in the virgin abdomen more aggressively. Should patients with virgin abdomen presenting with SBO be managed similar to patients with SBO resulting from postoperative adhesions? A retrospective analysis was conducted over a 5-year period that included 689 patients with SBO. A total of 9% of patients had a virgin abdomen, 13 patients had a previously known disease (IBD, malignancy), 75.5% had adhesions, and a newly diagnosed malignancy occurred in 10.2%. A similar rate of adhesions was found in patients with previous abdominal surgery with prevalence reported up to 80% if incarcerated external hernias were excluded. Therefore, a trial of nonoperative management may be justified [26]. Considering that the etiologies were similar with both operative and nonoperative groups, it is therefore safe to assume that the outcomes are similar. Butts and colleague studied 1036 patients with previous surgical adhesional SBO and examined the outcomes of patients with unexplained adhesions (no previous surgeries). Thirty-four patients were identified with no previous history of abdominal surgeries and showed that adhesions were clearly the most common cause of SBO. Patients with unexplained adhesional SBO were similar in demographics, clinical presentation, and initial laboratory test than with patients with abdominal surgical history SBO. There was no difference in any diagnostic delays and patient outcomes were similar to those patients with surgical history SBO [27].

*Recommendation*: In the absence of aberrant laboratory values, strangulation, and intra-abdominal sepsis, it is safe to offer a trial of nonoperative management to patients with no previous history of intra-abdominal surgery.

*Grade of recommendation*: B

#### 43.2.1.4 Are There Any Techniques/Agents That Have Been Shown to Decrease Intra-Abdominal Adhesion Formation Following Laparotomy?

There are a variety of technical methods used to minimize the formation of postoperative adhesions. One of the key surgical technical aspects is to reduce the amount of surgical trauma. Using electrocautery close to the bowel will cause adjacent tissue necrosis and contribute to robust adhesion formation as compared to sharp mechanical transection. The presence of foreign material that arise from gauze, sponges, starch powder, suture, debris from surgical drapes, gowns, masks, and many other items can elicit a peritoneal inflammation and be found in postoperative adhesions, demonstrating a causal relationship between the presence of foreign material and formation of adhesions [28]. Closure of the peritoneum does not offer benefit in reducing postoperative adhesion formation as seen in a prospective study by Kapustian and colleagues. They prospectively analyzed 533 patients undergoing primary cesarean sections, randomly assigning patients to peritoneal closure versus no peritoneal closure. They found that the nonclosure and closure groups were comparable with regard to the proportion of patients with adhesions at any site (60% vs. 51%). Their conclusion was that closure or nonclosure of the peritoneum at cesarean section did not lead to large differences in the adhesion rate [29]. Closure of the peritoneum layer does not necessary lead to an improved outcome overall. Closure of the fascia as a single layer as opposed to peritoneum as a separate layer offered no difference in wound complications, or dehiscence. Nonclosure of the peritoneum is safer, allowing the underlying viscera to remain under direct visualization during closure, and reduces operative time.

Studies evaluating laparoscopic to open surgery have revealed a lower rate of postoperative adhesions. Polymeneas et al. found a 44% rate of loose, easily separable adhesions between the gallbladder liver bed and the omentum or the duodenum after laparoscopic cholecystectomy, whereas after open cholecystectomy all patients (100%) had thick and extensive adhesions to the operative site [30]. Audebert and Gomel compared 125 patients with different prior laparoscopic procedures to 131 patients with previous horizontal suprapubic laparotomy and to 89 patients with previous midline laparotomy. The rates of umbilical adhesions were 1.6% after laparoscopy compared with 19.8% in those with a horizontal suprapubic laparotomy and 51.7% in those with a midline laparotomy [31]. A comparative analysis performed by Davies showed that from 2000 to 2011 patients undergoing laparoscopic lysis of adhesions were found to have a lower of rate postoperative morbidity and 30-day mortality as well as decrease perioperative contamination and lower ICU stays when compared to their open cohorts [32]. These studies have shown further support for performing laparoscopic adhesiolysis when feasible as it results in fewer adhesions when compared to open laparotomies. Laparoscopic adhesiolysis also results in decreased morbidity as it results in less hospital stay as well as decrease in morbidity.

There has been substantial investigation targeting a variety of mechanisms involved in adhesion formation. NSAIDs have been examined for their ability of reducing postoperative adhesions and their use has showed benefit in animal models [33–35]. Corticosteroids have also been examined with similar outcomes [36,37]. Other studies have examined agents that may interfere with the pathways of deposition and degradation of fibrin. The anticoagulants heparin and low molecular weight heparins (LMWH) have demonstrated a decrease in adhesion formation in animal studies [38,39]. The majority of these investigations that have reported success in using these various agents to prevent postoperative adhesions are limited to animal studies; similar results in humans are lacking.

Barrier devices have been utilized to separate the layers of the peritoneum and provide protection from adhesion formation. A barrier ideally should provide unrestricted coverage of the affected peritoneum. Various forms of barriers include polymer solutions and solid membranes of polysaccharides such as hyaluronic acid, cellulose, dextran, or chitosan. Various barriers currently FDA-approved include regenerated cellulose (Interceed®), expanded polytetrafluoroethylene (Preclude®), hyaluronic acid–carboxymethylcellulose (Seprafilm®), polylactide membrane (Surgiwrap®), and icodextrin solution (Adept®). Seprafilm is a nontoxic, nonimmunogenic, biocompatible material that was designed to reduce postoperative abdominal adhesion formation. It turns into a hydrophilic gel in approximately 24 h after placement and provides a protective coating around traumatized tissues for up to 7 days during remesothelialization. A recent meta-analysis studying the safety and efficacy of anti-adhesion products in 17 randomized trials in which primary outcome was the safety profile of anti-adhesion products as well as the reduction in the incidence, extent, and severity of adhesions. The data suggested that anti-adhesive products may be used safely; hyaluronic acid–carboxymethylcellulose membrane, reduced the incidence, extent, and severity of adhesions but without strong evidence of prevention of bowel obstruction [40].

There are studies that show the overall incidence of postoperative SBO was unchanged between patients treated with Seprafilm and controls [41]. The frequency of abdominal abscesses was slightly higher, although nonsignificant, while the incidence of fistulas, sepsis, and peritonitis occurred more frequently than controls (2% vs. <1%) and when wrapped around a fresh anastomosis had a higher frequency of anastomotic leaks (4% vs. 2%) [40].

*Recommendation*: There are a variety of methods that can be used to decrease the formation of postoperative abdominal adhesions, such as utilizing sharp dissection and minimize tissue trauma, reducing the amount of foreign body contamination within the surgical field, and employing minimally invasive surgical techniques if indicated. The use of barriers between the peritoneal layers seems logical; however, the improvement in postoperative adhesion formation observed has shown no impact on the rate of postoperative SBO.

*Grade of recommendation*: B

## 43.3 Adhesional SBO

### 43.3.1 Introduction

Intra-abdominal sepsis from bowel necrosis and bowel perforation secondary to strangulation is a devastating complication from bowel obstruction secondary to adhesions. Patients with adhesive bowel obstructions with no peritoneal signs or signs of intra-abdominal sepsis may undergo a trial of nonoperative management. Keenan retrospectively studied the effect of incremental delays in surgery on the 30-day postoperative outcomes of patients undergoing surgery for uncomplicated adhesive SBO. Of the 9297 patients included in the analysis, 46% received their operation after 3 days of hospitalization, while 22.5% received operation after 5 days. The 30-day postoperative mortality and overall morbidity were 4.4% and 29.6% respectively. Preoperative length of hospital stay of 3 or more days was associated with a higher risk of 30 day postoperative morbidity with a greater length of postoperative management for adhesive SBO [42].

### 43.3.2 Diagnosis of SBO

#### *43.3.2.1 What Does the Use of Water-Soluble Contrast Do?*

The role of water-soluble contrast medium in adhesive SBO in predicting the need for surgery, i.e., failure of conservative management, has been evaluated. Meglumine amidotrizoate (Gastrografin®) is the most commonly used water-soluble contrast agent and is a mixture of sodium diatrizoate and meglumine diatrizoate with an osmolarity of 1900 mosm/L. Gastrografin acts by causing an osmosis of water into the bowel lumen, decreasing the edema of the bowel wall that contributes to proximal bowel distention, increasing the pressure gradient across an obstructing region [43].

#### *43.3.2.2 Is the Early Use of Water-Soluble Contrast Indicated in the Diagnosis/Management of SBO?*

The use of Gastrografin has been studied for its use in the prediction of successful nonoperative management of SBO as well as assessing its therapeutic function in the resolution of SBO. Gaoussous et al. performed a retrospective analysis of 125 patients to assess whether a Gastrografin challenge test would decrease the rate of exploration in patients not meeting criteria for immediate operation. Patients with early SBO were given Gastrografin through an NGT. An abdominal radiograph was taken after 4–24 h to evaluate for transit of contrast to the colon. If contrast was present within the colonic lumen, there was a 99% chance that the obstruction would resolve without surgical intervention. Fifty-three patients received Gastrografin while 72 patients did not. There was a lesser rate of abdominal exploration (25% vs. 42%) and fewer complications (13% vs. 31%). There was a greater rate of exploration in patients with a failed challenge compared to those with a successful challenge (89% vs. 11%). Therefore, patients who failed the Gastrografin challenge test were much more likely to undergo an exploration [44]. In a prospective randomized trial, Choi et al. examined 124 patients with episodes of adhesive obstruction: 101 patients showed improvement within the initial 48 h and conservative management was continued; 35 patients showed no improvement. These were randomized to receive Gastrografin. Of the 19 patients to receive Gastrografin, there was complete resolution. The use of Gastrografin significantly reduced the need for surgery by 74% [45].

*Recommendation*: Water-soluble contrast agents such as Gastrografin have been shown to predict successful nonoperative management in patients who present with SBO.

*Grade of recommendation*: B

#### *43.3.2.3 Can CT Predict the Need for Operation in Patients with Incomplete SBO?*

Plain abdominal radiographs have proven to be diagnostic of SBO in only 67%–80% of patients [46]. Abdominal radiographs can be entirely normal in patients with complete, closed loop obstruction or strangulation associated with obstruction [47]. Computed tomography (CT) scan has a well-established role in the diagnosis of SBO since the first large published series showing its utility and efficacy [48]. CT findings of SBO include distended bowel loops proximal to collapsed loops, air-fluid levels, and a possible transition point. Studies have since proved the value of CT in confirming the diagnosis and revealing the cause of SBO, with a sensitivity of 94%–100% and an accuracy of 90%–95% [49]. Further reviews have shown that CT is highly accurate for diagnosing ischemic bowel with a sensitivity of 83%, specificity of 92%, positive predictive value of 79%, and a negative predictive value of 93% [50]. CT findings of slight thickening of the bowel wall, the "target sign," engorgement of the mesenteric vasculature, and mesenteric edema are all potential signs of early or reversible small bowel strangulation; bowel infarction or gangrene may be demonstrated by CT findings of high attenuation of the bowel wall, pneumatosis, hemorrhagic changes in the mesentery, gas in the portal vein, and poor or no enhancement of the bowel wall. Investigators, using of a combination of five highly specific findings, including poor enhancement of the bowel wall, a serrated beak, diffuse engorgement of mesenteric vasculature or mesenteric haziness, an unusual course of mesenteric vasculature, and a large amount of ascites, correctly identified 85% of patients with a strangulated SBO [51].

*Recommendation*: CT scan of the abdomen has the ability to identify SBO by specific findings and can use other specific findings to diagnose bowel ischemia and allow for surgical intervention. Following obstructive series, patients presenting with SBO should be evaluated with CT scan of the abdomen if clinically warranted.

*Grade of recommendation*: C

#### 43.3.2.4 Is There Any Difference between Stapled or Hand-Sewn Techniques for Bowel Anastomosis?

A meta-analysis was conducted to compare hand-sewn to stapled anastomosis which combined data from 13 randomized controlled trials comparing hand-sewn with stapled anastomoses in colon and rectal surgery. Overall, there were no significant differences between hand-sewn and stapled anastomoses for mortality, total, radiological, and clinical anastomotic leak rates, cancer recurrence rate, or wound infection rate. However, a significant difference existed favoring hand-sewn anastomoses for strictures and intraoperative technical problems [52]. The possibility of an overactive inflammatory response and higher collagen levels may be responsible for the increased stricture rate with stapled anastomoses [53]. Farrah et al. showed that in the emergency general surgery patient there was a difference in outcome between stapled versus hand-sewn anastomosis. A retrospective chart review analyzing 100 patients who underwent hand-sewn anastomosis versus 133 stapled anastomosis was reviewed. Operative times were shorter in stapled anastomosis (205 min hand-sewn vs. 193 min for stapled) as well increased anastomosis failure in stapled versus hand-sewn (15% vs. 6.1%). They showed that anastomotic failure rates were twice as likely with the stapled than hand-sewn anastomosis in the emergency general surgery patient [54] (Table 43.1).

*Recommendation*: Prospective randomized trials have shown no differences between hand-sewn and stapled anastomoses; however, the rate of postoperative stricture formation may be higher with stapled anastomoses. There were higher incidences of anastomotic failures in the emergency patient with the stapled technique versus the hand-sewn technique.

*Grade of recommendation*: B

**TABLE 43.1**

Chapter Questions Followed by Level of Evidence and Selected References

| Question | Answer | Grade | References |
|---|---|---|---|
| Does chewing gum shorten the duration of postoperative ileus? | Yes, chewing gum has been shown to decrease length of POI and LOS. | B | [4–6] |
| Does the use of selective opiate receptor inhibitors decrease duration of postoperative ileus? | Yes, it has an impact of both the duration of POI, tolerance of solid diet, and LOS, but unclear on cost/benefit ratio. | B | [7–15] |
| Which is more advantageous: open or laparoscopic adhesiolysis? | Performing laparoscopic adhesiolysis in the hands of an experienced surgeon provides improved outcomes conventional open adhesiolysis. | B | [20–23] |
| Should the sun set on an SBO? | In the absence of hard signs such as intra-abdominal sepsis, peritoneal examination findings, strangulation. It is safe to say that there is an increased risk of complications, LOS, and death in patients who are delayed by 4 or more days. | A | [24,25] |
| Should patients with SBO in the setting of a virgin abdomen be intervened on sooner? | In the absence of aberrant laboratory values, strangulation, intra-abdominal sepsis, it is safe to offer a trial of nonoperative management to patients with no previous history of intra-abdominal surgery. | B | [26,27] |
| Are there any techniques/agents that have been shown to decrease intra-abdominal adhesion formation following laparotomy? | Sharp dissection, minimizing tissue trauma, decreasing foreign bodies in surgical field, and barrier devices. | B | [28–41] |
| What does the use of water-soluble contrast do? | Causes an osmosis of water into the bowel lumen and decreases edema of the bowel wall which promotes proximal bowel distention and increases the pressure gradient across an obstructing region. | C | [43] |
| Is the early use of water-soluble contrast indicated in the diagnosis/management of SBO? | The use of water-soluble contrast has shown to predict the success of conservative management, but has not shown to decrease the need for operation. | B | [44,45] |
| Can CT predict the need for operation in patients with incomplete SBO? | CT scan can diagnose SBO and SBO-causing ischemia and the requirement for surgical intervention. | C | [46–51] |
| Is there any difference between stapled or hand-sewn techniques for bowel anastomosis? | There has been no difference shown between the two, however, stapled anastomoses have a higher rate of stricture. | B | [52–54] |

## References


1. Livingston EH, Passaro EP. Postoperative ileus. *Dig Dis Sci.* 1990;35:121–131.
2. Artinyan A, Nunoo-Mensah JW, Balasubramaniam S et al. Prolonged postoperative ileus-definition, risk factors, and predictors after surgery. *World J Surg.* 2008; 32(7):1495–1500.
3. Clevers GJ, Smout AJ. The natural course of postoperative ileus following abdominal surgery. *Neth J Surg.* 1989;41:97–99.
4. Asao T, Kuwano H, Nakamura J et al. Gum chewing enhances early recovery from postoperative ileus after laparoscopic colectomy. *J Am Coll Surg.* 2002;195:30–32.
5. Schuster R, Grewal N, Greaney GC et al. Gum chewing reduces ileus after elective open sigmoid colectomy. *Arch Surg.* 2006;141:174–176.
6. Li S, Liu Y, Peng Q et al. Chewing gum reduces postoperative ileus following abdominal surgery. *Gastroenterol Hepatol.* 2013;28(7):1122–1132.
7. Sternini C, Patierno S, Selmer IS et al. The opioid system in the gastrointestinal tract. *Neurogastroenterol Motil.* 2004;16(Suppl):3–16.
8. Schmidt WK. Alvimopan (ADL 8-2698) is a novel peripheral opioid antagonist. *Am J Surg.* 2001;182(Suppl):27–38.
9. Leslie JB. Alvimopan for the management of postoperative ileus. *Ann Pharmacother.* 2005;39:1502–1510.
10. Taguchi AT, Sharma N, Saleem RM et al. Selective postoperative inhibition of gastrointestinal opioid receptors. *N Engl J Med.* 2001;345:935–940.
11. Wolff BG, Michelassi F, Gerkin TM et al. Alvimopan, a novel, peripherally acting μ opioid antagonist. Results of a multicenter, randomized, double-blind, placebo-controlled, phase III trial or major abdominal surgery and postoperative ileus. *Ann Surg.* 2004;240:728–735.
12. Vaughan-Shaw PG1, Fecher IC, Harris S, Knight JS. A meta-analysis of the effectiveness of the opioid receptor antagonist alvimopan in reducing hospital LOS and time to GI recovery in patients enrolled in a standardized accelerated recovery program after abdominal surgery. *Dis Colon Rectum.* May 2012;55(5):611–620.
13. Harbaugh CM, Al-Holou SN, Bander TS, et al. A statewide, community-based assessment of alvimopan's effect on surgical outcomes. *Ann Surg.* Mar 2013;257(3):427–432.
14. Poston S, Broder MS, Gibbons MM et al. Impact of alvimopan (entereg) on hospital costs after bowel resection: Results from a large inpatient database. *P T.* Apr 2011;36(4):209–220.
15. Kauf TL, Svatek RS, Amiel G. Alvimopan, a peripherally acting μ-opioid receptor antagonist, is associated with reduced costs after radical cystectomy: Economic analysis of a phase 4 randomized, controlled trial. *J Urol.* Jun 2014;191(6):1721–1727.
16. Maciver AH, Mc Call M, Shapiro AM. Intra-abdominal adhesions: Cellular Mechanism and Strategies for Prevention. *Int J Surg.* 2011;9(8):589–594.
17. Menzies D, Parker M, Hoare R et al. Small bowel obstruction due to postoperative adhesions: Treatment patterns and associated costs in 110 hospital admissions. *Ann R Coll Surg Engl.* 2001;83:40–46.
18. Wysocki A, Pozniczek M, Kulawik J et al. Peritoneal adhesions as a cause of small bowel obstruction. *Przegl Lek.* 2003;60:32–35.
19. Van der Krabben AA, Dijkstra FR, Nieuwenhuijzen M et al. Morbidity and mortality of inadvertent enterotomy during adhesiotomy. *Br J Surg.* 2000;87:467–471.
20. Kelly KN1, Iannuzzi JC, Rickles AS. Laparotomy for small-bowel obstruction: First choice or last resort for adhesiolysis? A laparoscopic approach for small-bowel obstruction reduces 30-day complications. *Surg Endosc.* Jan 2014;28(1):65–73.
21. Lombaro S, Baum K, Filho JD. Should adhesive small bowel obstruction be managed laparoscopically? A National Surgical Quality Improvement Program propensity score analysis. *J Trauma Acute Care Surg.* Mar 2014;76(3):696–703.
22. Diamond MP, Freeman ML. Clinical implications of postsurgical adhesions. *Hum Reprod Update.* 2001;7:567–576.
23. Li MZ1, Lian L, Xiao LB. Laparoscopic versus open adhesiolysis in patients with adhesive small bowel obstruction: A systematic review and meta-analysis. *Am J Surg.* Nov 2012;204(5):779–786.
24. O'Leary EA, Desale SY, YI WS. Letting the sun set on small bowel obstruction: Can a simple risk score tell us when non-operative care is inappropriate? *Am Surg.* Jun 2014;80(6):572–579.
25. Schraufnagel D, Rajaee S, Millham FH. How many sunsets? Timing of surgery in adhesive small bowel obstruction: A study of the Nationwide Inpatient Sample. *J Trauma Acute Care Surg.* Jan 2013;74(1):181–187; discussion 187–189.
26. Beardsley C, Furtado R, Mosse C. Small bowel obstruction in the virgin abdomen: The need for a mandatory laparotomy explored. *Am J Surg.* Aug 2014;208(2):243–248.
27. Butt MU, Velmahos GC, Zacharias N. Adhesional small bowel obstruction in the absence of previous operations: Management and outcomes. *World J Surg.* Nov 2009;33(11):2368–2371.
28. Saxen L, Myllarniemi H. Foreign material and postoperative adhesions. *N Engl J Med.* 1968;279:200–202.
29. Kapustian V, Anteby EY, Gdalevich M. Effect of closure versus nonclosure of peritoneum at cesarean section on adhesions: A prospective randomized study. *Am J Obstet Gynecol.* Jan 2012;206(1):56.
30. Polymeneas G, Theodosopoulos T, Stamatiadis A et al. A comparative study of postoperative adhesion formation after laparoscopic vs open cholecystectomy. *Surg Endosc.* 2001;15:41–43.
31. Audebert AJ, Gomel V. Role of microlaparoscopy in the diagnosis of peritoneal and visceral adhesions and in the prevention of bowel injury associated with blind trocar insertion. *Fertil Steril.* 2000;73:631–635.
32. Davies SW, Gillen JR, Guidry CA. A comparative analysis between laparoscopic and open adhesiolysis at a tertiary care center. *Am Surg.* Mar 2014;80(3):261–269.

33. De Leon FD, Toledo AA, Sanfilippo JS et al. The prevention of adhesion formation by nonsteroidal anti-inflammatory drugs: An animal study comparing ibuprofen and indomethacin. *Fertil Steril.* 1984;41:639–642.
34. Guvenal T, Cetin A, Ozdemir H et al. Prevention of postoperative adhesion formation in rat uterine horn model by nimesulide: A selective COX-2 inhibitor. *Hum Reprod.* 2001;16:1932–1935.
35. Nishimura K, Nakamura RM, DiZerega GS. Ibuprofen inhibition of postsurgical adhesion formation: A time and dose response biochemical evaluation in rabbits. *J Surg Res.* 1984;36:115–124.
36. Maurer JH, Bonaventura LM. The effect of aqueous progesterone on operative adhesion formation. *Fertil Steril.* 1983;39:485–489.
37. Höckel M, Ott S, Siemann U et al. Prevention of peritoneal adhesions in the rat with sustained intraperitoneal dexamethasone delivered by a novel therapeutic system. *Ann Chir Gynaecol.* 1987;76:306–313.
38. Kutlay J, Ozer Y, Isık B et al. Comparative effectiveness of several agents for preventing postoperative adhesions. *World J Surg.* 2004;28:662–665.
39. Bahadir I, Oncel M, Kement M, at el. Intra-abdominal use of taurolidine or heparin as alternative products to an antiadhesive barrier (Seprafilm) in adhesion prevention: An experimental study on mice. *Dis Colon Rectum.* 2007;50:2209–2214.
40. Robb WB, Mariette C. Strategies in the prevention of the formation of postoperative adhesions in digestive surgery: A systematic review of the literature. *Dis Colon Rectum.* Oct 2014;57(10):1228–1240.
41. Fazio VW, Cohen Z, Fleshman JW et al. Reduction in adhesive small-bowel obstruction by Seprafilm® adhesion barrier after intestinal resection. *Dis Colon Rectum.* 2005;49:1–11.
42. Keenan JE, Turley RS, McCoy CC. Trials of nonoperative management exceeding 3 days are associated with increased morbidity in patients undergoing surgery for uncomplicated adhesive small bowel obstruction. *J Trauma Acute Care Surg.* Jun 2014;76(6):1367–1372.
43. Laerum F, Stordahl A, Aase S. Water-soluble contrast media compared with barium in enteric follow-through: Local effects and radiographic efficacy in rats with simple obstruction of the small bowel. *Acta Radiol.* 1988;29:603–610.
44. Gaoussous N, Eiken PW, Bannon MP, Zielinski MD. Enhancement of a small bowel obstruction model using the Gastrografin® challenge test. *J Gastrointest Surg.* Jan 2013;17(1):110–116; discussion 116–117.
45. Choi HK, Chu KW, Law WL. Therapeutic value of Gastrografin in adhesive small bowel obstruction after unsuccessful conservative treatment: A prospective randomized trial. *Ann Surg.* Jul 2002;236(1):1–6.
46. Maglinte DD, Balthazar EJ, Kelvin FM et al. The role of radiology in the diagnosis of small bowel obstruction. *AJR.* 1997;168:1171–1180.
47. Gough IR. Strangulating adhesive small bowel obstruction with normal radiographs. *Br J Surg.* 1978;65:431–434.
48. Megibow AJ, Balthazar EJ, Cho KC et al. Bowel Obstruction: Evaluation with CT. *Radiology.* 1991;180:313–318.
49. Maglinte DD, Gage SN, Harmon BH et al. Obstruction of the small intestine: Accuracy and role of CT in diagnosis. *Radiology.* 1993;188:61–64.
50. Mallo RD, Salem L, Lalani T et al. Computed tomography of ischemia and complete obstruction in small bowel obstruction: A systematic review. *J Gastrointest Surg.* 2005;9:690–694.
51. Ha HK, Kim JS, Lee MS et al. Differentiation of simple and strangulated small-bowel obstructions: Usefulness of known CT criteria. *Radiology.* 1997;204:507–512.
52. MacRae HM, McLeod RS. Handsewn vs. stapled anastomoses in colon and rectal surgery: A meta-analysis. *Dis Colon Rectum.* 1998;41:180–189.
53. Dziki AJ, Duncan MD, Harmon JW et al. Advantages of hand-sewn over stapled bowel anastomosis. *Dis Colon Rectum.* 1991;34:625–627.
54. Farrah JP, Lauer CW, Bray MS. Stapled versus hand-sewn anastomoses in emergency general surgery: A retrospective review of outcomes in a unique patient population. *J Trauma Acute Care Surg.* May 2013;74(5):1187–1192.

## Commentary on Small Bowel Surgery

*Gregory J. Jurkovich*

Ileus means a functional obstruction or alteration of motility of the GI tract. The term is Greek in origin, derived from *ileos* or *eilos*: to stop, hinder, bind, and roll up.

It is interesting that this chapter on small bowel surgery should begin with a discussion of ileus, but such is the problem this entity creates. Delayed transit and return of intestinal motility continues to be a significant source of anxiety on the part of patients and surgeons alike. It leads to concerns that some intra-abdominal error or catastrophe has or will soon occur; it puzzles the surgeon as he or she tries to be patient in letting "nature take its course," while nurses and families and the patient themselves feel they are being starved with no resolution in site. The surgeon hesitates to start parenteral nutrition, with good reason, thinking *soon* this ileus will resolve. By the time post of day 5 rolls around and the patient is still NPO, distended, no flatus, and uncomfortable, all involved it the care are wondering: "is there a problem here?" Next comes the NG tube reinserted, plain films of the abdomen showing distended small bowel with or without some air on the colon. A CT scan is not far to follow and the anxiety of the care rises.

As Drs Bustamante and Hong point out, a variety of agents have been used to stimulate intestinal utility. The dopamine-agonist metoclopramide (Reglan®) and low-dose erythromycin (a motilin agonist) are the two most widely used prokinetic agents, along with simple chewing gum*. The time frame for return of function does begin with small bowel, which may in fact never lose motility. This is why jejunal feedings can and should be started within 24 h postoperatively in the critically ill patient. Diabetes and a host of other chronic and largely idiopathic "delayed gastric emptying" syndromes can also cause delayed gastric emptying. As noted, the colon is the last to return synchronized motility, which is why the "passing of gas" is a sign that colonic myoelectrical activity has returned and the ileus is resolved.

The discussion of the opiate receptors in the small bowel, as well as the role of local anesthetic (not opioids) in epidural pain control is beneficial. What has never been investigated, to the best of my knowledge is: if starting an epidural postoperatively in someone with delayed return of function would have any benefit. The early ambulation of patients may be the most effective technique to limit a post-op ileus. Chewing gum appears to have about the same utility as the much more expensive mu-receptor antagonist alvimopan (Entereg®), which might serve to counter the effects of systemic opioids on the gut. With continued and growing interest in controlling health care costs in large and small ways, I question the widespread use of this agent, despite the moderate improvements detailed in the reported studies. The Food and Drug Administration approved Alvimopan for use in postoperative ileus in May 2008. Cisapride (serotonin receptor agonist) was once a popular agent as well for use in the resolution of post-op ileus and diabetic gastroperesis, but due to a high incidence of cardiac arrhythmias was withdrawn from use in the United States in 2000. Intravenous infusion of lidocaine during surgery and in the first 24 h post-op has also been used with success†.

To the list of causes of post-op ileus, I would also add significant retroperitoneal dissection or hematoma (e.g., pelvic fracture hemorrhage), which likely disrupts the reflex alpha- and beta-sympathetic stimulation (or cholinergic inhibition), as well as significant head and spinal cord injuries. The role of plasma motilin suppression post-op has also been suggested.

The likely role of lack of synergy in the sympathetic and parasympathetic nervous innervation to the gut has long been hypothesized. The parasympathetic (myenteric plexus) fibers are preganglionic, cholinergic receptors that are primarily excitatory. The sympathetic (celiac ganglion) fibers are postganglionic, adrenergic receptors, and largely inhibitory. It has been shown that various adrenergic receptor stimulations result in small bowel and colonic ileus. But in essence, the reason some people have a longer post-op ileus than others remains enigmatic.

Current best practices to minimize post-op ileus includes the use of epidural analgesia using diluted concentrations of local anesthetics, minimizing the use of opioids, aggressive control or prevention of nausea and vomiting, and early mobilization. Preventing edema from salt and fluid overloading is also key.

In general, parenteral nutritional support should be instituted in those patients who are unable to eat due to an ileus lasting longer than 5–7 days, those in whom acute weight loss is approaching or exceeding 10% lean body mass, or those in who presented malnourished or particularly hypercatabolic. This last category is often difficult to define.

The second major topic addressed in this chapter is adhesions involving the intestine. No good solution, prevention or resolution of intestinal adhesion formation has been developed, as is well outlined in this chapter. The advice to minimize unnecessary bowel

* Nguyen, NQ, Chapman MJ; Fraser RJ et al. Erythromycin is more effective than metoclopramide in the treatment of feed intolerance in critical illness. *Crit Care Med.* 2007;February;35(2):483–489.

† Herroeder S, Pecher S, Schonherr ME et al. Systemic lidocaine shortens length of hospital stay after colorectal surgery: A double-blinded randomized, placebo controlled trial. *Ann Surg.* 2007;246(2):192–200.

manipulation, observe good surgical technique, prevent foreign bodies (dust, lint, talc, etc.) from entering the wound are all important, and perhaps, inadequate attention is given to those simple tasks. The benefit of laparoscopic or minimally invasive approaches may simply be the avoidance of prolonged exposure of the gut to an unfiltered environment, and the limiting of the dissection to the area of interest only.

Barrier agents were once more popular, and widely used at the time of midline incision closure to prevent adhesions just beneath the incision. The rationale was that should re-exploration be required in the future, the bowel might not be stuck to the abdominal wall in this key area. However, the finding that hyaluronic acid-carboxymethycellulose (Seprafilm®) was associated with a higher anastomosis leak rate has curtailed the widespread use of these products.

The timing of operative intervention in the management of mechanical small bowel obstruction remains controversial. Current best national and international evidence-based guidelines are to decompress the bowel and wait 3–5 days for resolution, with care taken during the observation period to exclude gut strangulation or ischemia. The diagnosis of partial versus complete obstruction has been significantly aided by the use of oral contrast-enhanced CT imaging, as well discussed in this chapter. The need for operative intervention in the patient with signs and symptoms bowel ischemia is clear. Elevated WBC, fever, and abdominal tenderness are all indications for operating "before the sun sets," as the age-old adage advises. This adage is variably attributed to Charles L. Scudder, Surgeon in Chief at the Massachusetts General Hospital in 1908, and one of the founders of the American College of Surgeons. The challenge is in the patient who has a partial obstruction, or a near-complete obstruction that is being managed with NG suction, without signs of vascular gut compromise.

A recent review of the NSQIP database of 4163 patients demonstrated that for those patients operated on after more than 24 h of observation or nonoperative initial management, there was an increase in the risk of mortality (6.5% vs. 3.0%), infections (12.9% vs. 10%), sepsis (7.6% vs. 5.1%), septic shock (6.2% vs. 3.5%), and length of stay (8 days vs. 14 days)[*]. These results are also supported by a review of the National Inpatient Sampling database from 2009[†]. From approximately 8 million sample patients that year, they identified 27,000 patients admitted with the primary diagnosis of bowel obstruction. Like the NSQIP study, this 1 year national in-patient sample observed an increasing mortality and complication rate with delay of surgery. Of note, however, was the observation that only 5000 patients, or 18%, came to operation. Because 80% were apparently successfully managed nonoperatively, these authors concluded that 3–5 days of observation are acceptable, noting that 60% of patients are successfully managed nonoperatively within 3 days, 81% within 5 days, and 90% within 7 days.

Both of these studies are of course limited by the retrospective review of an administrative database, but they make a compelling argument that for some patients, the longer you wait, the greater the complications. But the enigma remains: what is the magic number of days we should be managing patients with bowel obstruction and no signs of intestinal ischemia? One sunset? Three sunsets? Five? Predicting and identifying those that need an operation immediately remains problematic.

The last point I will comment on is the fascinating observation that perhaps hand-sewing a bowel anastomosis is better than a stapled anastomosis. My goodness, if this is true, we may actually have to train people to sew. This observation should be attributed to the article by Susan Brundage from 1999[‡], subsequently expanded upon by the Western Trauma Association multicenter trials group[§]. I think the observation is real. Hand-sewn bowel anastomosis, in the patient likely to suffer bowel edema and ischemia, likely affords better control and lessens the likelihood of ischemic necrosis and leak.

* Teixeira PG, Karamanos E, Talving P et al. Early operation is associated with a survival benefit for patients with adhesive bowel obstruction. *Ann Surg*. 2013 September;258(3):459–465.

† Schraufnagel D, Rajaee S, Millham FH. How many sunsets? Timing of surgery in adhesive small bowel obstructions: A study of the Nationwide Inpatient Sample. *J Trauma Acute Care Surg*. 2013 January;74(1):181–187.

‡ Brundage SI, Jurkovich GJ, Grossman DC, Tong WC, Mack CD, Maier RV. Stapled versus sutured gastrointestinal anastomoses in the trauma patient. *J Trauma Acute Care Surg*. 1999 September;47(3):500–507.

§ Brundage SI, Jurkovich GJ, Hoyt DB et al. WTA Multi-institutional Study Group: Stapled versus sutured gastrointestinal anastomoses in the trauma patient: A multicenter trial. *J Trauma Acute Care Surg*. 2001 December;51(6):1054–1061.

# 44

# Evidence-Based Approach to Upper Gastrointestinal Bleeding

**Bruce A. Crookes and Margaret Dorlon**

**CONTENTS**



## 44.1 Introduction

Upper gastrointestinal (UGI) bleeding is a common cause for admission to the intensive care unit (ICU), and accounts for over 300,000 ICU admissions in the United States alone [1,2]. Optimal outcomes depend upon the rapid identification of the etiology of the hemorrhage and subsequent implementation of appropriate pharmacologic and procedural therapies.

The majority (80%–90%) of episodes of acute UGI bleeding are due to nonvariceal causes [3], with ulcer disease accounting for the majority of nonvariceal cases. Aside from ulcer disease, other etiologies of UGI bleeding include varices, Mallory–Weiss syndrome, vascular lesions, and inflammatory states of the upper GI tract. Despite advances in pharmacology and endoscopic therapies over the last several decades, all cause mortality has remained constant, ranging from 6% to 10% in most series [1,2,4], and up to 50% for variceal bleeding [5]. Medical comorbidities and the use of anticoagulants complicate treatment. Fortunately, over 80% of UGI bleeds stop spontaneously, but when bleeding continues or when the bleed occurs in the setting of a high-risk patient, prompt decisive management is required. Additionally, best practices should be used to prevent further bleeding episodes.

Initial guidelines for the management of UGI bleeding were published almost 20 years ago. Since that time, significant advancements in treatment and prophylaxis have been developed. UGI bleeding mortality rates have significantly decreased in the last three decades, most significantly in patients more than 65 years of age [6]. This chapter will review the current evidence, including recent practice guidelines, for the prevention and management of UGI bleeding.

## 44.2 What Is the Role of Medical Therapy in the Prevention of UGI Bleeds and How Successful Is It?

The type and use of medical prophylaxis is highly dependent on the potential etiology of an UGI bleed. In some cases, medical prophylaxis is the primary means of prevention, while in others, secondary prevention is the goal. As ulcer disease is the primary cause of the majority UGI bleeds, providers must identify the etiology of the ulceration. There are three principal causes: stress-related mucosal damage (SRMD), nonsteroidal anti-inflammatory drug (NSAID) use, and *Helicobacter pylori* infection.

Patients who are critically ill have a number of causes for ulcer formation, including decreased mucous secretion, altered GI motility, and mucosal ischemia [7]. These factors are especially prevalent in patients with large burns, head injury, coagulopathy, or those patients who require mechanical ventilation. Traditionally, antacids, sucralfate, or histamine-2 receptor antagonists (H2RA) have been used [7]. All have been shown to reduce bleeding episodes, but none have been shown to be clearly superior.

Cook et al. [8] found that the use of ranitidine conferred lower bleeding rates when compared to sucralfate.

Several other studies, however, have shown decreased mortality and pneumonia rates with sucralfate [7,9,10]. More recently, proton pump inhibitors (PPI) have been studied for stress ulcer prophylaxis. These agents are able to keep gastric pH >4 by suppressing acid secretion [7]. Conrad et al. [11], in a randomized double-blind study, found omeprazole to be more effective than cimetidine in preventing GI bleeding for critically ill patients. Omperazole was able to reduce the rate of bleeding from 6.8% to 4.5%, although neither pneumonia nor mortality rates were improved. Liu demonstrated in a randomized controlled trial (RCT) that omeprazole, when compared to cimetidine, significantly reduced the morbidity of stress-induced UGI bleeding in patients with intracerebral hemorrhage without increasing pneumonia risk [12]. Unfortunately, the study failed to show a decrease in 1-month mortality. Udd et al. [13] found that regular and high-dose omeprazole were equally effective for preventing peptic ulcer bleeding.

How should the intensivist medically manage patients whose UGI bleed is associated with NSAID use? Fortunately, pharmacotherapy is beneficial for preventing bleeding related to NSAIDs used for pain relief or cardiovascular disease. In fact, the prognosis for NSAID-associated UGI bleeding may be better than UGI bleeds from other causes: Chason observed that *H. pylori*-negative ulcers were associated with higher rates of rebleeding and poorer outcomes regardless of NSAID use [14].

After a bleeding episode, a review of the patient's current medications is paramount in the prevention of future UGI bleeds. Chan et al. [15], in a randomized placebo-controlled study found that patients with a history of bleeding ulcers have less frequent bleeding when esomeprazole was added to aspirin as opposed to changing to clopidogrel (0.7% as compared to 8.6%). Alternative drugs, such as COX-2 inhibitors, also can be used when NSAIDs are used for pain control in arthritis. A case-control study of 1600 patients who used NSAIDs, low-dose aspirin, antiplatelets, and anticoagulant medications within 2 weeks of endoscopy with endoscopically confirmed gastroduodenal ulcer disease showed that low-dose aspirin (odds ratio [OR] 1.8) and NSAIDs (OR 1.35) individually increased risk of bleeding, and a combination of low-dose aspirin and NSAIDs (OR 3.59) or low-dose aspirin and antiplatelet agents (OR 6.7) contributed to more profound bleeding rates [16]. Another study by Chan et al. [17] found that in patients who are *H. pylori* negative and taking nonaspirin NSAIDs, there was an additional reduction in upper GI bleeding (8.8%–0%) with the addition of esomeprazole after they were changed to celecoxib. Lai et al. [18] studied patients who were taking aspirin and *H. pylori* positive. After eradication therapy, patients were randomized to lansoprazole or placebo while continuing aspirin. The PPI group had an ulcer complication rate of 1.6% compared to 14.8% with placebo. Lim reviewed 500 patients with chronic kidney disease (CKD) and concluded that prophylactic low-dose PPI can reduce nonvariceal UGIB in dialysis patients receiving aspirin [19]. Other medications may put patients at higher risk of UGI bleeding: recent retrospective data suggest that selective serotonin reuptake inhibitors used to treat various psychiatric disorders are associated with almost a two-fold increase in risk of developing a UGI bleed, especially among patients with concurrent use of NSAIDs or antiplatelet drugs [20].

While acid suppression is the hallmark of prevention for ulcer-related bleeding, reduction in portal venous pressure is most effective for preventing esophageal bleeding. Beta-blockers are the main class of drugs that are used to accomplish this goal, having first been used in the 1980s after introduction by Lebrec et al. [21]. Lebrec found that patients with large varices were significantly less likely to bleed when nadolol was added as therapy for variceal hemorrhage, when compared with placebo [22]. Kiire similarly found that propranolol, as compared with placebo, significantly reduced bleeding when used in secondary prevention [23]. Other authors have investigated the use of beta-blockers to prevent the formation and growth of varices: Merkel and colleagues [24] found that the risk of variceal growth was decreased from 21% to 7% and 51% to 20%, at 1 and 5 years follow-up, respectively, when compared with placebo. Groszmann et al. [25], however, studied patients with cirrhosis and portal hypertension and were unable to show that beta-blockers prevented variceal formation. Additionally, recent studies have compared beta-blockers and endoscopic ligation as primary prophylaxis.

Other drugs, such as isosorbide mononitrate (IM), have also been investigated in the prevention of variceal bleeding. Angelico et al. [26] found that propranolol and IM provided similar protection against variceal bleeding. Long-term use of nitrates, however, has been linked to increased mortality. A review by Talwalkar and Kamath [27] showed that beta-blockers provide a 9% absolute risk reduction for primary prophylaxis and 21% reduction for secondary prevention. The authors also note that no individual trial has linked beta-blocker prophylaxis to improve survival, but a survival advantage has been demonstrated in meta-analysis [27].

Some authors have investigated the combination of beta-blockers and nitrates. Merkel et al. [28] demonstrated a decreased bleeding risk from 29% to 12% with a combination treatment. Some studies, however, have shown an increased rate of adverse events with combination treatments [27].

*Recommendations*:

1. PPI should be used as stress ulcer prophylaxis in critically ill patients to prevent GI bleeding.
2. Risk of ulcer formation for patients taking NSAIDs is significantly reduced with PPI or H2RA prophylaxis.
3. Beta-blockers can be used safely for primary prophylaxis from variceal bleeding and may slow the growth of small varices.

*Grade of recommendation*: 1. A, 2. A, 3. B

## 44.3 What Is the Role of Medical Therapy in Treating UGI Bleeds and How Effective Is It?

As mentioned in the introduction, most UGI bleeds stop spontaneously. However, clinicians should optimize patient outcomes through both pharmacologic and procedural interventions. UGI bleeds caused by ulcer disease are treated with acid suppression, just as in prevention. A review by Collins and Langman [29] in the mid-1980s found that H2RA drugs decreased rates of surgery and death in certain populations of patients with UGI bleeding, marking the dawn of a new era in the treatment of what was then a common problem.

Over the next decade, however, PPIs were introduced. Lanas et al. [30] found that omeprazole was superior to ranitidine in decreasing rebleeding episodes. No differences were found in mortality or units of blood transfused. Khuroo and colleagues [31] found that PPIs reduced ongoing bleeding from 36.4% to 10.9% and reduced the need for surgery as compared to placebo. Lau et al. [32] also found that PPI treatment was superior in preventing rebleeding after endoscopic treatment of ulcer bleeding. Daneshmend et al. [33], however, did not find that omeprazole reduced mortality, rebleeding, or transfusion requirements; these authors were only able to demonstrate a decrease in the endoscopic signs of bleeding with PPI treatment. Regional differences in patient populations may account for these differences, as one study was conducted in Europe and the other in Asia. Another study by Lau et al. [34] similarly found a decrease in the signs of recent bleeding with PPI treatment. Their study also demonstrated a decreased need for endoscopic therapy.

In addition to acid suppression, treating the etiology of the ulcer is imperative. This includes managing critical illness, limiting NSAID use, and treating *H. pylori* when appropriate. Riemann et al. [35] demonstrated that curative triple therapy with PPI was superior to maintenance therapy with H2RAs. Sung et al. [36], however, showed that medical therapy should not stand-alone: this study found that patients treated with both endoscopy and PPI were much less likely to rebleed than PPI treatment alone (1.1% compared to 11.6%).

Medical treatment of variceal bleeding differs from ulcer bleeding in that the therapeutic agents used are different in their mechanisms of action: the mainstays of the pharmacologic treatment of active variceal bleeding are vasoconstrictive and vasoactive drugs. Vasopressin and terlipressin are vasoconstrictive agents that have been shown to decrease active variceal bleeding. These drugs, however, can have significant side effects, including headache, pulmonary edema, and coronary vasoconstriction [37].

Octreotide is the main vasoactive drug used to treat variceal bleeding. It is a hormone analog of somatostatin that alters GI hormone signaling, decreases gastric and pancreatic secretions, and alters splanchnic blood flow. Multiple studies have demonstrated the superior efficacy of octreotide over vasopressin [37–39] for stopping active bleeding and preventing rebleeds. Despite this, no mortality benefit is gained. A meta-analysis by Gross et al. [40] found that vasoconstrictive therapy was only 68.7% successful, as compared to vasoactive therapy that was 75.9% successful. It should be kept in mind, however, that banding ligation is the most effective therapy and should be the primary intervention for stopping variceal bleeding [40].

Present authors have begun to examine the manipulation of the clotting cascade in the treatment of UGI bleeding: currently, there is a randomized controlled trial designed to examine the role of tranexamic acid in the management of acute UGI bleeding. The study of 8000 patients is powered to determine the mortality, morbidity, need for blood transfusion, and the need for surgical intervention when patients are given tranexamic acid or placebo [41].

*Recommendations*:

1. Proton pump inhibitors (PPI) should be preferentially used over H2RAs to reduce rebleeding episodes after successful endoscopic therapy.
2. In *H. pylori*-positive patients, eradication therapy should be employed.
3. Octreotide should be used to slow the rate of variceal bleeding, until definitive endoscopic therapy can be implemented.

*Grade of recommendation*: 1. A, 2. B, 3. B

## 44.4 What Is the Role of Endoscopy in Treating or for Prophylaxis in UGI Bleeds and How Successful Is It?

Endoscopy is beneficial in UGI bleeds because it can be simultaneously diagnostic and therapeutic, particularly in patients with no prior history of bleeding. Ulcer bleeding can be stopped or reduced with medical treatment as discussed previously, but multiple studies have shown that endoscopy confers further prevention of rebleeding [36,42]. Endoscopic findings of active bleeding or a visible vessel require treatment due to their high rates of rebleeding.

Ulcers with adherent clot are more controversial. Bini and Cohen [42] directly compared endoscopy with medical treatment in patients with adherent clot. These authors found that recurrent bleeding, mean hospital stay, transfusion requirements, and repeat endoscopy were significantly reduced with endoscopy.

Several methods are available to achieve endoscopic hemostasis, including adrenaline injection, laser therapy, and heater probes. No significant differences, however, have been found when these therapeutic modalities have been compared [2]. Similarly, Chung et al. [43] found that initial hemostasis was achieved equally by injection and heater probe. Yet, for ulcers with "spurting" vessels, combination treatment with injection and heater probe reduced the rate of surgery from 29.6% to 6.5%. Administration of pro-kinetics (erythromycin) before endoscopy in UGI bleeding has been shown to improve visualization of gastric mucosa and decrease the need for second endoscopy, the amount of blood transfusion required, and the duration of hospital stay [44].

There are patients that fail endoscopic treatment. Lau et al. [45] studied patients who had undergone successful initial endoscopic treatment and randomized them to surgery or repeat endoscopy if they rebleed. Over one-quarter of patients who were randomized to have repeat endoscopy still required salvage surgery [45].

While endoscopy is used solely for the treatment of ulcer disease, this intervention can be used for both the treatment of active bleeding and prophylaxis in patients with varices. Options for the endoscopic management of varices include injection sclerotherapy and banding ligation. Both techniques have been used for the control of acute hemorrhage: multiple studies, however, have found that ligation is superior to sclerotherapy [5,46,47].

Banding has a lower rebleeding rate and reduced complications. Stiegmann et al. [48] also showed a higher mortality rate in patients that had sclerotherapy used for the control of hemorrhage. Additionally, a meta-analysis by Gross et al. [40] demonstrated the superiority of endoscopic banding ligation over medical therapy in the treatment of acute variceal bleeding. The combination of banding and sclerotherapy has been evaluated as well: neither Laine et al. [49] nor Saeed et al. [50] were able to demonstrate additional benefit to combination therapy, and the latter study showed an increased complication rate with dual treatment.

While endoscopic banding is superior for the treatment of acute bleeding, the role of endoscopy and the type of treatment for prophylaxis is discordant and more divisive. van Buuren et al. [51] found that there was no difference in the number of episodes of bleeding when sclerotherapy was compared with no treatment. Villanueva et al. [54], however, found that combination medical therapy was more successful in preventing bleeding. Additionally, other trials have shown increased mortality rates with sclerotherapy, and these practices are not recommended [5]. Endoscopic banding has been widely studied for the prophylaxis of variceal bleeding. This technique is often compared with medical prophylaxis with beta-blockers alone or in combination with IM. A study by Wang et al. [52] found that combined medical (beta-blocker plus IM) and procedural therapies were equally effective for primary prophylaxis. Conversely, Sarin et al. [53] showed that banding reduced initial bleeding risk from 43% to 15% as compared to beta-blocker alone. Villanueva et al. [54] showed that combined medical therapy was superior for secondary prophylaxis without an all-cause mortality benefit. Lo et al. [55] published a series indicating that banding was better for secondary prevention, but that combined medical therapy improved overall survival. A meta-analysis by Gluud et al. [56] showed that banding ligation reduced bleeding episodes as compared to beta-blockers without any difference in morality. Wang et al. performed a randomized controlled trial to assess whether monthly versus biweekly endoscopic banding had any effect on rates of prevention of esophageal variceal bleeding, but found similar rebleeding rates between groups (17% in monthly group vs. 20% in biweekly group) [57].

*Recommendations*:

1. Endoscopic treatment should be used to stop active hemorrhage from ulcer disease and confers additional prevention of rebleeding episodes.
2. Endoscopic banding ligation is the treatment of choice for acute variceal hemorrhage and should be undertaken as soon as possible.
3. Banding ligation is an effective means of preventing variceal bleeding and can be used when medical prophylaxis cannot be tolerated.

*Grade of recommendation*: 1. A, 2. A, 3. B

**TABLE 44.1**

Upper GI Bleeds: Question Summary

| No. | Question | Answer | Grade | References |
|---|---|---|---|---|
| 1 | What is the role of medical therapy in the prevention of UGI bleeds? | PPI should be used as stress ulcer prophylaxis in critically ill patients to prevent GI bleeding. | A | [11–13] |
| | | Risk of ulcer formation for patients taking NSAIDs is significantly reduced with PPI or H2RA prophylaxis. | A | [15,17–19] |
| | | Beta-blockers can be used safely for primary prophylaxis from variceal bleeding and may slow the growth of small varices. | B | [21–27] |
| 2 | What is the role of medical therapy in treating active UGI bleeds? | Proton pump inhibitors should be preferentially used over H2RAs to reduce rebleeding episodes after successful endoscopic therapy. | A | [30–34] |
| | | In *H. Pylori-positive* patients, eradication therapy should be employed. | B | [35,36] |
| | | Octreotide should be used to slow the rate of variceal bleeding, until definitive endoscopic therapy can be implemented. | B | [37–40] |
| 3 | What is the role of endoscopy for treating or preventing UGI bleeds? | Endoscopic treatment should be used to stop active hemorrhage from ulcer disease and confers additional prevention of rebleeding episodes. | A | [2,36,42–45] |
| | | Endoscopic banding ligation is the treatment of choice for acute variceal hemorrhage and should be undertaken as soon as possible. | A | [5,40,46–50] |
| | | Banding ligation is an effective means of preventing variceal bleeding and can be used when medical prophylaxis cannot be tolerated. | B | [5,46,51–57] |
| 4 | What is the role for interventional radiology in treating UGI bleeds? | Angiography is safe and should be used in patients with massive UGI bleeding who are too ill to undergo an operation. | C | [59–65] |

## 44.5 What Is the Role of Interventional Radiology in Treating UGI Bleeds?

Angiography has been established as the primary therapy for many lower GI bleeds. Its role in UGI bleeding, however, is not as well defined. While there are many case reports of the use of angiography for the identification and control of bleeding from more obscure bleeding sources (such as small bowel diverticula or mesenteric aneurysms), the data for its use in the control of typical UGI hemorrhage is far from robust.

Angiography has been used since the 1970s for the control of GI hemorrhage for both diagnosis and therapy [58]. Defreyne et al. [59] published a series of patients with GI bleeding treated with angioembolization that showed patients with an upper GI source had higher rates of rebleeding, and a lower success rate, when compared to lower GI sources. Carreira et al. [60], however, showed that embolization was successful 90% of the time in a study with predominately upper GI bleeds. Other studies have found similar success rates [61,62]. Poultsides et al. published a series of patients with gastroduodenal hemorrhage that underwent embolization with a 94% technical, and 51% clinical success rate [63]. A 10-year retrospective review of 98 hemodynamically unstable (SBP <90 mmHg) patients who underwent super-selective angioembolization for UGI bleeding demonstrated technical and clinical success rates of 98% and 71%, respectively, of the initial bleeding episode and a 20% rebleeding rate within 30 days requiring additional intervention [64]. Most of these studies indicate that embolization should be used in patients with massive ongoing hemorrhage who cannot tolerate surgery due to medical co-morbidities. A meta-analysis of nine studies comparing emergency surgery versus transarterial embolization (TAE) suggests an increased risk of rebleeding with TAE and no difference in mortality rate, demonstrating that further study of TAE is necessary to establish the role of this technique in UGI bleeding [65] (Table 44.1).

*Recommendation*: Angiography should be used in patients with massive hemorrhage who are too ill to undergo an operation.

*Grade of recommendation*: C

## Disclaimer

There were no sources of funding or conflicts of interest in the writing of this chapter.

## References

1. Conrad SA. Acute upper gastrointestinal bleeding in critically ill patients: Causes and treatment modalities. *Crit Care Med.* 2002;30:S365–S368.

2. Barkun A, Bardou M, Marshall JK. Consensus recommendations for managing patients with nonvariceal upper gastrointestinal bleeding. *Ann Intern Med.* 2003;139:843–857.
3. Khamaysi I, Gralnek IM. Acute upper gastrointestinal bleeding (UGIB)—Initial evaluation and management. *Best Pract Res Clin Gastroenterol.* 2013;27:633–638.
4. Eisen GM, Dominitz JA, Faigel DO et al. An annotated algorithmic approach to upper gastrointestinal bleeding. *Gastrointest Endosc.* 2001;53:853–858.
5. Qureshi W, Adler DG, Davila R et al. ASGE Guideline: The role of endoscopy in the management of variceal hemorrhage, updated July 2005. *Gastrointest Endosc.* 2005;62:651–655.
6. Taefi A, Cho WK, Nouraie M. Decreasing trend of upper gastrointestinal bleeding mortality risk over three decades. *Dig Dis Sci.* 2013;58:2940–2948.
7. Cook DJ, Reeve BK, Guyatt GH et al. Stress ulcer prophylaxis in critically ill patients: Resolving discordant meta-analyses. *JAMA.* 1996;275:308–314.
8. Cook D, Guyatt G, Marshall J et al. A comparison of sucralfate and ranitidine for the prevention of upper gastrointestinal bleeding in patients requiring mechanical ventilation: Canadian Critical Care Trials Group. *N Engl J Med.* 1998;338:791–797.
9. Cook DJ, Reeve BK, Scholes LC. Histamine-2-receptor antagonists and antacids in the critically ill population: Stress ulceration versus nosocomial pneumonia. *Infect Control Hosp Epidemiol.* 1994;15:437–442.
10. Jung R, MacLaren R. Proton-pump inhibitors for stress ulcer prophylaxis in critically ill patients. *Ann Pharmacother.* 2002;36:1929–1937.
11. Conrad SA, Gabrielli A, Margolis B et al. Randomized, double-blind comparison of immediate-release omeprazole oral suspension versus intravenous cimetidine for the prevention of upper gastrointestinal bleeding in critically ill patients. *Crit Care Med.* 2005;33:760–765.
12. Liu BL, Li B, Zhang X et al. A randomized controlled study comparing omeprazole and cimetidine for the prophylaxis of stress-related upper gastrointestinal bleeding in patients with intracerebral hemorrhage. *J Neurosurg.* 2013;118:1115–1120.
13. Udd M, Miettinen P, Palmu A et al. Regular-dose versus high-dose omeprazole in peptic ulcer bleeding: A prospective randomized double-blind study. *Scand J Gastroenterol.* 2001;36:1332–1338.
14. Chason RD, Reisch JS, Rockey DC. More favorable outcomes with peptic ulcer bleeding due to Helicobacter pylori. *Am J Med.* 2013;126:811–818.
15. Chan FK, Ching JY, Hung LC et al. Clopidogrel versus aspirin and esomeprazole to prevent recurrent ulcer bleeding. *N Engl J Med.* 2005;352:238–244.
16. Kawasaki K, Kurahara K, Yanai S, Kochi S, Fuchigami T, Matsumoto T. Low-dose aspirin and non-steroidal anti-inflammatory drugs increase the risk of bleeding in patients with gastroduodenal ulcer. *Dig Dis Sci.* 2014;60(4):1010–1015.
17. Chan FK, Wong VW, Suen BY et al. Combination of a cyclo-oxygenase-2 inhibitor and a proton-pump inhibitor for prevention of recurrent ulcer bleeding in patients at very high risk: A double-blind, randomised trial. *Lancet.* 2007;369:1621–1626.
18. Lai KC, Lam SK, Chu KM et al. Lansoprazole for the prevention of recurrences of ulcer complications from long-term low-dose aspirin use. *N Engl J Med.* 2002;346:2033–2038.
19. Lim H, Kim JH, Baik GH et al. Effect of low-dose PPI on preventing upper gastrointestinal bleeding in chronic kidney disease patients receiving aspirin. *J Gastroenterol Hepatol.* 2014;30(3):478–484.
20. Jiang HY, Chen HZ, Hu XJ et al. Use of selective serotonin reuptake inhibitors and risk of upper gastrointestinal bleeding: A systematic review and meta-analysis. *Clin Gastroenterol Hepatol.* 2014;13(1):42–50.
21. Lebrec D, Nouel O, Bernuau J, Bouygues M, Rueff B, Benhamou JP. Propranolol in prevention of recurrent gastrointestinal bleeding in cirrhotic patients. *Lancet.* 1981;1:920–921.
22. Lebrec D, Poynard T, Capron JP et al. Nadolol for prophylaxis of gastrointestinal bleeding in patients with cirrhosis: A randomized trial. *J Hepatol.* 1988;7:118–125.
23. Kiire CF. Controlled trial of propranolol to prevent recurrent variceal bleeding in patients with non-cirrhotic portal fibrosis. *BMJ.* 1989;298:1363–1365.
24. Merkel C, Marin R, Angeli P et al. A placebo-controlled clinical trial of nadolol in the prophylaxis of growth of small esophageal varices in cirrhosis. *Gastroenterology.* 2004;127:476–484.
25. Groszmann RJ, Garcia-Tsao G, Bosch J et al. Beta-blockers to prevent gastroesophageal varices in patients with cirrhosis. *N Engl J Med.* 2005;353:2254–2261.
26. Angelico M, Carli L, Piat C et al. Isosorbide-5-mononitrate versus propranolol in the prevention of first bleeding in cirrhosis. *Gastroenterology.* 1993;104:1460–1465.
27. Talwalkar JA, Kamath PS. An evidence-based medicine approach to beta-blocker therapy in patients with cirrhosis. *Am J Med.* 2004;116:759–766.
28. Merkel C, Gatta A, Donada C et al. Long-term effect of nadolol or nadolol plus isosorbide-5-mononitrate on renal function and ascites formation in patients with cirrhosis: GTIP Gruppo Triveneto per l'Ipertensione Portale. *Hepatology.* 1995;22:808–813.
29. Collins R, Langman M. Treatment with histamine H2 antagonists in acute upper gastrointestinal hemorrhage: Implications of randomized trials. *N Engl J Med.* 1985;313:660–666.
30. Lanas A, Artal A, Blas JM, Arroyo MT, Lopez-Zaborras J, Sainz R. Effect of parenteral omeprazole and ranitidine on gastric pH and the outcome of bleeding peptic ulcer. *J Clin Gastroenterol.* 1995;21:103–106.
31. Khuroo MS, Yattoo GN, Javid G et al. A comparison of omeprazole and placebo for bleeding peptic ulcer. *N Engl J Med.* 1997;336:1054–1058.
32. Lau JY, Sung JJ, Lee KK et al. Effect of intravenous omeprazole on recurrent bleeding after endoscopic treatment of bleeding peptic ulcers. *N Engl J Med.* 2000;343:310–316.

33. Daneshmend TK, Hawkey CJ, Langman MJ, Logan RF, Long RG, Walt RP. Omeprazole versus placebo for acute upper gastrointestinal bleeding: Randomised double blind controlled trial. *BMJ*. 1992;304:143–147.
34. Lau JY, Leung WK, Wu JC et al. Omeprazole before endoscopy in patients with gastrointestinal bleeding. *N Engl J Med*. 2007;356:1631–1640.
35. Riemann JF, Schilling D, Schauwecker P et al. Cure with omeprazole plus amoxicillin versus long-term ranitidine therapy in *Helicobacter pylori*-associated peptic ulcer bleeding. *Gastrointest Endosc*. 1997;46:299–304.
36. Sung JJ, Chan FK, Lau JY et al. The effect of endoscopic therapy in patients receiving omeprazole for bleeding ulcers with nonbleeding visible vessels or adherent clots: A randomized comparison. *Ann Intern Med*. 2003;139:237–243.
37. Jenkins SA, Baxter JN, Corbett W, Devitt P, Ware J, Shields R. A prospective randomised controlled clinical trial comparing somatostatin and vasopressin in controlling acute variceal haemorrhage. *Br Med J (Clin Res Ed)*. 1985;290:275–278.
38. Hwang SJ, Lin HC, Chang CF et al. A randomized controlled trial comparing octreotide and vasopressin in the control of acute esophageal variceal bleeding. *J Hepatol*. 1992;16:320–325.
39. Corley DA, Cello JP, Adkisson W, Ko WF, Kerlikowske K. Octreotide for acute esophageal variceal bleeding: A meta-analysis. *Gastroenterology*. 2001;120:946–954.
40. Gross M, Schiemann U, Muhlhofer A, Zoller WG. Meta-analysis: Efficacy of therapeutic regimens in ongoing variceal bleeding. *Endoscopy*. 2001;33:737–746.
41. Roberts I, Coats T, Edwards P et al. HALT-IT—Tranexamic acid for the treatment of gastrointestinal bleeding: Study protocol for a randomised controlled trial. *Trials*. 2014;15:450.
42. Bini EJ, Cohen J. Endoscopic treatment compared with medical therapy for the prevention of recurrent ulcer hemorrhage in patients with adherent clots. *Gastrointest Endosc*. 2003;58:707–714.
43. Chung SS, Lau JY, Sung JJ et al. Randomised comparison between adrenaline injection alone and adrenaline injection plus heat probe treatment for actively bleeding ulcers. *BMJ*. 1997;314:1307–1311.
44. Theivanayagam S, Lim RG, Cobell WJ et al. Administration of erythromycin before endoscopy in upper gastrointestinal bleeding: A meta-analysis of randomized controlled trials. *Saudi J Gastroenterol*. 2013;19:205–210.
45. Lau JY, Sung JJ, Lam YH et al. Endoscopic retreatment compared with surgery in patients with recurrent bleeding after initial endoscopic control of bleeding ulcers. *N Engl J Med*. 1999;340:751–756.
46. Gimson AE, Ramage JK, Panos MZ et al. Randomised trial of variceal banding ligation versus injection sclerotherapy for bleeding oesophageal varices. *Lancet*. 1993;342:391–394.
47. Laine L, el-Newihi HM, Migikovsky B, Sloane R, Garcia F. Endoscopic ligation compared with sclerotherapy for the treatment of bleeding esophageal varices. *Ann Intern Med*. 1993;119:1–7.
48. Stiegmann GV, Goff JS, Michaletz-Onody PA et al. Endoscopic sclerotherapy as compared with endoscopic ligation for bleeding esophageal varices. *N Engl J Med*. 1992;326:1527–1532.
49. Laine L, Stein C, Sharma V. Randomized comparison of ligation versus ligation plus sclerotherapy in patients with bleeding esophageal varices. *Gastroenterology*. 1996;110:529–533.
50. Saeed ZA, Stiegmann GV, Ramirez FC et al. Endoscopic variceal ligation is superior to combined ligation and sclerotherapy for esophageal varices: A multicenter prospective randomized trial. *Hepatology*. 1997;25:71–74.
51. van Buuren HR, Rasch MC, Batenburg PL et al. Endoscopic sclerotherapy compared with no specific treatment for the primary prevention of bleeding from esophageal varices. A randomized controlled multicentre trial [ISRCTN03215899]. *BMC Gastroenterol*. 2003;3:22.
52. Wang HM, Lo GH, Chen WC et al. Comparison of endoscopic variceal ligation and nadolol plus isosorbide-5-mononitrate in the prevention of first variceal bleeding in cirrhotic patients. *J Chin Med Assoc*. 2006;69:453–460.
53. Sarin SK, Lamba GS, Kumar M, Misra A, Murthy NS. Comparison of endoscopic ligation and propranolol for the primary prevention of variceal bleeding. *N Engl J Med*. 1999;340:988–993.
54. Villanueva C, Minana J, Ortiz J et al. Endoscopic ligation compared with combined treatment with nadolol and isosorbide mononitrate to prevent recurrent variceal bleeding. *N Engl J Med*. 2001;345:647–655.
55. Lo GH, Chen WC, Lin CK et al. Improved survival in patients receiving medical therapy as compared with banding ligation for the prevention of esophageal variceal rebleeding. *Hepatology*. 2008;48:580–587.
56. Gluud LL, Klingenberg S, Nikolova D, Gluud C. Banding ligation versus beta-blockers as primary prophylaxis in esophageal varices: Systematic review of randomized trials. *Am J Gastroenterol*. 2007;102:2842–2848; quiz 1, 9.
57. Wang HM, Lo GH, Chen WC et al. Randomized controlled trial of monthly versus biweekly endoscopic variceal ligation for the prevention of esophageal variceal rebleeding. *J Gastroenterol Hepatol*. 2014;29:1229–1236.
58. Rahn NH III, Tishler JM, Han SY, Russinovich NA. Diagnostic and interventional angiography in acute gastrointestinal hemorrhage. *Radiology*. 1982;143:361–366.
59. Defreyne L, Vanlangenhove P, De Vos M et al. Embolization as a first approach with endoscopically unmanageable acute nonvariceal gastrointestinal hemorrhage. *Radiology*. 2001;218:739–748.
60. Carreira JM, Reyes R, Pulido-Duque JM et al. Diagnosis and percutaneous treatment of gastrointestinal hemorrhage: Long-term experience. *Rev Esp Enferm Dig*. 1999;91:684–692.

61. Toyoda H, Nakano S, Takeda I et al. Transcatheter arterial embolization for massive bleeding from duodenal ulcers not controlled by endoscopic hemostasis. *Endoscopy.* 1995;27:304–307.
62. Park MH, Park GS, Park SW et al. Clinical effectiveness of transcatheter arterial embolization for acute upper and lower non-variceal gastrointestinal bleeding. *Korean J Gastroenterol.* 2005;46:262–268.
63. Poultsides GA, Kim CJ, Orlando R III, Peros G, Hallisey MJ, Vignati PV. Angiographic embolization for gastroduodenal hemorrhage: Safety, efficacy, and predictors of outcome. *Arch Surg.* 2008;143:457–461.
64. Mejaddam AY, Cropano CM, Kalva S et al. Outcomes following "rescue" superselective angioembolization for gastrointestinal hemorrhage in hemodynamically unstable patients. *J Trauma Acute Care Surg.* 2013;75:398–403.
65. Beggs AD, Dilworth MP, Powell SL, Atherton H, Griffiths EA. A systematic review of transarterial embolization versus emergency surgery in treatment of major nonvariceal upper gastrointestinal bleeding. *Clin Exp Gastroenterol.* 2014;7:93–104.

## Commentary on Evidence-Based Approach to Upper Gastrointestinal Bleeding

*Mark A. Malangoni*

The management of acute upper gastrointestinal bleeding (UGIB) has evolved considerably over the past few decades. Operations for UGIB have become very uncommon as medical therapy and less invasive interventions have improved. The use of histamine type-2 receptor blockade and proton pump inhibitors has been shown to effectively reduce gastric acid production, and beta-blockers have been demonstrated to decrease portal pressure. Treating *H. pylori* infection when present has been demonstrated to be effective in reducing subsequent complications of peptic ulcer disease including bleeding. These treatments have become mainstays to prevent and manage UGIB related to peptic ulcer disease and esophageal varices.

Endoscopy has advanced from its early role strictly to improve diagnostic accuracy prior to operation to one of the effective interventions for acute bleeding with a corresponding reduction in operative management. Prospective studies have identified which ulcers are at high risk to rebleed, this has helped define when injection therapies are necessary. Similarly, acute bleeding of esophageal varices is now effectively treated with a combination of band ligation and portal pressure reduction.

This chapter captures the essence of the current management of UGIB. There are some areas where supplemental information is necessary. On rare occasion, UGIB will be due to gastrinoma (Zollinger–Ellison syndrome) and when this is suspected (unusual ulcer location, persistent rebleeding), a serum gastrin level should be measured and if diagnostic, the dosage of medical therapy should be increased substantially.

The authors have not addressed the operative management of UGIB, which often is resorted to when other treatments fail. In these cases, endoscopy usually has defined the source of bleeding, which is immensely helpful in planning the operation. Pinpointing the location of the site of bleeding allows the surgeon to rapidly open the stomach or pylorus to ligate the bleeding vessel, curtail blood loss, and restore cardiovascular homeostasis. The bleeding vessel in the ulcer base should be ligated using permanent suture with figure-of-eight technique. For duodenal ulcers, this should be done both superior and inferior to the bleeding point. Other points of ligation have been advocated by some, but I have found that necessary. Gastric ulcers can usually be effectively ligated with a single figure of eight suture.

There are some unusual lesions that cause UGIB. Dieulafoy's ulcers are located in the upper body of the stomach and can usually be treated with endoscopic injection. The occasional patient with UGIB due to a Mallory–Weiss tear usually stops bleeding spontaneously, but when bleeding persists, endoscopic management is usually effective.

Once operative control of bleeding has occurred, the dilemma is whether more needs to be done and, if so, what operation is best. Most surgeons would agree that truncal vagotomy with pyloroplasty is indicated along with suture ligation of a bleeding duodenal ulcer. The pyloroplasty should be at least 6 cm in length and most surgeons employ a Heinecke–Mikulicz closure. The phrenoesophageal ligament is then incised and the esophagus encircled by inserting a finger above the incision and bluntly dissecting the esophagus from the areolar tissues of the lower mediastinum. Having a nasogastric or orogastric tube in place facilitates identification of the esophagus and helps avoid esophageal injury. A drain is then placed around the esophagus for traction and the vagal nerves identified and transected. The anterior vagus nerve is located on the left anterolateral surface of the esophagus and the posterior nerve is located inferior and posterior on the patient's right side (8 o'clock). The posterior trunk is larger than the anterior nerve and sometimes is not included in the esophageal dissection. In this case, a thorough search in the area should be done. A 2 cm segment of each vagal trunk should be resected and sent for pathologic confirmation. Failure to divide both vagal trunks is associated with recurrent bleeding, usually at a later time and the posterior trunk is not identified more often. There are often additional branches of the anterior vagus that are evident on either immediately medial or lateral to the main trunk. When present, these braches should be divided.

Historically, truncal vagotomy and pyloroplasty has a rebleeding rate of <2% and an ulcer recurrence rate of about 8%–10%. However, these studies were done before current medical therapy was available and most believe that rebleeding is much lower when H2 receptor antagonists and PPIs are used postoperatively.

Wedge resection of a gastric ulcer is effective in most circumstances when nonoperative management has failed. Performing a vagotomy adds little to the short- or long-term results with this disease; avoiding vagotomy reduces postoperative gastric emptying problems. A bleeding Dieulafoys' ulcer that requires operation is treated with suture ligation and this is usually supplemented with acid-reducing medical therapy perioperatively.

Gastric resection for gastroduodenal ulcer disease is uncommonly needed and is usually reserved for reoperation, patients who require long-term NSAID therapy, and patients with a giant (>4 cm) duodenal ulcer. When resection is needed, antrectomy alone is effective for gastric ulcers and truncal vagotomy should be added for duodenal ulcers. Duodenal ulcers should not be resected. Failure to abide by this principle often leads to complications that result in additional complications. In contrast, gastric ulcers should always be resected unless resection would narrow the gastroesophageal junction. Restoration of gastrointestinal continuity is most commonly done with a gastrojejunostomy, particularly when a duodenal ulcer is present. Gastroduodenal anastomoses are usually reserved for when gastric ulcers are being treated in which case the duodenum is not inflamed and an anastomosis is safe. Performing a Kocher maneuver frees up the duodenum and helps reduce anastomotic tension.

The use of transjugular portosystemic shunts (TIPSs) has revolutionized the management of bleeding gastroesophageal varices and is second-line therapy following medication to reduce portal pressure. TIPSs reduce the incidence of UGI rebleeding from portal hypertension but are not useful when extrhepatic portal hypertension is present. Patients who have bleeding varices due to splenic vein thrombosis will respond to splenectomy if bleeding persists. There is no evidence that prophylactic splenectomy is indicated to treat gastric varices that have not bled.

The mortality of operations for acute UGIB due to bleeding varices can be high, which is not surprising, since these patients have almost invariably failed other interventions. H-graft portosystemic shunts are usually employed in this situation.

# 45

## *Peptic Ulcer Disease*

**Wayne H. Schwesinger**

**CONTENTS**



### 45.1 How Has the Surgery of Peptic Ulcer Disease Changed Over Time?

Few diseases in the Western society have been so dramatically transformed over time as peptic ulcer disease (PUD). Although rarely described in the early medical literature, its incidence reached epidemic proportions by the mid-1900s, then slowly began to decline [1,2]. From the beginning, operative therapy served as an important cornerstone in the management of PUD because the available medical measures were often ineffective. Landmark investigations by Beaumont, Pavlov, Dragsted, and Edkins, among others, served as the pathophysiological foundation on which many new surgical strategies for the management of PUD were developed. Though these operations appeared to be very effective at controlling both intractable and complicated PUD, they could be associated with significant short-term and long-term consequences.

Simultaneously, major progress was also being made with two different nonoperative approaches to the management of PUD: pharmacotherapy and flexible endoscopy. Antisecretory therapy, introduced in 1977, largely replaced both the Sippy diet and antacid therapy and a decade later was itself superseded by the introduction of the first proton pump inhibitor (PPI). In 1983, a specific infectious etiology for PUD was suggested by Warren and Marshall; within a decade, more than 1500 scientific articles were being published on the topic annually. The possibility of a medical cure with antibiotic therapy was quickly established.

As a result of these pharmacological advances and evolving endoscopic techniques, the profile of surgery for PUD has dramatically changed. A personal survey of a 20-year experience in two major teaching hospitals demonstrated an 80% decrease in the overall number of operations for PUD [3]. Currently, the most common indications for surgery are perforation and bleeding, whereas intractability has become nearly obsolete.

Other studies have demonstrated that patient demographics are also continuing to change. Patient hospitalized with PUD are now older, more frequently female, and more likely to have major comorbid conditions [4,5].

*Recommendation*: The number of operations performed for PUD has declined by >80% over the past two decades. The most common indications are perforation and bleeding. Operations for intractability are rare. Patients are generally older, sicker, and more often female.

*Grade of recommendation*: B

### 45.2 What Are the Major Risk Factors for PUD?

By the mid-twentieth century, it was generally agreed that gastric hyperacidity was the major cause of PUD. Thus, the commonly quoted aphorism: "no acid, no ulcer" [6]. Early speculations on the specific pathogenetic factors causing hyperacidity focused on the relative contributions of stress, smoking, familial predisposition, hormonal changes, aspirin intake, and dietary indiscretions.

A paradigm shift occurred when it was recognized that either *Helicobacter pylori* infection or nonsteroidal anti-inflammatory drug (NSAID) use could be implicated in most cases of peptic ulceration, albeit through entirely different mechanisms [7,8]. With *H. pylori* infection, a complex interaction occurs between bacterial virulence factors (cagA, cagPAI, vacA), host factors (interleukins, tumor necrosis factor-A, chemokines), and environmental factors (smoking, high salt intake) [9]. The result is a persistent chronic gastritis. The location of the infection in the stomach helps to determine the clinical course. Antral-dominant infections result in reduced somatostatin levels, hypergastrinemia, and gastric acid hypersecretion and can produce duodenal ulcers. Body-dominant infections are associated with mucosal atrophy and hypochlorhydria; this pattern may result in either benign gastric ulcers or malignancy.

The gastric mucosal injury caused by NSAIDs (including aspirin) results mostly from inhibition of the constitutive enzyme cyclo-oxygenase-1 (COX-1), a major product of arachidonic acid metabolism in the gastric mucosa. COX-1 is responsible for the release of prostacyclin, a potent cytoprotectant, and, when inhibited, allows gastric acid and other irritants to damage the mucosa. Another isoform, COX-2, is induced by inflammatory stimuli and has significant anti-inflammatory activity but fewer gastric side effects [10].

Importantly, a synergism can develop between the two major risk factors. In a meta-analysis of 25 related studies, the presence of *H. pylori* infection was found to increase the risk of PUD 3.5-fold in NSAID users compared with noninfected patients [11].

The category of idiopathic, non-NSAID, and non–*H. pylori* PUD can be accounted for by inaccurate *H. pylori* testing, covert NSAID use, or otherwise altered gastric physiology. Non-NSAID and non-*H. pylori* ulcers tend to occur in older and sicker patients and are associated with a higher recurrence rate [12]. Other causes of ulceration include Zollinger–Ellison syndrome, G-cell hyperplasia, Crohn's disease, cocaine abuse, and systemic mastocytosis.

*Recommendation*: In Western countries, PUD is primarily caused by *H. pylori* infection and NSAID use. Idiopathic causes include Zollinger–Ellison syndrome, G-cell hyperplasia, Crohn's disease, cocaine abuse, and systemic mastocytosis.

*Grade of recommendation*: A

## 45.3 What Is the Appropriate Therapy for *Helicobacter pylori*-Positive PUD?

In patients with PUD who are *H. pylori*-positive, eradication of the organism is indicated. In a Cochrane analysis of over 3900 patients in 34 trials, the ulcer healing rate after therapy was 75%–85% and the recurrence rate was 12%–14% [13]. First-line therapy as recommended in the Maastricht Consensus Report 2-2000 combines a PPI with clarithromycin and amoxicillin or metronidazole twice daily for 1–2 weeks [14]. Successful eradication can be achieved with initial treatment of 75%–90% of patients. Second-line rescue treatment with quadruple therapy typically combines a PPI with bismuth, metronidazole, and tetracycline.

Eradication should always be confirmed with either a urea breath test or a stool antigen. Antimicrobial resistance is the usual cause of repeated treatment failures, and cultures with sensitivities may be necessary to tailor treatment protocols in selected patients. The Helicobacter Antimicrobial Resistance Monitoring Program studied 347 clinical isolates and found that the highest rate of resistant strains occurred with metronidazole (25.1%) and clarithromycin (12.9%), whereas [15] amoxicillin resistance was uncommon (0.9%).

*Recommendation*: First-line therapy combines PPI + clarithromycin + amoxicillin or metronidazole and has a successful eradication rate of 78%–90%. Rescue therapies are available for nonresponders.

*Grade of recommendation*: A

## 45.4 In a Patient Suspected of Having a Bleeding Peptic Ulcer, What Should the Initial Approach Be?

Optimal management depends on a timely and accurate diagnosis and an adequate resuscitation, processes that should proceed concurrently. The initial clinical approach is determined in large part by the patient's presentation. A history of red blood or dark "coffee ground" emesis nearly always indicates an upper gastrointestinal (UGI) source. The rectal passage of black, digested blood (melanic stool) is also indicative of a lesion proximal to the ligament of Trietz. The passage of bright red blood per rectum usually suggests a primary colorectal source, but it also occurs in patients with upper tract lesions when the rate of bleeding is rapid and the transit time is brief.

A rapid assessment of the patient's hemodynamic and physical status can guide early therapy and appropriate triage. The presence of hemorrhagic shock, either compensated or decompensated, mandates aggressive fluid management with blood products and/or crystalloid. In addition, preexisting comorbidities such as cardiac disease or hepatic or renal dysfunction must be addressed to avoid deterioration. Specific coagulation abnormalities must also be rapidly corrected.

Endpoints for resuscitation include: normalization of blood pressure, restoration of hemoglobin concentration, correction of coagulopathies, and correction of end-organ dysfunction [16]. Such an aggressive and multifaceted approach is supported in the controlled study of Baradarian et al., in which intensive monitoring and early hemodynamic stabilization were provided by a specialized resuscitation group [17]. This resulted in a significant reduction in the associated mortality when compared with routine floor management.

During resuscitation, nasogastric tube placement is used to sample the contents of the stomach. In patients who present with a history of hematemesis, nasogastric aspiration of fresh, red blood indicates the presence of ongoing bleeding and is an independent predictor of poor clinical outcome when compared with aspiration of either clear or "coffee ground" material [18]. In bleeding patients who present with melena but without hematemesis, a bloody nasogastric aspirate provides strong evidence for a lesion in the UGI tract (specificity = 91%–95%) [19]. However, a negative aspirate is less reliable because it may fail to detect duodenal lesions (sensitivity = 42%–73%).

Nasogastric tubes can also be used for gastric lavage prior to endoscopy, but success is limited by the size of the tube and the presence of clots. Alternatively, prokinetic agents are able to effectively clear the stomach. Several randomized controlled clinical trials have documented that a pre-endoscopic bolus or infusion of erythromycin improves the quality of the subsequent endoscopic examination and reduces the need for repeat endoscopic procedures [20].

*Recommendation*: A rapid and accurate diagnosis and aggressive resuscitation should proceed simultaneously in patients thought to be bleeding from an UGI source.

*Grade of recommendation*: A

## 45.5 In Patients with Bleeding Ulcers, What Is the Current Role of Endoscopy?

Endoscopy is the definitive diagnostic study for UGI bleeding. In a multicenter study of 11,160 patients with nonvariceal UGI bleeding, endoscopy identified the bleeding site in 83% of cases. The most common finding was peptic ulcers (32%) with gastric ulcers more common than duodenal ulcers (54% vs. 37%) [21].

Risk stratification is another important function of endoscopy because it guides early management [22]. Patients with a clean-based ulcer or a nonprotruding pigmented spot are at low risk of rebleeding (5%) and generally require no further endoscopic interventions. Conversely, high-risk stigmata, such as an actively bleeding ulcer or an ulcer with a visible vessel, forecast a poor outcome with rebleeding rate of 55% and indicate the need for aggressive endoscopic therapy. Another subset of patients who have an ulcer with an adherent clot appears to be at an intermediate risk for rebleeding (22%) and benefits from removal of the clot and directed endoscopic therapy [23].

The optimal timing for endoscopy continues to be debated. It is generally agreed that patients who are actively bleeding or who are unstable require urgent endoscopy to prevent further deterioration. In the remaining patients, the recommended timing ranges from urgent to elective. Nonetheless, it is generally recommended that endoscopy be performed within 24 h.

Ulcer bleeding stops spontaneously in the majority of patients (80%–85%) [24]. In the remainder, endoscopic therapy has proven efficacious and cost-effective. By 1992, a meta-analysis of 30 randomized clinical trials was reported, in which a variety of endoscopic hemostatic techniques was compared to medical therapy alone [25]. The endoscopically treated group demonstrated significant reductions in further bleeding (odds ratio [OR] = 0.38; 95% confidence interval [CI] = 0.32–0.45), need for surgery (OR, 0.36; 95% CI, 0.28–0.45), and mortality (OR, 0.55; 95% CI, 0.40–0.76). Serious complications directly related to endoscopy were infrequent and included induced rebleeding (0.4%) and perforation (0%–0.9%).

Numerous studies since have compared the wide variety of available hemostatic techniques: injection, thermal, and mechanical. Overall, initial hemostasis rates range from 85% to 100% for all methods [26]. However, injection therapy alone, whether with dilute epinephrine, thrombin, polidocanol, or cyanoacrylate, is associated with a higher rebleeding rate and a more frequent need for surgery than when combined with any other therapy [27]. A Cochrane systematic review of 17 randomized studies concluded that dual therapy with epinephrine injection and any other technique reduces the further bleeding rate from 18.8% to 10.4%, emergency surgeries from 10.8% to 7.1%, and mortality from 5% to 2.5% without increasing the complication rate [28].

*Recommendation*: Endoscopy is the definitive diagnostic and prognostic study. It is also an effective therapeutic tool with initial hemostasis rates of 85%–100%

*Grade of recommendation*: A

## 45.6 What Is the Role of Pharmacotherapy in the Management of a Bleeding Peptic Ulcer?

Pharmacotherapy in patients with bleeding PUD significantly impacts outcome. PPI infusion when used as an adjunct to endoscopic therapy reduces the risk of further bleeding (OR = 0.49; 95% CI = 0.37–0.65) and decreases the need for surgery (OR = 0.61; 95% CI = 0.48–0.78) [29]. Such therapy should be initiated as early as possible. In a related randomized study, pre-endoscopic PPI was found to facilitate clot formation at the bleeding site and to reduce the need for further endoscopic therapy [30].

All patients who are found to be infected with *H. pylori* should receive oral eradication therapy as soon as practicable because the continued presence of *H. pylori* predicts rebleeding. Thus, in a meta-analysis of seven studies, successful eradication therapy was found to reduce rebleeding rates to 2.9% compared with 20% in the noneradicated group (OR = 0.17; 95% CI = 0.10–0.32) [31]. Furthermore, eradication therapy has been shown to be the most cost-effective pharmacologic approach to the bleeding patient [32].

In the absence of *H. pylori* infection, NSAID usage is commonly found to be a contributing cause of ulcer bleeding and may actually have more severe consequences. A single case–control study of this issue has demonstrated that NSAID-related bleeding when compared to matched *H. pylori*-positive cases is associated with an increased risk of rebleeding (32.4% vs. 13.3%; $p = 0.001$), an increased need for surgical therapy (15.2% vs. 4.8%; $p = 0.01$), and an increased mortality (15.2% vs. 3.8%; $p = 0.005$) [33].

*Recommendation*: When used as an adjunct to endoscopic therapy, PPIs reduce the risk of further bleeding and the need for surgery.

*Grade of recommendation*: A

## 45.7 Under What Circumstances Is an Operation Indicated for a Bleeding Peptic Ulcer? What Techniques Are Associated with the Lowest Rate of Rebleeding?

Surgical therapy is indicated in patients whose bleeding is not controlled by nonoperative measures [34]. The presence of exsanguinating hemorrhage or the lack of endoscopic support are self-evident indications for emergency operation. Recurrent bleeding after endoscopy is a more common (albeit less precise) indication. In 5%–20% of patients who undergo endoscopic hemostasis, bleeding continues or recurs, a finding that is associated with an increase in mortality of 5–16-fold over controls [35]. Risk factors identified by logistic regression analysis as independent predictors of rebleeding or mortality include advanced age, shock, comorbidities, size of ulcer, and presence of major stigmata of hemorrhage [36].

Most patients with rebleeding can benefit from a second-look endoscopy that provides additional hemostatic therapy. In a randomized trial comparing endoscopic retreatment with surgery, control of recurrent bleeding was achieved endoscopically in 35 of the 48 patients (72.9%) with fewer complications experienced than in the surgery alone group (7 vs. 16) [37]. Another randomized trial compared a scheduled second therapeutic endoscopy within 16–24 h after the initial endoscopy with a control group without a routine second endoscopy. The rate of recurrent bleeding was significantly lower in the second-look group (5% vs. 13.8%; $p = 0.03$), and a trend toward fewer operations for rebleeding was identified [38]. Thus, both selective and routine second-look endoscopy appear to favorably influencing the outcome of peptic ulcer bleeding.

Unsuccessful endoscopic retreatment manifest as persistent or recurrent bleeding should generally be addressed by operation. However, an informed choice concerning the most appropriate procedure is difficult because timely, relevant, and high-grade surgical evidence is rare. As a result, widely divergent opinions prevail. Only two small, controlled, randomized trials of different operative strategies have been reported since 1990—one from Great Britain and one from France. In the former, Poxon et al. [39] compared conservative surgery (ulcer oversewing or excision) with conventional surgery (vagotomy and pyloroplasty or gastric resection) and found a significant reduction in fatal rebleeding in the conventional surgery group. In the French study, Millat et al. [40] compared ulcer oversewing and vagotomy with a more aggressive protocol of gastric resection and Billroth I or Billroth II anastomosis. They found that the resection group had a significantly lower rate of recurrent bleeding. They concluded that gastric resection was the procedure of choice in the management of uncontrolled peptic bleeding. In contrast, a database audit of more than 900 patients from the Department of Veterans Affairs National Surgical Quality Improvement Program (NSQIP) demonstrated no differences in mortality, morbidity, or rebleeding rates when vagotomy and drainage was compared to vagotomy and gastric resection [41]. Notably, all operative techniques described in these studies were associated with a similar and relatively high mortality rate (Table 45.1).

Taken together, such sparse data provide little guidance for the surgeon faced with treating a patient who presents with hemorrhage refractory to nonoperative therapies. Based on the available literature and personal experience, the author prefers to oversew the bleeding vessel in duodenal ulcers with the addition of a truncal

**TABLE 45.1**

Controlled Randomized Trials of Surgical Management of Peptic Ulcer

| Author (Ref.) | Presentation | n | Operation | Recurrence (%) | Mortality (%) |
|---|---|---|---|---|---|
| Poxon et al. [39] | Hemorrhage | 62 | Oversewing/excision | 7 (11.3)* | 16 (26) |
| | | 67 | TV/P or TV/A | 4 (5.0) | 13 (19) |
| Millat et al. [40] | Hemorrhage | 58 | Oversewing/TV/P | 10 (17)* | 13 (22.4) |
| | | 60 | Resection | 2 (3) | 14 (23.3) |
| Boey et al. [52] | Perforation | 41 | Closure | 36.6 | 0 |
| | | 37 | Closure/PCV | 10.6* | 0 |
| Gutierrez de la Pena et al. [54] | Perforation | 117 | Closure | 7.1 | 4.3 |
| | | 90 | V/P | 4.4 | 4.4 |

*Abbreviations*: A, antrectomy; TV, truncal vagotomy, P, pyloroplasty; PCV, parietal cell vagotomy.
$^*p < 0.05$.

vagotomy and pyloroplasty. Bleeding gastric ulcers are managed with partial gastric resection but without vagotomy. In each situation, the patient should be tested for *H. pylori* infection and treated, if positive. Eradication of the organism must be confirmed.

An alternative strategy, transcatheter arterial embolization (TAE), was initially reserved for poor risk surgical candidates in highly specialized centers but is now more broadly available. In a recent audit by the National Health Service in Great Britain, TAE was shown to be very effective when used for endoscopically refractory ulcer bleeding and was safer than salvage surgery [42]. No prospective, randomized studies have been reported.

*Recommendations*: Surgery or TAE is indicated for peptic ulcer hemorrhage that is not controlled by endoscopic therapy or that recurs following apparently successful endoscopic therapy (5%–20%).

*Grade of recommendation*: A

When operation is used for peptic ulcer bleeding, combined partial gastric resection and vagotomy is associated with the lowest recurrence rate. However, this approach also has a higher rate of short-term and long-term postoperative complications. Vagotomy with oversewing of the ulcer is effective when combined with anti-*H. pylori* therapy in *H. pylori*-positive patients.

*Grade of recommendation*: A

## 45.8 What Approach Is Preferred for the Management of Perforated PUD?

Perforation is a potentially catastrophic complication of PUD that is usually heralded by the abrupt and dramatic onset of severe, mid-epigastric, or generalized abdominal pain. Because the large majority of perforations occur on the anterior aspect of the stomach or duodenum, pneumoperitoneum is present in the majority of cases and is readily detectable on plain abdominal films or computed tomography scan [43].

The therapy of ulcer perforation should address three separate but related issues: the perforation itself, its underlying cause, and the resultant peritonitis and sepsis. In the latter regard, initial management should include rapid fluid resuscitation, nasogastric tube drainage, and systemic antibiotic administration. There is less unanimity about the respective roles of operative and nonoperative therapies for the actual perforation and its associated pathogenetic factors.

Peptic ulcer perforation remains a highly morbid condition with a related mortality of 8%–30% [44]. Based on a number of multifactorial analyses, several predictors of postoperative complications and death have been consistently identified including: treatment delay, circulatory shock, and major concurrent illness [45]. Moreover, it has been suggested that these predictors can be used to stratify patients and to plan initial therapy. Using such an approach, Rahman et al. identified 84 high-risk patients in a cohort of 626 patients with perforated ulcer and managed them nonoperatively with peritoneal tube drainage [46]. They found a significant decrease in overall mortality compared with historical controls who had undergone conventional operative treatment (9.5% vs. 3.9%; $p < 0.0001$).

The use of nonoperative therapy for ulcer perforation remains controversial but appears to be gaining wider acceptance. Nonrandomized studies have generally indicated that nonoperative treatment of sealed perforations can result in a lower morbidity and mortality than with conventional surgical therapy [47–49]. However, nonoperative treatment fails in 16%–32% of perforated patients necessitating emergency operation. In a controlled, randomized trial, Crofts et al. compared initial nonoperative therapy with early operation in 83 patients with perforation [50]. No difference was noted in mortality (4.7% vs. 5.0%), but the hospital stay was 35% longer in the nonoperative group, and patients over 70 years of age were significantly less likely to respond to conservative measures. The mixed results with nonoperative therapy suggest that such an approach cannot be universally applied; however, its selective use, especially in high-risk patients, may be appropriate if a strict protocol and close follow-up can be ensured [51].

Specific operative strategies for the management of ulcer perforation have continued to evolve. Prior to recognition of the pathogenic roles of *H. pylori* and NSAIDs, studies comparing simple closure with definitive operations (vagotomy with or without resection) demonstrated a lower recurrence rate following the more aggressive approach [52,53] (Table 45.1). The authors reported an operative mortality of 0.9% and a recurrence rate of 7.4%. However, a more recent controlled randomized study comparing simple closure with vagotomy and pyloroplasty in over 200 patients failed to demonstrate an advantage in mortality or recurrence following the more definitive procedure [54].

In the current *Helicobacter* era, pharmacotherapy has largely replaced definitive surgery in the management of ulcer perforation. Worldwide, the prevalence of *H. pylori* infection in patients with perforated peptic ulcer is reported to range from 47% to 100% [55]. Persistence of the infection after perforation predicts recurrence of the ulcer, whereas successful eradication of the organism results in a significant reduction in recurrence rates. In a related study of patients followed for 18 months, ulcer recurrence was noted in 70% of patients with persistent infection but in only 19% of those in whom *H. pylori* was eradicated [56]. In a controlled, randomized trial comparing PPI therapy with anti-*Helicobacter* therapy following simple closure of the ulcer, the relapse rate was found to be significantly reduced in the anti-*Helicobacter* group after 1 year (4.8% vs. 38.1%; $p < 0.001$) [57].

These data suggest that the majority of patients with perforated peptic ulcers can be treated with simple closure of the ulcer when the procedure is combined with appropriate medical measures such as anti-*Helicobacter* therapy, PPI administration, or NSAID modulation. More definitive surgical approaches may be reserved for patients with recurrent ulcer disease or for perforations that are associated with hemorrhage or obstruction.

Successful closure of perforations can be achieved with either open or laparoscopic techniques. A recent meta-analysis of 1113 patients from 15 selected studies found that the laparoscopic approach required longer operating times but was associated with less postoperative analgesic use, a shorter hospital stay, and fewer wound infections [58]. A Cochrane review of three randomized studies concluded that open and laparoscopic repairs are equally safe and effective [59].

**TABLE 45.2**

Summary of Chapter Contents

| | Questions | Answers | Grade |
|---|---|---|---|
| 1 | How has the surgery of PUD changed over time? | The number of operations performed for PUD has declined by >80% over the past two decades. The most common indications are perforation and bleeding. Operations for intractability are rare. Patients are generally older, sicker, and more often female. | B |
| 2 | What are the major risk factors for PUD? | In Western countries, PUD is primarily caused by *H. pylori* infection and NSAID use. Idiopathic causes include Zollinger–Ellison syndrome, G-cell hyperplasia, Crohn's disease, cocaine abuse, and systemic mastocytosis. | A |
| 3 | What is the appropriate therapy for *H. pylori*–positive PUD? | First-line therapy combines PPI + clarithromycin + amoxicillin or metrinidazole and has a successful eradication rate of 78%–90%. Rescue therapies are available for nonresponders. | A |
| 4 | In a patient suspected of having a bleeding peptic ulcer, what should the initial approach be? | A rapid and accurate diagnosis and aggressive resuscitation should proceed simultaneously in patients thought to be bleeding from an UGI source. | A |
| 5 | In patients with bleeding ulcers, what is the current role of endoscopy? | Endoscopy is the definitive diagnostic and prognostic study. It is also an effective therapeutic tool with initial hemostasis rates of 85%–100%. | A |
| 6 | What is the role of pharmacotherapy in the management of a bleeding peptic ulcer? | When used as an adjunct to endoscopic therapy, PPIs reduce the risk of further bleeding and the need for surgery. | A |
| 7 | Under what circumstances is an operation indicated for a bleeding peptic ulcer? | Surgery is indicated for peptic ulcer hemorrhage that is not controlled by endoscopic therapy or recurs following apparently successful endoscopic therapy (5%–20%). | A |
| 8 | What surgical techniques are associated with the lowest rate of UGI rebleeding? | When used for peptic ulcer bleeding, combined partial gastric resection and vagotomy is associated with the lowest recurrence rate. However, this approach also has a higher rate of short-term and long-term postoperative complications. Vagotomy with oversewing of the ulcer is effective when combined with anti-*H. pylori* therapy in *H. pylori*-positive patients. | A |
| 9 | What approach is preferred for the management of perforated PUD? | Nonoperative therapy can be used in selected patients who are found to have a sealed perforation on contrast study. Patch closure is indicated in most patients. *H. pylori* should be eradicated when infection is present. The laparoscopic approach is being used with increased frequency. | B |

In another study using the NSQIP database from 2005 to 2009, 50 patients with perforation who underwent laparoscopic repair were compared with 50 case-matched open controls. Clinical outcomes were not different, but hospital length of stay was significantly shorter in the laparoscopic group [60] (Table 45.2).

*Recommendations*: Nonoperative therapy can be used in selected patients who are found to have a sealed perforation on contrast study. Patch closure is indicated in most patients. *H. pylori* should be eradicated when infection is present. The laparoscopic approach is being used with increased frequency.

*Grade of recommendation*: B

## References


1. Baron JSA. Hospital admission for peptic ulcer and indigestion in London and New York in the 19th and early 20th centuries. *Gut.* 2001:568–570.
2. Wang YR, Richter JE, Dempsey DT. Trends and outcomes of hospitalizations for peptic ulcer disease in the United States, 1993 to 2006. *Ann Surg.* 2010;251:51–58.
3. Schwesinger WH, Page CP, Sirinek KR, Gaskill HV, 3rd, Melnick G, Strodel WE. Operations for peptic ulcer disease: paradigm lost. *J Gastrointest Surg.* 2001;5:438–443.
4. Ohmann C, Imhof M, Ruppert C et al. Time-trends in the epidemiology of peptic ulcer bleeding. *Scand J Gastroenterol.* 2005;40:914–920.
5. Rockall TA, Logan RF, Devlin HB, Northfield TC. Incidence of and mortality from acute upper gastrointestinal haemorrhage in the United Kingdom. Steering Committee and members of the National Audit of Acute Upper Gastrointestinal Haemorrhage. *BMJ.* 1995;311:222–226.
6. Schwarz K. Uber penetricrende magen und jejunalgeschwur. *Beitr Klin Surg.* 1919:96.
7. Schwesinger WH, Edgar J. Poth Memorial Lecture. Is *Helicobacter pylori* a myth or the missing link? *Am J Surg.* 1996;172:411–417.
8. Chow DK, Sung JJ. Is the prevalence of idiopathic ulcers really on the increase? *Nat Clin Pract Gastroenterol Hepatol.* 2007;4:176–177.
9. Dixon MF. Pathophysiology of *Helicobacter pylori* infection. *Scand J Gastroenterol Suppl.* 1994;201:7–10.
10. Vane JR, Botting RM. Mechanism of action of nonsteroidal anti-inflammatory drugs. *Am J Med.* 1998;104:2S–8S; discussion 21S–22S.
11. Huang JQ, Sridhar S, Hunt RH. Role of *Helicobacter pylori* infection and non-steroidal anti-inflammatory drugs in peptic-ulcer disease: A meta-analysis. *Lancet.* 2002;359:14–22.
12. Peura DA. The problem of *Helicobacter pylori*-negative idiopathic ulcer disease. *Baillieres Best Pract Res Clin Gastroenterol.* 2000;14:109–117.
13. Ford AC, Delaney BC, Forman D, Moayyedi P. Eradication therapy for peptic ulcer disease in *Helicobacter pylori* positive patients. *Cochrane Database Syst Rev.* 2006:CD003840.
14. Malfertheiner P, Megraud F, O'Morain C et al. Current concepts in the management of *Helicobacter pylori* infection–the Maastricht 2–2000 Consensus Report. *Aliment Pharmacol Ther.* 2002;16:167–180.
15. Duck WM, Sobel J, Pruckler JM, et al. Antimicrobial resistance incidence and risk factors among *Helicobacter pylori*-infected persons, United States. *Emerg Infect Dis.* 2004;10:1088–1094.
16. Matlock JFM. Non-variceal upper GI hemorrhage: Doorway to diagnosis. *Gastrointest Endoscc.* 2005:112–117.
17. Baradarian R, Ramdhaney S, Chapalamadugu R et al. Early intensive resuscitation of patients with upper gastrointestinal bleeding decreases mortality. *Am J Gastroenterol.* 2004;99:619–622.
18. Aljebreen AM, Fallone CA, Barkun AN. Nasogastric aspirate predicts high-risk endoscopic lesions in patients with acute upper-GI bleeding. *Gastrointest Endosc.* 2004;59:172–178.
19. Adamopoulos AB, Baibas NM, Efstathiou SP et al. Differentiation between patients with acute upper gastrointestinal bleeding who need early urgent upper gastrointestinal endoscopy and those who do not. A prospective study. *Eur J Gastroenterol Hepatol.* 2003;15:381–387.
20. Carbonell N, Pauwels A, Serfaty L, Boelle PY, Becquemont L, Poupon R. Erythromycin infusion prior to endoscopy for acute upper gastrointestinal bleeding: A randomized, controlled, double-blind trial. *Am J Gastroenterol.* 2006;101:1211–1215.
21. Enestvedt BK, Gralnek IM, Mattek N, Lieberman DA, Eisen G. An evaluation of endoscopic indications and findings related to nonvariceal upper-GI hemorrhage in a large multicenter consortium. *Gastrointest Endosc.* 2008;67:422–429.
22. Laine L, Peterson WL. Bleeding peptic ulcer. *N Engl J Med.* 1994;331:717–727.
23. Kahi CJ, Jensen DM, Sung JJ et al. Endoscopic therapy versus medical therapy for bleeding peptic ulcer with adherent clot: A meta-analysis. *Gastroenterology.* 2005;129:855–862.
24. Sung J. Current management of peptic ulcer bleeding. *Nat Clin Pract Gastroenterol Hepatol.* 2006;3:24–32.
25. Cook DJ, Guyatt GH, Salena BJ, Laine LA. Endoscopic therapy for acute nonvariceal upper gastrointestinal hemorrhage: A meta-analysis. *Gastroenterology.* 1992;102:139–148.
26. Park CH, Lee SJ, Park JH, Park JH et al. Optimal injection volume of epinephrine for endoscopic prevention of recurrent peptic ulcer bleeding. *Gastrointest Endosc.* 2004;60:875–880.
27. Marmo R, Rotondano G, Piscopo R, Bianco MA, D'Angella R, Cipolletta L. Dual therapy versus monotherapy in the endoscopic treatment of high-risk bleeding ulcers: A meta-analysis of controlled trials. *Am J Gastroenterol.* 2007;102:279–289; quiz 469.
28. Vergara M, Calvet X, Gisbert JP. Epinephrine injection versus epinephrine injection and a second endoscopic method in high risk bleeding ulcers. *Cochrane Database Syst Rev.* 2007:CD005584.
29. Leontiadis GI, Sharma VK, Howden CW. Proton pump inhibitor therapy for peptic ulcer bleeding: Cochrane collaboration meta-analysis of randomized controlled trials. *Mayo Clin Proc.* 2007;82:286–296.

30. Lau JY, Sung JJ, Lee KK et al. Effect of intravenous omeprazole on recurrent bleeding after endoscopic treatment of bleeding peptic ulcers. *N Engl J Med.* 2000;343:310–316.
31. Gisbert JP, Khorrami S, Carballo F, Calvet X, Gene E, Dominguez-Munoz JE. *H. pylori* eradication therapy vs. antisecretory non-eradication therapy (with or without long-term maintenance antisecretory therapy) for the prevention of recurrent bleeding from peptic ulcer. *Cochrane Database Syst Rev.* 2004:CD004062.
32. Lai KC, Hui WM, Wong WM et al. Treatment of *Helicobacter pylori* in patients with duodenal ulcer hemorrhage—A long-term randomized, controlled study. *Am J Gastroenterol.* 2000;95:2225–2232.
33. Adamopoulos AB, Efstathiou SP, Tsioulos DI et al. Bleeding duodenal ulcer: Comparison between *Helicobacter pylori* positive and *Helicobacter pylori* negative bleeders. *Dig Liver Dis.* 2004;36:13–20.
34. Lau JY, Chung SC. Surgery in the acute management of bleeding peptic ulcer. *Baillieres Best Pract Res Clin Gastroenterol.* 2000;14:505–518.
35. Cowles RA, Mulholland MW. Surgical management of peptic ulcer disease in the Helicobacter era--management of bleeding peptic ulcer. *Surg Laparosc Endosc Percutan Tech.* 2001;11:2–8.
36. Rockall TA, Logan RF, Devlin HB, Northfield TC. Risk assessment after acute upper gastrointestinal haemorrhage. *Gut.* 1996;38:316–321.
37. Lau JY, Sung JJ, Lam YH et al. Endoscopic retreatment compared with surgery in patients with recurrent bleeding after initial endoscopic control of bleeding ulcers. *N Engl J Med.* 1999;340:751–756.
38. Chiu PW, Lam CY, Lee SW et al. Effect of scheduled second therapeutic endoscopy on peptic ulcer rebleeding: A prospective randomised trial. *Gut.* 2003;52:1403–1407.
39. Poxon VA, Keighley MR, Dykes PW, Heppinstall K, Jaderberg M. Comparison of minimal and conventional surgery in patients with bleeding peptic ulcer: a multicentre trial. *Br J Surg.* 1991;78:1344–1345.
40. Millat B, Hay JM, Valleur P, Fingerhut A, Fagniez PL. Emergency surgical treatment for bleeding duodenal ulcer: Oversewing plus vagotomy versus gastric resection, a controlled randomized trial. French Associations for Surgical Research. *World J Surg.* 1993;17:568–573; discussion 574.
41. de la Fuente SG, Khuri SF, Schifftner T, Henderson WG, Mantyh CR, Pappas TN. Comparative analysis of vagotomy and drainage versus vagotomy and resection procedures for bleeding peptic ulcer disease: Results of 907 patients from the Department of Veterans Affairs National Surgical Quality Improvement Program database. *J Am Coll Surg.* 2006;202:78–86.
42. Jairath V, Kahan BC, Logan RF et al. National audit of the use of surgery and radiological embolization after failed endoscopic haemostasis for non-variceal upper gastrointestinal bleeding. *Br J Surg.* 2012;99:1672–1680.
43. Chen CH, Huang HS, Yang CC, Yeh YH. The features of perforated peptic ulcers in conventional computed tomography. *Hepatogastroenterology.* 2001;48:1393–1396.
44. Svanes C, Salvesen H, Stangeland L, Svanes K, Soreide O. Perforated peptic ulcer over 56 years. Time trends in patients and disease characteristics. *Gut.* 1993;34:1666–1671.
45. Testini M, Portincasa P, Piccinni G, Lissidini G, Pellegrini F, Greco L. Significant factors associated with fatal outcome in emergency open surgery for perforated peptic ulcer. *World J Gastroenterol.* 2003;9:2338–2340.
46. Rahman MM, Islam MS, Flora S, Akhter SF, Hossain S, Karim F. Mortality in perforated peptic ulcer patients after selective management of stratified poor risk cases. *World J Surg.* 2007;31:2341–2344; discussion 2345–2346.
47. Donovan AJ, Vinson TL, Maulsby GO, Gewin JR. Selective treatment of duodenal ulcer with perforation. *Ann Surg.* 1979;189:627–636.
48. Berne TV, Donovan AJ. Nonoperative treatment of perforated duodenal ulcer. *Arch Surg.* 1989;124:830–832.
49. Marshall C, Ramaswamy P, Bergin FG, Rosenberg IL, Leaper DJ. Evaluation of a protocol for the non-operative management of perforated peptic ulcer. *Br J Surg.* 1999;86:131–134.
50. Crofts TJ, Park KG, Steele RJ, Chung SS, Li AK. A randomized trial of nonoperative treatment for perforated peptic ulcer. *N Engl J Med.* 1989;320:970–973.
51. Donovan AJ, Berne TV, Donovan JA. Perforated duodenal ulcer: An alternative therapeutic plan. *Arch Surg.* 1998;133:1166–1171.
52. Boey J, Branicki FJ, Alagaratnam TT et al. Proximal gastric vagotomy. The preferred operation for perforations in acute duodenal ulcer. *Ann Surg.* 1988;208:169–174.
53. Tsugawa K, Koyanagi N, Hashizume M et al. The therapeutic strategies in performing emergency surgery for gastroduodenal ulcer perforation in 130 patients over 70 years of age. *Hepatogastroenterology.* 2001;48:156–162.
54. Gutierrez de la Pena C, Marquez R, Fakih F, Dominguez-Adame E, Medina J. Simple closure or vagotomy and pyloroplasty for the treatment of a perforated duodenal ulcer: Comparison of results. *Dig Surg.* 2000;17:225–228.
55. Gisbert JP, Pajares JM. *Helicobacter pylori* infection and perforated peptic ulcer prevalence of the infection and role of antimicrobial treatment. *Helicobacter.* 2003;8:159–167.
56. Bose AC, Kate V, Ananthakrishnan N, Parija SC. *Helicobacter pylori* eradication prevents recurrence after simple closure of perforated duodenal ulcer. *J Gastroenterol Hepatol.* 2007;22:345–348.
57. Ng EK, Lam YH, Sung JJ, et al. Eradication of *Helicobacter pylori* prevents recurrence of ulcer after simple closure of duodenal ulcer perforation: Randomized controlled trial. *Ann Surg.* 2000;231:153–158.
58. Lunevicius R, Morkevicius M. Comparison of laparoscopic versus open repair for perforated duodenal ulcers. *Surg Endosc.* 2005;19:1565–1571.
59. Sanabria A, Villegas MI, Morales Uribe CH. Laparoscopic repair for perforated peptic ulcer disease. *Cochrane Database Syst Rev.* 2013;2:CD004778.
60. Byrge N, Barton RG, Enniss TM, Nirula R. Laparoscopic versus open repair of perforated gastroduodenal ulcer: A National Surgical Quality Improvement Program analysis. *Am J Surg.* 2013;206:957–962; discussion 962–963.

## Commentary on Peptic Ulcer Disease

*Frederick A. Moore*

Management of peptic ulcer disease (PUD) has changed drastically over my career. As a young surgeon at Denver General Hospital in the late 1980s, elective operations for intractable PUD and gastric outlet obstruction as well as emergency operations for bleeding and perforation were surprisingly common. We debated the optimal role of various procedures (including subtotal resection, vagotomy and antrectomy, vagotomy with pyloroplasty or gastroenterostomy and highly selective vagotomy) based on the indication and patient stability. We fretted over how to close the "difficult duodenal stump" and when to use a lateral duodenostomy tube. On teaching rounds, we discussed (1) different types of pyloroplasty (e.g., Heineke–Mikulicz, Finney and Jaboulay), (2) different ways to reconstruct after gastric resection (e.g., Billroth I, Billroth II, Hofmeister, Roux-en-y, Polya, etc.) and their relative advantages/disadvantages, (3) giant duodenal ulcer, (4) classic presentation of a "blown duodenal stump," (5) the Zollinger–Ellison syndrome, and (6) different types postgastrectomy syndromes (e.g., dumping, bile gastritis, afferent loop, efferent loop, etc.) and how they would be managed surgically. We were diligent in these discussions, because we were certain that there would be questions related to PUD on the in-service exams as well as the written and oral board exams. These operations and the associated discussions are now largely irrelevant in my current practice as an acute care surgeon. I occasionally operate for perforation, rarely for bleeding or obstruction, and never for intractability. Occasionally, I am called to assist my junior partners, because they have done so few of these operations. The manuscript nicely outlines the reasons for these changes including (1) the widespread use of new pharmacotherapy, (2) the expanded role of interventional endoscopy and interventional radiology, (3) the changing epidemiology of PUD where pathologic hyperacidity has been replaced by the *Helicobacter pylori* infection and nonsteroidal anti-inflammatory drug (NSAID) use as prime inciting events.

So what does a surgeon really need to know about PUD?

1. *The H. pylori story*: Most patients (over 90%) with PUD have an *H. pylori* infection and/or recent use of NSAIDs. The location of the *H. pylori* infection helps determine the clinical presentation. Antral dominant infection causes hyperacidity with duodenal ulcer, while body dominant infection causes mucosal atrophy with hypochlorhydria and gastric ulcers. NSAIDs can aggravate this pathophysiology by inhibiting constitutive COX-1, which decreases the local production cytoprotective prostacyline. The treatment of *H. pylori* includes a combination of a proton pump inhibitor (PPI) with clarithromycin (500 mg BID) and amoxicillin (1 g BID) or metronidazole (500 mg BID) for 10–14 days. Second-line rescue therapy treatment includes quadruple therapy, which combines a PPI with bismuth subsalicycle (2 tablets daily), metronidazole (250 mg QID), and tetracycline (500 mg QID) for 14 days. Eradication should always be confirmed with either a urea breath test or a stool antigen. Eradication rates with either regimen range from 75% to 90%.
2. *Management of upper gastrointestinal (GI) bleeding*: This has shifted to more aggressive endoscopy for risk stratification and therapeutic interventions. Resuscitation and correction of coagulopathy are key early interventions prior to endoscopy. PPI infusions should be started as early as possible. Stop NSAIDs and aspirin. Do not forget the *H. pylori* story. If rebleeding occurs after endoscopic intervention, repeat endoscopy (not surgery) is indicated. If bleeding cannot be controlled, interventional radiology embolization is an option in specialized centers. If you have to operate, what procedure should be performed is debatable. I agree with the author—be a minimalist: (a) wedge resection of gastric ulcers (if feasible) with no truncal vagotomy and (b) oversew the bleeding vessel within the duodenal ulcers with pyloroplasty and a truncal vagotomy. Again do not forget the *H. pylori* story.
3. *Treatment of perforated duodenal ulcer*: In this era of *H. pylori*, the treatment of a perforated PUD has been simplified. After volume resuscitation and antibiotic administration, go to the OR and perform open or laparoscopic repair with peritoneal washout. Usually the perforation is on the anterior surface of the postpyloric duodenum and is less than 5 mm in diameter. This is best closed with an omental patch. Attempts to close the hole directly can result in a bigger hole when the sutures pull through the inflamed tissue. Do not forget the *H. pylori* story. For patients who have clearly failed medical management or those who cannot afford, tolerate or comply with medical management, a highly selective vagotomy is reasonably definitive ulcer operation. Nonoperative management

of perforated PUD in selected patients is an option supported by the literature, but I rarely pursue this.

4. *Management of a perforated gastric ulcer*: These are commonly associated with NSAID use. In a stable patient, with a perforated ulcer on the greater curvature or in the body of the stomach are frequently amenable to wedge resection and this is a reasonable option. Perforated ulcers on the lesser curvature of the stomach, distal gastrectomy including the ulcer is usually required. Billroth I reconstruction is preferred and a vagotomy is not required. In the unstable patient, biopsy and omental patch closure can be life saving. Do not forget the *H. pylori* story.

# 46

## *Enterocutaneous Fistulas*

**Zachary M. Bauman, Edward B. Lineen, and Peter P. Lopez**

**CONTENTS**



Enterocutaneous fistulas (ECFs) represent a catastrophic problem for patients and continue to be complex and labor intensive for healthcare providers. In addition to the many physiologic and mental stressors the patients must endure, the development of ECFs also puts a strain on healthcare systems resulting in prolonged hospital stays, multiple readmissions, and increased resource consumption. Nutritional support, fluid and electrolyte management, wound care, frequent infections, chronic pain, and depression are just a few of the healthcare issues that require a significant amount of investment when managing these patients. Up to one-third of ECFs will close spontaneously when medically optimized, but for those patients whose ECF does not close spontaneously, surgery becomes necessary [1]. Unfortunately, definitive operative closure is only successful 75%–85% of the time [1].

The management of ECFs has improved significantly, resulting in decreased mortality rates, from 50% in the 1950s to approximately 5%–15% at present [2]. As many as 85% of ECFs present as a complication after abdominal surgery, providing further challenges to already compromised postoperative patients. Spontaneous fistulas usually result as a complication of inflammatory bowel disease, radiation, or cancer [2–4]. The general consensus is to withhold operative intervention until there has been resolution of most of the related metabolic complications and the abdominal cavity has become less hostile. As a clinician involved in the treatment of ECFs, it is important to have a step-wise approach to the management of ECFs (Table 46.1). Treatment decisions for the management of ECFs must be based around reducing patient morbidity and mortality, ultimately improving quality of life.

### 46.1 What Is the Definition of ECF?

A fistula is defined as an abnormal connection between two epithelized surfaces or between an epithelized organ and the exterior surface of the body. An ECF is specifically defined as an abnormal connection between the gastrointestinal tract and the skin. Most ECFs develop as a result of one of the following conditions: extension of bowel disease to surrounding structures, extension of disease of the surrounding structures to the bowel, unrecognized bowel injury, or breakdown of a gastrointestinal tract anastomosis [2]. ECFs may also form due to decreased blood supply to the bowel or from distended, weakened bowel due to delay in relieving a

**TABLE 46.1**

Management Phases for Enterocutaneous Fistulas

| Phase | Goal | Timing |
|---|---|---|
| Recognition/control of sepsis | Septic source control<br>Image-guided drainage vs. open drainage<br>Antibiotics<br>Resuscitation<br>Crystalloid vs. colloid vs. blood products | 1–2 days |
| Stabilization | Electrolyte hemostasis<br>Control of fistula drainage<br>Maintaining adequate source drainage | 2–7 days |
| Nutritional support | Enteral vs. parenteral feeding<br>Nutritional marker monitoring<br>Electrolyte monitoring | 2 days until fistula closure |
| Control of fistula output and wound care | Pharmacologic agents<br>Protective skin barriers<br>VAC therapy | 2 days until fistula closure |
| Decision | Investigation of source of fistula<br>Etiology, anatomy, drainage output<br>Duration of nonoperative management | 7 days until fistula closure |
| Definitive therapy | Planning operative approach<br>Resection of fistula with anastomosis<br>Secure abdominal wall closure<br>Feeding tube if needed | >4–5 months after fistula development |
| Healing | Continuation of nutritional support<br>Zinc supplementation | Postoperatively |

*Source:* Modified from Everson, AR and Fischer, JE, *J Gastrointest Surg*, 10, 455, 2006.

gastrointestinal tract obstruction. Furthermore, ECFs can form after repair of a ventral hernia with permanent mesh. ECF formation has been estimated as high as 10% from erosion of mesh into surrounding bowel [2]. ECFs can further be defined as postoperative or spontaneous. Postoperative ECFs account for 75%–85% of all fistulas whereas spontaneous fistulas account for 15%–25% of ECF occurrence [2–6]. Cancer and inflammatory bowel disease are the most common disease processes causing spontaneous ECF formation [2–6].

*Recommendations*: Postoperative ECFs are more common than spontaneous fistulas, often from unrecognized bowel injuries or anastomotic breakdown (Grade B). Permanent meshes have become more prevalent as sources for ECF development, so careful surgical decision-making should guide their use (Grade C).

## 46.2 What Are the Risk Factors for Developing an ECF?

Multiple preoperative patient factors can increase the likelihood of ECF development. These factors include infection, electrolyte abnormalities, malnutrition, anemia, hypothermia, poor oxygen delivery, and emergent procedures. For elective surgery, these factors should be optimized and tobacco use should be stopped prior to the operation. Ideally, albumin levels should be >3.3 g/dL and glucose levels should be well controlled. Nutritional status should be optimized using enteral immune-enhancing diets and, if needed, parenteral nutrition should be combined with enteral feeding to provide additional support [2,6]. Cardiac output, electrolytes, and anemia should be examined and corrected. Although controversy remains in the literature about preoperative bowel preparation (both mechanical and antibiotic), it will at least decrease the amount of enteric contents allowing for a cleaner anastomosis and less chance of postoperative infection and inflammation [7]. Last, intravenous antibiotics given within 1 h of incision will help decrease the rate of postoperative surgical site infections.

In patients requiring urgent or emergent surgical intervention, optimization of the above factors can be challenging. Patients who are hypotensive should be resuscitated with blood and intravenous fluids. Goal-directed endpoints for fluid resuscitation should be used to avoid harmful side-effects of fluid overload. Maintenance of cardiac output, temperature, and oxygenation will help improve overall outcomes.

Most importantly, however, is adherence to meticulous surgical technique. Hemostasis should be assured and prior to abdominal wall closure, the bowel should be thoroughly inspected. Recognized injuries should be repaired, as they represent areas of bowel weakness and a set-up for ECF formation.

*Recommendations*: Multiple factors contribute to the formation of ECFs, especially nutritional status, which should be optimized if possible (Grade B). Furthermore, attention to meticulous surgical technique will aid in better outcomes (Grade C).

## 46.3 How Are ECFs Classified?

Enterocutaneous fistulas are classified anatomically as external fistulas connecting a hollow visceral organ to the skin. Esophageal, duodenal stump, and jejunal fistulas with enteric defects less than 1 cm and tracts longer than 2 cm are favorable as they have high spontaneous closure rates. Gastric, lateral duodenal, ligament of Treitz, and ileal fistulas are much less likely to close spontaneously. Furthermore, fistulas resulting from adjacent abscesses, complete disruption of intestinal continuity, diseased and/or strictured bowel, obstructed bowel, or foreign bodies are unlikely to close spontaneously. Understanding the anatomic make-up of the ECF is important in the decision-making process. This information provides insight into the type and amount of intestinal fluid that will be lost from the ECF and if surgical closure will likely be required.

Enterocutaneous fistulas can also be classified based on physiologic output. Fistulas may be classified as low-output (<200 mL daily), moderate-output (200–500 mL daily), or high-output (>500 mL daily) [2–6]. Thorough monitoring of fistula output helps determine appropriate nutritional support, as intestinal fluid is rich in minerals, electrolytes, and protein. Loss of intestinal fluid through the ECF results in electrolyte imbalances and malnutrition that plague these patients until ECF resolution. Fistula output is also predictive of overall mortality [3]. Mortality rates up to 54% for patients with high-output fistulas and 16%–26% with low-output fistulas have been reported [3,8]. Unfortunately, the literature is still controversial on whether or not fistula output is directly related to spontaneous closure. Some studies suggest low-output fistulas are 2–3 times more likely to close spontaneously, while others lack this evidence [3,9,10].

*Recommendations*: Fistulas can be classified as low, medium, or high-output based on the amount of output daily (Grade B). Measures should be taken to aggressively monitor and slow output to decrease patient mortality (Grade C).

## 46.4 How Do ECFs Present Clinically?

An ECF begins with disruption of bowel wall integrity resulting in leakage of bowel contents into the abdominal cavity or from the surface of the body. Once this occurs, the postoperative clinical presentation follows a fairly distinct pattern. The patient usually experiences a feeling of malaise and overall does not progress as predicted [2–4]. The patient develops a fever around postoperative days 3–5 along with leukocytosis [2–4]. An ileus with abdominal distension and pain develops when the normal postoperative ileus should be resolving [2–4]. A wound infection may develop at this point, presenting either as superficial, deep, or as an intra-abdominal abscess. The infection is drained by opening the skin incision at the bedside or placement of an intra-abdominal drain.

*Recommendations*: A high suspicion for ECF development should be entertained if these symptoms are present in a postoperative patient in order to start the management and investigation process promptly (Grade C).

## 46.5 What Is the Best Method to Define ECF Anatomy?

Approximately 7–10 days after recognition of the fistula, the patient is usually stabilized and the fistula has matured to the point of supporting intubation with a small catheter. It is generally recommended that the patient undergo fistulography with water-soluble contrast. Much information can be obtained by performing a fistulogram such as the source of the fistula, the length and course of the fistula tract, its relationship to surrounding structures, the absence or presence of bowel continuity, the absence or present of distal obstruction, whether the bowel adjacent to the fistula is inflamed or strictured, and the presence or absence of an abscess cavity communicating with the fistula [3]. Computed tomography (CT) can also identify abscesses within the abdominal cavity and show the relationship of the fistula to surrounding organs. Unfortunately, CT is not always able to identify the exact location of the fistula.

*Recommendations*: Fistulography coupled with CT scanning provides the most accurate evaluation of an ECF to better develop the overall management plan (Grade C).

## 46.6 Medical Management

### 46.6.1 What Are the First Steps in ECF Management?

The management of ECFs is a complex problem that challenges even the most experienced clinicians. Not only can ECF lead to multiple hospitalizations, recurrent infections, deep vein thrombosis, complex wound care issues, severe malnutrition, and extreme deconditioning, they are mentally and emotionally taxing on both patients and clinicians. When approaching this complex disease, a detailed stepwise approach should be embraced (Table 46.1). A multidisciplinary team consisting of a surgeon, nutrition specialist or registered dietician, pharmacist, wound care nurse/enterostomal therapist, social worker, and physical therapist should be assembled. The ultimate goal for these patients is to restore continuity of the gastrointestinal tract while reducing morbidity and mortality.

Enterocutaneous fistulas are associated with a classic triad of complications including sepsis, malnutrition, and electrolyte and fluid abnormalities. Initially, these patients require control of their septic source while undergoing appropriate resuscitation and stabilization. Bowel contents outside the lumen lead to soft tissue infections, abscess formation, sepsis or peritonitis, and loss of skin integrity. Gaining control of fistula output and localized drainage of abscesses coupled with appropriate antibiotic selection is vital in managing ECFs. There is a 22-fold increase in mortality when an associated infectious complication accompanies the ECF [3,9,10].

The infectious source must be adequately drained and this drainage must be maintained. CT scanning should be used liberally assuring adequate drainage of abscesses. If deep abscesses are discovered, image-guided drainage can be utilized and closely monitored for the need for replacement with larger caliber drains. Antibiotics alone are rarely sufficient in resolving the infection and should only be used as an adjunct to adequate drainage. Initially, broad-spectrum empiric antibiotics should be administered and then tailored to the specific pathogens identified [11]. Operative intervention for source control is often prohibited by the patient's hostile abdomen and physiologic condition. Operating during this phase can lead to additional enterotomies, complete disruption of a created anastomosis, or conversion of a contained abscess into widespread intra-abdominal sepsis.

Septic patients further complicate the situation as they are severely hypercatabolic and unable to achieve positive nitrogen balances. This is often the case regardless of adequate nutritional support. Studies demonstrated that ECF patients with uncontrolled sepsis lost 2% of body protein stores daily even though they were receiving total parenteral nutrition (TPN) [3,12]. Controlling sepsis, while providing adequate nutritional support, is essential for management of ECF patients.

Restoration of intravascular volume and correction of multiple electrolyte deficiencies is also necessary. Aggressive crystalloid resuscitation may be required to account for septic third-spacing and continued fluid losses from the fistula. In the acute phase of resuscitation, the placement of a central venous catheter and arterial catheter coupled with ultrasonography can help guide fluid resuscitation [12]. These patients are usually dehydrated, anemic, and have low levels of serum oncotic proteins. Continued resuscitation should be carefully guided to avoid fluid overload leading to bowel wall edema and other complications.

*Recommendations*: Initial recognition and control of the septic source in a timely fashion is crucial for ECF patients to improve mortality (Grade B). Adequate drainage coupled with appropriate antibiotics will provide the best resolution of the patient's sepsis and hypermetabolic state (Grade B). Pitfalls include early surgical intervention which is prone to failure and often makes the ability to control the fistula worse. Inappropriate early reoperation also increases the risk of new fistulas as the metabolic problems and inflammatory state have not been treated. Aggressive intravascular volume resuscitation is required and should be carefully monitored to avoid the effects from fluid overload (Grade C).

### 46.6.2 What Is the Best Way to Provide Nutritional Support to ECF Patients?

Nutritional support is imperative in the care, stabilization, and rehabilitation of patients with ECFs. Prior to ECF development, these patients are usually malnourished due to their underlying disease process or surgical stressors. With the development of sepsis and an ECF, the metabolic demands increase substantially. Baseline nutritional needs in nonseptic patients are 20 kcal/kg/day of carbohydrates and fat and 0.8 g/kg/day of protein. These requirements can increase to 30 kcal/kg/day and 2.5 g/kg/day in the setting of sepsis and high-output fistulas [3,4,13,15]. Patients require a calorie–nitrogen ratio of 100:1 during severe catabolic states and when more stable, the calorie–nitrogen ratio increases to 150:1 [2,3,13].

Once septic complications resolve, the external loss of protein-rich enteric contents contributes to further malnutrition. This fluid loss results in dehydration and extreme electrolyte abnormalities. Colonic fistulas tend to be low-output, whereas small bowel fistulas tend to be moderate to high-output resulting in worse dehydration. The location of ECFs also affects the composition and amount of output. Nearly all fistulas have output high in potassium resulting in hypokalemia.

Traditionally, the Harris–Benedict equation along with patient stress factors have been used to provide a starting point for calculating the caloric and protein requirements for ECF patients. The caloric needs should be supplied through glucose and fat. Protein should not be used to meet basal metabolic requirements, rather for replenishing body protein needs and healing wounds [13]. Consultation with a nutritional specialist can be extremely helpful as it is important to address nutritional deficits early providing the best possible outcomes. Reversing the poor nutritional status of these patients depends on the ability to control the septic source and hypermetabolic state.

The route for nutritional delivery is based on caloric needs, fistula tract anatomy, and fistula output. Enteral feeding is physiologically preferred for nutritional support [2,3]. Enteral nutrition has shown to maintain bowel integrity as well as providing benefits regarding healing, repletion of nutrient stores, hepatic protein synthesis, hormonal function of the gut, and immune function [4,8]. It has long been recognized, however, that TPN is an integral part of ECF management. Occasionally, patients cannot tolerate enteral nutrition due to ileus, obstruction, or high fistula output [10,13,14]. Caution should be taken when utilizing TPN, as it is not without its own risks and drawbacks. TPN can be very costly as it must be made individually for the patient. This requires frequent lab work and long-term central venous access. If not carefully monitored, TPN can cause extreme electrolyte abnormalities, specifically hyperglycemia, and blood stream infections [15]. It is important to remember that the re-introduction of calories to patients who have severe malnutrition can lead to refeeding syndrome [4]. This disease process results in metabolic and electrolyte abnormalities, and arrhythmic abnormalities, which usually present within 2 days of caloric renourishment [4].

Nutritional status is an important predictor for mortality in patients with ECFs [5,6,13]. Serum albumin is the best marker to examine overall nutritional status [2,3]. Albumin levels <2.5 g/dL have been associated with mortality rates as high as 42% whereas those patients obtaining albumin levels ≥3.5 g/dL usually experience very small mortality rates if at all [16]. Any improvement in nutritional status of patients undergoing surgical closure of their fistula will aid by improving wound healing, enhancing the immune system, and preserving lean cell mass. Serum markers such as transferrin level, retinol-binding protein, and thyroxin-binding prealbumin have also been associated with predicting mortality in ECF patients [2,3].

*Recommendations*: The gut is always preferred for nutritional support, but if the patient cannot tolerate it, TPN is required for adequate caloric intake (Grade B). Fistula patients should be closely monitored to make adjustments in nutritional support as needed (Grade C). Serum albumin should be monitored with a goal to obtain levels ≥3.5 g/dL to improve overall mortality (Grade B).

### 46.6.3 What Is the Best Way to Decrease Fistula Output?

A number of strategies have been used to decrease fistula output. Initially, patients are restricted to nothing by mouth. Liquids and food are cautiously introduced to help with nutritional and electrolyte support as long as fistula output does not substantially increase. Medications such as $H_2$-receptor antagonists, proton-pump inhibitors, and sucralfate have been shown to decrease the volume and acidity of gastric secretions [2,3]. Although these medications have never been shown to improve fistula closure rates, decreasing gastric acid secretion allows for better control of electrolyte and acid–base imbalances [2,3]. Historically, nasogastric tubes have been used to help decrease fistula output. Unless the patient has an obstruction or prolonged ileus, this is now considered undesirable treatment as it can lead to other complications such as sinusitis, acid reflux, or esophageal strictures. Furthermore, antidiarrheal medication and bulking agents, such as psyllium, can help to control fistula output.

Somatostatin and its analog, octreotide, have frequently been utilized to help slow fistula production. Somatostatin inhibits the endocrine and exocrine secretion of many gastrointestinal hormones including gastrin, cholecystokinin, secretin, insulin, glucagon, and vasoactive intestinal peptide [17]. Furthermore, somatostatin inhibits gastric acid secretion, intestinal and gallbladder motility and contractility [17]. Theoretically, it makes sense that somatostatin would decrease ECF output and aid in spontaneous closure of ECFs; however, multiple studies have failed to demonstrate this process [3,18]. Occasionally, somatostatin may convert high-output fistulas to moderate or low-output fistulas; however, there has been little success using this medication to close ECFs [4]. Caution should be taken when using somatostatin as it can result in frequent hyperglycemia, a significant rebound effect when discontinued, and decreased blood supply to the gastrointestinal tract [3,18].

*Recommendations*: Bulking agents and medications that reduce gastric acid production can help decrease fistula output and maintain acid–base balances (Grade C). Somatostatin analogs should be used with caution as they may decrease fistula output but are not without their own side-effects (Grade C).

### 46.6.4 What Is the Best Way to Manage the ECF Wound?

Maintaining skin integrity surrounding the fistula is important in ECF management. Protecting or diverting the fistula output will decrease local irritation and infection and assure an intact abdominal wall aiding in complete abdominal closure should surgery be required. A variety of methods have been reported for management of fistula drainage including simple gauze dressings, skin barriers, pouches, and suction catheters. These methods work well for low-output fistulas but for more complicated fistulas, Karaya powder or seal, Stomahesive, glycerin, or ion exchange resins may be required. Using a large wound manager can be very helpful in protecting the skin for large, complex fistulas. A highly experienced, creative, and skilled enterostomal therapist can significantly contribute to patient care and improvement of quality of life.

Multiple studies have demonstrated that vacuum-assisted closure (VAC) dressings can help with effluent drainage management and promote wound healing through granulation tissue formation [3,19]. Furthermore, VAC dressings can simplify care by decreasing the number of dressing changes. There are concerns associated with the use of VAC dressings, however. Effluent trapped under the VAC dressing could potentiate further skin breakdown and infection. It has also been reported that negative pressure dressings applied to granulating bowel can cause additional ECFs [3]. Despite these concerns, VAC therapy continues to be an encouraging management option.

One of the most dangerous types of fistula is the entero-atmospheric fistula. This is a fistula where the bowel drains not to an epithelized surface but to a granulation plate on an open abdomen. The optimal treatment is to avoid this with all attempts made at early closure of the abdomen. However, after development, the principles remain the same with all resources used to control the output. Early skin grafting in order to assist in bag or wound manager control is essential, but again may be difficult and take multiple attempts at grafting. The grafting will not only help control the output, but also decrease the increased metabolic demands of the open abdomen.

*Recommendations*: Any method that will help control fistula effluent while protecting the skin should be utilized (Grade C). VAC dressing therapy is a promising management option and should be monitored closely when utilized (Grade C).

## 46.7 Surgical Management

### 46.7.1 When Is the Best Time to Provide Surgical Closure of an ECF?

Spontaneous ECF closure occurs in approximately 30% of patients. About 90% to 95% of those fistulas that will spontaneously resolve do so within the first 4–6 weeks [2,3]. Fistulas of the stomach, ileum, and ligament of Treitz as well as those associated with large abscesses, short fistula tracts, large openings in the bowel, damaged or strictured intestine, intestinal discontinuity, or distal obstruction are less likely to resolve spontaneously. Fistulas associated with cancer, inflammatory bowel disease, or radiation rarely close without surgical intervention.

Once the ECF has been appropriately investigated, planning for operative intervention begins. During this phase of care, the surgeon must balance adequacy of nutritional support, likelihood of spontaneous closure, and the technical feasibility of the procedure [2,3]. One of the biggest challenges of ECF management is patients who are constantly pushing clinicians to repair the ECF before surgery can safely be tolerated. Many elements must be taken into consideration at this stage, especially the timing of the operation. Studies suggest that patients with an ECF who are re-operated on within 10 days of the initial surgery or whose re-operation is delayed beyond 120 days have mortality rates of approximately 10%. Those patients who are operated on between 10 and 120 days of the initial surgery have mortality rates of approximately 20% [2,20]. Although mortality is decreased with early ECF operative intervention, it is wise to avoid operating during this time period. The risks of causing additional enterotomies or disrupting the previously created anastomosis are too great. Furthermore, the patient is rarely optimized at this time, specifically from a septic or nutritional standpoint. Instead, it is more prudent to continue to stabilize the patient by controlling and eradicating sepsis, controlling fistula output, correcting fluid and electrolyte deficiencies, and correcting nutritional deficits. Furthermore, by waiting to surgically close the ECF, time is allotted to allow the fistula to spontaneously close, avoiding an operation altogether. Before surgically addressing the ECF, the surgeon must have many open and honest discussions with the patient about the expected road ahead. Not until the patient has been adequately optimized can definitive surgical therapy be achieved.

*Recommendations*: Enterocutaneous fistulas should not be surgically corrected for at least 4–5 months and sometimes longer to allow for potential spontaneous closure and to medically optimize these patients for the best possible outcomes if surgery is required (Grade C).

### 46.7.2 What Is the Surgical Technique for Definitive Management of an ECF?

The operation for resolution of an ECF is extensive, requiring a significant time commitment and multiple resources. We recommend at least a 4–6 h block of time for the surgery itself, especially if abdominal wall reconstruction is required. Enteral feeding should be continued until the night before surgery, if possible. A mechanical bowel preparation can be given preceding the surgery. The patient and family should be adequately informed of the extensive nature of the surgery and recovery time.

The abdomen should be entered through a new incision away from the ECF in virgin tissue if possible. If a prior midline incision must be used to gain access into the abdomen, we recommend going above or below the previous incision, which may avoid creating enterotomies in bowel adherent to the abdominal wall. Once in the abdominal cavity, the viscera should be completely freed from each other through an extensive adhesiolysis. Freeing the viscera should be performed sharply and great care should be taken during this time to avoid injury to the bowel or any other organs. A thorough inspection of the abdominal cavity should be undertaken to ensure all abscesses and sources of obstruction have been identified and relieved to allow for success of a future anastomosis.

Working around and down to the portion of bowel containing the fistula allows evaluation of the adjacent structures and assessment of the length and viability of the remaining bowel. Once the ECF is taken down, the fistulous section of bowel is resected and a primary anastomosis is performed. The bowel anastomosis can be performed, with good success, either in a stapled or hand-sewn fashion. If multiple bowel loops are involved, the decision becomes whether to resect these multiple enterotomies as a single segment with one anastomosis or as several segments with several anastomoses. Usual preference is to perform one resection with one anastomosis if possible (as long as it does not cause significant bowel length loss) as this will decrease the risks of anastomotic complications. Once the resection is completed, the bowel surface must be carefully inspected making sure to repair any serosal tears and enterotomies [2,3]. If these injuries are not appropriately repaired, they can become sources of recurrent ECFs.

Once the gastrointestinal portion of the operation is complete, the next challenge is closure and possible reconstruction of the abdominal wall. Often the fistula takedown requires full-thickness resection of a portion of the abdominal wall. If this resection is small, then primary closure is usually adequate. However, if this resected portion is large, we recommend biologic mesh placement as these cases are at the least considered clean—contaminated and non-absorbable mesh should be avoided. If primary closure is unattainable,

**TABLE 46.2**

Summary of Recommendations for the Management of Enterocutaneous Fistulas

| Question | Answer | Grade | Refs. |
|---|---|---|---|
| What is the definition of ECF? | Abnormal connection between gastrointestinal tract and skin. More common in postoperative patients. | B, C | [2–6] |
| What are the risk factors for developing an ECF? | Infection, electrolyte abnormalities, malnutrition, anemia, hypothermia, poor oxygen delivery, emergent procedures, and poor surgical technique. | B, C | [2,6,7] |
| How are ECFs classified? | According to anatomic location and daily output (low, medium, or high). | B, C | [2–6,8–10] |
| How do ECFs present clinically? | Within 3–5 days from original abdominal surgery. Patients will not follow the normal postoperative progress and develop a fever, leukocytosis, and wound infection. | C | [2–4] |
| What is the best method to define ECF anatomy? | Fistulography with computed tomography. | C | [3] |
| What are the first steps in ECF management? | Recognition and drainage of septic source. Antibiotic administration. Intravascular volume restoration. | B, C | [3,9–12] |
| What is the best way to provide nutritional support to ECF patients? | Enteral nutrition is always preferred but if inadequate or not tolerated, parenteral nutrition should be used to supplement. Close monitor of serum albumin is needed to assess nutritional progression. | B, C | [2–5,8,10,13–16] |
| What is the best way to decrease fistula output? | $H_2$-blockers, proton-pump inhibitors, sucralfate, and bulking agents can help decrease fistula output. Somatostatin analogs may decrease fistula output but are not without side-effects. | C | [2–4,17,18] |
| What is the best way to manage the ECF wound? | Any method to manage the effluent from the ECF while protecting the skin. VAC therapy looks to be very promising. | C | [3,19] |
| When is the best time to provide surgical closure of an ECF? | Surgical closure after 120 days is associated with better mortality rates compared to earlier closure. This also allows for potential spontaneous closure of the ECF. | C | [2,3,20] |
| What is the surgical technique for definitive management of an ECF? | Enter virgin abdomen if possible. Thoroughly inspect all bowel for injuries and repair. Perform one anastomosis if possible. Continue aggressive nutritional support postoperatively and inform patient that recurrent ECFs are possible. | C | [2,3] |

a component separation can be performed to bring the abdominal fascia more midline to attain closure. This is often reinforced with an underlay utilizing biologic mesh. Surgical judgment must be used when performing a component separation during the first surgical attempt at ECF excision as performance of component separation limits many future options for incisional hernia repair.

Unfortunately, bowel anastomoses can break down and ECFs can recur. Whether the ECF is closed spontaneously or operatively, nutritional support is essential for appropriate healing and prevention of recurrent ECFs. The TPN should typically be continued, or restarted, postoperatively until the patient's postoperative ileus has resolved. Once the patient has reached adequate oral daily caloric intake, the TPN is slowly weaned.

*Recommendations*: Whatever surgical technique is utilized for closure, adherence to good surgical technique is mandatory and all bowel injuries should be identified and repaired (Grade C). Patients should be well informed of the anticipated recovery and the possibility of ECF recurrence (Grade C) (Table 46.2).

## 46.8 Conclusion

Enterocutaneous fistulas are a complex and undesired problem of the surgical patient population. A strong knowledge of the pathophysiology and risk factors for development of ECFs allows for early recognition and management. Once this complication occurs, a systematic, rational management protocol should be established to provide the best outcome. Sepsis control and resuscitation should occur early followed by aggressive nutritional support to reduce morbidity and mortality. After stabilization of the patient, adequate time should be allotted for spontaneous closure of the fistula. If definitive surgical intervention is required, detailed preoperative planning followed by meticulous execution of the procedure should be accomplished to ensure resolution of the ECF and a full recovery.

## References


1. Owen RM, Love TP, Perez SD et al. Definitive surgical treatment of enterocutaneous fistula. *JAMA Surg.* 2013;148(2):118–126.
2. Fischer JE, Everson AR. 2012. Chapter 146. *Gastrointestinal-Cutaneous Fistulas. Fischer's Mastery of Surgery*, 6th edn. Lippincott Williams & Wilkins: Philadelphia, PA, pp. 1564–1574.
3. Everson AR, Fischer JE. Current management of enterocutaneous fistulas. *J Gastrointest Surg.* 2006;10:455–464.
4. Manos LL, Wolfgang CL. 2014. The management of enterocutaneous fistulas. In: *Current Surgical Therapy*, 11th edn. Elsevier: Philadelphia, PA, pp. 142–145.
5. Martinez JL, Luque-de-Leon E, Blanco-Benavides R et al. Factors predictive of recurrence and mortality after surgical repair of enterocutaneous fistula. *J Gastrointest Surg.* 2012;16:156–164.
6. Martinez JL, Luque-de-Leon E, Mier J et al. Systematic management of postoperative enterocutaneous fistulas: Factors related to outcomes. *World J Surg.* 2008;32:436–443.
7. Zelhart MD, Hauch AT, Slakey DP et al. Preoperative antibiotic colon preparation: Have we had the answer all along? *J Am Coll Surg.* 2014;219(5):1070–1077.
8. Levy E, Frileux P, Cugnenc PH et al. High-output external fistulae of the small bowel: Management with continue enteral nutrition. *Br J Surg.* 1989;76:676–679.
9. Campos AC, Andrade DF, Campos GM. A multivariate model to determine prognostic factors in gastrointestinal fistulas. *J Am Coll Surg.* 1999;188:483–490.
10. Soeters PB, Ebeid AM, Fischer JE. Review of 404 patients with gastrointestinal fistulas: Impact of parenteral nutrition. *Ann Surg.* 1979;190:189–202.
11. Dellinger RP, Levy MM, Rhodes A et al. Surviving sepsis campaign: International Guidelines for Management of Severe Sepsis and Septic Shock: 2012. *Crit Care Med.* 2013;41(2):580–637.
12. Hill GL, Bourchier RG, Witney GB. Surgical and metabolic management of patients with enteral fistulas of the small intestine associated with Crohn's disease. *World J Surg.* 1988;12:191–197.
13. Polk TM, Schwab CW. Metabolic and nutritional support of the enterocutaneous fistula patient: A three phase approach. *World J Surg.* 2012;36:514–533.
14. Rose D, Yarborough MF, Canizaro PC, et al. One hundred and fourteen fistulas of the gastrointestinal tract treated with total parenteral nutrition. *Surg Gynecol Obstet.* 1986;163:345–350.
15. Berlana D, Barraquer A, Sabin P et al. Impact of parenteral nutrition standardization on costs and quality in adult patients. *Nutr Hosp.* 2014;30(2):351–358.
16. Fazio VS, Coutsoftides T, Steiger E. Factors influencing the outcome of treatment of small bowel cutaneous fistula. *World J Surg.* 1983;7:481–488.
17. Alivizatos V, Felekis D, Zorbalas A. Evaluation of the effectiveness of octreotide in the conservative treatment of post-operative enterocutaneous fistulas. *Hepatogastroenterology.* 2002;49:1010–1012.
18. Martineau P, Showed JA, Denis R. Is octreotide a new hope for enterocutaneous and external pancreatic fistulas closure? *Am J Surg.* 1996;172:386–395.
19. de Leon JM. Novel techniques using negative pressure wound therapy for the management of wounds with enterocutaneous fistulas in long-tern acute care facility. *J Wound Ostomy Continence Nurs.* 2013;40(5):481–488.
20. Osborn C, Fischer JE. How I do it: Gastrointestinal cutaneous fistulas. *J Gastrointest Surg.* 2009;13(11):2068.

## Commentary on Enterocutaneous Fistula

*James W. Davis*

The enterocutaneous or enteroatmospheric fistula is one of the most dreaded complications in abdominal surgery. These fistulas are difficult to manage and are incredibly taxing to the nursing staff, wound care specialist, and physician, but first and foremost, to the patient.

The preceding chapter has identified the key points in management: source and wound control, management of sepsis, electrolyte repletion, nutritional support, and eventual closure for the fistulas that remain open. Many of these patients will be referred or transferred to tertiary care centers (teaching hospitals) because of the intensity of care and expertise required to appropriately manage this problem. These patients frequently have long lengths of stay and a relatively high complication rate*.

Of note, there has been an increase in ECF with the increase in damage control surgery and temporary abdominal closure, and these fistulas have a lower rate of spontaneous closure*. Morbidity from wound complications in open abdomen patients can be as high as 25% and increases the longer the abdomen is left open, stressing the importance of early closure†.

### How Is the Fistula Managed?

Control of the fistula can be extremely challenging. Numerous approaches have been described; from irrigation and drainage systems that continually rinse the wound to suture of a condom catheter to the fistula to control the drainage to modified vacuum-assisted dressings, all with varying degrees of success. I have had success in some patients with large sized foley catheters with 30 mL balloons inserted into both sides of fistulas with control of the effluent and the ability to refeed the bilious drainage. Control of the fistula is generally an ongoing process that may require multiple different strategies rather than a discrete endpoint.

### What Is the "Best" Means of Nutritional Support?

Nutritional support is a vital part of success in managing ECF. Initially, total parenteral nutrition (TPN) may be required. If at all feasible, begin enteral feedings as soon as possible. Enteral nutrition, as noted in the chapter, is the preferred physiologic method for nutritional support with maintaining bowel integrity (and caliber), hepatic protein synthesis, and both improving and maintaining hormonal and immune function of the gut. The use of elemental diets and other specialty tube feeds with less complex proteins and medium chain triglycerides may allow for significant enteric absorption, even in relatively short segments of bowel. The use of fistulograms to study the location of the fistula can also allow the astute clinician to determine the appropriateness of a feeding catheter (even a simple Foley) placed distally to not only improve the patient's nutrition but to help maintain bowel integrity and size for eventual reconstruction. The use of various equations serves as a starting point to estimate caloric and protein requirements, but serial testing for transferrin, prealbumin, and albumin should be used along with indirect calorimetry (if available) to tailor and refine the protein and caloric goals.

### When and How Should Patients with Enterocutaneous Fistula Undergo Surgery?

Successful repair of ECF requires careful planning and optimization of all controllable factors. The major points are well made in the chapter. Interrogation of the fistula with a contrast study (fistulogram) is extremely important and cannot be substituted by a contrast CT scan. If there are multiple fistulas, each should have a contrast study done to help define anatomy. The patient's nutritional status should be stable with normal prealbumin and albumin levels. All electrolytes should be within normal range.

The timing of surgery has been widely debated. There is no prospective, randomized literature; the published reports are case series, retrospective reviews, and review articles. It is generally agreed that efforts at reconstructive surgery should occur after the inflammation has receded and the abdomen is "less hostile." The usual recommended time frame is 6–12 months from the last abdominal operation or wound closure. Simple clinical assessment of the patient provides important information. If the scar is still red, the abdomen is still likely inflamed. If the patient has a skin graft over the bowel and fascial defect, the examiner grasps and elevates the skin to see whether the underlying viscera is still adherent or only the skin is elevated.

The operation requires patience and meticulous technique and it may be best to plan that as the only procedure for the day. The entire GI tract needs to be carefully examined, requiring a complete adhesiolysis. The area of intestine with the ECF should be resected and a meticulous anastomosis performed. If there are

* Fischer PE, Fabian TC, Magnotti LJ et al. A ten year review of enterocutaneous fistulas after laparotomy for trauma. *J Trauma.* 2009;67:924–928.

† Miller RS, Morris JA Jr., Diaz JJ Jr., et al. Complications after 344 damage control open celiotomies. *J Trauma.* 2005;59:1365–1371.

multiple fistulas in a confined area, a single anastomosis is preferable. However, if there is concern for short gut, then multiple, careful anastomoses may be necessary. Most of the literature suggests equivalence in hand-sewn versus stapled anastomoses*. However, a recent retrospective study showed significantly higher leak rates for stapled anastomoses in emergency surgery†.

* Neutzling CB, Lustosa SA, Proenca IM et al. Stapled versus hand sewn methods for colorectal anastomosis surgery. *Cochrane Database Syst Rev.* 2012;15(2):CD003144.

† Farrah JP, Lauer CW, Bray MS et al. Stapled versus hand-sewn anastomoses in emergency general surgery: A retrospective review of outcomes in unique patient population. *J Trauma Acute Care Surg.* 2013;74:1187–1192.

Our institutional experience with numerous ECFs has been that simple repair of the area is not successful, and that there are more anastomotic leaks and strictures with stapled anastomoses than hand-sewn anastomoses. Our practice has then evolved to meticulous, 2-layer hand-sewn anastomoses for these procedures.

Closure of the abdominal wall may require a complex reconstruction, including component separation. If this is insufficient to close the defect, a biologic mesh may be used.

The management of ECF requires careful assessment, source and wound management, vigorous nutritional support, and a great deal of patience prior to meticulous surgical reconstruction.

# 47

# *Paraesophageal Hernia Repair*

**Abdul Alarhayem and Kent Van Sickle**

**CONTENTS**



## 47.1 Introduction

Hiatal hernias are characterized by the intrathoracic protrusion of elements of the abdominal cavity through a widened esophageal hiatus. They are anatomically classified into four types (I–IV). Types II–IV hernias are collectively referred to as paraesophageal hernias (PEH). Characterized by the presence of a hernia sac, these are true hernias that protrude through a defect in the phrenoesophageal membrane with a relative preservation of the posterolateral phrenoesophageal attachments around the gastroesophageal junction (GEJ) [1]. Of the paraesophageal hernias, more than 90% are Type III.

Hiatal hernias are traditionally classified according to the position of the GEJ:

- *Type I*: Classic sliding hiatal hernia in which the GE junction migrates cephalad through the esophageal hiatus due to a laxity in the phrenoesophageal membrane (which remains intact); accounts for >95% of hiatal hernias.
- *Type II*: True paraesophageal hernia in which the fundus herniates into the posterior mediastinum alongside a normally positioned GEJ.
- *Type III*: Combined or mixed hiatal hernia, in which both the GEJ and the fundus herniate into the thorax through the hiatus.
- *Type IV hernia*: Often described where all of the stomach and/or other viscera (i.e., colon, spleen, pancreas, etc.) herniate into the chest.

Although no consensus definition exists, it is widely accepted that giant PEHs are present when greater than 50% of the stomach resides within the chest.

## 47.2 Should All Paraesophageal Hernias Be Repaired?

The natural history of paraesophageal hernias is progressive enlargement such that eventually, the entire stomach herniates alongside the esophagus, with the pylorus juxtaposed to the gastric cardia, forming an intrathoracic upside-down stomach. The driving force for this progression is a positive intra-abdominal pressure combined with a negative intrathoracic pressure [2]. As more stomach moves up into the thorax, respiratory symptoms may predominate secondary to pulmonary compression [3].

Most patients with PEHs are asymptomatic. In symptomatic patients, the most common finding is gastritis and gastric ulceration. Symptoms of postprandial fullness, epigastric discomfort, and dysphagia are not infrequent. Serious complications include acute gastric hemorrhage, volvulus, obstruction, strangulation, and perforation.

Traditionally, prophylactic repair of asymptomatic PEHs had been favored secondary to a perceived high incidence of catastrophic complications (29%), and an exceedingly high mortality associated with emergent repair (17%) [4].

More recent studies have shown that the occurrence of such complications is infrequent, thus advocating for a censored observation policy in asymptomatic cases. In 1993, Allen and coworkers reported a large retrospective chart review series from the Mayo Clinic. Out of 147 patients, 23 patients were managed nonoperatively; 4/23 developed progression of their symptoms [5].

Stylopoulos and colleagues designed a Markov Monte Carlo decision analytic model and used it to determine if elderly asymptomatic, or minimally symptomatic, patients benefit from elective PEH repair. The model examined existing literature regarding mortality and hernia progression rates in patients who were 65 years old and asymptomatic.

They concluded that the mortality rate of emergency repair of PEHs was overestimated by early studies, likely only 5.4% versus the 17% quoted previously. They also estimated that the mortality rate of elective PEH repair likely was 1.4% whereas the annual likelihood of developing gastric complications from the hernias was only 1.1%. This analysis found that less than 1 in 5 asymptomatic patients aged 65 years and older, and less than 1 in 10 asymptomatic patients aged 85 years and older, benefit from elective PEH repair.

Even if an emergency operation is required, the burden of the procedure is not as severe as was previously thought [6].

Based on these data, prophylactic PEH repair in the absence of symptoms is rarely indicated. There remains little debate, however, that all symptomatic patients who are medically operable should undergo surgical treatment, particularly those with acute obstructive symptoms or volvulus [7].

*Recommendation*: The decision to surgically repair a PEH is based on the patient's overall medical status, symptomatic complaints, and the chance of incarceration/strangulation [8]. All symptomatic patients who are medically operable should be surgically treated. Routine elective repair of asymptomatic or minimally symptomatic paraesophageal hernias is not indicated (Grade B recommendation).

## 47.3 What Is the Best Approach to Repair PEH When Indicated?

The technique and approach to PEH repair continues to be one of the most controversial topics in the surgical literature. The three approaches for PEH repair are (1) transthoracic, (2) transabdominal, and (3) laparoscopic.

Traditionally, PEH repair was conducted through a thoracotomy or laparotomy. The morbidity (postoperative pain, pulmonary complications) and increased hospital length of stay associated with the transthoracic approach have rendered it obsolete except in select circumstances. In the setting of a shortened esophagus, the transthoracic approach offers a relatively easy dissection with an enhanced ability to fully mobilize the esophagus, allowing for a tension-free repair while minimizing the need for a lengthening procedure. Even if a lengthening procedure were needed, it is generally easier with the thoracic approach [9,10].

Compared to a thoracic approach, dissection of the mediastinal esophagus is significantly more difficult through a midline laparotomy. Nevertheless, the open abdominal approach enables improved reduction of volvulus, especially with giant PEHs, and permits gastropexy or gastrostomy to be performed, with a reduced chance of recurrent volvulus [10,11].

Contemporary authors comparing transabdominal to transthoracic access for PEH repair have concluded that outcomes are equivalent [7].

Although there are no randomized trials comparing the different approaches, laparoscopic repair has emerged as the standard of care in the elective setting, mainly due to a reduced rate of perioperative morbidity and shorter hospital length of stay.

Even in patients presenting with obstruction or gangrene, utilization of the laparoscopic approach may be associated with improved outcomes compared with open repair [12]. In the setting of perforation and gross peritoneal contamination, however, an open transabdominal approach is advocated [13].

Laparoscopic PEH repair is associated with decreased postoperative morbidity and affords superior visualization of the hiatus and mediastinum, allowing for better distal esophageal mobilization [14].

Recurrence rates between laparoscopic and open approaches have not been compared in randomized trial. Geha et al. reported follow-up for 100 consecutive patients undergoing open repair. A total of 82 patients underwent transabdominal repair with frequent use of gastropexy. There were no recurrences in the entire cohort [17].

Rathore et al. published a meta-analysis of nonrandomized series of laparoscopic PHH repair. In 965 patients with follow-up beyond 6 months, the overall recurrence rate was 10.2%. Among those patients formally evaluated with a contrast esophagogram postoperatively, 25.5% had recurrence. Lower recurrence rates were noticed in those who underwent an esophageal lengthening procedure with a Collis–Nissen gastroplasty versus those who did not (0% vs. 12%) [18]. Given the high recurrence rates following Lap PEH repair

(25.5%), the authors recommended mandatory follow-up esophagograms at 1 year.

Nguyen et al. retrospectively compared 2069 laparoscopic and 657 open repair of PHH. For elective procedures, utilization of laparoscopic repair was 81% and was associated with a shorter hospital stay (3.7 vs. 8.3 days, $p < 0.01$), less requirement for intensive care unit care, and lower overall complications. In patients presenting with obstruction or gangrene, utilization of laparoscopic repair was 57% and was similarly associated with improved outcomes compared with open repair [12].

Despite the wide adoption and good results of laparoscopic repair of PHH, a recent international survey of members of Cardio Thoracic Surgery Network revealed only 48% of members repair PHH laparoscopically, while 35% perform thoracotomy, and 17% perform laparotomy [11]. Critics of the laparoscopic approach cite higher recurrence rates compared to the open approach, stating this may be due to an overestimation of intra-abdominal esophageal length in the setting of diaphragmatic elevation from pneumoperitoneum [15,16].

*Recommendation*: Laparoscopic PEH repair is the preferred approach for the majority of PEHs. It is as effective as open transthoracic/transabdominal repair, and is associated with a reduced rate of perioperative morbidity and shorter hospital length of stay (Grade C recommendation).

## 47.4 What Operative Strategies Have Been Shown to Minimize Recurrence Rates Following PEH Repair?

Regardless of the approach, the tenets for a successful repair of PEH are tension-free reduction of hernia contents into the subdiaphragmatic position, removal of the hernia sac, and closure of the hiatal defect. Most surgeons also agree that performing an antireflux procedure is an important element of a successful PEH repair. The role of fixation of the stomach below the diaphragm with gastropexy or gastrostomy is debated [11].

### 47.4.1 Hernia Sac Resection

PEHs are characterized by widening of the esophageal hiatus with the development of a true peritoneal lined hernia sac into which the greater part of the stomach migrates. Resection of the entire hernia sac is arguably the most technically demanding part of PEH repair. However, leaving the sac in place is clearly associated with a higher rate of recurrence. Edye et al. prospectively compared laparoscopic repair with and without excision of the hernia sac. About 5 of 25 operations without sac excision suffered hernia recurrence during a 38-month follow-up period. No recurrences were reported at 15-month follow-up for the 30 patients whose PEH repair procedure included hernia sac excision [19].

The hernia sac should thus be dissected circumferentially from the mediastinal structures, and then preferably excised. Sac dissection is thought to release the tethering of the esophagus, thus facilitating intraoperative reduction of the hernia and decreasing early recurrence. Even when the sac cannot be completely excised safely, a partial sac excision should be performed.

### 47.4.2 Reinforced Crural Repair

Unacceptably high recurrence rates (>42%) associated with primary sutured crural repair have prompted many surgeons to advocate reinforcing crural repairs with mesh. Mesh is usually applied in an onlay fashion after primary crural closure or used as an interposition bridge when crural approximation is not possible. Three prospective randomized controlled trials reported decreased short-term recurrence rates with mesh crural reinforcement. There are inadequate long-term data on which to base a recommendation either for or against the use of mesh at the hiatus.

The first RCT studied patients with hiatal defects >8 cm. With a mean follow-up of 3.3 years, radiographic recurrence was significantly higher in patients undergoing primary crural repair alone versus those whose crural repair was reinforced with an onlay PTFE mesh (22% vs. 0%). No mesh-related complications during the study period were reported [20]. Similar findings were reported by another RCT in patients with hernia defects >5 cm (26% recurrence rate in patients undergoing primary crural repair vs. 8% mesh reinforced crural repair) [21].

Oelschlager and coworkers demonstrated similar short-term results using bioprosthetic mesh with no mesh-related complications reported. This improvement in recurrence rates however was not seen at 4 years. The findings of the follow-up study must be interpreted with caution given a significant drop-out rate and the lack of uniform radiographic evaluation [22].

Mesh erosion is arguably the most feared complication when using mesh reinforced crural repair. Although rare, it is catastrophic and may require an esophagectomy. Theoretically, it is more likely to be seen when mesh comes in direct contact with the esophagus, like when mesh is used to bridge a large crural defect. Although no data exist, this practice should be avoided.

*Recommendation*: During PEH repair, the hernia sac should be dissected away from mediastinal structures and preferably excised (Grade C).

The use of mesh for reinforcement of large hiatal hernia repairs leads to decreased short-term recurrence rates. Long-term data on which to base a recommendation either for or against the use of mesh at the hiatus are lacking (Grade C).

Although no prospective data exist, a lengthening gastroplasty reduces the rate of recurrent herniation when esophageal shortening is encountered (Grade C).

## 47.5 Is There a Role for Esophageal Lengthening Procedures during Paraesophageal Hernia Repair?

Decades of experience with open and laparoscopic PEH repairs have established certain principles as essential for a successful tension-free repair.

One of these defining aspects is establishing a 2.5–3 cm intra-abdominal esophagus. Extensive hernia sac resection, high mediastinal dissection, and esophageal mobilization may all be employed in bringing the GEJ at least 2.5 cm below the hiatus without tension. If such strategies are unsuccessful, most reports would agree that this constitutes a shortened esophagus, and a Collis gastroplasty should be attempted [23].

Although the precise incidence of esophageal shortening in PEH is unknown, with reports ranging from 0% to 60%, its true burden is probably close to 10%.

Intrinsic shortening of the esophagus is invariably encountered in the setting of GERD, where repeated cycles of acid or alkali injury result in chronic periesophageal inflammation and fibrosis. Longitudinal contraction of collagen in the fibrous tissue results in a shortened esophagus.

Although certain preoperative findings may raise the index of suspicion for a short esophagus (e.g., Giant hiatal hernia, longstanding GERD), no imaging or endoscopic modality has been found to be superior to surgeon assessment in predicting intra-abdominal esophageal length intraoperatively [23].

At a median follow-up of 58 months, Oelschlager described a 54% radiologic recurrence rate even with the use of a biologic mesh. Only 5/108 (4.6%) of patients in this group underwent a Collis gastroplasty [22].

At a median of 22 postoperative months, Luketich and colleagues reported a radiographic recurrence of 15.7% after 662 laparoscopic giant PEH repairs; interestingly 63% of these repairs included a Collis gastroplasty [24].

Although no prospective data exists, there is general agreement that a lengthening gastroplasty reduces the rate of recurrent herniation following repair of PEH when esophageal shortening is encountered [25,26].

*Recommendation*: At the completion of the hiatal repair, the intra-abdominal esophagus should measure at least 2–3 cm in length to decrease the risk of recurrence (Grade C).

## 47.6 Is There Evidence Supporting Routine Fundoplication in Patients Undergoing Laparoscopic PEH Repair?

High-level evidence supporting the practice of routine fundoplication in all PEH repairs is lacking; nevertheless, expert opinion suggests a fundoplication be performed when feasible.

The benefits of a fundoplication are thought to be two-fold; they help reduce postoperative reflux and may decrease recurrence rates.

The extensive dissection necessary to fully mobilize the esophagus and dissect the hernia sac is thought to render the GEJ incompetent, resulting in postoperative reflux. This has been reported as high as 65% in patients who did not receive a fundoplication [27,28]. A fundoplication may reestablish a "lower esophageal sphincter" mechanism.

A fundoplication may also buttress the repair and anchor the stomach intra-abdominally, theoretically reducing the likelihood of recurrence [7,29].

As with fundoplication done for GERD, gas-bloat syndrome and dysphagia are the most frequent postoperative complications. These complications usually improve 3–6 months after surgery [30].

One recent case-controlled study of 46 patients compared laparoscopic PEH repair with and without fundoplication (Lap Nissen over a 56F bougie). Findings were of increased dysphagia with fundoplication, and of reflux symptoms in the group without fundoplication [31].

*Recommendation*: High-level evidence supporting the practice of routine fundoplication is lacking; nevertheless, most surgeons consider it essential during PEH repair to reduce recurrence and minimize reflux symptoms (Grade C).

## 47.7 What Are the Options for High-Risk Patients with Symptomatic PEH?

Hernia reduction and gastropexy alone without cruroplasty or sac excision has been described in high-risk symptomatic patients.

**TABLE 47.1**
Clinical Questions

| Question | Answer | Level of Evidence | Grade of Recommendation | References |
|---|---|---|---|---|
| Should all paraesophageal hernias be repaired? | The decision to surgically repair a PEH is based on the patient's overall medical status, symptomatic complaints, and the risk of incarceration or strangulation.<br>All symptomatic patients who are medically operable should be surgically treated.<br>Routine elective repair of asymptomatic PEHs is not indicated. | 2B | B | [3–8] |
| What is the best approach to repair PEH when indicated? | Laparoscopic PEH repair is the preferred approach for the majority of PEHs. It is as effective as open transthoracic and transabdominal repair, and is associated with reduced perioperative morbidity and a shorter hospital length of stay | 2C | C | [10–18] |
| What operative strategies have been shown to minimize recurrence rates following PEH repair? | During PEH repair, the hernia sac should be dissected away from mediastinal structures and preferably excised.<br>The use of mesh reinforcement with large hiatal hernia repairs leads to decreased short-term recurrence rates. Long-term data on which to base a recommendation either for or against the use of mesh at the hiatus are lacking | 3B<br>2B | C<br>C | [20–22] |
| Is there a role for esophageal lengthening procedures during PEH repair? | At the completion of the hiatal repair, the intra-abdominal esophagus should measure at least 2–3 cm in length to decrease the risk of recurrence. Although no prospective data exists, a lengthening gastroplasty reduces the rate of recurrent herniation when esophageal shortening is encountered | 3A | C<br>C | [22–26] |
| Is there evidence supporting routine fundoplication in patients undergoing laparoscopic PEH repair? | High-level evidence supporting the practice of routine fundoplication is lacking; nevertheless, most surgeons consider it essential during PEH repair to reduce recurrence and minimize reflux symptoms. | 4 | C | [27–31] |
| What options are there for high-risk patients with symptomatic PEH? | Hernia reduction with gastropexy alone and no hiatal repair may be a safe alternative in high-risk patients but may be associated with high recurrence laparoscopic-assisted endoscopic hernia reduction with PEG tube placement may be useful in the symptomatic patient with prohibitive surgical risk | 4<br>4 | C<br>C | [32–34] |

Radiological recurrence is exceedingly high (22% at 3 months) compared to formal repair. Based on these findings, gastropexy alone is not recommended when other options are present [32,33].

In symptomatic patients who are too frail to undergo any laparoscopic attempt at PEH repair, Kercher et al. studied the role of laparoscopic-assisted endoscopic hernia reduction with placement of two percutaneous endoscopic gastrostomy (PEG) tubes to secure the stomach to the anterior abdominal wall. Ideally fit for the emergency setting, this procedure prevents the occurrence of a gastric volvulus and a formal hernia repair can be performed later, if needed [34] (Table 47.1).

*Recommendation*: Hernia reduction with gastropexy alone and no hiatal repair may be a safe alternative in high-risk patients but may be associated with high recurrence rates (Grade C). Laparoscopic-assisted endoscopic hernia reduction with PEG tube placement may be useful in the symptomatic patients with prohibitive surgical risk (Grade C).

## References


1. Kahrilas PJ, Pandolfino JE. *Hiatus hernia*. GI Motility online, 2006.
2. Landreneau RJ, Del Pino M, Santos R. Management of paraesophageal hernias. *Surg Clin N Am*. 2005;85(3):411–432.
3. Low DE, Simchuk EJ. Effect of paraesophageal hernia repair on pulmonary function. *Ann Thorac Surg*. 2002;74(2):333–337; discussion 337.
4. Skinner DB, Belsey RH. Surgical management of esophageal reflux and hiatus hernia. Long-term results with 1,030 patients. *J Thorac Cardiovasc Surg*. 1967;53(1):33–54.
5. Allen MS, Trastek VF, Deschamps C et al. Intrathoracic stomach. Presentation and results of operation. *J Thorac Cardiovasc Surg*. 1993;105(2):253–258; discussion 258–259.
6. Stylopoulos N, Gazelle GS, Rattner DW. Paraesophageal hernias: Operation or observation? *Ann Surg*. 2002;236(4): 492–500; discussion 500–501.
7. Kohn GP, Price RR, DeMeester SR et al. Guidelines for the management of hiatal hernia. *Surg Endosc*. 2013;27(12):4409–4428.

8. Sheff SR, Kothari SN. Repair of the giant hiatal hernia. *J Long Term Eff Med Implants.* 2010;20(2):139–148.
9. Davis SS, Jr. Current controversies in paraesophageal hernia repair. *Surg Clin N Am.* 2008;88(5):959–978.
10. Callender GG, Ferguson MK. 2007. Giant paraesophageal hernia: Thoracic, open abdominal, or laparoscopic approach. In: *Difficult Decisions in Thoracic Surgery.* Springer: London, pp. 343–349.
11. Schieman C, Grondin SC. Paraesophageal hernia: Clinical presentation, evaluation, and management controversies. *Thorac Surg Clin.* 2009;19(4):473–484.
12. Nguyen NT, Christie C, Masoomi H et al. Utilization and outcomes of laparoscopic versus open paraesophageal hernia repair. *Am Surg.* 2011;77(10):1353–1357.
13. Bawahab M, Mitchell P, Church N et al. Management of acute paraesophageal hernia. *Surg Endosc.* 2009;23(2): 255–259.
14. Draaisma W, Gooszen HG, Tournoij E et al. Controversies in paraesophageal hernia repair; a review of literature. *Surg Endosc Other Intervent Techniq.* 2005;19(10): 1300–1308.
15. Latzko M, Borao F, Squillaro A et al. Laparoscopic repair of paraesophageal hernias. *JSLS.* 2014;18(3).
16. Hashemi M, Peters JH, DeMeester TR et al. Laparoscopic repair of large type III hiatal hernia: Objective followup reveals high recurrence rate. *J Am Coll Surg.* 2000;190(5): 553–560; discussion 560–561.
17. Geha AS, Massad MG, Snow NJ et al. A 32-year experience in 100 patients with giant paraesophageal hernia: The case for abdominal approach and selective antireflux repair. *Surgery* 2000;128(4):623–630.
18. Rathore MA, Andrabi SI, Bhatti MI et al. Metaanalysis of recurrence after laparoscopic repair of paraesophageal hernia. *JSLS.* 2007;11(4):456–460.
19. Edye M, Salky B, Posner A et al. Sac excision is essential to adequate laparoscopic repair of paraesophageal hernia. *Surg Endosc.* 1998;12(10):1259–1263.
20. Frantzides CT, Madan AK, Carlson MA et al. A prospective, randomized trial of laparoscopic polytetrafluoroethylene (PTFE) patch repair vs simple cruroplasty for large hiatal hernia. *Arch Surg.* 2002;137(6):649–652.
21. Granderath FA, Schweiger UM, Kamolz T et al. Laparoscopic Nissen fundoplication with prosthetic hiatal closure reduces postoperative intrathoracic wrap herniation: Preliminary results of a prospective randomized functional and clinical study. *Arch Surg.* 2005;140(1):40–48.
22. Oelschlager BK, Pellegrini CA, Hunter JG et al. Biologic prosthesis to prevent recurrence after laparoscopic paraesophageal hernia repair: Long-term follow-up from a multicenter, prospective, randomized trial. *J Am Coll Surg.* 2011;213(4):461–468.
23. Horvath KD, Swanstrom LL, Jobe BA. The short esophagus: Pathophysiology, incidence, presentation, and treatment in the era of laparoscopic antireflux surgery. *Ann Surg.* 2000;232(5):630–640.
24. Luketich JD, Nason KS, Christie NA et al. Outcomes after a decade of laparoscopic giant paraesophageal hernia repair. *J Thorac Cardiovasc Surg.* 2010;139(2):395–404, 404.e1.
25. Darling G, Deschamps C. Technical controversies in fundoplication surgery. *Thorac Surg Clin.* 2005;15(3): 437–444.
26. Parekh KR, Iannettoni MD. 2007. Lengthening gastroplasty for managing giant paraesophageal hernia. In: *Difficult Decisions in Thoracic Surgery.* Springer: London, pp. 318–322.
27. Pearson F, Cooper JD, Ilves R et al. Massive hiatal hernia with incarceration: A report of 53 cases. *Ann Thorac Surg.* 1983;35(1):45–51.
28. Ponsky J, Rosen M, Fanning A et al. Anterior gastropexy may reduce the recurrence rate after laparoscopic paraesophageal hernia repair. *Surg Endosc Other Intervent Techniq.* 2003;17(7):1036–1041.
29. Wu J, Dunnegan D, Soper N. Clinical and radiologic assessment of laparoscopic paraesophageal hernia repair. *Surg Endosc.* 1999;13(5):497–502.
30. Richter JE. Gastroesophageal reflux disease treatment: Side effects and complications of fundoplication. *Clin Gastroenterol Hepatol.* 2013;11(5):465–471.
31. Morris-Stiff G, Hassn A. Laparoscopic paraoesophageal hernia repair: Fundoplication is not usually indicated. *Hernia.* 2008;12(3):299–302.
32. Rosenberg J, Jacobsen B, Fischer A. Fast-track giant paraoesophageal hernia repair using a simplified laparoscopic technique. *Langenbeck's Arch Surg.* 2006;391(1):38–42.
33. Agwunobi A, Bancewicz J, Attwood S. Simple laparoscopic gastropexy as the initial treatment of paraoesophageal hiatal hernia. *Br J Surg.* 1998;85(5):604–606.
34. Kercher KW. Minimally invasive management of paraesophageal herniation in the high-risk surgical patient. *Am J Surg.* 2001;182(5):510–514.

## Commentary on Paraesophageal Hernia Repair

*J. David Richardson*

The diagnosis of paraesophageal hernias seems to be encountered with increasing frequency, whether due to improved recognition or an actual increase in our aging population. Prior to the laparoscopic era, most of these hernias were repaired with an open abdominal approach and the standard mantra was that the diagnosis of this lesion mandated operative treatment[*†]. With the advent of minimally invasive procedures, a laparoscopic approach for repair has become much more common and some would argue it should be the standard of care[‡§¶**]. Several studies have demonstrated the efficacy and safety of this approach. However, with the exception of the acceptance of laparoscopic repair, virtually all other aspects of paraesophageal hernia repair have some elements of controversy associated with it. Despite the acceptance of laparoscopic repair, there are those who question its routine use[††]. These issues are discussed in the following.

### Operative Repair versus Observation

Elective repair of paraesophageal hernias was recommended routinely even in asymptomatic patients until a decade or so ago. In the past few years, the recommendation for universal repair has been challenged[‡‡]. A decision analysis model was studied from 20 pooled reports comparing elective repair versus watchful waiting with the outcome assessed being quality-adjusted life years. This model demonstrated observations benefited 83% of patients[§§]. The authors concluded watchful waiting was an effective strategy for most asymptomatic or minimally systematic patients.

At the present time, symptomatic patients should be offered a laparoscopic repair. Patients with "giant hernias" usually defined as having over one-third of the stomach in the chest are often offered repair because of the tendency for ongoing herniation. In my experience, patients with hernias that are undergoing organoaxial rotation should be offered repair because of the high risk of strangulation. Despite the improvements in operative repair, patients who develop gastric necrosis have an extremely high mortality rate.

### Aspects of Operative Techniques

While elements of operative repair are generally widely accepted, i.e., laparoscopic approach and the necessity for crural repair, other features of the repair remain unsettled. These include (1) use of mesh reinforcement of the crural repair, (2) the use of a fundoplication in those patients; (3) the management of a shortened esophagus; and (4) the appropriateness of adding a gastropexy or gastrostomy.

In all areas of potential controversy, most of the clinical decisions must be based on empiric or observational evidence as large definitive randomized trials are generally lacking. Several large series of repairs performed without mesh or biologic material have shown a low recurrence rate or only sliding hernias requiring no treatment. Numerous studies have noted satisfactory results with mesh or biologics (such as acellular dermis)[¶¶***]. The limitations of these reports are generally similar: (1) nonrandomized; (2) relatively short follow-ups, and (3) a nonuniform definition of recurrence. Use of mesh has a theoretic (and likely real albeit low) risk of gastric or esophageal erosion. Biologics are expensive and few long-term experiences are available. There have been two randomized studies on the use of mesh versus a hiatal closure alone. One study of 72 patients compared a PTFE closure to cruroplasty alone and noted less recurrence in patients with the use of prosthetic reinforcement[‡‡]. A larger multicenter, prospective randomized trial with longer follow-up was reported in 2011. Those authors

* Hill LD. Incarcerated paraesophageal hernias: A surgical emergency. *Am J Surg.* 1973;126:206–209.

† Geha AS, Massad MG, Snow NJ, Bave AE. A 32-year experience in 100 patients with giant paraesophageal hernia: The case for abdominal approach and selective antireflux repair. *Surgery.* 2000 October;128(4):623–630.

‡ Luketich JD, Raja S, Fernando HC et al. Laparoscopic repair of giant paraesophageal hernia: 100 consecutive cases. *Ann Surg.* 2000;232:608–618.

§ Pierre AF, Luketich JD, Fernardo HS et al. Results of laparoscopic repair of giant paraesophageal hernias: 200 consecutive cases. *Ann Thorac Surg.* 2002;74:1909–1915.

¶ Metha S, Boddy A, Rhodes M. Review of outcome after laparoscopic paraesophageal hernia repair. *Surg Laparosc Endogc.* 2006;16:301–306.

** Edye MB, Canin-Endres J, Gattorno F, Salky BA. Durability of laparoscopic repair of paraesophageal hernia. *Ann Surg.* 1998;228: 528–535.

†† Low DE, Unger T. Open repair of paraesophageal hernias: Reassessment of subjective and objective outcomes. *Ann Thorac Surg.* 2005;80:287–294.

‡‡ Allen MS, Trastek VF, Deschamps C, Pairolero PC. Intrathoracic stomach: Presentation and results of operation. *J Thorac Cardiovasc Surg.* 1993 February;105(2):253–258; discussion 258–259.

§§ Stylopoulos N, Gazelle GS, Rattner DW. Paraesophageal hernia: Operation or observation. *Ann Surg.* 2002;236:492–500.

¶¶ Frantzides CT, Madan AK, Carlson MA, Stavropoulos GP. A prospective randomized trial of laparoscopic PTFE patch repair vs. simple cruroplasty for large hiatal hernia. *Arch Surg.* 2002;137:649–656.

*** Oelschlager BK, Pelligrini CA, Hunter JC et al. Biologic prostheses to prevent recurrence after laparoscopic paraesophageal hernia repair: Long-term follow-up from a multicenter, prospective, randomized trial. *J Am Coll Surg.* 2011;213:461–468.

noted there were few mesh complications but discerned no benefit in terms of prevention of recurrence with the incidence of recurrence being virtually identical with a mean follow-up of 58 months. A decision analysis study examined multiple reports and concluded this was little difference in outcome between the two methods[§§]. In my experience, I rely on crural closure alone if the closure appears adequate. If on the other hand, the crura cannot be adequately reapproximated (as is often the case with very large hernias), I would use a s

The issue of whether a fundoplication should be added is not settled and large series produce differing results. Most reviews now favor the addition of a fundoplication although there is a reported variance between total wraps (Nissen) and partial wraps such as a Toupet fundoplication. Metha and associates analyzed 20 studies with paraesophageal hernia repair and noted 94% of the 1415 patients had an antireflux procedure[‡]. In my opinion, one can find literature to support either approach. I added a fundoplication in all repairs—a complete wrap if swallowing was normal and a partial wrap in the uncommon patient with a suspected motility disorder.

The shortened esophagus presents a challenge[*]. Many hernias that appear to have a short esophagus on radiographs actually have adequate length after hernia reduction. However, in some patients, the esophagus is foreshortened and a gastric lengthening procedure is recommended—usually a Collis–Nissen repair. In my experience, this is not a procedure to be undertaken by a novice laparoscopic surgeon.

At one time, authors recommended a gastropexy be performed by suturing the greater curvature of the stomach to the abdominal wall with the hope of preventing a recurrence. A tube gastrostomy could accomplish the same objective. Some recent series have abandoned this addition with few, if any, reported problems caused by the omission of this feature[†‡]. Ponsky believed that an anterior gastropexy could reduce the recurrence rate after laparoscopic paraesophageal hernia repair[§]. I would caution that there is one situation where a gastropexy or gastrostomy should be added; i.e., patients with long-standing organoaxial rotation of the stomach in the chest may continue to have a tendency toward gastric torsion even when the stomach is reduced. I treated two referral patients who had functional obstruction after a repair because of intra-abdominal gastric volvulus. This is likely uncommon, but in large hernias with a rotated stomach, consider adding a gastropexy or gastrostomy. While it is difficult to suggest this is "evidence based," there are numerous case reports of recurrent gastric volvulus corrected by gastropexy.

#### The Issue of Recurrence Rate and Does It Matter

Davis has nicely outlined the many controversies involved in the management of paraesophageal hernias[¶] . In addition to the aforementioned issues, the one which is most problematic is that of recurrence of the hernia after repair. Several reports have noted very low recurrence rates (particularly with short-term follow-up while others have noted a high recurrence rate[†‡‡‡**]. Rathore and associates noted a 25.5% recurrent rate after laparoscopic repair but noted a lengthening procedure, when added, decreased rate of herniation[††]. One recent review of hernia repair both emergently and electively had an 8.3 recurrence rate when performed by an open technique versus a 25% when done laparoscopically. Metha et al. noted a 26.9% combined recurrence rate in 20 studies[‡‡]. Others have noted an open approach might be superior in preventing recurrence but low morbidity favors a laparoscopic approach[§§].

A question to be considered is whether a radiologically diagnosed hernia really matters. If the patient has a large remnant of the stomach in the chest, it is likely important, but if a small portion of fundus herniates in a sliding fashion and the patient is asymptomatic, such a recurrence may be of little consequence.

* Obeid NM, Velanovich V. The choice of primary repair or mesh repair for paraesophageal hernia: A decision analysis based on utility scores. *Ann Surg.* 2013;257:655–656.

† Luketich JD, Raja S, Fernando HC et al. Laparoscopic repair of giant paraesophageal hernia: 100 consecutive cases. *Ann Surg.* 2000;232:608–618.

‡ Pierre AF, Luketich JD, Fernardo HS et al. Results of laparoscopic repair of giant paraesophageal hernias: 200 consecutive cases. *Ann Thorac Surg.* 2002;74:1909–1915.

§ Swanstrom LL, Marcus DR, Galloway GO. Laparoscopic Collis gastroplasty is the treatment of chronic for the shortened esophagus. *Am J Surg.* 1996;171:477–481.

¶ Davis SS Jr. Current controversies in paraesophageal hernia repair. *Surg Clin North Am.* 2008;88:959–978.

** Edye MB, Canin-Endres J, Gattorno F, Salky BA. Durability of laparoscopic repair of paraesophageal hernia. *Ann Surg.* 1998;228: 528–535.

†† Rathore MA, Andrabi SIH, Bhatti MI et al. Metaanalysis of recurrence after laparoscopic repair of paraesophageal hernia. *J Soc Laparoendosc Surg.* 2007;11:456–460.

‡‡ Metha S, Boddy A, Rhodes M. Review of outcome after laparoscopic paraesophageal hernia repair. *Surg Laparosc Endogc.* 2006;16:301–306.

§§ Low DE, Unger T. Open repair of paraesophageal hernias: Reassessment of subjective and objective outcomes. *Ann Thorac Surg.* 2005;80:287–294.

# 48

## Appendicitis: Evidence-Based Medicine

**Elizabeth A. Lax and Peter P. Lopez**

**CONTENTS**



### 48.1 Introduction

Acute appendicitis remains the most common intra-abdominal surgical emergency requiring an operation. The lifetime risk of developing appendicitis is around 7%–12%; however, the lifetime rate of an appendectomy is 12% for men and 25% for women. Appendicitis can occur at any age but is most frequently seen in patients in their second and fourth decade of life, with a mean age of 31.3 and a median age of 22 years [1].

Early reports describe a potentially lethal inflammatory disease process of the right lower quadrant (RLQ), known then as "perityphlitis." In 1886, Reginald Fitz [2] first described this inflammatory disease process of the right lower quadrant as appendicitis, including the clinical sequelae of abscess formation and perforation. Even today, the diagnosis of acute appendicitis remains a challenging clinical entity. This condition is more difficult to diagnose at the extremes of age: in the very young and elderly because of a lack of history, late presentation and often less than impressive physical examination. The diagnoses can also be challenging in women of childbearing age who have a wider list of differential diagnoses.

The timely and accurate recognition of patients requiring urgent surgical and nonsurgical management continues to be the overriding principle in the workup and treatment of patients with suspected appendicitis. Delays in the diagnosis and treatment of appendicitis can result in an increased morbidity and mortality. Krajewski and associates recently published a retrospective review that shows a significant, inverse relationship between economic status and perforated appendicitis. This study compared data between health systems in Canada and the United States, revealing that rates of perforated appendicitis in American patients (but not in Canada, where healthcare is universal) increased as income level decreases [3].

In this chapter, we try to answer a few common issues that clinicians face when dealing with the diagnosis and management of acute appendicitis. Important questions to consider in the care of a patient with appendicitis include how to make an accurate diagnosis, whether to treat it medically or surgically, and whether to proceed surgically with an open or laparoscopic approach. The answers to these questions are based on an evidence base review of the literature.

## 48.2 What Clinical Signs and Symptoms Are Most Reliable to Rule In or Out Appendicitis?

The history and physical examination continues to be the most reliable predictor for the diagnosis of appendicitis [4]. But there is an old adage that only about 25% of patients have the classic presentation and, therefore, 75% have an atypical presentation. By performing a thorough history and physical examination, an experienced clinician can accurately diagnose acute appendicitis in the majority of cases [5]. A typical patient will present with vague abdominal pain (usually epigastric region) followed by anorexia, nausea, with or without vomiting. The pain then shifts to the RLQ as the inflammation of the appendix progresses to involve the overlying peritoneum. Common symptoms of appendicitis include the following: periumbilical abdominal pain and anorexia in nearly 100% of cases, nausea in 90%, and migration of pain from the periumbilical area to the RLQ around 50% of the time [6]. Lee and Ho [7] reported that the most reliable symptom in making the diagnosis of appendicitis is the classic pattern of migratory abdominal pain from periumbilical to the RLQ. Occasionally, patients will complain of dysuria, hematuria, urgency and frequent urination, diarrhea or constipation from inflammation adjacent to the ureter, bladder and colon and rectum. As all clinicians have found out, these clinical features are not entirely reliable. However, the history and physical examination continues to remain the most reliable indicator for appendicitis. Most patients with appendicitis except the very young, very old, and those who are neurologically impaired, will have some degree of tenderness on palpation of the abdomen. In more than 95% of patients with acute appendicitis, the sequence of symptoms was anorexia, followed by abdominal pain, and then vomiting [8]. In 1996, a meta-analysis performed by Wagner et al. [9] reported the sensitivity, specificity, and positive likelihood ratio with a 95% confidence interval for findings on the clinical examination characteristic of appendicitis. They reported the sensitivity, specificity, and positive likelihood ratio for RLQ pain (0.81, 0.53, 7.31–8.46); fever (0.67, 0.79, 1.94); and anorexia (0.68, 0.36, 1.27).

Physical examination findings are determined by the anatomic position of the inflamed appendix and whether it has ruptured. A retrocecal appendix can give rise to tenderness in the right flank or right upper quadrant (RUQ), whereas a pelvic appendix can give rise to little abdominal tenderness but pain on rectal examination. A patient who presents with uncomplicated appendicitis may present with a slight elevation in temperature (by 1°C or 1.8°F) and a slight elevation in heart rate; otherwise, vital signs are normal. Patients with peritonitis will prefer to lie still, as any motion will tend to worsen their pain. If the appendix lies in the classic anterior position, abdominal pain will be maximal at McBurney's point, with rebound tenderness elucidated in the RLQ [10]. Palpation of the left lower quadrant (LLQ) may cause RLQ pain, also known as Rovsing's sign.

Deviations from these commonly associated physical findings usually are related to the anatomic position of the inflamed appendix. The common anatomic locations of the appendix include: paracolic (the appendix lies in the right paracolic gutter lateral to the cecum), retrocecal (the appendix lies posterior to the cecum and may be partially or totally extraperitoneal), preileal (the appendix is anterior to the terminal ileum), postileal (the appendix is posterior to the ileum), promontoric (the tip of the appendix lies in the vicinity of the sacral promontory), pelvic (the tip of the appendix lies in or toward the pelvis), and subcecal (the appendix lies inferior to the cecum) [11]. Wakeley [12] performed a postmortem analysis of 10,000 cases and described the frequency of the location of the appendix as follows: retrocecal, 65.3%; pelvic, 31%; subcecal, 2.3%; preileal, 1%; and right paracolic and postileal, 0.4%. When the appendix occupies an unusual location the diagnosis of appendicitis can be more difficult and may contribute to delays in presentation, diagnosis, and treatment.

*Recommendation*: Abdominal pain localized to the epigastrium or periumbilical area radiating to the RLQ and associated with anorexia and nausea are the most reliable diagnostic symptoms for acute appendicitis (Grade B recommendations).

## 48.3 What Is the Best Laboratory Test to Help Make the Diagnosis of Appendicitis?

The use of laboratory values in diagnosing appendicitis has been disappointing as no one test has been found to be highly sensitive and specific. White blood cell (WBC) count was found to be of limited value for making the diagnoses of appendicitis in one study [13]. On the other hand, Andersson et al. concluded a leukocytosis was actually more diagnostic of advanced or complicated appendicitis than noncomplicated acute cases [14]. The sensitivity of an elevated WBC above 10,000 cells/μL for acute appendicitis is 70%–90%, but the specificity is very low [15]. A value greater than 18,000 cells/μL suggests complicated appendicitis with either gangrene or perforation. The diagnostic value of C-reactive protein and erythrocyte sedimentation rate in diagnosing appendicitis has been both controversial and disappointing [16]. A recent paper by Yang et al. [17] found the use of WBC and C-reactive protein individually or together had a high sensitivity to differentiate patients with appendicitis but a very low specificity. In another study in adults, the finding of a normal white blood cell count and a normal C-reactive protein level was highly predictive of no appendicitis [18]. Other studies have shown that inflammatory cytokines and acute-phase reaction proteins such as interleukin-6 (IL-6), tumor necrosis factor (TNF-alpha), lipopolysaccharide-binding protein, alpha1-glycoprotein (alpha1GP), and endotoxin are also elevated in this patient population. The result of many of these studies is that these inflammatory markers are elevated in appendicitis (high sensitivity) but that many are not specific enough to reliably diagnose the disease [19–21]. In a study by Lycopoulou et al. [22] reported the sensitivity and specificity of the use of white blood cell count (WBC) >10, [75% and 76%], C-reactive protein (CRP) >10 mg/L, [62% and 94%], and serum amyloid protein (SSA) >45 mg/L, [86% and 83%], in diagnosing acute appendicitis in children. Procalcitonin was found to be increased in rare cases of severe inflammation after appendiceal perforation and gangrenous appendicitis, but because of its low sensitivity, it cannot be recommended for the diagnosis of acute appendicitis [23].

*Recommendation*: Overall, laboratory markers of acute inflammation in acute appendicitis remain highly sensitive but relatively nonspecific when it comes to making the diagnosis of acute appendicitis. No one test has been found to be both highly sensitive and specific to reliably diagnose acute appendicitis. (Grade B recommendations).

## 48.4 Does Giving Pain Medicine to a Patient with Suspected Appendicitis Decrease the Ability to Make the Diagnosis of Appendicitis?

It has been taught that patients with abdominal pain should not receive narcotics for fear of masking a surgical condition, such as appendicitis in patients who present with acute abdominal pain. In a retrospective study by Aydelotte et al. [24] charts were reviewed on 75 patients diagnosed with acute appendicitis confirmed intra-operatively. A total of 10 men and 14 women received narcotics prior to surgical evaluation, and 28 men and 14 women were not given narcotics prior to surgical evaluation. In this study, there was no statistically significant difference between the two groups of patients in regard to length of hospital stay, time to operation, complication rate, perforation rate, or negative appendectomy rate. The authors concluded that the administration of narcotics before evaluation of the patient by a surgeon for acute appendicitis had no effect on patient outcomes. Attard and his group assessed the safety of early pain relief in patients with acute abdominal pain and found that the use of analgesia did not affect the diagnostic work up of these patients [25]. A matched case–control study was performed in an emergency room (ER) setting to determine if early use analgesia led to a delay in the treatment of patients with acute appendicitis [26]. The authors found that there was no delay in treatment with opiates, but there appears to be a delay in treatment with the use of nonsteroidal anti-inflammatory analgesia. A prospective randomized double-blind study of parenteral tramadol analgesic use versus placebo in 68 emergency department (ED) patients with RLQ pain resulted in significant levels of pain control without concurrent normalization of abdominal pain [27]. In another prospective, double-blind study in ED patients with undifferentiated abdominal pain, patients were randomized to receive placebo or morphine sulfate (MS) [28]. Diagnostic accuracy, however, did not differ between MS and control groups (64.2% vs. 66.7%). These results support the practice of early provision of analgesia to patients with undifferentiated abdominal pain. A prospective double-blind crossover study by Wolfe and associates [29] also evaluated administration of morphine to the suspected appendicitis patient and its impact on their physical examination. The authors concluded that patients with signs of appendicitis who received morphine had significant improvement in their pain but were without changes in their physical examination. In the pediatric population, the findings were consistent as well. Another prospective randomized study performed in children with a presumptive diagnosis of appendicitis was randomized to receive parenteral morphine sulfate or placebo [30]. The authors found no difference in the time to surgical decision and no decrease in pain at 30 min between morphine at a dose of 0.1 mg/kg and placebo. A separate randomized study in children with acute abdominal pain concluded morphine was found to effectively reduce the intensity of pain and did not seem to impede the diagnosis of appendicitis [31].

*Recommendation*: Giving pain medicine to adults and children suspected of acute appendicitis does not adversely affect the ability to diagnosis appendicitis. Analgesia should not be withheld pending clinical investigation in patients with suspected acute appendicitis (Grade B recommendation).

## 48.5 What Is the Best Diagnostic Imaging Modality to Diagnose Acute Appendicitis?

Many different radiologic modalities have been used to diagnose acute appendicitis. The optimal radiologic technique used to diagnose acute appendicitis should be accurate, quick, safe, readily available, and cost-efficient and should provide little risk or discomfort to the patient. The use of abdominal US and computed tomography has proven extremely useful in diagnosing this disease. However, routine use of these modalities in all patients with suspected appendicitis is not well established [32]. Despite the recent increase in their use, these tests have not consistently increased the diagnostic accuracy of making the diagnosis of acute appendicitis in all patient populations.

The use of plain radiography for diagnosing acute gastrointestinal diseases has been around since the early 1900s. The appearance of an opaque fecalith in the RLQ is often quoted as being the hallmark radiographic finding in acute appendicitis, but fewer than 5%–8% of patients present with this finding [33]. Other common but nonspecific findings on plain films include localized paralytic ileus, loss of the cecal shadow, blurring of the right psoas muscle, and rightward scoliosis of the lumbar spine [34]. In a recent study of 821 consecutive patients hospitalized for suspected appendicitis, no individual radiographic finding was highly sensitive or specific in ultimately making the diagnosis of appendicitis [35]. Plain abdominal radiographs may be indicated when other acute abdominal conditions, such as gastric or duodenal perforation, intestinal obstruction, or ureteral calculus, are part of the differential as the cause of RLQ abdominal pain [36]. Overall, plain abdominal radiographs are not cost-effective and lack both sensitivity and specificity in the diagnosis of appendicitis.

Deutsch and Leopold [37] first visualized the inflamed appendix using ultrasound (US) in 1981. Ultrasound has become a more frequently used radiologic test to rule appendicitis in children and pregnant women because of concerns exposure to ionizing radiation from computed tomography (CT) scans. Its accuracy in diagnosing appendicitis has been hampered by the interference of the US image by overlying bowel gas, the slow development of a transducer with enough spatial resolution to pick up small structures such as the appendix as well as the highly variable operator-dependent interpretation and technical expertise at individual hospitals [38]. With the advancement in US technology and the use of the graded compression technique when scanning the RLQ, the ability to visualize the appendix has improved. The graded compression technique involves applying steady, gradual pressure to the RLQ in an effort to collapse normal bowel and eliminate bowel gas in the area in order to visualize the appendix. The inflamed appendix when seen by US commonly includes the following findings: an appendix of 7 mm or more in anteroposterior diameter, an immobile, thick-walled, noncompressible luminal structure seen in cross section referred to as a target lesion, or the presence of an appendicolith, a blind-ending structure consisting of anechoic lumen surrounded by mucosa and a hypoechoic thickened wall adjacent to the cecum [39]. Despite these well-described US findings, there is no evidence-based standard of findings by which an individual radiologist can use to make the diagnosis of appendicitis. In a prospective study by Rettenbacher et al. [40] using US to diagnose appendicitis, the authors used six different US findings. Unfortunately, they did not state the number of these findings necessary to make their diagnosis of appendicitis. In a recent systemic review of the use of US to diagnose acute appendicitis in adults and adolescent patients, the accuracy of using graded compression US was reported to have an overall sensitivity of 0.86 (CI: 0.83–0.88) and a specificity of 0.81 (CI: 0.78–0.84) with a positive likelihood ratio 5.8 (CI: 3.5–9.5) [41].

Ultrasound is most reliable in centers with considerable experience using this modality to diagnose acute appendicitis. In a meta-analysis looking at the sensitivity and specificity of US in diagnosing appendicitis in adults and children, for US in children 88% sensitivity and 94% specificity, and for US in adults 83% sensitivity and 93% specificity was reported [42]. In another study reporting on the sensitivity and specificity of US in making the diagnosis of appendicitis in adults and children, it was reported an overall 83% sensitivity and 98% sensitivity [43]. The reported sensitivity and specificity of US in diagnosing acute appendicitis in pregnant patients was 66%–100% and 95%–96%, respectively [44]. However, it is recommended that if an US is negative or inconclusive in a pregnant patient with a suspected diagnosis of appendicitis another imaging study, such as CT or magnetic resonance imaging (MRI) should be performed [45].

Computed tomography (CT) has been used as a diagnostic modality for acute abdominal pain since it became available in the late 1970s. Helical CT scans have excellent resolution, are widely available, are operator independent and are easy to interpret making them often the preferred diagnostic test to rule out appendicitis. Findings strongly suggestive of acute appendicitis on standard abdominal CT scan include (1) a thick wall (>2 mm), often with "targeting" (concentric thickening of the inflamed appendix wall); (2) increased diameter of the appendix (>7 mm); (3) an appendicolith; (4) a phlegmon or abscess; or (5) free fluid [46]. Stranding of the adjacent fatty tissues in the RLQ is also commonly associated. The top four CT findings suggestive of appendicitis are an enlarged appendix, appendiceal wall thickening, appendiceal wall enhancement and periappendiceal fat stranding [47,48]. If air is seen in the appendix or if the appendiceal lumen is filled with contrast and there are no other abnormalities seen on CT, these findings virtually eliminate appendicitis as the diagnosis. It has been thought that appendicitis could not be excluded if the appendix was not visualized on CT scan. A more recent report, however, concluded that nonvisualization of the appendix on a CT scan was negative for appendicitis in 98% of cases [49]. Computed tomography is also useful in diagnosing an appendiceal abscess and can used to guide percutaneous drainage. CT can also be helpful in diagnosing other causes of acute abdominal pain in patients suspected of acute appendicitis.

The performance of CT scans to evaluate RLQ pain has increased considerably since Rao and colleagues [50] reported an accuracy rate of 98% with administration of rectal contrast in diagnosing acute appendicitis. Rao also reported that the use of CT at his institution decreased the rate of removal of a normal appendix from 20% before the introduction of CT scanning to 7% after [51]. Other authors have not found CT to be as accurate. Perez et al. [52] found the accuracy of CT in diagnosing appendicitis to be 80%. Morris et al. [53] reported a diagnostic accuracy of 90% at their institution. In a study performed by Holloway and associates [54], using a well-defined CT imaging protocol as an adjunct to the clinical diagnosis of acute appendicitis, they found the accuracy of CT to be 97.8% with a negative appendectomy rate of 3%. These same authors also reported on 104 patients who underwent appendectomy without their CT protocol who had a negative appendectomy rate of 12.5%. In a retrospective review of CT use in the pediatric population suspected of appendicitis, a normal appendix was removed in 7% of children who underwent CT prior to appendectomy, 11% with use of the US prior to appendectomy and an 8% negative appendectomy rate when no preoperative radiologic study was performed [55]. In a recent retrospective study, the use of preoperative CT scans only decreased the negative appendectomy rate for the women of childbearing age (women 45 years and younger) [56]. Livingston et al. [57] found that the rate of nonperforated appendicitis increased since 1995 with the liberal use of CT scans and laparoscopic surgery, but the rate of perforated appendicitis also increased during the same period. Krajewski et al. [58] showed that the incidence of perforated appendicitis was higher for lower socioeconomic patients than that of the patients in the higher socioeconomic group in the United States from 2001 to 2005 but that the authors found no difference in perforated appendicitis rates between the lower and higher socioeconomic patients in Canada.

Although many studies have found CT to be accurate in diagnosing acute appendicitis, there is still controversy regarding the optimal technique. Three common techniques used include a focused appendiceal CT using rectally administered contrast, the unenhanced or the use of oral and/or intravenous contrasted CT of the abdomen and pelvis. Every institution has their own preference to which version they prefer to use to diagnose appendicitis, all of which seem to have the same reported accuracy [59,60].

In a systemic review performed by van Redan et al. [61] comparing graded compression US to computed tomography in the diagnosis of appendicitis, the authors found the respective mean sensitivities for CT and graded compression US were 91% (95% CI: 84%, 95%) and 78% (95% CI: 67%, 86%) ($p < 0.017$) and the respective mean specificities for CT and graded compression US were as follows: 90% (95% CI: 85%, 94%) and 83% (95% CI: 76%, –88%) ($p < 0.037$). Calculated positive LRs for CT and graded compression US were 9.29 (95% CI: 6.86, 12.58) and 4.5 (95% CI: 3.03, 6.68), respectively ($p = 0.011$). The authors concluded from their meta-analysis of head-to-head comparison studies in patient populations with a high prevalence of appendicitis, CT was found to have a better test performance than did graded compression US in making the diagnosis. The authors recommend the use of CT in patients suspected of acute appendicitis.

Should CT be used routinely in the diagnostic evaluation of patients suspected of appendicitis? Because of the increasing reports of excellent accuracy rates of CT diagnosing appendicitis, some have called for the routine use of CT for all patients with possible appendicitis [52,62–64]. Others have questioned the need for routine use of CT for all patients especially those with classic clinical presentations. McCay and Shepherd [65] recommend only ordering CT on patients presenting to the emergency room suspected of having appendicitis if their Alvarado score [66] is between 4 and 6. For a score of less than 3, no CT or US was recommended as appendicitis was doubtful. The authors do, however, recommend a surgical consult for an Alvarado score of 7 or more. In a prospective randomized study of patients presenting to the emergency room for possible appendicitis comparing clinical assessment versus CT, the reported diagnostic accuracy was 90% for clinical assessment and 92% for CT [67]. The authors concluded that clinical assessment unaided by CT reliably identifies patients with acute appendicitis who need an operation. They do not advocate the routine use of CT for diagnosis of suspected appendicitis. In a prospective randomized study performed in women of childbearing age who presented to the emergency room with the suspected diagnosis of appendicitis, each was randomized to the clinical assessment only arm or the CT arm [68]. In this study, the reported accuracy for the diagnosis of appendicitis was 93% for both clinical assessment and CT. The authors concluded that a CT scan is as good as clinical assessment alone and reliably identifies women of childbearing age who need an appendectomy. In a recent retrospective study, the negative appendectomy rate for patients who had a CT scan prior to appendectomy was 6%. The negative appendectomy rate was unchanged for patients who underwent an appendectomy based on clinical examination alone [69]. The study also found that preoperative CT scans increased the appendectomy rate only in patients with a low clinical suspicion of appendicitis. In a retrospective study in children reported by Martin and associates [70], the liberal use of CT scans did not decrease the negative appendectomy rate. In conclusion, the selective use of CT scans seems more appropriate in diagnosing suspected appendicitis. This study should be reserved as an adjunct in clinical settings in which other sources of pathology other than appendicitis may cause pain or the clinical history alone is not helpful in making the diagnosis.

Magnetic resonance imaging (MRI) for the evaluation of acute appendicitis has been performed more frequently recently in order to avoid the risks associated with ionizing radiation. MRI has become a frequently performed test in pregnant women and children with symptoms of appendicitis and a nondiagnostic US [71]. MRI has good resolution and has been shown to be accurate in diagnosing acute appendicitis [72]. MRI is considered positive for acute appendicitis when the appendix is enlarged (>7 mm), the appendiceal wall is thicker than 2 mm, or there are signs of inflammatory changes surrounding the appendix, such as fat stranding, phlegmon, or abscess formation [73]. MRI has been shown to be safe and reliable in diagnosing acute appendicitis in pregnant patients [74,75]. No IV contrast should be given to pregnant patients because gadolinium is a category C drug and potentially teratogenic.

In a recent multicenter diagnostic study of MRI in patients with suspected appendicitis, authors suggest that if MRI is found to be sufficiently accurate in the general population of patients with suspected appendicitis, MRI could replace CT in some or all patients. This could limit or obviate the ionizing radiation exposure and decrease the risk of contrast medium-induced nephropathy with CT [76]. Limitations to the use of MRI are: it is a more expensive test, it is not always widely available, images can be degraded by motion, and a specialist needs to interpret the MRI images. Until these limitations can be overcome, MRI should not be a first line test to rule out appendicitis.

*Recommendation*: The most accurate imaging modality for making the diagnosis of appendicitis is computed tomography. The routine use of performing CT on all patients suspected of appendicitis cannot be recommended (Grade B recommendation).

## 48.6 Does Giving Antibiotics to Patients with Appendicitis Who Undergo Appendectomy Decrease Postoperative Infectious Complications?

Appendicitis, once diagnosed, is usually followed by an appendectomy. Antibiotics should be given as soon as the diagnosis is suspected. The bacteria that populate the appendix are similar to the bacterial flora of the colon. The antibiotics chosen for patients with appendicitis should provide coverage for gram-negative and gram-positive aerobic and anaerobic bacteria, along with anaerobes. *Bacteriodes fragilis* and *Escherichia coli* are the two most common organism grown from peritoneal cultures after acute appendicitis.

Acute appendicitis is a polymicrobial infection. In 1938, William Altemeier isolated at least four different organisms per specimen in patients with perforated appendicitis [77]. More recent reports demonstrate on average up to 12 organisms per specimen from patients with gangrenous or perforated appendicitis [78]. Few bacteria are cultured from the peritoneal fluid of patient's with acute appendicitis only; however, bacteria are recovered from peritoneal fluid in over 80% patients with a gangrenous or perforated appendix. Two common postoperative complications following appendectomy are wound infections and intra-abdominal abscesses. Prior to the use of antibiotics, there was a 10%–40% rate of wound infections and intra-abdominal abscesses after appendectomy [79,80].

All patients undergoing appendectomy for acute appendicitis should receive antibiotics preoperatively [81]. The use of antibiotics to reduce postoperative morbidity following appendectomy has been studied. Gorbach in his review of antimicrobial prophylaxis for appendectomy reported a reduction in the rate of postoperative infectious complication in all operations for acute appendicitis and especially in patients with perforated and/or gangrenous appendicitis [82]. In another analysis of clinical studies by Pottecher et al. [83], they reported that a single preoperative dose of systemic antibiotic reduced the postoperative sepsis rates after appendectomy. They also reported that if the appendix was perforated then antibiotic therapy should last longer than one dose and should not be considered prophylaxis but treatment. In a study by Mui et al., a single dose of preoperative antibiotics was found to be adequate for the prevention of postoperative infective complications in patients with nonperforated appendicitis [84]. Another study also supported the fact that only one preoperative dose of antibiotic is needed to prevent postoperative infectious complications in patients with nonperforated appendicitis and the use of any further postoperative antibiotics does not decrease the rate of surgical site infections (SSI) [85]. Patients with perforated and complicated appendicitis can be treated with antibiotics for 5–7 days [86].

Anderson et al. performed a meta-analysis of randomized or controlled clinical trials investigating the use of antibiotics versus placebo for patients with suspected appendicitis who underwent an appendectomy [87]. The authors evaluated 45 studies with

9576 patients. Their outcome measures were wound infection, intra-abdominal abscess, hospital length of stay, and mortality. They concluded that the use of antibiotics is superior to placebo in preventing wound infection and intra-abdominal abscesses in patients with acute, gangrenous, and perforated appendicitis. They were unable to determine from their analysis the optimal duration of antibiotic treatment for complicated cases. The authors found that a single dose of antibiotics may have the same impact as multiple doses, although it is best to administer the first dose of antibiotics preoperatively. The choice of antibiotic selection should be based on the bacteriology of appendix and provide coverage for gram-negative, gram-positive, and anaerobic organisms. The optimal duration of antibiotics in complicated appendicitis is unclear. A recent retrospective study examined 52 patients with complicated appendicitis. They report that there is no significant difference in postoperative abscess development among patients who received over 24 h of postoperative antibiotics compared with those who received 24 h or less of antibiotics. They conclude that postoperative antibiotics may not provide a significant benefit for preventing intra-abdominal abscesses [88]. A second retrospective study included 266 patients, 78 with complicated and 188 with noncomplicated appendicitis. They concluded that antibiotic therapy postoperatively for noncomplicated appendicitis showed no significant advantage in preventing postoperative intra-abdominal infections. They also conclude that prolonged postoperative intravenous antibiotics for complicated appendicitis that lasts beyond 5 days did not improve the incidence of intra-abdominal infections [89]. Larger prospective trials will be needed to confirm these conclusions.

A recent prospective study by Fraser and colleagues of pediatric patients with perforated appendicitis examined early transition to oral antibiotics in comparison to a traditional 5-day intravenous antibiotic course. Patients were transitioned to oral antibiotics as soon as they tolerated a diet and discharged, to complete a total 7-day regimen of IV/PO antibiotics. This group had no increased morbidity compared to the group receiving 5 days of IV antibiotics [90].

*Recommendation*: Antibiotic prophylaxis is effective in preventing postoperative wound infections and intra-abdominal abscesses. For nonperforated appendicitis, the one-time preoperative dose of antibiotic seems to be sufficient to decrease infectious complications. The optimal duration of administration of antibiotic for complicated appendicitis seems to be 5–7 days but needs to be further evaluated (Grade B recommendation).

## 48.7 What Operation Is Better for Treating Acute Appendicitis: Laparoscopic or Open Appendectomy?

The treatment for acute appendicitis has been to perform an appendectomy through a RLQ incision since its introduction by McBurney [91] in 1894. The first laparoscopic appendectomy was performed by Semm [92] in 1983. This new surgical technique was slow to be accepted because the standard open technique provided excellent therapeutic efficacy combined with its low morbidity and mortality rates. The use of laparoscopic appendectomy varies considerably. It seems that the most important determinate of whether a patient will have an open or laparoscopic appendectomy is the preference or experience of the treating surgeon, which may vary significantly even within an institution [93]. During the traditional open appendectomy technique performed through a muscle splitting incision in the RLQ, the appendix is usually ligated with an absorbable suture. Inversion of the appendiceal stump has been advocated to prevent leakage and fistulization, but studies have shown no difference in complication rates between inversion and simple ligation of the appendiceal stump [94]. The peritoneal cavity is typically irrigated after an appendectomy. The skin incision is normally closed without complications, although if the wound is grossly contaminated, one may consider delayed primary closure or simply allow the wound to heal by secondary intention [95]. Leaving an intraperitoneal drain has not been shown to be useful even in cases of a perforated appendix [96].

Is laparoscopic appendectomy better than open appendectomy? The answer to this question depends on the outcomes being measured. Over the last 20 years, various studies have looked at duration of operation, cost of operation, cost of hospitalization, length of hospital stay, the time to return to work, and postoperative pain often with conflicting results [97–100]. Although many of the randomized controlled trials comparing laparoscopic and open appendectomy are plagued by several biases, they represent the best evidence available.

Two early meta-analysis of laparoscopic versus open appendectomy for acute appendicitis have confirmed the benefit of the laparoscopic approach in relation to less pain, a faster recovery, and a lower incidence of wound infections compared to open appendectomy [101,102]. As surgeons become more skilled in minimally invasive surgical techniques, the incidence of laparoscopic appendectomy has become more common [103]. Reported complications after laparoscopic appendectomy include injury to bowel, bladder, and ureter, bleeding from epigastric vessels, iliac vessels, and mesentery, appendiceal stump leak, wound infection, and intra-abdominal abscess. One of the reported complications of laparoscopic appendectomy is recurrent appendicitis. This entity known as stump appendicitis occurs when the surgeon fails to remove the appendix at the base of the cecum, thus leaving a stump of appendix that can become infected causing recurrent appendicitis [104].

The Cochrane Library published a systemic review of randomized clinical trials comparing open with laparoscopic appendectomy in 2010 [105]. This review included randomized clinical trials comparing laparoscopic appendectomy (LA) versus open appendectomy (OA) in adults and children. The authors included 67 studies, of which the majority of (56) studies compared laparoscopic (with or without diagnostic laparoscopy) versus open appendectomy in adults. The authors reported that wound infections were less likely after LA than after OA (OR: 0.43; CI: 0.34–0.54), but the incidence of intra-abdominal abscess was increased after LA (OR: 1.87; CI: 1.19–2.93). The duration of LA was 10 min (CI: 6–15) longer to perform than OA. Pain on postoperative day 1 was reduced by 8 mm (CI: 5–11 mm) on a 100 mm visual analog scale (VAS) after LA compared to OA. Hospital stay was shortened by 1.1 day (CI: 0.7–1.5) after LA. Return to normal activity, work, and sports occurred earlier after LA than after OA. While the operation costs of LA were significantly higher, the costs outside the hospital were reduced. Diagnostic laparoscopy reduced the risk of a negative appendectomy, but this effect was stronger in fertile women (RR: 0.2; CI: 0.11–0.34) as compared to unselected adults (RR: 0.37; CI: 0.13–1.01). The authors concluded that in clinical settings where surgical expertise and equipment are available and affordable, laparoscopic appendectomy seems to hold various advantages over open appendectomy. They recommend LA be done for patients with suspected appendicitis especially in young patients, female patients, obese patients, and employed patients.

The role of laparoscopy between male and female patients is an area that needs further exploration and strict protocols for the choice of technique do not exist. The diagnosis of abdominal pain is variable between the genders, especially in females of childbearing age where the differential includes ovarian cysts, pelvic infection, ectopic pregnancy, and appendicitis. A review was recently published which included 12 studies and 1020 patients, eight studies compared laparoscopy versus open appendectomy, and four compared laparoscopy with a "wait and see" approach. They conclude that laparoscopy was superior to both open appendectomy and a "wait and see" strategy, in the ability to make specific diagnoses prior to discharge, as well as attributing to shorter hospital stays and earlier return to work in female patients of childbearing age [106]. Early laparoscopy in females with abdominal pain can lead to a more accurate diagnosis allowing for timely treatment and possible avoidance of other disease-associated complications.

Conversely, using laparoscopic technique in males may not always be necessary. A 1996 study examined 100 males between 16 and 65 years old and randomized patients to laparoscopic and open appendectomy groups and compared them on the basis of clinical parameters, postoperative complications, and length of stay. They reported that laparoscopic appendectomy versus open appendectomy required longer anesthetic (72.5 vs. 55 min) and operative times (45 vs. 25 min), and no significant difference was found in recovery of bowel function (24.7 vs. 21 h) and length of stay (4.9 vs. 5.3 days). They conclude that there is no significant advantage to using laparoscopic technique in male patient population and that it should be reserved for obese patients and males with an uncertain diagnosis [107].

Traditional open appendectomy performed on obese patients may require a larger skin incision, potentially resulting in more postoperative pain and higher potential for wound complications [108]. In obese individuals, laparoscopic appendectomy is a potentially easier technique that avoids a large and deep incision and can lead to improved wound outcomes. It has been reported that laparoscopy is superior to open appendectomy for obese patients (body mass index ≥30) based on clinical outcomes which include length of stay and wound complication rates [109]. A recently published review examined the outcomes of 13,330 patients with body mass index ≥30 who underwent either laparoscopic or open appendectomy. Laparoscopic technique was associated with a 57% reduction in overall morbidity (OR: 0.43; 95% CI: 0.36–0.52), a 53% reduction in risk (OR: 0.47; 95% CI: 0.32–0.65), a 1.2 days shorter length of stay (mean difference 1.2 days; 95% CI: 0.98–1.42). Confirming previous studies, they conclude that for the obese population laparoscopic appendectomy is not only safe but also superior based on clinical outcomes [110].

In considering elderly patients, the differential diagnosis of abdominal pain is variable and extends to include perforated diverticulitis as well as neoplastic processes. There is also difficultly in making early and accurate diagnosis in elderly patients. One study retrospectively examined 10 years of data that included patients with appendicitis who were 60 years old and older. They reported that only 26% of elderly patients have typical symptoms and one-third delay seeking medical care [111]. When comparing age groups, elderly patients with acute appendicitis have significantly increased rates of perforation attributed to presentation delay and increased morbidity and mortality [112]. Given the fact that elderly patients with appendicitis have increased perforation rates that are likely attributable to a delay in presentation, a question is raised as to whether laparoscopic appendectomy has an advantage in the treatment of this patient population. One meta-analysis included six studies and a total of 4,398 laparoscopic and 11,454 open appendectomies in older patients. Laparoscopic technique was associated with significant reductions in postoperative mortality (pooled OR: 0.24; 95% CI: 0.15–0.37), postoperative complications (pooled OR: 0.61; 95% CI: 0.50–0.73), and the length of hospital stay (−0.51 days; 95% CI: −0.64 to −0.37 days). When comparing operative time, postoperative wound infection, and intra-abdominal collection, no significant difference was found between groups [113]. A second recently published study examined the Nation Wide Inpatient Database including 65,464 patients and evaluating the outcomes of laparoscopic versus open in perforated and nonperforated appendicitis in patients 65 years of age and older. In nonperforated appendicitis, laparoscopy had lower overall complication rates (15.82% vs. 23.49%), in-hospital mortality (0.39% vs. 1.31%), and mean length of stay (3.0 vs. 4.8 days) when compared with open appendectomy. Results were similar when comparing patients with perforated appendicitis. They reported that laparoscopy was associated with lower overall complication rate (36.27% vs. 46.92%), in-hospital mortality (1.4% vs. 2.63%), and shorter mean LOS (5.8 vs. 8.7 days, $p < 0.01$). The authors conclude that laparoscopic appendectomy can be performed safely and has advantages of shorter length of stay and decreased complications when compared with open appendectomy. Elderly patients that present with right iliac fossa pain can safely undergo laparoscopic appendectomy with good outcomes, and it should be considered first-line treatment for both perforated and nonperforated appendicitis [114].

*Recommendation*: The data support performing both open and laparoscopic appendectomy for patients with acute appendicitis if the surgical expertise and equipment are available. The literature supports the consideration of a laparoscopic approach especially in female patients of childbearing age, obese patients, and elderly patients. Open appendectomy may be the preferred method of appendectomy in male aged 18–65 with a BMI of less than 30 (Grade B recommendation).

## 48.8 Is Interval Appendectomy Necessary?

Patients presenting with a periappendiceal mass or abscess diagnosed preoperatively by physical examination or imaging studies can be treated with antibiotics with the potential of having their periappendiceal abscess drained by image-guided percutaneous catheter [115]. With the increased use of computed tomography (CT) in the workup of acute appendicitis, the ability to identify complicated appendicitis preoperatively has allowed for the utilization of initial nonoperative therapy [116]. Generally, antibiotics for 7–14 day with or without catheter drainage have been necessary to treat those patients. An interval appendectomy has been advocated after the abscess and surrounding inflammation have resolved, usually 6–8 weeks after initial nonoperative treatment to prevent recurrent appendicitis and to treat other tumor pathology of the cecum and appendix [117]. Alternative treatment options of complicated appendicitis have included early aggressive resection [118], or initial conservative treatment with interval appendectomy only if symptoms recur [119,120]. Immediate appendectomy may be technically demanding because of the distorted anatomy and the challenges faced when closing an inflamed/necrotic appendiceal stump. Many times the immediate exploration ends up with an ileocecal resection or a right-sided hemicolectomy due to inflammation distorting the tissue planes or a suspicion of malignancy. Following successful nonsurgical treatment of a periappendiceal mass, the need for interval appendectomy has recently been questioned as the risk of recurrence is relatively small (0.2%–7%) [121,122].

In two other recent retrospective studies, it was found that children presenting with complicated appendicitis could be successfully treated with conservative treatment followed by appendectomy [123,124]. Roach et al. [125] concluded from their data that children who presented with prolonged symptoms and a discrete appendiceal abscess or phlegmon, drainage and performance of a delayed appendectomy should be the treatment of choice. In another study, children with complicated appendicitis were initially treated nonoperatively and then had a laparoscopic interval appendectomy, the conclusion was that the surgery could be safely performed, was associated with a shorter hospital stay, with minimal morbidity, analgesia, and scarring. These authors recommended that interval laparoscopic appendectomy be routinely performed because it eliminates the risk of recurrent appendicitis and serves to excise undiagnosed carcinoid tumors [126]. Another group compared initial laparoscopic appendectomy versus initial nonoperative management and interval appendectomy for complicated appendicitis in children in a randomized prospective study [127]. These authors found that the initial laparoscopic surgery took longer but that the overall days in the hospital, infection rates, and total costs did not differ between the two treatment strategies.

In a large retrospective study performed by Kaminski et al. [128], 32,938 patients were hospitalized with acute appendicitis. Emergency appendectomy was performed in 31,926 (97%) patients. Nonoperative treatment was used initially in 1,012 patients (3%). Of these, 148 (15%) had an IA and the remaining 864 (85%) did not. In their study, only 39 patients (5%) had recurrence of appendicitis after a median follow-up of 4 years. Males were more likely to have recurrence of their symptoms than females. Median length of hospital stay was 4 days for the admission for recurrent appendicitis compared with 6 days for the IA admission. The authors concluded that they cannot justify the practice of routine interval appendectomy after initial successful nonoperative treatment of appendicitis based on the observation that most patients undergo appendectomy initially, and those who are treated nonoperatively have a low recurrence rate of appendicitis. In a similar retrospective study in children reported by Paupong et al. [129], there were 6439 patients, of which 6367 (99%) underwent initial appendectomy for acute appendicitis. Seventy-two (1%) patients were initially managed nonoperatively and 11 patients had IA. Of the remaining 61 patients without IA, five (8%) developed recurrent appendicitis. The authors concluded that since recurrent appendicitis is rare in children after successful nonoperative treatment of perforated appendicitis, performance of routine interval appendectomy is not necessarily indicated.

Adult patients who present with an appendiceal mass in the RLQ are commonly managed nonoperatively and then scheduled for an interval appendectomy following resolution of the inflammatory appendiceal mass. This mass could represent a perforated appendix, complicated Crohn's disease or a perforated colon cancer. Tekin et al. [130] reported their experience with not performing routine interval appendectomy after successful treatment of an appendiceal mass. Four patients (4%) in their series had another diagnosis found for their appendiceal mass (two cecal cancers, one cecal diverticulitis, and one Crohn's disease). The recurrence rate of appendicitis in their series was 14.6% with most recurrences happening in the first 6 months after initial presentation. Patients who present with recurrent symptoms should undergo interval appendectomy. They concluded that routine interval appendectomy after initial successful conservative treatment is not justified but they recommend that a protocol should be developed for the management of patients presenting with an appendiceal mass. Similar recommendations were reported by Lai et al. [131]. In their study, five patients were found to have colon cancer, and the rate of recurrent appendicitis was 25.5% with 83% of patients present with recurrent symptoms within 6 months of their initial presentation. They recommend that adult patients who recover from conservative treatment of an appendiceal mass should undergo colonoscopy to detect any underlying disease and interval appendectomy should only be offered to patients who present with recurrent symptoms.

Stevens and de Vries [132] reported on their experience of performing an interval appendectomy only after symptoms developed rather than routinely offering it to their patients with complicated appendicitis. They concluded that the rate of appendectomies performed dropped by 63% and the total length of hospital stay also decreased by 4 days. A group from China reported that by performing an interval appendectomy only after symptoms develop was more cost-effective than performing routine interval appendectomy [133]. In their study, the authors showed that performance of routine interval appendectomy would increase the cost per patient by 38% compared with follow-up and appendectomy after recurrence of symptoms. It is important to also consider patients, such as military personnel, who have undergone nonoperative management of appendicitis and who will, in the future, be in an environment with limited access to medical and surgical care. With recurrent symptoms, these patients risk future development of complications and even death; therefore, this select population benefit from the performance of interval appendectomy.

In a systemic review of the nonsurgical treatment of appendiceal abscess or phlegmon, the need for an interval appendectomy was evaluated [134]. Findings from the meta-analysis: nonsurgical treatment fails in 7.2% of cases (CI: 4.0–10.5), the risk of recurrent symptoms is 7.4% (CI: 3.7–11.1), the risk of finding malignant disease is 1.2% (CI: 0.6–1.7), and the risk of finding an important benign disease is 0.7% (CI: 0.2–11.9) during follow-up. From their meta-analysis (mainly from retrospective studies), the authors support the practice of nonsurgical treatment without interval appendectomy in patients with appendiceal abscess or phlegmon. Another recent systemic review has confirmed that nonoperative management of complicated appendicitis will be successful in the majority of cases with a low incidence of recurrent symptoms. As a result, the routine use of interval appendectomy is no longer justified [135].

*Recommendation*: The routine performance of interval appendectomy after nonoperative treatment of complicated acute appendicitis is not supported. Interval appendectomy should be performed when patients present with recurrent symptoms. Patients presenting with an appendiceal mass managed conservatively should undergo further workup to rule out other pathology for their mass (Grade B recommendation).

## 48.9 Should Antibiotic Treatment Replace Appendectomy for Acute Appendicitis?

Nonoperative treatment of acute appendicitis with antibiotics alone has been reported to be successful [136,137]. Andersson writes that an increasing amount of circumstantial evidence suggests that not all patients with appendicitis will progress to perforation and that resolution may be a common event [138,139]. Other evidence of resolving appendicitis are reports of a history of recurrence, obviously a consequence of spontaneous resolution, which can be found in up to 6.5% of patients not operated on for appendicitis [140]. In the past, appendectomy has been associated with higher morbidity and mortality especially in older patients, those with perforation and sepsis, and those who have a normal appendix at the time of appendectomy. A wide range of recurrence rates have been reported. One study reported recurrent symptoms of appendicitis up to 70% at 1 year in patients who had received antibiotic treatment alone for their acute appendicitis [141,142]. A second study reported an 11% recurrence rate [143]. Further randomized controlled trials (RCTs) are required to gain an understanding of true recurrence rates after antibiotic therapy as first-line treatment.

In 1995, Eriksson and Granstrom [144] reported a randomized controlled trial of appendectomy versus antibiotics alone in 40 patients suspected to have appendicitis, who presented with abdominal pain for less than 72 h. Twenty patients underwent surgery and 20 patients received intravenous antibiotics for 2 days, followed by an 8-day course of oral antibiotics. The authors concluded that antibiotic treatment in patients with acute appendicitis was as effective as surgery. However, they reported a 15% negative appendectomy rate for the surgery group and a 40% recurrence rate of appendicitis that led to appendectomy within 1 year of treatment in the nonoperative group. A recent multicenter trial randomly allocated 252 male patients (age 18–50) to either antibiotic treatment (intravenous cefotaxime and tinidazole for 2 days followed by oral ofloxacin and tinidazole for 10 days) or appendectomy for acute, uncomplicated appendicitis. The trial concluded that antibiotic treatment could serve as an alternative to appendectomy [145]. The complication rate among the surgery group was 14% (17/124), mainly wound infections. Of the 128 patients enrolled in the antibiotic group, 15 patients (12%) were operated on within the first 24 h due to lack of improvement in symptoms and apparent local peritonitis. The operation showed that seven of these patients (5%) had a perforation of their appendix. The rate of recurrence of appendicitis in the antibiotic group was 14%. In another meta-analysis of antibiotic therapy versus appendectomy for acute appendicitis, the authors concluded that even though antibiotics may be used as primary treatment for selected patients with uncomplicated appendicitis, they do not feel that this treatment should supersede appendectomy at the present time [146]. They found selection bias and crossover to surgery in the RCTs suggest that appendectomy is still the gold standard therapy for acute appendicitis.

A total of 113 patients were successfully treated with antibiotics and were sent home for oral antibiotic therapy for 10 days. The recurrence rate within 1 year was 15% (16 patients) in the group treated with antibiotics. Overall, the success rate of conservative management of acute appendicitis with antibiotics is ~70% at best for male patients with unequivocal clinical and laboratory signs of uncomplicated appendicitis. In another recent randomized clinical trial of antibiotic therapy versus appendectomy for acute appendicitis in unselected patients, the authors concluded that antibiotic treatment appears to be a safe first-line therapy in unselected patients with appendicitis [147]. In this study, only 52% of patients randomized to antibiotics followed through. In both of these studies, the conclusions have, however, been made on the basis of only 1 month to 1 year of follow-up data. Another recently published meta-analysis of six studies and 1201 patients reported that 6.9% ± 4.4% patients treated with antibiotics alone failed treatment and required appendectomy, and acute appendicitis recurred in 14.2% ± 10.6% of patients. They concluded that antibiotic therapy lead to an avoidance of surgical risk and morbidity and is a safe treatment option for patients with uncomplicated appendicitis [148].

The most recent meta-analysis published by Varadhan et al. [149] explored the efficacy of antibiotic treatment compared with appendectomy and includes four trials and 900 patients. They conclude that using antibiotic therapy as first-line treatment is worthy of consideration for all patients with early uncomplicated appendicitis and report a success rate of 63% at 1 year and a relative risk reduction in 31% for antibiotic treatment of uncomplicated cases compared with appendectomy. The NOTA (nonoperative treatment for acute appendicitis) study is the most recent prospective study published concerning this subject. A total of 159 patients with suspected appendicitis underwent observation and received a course of amoxicillin/clavulanate. Follow-up was conducted at set intervals up to 2 years. Initial assessment of patients included the use of clinical assessment scores such as Alvarado score. Ultrasound and CT scans were not part of routine work up and were obtained at the discretion of the consultant surgeon, 73% of enrolled patients received US, and 17% received CT imaging. Failure rates at 7 days were 11.9%, recurrence rates after 2 years were 13.8%, and overall efficacy rate of nonoperative treatment was 83%. The authors stress the importance of initial accurate clinical diagnosis and conclude that for select patients with suspected uncomplicated appendicitis initial antibiotic therapy is cost-effective as well as safe and efficacious [150].

Conservative management of acute appendicitis remains a controversial topic despite multiple studies exploring the efficacy of antibiotics as first-line therapy. Selection bias and crossover to surgery in RCT as well as inconsistencies of diagnostic methods used and a predominance of male patients have been suggested. These protocol differences among major studies create an inability for subgroup analysis making it difficult to draw conclusions on the effectiveness of antibiotic therapy compared with appendectomy. The Cochrane Library published a systemic review of randomized clinical trials comparing appendectomy versus antibiotic treatment for acute appendicitis. This study included five trials with a total of 901 patients. Results were evaluated using a noninferiority analysis to compare antibiotic treatment to appendectomy. The authors reported that 73.4% (95% CI: 62.7–81.9) of patients who were treated with antibiotics as compared to 97.4% (95% CI: 94.4–98.8) of patients who underwent appendectomy had complete relief of symptoms within 2 weeks and remained without major complications for up to 1 year. Statistical analysis did not support antibiotic treatment as being noninferior to appendectomy, and therefore, the authors concluded that appendectomy remains the gold standard of treatment for patient presenting with acute appendicitis [151].

The continued lifetime risk of, and the associated morbidity and mortality of, nonoperative treatment with antibiotics only for acute appendicitis remain unknown and need to be investigated. The recommendation of antibiotic treatment as an alternative to the surgical treatment of acute appendicitis cannot be recommended at this time (Table 48.1) [152].

*Recommendation*: Although antibiotics may be used as primary treatment for selected patients with early uncomplicated appendicitis, surgery continues to remain

**TABLE 48.1**

Clinical Questions Summary

| Question | Answer | Level of Evidence | Grade of Recommendation | References |
|---|---|---|---|---|
| What clinical signs and symptoms are most reliable to rule in or out appendicitis? | Abdominal pain localized to the epigastrium or periumbilical area radiating to the right lower quadrant and associated with anorexia and nausea are the most reliable diagnostic symptoms for acute appendicitis. | 4 | Grade B | [4–12] |
| What is the best laboratory test to help make the diagnosis of appendicitis? | Overall laboratory markers of acute inflammation in acute appendicitis remain highly sensitive but relatively nonspecific when it comes to making the diagnosis of acute appendicitis. No one test has been found to be both highly sensitive and specific for acute appendicitis. | 2B | Grade B | [13–23] |
| Does giving a patient with suspected appendicitis pain medicine decrease the ability to make the diagnosis of appendicitis? | Giving pain medicine to adults and children suspected of acute appendicitis does not adversely affect the ability to diagnose appendicitis. Analgesia should not be withheld pending clinical investigation with suspected acute appendicitis. | 3B | Grade B | [24–31] |
| What is the best diagnostic imaging modality to diagnose acute appendicitis? | The most accurate imaging modality for making the diagnosis of appendicitis is computed tomography (CT). The routine use of performing CT on all patients suspected of appendicitis cannot be recommended. | 2B | Grade B | [32–76] |
| Does giving antibiotics to patients with appendicitis who undergo appendectomy decrease postoperative complication rates? | Antibiotic prophylaxis is effective in preventing postoperative wound infections and intra-abdominal abscesses. For nonperforated appendicitis, the one-time preoperative dose of antibiotic seems to be sufficient to decrease infection complications. The optimal duration of administration of antibiotics for complicated appendicitis seems to be 5–7 days but needs to be further evaluated. | 2B | Grade B | [77–90] |
| What operation is better for treating acute appendicitis: laparoscopic or open appendectomy? | The data support performing both open and laparoscopic appendectomy for patients with acute appendicitis if the surgical expertise and equipment are available. The literature supports the consideration of laparoscopic approach especially in female patients of childbearing age, obese patients, and elderly patients. Open appendectomy may be the preferred method of appendectomy in males aged 18–65 with a BMI of less than 30. | 2B | Grade B | [91–114] |
| Is interval appendectomy necessary? | The routine performance of interval appendectomy after nonoperative treatment of complicated acute appendicitis is not supported. Interval appendectomy should be performed when patients present with recurrent symptoms. Patients presenting with an appendiceal mass managed conservatively should undergo further workup to rule out other pathology for their mass. | 3B | Grade B | [115–135] |
| Should antibiotic treatment replace appendectomy for acute appendicitis? | Although antibiotics may be used as primary treatment for selected patients with uncomplicated appendicitis, surgery continues to remain the primary treatment option for the treatment of acute appendicitis. | 3B | Grade B | [136–152] |

the primary treatment option for the treatment of acute appendicitis (Grade B recommendation).

## References


1. Addiss DG, Schaffer N, Fowler BS et al. The epidemiology of appendicitis and appendectomy in the United States. *Am J Epidemiol*. 1990;132:910.
2. Fitz RH. Perforating inflammation of the vermiform appendix: With special reference to its early diagnosis and treatment. *Trans Assoc Am Phys*. 1886;1:107.
3. Krajewski SA, Hameed SM, Smink DS, Rogers SO, Jr. Access to emergency operative care: A comparative study between the Canadian and American health care systems. *Surgery*. Aug 2009;146(2);300–307.
4. Bergeron E, Richer B, Gharib R, Giard A. Appendicitis a place for clinical judgement. *Am J Surg*. 1999;177:460–462.
5. Silen W. 1996. *Cope's Early Diagnosis of the Acute Abdomen*, 19th edn. Oxford University Press: New York.
6. Shelton T, McKinlay R, Schwartz RW. Acute appendicitis: Current diagnosis and treatment. *Curr Surg*. 2003;60(5):502–505.
7. Lee SL, Ho HS. Acute appendicitis: Is there a difference between children and adults? *Am Surg*. 2006;72:409–413.
8. Jaffe BM, Berger DH. 2010. The Appendix. In: *Schwartz's Principles of Surgery*, 9th edn. McGraw-Hill.
9. Wagner J, McKinney WP, Carpenter JL. Does this patient have appendicitis? *JAMA*. 1996;276:1589.
10. McBurney C. Experience with early operative interference in cases of disease of the vermiform appendix. *NY State Med J*. 1889;50:676.
11. Prystowsky JP, Pugh CM, Nagle AP. Appendicitis. *Curr Prob Surg*. 2005;42(10):685–742.
12. Wakeley CP. The position of the vermiform appendix as ascertained by an analysis of 10,000 cases. *J Anat*. 1933;67:277–283.
13. Vermeulen B, Morabia A, Unger PF. Influence of white blood cell count on surgical decision making in patients with abdominal pain in the right lower quadrant. *Eur J Surg*. 1995;161:483.
14. Andersson RE, Hugander AP, Ghazi SH, Ravn H, Offenbartl SK, Nystrom PO, Olaison GP. Diagnostic value of disease history, clinical presentation, and inflammatory parameters of appendicitis. *World J Surg*. 1999;23:133–140.
15. Hoffmann J, Rausmussen O. Aids in the diagnosis of acute appendicitis. *Br J Surg*. 1989;76:774.
16. Jaye DL, Waites KB. Clinical applications of C-reactive protein in pediatrics. *J Pediatr Infect Dis J*. 1997;16:735.
17. Yang HR, Wang YC, Chung PK et al. Laboratory tests in patients with acute appendicitis. *ANZ J Surg* Jan–Feb 2006;76(1–2):71–74.
18. Sengupta A, Bax G, Paterson-Brown S. White blood cell count and C-reactive protein measurement in patients with possible appendicitis. *Ann R Coll Surg Engl*. Sep 2009;91(2):113–115.
19. Sack U, Biereder B, Elouahidi T et al. Diagnostic value of blood inflammatory markers for detection of acute appendicitis in children. *BMC Surg*. 2006;6:15.
20. Paajanen H, Mansikka A, Laato M et al. Novel serum inflammatory markers in acute appendicitis. *Scand J Clin Lab Invest*. 2002;62(8):579–584.
21. Yildirim O, Solak C, Kocer B et al. The role of serum inflammatory markers in acute appendicitis and their success in preventing negative laparotomy. *J Invest Surg*. 2006;19(6):345–352.
22. Lycopoulou L, Mamoulakis C, Hantzi E et al. Serum amyloid A protein levels as a possible aid in the diagnosis of acute appendicitis in children. *Clin Chem Lab Med*. 2005;43(1):49–53.
23. Sand M, Trullen XV, Bechara FG et al. A prospective bicenter study investigating the diagnostic value of procalcitonin in patients with acute appendicitis. *Eur Surg Res*. 2009;43(3):291–297.
24. Aydelotte JD, Collen JF, Martin R. Analgesic administration prior to surgical evaluation for acute appendicitis. *Curr Surg*. 2004;61(4):373–375.
25. Attard AR, Corlett MJ, Kinder NJ et al. Safety of early pain relief for acute abdominal pain. *Br Med J*. 1992;30:554–556.
26. Frei SP, Bond WF, Bazuro RK et al. Is early analgesia associated with delayed treatment of appendicitis? *Am J Emerg Med*. Feb 2008;26(2):176–180.
27. Manadevan M, Graff L. Prospective randomized double blind study of analgesic use for ED patients with right lower quadrant abdominal pain. *Am J Emerg Med* 2000;18:753–756.
28. Thomas SH, Silen W, Cheema F, Reisner A, Aman S, Goldstein JN, Kumar Am, Stair TO. Effects of morphine analgesia on diagnostic accuracy in emergency department patients with abdominal pain: A prospective, randomized trial. *J Am Coll Surg*. 2003;196:18–31.
29. Wolfe JM, Smithline HA, Phipen S, Montano G, Grab JL, Fiallo V. Does morphine change the physical examination in patients with acute appendicitis? *Am J Emerg Med*. 2004;22:280–285.
30. Bailey B, Bergeron S, Gravel J, Bussieres JF, Bensoussan A. Efficacy and impact of intravenous morphine before surgical consultation in children with right lower quadrant pain suggestive of appendicitis: A randomized controlled trial. *Ann Emerg Med*. 2007;50:371–378.
31. Green R, Bulloch B, Kabani A, Hancock BJ, Tenenbein M. Early analgesia for children with acute abdominal pain. *Pediatrics*. 2005;116:978–983.
32. Old JL, Dusing RW, Yap W, Dirks J. Imaging for suspected appendicitis. *Am Fam Phys*. 2005;71:71–78.
33. Berry J JR, Malt RA. Appendicitis near its centenary. *Ann Surg*. 1984;200:567–575.
34. Graffeo CS, Counselman FL. Appendicitis. *Emerg Med Clin North Am*. 1996;14:653–671.
35. Rao PM, Rhea JT, Rao JA, Conn AK. Plain abdominal radiography in clinically suspected appendicitis: Diagnostic yield, resource use, and comparison with CT. *Am J Emerg Med*. 1999;17:325–328.
36. Boleslawski E, Panis Y, Benoist S, Denet C, Mariani P, Valleur P. Plain abdominal radiography as a routine procedure for acute abdominal pain of the right lower quadrant: Prospective evaluation. *World J Surg*. 1999;23:262–264.

37. Deutsch A, Leopold GR. Ultrasonic demonstration of the inflamed appendix: Case report. *Radiology.* 1981;140:163–164.
38. Prystowsky JB, Pugh CM, Nagle AP. Current problems in surgery: Appendicitis. *Curr Prob Surg.* 2005;42(10):688–742.
39. Adams DH, Fine C, Brooks DC. High-resolution real-time ultrasonography. A new tool in the diagnosis of acute appendicitis. *Am J Surg.* 1988;155:93–97.
40. Rettenbacher T, Hollerweger A, Macheiner P et al. Presence or absence of gas in the appendix: Additional criteria to rule out or confirm acute appendicitis-evaluation with US. *Radiology.* 2000;214:183–187.
41. Terasawa T, Blackmore CC, Bent S. Systemic review: Computed tomography and ultrasonography to detect acute appendicitis in adults and adolescents. *Ann Inter Med.* 2004;141(7):537.
42. Doria AS, Moineddin R, Kellenberger CJ et al. US or CT for diagnosis in children and adults? A meta-analysis. *Radiology.* Oct 2006;241(1):83–94.
43. Johansson EP, Rydh A, Rilund KA. Ultrasound, computed tomography, and laboratory findings in the diagnosis of appendicitis. *Acta Radiol.* Apr 2007;48(3):267–273.
44. Patel SJ, Reede DL, Katz DS et al. Imaging the pregnant patient for nonobstretric conditions: Algorithms and radiation dose considerations. *Radiographics.* 2007;27(6):1705–1722.
45. Parks NA, Schroeppel TJ. Update on imaging for acute appendicitis. *Surg Clin N Am.* 2011;91:141–154.
46. Melton GB, Duncan MD. 2008. Acute appendicitis. In: Cameron JL (ed.). *Current Surgical Therapy,* 9th edn. Mosby: Philadelphia, PA, pp. 257–261.
47. Choi D, Park H, Lee YR, Kook SH, Kim SK, Kwag HJ, Chung EC. The most useful findings for diagnosing acute appendicitis in contrast enhanced helical CT. *Acta Radiol.* 2003;44:574–582.
48. Hansen AJ, Young SW, De Petris G et al. Histologic severity of appendicitis can be predicted by computed tomography. *Arch Surg.* 2004;139:1304–1308.
49. Ganguli S, Raptopoulos V, Komlos F, Siewert B, Kruskal J. Right lower quadrant pain: Value of the nonvisualized appendix in patients at multidetector CT. *Radiology.* 2006;241(1):175–180.
50. Rao PM, Rhea JT, Novelline RA et al. Effect of computed tomography of the appendix on treatment of patients and use of hospital resources. *N Engl J Med.* 1998;338:141–146.
51. Rao PM, Rhea JT, Rattner DW et al. Introduction of appendiceal CT: Impact on negative appendectomy and appendiceal perforation rates. *Ann Surg.* 1999;229:339–344.
52. Perez J, Barone JE, Wilbanks TO, Jorgensson D, Corvo PR. Liberal use of computed tomography scanning does not improve the diagnostic accuracy in appendicitis. *Am J Surg.* 2003;185:194–197.
53. Morris KT, Kavanagh M, Hansen P, Whiteford MH, Deveney K, Standage B. The rational use of computed tomography scans in the diagnosis of appendicitis. *Am J Surg.* 2002;183:547–550.
54. Holloway JA, Westerbuhr LM, Chain J, Forney GA, White TW, Hughes RJ, Blankenship JD. Is appendiceal computed tomography in a community hospital helpful? *Am J Surg.* 2003;186:682–684.
55. Patrick DA, Janik JE, Janik JS Bensard DD, Karrer FM. Increased CT scan utilization does not improve the diagnostic accuracy of appendicits in children. *J Pediatr Surg.* 2003;38:659–662.
56. Coursey CA, Nelson RC, Patel MB et al. Making the diagnosis of acute appendicitis: Do more preoperative scans mean fewer negative appendectomies? A 10-year study. *Radiology.* 2010;254(2):460–468.
57. Livingston EH, Woodward WA, Sarosi GA, Haley RW. Disconnect between incidence of nonperforated and perforated appendicitis: Implications for pathophysiology and management. *Ann Surg.* Jun 2007;245(6):888–892.
58. Krajewski SA, Hameed SM, Smink DS, Rodgers SO, Jr. Access to emergency care: A comparative study between the Canadian and American health care systems. *Surgery.* Aug 2009;186(2):300–307.
59. Guiliano V, Guiliano C, Pinto F et al. CT method for visualization of the appendix using fixed oral dosage of diatrizoate clinical experience in 525 cases. *Emerg Radiol.* 2005;190:1300–1306.
60. Weltman DI, Yu J, Krumenacker J et al. Diagnosis of acute appendicitis: Comparison of 5- and 10- mm CT sections in the same patient. *Radiology.* 2000;216:172–177.
61. Van Randen A, Bipat S, Zwindermann AH, Ubbink DT, Stoker J, Boermeester MA. Acute appendicitis: Meta-analysis of diagnostic performance of ct and graded compression US related to prevalence of disease. *Radiology.* 2008. Aug 5 Epub ahead of print.
62. Peck J, Peck A, Peck C et al. The clinical role of noncontrast helical computed tomography in the diagnosis of appendicitis. *Am J Surg.* 2000;180:133–136.
63. Rhea JT, Rao PM, Novelline RA, McCabe CJ. A focused appendiceal CT technique to reduce the cost of caring for patients with clinically suspected appendicitis. *AJR.* 1997;169:113–118.
64. Pena BM, Taylor GA, Lund DP, Mandl KD. Effect of computed tomography on patient management and costs in children with suspected appendicitis. *Pediatrics.* 2001;107:1231.
65. McKay R, Shepherd J. The use of the clinical scoring system by Alvardo in the decision to perform computed tomography for acute appendicitis in the ED. *Am J Emerg Med.* 2007;25:489–493.
66. Alvarado A. A practical score for early diagnosis of acute appendicitis. *Ann Emerg Med.* 1986;15:557–565.
67. Hong JJ, Cohn SM, Ekeh AP et al. A prospective randomized study of clinical assessment versus computed tomography for the diagnosis of acute appendicitis. *Surg Infect (Larchmt).* 2003;3:231–239.
68. Lopez PP, Cohn SM, Popkin CA et al. The use of computed tomography scan to rule out appendicitis in women of childbearing age is as accurate as clinical exam: A prospective randomized trial. *Am Surg.* 2007;73:1232–1236.
69. Petrosyan M, Estrada J, Chan S, Somers S et al. CT scan in patients with suspected appendicitis: Clinical implications for the acute care surgeon. *Eur Surg Res.* 2008;40:211–219.
70. Martin AE, Vollman D, Adler B, Caniano DA. CT scans may not reduce the negative appendectomy rate in children. *J Pediatr Surg.* 2004;39:886–890.

71. Singh A, Danrad R, Hahn PF et al. MR imaging of the acute abdomen and pelvis: Acute appendicitis and beyond. *Radiographics*. 2007;27:1419–1431.
72. Cobben L, Groot I, Kingma L et al. A simple MRI protocol in patients with clinically suspected appendicitis: Results in 138 patients and effect on outcome of appendectomy. *Eur Radiol*. 2009;19:1175–1183.
73. Tkacz JN, Anderson SA, Soto J. MR imaging in gastrointestinal emergencies. *Radiographics*. 2009;29:1767–1780.
74. Tannus JF, Dagoglu G, Oto A. Magnetic resonance imaging of maternal diseases of the abdomen and pelvis in the pregnant patient. *Am J Perinatol*. 2008;25:605–610.
75. Beddy P, Keogan MT, Sala E, Griffin N. Magnetic resonance imaging for the evaluation of acute abdominal pain in pregnancy. *Semin Ultrasound CT MR*. 2010;31:433–441.
76. Leeuwenburgh MM, Lameris W, van Randen A et al. Optimizing imaging in suspected appendicitis (OPTIMAP-Study): A multicenter diagnostic accuracy study of MRI in patients with suspected acute appendicitis. *Study protocol BMC Emerg Med*. 2010;20:10–19.
77. Altmeier WA. The bacterial flora of acute perforated appendicitis with peritonitis. A bacteriological study based upon a hundred cases. *Ann Surg*. 1938;107:517–528.
78. Bennion RS, Thompson JE, Jr., Baron EJ, Finegold SM. Gangrenous and perforated appendicitis with peritonitis: Treatment and bacteriology. *Clin Ther*. 1990;12 suppl C:31–44.
79. Fischer AC. 2001. In: Cameron JL, ed. *Acute Appendicitis Current Surgical Therapy*, 7th edn. Mosby: Philadelphia, PA, pp. 267–272.
80. Almqvist P, Leandoer L, Tornqvist A. Timing of antibiotic treatment in non-perforated gangrenous appendicitis. *Eur J Surg*. 1995;161:431–433.
81. Bauer T, Vennitis B, Holm B et al. Antibiotic prophylaxis in acute non-perforated appendicitis. The Danish Multicenter Study Group III. *Ann Surg*. 1989;209:307–311.
82. Gorbach SL. Antimicrobial prophylaxis for appendectomy and colorectal surgery. *Rev Infect Dis*. Sept–Oct 1991;13 Suppl 10:15–20.
83. Pottecher T, Gogny E, Pain L. Antibiotic prophylaxis and appendectomy.
84. Mui LM, Ng CS, Wong SK et al. Optimum duration of prophylactic antibiotics in acute non-perforated appendicitis. *ANZ J Surg*. Jun 2005;75(6):425–428.
85. Le D, Rusin W, Hill B, Langell J. Post-operative antibiotic use in non-perforated appendicitis. *Am J Surg*. Dec 2009;198(6):748–752.
86. Solomkin JS, Mazuski JE, Bradley JS et al. Diagnosis and management of complicated intra-abdominal infection in adults and children: Guidelines by the Surgical Infection Society and the Infectious Diseases Society of America. *Clin Infect Dis*. 2010;50:133–164.
87. Andersen BR, Kallehave FL, Andersen HK. Antibiotics versus placebo for prevention of postoperative infection after appendectomy. *Cochrane Database Syst Rev*. 2005;(3):CD001439.
88. Kimbrell AR, Novosel TJ, Collins JN et al. Do postoperative antibiotics prevent abscess formation in complicated appendicitis?. *Am Surg*. 2014;80(9):878–883.
89. Hughes MJ, Ewen H, Simon P-B. Post-operative antibiotics after appendectomy and post-operative abscess development: A retrospective analysis. *Surg Infect*. 2013;14(1):56–61.
90. Fraser JD, Aguayo P, Leys CM et al. A complete course of intravenous antibiotics vs a combination of intravenous and oral antibiotics for perforated appendicitis in children: A prospective, randomized trial. *J Ped Surg*. Jun 2010;45(6):1198–1202.
91. McBurney C. The incision made in the abdominal wall in cases of appendicitis, with description of a new method of operating. *Ann Surg*. 1894;20:38.
92. Semm K. Endoscopic appendectomy. *Endoscopy*. 1983;15:59–64.
93. Cervini P, Smith LC, Urbach DR. The surgeon on call is a strong factor determining the use of a laparoscopic approach for appendectomy. *Surg Endosc*. 2002;16:1774–1777.
94. Street D, Bodai BI, Owens LJ et al. Simple ligation vs. stump ligation in appendectomy. *Arch Surg*. 1988;123:689.
95. Cohn SM, Giannotti G, Ong AW et al. Prospective randomized trial of two wound management strategies for dirty abdominal wounds. *Ann Surg*. 2001;233:409–413.
96. Greenall MJ, Evans M, Pollack AV. Should you drain a perforated appendix? *Br J Surg*. 1978;65:880.
97. Kum CK, Ngoi SS, Goh PMY et al. Randomized controlled trial comparing laparoscopic and open appendectomy. *Br J Surg*. 1993;80:1599–1600.
98. Martin LC, Puente I, Sosa JL et al. Open versus laparoscopic appendectomy. *Ann Surg*. 1995:222:256–262.
99. Minne L, Burnell A, Ratzer E et al. Laparoscopic vs open appendectomy. *Arch Surg*. 1997;132:708–712.
100. Hellberg A, Rudberg C, Kullman E et al. Prospective randomized multicenter study of laparoscopic versus open appendectomy. *Br J Surg*. 1999;86:48–53.
101. Sauerland S, Lefering R, Holthausen U et al. 1998. A meta-analysis of studies comparing laparoscopic with conventional appendectomy. In: Krahenbuhl L, Frei E, Klaiber Ch et al., eds., *Acute Appendicitis: Standard Treatment or Laparoscopic Surgery?* Krager: Basel, Germany, pp. 109–114.
102. Golub R, Siddiqui F, Pohl D. Laparoscopic versus open appendectomy: A meta-analysis. *J Am Coll Surg*. 1998;186:545–553.
103. Paterson HM, Qadan M, de Luca SM et al. Changing trends in surgery for acute appendicitis. *Br J Surg*. 2008;95:363–368.
104. Milne AA, Bradbury AW. "Residual" appendicitis following incomplete laparoscopic appendicectomy. *Br J Surg*. 1996;83:217.
105. Sauerland S, Jaschincki, T., Neugebauer EAM. Laparoscopic versus open laparoscopic surgery for suspected appendicitis. *Cochrane Database Syst Rev*. 2010;Issue 10. Art No.: CD001546.
106. Gaitán HG, Ludovic R, Cindy F. Laparoscopy for the management of acute lower abdominal pain in women of childbearing age. *Cochrane Database Syst Rev*. 2011;1.
107. Mutter D, Vix M, Bui A et al. Laparoscopy not recommended for routine appendectomy in men: Results of a prospective randomized study. *Surgery*. 1996;120(1):71–74.

108. Ricca R, Schneider JJ, Brar H et al. Laparoscopic appendectomy in patients with a body mass index of 25 or greater: Results of a double blind, prospective, randomized trial. *JSLS.* 2007;11(1):54–58.
109. Corneille MG, Steigelman MB, Myers JG et al. Laparoscopic appendectomy is superior to open appendectomy in obese patients. *Am J Surg.* 2007;194(6):877–881.
110. Mason RJ, Moazzez A, Moroney JR, Katkhouda N. Laparoscopic vs open appendectomy in obese patients: Outcomes using the American College of Surgeons National Surgical Quality Improvement Program database. *J Am Coll Surg.* 2012;215:88–99; discussion 99–100.
111. Storm-Dickerson TL, Horattas MC. What have we learned over the past 20 years about appendicitis in the elderly? *Am J Surg.* 2003;185(3):198–201.
112. Kraemer M, Franke C, Ohmann C, Yang Q. Acute Abdominal Pain Study Group. Acute appendicitis in late adulthood: Incidence, presentation, and outcome: Results of a prospective multicenter acute abdominal pain study and a review of the literature. *Langenbecks Arch Surg.* 2000;385(7):470–481.
113. Southgate E, Vousden N, Karthikesalingam A, Markar SR, Black S, Zaidi A. Laparoscopic vs open appendectomy in older patients. *Arch Surg.* 2012;147:557–562.
114. Masoomi H, Mills S, Dolich MO, Ketana N, Carmichael JC, Nguyen NT, Stamos MJ. Does laparoscopic appendectomy impart an advantage over open appendectomy in elderly patients? *World J Surg.* 2012;36:1534–1539.
115. Von Sonnenberg E, Wittich GR, Casola G et al. Periappendiceal abscesses: Percutaneous drainage. *Radiology.* 1987;163:23–26.
116. Frei SP, Bond WF, Bazuro RK et al. Appendicitis outcomes with increased computed tomographic scanning. *Am J Emerg Med.* 2008;26:39.
117. Nitecki S, Assalia A, Schein M. Contemporary management of Appendiceal mass. *Br J Surg.* 1993;30:18.
118. Thompson JE, Jr., Bennion RS, Schmit PJ et al. Cecetomy for complicated appendicitis. *J Am Coll Surg.* 1994;179:135.
119. Adalla SA. Appendiceal mass: Interval appendectomy should not be the rule. *Br J Clin Pract.* 1996;50:168.
120. Ein SH, Shandling B. Is interval appendectomy necessary after rupture of an appendiceal mass? *J Pediatr Surg.* 1996;31:849.
121. Nguyen DB, Silen W, Hodin RA. Interval appendectomy in the laparoscopic era. 1999;3:189–193.
122. Andersson RE, Petzhold MG. Nonsurgical treatment of appendiceal abscess or phlegmon: A systematic review and meta-analysis. *Ann Surg.* 2007;246:741–748.
123. Roach JP, Patrick DA, Bruny JL, Allshouse MJ, Karrer FM, Ziegler MM. Complicated appendicitis in children: A clear role for drainage and delayed appendectomy. *Am J Surg.* 2007;194:769–772.
124. Bufo AJ, Shah RS, Li MH, Cyr NA, Hollabaugh RS, Hixson SD, Schropp KP, Lasater OE, Joyner RE, Lobe TE. Interval appendectomy for perforated appendicitis in children. *J Laparoendosc Adv Surg Tech A.* Aug 1998;8(4):209–214.
125. Roach JP, Patrick DA, Bruny JL, Allshouse MJ, Karrer FM, Ziegler MM. Complicated appendicitis in children: A clear role for drainage and delayed appendectomy. *Am J Surg.* 2007;194:769–772.
126. Owen A, Moore O, Marven S, Roberts J. Interval laparoscopic appendectomy in children. *J Laparoendosc Adv Surg Tech A.* 2006;16:308–311.
127. St Peter SD, Aguayo P, Fraser JD et al. Initial laparoscopic appendectomy versus initial nonoperative management and interval appendectomy for perforated appendicitis with abscess: A prospective, randomized trial. *J Pediatr Surg.* Jan 2010;45(1):236–240.
128. Kaminski A, Liu IL, Appelbaum H, Lee SL, Haigh PI. Routine interval appendectomy is not justified after initial nonoperative treatment of acute appendicitis. *Arch Surg.* 2005;140(9):897–901.
129. Paupong D, Lee SL, Haigh PI, Kaminski A, Lui IL, Applebaum H. Routine interval appendectomy in children is not indicated. *J Pediatr Surg.* 2007;42(9): 1500–1503.
130. Tekin A, Kurtoglu HC, Can I, Oztan S. Routine interval appendectomy is unnecessary after conservative treatment of appendiceal mass. *Colorectal Dis.* Jun 2008;10(5): 465–468.
131. Lai HW, Loong CC, Chiu JH et al. Interval appendectomy after conservative treatment of an appendiceal mass. *World J Surg.* Mar 2006;30(3):352–357.
132. Stevens CT, de Vries JE. Interval appendectomy as indicated rather than as routine therapy: Fewer operations and shorter hospital stays. *Ned Tijdschr Geneeskd.* Mar 2007;151(13):759–763.
133. Lai HW, Loong CC, Wu CW, Lui WY. Watchful waiting versus interval appendectomy for patients who recovered from acute appendicitis with tumor formation: A cost-effectiveness analysis. *J Chin Med Assoc.* Sep 2005; 68(9):431–434.
134. Andersson RE, Petzold MG. Nonsurgical treatment of appendiceal abscess or phlegmon: A systemic review and meta-analysis. *Ann Surg.* 2007;246:741–748.
135. Deakin DE, Ahmed I. Interval appendectomy after resolution of adult inflammatory appendix mass—Is it necessary? *Surgeon.* 2007;5:45–50.
136. Groetsch Sm, Shaughnessy JM. Medical management of acute appendicitis: A case report. *J Am Board Fam Pract.* May–Jun 2001;14(3):225–226.
137. Salim AS, Ahmed TM. Antibiotic treatment of acute appendicitis—Initial observations. *Saudi Med J.* 2001;22; 643–644.
138. Migraine S, Atri M, Bret PM, Lough JO, Hinchey JE. Spontaneously resolving acute appendicitis: Clinical and sonographic documentation. *Radiology.* 1997;205:55–58.
139. Andersson RE. The natural history and traditional management of appendicitis revisited: Spontaneous resolution and predominance of prehospital perforations imply that a correct diagnosis is more important than an early diagnosis. *World J Surg.* 2007;31: 86–92.
140. Barber MD, McLaren J, Rainey JB. Recurrent appendicitis. *Br J Surg.* 1997;84:110–112.
141. Humes DJ, Simpson J. Acute appendicitis. *BMJ.* 2006;333:530–534.
142. Cobben LP, de Van Otterloo AM, Puylaert JB. Spontaneously resolving appendicitis: Frequency and natural history in 60 patients. *Radiology.* 2000;215:349–352.

143. Hansson J, Körner U, Ludwigs K et al. Antibiotics as first-line therapy for acute appendicitis: Evidence for a change in clinical practice. *World J Surg.* 2012;36(9):2028–2036.
144. Eriksson S, Granstrom L. Randomized controlled trial of appendectomy versus antibiotic therapy for acute appendicitis. *Br J Surg.* 1995;82:166–169.
145. Styrud J, Eriksson S, Nilsson I, Ahlberg G, Haapaniemi S, Neovius G, Rex L, Badume I, Granström L. Appendectomy versus antibiotic treatment in acute appendicitis: A prospective multicenter randomized controlled trial. *World J Surg.* 2006;30:1033–1037.
146. Varadhan KK, Humes DJ, Neal KR, Lobo DN. Antibiotic therapy versus appendectomy for acute appendicitis: A meta-analysis. *World J Surg.* Feb 2010;34(2):199–209.
147. Hansson J, Komer U, Khorram-Manesh A et al. Randomized clinical trial of antibiotic therapy versus appendectomy as primary treatment of acute appendicitis in unselected patients. *Br J Surg.* May 2009;(5): 473–481.
148. Liu K, Louis F. Use of antibiotics alone for treatment of uncomplicated acute appendicitis: A systematic review and meta-analysis. *Surgery.* 2011;150(4):673–683.
149. Varadhan KK, Keith RN, Dileep NL. Safety and efficacy of antibiotics compared with appendicectomy for treatment of uncomplicated acute appendicitis: Meta-analysis of randomised controlled trials. *BMJ.* 2012;344.
150. Di Saverio S, Sibilio A, Giorgini E et al. The NOTA Study (Non Operative Treatment for Acute Appendicitis): Prospective study on the efficacy and safety of antibiotics (amoxicillin and clavulanic acid) for treating patients with right lower quadrant abdominal pain and long-term follow-up of conservatively treated suspected appendicitis. *Ann Surg.* 2014;260(1):109–117.
151. Wilms IM, De Hoog DE, de Visser DC, Janzing HM. Appendectomy versus antibiotic treatment for acute appendicitis. *Cochrane Database Syst Rev.* 2011;11.
152. Soreide K. Should antibiotic treatment replace appendectomy for acute appendicitis? *Nat Clin Pract Gastroenterol Hepatol.* 2007;4:584–585.

## Commentary on Appendicitis: Evidence-Based Medicine

*Donald E. Fry*

My first experience with appendectomy for appendicitis was in 1970 as a third year medical student. The diagnosis was made strictly by the physical examination by the surgeon. No antibiotics were given before or after the operation. A four-inch incision was made with a traditional McBurney incision. The appendiceal mesentery was divided between surgical clamps and tied with silk ligatures. The appendiceal base was divided between straight clamps with a surgical knife. The appendiceal stump was ligated with a suture of chromic catgut, and then inverted with a figure-of-eight silk ligature. The skin incision was closed with interrupted silk. The patient went home on the second postoperative day.

My career final appendectomy for appendicitis was performed after the patient had a complete abdominal computed tomography, despite my subsequent examination that was classic for acute appendicitis. The patient received a generous dose of piperacillin-tazobactam preoperatively. The operation was performed laparoscopically. The mesentery and appendix were divided with staple cartridges. The port sites were closed with staples. The resident had to be chastised about the inappropriateness of giving postoperative antibiotics. The patient was discharged on the first postoperative day.

The changes in diagnosis and management of the abdominal surgical patient over the last several decades have been numerous, and acute appendicitis is a microcosm of these changes. With changing management and new technology inevitably comes the controversies and debates about "out with the old and in with the new." The questions posed about the diagnosis and management of acute appendicitis in this chapter provides an excellent platform for the discussion about "something old, something new."

### What Clinical Signs and Symptoms Are Most Reliable for the Diagnosis of Appendicitis?

This chapter reinforces the value of a history and well done physical examination of the abdomen when appendicitis is a legitimate consideration for the patient. A 16–40-year-old male with poorly defined midabdominal pain and nausea over the preceding 12–24 h that has migrated to the right lower quadrant and has rebound tenderness on palpation has acute appendicitis. The chapter appropriately identifies the variability of the anatomic location of the appendix and how that can account for unusual presentations. Sensitivity and understanding of the unusual presentations, and the particularly difficult diagnosis in the female of reproductive age are appropriately emphasized and the merits of imaging studies to assist in these circumstances are understood. However, clear and straightforward presentations of the disease should permit the confident clinician to proceed with definitive treatment of the disease.

### What Is the Best Laboratory Test to Help Make the Diagnosis of Appendicitis?

Relative to laboratory studies, another way to conclude this section of the chapter is to say that nothing really works in the difficult case. Seldom have I found that laboratory findings were of significance in the clinical setting where the patient did have the physical findings detailed in section "What clinical signs and symptoms are most reliable for the diagnosis of appendicitis?." It is important to remember that fever, leukocytosis, C-reactive protein, and even procalcitonin are systemic expressions of the activated inflammatory response. Abnormalities of laboratory biomarkers commonly will indicate that something is amiss, but appendicitis may not be it. The more interesting patient is the acute or ruptured appendicitis patient that does not have any abnormalities of these biomarkers. *The activation of the inflammatory response is host dependent and not disease dependent.* The good history and physical examination always trumps the laboratory results.

### Does Giving a Patient with Suspected Pain Medicine Decrease the Ability to Make the Diagnosis?

The authors correctly identify the lack of evidence that pain medications may blunt findings of acute appendicitis. My experience is that Americans have psychological dependence upon taking nonsteroidal anti-inflammatory drugs (NSAIDs). NSAID consumption in the United States is likely measured in tonnage per week. While the chapter focuses on analgesics given once the patient arrives in the healthcare facility, the reality is that it is the unusual patient that has not taken something including some of mom's leftover codeine-NSAID combination from her last illness. I would concur with the authors' conclusion and would suggest that it is the unusual patient that will have symptoms influenced by pain medications when appendicitis is the real diagnosis.

### What Is the Best Imaging Modality to Diagnose Acute Appendicitis?

The authors conclude in this chapter that CT scanning is the best imaging modality for the patient with suspected appendicitis, and I would agree with that conclusion. The use of rectal contrast I believe enhances the accuracy of the CT. Conventional x-rays of the abdomen offer little and ultrasound imaging for appendicitis becomes fraught with interpretation problems. The radiation exposure of CT scanning is getting some attention at present and I have seen estimates that one abdominal CT may expose the patient to 100× the radiation exposure of a chest x-ray. Thus, the MRI scan may well supplant the CT when cost for performance becomes less.

The most important part of this discussion is should CT imaging be employed in every case. CT scanning should not be used in every case, The classic case of migrating abdominal pain into the right lower quadrant in the patient with recent onset anorexia and nausea, who also has rebound tenderness in the right lower quadrant, needs an appendectomy. In the era of laparoscopic appendectomy, this is easily done without appreciable morbidity, pain, or temporary disability. The diagnosis will rarely be wrong and the younger patient, especially women of reproductive age, will avoid the radiation exposure.

### Does Giving Antibiotics to Patients with Appendicitis Who Undergo Appendectomy Decrease Postoperative Infectious Complications?

If diagnostic accuracy permitted the identification of every patient with perforative or gangrenous appendicitis, then those with simple acute appendicitis in the era of laparoscopic appendectomy could safely avoid any antibiotics. A single dose of whatever (piperacillin-tazobactam, or cefazolin-metronidazole, or ertapenem) will provide wound coverage until operative findings dictate whether antibiotics need to be continued after the operation. With gangrene, perforation, or abscess, the antibiotics should be continued but probably not for 5–7 days. When the patient is passing stools, ambulating to the bathroom, and eating food; then stop the antibiotics. *C. difficile* is alive and well and early cessation of systemic drugs when gut function has resumed is in the patient's best interest.

### What Operation Is Better for Treating Acute Appendicitis: Laparoscopic or Open Appendectomy?

The answer to this question is to do what is in the patient's best interest. I would certainly prefer a laparoscopic operation if it were my personal appendicitis. Most patients with appendicitis can be started with the laparoscopic approach and converted to an open operation depending upon operative findings. Arguments about length of operation and length of hospitalization between the two methods are pretty meaningless: laparoscopic appendectomy is less painful and patients return to full activity faster. As this chapter points out, female and overweight patients are best served by laparoscopic appendectomy. For patients with severe sepsis from perforation, open appendectomy may be best to avoid the application of pressure pneumoperitoneum to a septic peritoneal cavity. Open surgical incisions are often left open for the mythical delayed primary closure. All are usually closed by secondary intention. The dogma of using delayed primary closure has been challenged by Brasel et al.*. More evidence is needed to evaluate the true merits of leaving surgical wounds open, versus local strategies (topical antimicrobials, wound wicks, etc.) that may obviate the open wound.

### Is Interval Appendectomy Necessary?

The evidence presented by the authors is convincing that interval appendectomy is not necessary. Conventional wisdom would dictate that if a patient had an initial episode of acute appendicitis, then they should be at increased risk for a second episode. One would expect that scarring and deformity of the appendix should make this so. With modest experience in interval appendectomies, I have been impressed at the normal anatomic appearance of the appendix at these interval procedures. If patients have recurrent symptoms, then interval appendectomy would appear to be justified.

### Should Antibiotic Treatment Replace Appendectomy for Acute Appendicitis?

The use of antibiotics for the treatment of acute appendicitis would appear to me to be a suspension of common sense. With acute appendicitis in the current environment, a laparoscopic appendectomy fixes the pathologic condition and sends the patient back home the following day. A 7–10-day course of antibiotics with much of that being administered in the hospital hardly seems to be cost-effective care. Furthermore, the patient still has the appendix for future additional episodes. Gangenous and perforated acute appendicitis is not always defined at the time of presentation and the antibiotic management of these cases can turn into issues of complications and lengthy stay at the hospital. Obviously, if the patient has an appendiceal phegmon that is identified by a mass on physical examination or by CT scan, then antibiotic management is in the patient's best interest.

In conclusion, this chapter provides an excellent insight into current diagnosis and management of acute appendicitis. Changes of the next 40–50 years in management will be most interesting.

---

* Brasel KJ, Borgstrom DC, Weigelt JA. Cost-utility of contaminated appendectomy wounds. *J Am Coll Surg*. 1997;184:23–30.

# 49

# *Lower Gastrointestinal Bleeding*

**Rachel E. Beard and Steven D. Schwaitzberg**

**CONTENTS**



## 49.1 Introduction

The diagnosis of lower gastrointestinal bleeding (LGIB) begins with two basic principles. First, the surgeon must have a clear picture of the nature of the blood loss differentiating bright red blood per rectum (BRBPR) from maroon stool and these from true melena. This gives the physician a first-order approximation as to the site of bleeding leading to the second principle, which is to rule out an upper gastrointestinal source very early in the workup. There are classic challenges for selecting the best therapeutic option for a given patient that require surgeons to make thoughtful choices based on the available data in the context of the status of individual patients. The other realization that must be confronted is that each hospital is different in terms of resource availability. Nuclear medicine or angiographic expertise may be limited to weekdays during business hours or not available at all in some settings. These realities force surgeons to have intimate familiarity of the effectiveness of all the diagnostic and therapeutic options required in the diagnosis and management of LGIB. This is particularly challenging since the nature of the clinical problem does not lend itself easily to randomized controlled trials. Review of the available literature reveals few prospective studies as well.

## 49.2 What Is the Diagnostic Accuracy of Technetium-99m (Tc-99m) Sulfur Colloid Injection versus Tc-99m Tagged Red Cells?

In 1982, Alavi reported on the utility of intravenous administration of Tc-99m sulfur colloid [1] (level 4 evidence). His group cited potential hemorrhage detection at bleeding rates as low as 0.5 mL/min allowing for detection even in patients with negative arteriography. In 1983, Winn retrospectively reviewed 63 patients studied with this technique [2] (level 4 evidence). He found that the likelihood of a positive arteriogram was 15% when Tc-99m sulfur colloid was negative. Miskowak demonstrated 85% sensitivity and 100% specificity when technetium-labeled red cells were used to diagnose LGIB [3] (level 4 evidence). Markisk found similar accuracy (91%) and no occurrence of positive angiography when scintigraphy was negative [4] (level 4 evidence). An early comparative study is that of Siddiqui and colleagues who performed a comparison of Tc-99m sulfur colloid (SC) and Tc-99m tagged RBC scintigraphy in 27 patients prospectively [5] (level 1b evidence). They found far greater sensitivity in the tagged red cell group with 70% of the studies destined to be positive diagnostic in the first hour, although animal studies demonstrated similar sensitivity for both techniques [6]. Some retrospective studies demonstrate similar rates of detection of bleeding with Tc-99m SC and Tc-99m tagged RBC scintigraphy (24% vs. 28%, respectively), and suggest that the simpler and quicker Tc-99m is more useful in clinical practice [7] (level 4 evidence). However, the majority of studies have shown that when compared to Tc-99m SC, Tc-99-labeled RBCs are more sensitive, though somewhat less specific, are useful as a screen for angiography since contrast studies are rarely positive in scintigraphy-negative patients [7–17] (level 4 evidence). It is pointed out in nearly all of these studies that the anatomic accuracy of Tc-99-labeled positive scan is in the 70%–85% range. Recent studies suggest that the rate of accurate localization of a bleeding site may be even lower (39%–48%), and suggest using criteria such as greater than 2u PRBC transfused as selection criteria for patients to scan [18,19] (level 4 evidence). Rapid transit of tagged hemorrhaged red cells within the lumen of the colon is cited for this discrepancy, and because of this and the fact that many scans performed are negative, Levy pointed out that the resection site utility of Tc-99-labeled RBCs is a small percentage of all scans performed [21] (level 4 evidence). Ng suggests that the angiographic yield could be further refined by selecting only patients whose scintigraphy is positive early after injection [22] (level 4 evidence).

*Recommendation*: Tc-99-labeled RBCs appear to demonstrate superior sensitivity to Tc-99 sulfur colloid injection in the detection of LGIB (Grade B Recommendation). Angiography is not indicated when scintigraphy is negative (Grade C Recommendation). The utility of Tc-99-labeled RBC scanning is limited by the poor predictive value of the anatomic location of bleeding, therefore positive scans should be followed up with further localization studies to improve anatomic accuracy (Grade C Recommendation).

## 49.3 What Is the Diagnostic Accuracy of Colonoscopy, Radionuclide Scanning, Computed Tomography (CT), and Angiography in the Setting of LGIB?

Neither scintigraphy nor angiography alone is a sufficient guide for surgical resection. Hunter pointed that as many as 42% of patients could have an undesirable result if a limited surgical procedure was planned on the basis of Tc-99-labeled RBCs alone [23] (level 4 evidence). Whitaker demonstrated that angiography alone is also of limited sensitivity and specificity [24] (level 4 evidence). As noted above, the yield can be improved with pre-angiography scintigraphy. Furthermore, surgical site resection utility of angiography was noted to be low in a retrospective study by Cohn in 1998 [25] (level 4 evidence) where only 12% of the angiograms were useful in selecting the site of colon resection, noting an 11% complication rate from angiography.

Angiography and panendoscopy were first compared in 55 patients in 1976 with comparable accuracy [26] (level 3b evidence). Chaudhry studied 85 patients where unprepped colonoscopy was performed as the initial evaluation in cases of suspected LGIB. They concluded that this method was 95% sensitive and allowed for concomitant therapeutic control in 63% of the patients with active bleeding. In addition, they were able to diagnose that the source of bleeding was proximal to the ileocecal valve in 10% of the total patients studied [27] (level 4 evidence). Early colonoscopy is associated with shorter hospitalizations [28] (level 4 evidence). Haykir evaluated the diagnostic accuracy of MR colonography and CT colonography with conventional colonoscopy. MR was slightly more accurate than CT and close to conventional colonoscopy in sensitivity with discovery of the lesion 96% of the time [29] (level 3b evidence).

Computed tomography has been increasingly utilized to evaluate LGIB. Several authors have studied computed tomographic angiography (CTA) and found this method to be 70%–80% sensitive and 100% specific for evaluating colonic angiodysplasia and other GI sources [30–32] (level 4 evidence). Jaeckle evaluated the accuracy of multi-detector row helical CT (MDCT) for detection and localization of hemorrhage. They found MDCT to be 92% accurate with ongoing bleeding frequently demonstrated [33] (level 4 evidence). In a prospective study of 26 patients for massive GI bleeding, Yoon demonstrated that arterial phase MDCT was about 90% sensitive, 99% specific with an overall accuracy rate of 88%. The negative predictive value was 98%, suggesting formal angiography would not be indicated in MDCT-negative studies [34] (level 3b evidence). This test was found to be readily available and sufficiently sensitive for Duchesne and others to recommend MDCT as the initial screen for LGIB especially in light of its rapidity and noninvasiveness [35,36] (level 4–5 evidence). Wu performed a meta-analysis of 9 studies with 198 patients comparing the accuracy of CTA to other modalities including endoscopy, colonoscopy, angiography, and surgery, and determined that CT is cost-effective and accurate at diagnosing the location of acute GI bleeding, with a pooled sensitivity of 89% and specificity of 85% [37] (level 3a evidence).

*Recommendation*: Colonoscopy when available is the most accurate method of diagnosing LGIB and is the gold standard against which other studies are measured, offering control of bleeding from some lesions as well (Grade C Recommendation). Scintigraphy may offer valuable information for angiographic screening but is insufficient for operative planning alone (Grade C Recommendation). MDCT is highly sensitive and specific at detecting ongoing GI bleeding, and its rapidity, cost-effectiveness, and noninvasiveness make it an ideal first-line test to direct further management (Grade C recommendation).

## 49.4 What Is the Ideal Single Test in the Setting of LGIB?

The critical purpose for performing diagnostic testing in LGIB is to rule out the presence of bleeding above the ileocecal valve which has been noted above to be as high as 9% of patients presenting for evaluation [20,33]. Chaudhry and colleagues suggest that colonoscopy is an accurate single-stage evaluation for LGIB [33] (level 4 evidence). Since this is an invasive procedure, it may not always be readily available. It has been demonstrated that the yield from angiography for all comers is low [27] (level 4 evidence). Furthermore in this potentially volume-depleted population, the incidence of complications from contrast angiography has been underappreciated [25] (level 4 evidence). The positive predictive value of either scintigraphy or MDCT is sufficient to utilize either of these tests prior to angiography [16–18,30,31] (level 4 evidence). One randomized controlled trial comparing urgent colonoscopy to angiographic intervention with expectant colonoscopy found that though a definite source of bleeding was found more often in the urgent colonoscopy group, there was no difference in outcomes including mortality, hospital stay, transfusion requirement, and rebleeding [38] (level 1b evidence).

*Recommendation*: Colonoscopy is the ideal single test in the face of LGIB. Compared to angiography, colonoscopy is better at identifying a source of bleed, though it may not improve clinical outcomes (Grade B recommendation). In the event this is not available and an intervention is required, scintigraphy or MDCT should be performed to rule out proximal sources in the small bowel prior to angiographic embolization/vasopressin or surgical resection.

## 49.5 What Is the Preferred Timing of Colonoscopy for LGIB and the Effect on Clinical Outcomes?

Retrospective studies demonstrate that colonoscopy during hospitalization for LGIB is associated with increased likelihood of discharge, and that an early colonoscopy (within 24 h of admission) predicted earlier hospital discharge [39,40] (level 4 evidence). A nationwide cross-sectional study also examined this issue and also demonstrated that colonoscopy within the first 24 h of hospitalization is associated with a statistically significantly decreased length of hospital stay (2.9 vs. 4.6 days, $p < 0.001$), decreased need for blood transfusion (45% vs. 54%, $p < 0.001$), and decreased hospitalization costs ($22,123 vs. $28,749, $p < 0.001$), though no difference in mortality was observed [41] (level 4 evidence). A subsequent 2010 trial randomized 72 LGIB patients to either urgent (within 12 h of presentation) or elective (36–60 h after presentation) colonoscopy and no differences in rebleeding, transfusions, length of stay, or hospital charges was observed; however, the small study size and suggestion of more severe bleeding in the urgent colonoscopy arm patients make it difficult to draw conclusions from this study [42] (level 2b evidence).

*Recommendation*: Colonoscopy performed early in the clinical course may lead to decreased length of hospital stay and hospitalization costs, however, there is insufficient evidence to suggest that it has an impact on clinical outcomes (Grade C recommendation).

## 49.6 What Is the Clinical Effectiveness of Intra-Arterial Vasopressin Infusion versus Transcatheter Embolization?

Athanasoulis reported successful cessation of bleeding in 22 of 24 patients (92%) with hemorrhage from colonic diverticulosis utilizing selective intra-arterial vasopressin [44] (level 4 evidence), 14 of these 24 patients underwent surgical resection (58%) for persistent hemorrhage, early rebleeding, late rebleeding or planned resection. Similar control has been reported by others [45] (level 4 evidence). In a 3 year review of medically compromised patients utilizing intra-arterial vasopressin, a 63% success rate in controlling colonic hemorrhage was demonstrated. Rebleeding occurred in 16% of these patients with high morbidity and mortality [46] (level 4 evidence). Browder found similar results with 90% of patients controlled with intra-arterial vasopressin but a 50% rebleed

**TABLE 49.1**

Question Summary

| Question | Answer | Grade of Recommendation | Level of Evidence | References |
|---|---|---|---|---|
| What is the diagnostic accuracy of Tc-99 sulfur colloid injection versus Tc-99 tagged red cells? | Tc-99-labeled RBCs appear to demonstrate superior sensitivity to Tc-99 sulfur colloid injection in the detection of LGIB. | B | 1b | [5] |
| | Angiography is not indicated when scintigraphy is negative. | C | 4 | [7–20] |
| | The utility of Tc-99-labeled RBC scanning limited by the poor predictive value of the anatomic location of bleeding, therefore positive scans should be followed up with further localization studies to improve anatomic accuracy. | C | 4 | [18–22] |
| What is the diagnostic accuracy of colonoscopy, radionuclide scanning, and angiography in the setting of LGIB? | Colonoscopy when available is the most accurate method of diagnosing LGIB and is the gold standard against which other studies are measured offering control of some lesions as well. | C | 4 | [27–29] |
| | Scintigraphy may offer valuable information for angiographic screening but is insufficient for operative planning alone. | C | 4 | [11–25] |
| | MDCT is highly sensitive and specific at detecting ongoing GI bleeding, and its rapidity, cost-effectiveness, and noninvasiveness make it an ideal first-line test to direct further management. | C | 3a, 3b, 4, 5 | [26,27,35–37] |
| What is the ideal single test in the setting of LGIB? | Colonoscopy is the ideal single test in the face of LGIB. Compared to angiography, upfront colonoscopy is better at identifying a source of bleeding, though it may not improve clinical outcomes. | B | 1b, 4 | [20,24,28,33,38] |
| | In the event this is not available and an intervention is required, scintigraphy or MDCT should be performed to rule out proximal sources in the small bowel prior to angiographic embolization/vasopressin or surgical resection. | C | 4 | [16–18,25–27,33] |
| What is the preferred timing of colonoscopy for LGIB and the effect on clinical outcomes? | Colonoscopy performed early in the clinical course may lead to decreased length of hospital stay and hospitalization costs, however, there is insufficient evidence to suggest that it has an impact on clinical outcomes. | C | 2b, 4 | [39–42] |
| What is the clinical effectiveness intra-arterial vasopressin infusion versus transcatheter embolization? | The major drawbacks of vasopressin therapy are coronary ischemia and rebleeding after cessation of therapy. Cessation of bleeding occurs in up to 90% of patients. Some studies have shown significant rebleeding after therapy is stopped. | No recommendations | 4 | [43–47] |
| | On the other hand, embolic therapy shows a similar rate of initial hemorrhage control with less early rebleeding, however, there is about a 10% risk of significant colon ischemia. Super-selective embolism has not eliminated ischemia as a risk. | | 4 | [45,48–51,56] |
| | The late rebleeding risk is 10%–15% with either technique. | | 4 | [52] |
| What are the criteria for surgical intervention in LGIB and what operation should be done? | Patients who bleed two or more units of blood should receive an evaluation to localize the source of bleeding expeditiously. | C | 4 | [57,60] |
| | Stable patients without massive bleeding should not be considered for surgery as many of these episodes will resolve either spontaneously or with less invasive therapies such as barium enema. | C | 4 | [68–73] |
| | Persistent bleeding with true anatomic localization may allow for segmental resection otherwise subtotal colectomy with ileorectostomy should be performed. | C | 4 | [29,59–66,74] |
| | If transfusion requirement is approaching 10 units, surgery should be seriously considered. Other factors, such as hypotension on presentation, the presence of comorbidities, and localization of left-sided bleeding should prompt consideration for earlier operative therapy, as complications of urgent surgery may be unacceptably high. | C | 4 | [66–68,74–76] |

rate upon cessation of therapy [47] (level 4 evidence). Other authors have reported lower success rates in the 35% range with this technique [43] (level 4 evidence). Similarly, there are numerous series reporting of control of LGIB with intra-arterial embolization with similar or better success to vasopressin; however, nearly all of these reported a higher incidence of complication of the therapy (i.e., the embolus vs. the pharmacologic agent) with embolization, most notably colonic necrosis [45,48–51] (level 4 evidence). Gomes compared these techniques in a single hospital retrospective review and found similar rates of hemorrhage control but a higher rate of rebleeding in the vasopressin group [52] (level 4 evidence).

Patel and Nawawi have recently advocated "super"-selective embolization to minimize colonic ischemia with good hemorrhage control in a small series [51,53,54] (level 4 evidence). Preclinical data in a porcine model support the theory that "super"-selective embolization may enhance the safety of this technique [46]. Burgess and Kickuth, however, reported colonic necrosis even with this technique [54–56] (level 4 evidence).

*Recommendation*: The major drawbacks of vasopressin therapy are coronary ischemia and rebleeding after cessation of therapy. Cessation of bleeding occurs in up to 90% of patients. Some studies have shown significant rebleeding after therapy is stopped. On the other hand, embolic therapy shows a similar rate of initial hemorrhage control with less early rebleeding, however, there is about a 10% risk of significant colon ischemia. Superselective embolization techniques have not entirely eliminated ischemia as a risk. The late rebleeding risk is 10%–15% with either technique (no recommendations).

## 49.7 What Are the Criteria for Surgical Intervention in LGIB and What Operation Should Be Done?

The desire to localize bleeding must be tempered with the need to make timely surgical intervention. The benefit of extensive preoperative testing must be balanced against the impact of delayed care [57] (level 4 evidence). In the case of LGIB, it is warranted to avoid colonic resection for sources proximal to the ileocecal valve [57]. Localization of massive LGIB lowers perioperative mortality when compared to blind resection, but even with appropriate localization, mortality remains in the 8%–18% range [43,47,58] (level 4 evidence). Ideally surgical resection for LGIB should be limited to patients likely to continue to bleed or rebleed and localized to the bleeding segment [59,60]. Authors have disagreed about the morbidity of emergent subtotal colon resection (SCR) for bleeding that is not localizable. The majority of studies suggest SCR, which allows for the preservation of continence, is well tolerated and associated with a low rebleeding rate [29,61–64] (level 4 evidence) though a few studies demonstrate a high morbidity (20%–42%) and mortality (17%–33%), primarily due to sepsis as a sequelae of anastomotic leak [65–67] (level 4 evidence).

Not every patient with LGIB requires colonic resection. MacGuire showed that bleeding stopped spontaneously in 75% of episodes, and that number rose to 99% in cases where less than four units of blood were transfused over 24 h. Conversely, among patients who received more than four units in 24 h, 60% required emergency surgery [68] (level 4 evidence). In retrospective series where the average transfusion requirement was three units or less as many as 97% of patients could be managed nonoperatively [69–71] (level 4 evidence). Therapeutic barium enema has been used in first episode of diverticular bleeding with good effect allowing some patients to avoid resection, and has been shown to be as effective as endoscopic therapy for the prevention of recurrent diverticular bleeding [72,73] (level 4 evidence).

Authors have varied on recommendations to resect based on transfusion requirements. Patients presenting to the emergency department with hypotension should be considered for earlier resection [74] (level 4 evidence). Earlier resection (6–9 units) was associated with lower perioperative mortality [66,75] (level 4 evidence). The presence of comorbidities including diabetes and gouty arthritis has been shown to potentially increase the risk of urgent surgery and it may be appropriate to operate on these patients earlier in an attempt to reduce perioperative morbidity [67] (level 4 evidence). Some studies also suggest that segmental resections for left-sided disease have increased morbidity and mortality as compared to right-sided disease [76] (level 4 evidence).

*Recommendation*: Patients who bleed two or more units of blood should receive an evaluation to localize the source of bleeding expeditiously (Grade C recommendation). Stable patients without massive bleeding should not be considered for surgery as many of these episodes will resolve either spontaneously or with less invasive therapies such as barium enema (Grade C recommendation). Persistent bleeding with true anatomic localization may allow for segmental resection otherwise subtotal colectomy with ileorectostomy should be performed (Grade C recommendation). If transfusion requirement is approaching 10 units, surgery should be seriously considered. Other factors, such as hypotension on presentation, the presence of comorbidities, and localization of left-sided bleeding should prompt consideration for earlier operative therapy, as complication rates of urgent surgery may be unacceptably high (Grade C recommendation) (Table 49.1).

## References


1. Alavi A. Detection of gastrointestinal bleeding with 99mTc-sulfur colloid. *Semin Nucl Med.* 1982;12:126–138.
2. Winn M, Weissmann HS, Sprayregen S, Freeman LM. The radionuclide detection of lower gastrointestinal bleeding sites. *Clin Nucl Med.* 1983;8:389–395.
3. Miskowiak J, Nielsen SL, Munck O. Scintigraphic diagnosis of gastrointestinal bleeding with 99mTc-labeled blood-pool agents. *Radiology.* 1981;141:499–504.
4. Markisz JA, Front D, Royal HD, Sacks B, Parker JA, Kolodny GM. An evaluation of 99mTc-labeled red blood cell scintigraphy for the detection and localization of gastrointestinal bleeding sites. *Gastroenterology.* 1982;83:394–398.
5. Siddiqui AR, Schauwecker DS, Wellman HN, Mock BH. Comparison of technetium-99m sulfur colloid and in vitro labeled technetium-99m RBCs in the detection of gastrointestinal bleeding. *Clin Nucl Med.* 1985;10:546–549.
6. Thorne DA, Datz FL, Remley K, Christian PE. Bleeding rates necessary for detecting acute gastrointestinal bleeding with technetium-99m-labeled red blood cells in an experimental model. *J Nucl Med.* 1987;28:514–520.
7. Ponzo F, Zhuang H, Liu FM, Lacorte LB, Moussavian B, Wang S, Alavi A. Tc-99m sulfur colloid and Tc-99m tagged red blood cell methods are comparable for detecting lower gastrointestinal bleeding in clinical practice. *Clin Nucl Med.* 2002;27:405–409.
8. Friedman HI, Hilts SV, Whitney PJ. Use of technetium-labeled autologous red blood cells in detection of gastrointestinal bleeding. *Surg Gynecol Obstet.* 1983;156:449–452.
9. Rosenkilde Olsen P, Nielsen L, Dyrbye M, Kuld Hansen L. Colorectal bleeding localized with gamma camera. *Acta Chir Scand.* 1983;149:793–795.
10. Orecchia PM, Hensley EK, McDonald PT, Lull RJ. Localization of lower gastrointestinal hemorrhage. Experience with red blood cells labeled in vitro with technetium Tc 99m. *Arch Surg.* 1985;120:621–624.
11. Bearn P, Persad R, Wilson N, Flanagan J, Williams T. 99mTechnetium-labelled red blood cell scintigraphy as an alternative to angiography in the investigation of gastrointestinal bleeding: Clinical experience in a district general hospital. *Ann R Coll Surg Engl.* 1992;74:192–199.
12. Wang CS, Tzen KY, Huang MJ, Wang JY, Chen MF. Localization of obscure gastrointestinal bleeding by technetium 99m-labeled red blood cell scintigraphy. *J Formos Med Assoc.* 1992;91:63–68.
13. Dusold R, Burke K, Carpentier W, Dyck WP. The accuracy of technetium-99m-labeled red cell scintigraphy in localizing gastrointestinal bleeding. *Am J Gastroenterol.* 1994;89:345–348.
14. Rantis PC, Jr., Harford FJ, Wagner RH, Henkin RE. Technetium-labelled red blood cell scintigraphy: Is it useful in acute lower gastrointestinal bleeding? *Int J Colorectal Dis.* 1995;10:210–215.
15. Dolezal J, Vizd'a J, Bures J. Detection of acute gastrointestinal bleeding by means of technetium-99m in vivo labelled red blood cells. *Nucl Med Rev Cent East Eur.* 2002;5:151–154.
16. Howarth DM, Tang K, Lees W. The clinical utility of nuclear medicine imaging for the detection of occult gastrointestinal haemorrhage. *Nucl Med Commun.* 2002;23:591–594.
17. Emslie JT, Zarnegar K, Siegel ME, Beart RW, Jr. Technetium-99m-labeled red blood cell scans in the investigation of gastrointestinal bleeding. *Dis Colon Rectum.* 1996;39:750–754.
18. Gutierrez C, Mariano M, Vander Laan T, Wang A, Faddis DM, Stain SC. The use of technetium-labeled erythrocyte scintigraphy in the evaluation and treatment of lower gastrointestinal hemorrhage. *Am Surg.* 1998;64:989–992.
19. Olds GD, Cooper GS, Chak A, Sivak MV, Jr., Chitale AA, Wong RC. The yield of bleeding scans in acute lower gastrointestinal hemorrhage. *J Clin Gastroenterol.* 2005;39:273–277.
20. Tabiban JH, Wong Kee Song LM, Enders FB, Aquet JC, Tabiban A. Technetium-labeled erythrocyte scintigraphy in acute gastrointestinal bleeding. *Int J Colorectal Dis.* 2013;28:1099–1105.
21. Levy R, Barto W, Gani J. Retrospective study of the utility of nuclear scintigraphic-labelled red cell scanning for lower gastrointestinal bleeding. *ANZ J Surg.* 2003;73:205–209.
22. Ng DA, Opelka FG, Beck DE et al. Predictive value of technetium Tc 99m-labeled red blood cell scintigraphy for positive angiogram in massive lower gastrointestinal hemorrhage. *Dis Colon Rectum.* 1997;40:471–477.
23. Hunter JM, Pezim ME. Limited value of technetium 99m-labeled red cell scintigraphy in localization of lower gastrointestinal bleeding. *Am J Surg.* 1990;159:504–506.
24. Whitaker SC, Gregson RH. The role of angiography in the investigation of acute or chronic gastrointestinal haemorrhage. *Clin Radiol.* 1993;47:382–388.
25. Cohn SM, Moller BA, Zieg PM, Milner KA, Angood PB. Angiography for preoperative evaluation in patients with lower gastrointestinal bleeding: Are the benefits worth the risks? *Arch Surg.* 1998;133:50–55.
26. Butler ML, Johnson LF, Clark R. Diagnostic accuracy of fiberoptic panendoscopy and visceral angiography in acute upper gastrointestinal bleeding. *Am J Gastroenterol.* 1976;65:501–511.
27. Chaudhry V, Hyser MJ, Gracias VH, Gau FC. Colonoscopy: The initial test for acute lower gastrointestinal bleeding. *Am Surg.* 1998;64:723–728.
28. Strate LL, Syngal S. Predictors of utilization of early colonoscopy vs. radiography for severe lower intestinal bleeding. *Gastrointest Endosc.* 2005;61:46–52.
29. Haykir R, Karakose S, Karabacakoglu A, Sahin M, Kayacetin E. Three-dimensional MR and axial CT colonography versus conventional colonoscopy for detection of colon pathologies. *World J Gastroenterol.* 2006;12:2345–2350.
30. Junquera F, Quiroga S, Saperas E et al. Accuracy of helical computed tomographic angiography for the diagnosis of colonic angiodysplasia. *Gastroenterology.* 2000;119:293–299.

31. Ernst O, Bulois P, Saint-Drenant S, Leroy C, Paris JC, Sergent G. Helical CT in acute lower gastrointestinal bleeding. *Eur Radiol.* 2003;13:114–117.
32. Yamaguchi T, Yoshikawa K. Enhanced CT for initial localization of active lower gastrointestinal bleeding. *Abdom Imaging.* 2003;28:634–636.
33. Jaeckle T, Stuber G, Hoffmann MH, Jeltsch M, Schmitz BL, Aschoff AJ. Detection and localization of acute upper and lower gastrointestinal (GI) bleeding with arterial phase multi-detector row helical CT. *Eur Radiol.* 2008;18:1406–1413.
34. Yoon W, Jeong YY, Shin SS et al. Acute massive gastrointestinal bleeding: Detection and localization with arterial phase multi-detector row helical CT. *Radiology.* 2006;239:160–167.
35. Duchesne J, Jacome T, Serou M et al. CT-angiography for the detection of a lower gastrointestinal bleeding source. *Am Surg.* 2005;71:392–397.
36. Lee S, Welman CJ, Ramsay D. Investigation of acute lower gastrointestinal bleeding with 16- and 64-slice multidetector CT. *J Med Imaging Radiat Oncol.* 2009;53:56–63.
37. Wu LM, Xu JR, Yin Y, Qu XH. Usefulness of CT angiography in diagnosing acute gastrointestinal bleeding: A meta-analysis. *World J Gastroenterol.* 2010:3957–3963.
38. Green BT, Rockey DC, Portwood G et al. Urgent colonoscopy for evaluation and management of acute lower gastrointestinal hemorrhage: A randomized controlled trial. *Am J Gastroenterol.* 2005;100:2395–2402.
39. Schmulewitz N, Fisher DA, Rockey DC. Early colonoscopy for acute lower GI bleeding predicts shorter hospital stay: A retrospective study of experience in a single center. *Gastrointest Endosc.* 2003;58:841–846.
40. Strate LL, Syngal S. Timing of colonoscopy: Impact on length of hospital stay in patients with acute lower intestinal bleeding. *Am J Gastroenterol.* 2003;98:317–322.
41. Navaneethan U, Njei B, Venkatesh PG, Sanaka MR. Timing of colonoscopy and outcomes in patients with lower GI bleeding: A nationwide population-based study. *Gastrointest Endosc.* 2014;79:297–306.
42. Laine L, Shah A. Randomized trial of urgent vs. elective colonoscopy in patients hospitalized with lower GI bleeding. *Am J Gastroenterol.* 2010;105:2636–2641.
43. Leitman IM, Paull DE, Shires GT, 3rd. Evaluation and management of massive lower gastrointestinal hemorrhage. *Ann Surg.* 1989;209:175–180.
44. Athanasoulis CA, Baum S, Rosch J et al. Mesenteric arterial infusions of vasopressin for hemorrhage from colonic diverticulosis. *Am J Surg.* 1975;129:212–216.
45. Waltman AC. Transcatheter embolization versus vasopressin infusion for the control of arteriocapillary gastrointestinal bleeding. *Cardiovasc Intervent Radiol.* 1980;3:289–295.
46. Sherman LM, Shenoy SS, Cerra FB. Selective intra-arterial vasopressin: Clinical efficacy and complications. *Ann Surg.* 1979;189:298–302.
47. Browder W, Cerise EJ, Litwin MS. Impact of emergency angiography in massive lower gastrointestinal bleeding. *Ann Surg.* 1986;204:530–536.
48. Rahn NH, 3rd, Tishler JM, Han SY, Russinovich NA. Diagnostic and interventional angiography in acute gastrointestinal hemorrhage. *Radiology.* 1982;143:361–366.
49. Rosenkrantz H, Bookstein JJ, Rosen RJ, Goff WB, 2nd, Healy JF. Postembolic colonic infarction. *Radiology.* 1982;142:47–51.
50. Patel TH, Cordts PR, Abcarian P, Sawyer MA. Will transcatheter embolotherapy replace surgery in the treatment of gastrointestinal bleeding? *Curr Surg.* 2001;58:323–327.
51. DeBarros J, Rosas L, Cohen J, Vignati P, Sardella W, Hallisey M. The changing paradigm for the treatment of colonic hemorrhage: Superselective angiographic embolization. *Dis Colon Rectum.* 2002;45:802–808.
52. Gomes AS, Lois JF, McCoy RD. Angiographic treatment of gastrointestinal hemorrhage: Comparison of vasopressin infusion and embolization. *AJR.* 1986;146:1031–1037.
53. Nawawi O, Young N, So S. Superselective coil embolization in gastrointestinal haemorrhage: Early experience. *Australas Radiol.* 2006;50:21–26.
54. Kickuth R, Rattunde H, Gschossmann J, Inderbitzin D, Ludwig K, Triller J. Acute lower gastrointestinal hemorrhage: Minimally invasive management with microcatheter embolization. *J Vasc Interv Radiol.* 2008;19:1289–1296 e2.
55. Chin AC, Singer MA, Mihalov M et al. Superselective mesenteric embolization with microcoils in a porcine model. *Dis Colon Rectum.* 2002;45:212–218.
56. Burgess AN, Evans PM. Lower gastrointestinal haemorrhage and superselective angiographic embolization. *ANZ J Surg.* 2004;74:635–638.
57. Rozycki GS, Tremblay L, Feliciano DV et al. Three hundred consecutive emergent celiotomies in general surgery patients: Influence of advanced diagnostic imaging techniques and procedures on diagnosis. *Ann Surg.* 2002;235:681–688; discussion 8–9.
58. Kouraklis G, Misiakos E, Karatzas G, Gogas J, Skalkeas G. Diagnostic approach and management of active lower gastrointestinal hemorrhage. *Int Surg.* 1995;80:138–140.
59. So JB, Kok K, Ngoi SS. Right-sided colonic diverticular disease as a source of lower gastrointestinal bleeding. *Am Surg.* 1999;65:299–302.
60. Strate LL, Saltzman JR, Ookubo R, Mutinga ML, Syngal S. Validation of a clinical prediction rule for severe acute lower intestinal bleeding. *Am J Gastroenterol.* 2005;100:1821–1827.
61. Renzulli P, Maurer CA, Netzer P, Dinkel HP, Buchler MW. Subtotal colectomy with primary ileorectostomy is effective for localized diverticular hemorrhage. *Langenbecks Arch Surg.* 2002;387:67–71.
62. Baker R, Senagore A. Abdominal colectomy offers safe management for massive lower GI bleed. *Am Surg.* 1994;60:578–581; discussion 82.
63. Farner R, Lichliter W, Kuhn J, Fisher T. Total colectomy versus limited colonic resection for acute lower gastrointestinal bleeding. *Am J Surg.* 1999;178:587–591.
64. Field RJ, Sr., Field RJ, Jr., Shackleford S. Total abdominal colectomy for control of massive lower gastrointestinal bleeding. *J Miss State Med Assoc.* 1994;35:29–33.

65. Setya V, Singer JA, Minken SL. Subtotal colectomy as a last resort for unrelenting, unlocalized, lower gastrointestinal hemorrhage: Experience with 12 cases. *Am Surg.* 1992;58:295–299.
66. Plummer JM, Gibson TN, Mitchell DI, Herbert J, Henry T. Emergency subtotal colectomy for lower gastrointestinal haemorrhage: Over-utilised or under-estimate? *Int J Clin Pract.* 2009;63:865–868.
67. Chen CY, Wu CC, Jao SW, Pai L, Hsiao CW. Colonic diverticular bleeding with comorbid diseases may need elective colectomy. *J Gastrointest Surg.* 2009;13:516–520.
68. McGuire HH, Jr. Bleeding colonic diverticula. A reappraisal of natural history and management. *Ann Surg.* 1994;220:653–656.
69. Bokhari M, Vernava AM, Ure T, Longo WE. Diverticular hemorrhage in the elderly—Is it well tolerated? *Dis Colon Rectum.* 1996;39:191–195.
70. Al Qahtani AR, Satin R, Stern J, Gordon PH. Investigative modalities for massive lower gastrointestinal bleeding. *World J Surg.* 2002;26:620–605.
71. Buttenschoen K, Buttenschoen DC, Odermath R, Beger HG. Diverticular disease-associated hemorrhage in the elderly. *Langenbecks Arch Surg.* 2001;386:8–16.
72. Koperna T, Kisser M, Reiner G, Schulz F. Diagnosis and treatment of bleeding colonic diverticula. *Hepatogastroenterology.* 2001;48:702–705.
73. Fujimoto A, Sato S, Kurakata H, Nakano S, Igarashi Y. Effectiveness of high-dose barium enema filling for colonic diverticular bleeding. *Colorectal Dis.* 2011;13:896–898.
74. Rios A, Montoya MJ, Rodriguez JM et al. Severe acute lower gastrointestinal bleeding: Risk factors for morbidity and mortality. *Langenbecks Arch Surg.* 2007;392:165–171.
75. Clarke CS, Afifi AY. Impact of blood transfusion on outcome in patients admitted for gastrointestinal hemorrhage. *Curr Surg.* 2000;57:493–496.
76. Oh HK, Han EC, Ha HK, Choe EK, Moon SH, Ryoo SB, Jeong SY, Park KJ. Surgical management of colonic diverticular disease: Discrepancy between right- and left-sided diseases. *World J Gastroenterol.* 2014:20:10115–10120.

## Commentary on Lower Gastrointestinal Bleeding

*Mark Y. Sun and Robert D. Madoff*

Although it is conceptually simple, lower gastrointestinal bleeding (LGIB) can be one of the most frustrating, and therefore difficult, problems commonly encountered in clinical practice. Unfortunately, despite the many advances in medical and surgical technology over the last few decades, their impact on the management and subsequent success in the treatment of LGIB has to date been very limited.

Just like in real estate, the three most important factors in the treatment of GI bleeding are location, location, and location. Once the site of the bleeding has been accurately identified, treatment becomes relatively straightforward. Whether it is through an angiographic, endoscopic, surgical, or combined approach, in almost all cases, the bleeding is eventually controlled. Unfortunately, accurate identification of the bleeding site can be an elusive goal, and not uncommonly, imaging can actually be misleading.

It is important to rule out an upper GI bleed in cases where the source remains unclear. Although the patient's history often suggests about the general area of the GI tract that is bleeding, rapid hemorrhage can make an upper GI source appear to be lower due to the rapid transit of fresh red blood. If the source of bleeding in the lower GI tract is doubtful, an upper endoscopy, push enteroscopy, or capsule endoscopy should be performed prior to any surgical intervention.

Anal bleeding is an uncommon source of severe LGIB but should be excluded by anoscopy. Severe anal hemorrhage is most commonly seen in the setting of portal hypertension, with anal varices (not hemorrhoids!) as the cause. These are best treated by a transjugular intrahepatic portosystemic shunt (TIPS). When TIPS is not feasible or contraindicated, the varices should be oversewn in the operating room. Hemorrhoidectomy is contraindicated, and may result in uncontrollable bleeding.

The management of LGIB is truly a team effort. The surgeon, gastroenterologist, radiologist, and nursing staff must all work in concert to effectively diagnose and treat the problem. In many cases, deficiencies in individual hospital system processes are responsible for the failure to accurately identify the source. Too often a nuclear study is obtained, which shows active bleeding, but angiography is unavailable directly afterward. Or a patient starts to bleed in the middle of the night and resources to perform a colonoscopy are not available. In order to efficiently identify the source of bleeding, all the team members must make it a priority and communication among the team is of paramount importance.

Colonoscopy is, at present, the best means of both identifying and treating the majority of LGIB. In hemodynamically stable patients, we generally perform a full bowel prep, as this allows for an easier and more complete exam and higher chance of success. Performing an unprepped colonoscopy presents its own inherent difficulties, but one advantage of the unprepped exam is the ability to identify a transition area between bloody and nonbloody stool that can at least narrow down the location of the bleed. If a site of bleeding is identified, it should be treated endoscopically and also marked for potential surgical resection with an India ink tattoo in case bleeding recurs.

Although radionuclide scans and angiography have always held prominent positions in the LGIB algorithm, these studies should be considered adjuncts to colonoscopy and not the primary mode of diagnosis. Radionuclide scans must be interpreted with caution, especially when there is a long delay between images. Many surgeons have been misled by the appearance of intraluminal activity in one segment of the colon when the actual bleeding site is elsewhere. It is important to remember that bowel contents can move both anterograde and retrograde, so the actual bleeding site can be either proximal or distal to a delayed image. Blushes that occur early after injection and move anterograde on images taken at short time intervals are the most reliable. Many institutions require a positive radionuclide scan before proceeding to angiography because of its greater sensitivity to detect active bleeding. The interventional radiologist should be informed whenever a nuclear medicine scan is being performed for bleeding so that the patient can proceed directly to angiography if the scan is positive. We have found delayed angiography after a positive nuclear study to be of limited utility, because the bleeding often stops in the interim. Unfortunately, negative angiograms subject the patient to the same risks of arterial puncture and intravenous contrast as positive studies, and should the patient rebleed in the short term, the angiogram option is foreclosed due to the risk of contrast-induced acute kidney injury. The one situation where angiography may have an advantage over colonoscopy is with brisk hemorrhage. Bowel preparation is impossible, and endoscopic visualization can be extremely difficult in the face of severe bleeding. Under these circumstances, an angiography is more likely to be positive and a definitive therapeutic intervention can often be performed.

Operative intervention based solely on a radionuclide scan should be avoided, as the diagnostic accuracy of this study is too low to justify the significant risk of recurrent bleeding should a segmental resection be performed. Localization is far more convincing when a positive angiogram confirms the radionuclide scan findings.

As pointed out by Drs. Beard and Schwaitzberg, CT angiogram represents a widely available, accurate, and cost-effective alternative. Single photon emission computed tomography/computed tomography (SPECT/CT) should be considered, especially in the case of recurrent intermittent LGIB, as the fused images provide greater anatomic accuracy than conventional scintigraphy.

If emergency surgery is required without adequate localization of the bleeding site, total abdominal colectomy with or without an ileo-rectal anastomosis is almost always the correct choice. "Blind" segmental resection risks removal of the wrong bowel segment and is associated with a high risk of persisting bleeding, a dangerous circumstance when patients are brought urgently to the operating room, because they are too unstable for further diagnostic testing. For patients with recurrent but not life-threatening bleeding, it is preferable to keep them under close observation to allow repeated evaluation, or to consider provocative testing.

In the final analysis, lower gastrointestinal bleeding remains mainly a nonsurgical problem. Most cases are not life threatening and the bleeding stops on its own with supportive care. However, surgeons should always be involved in LGIB management from the outset, rather than being brought in when only the situation has become emergent, because the patient is unstable. The judgment to proceed with surgery should be made with the concurrence of the patient, surgeon, and medical team. Each case should be decided on an individual basis and not blindly based solely upon the number of units of blood that have been transfused. Additional factors to be considered include the age and general health of the patient, the patient's medical stability, underlying comorbidity, the presence of underlying clotting disorders or need for long-term anticoagulation, difficulties with cross-matching (e.g., due to multiple antibodies) or patient's unwillingness to accept transfusion (e.g., a Jehovah's Witness), and the patient's goals and willingness to undergo surgery. In general, surgery must paradoxically be considered earlier for patients who are the least optimal candidates: for example, an individual with severe coronary artery disease who may not tolerate severe recurrent bleeding, or for patients who refuse transfusion or are difficult to cross-match. A frank discussion should be undertaken to discuss not only the operative risks, but also future functional issues related to an ileo-rectal anastomosis or ileostomy, particularly in elderly patients.

# 50

## *Diverticular Disease of the Colon*

**Mary Stuever and Akpofure Peter Ekeh**

**CONTENTS**



Diverticular disease of the colon is a common condition, predominant in Western societies, that generates a significant socioeconomic burden. Its prevalence is age-related, affecting only 5% of individuals aged 30–39 years old, but involving two-thirds of adults over the age of 85—who are found to have colonic diverticula [1]. Recent United States (U.S.) population-based studies reveal that diverticular disease is the sixth most frequent outpatient gastrointestinal diagnosis, with 2.6 million emergency department visits annually. It accounts for the most common inpatient gastrointestinal diagnosis with 283,355 yearly hospitalizations at a cost of $2.7 billion dollars [2].

Acute diverticulitis is the most frequent complication arising from the presence of colonic diverticula. The incidence of diverticulitis has historically ranged from 10% to 25% with the sigmoid colon being affected in 95% of cases [3]. Diverticulitis is further classified into uncomplicated and complicated disease. Patients with uncomplicated disease typically present with abdominal pain, fever, nausea, and vomiting. These cases are managed nonoperatively, often in the outpatient setting, with bowel rest and antibiotics. Most patients recover without further episodes. Approximately one-third of patients treated for acute diverticulitis will experience a second attack, and a third attack will occur in roughly another third of this population. A 2013 study by Shahedi et al. at the Veterans Affairs Greater Los Angeles Healthcare System identified 2222 patients with diverticulosis, and followed them over an 11-year period with the goal of determining the rate of development of acute diverticulitis. Only a small proportion of individuals with diverticulosis went on to develop acute diverticulitis—4% in this study [4].

Complicated diverticulitis refers to cases in which patients present with an abscess, perforation, stricture, fistula formation, or sepsis. Approximately 22% of patients admitted for diverticulitis will undergo surgery for management of their complicated disease [5].

The methods of management of diverticulitis in the acute and elective setting subsequent to hospital discharge have evolved over the last few decades. Several of the commonly accepted standards and guidelines have required revision as larger studies, randomized trials, and the increasing use of laparoscopic surgery are changing the landscape.

We will review the existing evidence in the literature regarding the management of colonic diverticular disease, ranging from indications for operative management, the importance of age in operative decision-making, methods of operative management, the role of laparoscopy, and the prevention and management of recurrent attacks.

## 50.1 What Is the Appropriate Indication for Elective Sigmoid Resection after Uncomplicated Diverticulitis?

The need for surgical or other adjunct intervention in complicated diverticulitis is generally not disputed. The appropriate indications for surgical intervention after uncomplicated acute diverticulitis on the other hand has for several years been vigorously debated. The primary purpose of surgical intervention after acute attacks of diverticulitis is the prevention of recurrence, as well as the amelioration of the accompanying morbidity. Consequently, recommendations are generally based on the risk of recurrence and the severity of subsequent attacks. Most studies assessing risk of repeat attacks are retrospective studies and have very wide variability of follow up, making it difficult to establish an accurate recurrence rate.

Historically, clinical practice patterns and recommendation guidelines have proposed elective colon resection after two or more acute attacks of diverticulitis successfully treated medically; or after a single attack occurring in a patient less than 40 years of age. The recommendation for surgery following two attacks in older patients was based primarily on dated case series data indicating significant recurrence rates after medically managed acute diverticulitis. Parks in 1969 published a review of 455 patients admitted with acute diverticulitis. Of the patients treated medically, 24.6% subsequently had a second attack and 3.8% a third [6]. Furthermore, the paper suggested medical management was less effective for symptom control with subsequent bouts. Makela et al. similarly showed recurrences of 22% of patients with diverticulitis managed medically and complications seen in 50% of patients who presented with a second attack [7].

More recent series have challenged the prevalence of recurrence and the severity of subsequent attacks stated in the older literature. A large series involving over 3000 patients showed 13.3% of them had a single recurrence and only 3.9% had a second episode [8]. This is lower than reported in older studies with a longer follow-up period than any of the prior studies completed (8.9 years). Another recent retrospective review showed that only 2.7% of patients who presented emergently with acute diverticulitis and required surgery had a prior history of medical management and a majority of the cases were initial presentations [9]. Chapman et al. found multiple episodes of diverticulitis are not associated with increased risk of mortality or poor outcomes from complicated diverticulitis [10].

A prospective study of 934 patients by Ritz et al. revealed the incidence of perforation to be 25% during the first episode, 13% during the second episode, and 6% in the third [11]. Shaikh and Krukowski demonstrated only 19% of conservatively managed patients eventually underwent elective surgical resection, and the need for emergent surgery was 5% [12]. These studies challenge the notion that complications are directly related to or worsen with an increased number of episodes.

Hsiao et al. highlighted the role of individual patient variables in a retrospective review. Their study involving 246 patients revealed that independent patient comorbidities such as diabetes, cardiovascular disease, gouty arthritis, smoking, and aspirin or NSAID use were independent risk factors for the need for urgent colectomy in patients with diverticulitis. They found that addition consideration needed to be given immunocompromised patients, such as patients with kidney failure, organ transplants, and those using corticosteroids, as this subset of patients were more often diagnosed with complicated diverticulitis [13].

Results from an American College of Surgeons National Surgical Quality Improvement Project database study from 2005 to 2010 identified morbid obesity as an independent risk factor. In this review of 10,952 patients undergoing surgery for diverticulitis, morbidly obese patients were found to be on average 10 years younger and more likely to require emergency surgery, ostomy creation, and undergo procedures without a primary anastomosis (PA) [14].

Quality of life is considered to be an important factor for patients with regard to surgical intervention. A 2013 retrospective cohort study revealed that elective resection improved the quality of life based on visual analog scales and reduced abdominal pain in up to 89.3% and 87.5% of patients, respectively [15]. This study among others indicates the importance of considering amelioration of chronic symptoms in the decision-making process for elective surgery for diverticular disease.

The most current American Society of Colon and Rectal Surgeons recommendations addressing the management of uncomplicated diverticular disease, based on an exhaustive review of the literature, indicate that the decision to recommend elective sigmoid colectomy after recovery from uncomplicated acute diverticulitis should be individualized. These recommendations supplant prior ones that proposed elective surgery after two attacks. Factors such as risks of operative therapy, the overall patient medical condition, effects on lifestyle imposed by recurrent attacks, inability to exclude carcinoma, severity of the attacks, as well as chronicity of symptoms need to be considered in making a decision for surgery [16].

*Recommendation*: Though elective sigmoid resection has been traditionally recommended after two attacks of uncomplicated diverticulitis, a case-by-case determination of the need for operative management is necessary.

Given the strength of these recommendations, there is no basis for the prior conventional decision to routinely proceed to an elective colectomy after two episodes of uncomplicated diverticulitis (Grade C, level IIb).

## 50.2 Should Younger Patients (<40–50 Years) Undergo Elective Sigmoid Colon Resection after a Single Attack of Acute Diverticulitis?

Of all patients admitted with the diagnosis of diverticulitis, 18%–34% are younger than 50 years of age [17]. Traditional clinical practice and expert guidelines have advocated elective sigmoid colectomy after the first attack of uncomplicated diverticulitis in patients less than 40 years of age. This recommendation is based on multiple case series and retrospective studies from the 1960s and 1970s demonstrating more virulent presentations and more recurrences in patients less than 40. Studies confirming this notion, and others challenging this have appeared in the literature—all similarly retrospective.

More recent retrospective cohort studies have compared rates of complication and operation in younger patients to those of older patients. Older literature has shown that younger patients develop more subsequent complications, have more recurrences and that the disease displays a more aggressive course compared with older cohorts. Newer studies have rendered this concept outdated. Ünlü et al. revealed in a retrospective cohort study of 1441 patients that younger age is not associated with more severe disease or higher incidence of recurrence [17]. In a prospective study published in 2002 by Biondo et al. evaluating 327 patients, no difference in recurrence or the need for emergent operation was found when accounting for age as the primary indicator for surgical decision making [18]. Ritz in a prospective study of over 1000 consecutive admissions of patient with acute diverticulitis failed to demonstrate increased aggression or a higher risk of perforation in younger patients [19].

*Recommendation*: Given the more recent data, no specific evidence-based recommendations can be made with regard to the specific indications for surgery after an uncomplicated attack of acute diverticulitis in younger patients. As with the rest of this population, individualized decisions based on patient's circumstance will need to be made prior to proceeding with surgery. In young patients, the high risk of recurrent disease is an actual reflection of higher accumulated risk due to higher life expectancy. There is no evidence that younger patients should be managed differently than older patients based upon age alone (Grade C, level IIb).

## 50.3 Are There Any Evidence-Based Dietary Recommendations to Prevent the Recurrence of Acute Uncomplicated Diverticulitis? Is the Practice of Prohibiting the Intake of "Seeds," Popcorn, etc., after an Acute Episode Valid?

Fiber intake is a significant dietary factor in preventing and reducing recurrence of diverticulitis. The progression of colonic diverticular disease has paralleled the drop in dietary fiber consumption in the United States, Europe, and Asia.

A number of studies have highlighted the benefits of fiber intake in the prevention and recurrence of diverticular disease. The original observations of the effect of fiber were published several years ago by Burkitt, based on his experiences in some rural parts of Africa. He compared colonic transit times and stool weight in three populations with low, mixed, and high residue diets. Colonic transit time was decreased and stool weight was increased in patients with high residue diets. He further obtained epidemiological data from various countries, noting the very low prevalence of diverticular disease in populations with high residue diets compared to those with low and mixed residue diets [20].

A prospective cohort questionnaire-based study with a 4-year follow-up by Aldoori et al. evaluated the effect of various diets on the incidence of diverticular disease. The participants reporting diets high in fruit and vegetable fiber had a significantly lower incidence of symptomatic diverticulitis. Diets high in fat and red meat were also noted to augment the risk [21]. These findings are consistent with findings from a Greek study in patients with radiologically confirmed diverticulitis. Patients with diverticulitis were demonstrated to have a lower intake of fiber and higher intake of red meat [22].

Other studies give further credence to the clinical recommendation to increase fiber intake after acute attacks of diverticulitis as a means to lower recurrence rates. Brodribb demonstrated in a randomized controlled trial with fiber versus placebo that fiber improved symptoms of dyspepsia, bowel dysfunction, and pain in patients with symptomatic diverticular disease [23]. This is in line with a similarly dated randomized controlled crossover trial, by Taylor also performed in the 1970s, comparing bran tablets (18 g/day) with a high-roughage diet and a laxative. The bran group was found to have better results in improving symptom score, stool weight, transit time, and motility [24]. Lahner in a randomized controlled trial also demonstrated that high fiber diet and/or high fiber diet plus probiotic administration decreased abdominal pain symptoms by two-thirds [25]. An additional prospective cohort study of 47,033 people by Crowe et al. in 2011 demonstrated that higher fiber intake was a factor associated with a decreased risk of hospitalization for diverticular disease [26].

The advice given against the consumption of popcorn, seeds, and nuts in an attempt to prevent obstruction of diverticula and subsequent inflammation has no basis in the medical literature. Strate et al. in a prospective cohort study of male health professionals in 2008 demonstrated that dietary nuts, corn, and seeds were not associated with an increased risk of diverticulitis or diverticular bleeding [27].

*Recommendation*: Dietary fiber can play a role in both the prevention of initial and recurrent attacks of diverticulitis. Patients should be advised to increase their fiber content in their diet after a bout of uncomplicated diverticulitis (Grade A, level IIb).

## 50.4 What Is the Optimal Operation for Patients Requiring Surgery for Acute Complicated Diverticulitis? Is Performing a Primary Anastomosis an Option?

In his 1978 paper on the treatment of diverticulitis, Hinchey divided acute diverticulitis into four classes, now referred to as the Hinchey stages I–IV, with worse clinical features and mortality with each successive stage [28]. Stage IV disease involves feculent peritonitis and was described to be accompanied with a high mortality. This staging system has been widely adopted to provide a standard for comparison of the severity of disease.

The operative management of complicated acute diverticulitis has evolved over time. Historically, staged operations were commonly performed involving the initial closure of the perforation with a proximal diversion (ileostomy or transverse colostomy) with subsequent delayed resection of the diseased portion and anastomosis. This approach has been replaced by the Hartmann operation—resection of the acutely inflamed bowel, including the perforated portion of colon and a proximal end colostomy. This approach is still widely utilized for Hinchey class III and IV stages, and is the standard management for feculent peritonitis. While this is the standard practice, over time only 45% of patients with end colostomies have them reversed, not to mention the inherent risk of colostomy take down operations [29].

More recently, more authors have published data on the use of primary resection and anastomosis in patients with perforated sigmoid diverticulitis. Alizai et al. studied 98 patients, 72 undergoing Hartmann's procedure and 26 receiving a PA with a defunctioning stoma. In the PA group, 85% of patients had their stoma reversed, while this occurred only in 58% of the HP patients ($p = 0.046$). The 30-day mortality was 12% in the PA group and 25% in the HP group ($p = 0.167$) [30].

Oberkoffer et al. conducted a randomized controlled trial involving four centers comparing PA with diverting ileostomy to Hartmann's procedure. This study limited to 62 patients equally divided in both groups showed no significant differences in mortality or morbidity between both cohorts. The stoma reversal rate was higher after PA with ileostomy, 90% versus 58% $p = 0.005$. Additionally, serious complications (0% vs. 20%, $p = 0.046$), operating time (73 vs. 183 min, $p < 0.001$), hospital stay (6 vs. 9 days, $p = 0.016$), and in-hospital costs ($16,717 vs. $24,014) were reduced in the PA group. Total overall complications (80% HP vs. 84% PA), however, demonstrate no benefit of PA over HP, and confirm that perforated Hinchey III and IV diverticulitis carries a high morbidity regardless of approach [31].

Jafferji et al.'s review of 136 patients who underwent surgical resection for acute complicated diverticulitis determined that the surgeon not the patient determines the surgical approach. Noncolorectal surgeons performed more Hartmann procedures than the colorectal surgeons (68.3% vs. 40.9%, $p = 0.01$) despite similar demographics. Length of stay, time to stoma reversal, ICU days, and postoperative complications were lower among colorectal surgeons (43.2% vs. 16.7, $p = 0.02$). They concluded that in spite of patient-specific factors, the surgeon could be a potent predictor in the type of operation performed [32].

*Recommendation*: Primary resection of the inflamed colon (with or without PA) is the optimal method of treating complicated sigmoid diverticulitis. PA of the colon at the initial operation with the consideration of a defunctioning ileostomy in more advanced Hinchey is a feasible option (Grade C, level IIb).

## 50.5 What Is the Role of Laparoscopy in Acute Complicated Diverticulitis? Is There a Role for Laparoscopic Lavage or Laparoscopic Resection in the Emergent Setting?

With the increasing use of laparoscopic surgery, there has been a concomitant increase in the use of laparoscopic techniques to manage complicated diverticulitis in acute and elective settings. Laparoscopic lavage for acute perforations followed by elective laparoscopic resection is one of the techniques that have been increasingly heralded.

To date, most studies evaluating laparoscopic management of complicated diverticulitis have been limited to retrospective chart reviews [33]. Originally described in 1996, laparoscopic lavage has since then been touted as a promising alternative to acute sigmoid resection in multiple case series [34]. Bretagnol studied 24 patients with perforated sigmoid diverticulitis who were managed with laparoscopic washout followed by elective laparoscopic resection at a later date, demonstrating no mortality, an 8% morbidity, and a conversion to open rate on the follow up surgery of 16% [35]. Laparoscopic lavage is not recommended in Hinchey Class IV diverticulitis as the presence of feculent perforation should lead to a colectomy in the acute setting.

There are at least four ongoing randomized prospective trials in Europe designed to define clearly the role of laparoscopic lavage in acute complicated diverticulitis. These are the SCANDIV & DILALA trials (Scandinavia), LADIES trial (Netherlands), and the LapLAND trial (Ireland) [33]. Preliminary results from the Dutch LADIES trial found the control of sepsis in 31 of 38 patients in the laparoscopic lavage arm, four deaths, and a morbidity rate of 32%. Sepsis was controlled in 31 of 38 patients, 17 developed complications, and three patients underwent subsequent sigmoid resection for recurrent diverticulitis [36]. These studies all have different primary end points and when completed, will offer further valuable information into the optimal role of laparoscopic lavage.

A few studies have described a role for laparoscopic resection in the emergent setting. Zdichavsky et al. performed a retrospective review of a combined cohort of patients with acute and recurrent diverticulitis who underwent laparoscopic sigmoid colon resection—almost equally divided in the series of 197 patients. Minor complications occurred in 14.3% of acute cases and in 7.5% of elective cases and major complications in 2.2% of acute cases and 4.3% of elective cases. No anastomotic leaks or mortality occurred in either group. The combination of two distinctly different populations makes definitive conclusion difficult from this study [37].

*Recommendation*: Laparoscopic lavage of Hinchey stage III is a consideration in acute diverticulitis requiring operative therapy; however, the results of ongoing prospective studies are needed before definitive recommendations can be made (Grade C).

## 50.6 Is Elective Laparoscopic Colectomy Equivalent or Superior to Open Colectomy for Diverticular Disease? Is the Overall Cost Different?

A clear role for a laparoscopic approach in the management of colon cancer was established by a multi-institutional randomized prospective trial demonstrating non-inferiority in recurrence rates as well as a shorter length of stay and less use of parenteral narcotics in the laparoscopic group by the COST trial [38].

In an attempt to further define the role of laparoscopic surgery in the management of complicated diverticulitis, the SIGMA trial compared laparoscopic with open colon resection. There was randomization of 104 patients to open versus laparoscopic elective sigmoid colon resection. The patients in both groups were comparable. The laparoscopic resections had less intraoperative blood loss, less major complications, less postoperative pain, shorter length of stay, and better post-op quality of life on SF-36 questionnaires. The open resections took less operative time [39].

A number of retrospective chart reviews have supported the improved outcomes for patients managed with laparoscopic surgery seen in the SIGMA trial. Letarte et al. found overall morbidity was lower in laparoscopic colon resection (16% vs. 55%) as well as the length of stay and mean time to diet resumption [40]. De Magistris et al. showed lower morbidity when utilizing an exclusive laparoscopic approach for moderate and severe complicated diverticulitis [41].

Compared with the open procedure, a number of retrospective studies found no difference in complication rates or mortality when comparing laparoscopic to open surgery [42]. Furthermore, quicker return to diet, shorter time to first bowel movement, reduced length of hospital stay, and reduced estimated blood loss have been consistently reported in favor of laparoscopic operations [43–46]. Laparoscopic sigmoidoscopy however in most series had longer operative time although typically a shorter length of stay and charges [44,45].

Studies examining cost per case report an overall reduction with laparoscopic sigmoid colectomies—possibly related to the reduced length of stay [47].

Naguib et al. in a retrospective cohort demonstrated challenges of laparoscopic colorectal surgery for diverticular disease, concluding that these techniques were not suitable for the early part of the learning curve. Comparing patients who had resections for diverticular disease versus malignant disease showed a higher conversion rate (27.3% vs. 9.9%), longer operating times (250 vs. 196 min), and longer length of stays (6 vs. 4 days) (Tables 50.1 and 50.2) [48].

**TABLE 50.1**

Clinical Questions

| Question | Answer | Grade of Recommendation | References |
|---|---|---|---|
| What is the appropriate indication for elective sigmoid resection after uncomplicated diverticulitis? | A case-by-case determination of the need for operative management is necessary. There is no basis for routine resection after two episodes of diverticulitis. | C | [6–16] |
| Should younger patients (<40–50 years) undergo elective sigmoid colon resection after a single attack of acute diverticulitis? | Individualized decisions based on patient's circumstance will need to be made prior to proceeding with surgery. There is no evidence that younger patients should be managed differently based on age alone. | C | [16–19] |
| Are there any evidence-based dietary recommendations to prevent the recurrence of acute uncomplicated diverticulitis? | Dietary fiber can play a role in both the prevention of initial and recurrent attacks of uncomplicated diverticulitis. Patients should be advised to increase fiber content in their diet after an episode of uncomplicated diverticulitis. | A | [20–27] |
| Is the practice of prohibiting the intake of "seeds," popcorn, etc., after an acute episode valid? | There is no basis in medical literature that prohibiting certain foods prevents episodes of diverticulitis. | A | [27] |
| What is the optimal operation for patients requiring surgery for complicated acute diverticulitis? | Primary resection of the inflamed colon (with or without PA) is appropriate in the selected patient. | A | [28–33] |
| Is performing a PA an option? | | B | [28–33] |
| What is the role of laparoscopy in acute complicated diverticulitis? | Laparoscopic management of acute diverticulitis is an evolving field with great promise, yet no randomized control trials have been completed. | C | [33–40] |
| Is there a role for laparoscopic lavage or laparoscopic resection in the emergent setting? | There are at least four ongoing randomized prospective trials evaluating the role of laparoscopic washout for management of acute diverticulitis. These trials will offer further information. | C | [34–36] |
| Is laparoscopic colectomy equivalent or superior to open colectomy for diverticular disease? Is the overall cost different? | Laparoscopic colon resection is a safe and effective approach for the elective treatment of patients with diverticular disease. | A | [42–47] |

**TABLE 50.2**

Levels of Evidence

| Subject | Year | Reference | Level of Evidence | Strength of Recommendation | Findings |
|---|---|---|---|---|---|
| Indication for elective colectomy after uncomplicated diverticulitis | 2011 | [12] | IIb | B | Medical management of diverticulitis is appropriate. However, 19% of conservatively managed patients undergo resection, 5% of patients require emergency surgery. |
| Elective colectomy in younger patients | 2013 | [17] | IIb | B | Age is not associated with more severe disease or higher incidence of recurrence. |
| Dietary fiber intake and risk of diverticulitis | 1994 | [21] | IIb | B | Diets high in fruit and vegetable fiber had a significantly lower incidence of symptomatic diverticulitis |
| PA for sigmoid diverticulitis | 2013 | [16] | IIb | B | Primary resection and anastomosis (with diverting ileostomy) can be considered in low-risk patients (Hinchey Stage I and II) with acute diverticulitis. |
| Laparoscopy for diverticular disease | 2005 | [39] | IIb | B | Laparoscopy associated with quicker return to diet, shorter time, and reduced length of hospital stay |

*Recommendation*: Laparoscopic colon resection is a safe and effective approach for the elective treatment of patients with diverticular disease demonstrating no increased morbidity and a shorter hospital stay, quicker resumption of bowel function, and reduced blood loss. It is appropriate for elderly patients (Grade C, level IIb).

## References


1. Pogacnik JS, Messaris E, Deiling SM, Connelly TM, Berg AS, Stewart DB, McKenna KJ, Poritz LS, Koltun WA. Increased risk of incisional hernia after sigmoid colectomy for diverticulitis compared with colon cancer. *J Am Coll Surg*. 2014;218:920–928.
2. Peery AF, Sandler RS. Diverticular disease: Reconsidering conventional wisdom. *Clin Gastroenterol Hepatol*. 2013;11:1532–1537.
3. Anania G, Vedana L, Santini M, Scagliarini L, Giaccari S, Resta G, Cavallesco G. Complications of diverticular disease: Surgical laparoscopic treatment. *G Chir*. 2014;35:126–128.
4. Shahedi K, Fuller G, Bolus R et al. Long-term risk of acute diverticulitis among patients with incidental diverticulosis found during colonoscopy. *Clin Gastroenterol Hepatol*. 2013;11:1609–1613.
5. Morris AM, Regenbogen SE, Hardiman KM, Hendren S. Sigmoid diverticulitis: A systematic review. *JAMA*. 2014;311:287–297. Review.
6. Parks TG. Natural history of diverticular disease of the colon. A review of 521 cases. *BMJ*. 1969;4:639–645.
7. Makela J, Vuolio S, Kiviniemi H, Laitinen S. Natural history of diverticular disease: When to operate? *Dis Colon Rectum*. 1998;41:1523–1528.
8. Broderick-Villa G, Bruchette RJ, Collins JC et al. Hospitalization for acute diverticulitis does not mandate routine elective colectomy. *Arch Surg*. 2005;140:576–581.
9. Somasekar K, Foster ME, Haray PN. The natural history of diverticular disease: Is there a role for elective colectomy? *J R Coll Surg Edinb*. 2002;47:481–484.
10. Chapman JR, Dozois EJ, Wolff BG et al. Diverticulitis: A progressive disease? Do multiple recurrences predict less favorable outcomes? *Ann Surg*. 2006;243:876–883.
11. Ritz JP, Lehmann KS, Frericks B et al. Outcome of patients with acute sigmoid diverticulitis: Multivariate analysis of risk factors for free perforation. *Surgery* 2011;149:606–613.
12. Shaikh S, Krukowski ZH. Outcome of a conservative policy for managing acute sigmoid diverticulitis. *Br J Surg*. 2007;94:876–879.
13. Hsiao KC, Wann JG, Lin CS, Wu CC, Jao SW, Yang MH. Colonic diverticulitis with comorbid diseases may require elective colectomy. *World J Gastroenterol*. 2013;21:6613–6617.
14. Bailey MB, Davenport DL, Procter L, McKenzie S, Vargas HD. Morbid obesity and diverticulitis: Results from the ACS NSQIP dataset. *J Am Coll Surg*. 2013;217:874–880.
15. van de Wall BJ, Draaisma WA, van Iersel JJ, Consten EC, Wiezer MJ, Broeders IA. Elective resection for ongoing diverticular disease significantly improves quality of life. *Dig Surg*. 2013;30:190–197.
16. Feingold D, Steele SR, Lee S, Kaiser A et al. Practice parameters for the treatment of sigmoid diverticulitis. *Dis Colon Rectum*. 2014;57:284–294.
17. Ünlü Ç, van de Wall BJ, Gerhards MF, Wiezer M, Draaisma WA, Consten EC, Boermeester MA, Vrouenraets BC. Influence of age on clinical outcome of acute diverticulitis. *J Gastrointest Surg*. 2013;17:1651–1656.
18. Biondo S, Parés D, Martí Ragué J, Kreisler E, Fraccalvieri D, Jaurrieta E. Acute colonic diverticulitis in patients under 50 years of age. *Br J Surg*. 2002;89:1137–1141.
19. Ritz JP, Lehmann KS, Stroux A et al. Sigmoid diverticulitis in young patients—A more aggressive disease than in older patients? *J Gastrointest Surg*. 2011;15:667–674.
20. Burkitt DP, Walker AR, Painter NS. Effect of dietary fibre on stools and the transit-times, and its role in the causation of disease. *Lancet*. 1972;7792:1408–1412.
21. Aldoori WH, Giovannucci EL, Rimm EB, Wing AL, Trichopoulos DV, Willett WC. A prospective study of diet and the risk of symptomatic diverticular disease in men. *Am J Clin Nutr*. 1994;60:757–764.
22. Manousos O, Day NE, Tone A, Papadimitriou C, Kapetanakis A, Polychronopoulou-Trichopoulou A, Trichopoulos D. Diet and other factors in the aetiology of diverticulosis: An epidemiological study in Greece. *Gut*. 1985;26:544–549.
23. Brodribb AJ. Treatment of symptomatic diverticular disease with a high-fiber diet. *Lancet*. 1977;1:664–666.
24. Taylor I, Duthie HL. Bran tablets and diverticular disease. *Br Med J*. 1976;24:988–990.
25. Lahner E, Esposito G, Zullo A, Hassan C, Cannaviello C, Paolo MC, Pallotta L, Garbagna N, Grossi E, Annibale B. High-fibre diet and Lactobacillus paracasei B21060 in symptomatic uncomplicated diverticular disease. *World J Gastroenterol*. 2012;18:5918–5924.
26. Appleby PN, Allen NE, Key TJ. Diet and risk of diverticular disease in Oxford cohort of European Prospective Investigation into Cancer and Nutrition (EPIC): Prospective study of British vegetarians and non-vegetarians. *BMJ*. 2011;343:d4131.
27. Strate LL, Liu YL, Syngal S, Aldoori WH, Giovannucci EL. Nut, corn, and popcorn consumption and the incidence of diverticular disease. *JAMA*. 2008;300:907–914.
28. Hinchey EJ, Schaal PG, Richards GK: Treatment of perforated diverticular disease of the colon. *Adv Surg*. 1978;12:85–109.
29. Studer P, Schnüriger B, Umer M, Kröll D, Inderbitzin D, Candinas D. Laparoscopic versus open end colostomy closure: A single-center experience. *Am Surg*. 2014;80:361.
30. Alizai PH, Schulze-Hagen M, Klink CD, Ulmer F, Roeth AA, Neumann UP, Jansen M, Rosch R. Primary anastomosis with a defunctioning stoma versus Hartmann's procedure for perforated diverticulitis—A comparison of stoma reversal rates. *Int J Colorectal Dis*. 2013;28:1681–1688.

31. Oberkofler CE, Rickenbacher A, Raptis DA et al. A multicenter randomized clinical trial of primary anastomosis or Hartmann's procedure for perforated left colonic diverticulitis with purulent or fecal peritonitis. *Ann Surg.* 2012;256:819–826.
32. Jafferji MS, Hyman N. Surgeon, not disease severity, often determines the operation for acute complicated diverticulitis. *J Am Coll Surg.* 2014;218:1156–1161.
33. McDermott FD, Collins D, Heeney A, Winter DC. Minimally invasive and surgical management strategies tailored to the severity of acute diverticulitis. *Br J Surg.* 2014;101:e90–e99. Review.
34. O'Sullivan GC, Murphy D, O'Brien MG, Ireland A. Laparoscopic management of generalized peritonitis due to perforated colonic diverticula. *Am J Surg.* 1996;171:432–434.
35. Bretagnol F, Pautrat K, Mor C, Benchellal Z, Huten N, Calan L. Emergency laparoscopic management of perforated sigmoid diverticulitis: A promising alternative to more radical procedures. *ACS.* 2008;1072–7515.
36. Swank HA, Mulder IM, Hoofwijk AG et al. Dutch Diverticular Disease Collaborative Study Group. Early experience with laparoscopic lavage for perforated diverticulitis. *Br J Surg.* 2013;100:704–710.
37. Zdichavsky M, Kratt T, Stüker D, Meile T, Feilitzsch MV, Wichmann D, Königsrainer A. Acute and elective laparoscopic resection for complicated sigmoid diverticulitis: Clinical and histological outcome. *J Gastrointest Surg.* 2013;17:1966–1971.
38. Clinical Outcomes of Surgical Therapy Study Group. A comparison of laparoscopically assisted and open colectomy for colon cancer. *N Engl J Med.* 2004;350:2050–2059.
39. Klarenbeek BR, Veenhoff AA, Bergamaschi R et al. Laparoscopic sigmoid resection for diverticulitis decreases major morbidity rates: A randomized control trial: Short-term results of the Sigma Trial. *Ann Surg.* 2009;249:39–44.
40. Letarte F, Hallet J, Drolet S, Charles Grégoire R, Bouchard A, Gagné JP, Thibault C, Bouchard P. Laparoscopic emergency surgery for diverticular disease that failed medical treatment: A valuable option? Results of a retrospective comparative cohort study. 2013;56:1395–1402.
41. De Magistris L, Arru L, De Blasi V, Poulain V, Lens V, Mertens L, Goergen M, Azagra JS. Management of acute diverticulitis in a tertiary care institution. *Bull Soc Sci Med Grand Duche Luxemb.* 2013;25–32.
42. Gonzalez R, Smith CD, Mattar SG, Venkatesh KR, Mason E, Duncan T, Wilson R, Miller J, Ramshaw BJ. Laparoscopic vs open resection for the treatment of diverticular disease. *Surg Endosc.* 2004;18:276–280.
43. Alves A, Panis Y, Slim K, Heyd B, Kwiatkowski F, Mantion G; Association Français de Chirurgie: French multicentre prospective observational study of laparoscopic versus open colectomy for sigmoid diverticular disease. *Br J Surg.* 2005;92:1520–1525.
44. Lawrence DM, Pasquale MD, Wasser TE. Laparoscopic versus open sigmoid colectomy for diverticulitis. *Am Surg.* 2003;69:499–503.
45. Dwivedi A, Chahin F, Agrawal S, Chau WY, Tootla A, Tootla F, Silva YJ. Laparoscopic colectomy vs open colectomy for sigmoid diverticular disease. *Dis Colon Rectum.* 2002;45:1309–1314.
46. Senagore AJ, Duepree HJ, Delaney CP, Dissanaike S, Brady KM, Fazio VW. Cost structure of laparoscopic and open sigmoid colectomy for diverticular disease: Similarities and differences. *Dis Colon Rectum.* 2002;45:485–490.
47. Liberman MA, Phillips EH, Carroll BJ, Fallas M, Rosenthal R. Laparoscopic colectomy vs traditional colectomy for diverticulitis. Outcome and costs. *Surg Endosc.* 1996;10:158.
48. Naguib N, Masoud AG. Laparoscopic colorectal surgery for diverticular disease is not suitable for the early part of the learning curve. A retrospective cohort study. *Int J Surg.* 2013;11(10):1092–1096.

## Commentary on Diverticular Disease of the Colon

*Matthew O. Dolich*

There is perhaps no better disease process to display the transformative power of evidence-based medicine than the entity of colonic diverticular disease. As I completed my surgery residency training in the mid-1990s, I came of age knowing certain surgical "truths" based on the conventional wisdom of the day, and I practiced accordingly. I knew that younger adults with an initial bout of uncomplicated diverticulitis should be cooled down, and be scheduled for elective colon resection in short order for fear of the more virulent nature of this disease in young people. I knew that older adults should certainly have the sigmoid colon removed after two uncomplicated episodes. I understood intuitively that Hartmann's procedure was the only safe option when I was forced to operate in the setting of acute or perforated sigmoid diverticulitis. I did not question the fact that Henri Hartmann described this procedure for patients suffering from a completely different malady—namely obstructing cancer of the sigmoid colon. Perhaps most sadly, I reinforced the words of a well-intentioned internist with my own grandmother, instructing her to avoid seeds, nuts, tomatoes, and cucumbers for fear of stirring up her diverticular demons.

Over the course of my career, based on these assumptions, I have operated on people who, in retrospect, did not need surgery. In doing so, I most certainly incurred complications that need not have occurred at all. I have done big operations when smaller ones would have sufficed. I have created stomas that might have been avoided. And I unwittingly deprived my grandmother of some of her favorite foods in the final years of her life.

The authors do an excellent job of busting many myths about diverticular disease and reviewing best practice based on the available scientific evidence. While the indications for urgent or emergent surgical intervention and fecal diversion remain in some patients with complicated diverticulitis and peritonitis or septic shock, the landscape has changed for a great many patients with less dramatic manifestations of diverticular disease. From a big picture standpoint, it is important to note that less than 5% of people with colonic diverticulosis ever develop acute diverticulitis, and of those that do, more than 75% do not require surgery. Of those patients that do ultimately require surgery, up to a third have ongoing symptoms after bowel resection.

### Young Patients with Diverticular Disease

While conventional wisdom held that patients younger than 40 years of age should have an elective colectomy after a single bout of diverticular disease, that recommendation has not been proved by recent evidence, which suggests that age should not be used as a criterion to determine the need for surgery. In my current practice, we routinely follow patients in their 30s expectantly after a bout of acute diverticulitis.

### Patients with Recurrent Acute Diverticulitis

Traditionally, these patients have been referred for elective colon resection after two or more "attacks." These recommendations were based on the unfounded belief that recurrence rates are high and the incidence of complications even higher. As it turns out, the overall risk of recurrence is relatively low, even after a bout of complicated diverticular disease. It is interesting to note that paradoxically, the incidence of perforation actually seems to decrease with recurrent episodes of acute diverticulitis. Treatment is best individualized based on recurrent symptoms balanced against perioperative morbidity.

### Dietary Restrictions

The idea that large particulate residue in the colon might obstruct a diverticular lumen or otherwise irritate diverticula has intuitive appeal but no foundation in scientific evidence.

### Primary Anastomosis versus Fecal Diversion

The morbidity and mortality associated with Hartmann's procedure should not be underestimated. Despite the initial intent for "temporary" end-colostomy, many of these stomas become permanent. Those patients that do undergo colostomy reversal typically require extensive laparoscopic or open enterolysis and are subject to the not infrequent complications of ileus, infection, and venous thromboembolism. The evidence seems to indicate that when operating on recalcitrant or smoldering diverticulitis of lower Hinchey grade, primary anastomosis can be considered as an option, particularly in patients at low risk for perioperative morbidity. Conversely, if the surgeon's assessment is that an anastomotic leak might pose a prohibitive risk, fecal diversion should be done. Primary colo-colonic anastomosis with proximal diverting loop ileostomy remains a good option that avoids some of the morbidity associated with reversal of a Hartmann procedure.

## Laparoscopy in the Setting of Acute Diverticulitis

My experience with this technique has been positive, echoing the sentiments of the authors based on the limited data available. As a confirmed skeptic, I was a late adopter, but I recall my first experience about 5 years ago. An obese woman in her mid-50s with perforated diverticulitis and purulent peritonitis was admitted via the emergency room, and we quickly decided that she needed surgery. We performed laparoscopic lavage and placed a single closed-suction drain. A large amount of pus was easily suctioned from her pelvis and the phlegmon involving the sigmoid colon was left alone. The operation took less than 45 min. By morning, she felt dramatically better and she was discharged home that evening. Obviously, my experience is anecdotal, and I eagerly await the results of the ongoing prospective trials in Europe. The question of whether to recommend elective laparoscopic colectomy after successful laparoscopic peritoneal lavage remains a valid one. It does seem clear that patient selection is a key element for successful application of laparoscopy in acute diverticulitis. Patients with Hinchey class III disease appear to be the best candidates, as purulence is evacuated without difficulty and the diverticular perforation has either sealed or is drained with relative ease. Patients with Hinchey IV disease and feculent peritonitis seem more prone to failure and usually require more aggressive therapy in the form of colon resection. Most patients with Hinchey I or II disease may be treated without surgery, but may require percutaneous drainage of pericolonic or pelvic abscesses by interventional radiology.

# 51

# *Large Bowel Obstruction*

**Heather Norman and John J. Hong**

**CONTENTS**



Large bowel obstruction is a life-threatening condition that can present as a result of a variety of mechanisms. It can be complex in the sense that there are a wide range of causes that have different management and treatment decisions. Knowledge of anatomy, physiology, surgical treatment options, and critical care are all vital in managing this disease entity. Patients can present with significant physiologic derangements and early identification, and prompt intervention is necessary. Bowel obstructions can be classified in a number of ways, but the treatment philosophy is the same no matter what classification system is used: resuscitation and supportive measures followed by definitive therapy, most often in the form of surgery. Surgical decision making can sometimes be challenging, given the paucity of level 1 evidence. This chapter presents the most up-to-date and applicable research. Recent review articles were also used to support some of the points presented in other retrospective and prospective evaluations.

## 51.1 How Does Colonic Obstruction Present?

The presentation of colonic obstruction depends on the degree of intestinal luminal narrowing, duration of the obstruction, and etiology of the obstruction. The inciting pathologic process will often dictate the patient's presentation. Common symptoms include abdominal distention, nausea and vomiting, and crampy or colicky abdominal pain. They may present with constipation, obstipation, or diarrhea. Presence and severity of symptoms are related to the level of obstruction.

Other symptoms such as hypotension and tachycardia may be present secondary to dehydration or sepsis (from perforation, bowel ischemia, etc.).

In a prospective observational study of 150 adult patients admitted with acute mechanical bowel obstruction to a surgical specialty hospital in Greece over a 2-year period, it was noted that 24% of patients had a large bowel obstruction.

*Recommendation*: Absence of passage of flatus (90%) and/or feces (80.6%) and abdominal distension (65.3%) were the most common symptoms and physical findings, respectively. These percentages are for all patients admitted with mechanical bowel obstruction [1] (Grade C recommendation).

## 51.2 What Are the Causes of Large Bowel Obstruction?

A variety of classification schemes have been derived to organize the causes of large bowel obstruction. A comprehensive and simple outline is illustrated in Current

Therapy in Colon and Rectal Surgery [2]. Categories include (1) lesions extrinsic to the bowel wall, (2) lesions intrinsic to the bowel wall, (3) lesions within bowel lumen, and (4) bowel torsion. Lesions extrinsic to the bowel include compression due to tumor or abscess, hernia, and postoperative adhesions. Lesions intrinsic to the bowel wall would encompass tumor, inflammatory bowel disease, endometriosis, ischemia, or stricture. Lesions within the bowel lumen (intramural) would comprise foreign bodies, gallstone obstruction, intussusceptions, or fecal impaction. Bowel torsion essentially refers to volvulus, either cecal or sigmoidal and, less commonly, transverse colon, and splenic flexure.

By far, neoplasm represents the most common cause of colonic obstruction. In fact, the incidence of mechanical obstruction in patients with colorectal cancer is 14%–34% based on multiple studies. Sigmoid cancer accounted for 15 (75%) of the 20 patients with obstruction due to a large bowel cancer in the study by Markogiannakis et al. [1], whereas 2 (10%) patients had an ascending colon cancer, 1 (5%) had a descending colon cancer, and 1 (5%) had a rectal cancer. Ovarian cancer has a similarly high reported incidence.

Hernias account for less than 3% of patients who present with a large bowel obstruction. However, they do have a significant clinical impact. Hernias causing obstruction are associated with ischemia, necrosis, and perforation at a higher rate than other causes of obstruction [1]. Hernias comprise one of the main causes of extrinsic large bowel obstruction.

Colonic volvulus is responsible for roughly 5% of large bowel obstruction in the United States. This occurs when part of the colon rotates on its mesentery, leading to colonic obstruction and subsequent venous congestion and obstruction of arterial inflow. Sigmoid volvulus is most common, accounting for up to 75% of all colonic volvulus cases. Second most common is cecal volvulus, followed by transverse colon and splenic flexure.

Colonic pseudo-obstruction, or Ogilvie syndrome, should be viewed as a separate disease entity. It involves massive colonic dilation without true mechanical obstruction. The etiology is thought to be related to autonomic imbalance leading to a disturbance of the efferent parasympathetic output of the sacral spinal segments S2–S4 to the distal colon. Initial therapy is similar to mechanical obstruction with fluid resuscitation, nil per os (NPO) and possibly decompression in the form of nasogastric suction and/or rectal tube decompression. However, it is imperative to exclude true colonic obstruction as the subsequent management strategies can vary widely.

*Recommendation*: Large bowel cancer, adhesions, retroperitoneal tumors, and hernias were the most common causes of large bowel obstruction. Hernias, adhesions, strictures, endometriosis, ingested foreign bodies, phytobezoars, gallstones, and rectal foreign bodies have all been found to cause large bowel obstruction (Grade C recommendation).

## 51.3 What Is the Proper Diagnostic Evaluation?

A thorough laboratory evaluation is useful in determining the patient's overall clinical status and may suggest intestinal ischemia, necrosis, or perforation. Although no level 1 evidence can be found to support the routine ordering of certain laboratory tests, it is well known that patients with colonic obstruction often present with multiple metabolic derangements requiring correction prior to surgical intervention. A basic metabolic panel and complete blood count should be done to evaluate for electrolyte imbalances, anemia, and leukocytosis. Other useful laboratory values include a lactate if there is concern for ischemia and a coagulation panel for operative preparation. Given that the most common cause of large bowel obstruction is cancer, a baseline carcinoembryonic antigen level may be reasonable. A single upright chest radiograph may be useful to screen for free air if there is a high suspicion for obstruction with perforation.

In terms of options for confirming a radiographic diagnosis of large bowel obstruction, several studies have been used. Often, a plain abdominal radiograph can confirm the diagnosis, and is said to have 84% sensitivity and 72% specificity in diagnosing large bowel obstruction [3].

A water-soluble contrast enema is another option that may be utilized to establish a diagnosis. This has a sensitivity of 96% and a specificity of 98% [3]. However, CT scanners are now readily available in most hospitals and can be accessed for diagnostic purposes in a timely fashion. In a single institution review over 7 years, it was noted that multidetector CT imaging was more accurate in making the diagnosis of large bowel obstruction than was contrast enema. CT imaging also allowed for the evaluation of other disease processes and, in the case of suspected neoplasm, metastatic disease, and was more readily available [4]. In contrast, Cappell and Batke [3] state that the sensitivity and specificity of abdominopelvic CT in diagnosing large bowel obstruction is 90%.

*Recommendation*: It is the opinion of the authors that even though multidetector CT imaging has a comparable diagnostic capability to water-soluble enema, CT is preferable due to its ability to evaluate for other disease and its availability. Likewise, this modality is quickly interpreted, allows for studying the extent of the primary process, and can be combined with water-soluble enemas if necessary [15] (Grade C recommendation).

## 51.4 Management

Once a patient is diagnosed with a large bowel obstruction, the mainstays of treatment are resuscitation with correction of electrolyte disturbances when possible, followed by relief of obstruction—usually in the form of surgery. The patient should be made NPO. There is level 2 evidence that hydration of over 1 L/day may be associated with less nausea [5]. This was based on a randomized trial of 15 patients with inoperable malignant bowel obstructions. This will also have the desired effect of correcting dehydration and the metabolic abnormalities that can come with that. In some cases, decompression with nasogastric tube or colorectal tube may be warranted. Careful attention to antibiotic and prophylactic (deep venous thrombosis and gastrointestinal) regimens is needed [2].

To date, there is little level 1 evidence comparing one operative approach to another. With the gaining popularity of colonic stents, it is feasible that fewer large bowel obstructions will be taken emergently to the OR. If there is concern over ischemia or perforation, the patient has not clinically improved, or cecal diameter is increasing, laparotomy should be performed [6]. Since most cases of colonic obstruction are due to colon cancer, we will elaborate more thoroughly on this topic. In any case, it is incumbent upon the operating surgeon to thoroughly evaluate the remaining colon for synchronous lesions.

## 51.5 What Is the Preferred Operative Approach?

### 51.5.1 Operative Management of Obstructing Colon Cancer

The debate over management in obstructing colorectal cancer is centered on two issues: non-operative management using stents, and whether or not to perform a primary anastomosis. The role of stenting in colonic obstruction will be covered later in the chapter. In right-sided colon cancer, a right hemicolectomy should be performed [3]. The distal resection margin may include the right branch of the middle colic, especially if the cancer is located at the hepatic flexure [2]. In stable patients, this can be done with a primary anastomosis. Patients who are unstable, have perforation with peritonitis, or have distended bowel should have an ileostomy performed [3]. An article by Stoyanov et al. [7] looked at 232 cases of obstructing colorectal cancer requiring urgent surgical intervention. One hundred and sixty tumors were located in the colon and the remaining 72 had obstructing rectal lesions. In this group, there was a 25% mortality rate. It was noted that there was a higher mortality in the primary anastomosis group [18]. A second series retrospectively reviewed the records of 23 patients with obstructing lesions of the left colon [16]. The patients underwent different surgical procedures: 14 underwent one-stage colonic resection with intraoperative colonic lavage ($n$ = 10) or subtotal colectomy ($n$ = 4), which comprised the resection and primary anastomoses group. Nine patients underwent staged resection with either Hartmann's or loop colostomy and comprised the staged resection group. There was one case of anastomotic dehiscence in resection and primary anastomoses group and two cases in staged resection group. The authors concluded that a one-stage procedure is safe and may be indicated for the management of the majority of cases [8]. For those patients who present with disseminated disease, a palliative resection should be performed. For recurrent disease, a bypass procedure or proximal stoma is most appropriate [3].

*Recommendation*: Stomas are preferred for patients with recurrent disease or for palliative resections. A primary anastomosis can be performed for obstructing colon lesions (Grade C recommendation).

### 51.5.2 Operative Management of Other Causes

Benign strictures can be treated by segmental resection. Preoperative screening colonoscopy is warranted to rule out malignancy. However, this may not be feasible in cases of complete obstruction. Strong consideration must be given to diverting colostomy in the presence of a radiation-induced stricture. Radiation history does not thoroughly exclude a primary anastomosis [3]. There is also literature that supports the use of endoscopic balloon dilation for the treatment of benign strictures, either from inflammatory bowel disease or surgical anastomoses. This is most successful when stricture length is equal or less than 4 cm [9].

Operative management of volvulus depends on the type. Sigmoid volvulus is typically treated with endoscopic decompression followed by semielective surgery in the form of sigmoidectomy and primary anastomosis. Patients with cecal volvulus, on the other hand, classically go directly to the operating room secondary to the high failure rate of colonic decompression [9]. Right hemicolectomy is the standard operative choice. For an extremely debilitated patient with extensive comorbidities in which it is felt operative risk is prohibitive, a cecostomy is an option. In cases with extensive peritoneal contamination or nonviable bowel, it may be warranted to forego a primary anastomosis and proceed with an ostomy.

In summary, multiple operative approaches are available to the operating surgeon. The decision on which, if any, procedure is to be performed, is based on the preoperative imaging studies, the clinical status of the patients and the disease process causing the obstruction. Since the overwhelming majority of colonic obstruction cases are due to colon cancer, standard oncologic operative technique is imperative. It is our opinion that hemodynamically compromised patients, those with gross peritonitis, grossly overdistended bowel, palliative procedures, and patients with previous radiation are candidates for diverting ostomy. If none of the above conditions are met, performing a primary anastomosis is reasonable. On table colonic lavage does not appear to add any benefit [3,10] (Grade C recommendation).

## 51.6 What Is the Role of Laparoscopy in the Treatment of Large Bowel Obstruction?

Gash et al. did a prospective electronic database review between April 2001 and June 2009 looking at the outcomes in consecutive patients presenting with large bowel obstruction who were treated with laparoscopic resectional surgery. In their study, 24 patients underwent laparoscopic surgery secondary to cancer [11] and diverticulosis [12]. There were two conversions. The transition time to a normal diet was 24 h and the median hospital stay was 3 days. There were complications in 25% of the patients.

*Recommendation*: Based on these results, the authors concluded that laparoscopic surgery in acute colonic obstruction is safe and feasible [13]. However, further studies are needed as this was a fairly small study (Grade C recommendation).

## 51.7 Are There Any Nonoperative Options?

Great advances have been made in the nonoperative treatment of large bowel obstruction. Traditionally surgery was the treatment of choice. The current widespread use and technical advancements of endoscopy have expanded the available armamentarium to treat this disease. The current options for nonoperative management include photodynamic therapy, electrocoagulation, laser coagulation, and balloon dilatation. However, the endoluminal stent has made the most significant impact on the nonoperative treatment of colonic obstruction. Given that patients with large bowel obstruction have a significant morbidity and mortality from diverting colostomy (16% and 5%, respectively), stents have become an acceptable treatment option for those patients with inoperable disease and for those who are poor surgical candidates [10,14,15]. As such, level 1 evidence to justify the use of laser coagulation and the other aforementioned methods is scarce. Articles are now appearing frequently on the benefits of colonic stents. We will explore the indications, applications, and complications here. Outcomes for colonic stenting will be covered in the next section.

The minimally invasive nature of colonic stents makes them a perfect adjunct for treating large bowel obstruction in poor surgical candidates and those needing palliative treatment from obstructing cancer. Benign strictures are also being treated by stenting [10]. Some tout the widespread applicability of colonic stenting [10]. To these authors, colonic stenting is indicated in all patients when technically feasible, thus allowing a one-stage procedure while also allowing full evaluation of disease extent [10,16].

The most recent series published in *Colorectal Disease* highlights 63 patients referred for large bowel obstruction [8]. A prospective database was evaluated. Sixty-three patients had 71 stenting procedures performed. Thirty-two patients had metastatic disease discovered during their evaluation. Extrinsic compression caused seven strictures. The indication for stenting was palliation in 56 patients and served as a bridge to a one-stage procedure in 7 patients. Technical success was achieved 91% of the time. Obstructive symptoms were relieved in 89%. Twenty-four percent of the patients had complications including overgrowth (8%), migration (6%), fistulation (4%), stent fracture (3%), tenesmus (3%), and fecal urgency (1%). No procedure-related deaths occurred, and there were no technical failures for lesions proximal to the descending colon. The authors concluded that combination of endoscopic/fluoroscopic colorectal stenting is effective and safe [8]. Dauphine and colleagues [17] retrospectively reviewed 26 patients with malignant obstruction who underwent colonic stenting. The indications, success, and complication rates are mirrored in other studies. Fourteen patients had palliative procedures performed. Twelve patients had colonic stents placed as a bridge to surgery. First attempts were successful in 22 patients. In the remaining four individuals, three required emergency surgery, and one was successfully stented at the second attempt. Seventy-five percent of patients in the bridge-to-surgery group went on to elective colon resection. There was a 29% reobstruction rate and one (9%) stent migration. Patency was maintained in nine (64%) patients who underwent palliative treatment. Based on this, the authors concluded that colonic stents achieve immediate nonoperative decompression that is both safe and effective. Stenting is also a useful adjunct allowing elective resection in the majority of resectable cases [8]. A Cochrane review article published by Trompetas [18] found that colonic stenting is the best option for palliation or as a bridge to surgery. Using stents reduces morbidity, mortality, and colostomy rates. Stenting, depending on the healthcare system, is likely to be cost-effective [18]. The literature focuses on descending colon, sigmoid, and rectal obstruction. As such, more information is needed on the applicability of stenting with regards to right colon and transverse lesions.

Colonic stenting is the most widely accepted method of nonoperative treatment. However, its use is limited by the small number of trained physicians and centers performing the procedure and its utility, at this point, seems to be most pronounced in treating rectal, sigmoid, left, and distal transverse colon lesions. Stenting allows for the relief of obstruction, for full evaluation of the primary process, and can allow for a one-stage procedure. The complication rate is very low. Stenting is particularly helpful in those where treatment is palliative and for patients who are stable and can undergo resuscitation and primary disease evaluation as a bridge to a single operation [8,10,18].

*Recommendation*: Colonic stenting can be used as a bridge to surgery or as a palliative option. The success rate for relieving obstruction is around 90%. Three-quarters of patients in which colonic stents are used as a bridge to surgery will go on to elective resection (Grade B recommendation).

## 51.8 What Is the Preferred Management for Colonic Pseudo-Obstruction: Observation versus Medical or Endoscopic Decompression?

As mentioned previously, colonic pseudo-obstruction, or Ogilvie syndrome, is a functional disorder of the colon involving significant colonic dilation without evidence of true mechanical obstruction. Initial therapy is similar to mechanical obstruction: fluid resuscitation, NPO, enteric decompression, and minimization of contributing factors such as narcotics and other implicated medications. Supportive measures and observation is recommended as the initial treatment in all colonic pseudo-obstruction patients according to a review by Saunders and Kimmey [19]. Further intervention in the form of pharmacologic or endoscopic decompression should be considered in patients who are not showing signs of improvement after 24–48 h or have significant cecal dilation (over 10 cm) of greater than 3–4 days.

The next therapy of choice is neostigmine. Neostigmine is a reversible acetylcholinesterase inhibitor that indirectly stimulates muscarinic and nicotinic receptors thus improving colonic activity and motility. In a randomized, double-blind, placebo-controlled trial by Ponec et al., patients with acute colonic pseudo-obstruction with a cecal diameter greater than 10 cm and no response after 24 h of conservative therapy were given either 2 mg of neostigmine or saline infusion over 3–5 min. A clinical response was observed in 91% of patients who received neostigmine compared to 0% of those receiving saline infusion [20] (Grade B recommendation).

Colonic decompression is reserved for those who have cecal distension greater than 10 cm who are not improving after 24–48 h of supportive therapy and who have contraindications to neostigmine, such as renal insufficiency (serum creatinine greater than 3 mg/dL), uncontrolled cardiac arrhythmias, severe bronchospasm, and pregnancy. Of note, however, there have been no trials that directly compare endoscopic decompression with neostigmine. One other controversial issue is whether mucosal ischemia is a contraindication to colonic decompression. Traditionally, mucosal ischemia identified on endoscopy has been an indication to proceed with surgery. To date, however, there is no level 1 evidence to support or contest this. There are case reports of patients with mucosal ischemia being managed successfully with endoscopic decompression [21]. Given the lack of evidence, this should be reserved for patients who have no evidence of peritonitis and are poor operative candidates (Grade C recommendation).

Surgical treatment of colonic pseudo-obstruction is typically reserved for patients with perforation, mucosal ischemia with peritonitis, or those who fail decompressive therapy. Cecostomy may be performed for patients without perforation or ischemia, with segmental resection or subtotal colectomy being options for the latter depending on the extent of the disease [21].

*Recommendation*: Initial management is supportive, followed by either pharmacologic or endoscopic decompression. Surgery is reserved for peritonitis, perforation, or failure of above therapies (Grade B recommendation).

## 51.9 What Are the Outcomes?

The outcomes for patients presenting with large bowel obstruction vary depending on the cause and whether or not the patient has compromised bowel at the time

**TABLE 51.1**

Clinical Question Summary

| Question | Answer | Grade | References |
|---|---|---|---|
| How does colonic obstruction present? | Absence of passage of flatus (90%) and/or feces (80.6%) and abdominal distension (65.3%) were the most common symptoms and physical finding, respectively. | C | [1] |
| What are the causes of large bowel obstruction? | Large bowel cancer, adhesions, retroperitoneal tumors, and hernias were the most common causes of large bowel obstruction. Hernias, adhesions, strictures, endometriosis, ingested foreign bodies, phytobezoars, gallstones, and rectal foreign bodies have all been found to cause large bowel obstruction. | C | [1,2,24–26] |
| What is the proper diagnostic evaluation? | CT imaging is more accurate in making the diagnosis of large bowel obstruction than was contrast enema. CT imaging also allows for the evaluation of other disease processes, and is more readily available. | C | [4] |
| What is the preferred operative approach? | Stomas are preferred for patients with recurrent disease or for palliative resections. A primary anastomosis can be performed for obstructing colon lesions. | C | [3,22,23] |
| What is the role of laparoscopy in LBO? | Laparoscopic surgery in LBO is safe and feasible and may reduce hospital length of stay. | C | [13] |
| Are there any nonoperative options? | Colonic stenting can be used as a bridge to surgery or as a palliative option. The success rate for relieving obstruction is around 90%. Three-quarters of patients in which colonic stents are used as a bridge to surgery will go on to elective resection. | B | [16–18,28] |
| What is the preferred management for colonic pseudo-obstruction? | Initial management is supportive, followed by either pharmacologic or endoscopic decompression. Surgery is reserved for peritonitis, perforation, or failure of above therapies. | B | [14,20,21] |
| What are the outcomes? | Mortality rates for patients presenting with large bowel obstruction are 20%–25%. If colonic stenting is available, the mortality rate can be significantly reduced. | B | [7,16,23,27] |

of operation. Outcomes for some causes of large bowel obstruction were alluded to in their corresponding section. Mortality rates for those presenting with large bowel obstruction from colon cancer range from 5% to 25%. The mortality rates for those needing urgent operative Hartmann's procedure are similar [13,19]. The mortality rate increases with findings of necrosis and perforation. Incarcerated hernias are more likely to cause necrosis or perforation [1]. A study by Zorcolo et al. [28] retrospectively reviewed the records of 323 patients who presented acutely and underwent surgery over a 10-year period. The etiology of obstruction was left-sided colorectal cancer and diverticular disease. The aim of the review was to identify a difference in outcome of resection and primary anastomosis with Hartmann's procedure. Primary anastomosis was performed in 176 (55.7%) patients with a 30-day mortality of 5.7%. Nine (5.1%) patients had anastomotic breakdown. Hartmann's resection was associated with a higher incidence of systemic and surgical morbidity (39.5% and 24.3%, respectively). Mortality from primary anastomosis (5.7%) compared favorably with those undergoing Hartmann's resections (20.4%).

As mentioned previously, colonic stenting has the ability to convert an emergency procedure to an elective procedure with the ability to have a colon prep and evaluate the patient for other systemic disease. The aforementioned studies reveal a lower morbidity and mortality when colonic stents are used as a bridge to a single surgical procedure (Grade B recommendation).

*Recommendation*: Mortality rates for patients presenting with large bowel obstruction are 20%–25%. If colonic stenting is available, the mortality rate can be significantly reduced (Grade B recommendation) (Table 51.1).

In summary, colonic obstruction is a complex disease entity attributable to a large variety of causes, which may have unique operative strategies. Nevertheless, the treatment philosophy is the same no matter what the underlying cause: aggressive resuscitation followed by relief of the obstruction. Early recognition and prompt surgical consultation are crucial in limiting the morbidity and mortality of this disease process.

## References

1. Markogiannakis H, Messaris E, Dardamanis D et al. Acute mechanical bowel obstruction: Clinical presentation, etiology, management and outcome. *World J Gastroenterol*. 2007;13:432–437.
2. Fazio V, Church J, Delaney C. 2004. *Current Therapy in Colon and Rectal Surgery*. 2nd ed. Mosby: St. Louis, MO.

3. Cappell MS, Batke M. Mechanical obstruction of the small bowel and colon. *Med Clin North Am.* 208;92:575–597.
4. Jacob SE, Lee SH, Hill J. The demise of the instant/unprepared contrast enema in large bowel obstruction. *Colorectal Dis.* November 12, 2007 [Epub ahead of print].
5. Mercadante S, Ripamonti C, Casuccio A, Zecca E, Groff L. Comparison of octreotide and hyocine butylbromide in controlling gastrointestinal symptoms due to malignant inoperable bowel obstruction. *Support Care Cancer.* May 2000;8(3):188–191.
6. Lopez-Kostner F, Hool GR, Lavery IC. Management and causes of acute large bowel obstruction. *Surg Clin North Am.* 1997;77:1265–1290.
7. Stoyanov H, Julianov A, Valtchev D et al. Results of the treatment of colorectal cancer complicated by obstruction. *Wien Klin Wochenschr.* 198;110:262–265.
8. Finan PJ, Campbell S, Verma R et al. The management of malignant large bowel obstruction: ACPGBI position statement. *Colorectal Dis.* 2007;9(4):1–17.
9. Small AJ, Young-Fadok TM, Baron TH. Expandable metal stent placement for benign colorectal obstruction: outcomes for 23 cases. *Surg Endosc.* 2008;22:454–462.
10. Raveenthiran V. Restorative resection of unprepared left colon in gangrenous vs viable sigmoid volvulus. *Int J Colorectal Dis.* 2004;19:258–263.
11. Chueng HYS, Chung CC, Chieng WW, Wong JCH, Yau KKK, Li MKW. Endolaparoscopic approach vs conventional open surgery in the treatment of obstructing left-sided colon cancer. *Arch Surg.* 2009;144(12):1127–1132.
12. De Giorgio R, Knowles CH. Acute colonic pseudo-obstruction. *Br J Surg.* 2009;96:229–239.
13. Gash K, Chambers W, Ghosh A, Dixon AR. The role of laparoscopic surgery for the management of acute large bowel obstruction. *Colorectal Dis.* March 2011;13(3):263–266.
14. Lopera JE, Ferral H, Wholey Met al. Treatment of colonic obstructions with metallic stents: Indications, technique, and complications. *Am J Roentgenol.* 1997;169:1285–1290.
15. Seymour K, Johnson R, Marsh R, Corson J. Palliative stenting of malignant large bowel obstruction. *Colorectal Dis.* 2002,4:240–245.
16. Baraza W, Lee F, Brown S, Hurlstone DP. Combination endoradiological colorectal stenting: A prospective 5-year clinical evaluation. *Ann Surg Oncol.* 2002;9:574–579.
17. Dauphine CE, Tan P, Beart RW Jr, Vukasin P, Cohen H, Corman ML. Placement of self-expanding stents for acute malignant large-bowel obstruction: A collective review. *Ann Surg Oncol.* July 2002;9(6):574–579.
18. Trompetas V. Emergency management of malignant acute left-sided colonic obstruction. *Ann R Coll Surg Engl.* April 2008;90(3):181–186.
19. Saunders MD, Kimmey MD. Systematic review: Acute colonic pseudo-obstruction. *Aliment Pharmacol Ther.* 2005;22:917–925.
20. Ponec RJ, Saunders MD, Kimmey MB. Neostigmine for the treatment of acute colonic pseudo-obstruction. *N Engl J Med.* 1999;341(3):137–141.
21. Florto JJ, Schoen RE, Brandt LF. Pseudo-obstruction associated with colonic ischemia: successful management with colonoscopic decompression. *Am J Gastroenterol.* 1991;86:1472–1476.
22. De Aguilar-Nascimento JE, Caporossi C, Nascimento M. Comparison between resection and primary anastomosis and staged resection in obstructing adenocarcinoma of the left colon. *Arq Gastroenterol.* 2002;39:240–45.
23. Zorcolo L, Covotta L, CarloMagno Net al. Safety of primary anastomosis in emergency colo-rectal surgery. *Colorectal Dis.* 2003;5:262–269.
24. Jenkins JT, Taylor AJ, Behrns KE. Secondary causes of intestinal obstruction: Rigorous preoperative evaluation is required. *Am Surg.* 2000;66:662–666.
25. Varras M, Kostopanagiotou E, Katis K et al. Endometriosis causes extensive intestinal obstruction simulating carcinoma of the sigmoid colon: A case report and review of the literature. *Eur J Gynaecol Oncol.* 2002;23:353–357.
26. Efrati Y, Freud E, Serour F, Klin B. Phytobezoar-induced ileal and colonic obstruction in childhood. *J Pediatr Gastroenterol Nutr.* 1997;25:214–216.
27. Hennekine-Mucci S, Tuech JJ, Brehant O et al. Management of obstructed left colon carcinoma. *Hepatogastroenterology.* 2007;54:1098–1101.
28. Harrison ME, Anderson M, Appalaneni V et al. The role of endoscopy in the management of patients with known and suspected colonic obstruction and pseudo-obstruction. *GI Endosc.* 2010;71(4):669–679.

## Commentary on Large Bowel Obstruction

*Martin A. Schreiber*

The authors of this evidenced-based paper have very nicely summarized the etiology, workup, management, and outcome of large bowel obstruction. There are a few points I would like to emphasize. In terms of the workup, the authors have described plain films, water-soluble enema, and multidetector CT as the primary modalities. I think it is important to emphasize that CT performed with water-soluble rectal contrast allows one to characterize the degree of colonic obstruction as well as the degree of proximal dilatation while providing much more information about the intra-abdominal contents. This is particularly important in the colonic stenting era, because information concerning local invasion and distant metastatic spread in malignant processes is provided. The decision to stent a colon cancer for palliation requires this type of information so that CT becomes a very important modality in decision making.

In terms of the etiologies of large bowel obstruction, the authors have failed to mention diverticulitis. In fact, diverticulitis is frequently cited as the third most common cause of large bowel obstruction following neoplasm and volvulus*. Complete large bowel obstruction secondary to diverticulitis has traditionally been treated with sigmoid resection and proximal colostomy. Resection with on-table preparation followed by primary anastomosis with or without proximal diversion has also been reported†‡.

The authors have described the management of large bowel obstruction and have focused on the debate between primary anastomosis and diversion. Based on the literature, they have concluded that patients who are unstable, have a perforation with peritonitis or distended bowel should be diverted. While I agree with this in general, I also believe that there is a third option for the management of these patients, which encompasses a damage control approach§. Truly unstable patients may benefit from an abbreviated surgical procedure that includes amelioration of the obstruction and stapling of the bowel ends while leaving the abdomen open. The patient is then taken to the ICU for correction of physiologic abnormalities including stabilization of the hemodynamic status and correction of acidosis, coagulopathy, and hypothermia. Once these goals are achieved, the patient is returned to the operating room for primary anastomosis or diversion and closure of the abdomen.

I think the most important advances described in this chapter relate to the nonoperative management of strictures and malignant obstruction. Balloon dilatation of strictures provides an endoscopic method of treating strictures and stenting of malignant obstructions provides a method to either palliate patients with advanced disease or turn multistage procedures into single stage procedures. Traditionally, palliation of colon cancer patients with metastatic or unresectable disease has been associated with extremely high morbidity and mortality. Stenting is a much less morbid option for palliation and has the potential to improve the quality of life.

---

* Webb AL, Fink AS. 2011. Large Bowel Obstruction; Current Surgical Therapy, 10th edn. Elsevier: Philadelphia, PA, pp. 154–157.

† McCafferty MH, Roth L, Jorden J. Current management of diverticulitis. *Am Surg.* 2008;74:1041–1049.

‡ Edward CL, Murray JJ, Coller JA et al. Intraoperative colonic lavage in nonelective surgery for diverticulitis. *Dis Colon Rectum.* 1997;40:669–674.

§ Kafka-Ritsch R, Birkfeliner F, Perathoner A et al. Damage control surgery with abdominal vacuum and delayed bowel reconstruction in patients with perforated diverticulitis hinchey III/IV. *J Gastrointest Surg.* 2012;16:1915–1922.

# 52

# *Acute and Chronic Mesenteric Ischemia*

**Ramon F. Cestero**

**CONTENTS**



Mesenteric ischemic syndromes remain a challenging and morbid spectrum of surgical diseases, despite advances in surgical critical care, diagnostic imaging, and minimally invasive techniques. The mesenteric ischemic syndromes include acute mesenteric ischemia (AMI) of all causes, chronic mesenteric ischemia (CMI), mesenteric venous thrombosis (MVT), and nonocclusive mesenteric ischemia (NOMI). While lower extremity and carotid occlusive diseases may be more common, mesenteric ischemia carries higher morbidity and mortality rates. Delay in diagnosis is common and is the most serious shortcoming in current treatment of mesenteric ischemia. In one retrospective analysis, only one-third of patients with mesenteric ischemia were correctly diagnosed before surgery or death [1]. Early diagnosis of mesenteric ischemia is a challenge, but the entity must be considered if acceptable outcomes are desired.

Q: What is the ideal mode of imaging in the diagnosis of acute or chronic mesenteric ischemia?

*Duplex ultrasound*: Transabdominal duplex examination performed in a competent vascular laboratory offers an accurate, noninvasive method of splanchnic vascular assessment, especially for screening in the ambulatory population. In a prospective validation study in which duplex was paired with angiography, a peak systolic velocity (PSV) of ≥275 cm/s in the superior mesenteric artery (SMA) and ≥200 cm/s in the celiac artery (CA) was predictive of a 70%–100% stenosis with sensitivity of 92% and specificity of 96% for the SMA and sensitivity of 87% and specificity of 80% for the CA [2] (Level Ib evidence). Stenosis of the superior mesenteric artery >50% or occlusion may be predicted by an end-diastolic velocity (EDV) ≥45 cm/s. Celiac artery stenosis may be highly predicted by a finding of reversed flow in the common hepatic artery [3]. Postprandial duplex was not found to increase the sensitivity of the examination [4]. Duplex is significantly limited in several ways, however: Duplex ultrasound has not been evaluated in the setting of acute mesenteric ischemia, nor can it interrogate mesenteric vessels distal to the proximal main vessel, where emboli may lodge. Ultrasound findings must be interpreted in light of the patient's clinical scenario, since significant stenoses and occlusions of the mesenteric vessels can occur in the asymptomatic patient.

*Angiography*: Formal contrast angiography is considered the gold standard for diagnosis of acute mesenteric ischemia (AMI). Anteroposterior and lateral aortic views demonstrate the origins of the mesenteric arteries and are diagnostic of stenoses or occlusions. Case series report sensitivity of 74%–100% and specificity of 100% in the diagnosis of AMI [5]. Catheter access to the mesenteric vessels can also be obtained, allowing endovascular therapy of the offending lesion.

*CT Angiography*: Although early studies of CT angiography (CTA) yielded less than encouraging results, more recent reviews using multidetector row CT angiography seem to indicate an acceptable sensitivity of 96% and specificity of 94% [6]. A recent systematic review and meta-analysis of eight studies investigating the sensitivity and specificity of CT for the diagnosis of mesenteric ischemia reported a pooled sensitivity and specificity of 94% and 95%, respectively [7]. CT angiography may also yield additional information about the condition of the bowel, assisting in the decision of whether to perform laparotomy. Mesenteric venous thrombosis can also be reliably diagnosed on CTA, with a sensitivity of 100% for acute MVT and 93% for chronic MVT [8]. In summary, CT angiography may be considered as one of the first-line studies in mesenteric ischemic syndromes (Level 3b).

*MRA*: MRA in the setting of acute mesenteric ischemia is of limited value. MRA has been compared with digital subtraction angiography in the setting of chronic mesenteric ischemia only in small retrospective series [9,10]. Postprocedural imaging may be better using CTA rather than MRA, because of faster acquisition times, better resolution, and the improved ability to visualize flow through metallic stents [11] (Level 3b evidence in CMI).

A: For chronic mesenteric ischemia, duplex ultrasound, CTA, and MRA offer acceptable results, with angiography as a potential confirmatory step. In acute mesenteric ischemia, only CTA or invasive angiography have been studied and both are reliable (Grade B recommendation).

Q: Can endovascular therapy be recommended for acute thrombo-embolic mesenteric ischemia?

It is generally agreed that endovascular therapy has a limited role in the setting of AMI with peritonitis, in which case laparotomy is indicated. However, in that subset of patients with suspected early (and thus potentially reversible) mesenteric ischemia, some have advocated angiography with catheter-based therapy of the arterial lesion. In a review of 48 total published cases of thrombolysis in the setting of acute thromboembolic mesenteric ischemia from 1979 to 2002, technical success was achieved in 43 cases, but clinical success (defined as freedom from death or laparotomy) was seen in only 30 of 48 patients. Mortality in this highly select series of patients managed with combination of catheter-directed thrombolysis and surgery was 10.4% [12].

Reports of successful endovascular approaches to AMI have increased in the last decade, however. Schermerhorn et al. [13] evaluated the Nationwide Inpatient Sample from 1988 to 2006 and reported that 35% of patients presenting with AMI underwent angioplasty and stenting, while only 65% were treated with embolectomy, surgical bypass, or endarterectomy. The mortality rate was 16% for those undergoing endovascular therapy versus 39% for open revascularization ($p < 0.001$) despite patients in the endovascular group being older with more comorbidities. In another retrospective study evaluating endovascular versus traditional approaches to AMI, Arthurs et al. [14] reported 56 of 70 patients who underwent initial endovascular treatment. Patients managed with endovascular interventions had a high success rate with only 9 of 56 treatment failures and lower in-hospital mortality (36%) versus traditional open surgical therapy (50%, $p < 0.05$).

Although recent publications describing successful endovascular approaches to AMI are encouraging, no randomized comparison of open surgery versus endovascular therapy exists for the treatment of patients with acute mesenteric ischemia (Level 4 evidence).

A: No head-to-head comparison exists comparing open surgery with endovascular treatment for acute thromboembolic mesenteric ischemia. Selective thrombolysis may be attempted, mandating postprocedure observation for signs of intestinal infarction (Grade C recommendation).

Q: Does evidence favor open bypass or catheter-based endovascular intervention for chronic mesenteric ischemia?

Many small case series of percutaneous angioplasty and/or stenting (PAS) have reported short-term results at least consistent with, if not less morbid than, open revascularization (OR) [15–18]. Primary and primary-assisted patency rates are consistently lower than in large series of patients undergoing open revascularization [19]. One case–control study attempted to compare similar cohorts of patients undergoing OR versus PAS. In-hospital morbidity and mortality were not different between the groups, but PAS was associated with statistically significantly decreased 1-year primary patency (58% vs. 90%, $p < 0.001$) and primary-assisted patency (65% vs. 96%, $p < 0.001$), and the need for earlier reintervention [20] (Level 3b evidence).

A: Percutaneous angioplasty and stenting seem to offer greater patient convenience at the expense of diminished long-term patency. Both open and endovascular techniques can be safely offered to patients, but open surgery remains the gold standard (Grade B recommendation).

Q: Should open revascularization for CMI include single or multiple vessel reconstruction?

In multiple retrospective case series, no statistically significant difference in either primary patency or mortality has been shown between single (SMA) and multiple vessel reconstruction [19,21,22] (Level 4 evidence, case series). Choice of revascularization technique is typically tailored to the patient's anatomy and physiologic state at surgery.

A: The data are inconclusive. Choice of open revascularization technique may be tailored to the patient (Grade C recommendation).

Q: What is the ideal treatment for acute mesenteric venous thrombosis?

Mesenteric venous thrombosis (MVT) accounts for 5%–15% of presentations of mesenteric ischemic syndromes. The mainstay of treatment has historically been immediate heparin anticoagulation with observation for signs of development of intestinal infarction, which then mandates abdominal exploration with resection of involved bowel. Mortality ranges from 15% to 50% [23,24]. Some small but promising case series have been reported describing transhepatic or transjugular intrahepatic portal venous catheter access with thrombolysis of the portal vein and SMV, with low mortality rates (0%–9%) [25,26]. At this time, in the absence of trials comparing standard

**TABLE 52.1**
Clinical Questions

| Question | Answer | Grade of Recommendation | References |
|---|---|---|---|
| What is the ideal mode of imaging in CMI and AMI? | AMI—angio or CTA<br>CMI—duplex, angio, CTA, MRA | B | [2–11] |
| Endovascular therapy for AMI? | Selective thrombolysis in early AMI | C | [12–14] |
| Open or endovascular treatment for CMI? | Open has better patency, both may be offered safely | B | [15–20] |
| Single or multivessel open reconstruction? | Equivalent, may be tailored to patient | C | [19,21,22] |
| How to treat mesenteric venous thrombosis? | Anticoagulation ± surgery for peritonitis; catheter-directed thrombolysis may be safe | C | [23–26] |
| How to treat NOMI? | Catheter-directed vasodilators ± surgery for peritonitis | C | [27–30] |

**TABLE 52.2**
Levels of Evidence

| Subject | Year | References | Level of Evidence | Strength of Recommendation | Findings |
|---|---|---|---|---|---|
| Duplex vs. angio in CMI | 1997 | [2] | Ib | B | Duplex sens/spec is 92% and 96% for SMA and 87% and 80% for CA |
| CT angiography | 2003, 2013 | [6,7] | IIIb | B | Improved sens/spec when examining a constellation of findings |
| MRA for CMI | 1997, 2001 | [9,10] | IIIb | B | |
| Thrombolysis for AMI | 2005 | [12] | IV | C | Thrombolysis ± laparotomy may be attempted for thromboembolic AMI |
| OR vs. PAS for CMI | 2007 | [20] | IIIB | B | OR more durable, similar M&M |
| Single or multivessel open reconstruction | 1994, 2002, 1992 | [19,21,22] | IV | C | No difference in single and multiple vessel open reconstruction |
| Catheter-directed thrombolysis for MVT | 2005 | [25,26] | IV | C | Case series describe thrombolysis for venous thrombosis |
| Vasodilator therapy for NOMI | 1984, 1995, 1977, 2007 | [27–30] | IV | C | Case series describe vasodilator therapy for NOMI |

management with selective mesenteric venous thrombolysis, no strong recommendations can be made.

A: Systemic anticoagulation with serial observation for signs of bowel infarction. If resources allow, catheter-directed mesenteric venous thrombolysis may be considered (Grade C recommendation).

Q: What is the ideal treatment for nonocclusive mesenteric ischemia (NOMI)?

NOMI can be a diagnostic and therapeutic challenge, since patients who develop NOMI may be in no condition for an operation or an extended visit to the angiography suite. Vasopressors, cocaine use, diuretics, and digitalis have all been implicated as contributing factors in NOMI, and may exacerbate ischemia in the presence of preexisting atherosclerotic lesions of the mesenteric circulation or in low-flow states such as congestive heart failure (CHF), hemodialysis, or myocardial infarction. Vigorous treatment of the underlying cause of low cardiac output remains the cornerstone of treatment of patients suspected of having NOMI (Level 4 evidence).

Four small case series totaling 42 patients utilizing intra-arterial infusion of vasodilators (papaverine hydrochloride or tolazoline) or intravenous prostaglandin E2 as an adjunct to surgery demonstrated a mortality of 0%–55%, compared with historic rates of mortality of 70% or more for NOMI [27–30] (Level 4 evidence, case series).

A: In patients with NOMI who do not respond to systemic supportive therapy, early angiography with intra-arterial infusion of vasodilators (typically papaverine) and selective laparotomy for gut infarction can be cautiously recommended (Grade C recommendation) (Tables 52.1 and 52.2).

## References

1. Mamode N, Pickford I, Leiberman P. Failure to improve outcome in acute mesenteric ischaemia: Seven-year review. *Eur J Surg.* 1999;165(3):203–208.
2. Nicoloff AD, Williamson WK, Moneta GL et al. Duplex ultrasonography in evaluation of splanchnic artery stenosis. *Surg Clin North Am.* 1997;77(2):339–355.

3. Zwolak RM, Fillinger MF, Walsh DB et al. Mesenteric and celiac duplex scanning: A validation study. *J Vasc Surg.* 1998;27(6):1078–1087; discussion 1088.
4. Gentile AT, Moneta GL, Lee RL et al. Usefulness of fasting and postprandial duplex ultrasound examinations for predicting high-grade superior mesenteric artery stenosis. *Am J Surg.* 1995;169(5):476–479.
5. Brandt LJ, Boley SJ. AGA technical review on intestinal ischemia. American Gastrointestinal Association. *Gastroenterology.* 2000;118(5):954–968.
6. Kirkpatrick ID, Kroeker MA, Greenberg HM. Biphasic CT with mesenteric CT angiography in the evaluation of acute mesenteric ischemia: Initial experience. *Radiology.* 2003;229(1):91–98.
7. Cudnik MT, Darbha S, Jones J et al. The diagnosis of acute mesenteric ischemia: A systematic review and meta-analysis. *Acad Emerg Med.* 2013;20(11):1087–1100.
8. Rhee RY, Mendonca CT, Petterson TM et al. Mesenteric venous thrombosis: Still a lethal disease in the 1990s. *J Vasc Surg.* 1994;20(5):688–697.
9. Meaney JF, Prince MR, Nostrant TT et al. Gadolinium-enhanced MR angiography of visceral arteries in patients with suspected chronic mesenteric ischemia. *J Magn Reson Imag.* 1997;7(1):171–176.
10. Carlos RC, Stanley JC, Stafford-Johnson D et al. Interobserver variability in the evaluation of chronic mesenteric ischemia with gadolinium-enhanced MR angiography. *Acad Radiol.* 2001;8(9):879–887.
11. Shih MC, Angle JF, Leung DA et al. CTA and MRA in mesenteric ischemia: Part 2, Normal findings and complications after surgical and endovascular treatment. *AJR.* 2007;188(2):462–471.
12. Schoots IG, Levi MM, Reekers JA et al. Thrombolytic therapy for acute superior mesenteric artery occlusion. *J Vasc Interv Radiol.* 2005;16(3):317–329.
13. Schermerhorn ML, Giles KA, Hamdan AD et al. Mesenteric revascularization: Management and outcomes in the United States, 1988–2006. *J Vasc Surg.* 2009;50(2):341–348;e1.
14. Arthurs ZM, Titus J, Bannazadeh M et al. A comparison of endovascular revascularization with traditional therapy for the treatment of acute mesenteric ischemia. *J Vasc Surg.* 2011;53(3):698–704; discussion 704–705.
15. Sharafuddin MJ, Olson CH, Sun S et al. Endovascular treatment of celiac and mesenteric arteries stenoses: Applications and results. *J Vasc Surg.* 2003;38(4):692–698.
16. Kasirajan K, O'Hara PJ, Gray BH et al. Chronic mesenteric ischemia: Open surgery versus percutaneous angioplasty and stenting. *J Vasc Surg.* 2001;33(1):63–71.
17. Landis MS, Rajan DK, Simons ME et al. Percutaneous management of chronic mesenteric ischemia: Outcomes after intervention. *J Vasc Interv Radiol.* 2005;16(10):1319–1325.
18. AbuRahma AF, Stone PA, Bates MC et al. Angioplasty/stenting of the superior mesenteric artery and celiac trunk: Early and late outcomes. *J Endovasc Ther.* 2003;10(6):1046–1053.
19. Park WM, Cherry KJ, Jr., Chua HK et al. Current results of open revascularization for chronic mesenteric ischemia: A standard for comparison. *J Vasc Surg.* 2002;35(5):853–859.
20. Atkins MD, Kwolek CJ, LaMuraglia GM et al. Surgical revascularization versus endovascular therapy for chronic mesenteric ischemia: A comparative experience. *J Vasc Surg.* 2007;45(6):1162–1171.
21. Gentile AT, Moneta GL, Taylor LM et al. Isolated bypass to the superior mesenteric artery for intestinal ischemia. *Arch Surg.* 1994;129(9):926–931; discussion 931–932.
22. McAfee MK, Cherry KJ, Naessens JM et al. Influence of complete revascularization on chronic mesenteric ischemia. *Am J Surg.* 1992;164(3):220–224.
23. Chang RW, Chang JB, Longo WE. Update in management of mesenteric ischemia. *World J Gastroenterol.* 2006;12(20):3243–3247.
24. Kumar S, Sarr MG, Kamath PS. Mesenteric venous thrombosis. *N Engl J Med.* 2001;345(23):1683–1688.
25. Kim HS, Patra A, Khan J et al. Transhepatic catheter-directed thrombectomy and thrombolysis of acute superior mesenteric venous thrombosis. *J Vasc Interv Radiol.* 2005;16(12):1685–1691.
26. Hollingshead M, Burke CT, Mauro MA et al. Transcatheter thrombolytic therapy for acute mesenteric and portal vein thrombosis. *J Vasc Interv Radiol.* 2005;16(5):651–661.
27. Clark RA, Gallant TE. Acute mesenteric ischemia: Angiographic spectrum. *AJR.* 1984;142(3):555–562.
28. Ward D, Vernava AM, Kaminski DL et al. Improved outcome by identification of high-risk nonocclusive mesenteric ischemia, aggressive reexploration, and delayed anastomosis. *Am J Surg.* 1995;170(6):577–580; discussion 580–581.
29. Boley SJ, Sprayregan S, Siegelman SS et al. Initial results from an aggressive roentgenological and surgical approach to acute mesenteric ischemia. *Surgery.* 1977;82(6):848–855.
30. Mitsuyoshi A, Obama K, Shinkura N et al. Survival in nonocclusive mesenteric ischemia: Early diagnosis by multidetector row computed tomography and early treatment with continuous intravenous high-dose prostaglandin E(1). *Ann Surg.* 2007;246(2):229–235.

## Commentary on Acute and Chronic Mesenteric Ischemia

*Michael J. Sise*

Mesenteric ischemia remains a potentially lethal disease, which requires prompt recognition and effective treatment for successful management[*†]. Unfortunately, delay in diagnosis is very common. Both acute and chronic mesenteric ischemia present in the setting of significant comorbidities and the symptoms of both often mimic other gastrointestinal diseases. The acute mesenteric ischemic syndromes usually occur in the setting of cardiac embolic disease or critical illness with low mesenteric blood flow[‡]. Chronic mesenteric ischemia occurs in the setting of diffuse atherosclerotic occlusive disease and is insidious in onset. A high index of suspicion is the best approach to make the diagnosis in a timely fashion. Despite significant advances in the treatment of vascular occlusive disease, the mortality of mesenteric ischemia remains very high.

Overall, the pathophysiology of acute mesenteric occlusion includes cardiac source embolism in 50%, acute thrombotic occlusion of pre-existing stenotic vessels in 20%, nonocclusive mesenteric vasoconstriction in the setting of critical illness in 20%, and mesenteric venous thrombosis in 10%[§¶]. Symptomatic chronic mesenteric atherosclerotic occlusive disease is not uncommon. Usually, the gradual stenosis and growth of collaterals make symptoms of chronic postprandial pain and weight loss rare[**]. Single mesenteric vessel proximal atherosclerotic occlusion is usually well tolerated because of collateral flow. Asymptomatic total proximal occlusion of all three mesenteric arteries and adequate gut blood supply from internal iliac arteries via hemorrhoidal branches, marginal artery of Drummond, and gastroduodenal arteries have been documented with arteriography. Symptoms in chronic disease require mutlivessel disease with inadequate collaterals[§††].

The classic clinical presentation of acute intestinal ischemia in a patient with atrial fibrillation and cardiac embolic occlusion of the superior mesenteric artery with sudden onset of pain out of proportion to findings and profound leukocytosis occurs in less than half of all cases of acute mesenteric ischemia[†‡]. More commonly, acute ischemia causes a slower onset of initial pain followed at variable intervals by evidence of bowel necrosis with peritonitis and systemic effects. However, profound leukocytosis remains common and should prompt to inclusion of mesenteric ischemia in the differential diagnosis whenever the white blood count exceeds 20,000 in a patient with abdominal pain[†]. Acute thrombosis superimposed on chronic mesenteric occlusive ischemia is usually preceded by postprandial pain, fear of food, and weight loss[§].

Mesenteric venous thrombosis causes an insidious onset of initially vague symptoms, which worsen progressively over time[‡‡§§]. In patients with inherited hypercoagulability, it may occur spontaneously or after a brief episode of gastroenteritis or other illness. In contrast, mesenteric venous thrombosis from acquired hypercoagulability may occur in conjunction with abdominal or multisystem trauma, intra-abdominal inflammation, or oral contraceptives. Nonocclusive acute mesenteric ischemia from vasoconstriction occurs in the setting of critical illness with reduced cardiac output with or without pre-existing mesenteric arterial stenosis. It usually is insidious in onset and often difficult to diagnose in the critical care setting, because it is associated with vague symptoms or undetectable symptoms in the intubated patient[**††].

An early diagnosis of either acute or chronic mesenteric ischemia in patients at risk requires a promptly performed CT scan of the abdomen with intravenous contrast[¶¶***]. This exam effectively evaluates mesenteric arterial and venous patency, perfusion of the bowel, and will indicate if one of the other possible etiologies of clinical findings is present. Early CT scanning allows both timely diagnosis before significant bowel compromise occurs and makes appropriate interventions more likely to succeed. Although it may be effective in the hands of a skilled technician, few centers have extensive experience with Duplex scanning for mesenteric arterial and venous occlusive diseases. Catheter angiography of

* Wyers MC. Acute mesenteric ischemia: Diagnostic approach and surgical treatment. *Semin Vasc Surg*. 2010;23:9–20.

† Kougias P, Lau D, El Sayed FH et al. Determinants of mortality and treatment outcome following surgical interventions for acute mesenteric ischemia. *J Vasc Surg*. 2007;46:467–474.

‡ Schoots IG, Koffeman GI, Legemate DA et al. Systematic review of survival after acute mesenteric ischemia according to disease aetiology. *Br J Surg*. 2004;91:17–27.

§ Oldenburg WA, Louis Lau LL, Rodenberg TL et al. Acute mesenteric ischemia. *Arch Intern Med*. 2004;164:1054–1062.

¶ McKinsey JF, Gewertz BL. Acute mesenteric ischemia. *Surg Clin North Am*. 1997;77:307–318.

** Moore WS. Visceral ischemic syndromes. In: Moore WS, ed. *Vascular and Endovascular Surgery*, 7th edn. Saunders: New York, 2005.

†† Hansen KJ, Wilson DB, Craven TE, Pearce JD. Mesenteric artery disease in the elderly. *J Vasc Surg*. 2004;40:45–52.

‡‡ Boley SJ, Kaleya RN, Brandt LJ. Mesenteric venous thrombosis. *Surg Clin North Am*. 1992;72:183–201.

§§ Rhee RY, Gloviczki P, Mendonca CT et al. Mesenteric venous thrombosis: Still a lethal disease in the 1990s. *J Vasc Surg*. 1994;20:688–697.

¶¶ Horton KM, Fishman EK. Multidetector CT angiography in the diagnosis of mesenteric ischemia. *Radiol Clin North Am*. 2007;45:275–288.

*** Cikrit DF, Harris VJ, Hemmer CG et al. Comparison of spiral CT scan and arteriography for evaluation of renal and visceral arteries. *Ann Vasc Surg*. 1996;10:109–116.

the mesenteric vessels has diminished in importance for diagnosis with the availability of CT angiography. The time saved with immediately available CT imaging leads to both effective endovascular techniques and open surgical approaches.

The treatment for cardiac source emboli remains prompt exploratory laparotomy and superior mesenteric artery thrombectomy[§*]. Thrombolytic therapy is yet to be widely used or proved effective in acute mesenteric ischemia. For chronic disease, the need for open revascularization has markedly diminished with the advances made in endovascular techniques[†‡]. The need for arterial bypass is exceptionally uncommon if prompt CT scanning occurs and timely endovascular therapy is used in patients with acute thrombosis of a pre-existing stenosis[§]. For the patient with threatened bowel necrosis who needs to undergo exploratory laparotomy bypass is not always needed. A blended approach with a digital C-arm, a fluoroscopy-capable operating room table, a cart with the appropriate supplies, and a colleague with catheter and imaging skills (interventional radiologist or vascular surgeon) can create a "hybrid OR" in almost any operating room.

With the steady decrease in open vascular surgical procedures, fewer and fewer surgeons with extensive experience in mesenteric arterial reconstruction remain in practice. This expertise has become a precious commodity. Exposure and bypass of the proximal mesenteric vessels should only be undertaken by experienced surgeons[¶**]. Effective planning with a capable colleague on call for these uncommon surgical emergencies is essential to successful management.

Mesenteric venous thrombosis requires anticoagulation and bowel rest. Worsening symptoms mandate exploratory laparotomy[††‡‡]. Portal vein or mesenteric vein thrombectomy is extremely dangerous and not recommended[†]. Direct transjugular and transhepatic thrombolytic therapy early in the disease may be helpful but requires sufficient endovascular expertise. It has not been conclusively proven better than anticoagulation and bowel rest. The mainstay of treatment of nonocclusive mesenteric ischemia remains adequate fluid resuscitation, avoiding systemic vasoconstrictors, and selective use of catheter directed vasodilators[†].

Prompt recognition, rapid diagnosis, and early and effective intervention remain essential to the successful management of acute and chronic mesenteric ischemia. Preparation with effective planning, experienced surgical and interventional radiology colleagues on call and available is extremely important at all centers who manage acute care surgical emergencies.

* Ryer EJ, Manju Kalra M, Oderich GS et al. Revascularization for acute mesenteric ischemia. *J Vasc Surg.* 2012;55:1682–1689.

† Kasirajan K, O'Hara PJ, Gray BH et al. Chronic mesenteric ischemia: Open surgery versus percutaneous angioplasty and stenting. *J Vasc Surg.* 2001;33:63–71.

‡ Matsumoto AH, Angle JF, Spinosa DJ et al. Percutaneous transluminal angioplasty and stenting in the treatment of chronic mesenteric ischemia: Results and long-term follow up. *J Am Coll Surg.* 2002;194:S22–S31.

§ Schermerhorn ML, Giles KA, Hamdan AD et al. Mesenteric revascularization: Management and outcomes in the United States 1988–2006. *J Vasc Surg.* 2009;50:341–348.

¶ Moore WS. Visceral ischemic syndromes. In: Moore WS, ed. *Vascular and Endovascular Surgery*, 7th edn. Saunders: New York, 2005.

** Ryer EJ, Manju Kalra M, Oderich GS et al. Revascularization for acute mesenteric ischemia. *J Vasc Surg.* 2012;55:1682–1689.

†† Boley SJ, Kaleya RN, Brandt LJ. Mesenteric venous thrombosis. *Surg Clin North Am.* 1992;72:183–201.

‡‡ Rhee RY, Gloviczki P, Mendonca CT et al. Mesenteric venous thrombosis: Still a lethal disease in the 1990s. *J Vasc Surg.* 1994;20:688–697.

# 53

## *Ogilvie's Syndrome and Colonic Volvulus*

**Ramon F. Cestero**

**CONTENTS**



### 53.1 Ogilvie's Syndrome

#### 53.1.1 History and Pathogenesis

Ogilvie's syndrome, or colonic pseudo-obstruction, was first described by W.H. Ogilvie in 1948. It is manifested by dilatation of the colon with obstructive symptoms in the absence of mechanical obstruction. Ogilvie's syndrome has been reported in relation to various conditions, but two large retrospective studies have shown that the most common predisposing conditions are trauma (34%), cardiac disease (10%–18%), and infectious etiologies (10%) [1,2]. Although multiple review articles have proposed credible hypotheses associating colonic pseudo-obstruction with imbalances in colonic sympathetic and parasympathetic innervation, no direct evidence exists to support such claims [1,3,4].

While there are well over 1000 articles that have been published regarding Ogilvie's syndrome since its original description, the vast majority of these are simple case reports, uncontrolled case series, and narrative reviews. The level I, II, and III data are unfortunately sparse. The important articles are summarized in Table 53.1.

### 53.2 What Is the Best Method to Diagnose Ogilvie's Syndrome?

Acute colonic pseudo-obstruction presents with abdominal pain, nausea and/or vomiting, abdominal distension, and failure to pass stool and flatus in up to 60% of patients [2,5]. The differential diagnosis includes mechanical obstruction and possible toxic megacolon due to *Clostridium* difficile infection.

Plain abdominal films typically show various degrees of colonic dilatation, mainly involving the proximal colon, and chest x-rays may reveal free air, suggesting perforation. Although plain films may be suggestive of a diagnosis of Ogilvie's syndrome, in all cases mechanical obstruction must be ruled out by either a water-soluble contrast enema (WSCE) or CT scan to differentiate mechanical obstruction from pseudo-obstruction. Although WSCE [6] has a higher sensitivity and specificity (96% and 98%, respectively) compared to CT with intravenous contrast [7] (sensitivity and specificity of 91%), no direct comparison has been made between these two imaging techniques. CT scan offers the additional advantage of providing information regarding the bowel diameter and mucosal viability and inflammatory or ischemic changes.

**TABLE 53.1**

Summary of Pertinent Articles Regarding Ogilvie's Syndrome

| Ref. No. | Year | Comment |
|---|---|---|
| *Treatment of Ogilvie's Syndrome with Neostigmine* | | |
| 10 | 2005 | Systematic review. |
| 18 | 2010 | ASGE[a] Standards of Practice. Review of the topic with good recommendations. |
| 17 | 1992 | Original report of neostigmine use. |
| 25 | 1999 | PRCT[b] of 21 patients. Good results with neostigmine treatment. |
| 27 | 2001 | PRCT with 30 patients. |
| 26 | 2000 | PRCT of 11 patients. |
| 4 | 2009 | Systematic review of the pharmacologic treatment. |
| *Role of Colonoscopy in the Treatment of Ogilvie's Syndrome* | | |
| 28 | 1996 | 50 patients from Mayo Clinic with 88% success rate. |
| 29 | 1992 | 45 patients treated with colonoscopy. |
| 30 | 1982 | 22 patients treated. |
| 31 | 1983 | 44 patients treated over 8 years. |
| 32 | 1984 | 22 patients decompressed. |
| 33 | 1997 | 28 patients added to the literature. |
| *Prevention of Recurrence of Ogilvie's Syndrome* | | |
| 37 | 2006 | PRCT of Polyethylene glycol vs. placebo to prevent recurrence. |

[a] ASGE—American Society for Gastrointestinal Endoscopy.
[b] PRCT—Prospective randomized controlled trial.

## 53.3 What Is the Initial Management in the Treatment of Ogilvie's Syndrome?

All treatments for Ogilvie's syndrome are predicated on the finding that the patient does not have peritoneal signs or peritonitis. While the risk of spontaneous perforation is low (3%), the mortality rate in the setting of ischemia or perforation is 40%–50%, compared to a 15% mortality rate when ischemia or perforation do not occur [1,2,5,8,9]. The risk of perforation seems to vary with the duration of symptoms, progression of disease process, and cecal diameter of more than 12 cm [10]. In a retrospective analysis of 400 patients, mortality increased twofold when cecal diameter was 14 cm or greater [5].

Multiple studies have shown up to 96% resolution with conservative measures alone [11–17], and these measures are described and recommended in both the 2002 and 2010 consensus panel/treatment guideline statements from the American Society for Gastrointestinal Endoscopy [12,18]. Conservative measures include nasogastric tube placement, correction of electrolyte abnormalities (particularly potassium and magnesium), optimal body positioning, serial abdominal examinations and radiographs, discontinuation of potentiating drugs, rectal tube placement, enemas, and exclusion of mechanical obstruction by radiologic studies. Optimal body positioning is described as either prone positioning with the hips elevated on a pillow or the knee-chest position with the hips held high; both maneuvers will often help with the evacuation of flatus [12].

*Recommendation*: Essentially all of the current and historical studies on acute colonic pseudo-obstruction attempt a 24–48 h period of conservative, noninterventional treatment. Given the overall preponderance of successful studies, a trial of conservative management, in the absence of signs of peritoneal inflammation, carries a Category A recommendation.

## 53.4 What Is the Role of Neostigmine in Ogilvie's Syndrome?

Saunders and Kimmey, in a systematic review of acute colonic pseudo-obstruction, recommend intervention for patients with a cecal diameter >10 cm present for 3–4 days who have not responded to 24–48 h of conservative treatment [10]. Interventions to relieve acute colonic pseudo-obstruction can be divided into two broad categories: prokinetic medications and instrumentations (endoscopic and surgical).

Prokinetic agents such as erythromycin, metoclopramide, and cisapride have been used but do not have any level I, II, or III data to support their use [12].

Neostigmine remains the only well studied drug for the treatment of acute colonic pseudo-obstruction.

Neostigmine was first reported by Hutchinson et al. [17] in 1992, and since that time several nonrandomized studies have been reported [19–24]. In 1999, Ponec and coauthors reported a randomized control trial showing excellent results using neostigmine for the treatment of acute colonic pseudo-obstruction [25]. Even though this trial had small numbers (21 patients), 10 of 11 patients randomized to receive neostigmine responded to therapy, and none of the 10 patients randomized to placebo showed benefit. Interestingly, all eight placebo patients in whom neostigmine was subsequently administered under open-label experienced a positive response.

In 2000, Amaro and Rogers reported a prospective randomized blinded trial of neostigmine compared with placebo in patients unresponsive to conservative measures [26]. In this study, neostigmine was administered as 2 mg IV over 3–5 min. Ten of eleven patients treated with neostigmine resolved the colonic ileus compared to none in the placebo-treated patients. Nonresponders were eligible for treatment with unblinded neostigmine. Eight patients were treated in this group (seven from the placebo group and the one neostigmine nonresponder). Seven patients responded to the neostigmine therapy, with only a single patient from the original placebo group not responding.

In 2001, van der Spoel and colleagues randomized 30 critically ill patients with colonic ileus to treatment with neostigmine [27]. Nonresponders in each group were treated subsequently in a crossover manner with either neostigmine or placebo. Placebo was ineffective in causing passage of stool, and neostigmine led to defecation in 19 of 24 patients treated. Interestingly, neostigmine in this study was given as a continuous infusion of 0.4–0.8 mg/h instead of slow bolus treatment as in other studies.

A recent systematic review by De Giorgio et al. [4] has summarized the current evidence for neostigmine use and recommends neostigmine as the drug of choice for acute colonic pseudo-obstruction. Despite the effectiveness of this medication, due to its parasympathomimetic effects it can lead to bronchospasm, bradycardia, and hypotension. Risk can be minimized by reducing the dose to 1 mg versus 2 mg, or by selecting an intravenous infusion rather than bolus administration.

*Recommendation*: Given the level I and III evidence available including prospective trials, systematic reviews, and consensus statements, neostigmine should be considered the drug of choice for the treatment of acute colonic pseudo-obstruction unresponsive to conservative treatment. With the relative paucity of negative data regarding the use of neostigmine for the treatment of acute colonic pseudo-obstruction, this deserves a Category A recommendation.

## 53.5 What Is the Role of Colonoscopy in Ogilvie's Syndrome?

Multiple retrospective studies have shown the safety and efficacy of colonoscopic decompression [28–33], and initial success after colonoscopy has been reported between 61% and 95%. However, the efficacy of colonoscopy in acute colonic pseudo-obstruction has not been assessed in randomized clinical trials, and no studies have directly compared neostigmine with endoscopic therapy.

Despite the lack of level I data supporting colonoscopic decompression, endoscopy does provide the ability to directly inspect the mucosa and bowel viability. With a perforation risk of up to 2% [1,28], it is recommended that this procedure is performed by experienced endoscopists.

*Recommendation*: Based on a moderate number of retrospective studies, colonoscopic decompression of patients not responding to conservative measures deserves a Category C recommendation.

## 53.6 Can Recurrence of Ogilvie's Syndrome Be Prevented?

After colonoscopic decompression, up to 20% of patients may require a subsequent colonoscopy due to recurrence of Ogilvie's [28,31], although reports of ultimate success after one or more procedures are as high as 88% [34]. Placement of a colonic decompression tube may reduce the recurrence of Ogilvie's after initial decompression, since two nonrandomized studies have shown reduced rates of recurrence after placement of a tube compared to colonoscopy alone [35,36].

A randomized controlled trial of patients with Ogilvie's syndrome evaluated the effect of polyethylene glycol (PEG) electrolyte balanced solution on the relapse rate of the syndrome after initial resolution with neostigmine or endoscopic decompression [37]. Thirty patients were randomized to receive either PEG or placebo after resolution of the pseudo-obstruction. Patients who underwent PEG therapy experienced a significant decrease in recurrent cecal dilatation (33% in placebo versus none in PEG group), increase in stool and flatus evacuations, a reduction in abdominal circumference, and a significant decrease in cecal and colonic diameter. Although this study was prospective and randomized in nature, the small number of patients and short follow-up limits its applicability.

*Recommendations*: Due to lack of level I data and few retrospective studies, placement of a rectal tube during endoscopic decompression can only be given a Category C recommendation. Similarly, based on limited level I data, administration of PEG after initial resolution of pseudo-obstruction receives a Category C recommendation.

## 53.7 Colonic Volvulus

There are no prospective randomized trials evaluating sigmoid or cecal colonic volvulus published within the last 10 years. There is one published randomized controlled trial from 1993 that compared various treatments for sigmoid volvulus [38], but this study has limited usefulness due to its small sample size, unclear method of randomization, and poor study design.

Initial management of uncomplicated colonic volvulus is endoscopic decompression, and since endoscopic derotation is complicated by recurrence in 18%–90% of patients, definitive surgery is recommended within a few days of the initial procedure [39]. Elective surgical options include sigmoid resection and primary anastomosis or colostomy and Hartmann's procedure.

A number of retrospective articles have compared resection with primary anastomosis versus resection and colostomy [40–48], and these are summarized in Table 53.2.

Throughout these retrospective studies there are varying degrees of heterogeneity among the patient

**TABLE 53.2**

Resection with Primary Anastomosis vs. Colostomy or Pexy in the Literature

| Ref. No. | No. PA[a] | No. HC[b] | No. Pexy[c] | Comment |
|---|---|---|---|---|
| 40 | 21 | | | Single surgeon experience; no anastomotic failures or deaths. No intra-operative lavage. |
| 41 | 91 | 45 | | No difference between groups for mortality or complications. |
| 42 | 51 | 146 | 56 | Several groups; no difference between PA and HC. 15% mortality and 37 overall complication rates. Almost 7% recurrence with pexy alone. |
| 43 | 9 | 16 | 7 | HC group more complications and comorbidities than PA group. Sigmoidopexy had high recurrence rate. Only reviewed abstract due to language. |
| 44 | 44 | 33 | 7 | Mortality varied not with procedure but with colon viability. |
| 45 | 57 | | | Compared PA in gangrenous and viable bowel. High leak rate 27% and 15%. |
| 46 | 197 | | | 1% anastomotic leak and 1% mortality. |
| 47 | 13 | 37 | | Mortality 31% PA vs. 5% HC; morbidity similar. Article in French so only abstract for review. |
| 48 | 57 | 49 | | 6% mortality (11% if gangrenous bowel), four leaks. No decompression performed preoperation. |
| Total patients | 540 | 326 | 70 | |

[a] PA—Primary anastomosis.
[b] HC—Hartmann's type procedure (resection with colostomy).
[c] Pexy—Fixation of the volvulized portion of the colon.

**TABLE 53.3**

Clinical Questions—Ogilvie's Syndrome

| Question | Answer | Grade of Recommendation |
|---|---|---|
| What is the best method to diagnose Ogilvie's Syndrome? | CT scan or water-soluble contrast enema | C |
| Initial management of Ogilvie's Syndrome? | Conservative management for 24–48 h if no peritonitis or ischemia. | A |
| Role of neostigmine in Ogilvie's Syndrome? | Neostigmine should be considered the drug of choice in patients unresponsive to conservative treatment. | A |
| Role of colonoscopy in Ogilvie's Syndrome? | May be useful in patients unresponsive to conservative therapy; allows assessment of bowel mucosa and viability. | C |
| Can recurrence of Ogilvie's be prevented? | Administration of polyethylene glycol (PEG) may prevent recurrence after either neostigmine or colonoscopic decompression. Placement of a rectal tube after colonoscopic decompression may be helpful. | C |
| Sigmoid resection and primary anastomosis or colostomy and Hartmann's procedure in colonic volvulus? | Resection and primary anastomosis are safe and result in improved outcomes compared to colostomy and Hartmann's procedure. | C |

groups, mainly in terms of preoperative decompression and on-table lavage. The mortality rates in these series vary widely from 1% to over 30%, and the reported anastomotic leak rates have a similar degree of variability (0%–27%). Literature reviews have shown that overall there is significantly higher mortality associated with colostomy (25%–50%) compared with resection and anastomosis (8%–13%) [49,50] (Table 53.3).

*Recommendations*: Due to the significant lack of randomized controlled trials on this topic, it is difficult to make any definitive recommendations. Retrospective data and systematic reviews suggest that resection and primary anastomosis are safe and result in improved outcomes compared to colostomy and Hartmann's procedure, and therefore can be given a Category C recommendation.

## References


1. Batke M, Cappell MS. Adynamic ileus and acute colonic pseudo-obstruction. *Med Clin North Am*. 2008;92(3):649–670, ix.
2. Wegener M, Borsch G. Acute colonic pseudo-obstruction (Ogilvie's syndrome). Presentation of 14 of our own cases and analysis of 1027 cases reported in the literature. *Surg Endosc*. 1987;1(3):169–174.
3. Saunders MD. Acute colonic pseudo-obstruction. *Gastrointest Endosc Clin N Am*. 2007;17(2):341–360, vi–vii.
4. De Giorgio R, Knowles CH. Acute colonic pseudo-obstruction. *Br J Surg*. 2009;96(3):229–239.
5. Vanek VW, Al-Salti M. Acute pseudo-obstruction of the colon (Ogilvie's syndrome). An analysis of 400 cases. *Dis Colon Rectum*. 1986;29(3):203–210.
6. Chapman AH, McNamara M, Porter G. The acute contrast enema in suspected large bowel obstruction: Value and technique. *Clin Radiol*. 1992;46(4):273–278.
7. Beattie GC, Peters RT, Guy S et al. Computed tomography in the assessment of suspected large bowel obstruction. *ANZ J Surg*. 2007;77(3):160–165.
8. Rex DK. Acute colonic pseudo-obstruction (Ogilvie's syndrome). *Gastroenterologist*. 1994;2(3):233–238.
9. Rex DK. Colonoscopy and acute colonic pseudo-obstruction. *Gastrointest Endosc Clin N Am*. 1997;7(3):499–508.
10. Saunders MD, Kimmey MB. Systematic review: Acute colonic pseudo-obstruction. *Aliment Pharmacol Ther*. 2005;22(10):917–925.
11. Sloyer AF, Panella VS, Demas BE et al. Ogilvie's syndrome. Successful management without colonoscopy. *Dig Dis Sci*. 1988;33(11):1391–1396.
12. Eisen GM, Baron TH, Dominitiz JA et al. Acute colonic pseudo-obstruction. *Gastrointest Endosc*. 2002;56(6):789–792.
13. Wanebo H, Mathewson C, Conolly B. Pseudo-obstruction of the colon. *Surg Gynecol Obstet*. 1971;133(1):44–48.
14. Meyers MA. Colonic ileus. *Gastrointest Radiol*. 1977;2(1):37–40.
15. Bachulis BL, Smith PE. Pseudoobstruction of the colon. *Am J Surg*. 1978;136(1):66–72.
16. Baker DA, Morin ME, Tan A et al. Colonic ileus. Indication for prompt decompression. *JAMA*. 1979;241(24):2633–2634.
17. Hutchinson R, Griffiths C. Acute colonic pseudo-obstruction: A pharmacological approach. *Ann R Coll Surg Engl*. 1992;74(5):364–367.
18. Committee ASoP, Fisher L, Lee Krinsky M et al. The role of endoscopy in the management of patients with known and suspected colonic obstruction and pseudo-obstruction. *Gastrointest Endosc*. 2010;71(4):669–679.
19. Loftus CG, Harewood GC, Baron TH. Assessment of predictors of response to neostigmine for acute colonic pseudo-obstruction. *Am J Gastroenterol*. 2002;97(12):3118–3122.
20. Stephenson BM, Morgan AR, Salaman JR et al. Ogilvie's syndrome: A new approach to an old problem. *Dis Colon Rectum*. 1995;38(4):424–427.
21. Trevisani GT, Hyman NH, Church JM. Neostigmine: Safe and effective treatment for acute colonic pseudo-obstruction. *Dis Colon Rectum*. 2000;43(5):599–603.
22. Turegano-Fuentes F, Munoz-Jimenez F, Del Valle-Hernandez E et al. Early resolution of Ogilvie's syndrome with intravenous neostigmine: A simple, effective treatment. *Dis Colon Rectum*. 1997;40(11):1353–1357.
23. Paran H, Silverberg D, Mayo A et al. Treatment of acute colonic pseudo-obstruction with neostigmine. *J Am Coll Surg*. 2000;190(3):315–318.
24. Abeyta BJ, Albrecht RM, Schermer CR. Retrospective study of neostigmine for the treatment of acute colonic pseudo-obstruction. *Am Surg*. 2001;67(3):265–268; discussion 268–269.
25. Ponec RJ, Saunders MD, Kimmey MB. Neostigmine for the treatment of acute colonic pseudo-obstruction. *N Engl J Med*. 1999;341(3):137–141.
26. Amaro R, Rogers AI. Neostigmine infusion: New standard of care for acute colonic pseudo-obstruction? *Am J Gastroenterol*. 2000;95(1):304–305.
27. van der Spoel JI, Oudemans-van Straaten HM, Kuiper MA et al. Neostigmine resolves critical illness-related colonic ileus in intensive care patients with multiple organ failure—A prospective, double-blind, placebo-controlled trial. *Intensive Care Med*. 2001;27(5):822–827.
28. Geller A, Petersen BT, Gostout CJ. Endoscopic decompression for acute colonic pseudo-obstruction. *Gastrointest Endosc*. 1996;44(2):144–150.
29. Jetmore AB, Timmcke AE, Gathright BJ, Jr. et al. Ogilvie's syndrome: Colonoscopic decompression and analysis of predisposing factors. *Dis Colon Rectum*. 1992;35(12):1135–1142.
30. Nivatvongs S, Vermeulen FD, Fang DT. Colonoscopic decompression of acute pseudo-obstruction of the colon. *Ann Surg*. 1982;196(5):598–600.
31. Strodel WE, Norstrant TT, Eskhauser FE et al. Therapeutic and diagnostic colonoscopy in nonobstructive colonic dilatation. *Ann Surg*. 1983;197(4):416–421.

32. Bode WE, Beart RW, Spencer RJ et al. Colonoscopic decompression for acute pseudoobstruction of the colon (Ogilvie's syndrome). Report of 22 cases and review of the literature. *Am J Surg.* 1984;147(2):243–245.
33. Farinon AM, Stroppa I, Torquati A et al. Acute pseudo-obstruction of the colon (Ogilvie's syndrome): Advances in management. *Ann Ital Chir.* 1997;68(3):331–336; discussion 337–338.
34. Saunders MD. Acute colonic pseudo-obstruction. *Best Pract Res Clin Gastroenterol.* 2007;21(4):671–687.
35. Harig JM, Fumo DE, Loo FD et al. Treatment of acute nontoxic megacolon during colonoscopy: Tube placement versus simple decompression. *Gastrointest Endosc.* 1988;34(1):23–27.
36. Lavignolle A, Jutel P, Bonhomme J et al. Ogilvie's syndrome: Results of endoscopic exsufflation in a series of 29 cases. *Gastroenterol Clin Biol.* 1986;10(2):147–151.
37. Sgouros SN, Vlachogiannakos J, Vassilliadis K et al. Effect of polyethylene glycol electrolyte balanced solution on patients with acute colonic pseudo obstruction after resolution of colonic dilation: A prospective, randomised, placebo controlled trial. *Gut.* 2006;55(5):638–642.
38. Bagarani M, Conde AS, Longo R et al. Sigmoid volvulus in west Africa: A prospective study on surgical treatments. *Dis Colon Rectum.* 1993;36(2):186–190.
39. Raveenthiran V, Madiba TE, Atamanalp SS et al. Volvulus of the sigmoid colon. *Colorectal Dis.* 2010;12(7 online):e1–e17.
40. Sule AZ, Iya D, Obekpa PO et al. One stage procedure in the management of acute sigmoid volvulus without colonic lavage. *Surgeon.* 2007;5(5):268–270.
41. Akcan A, Akyildiz H, Artis T et al. Feasibility of single-stage resection and primary anastomosis in patients with acute noncomplicated sigmoid volvulus. *Am J Surg.* 2007;193(4):421–426.
42. Oren D, Atamanalp SS, Aydinli B et al. An algorithm for the management of sigmoid colon volvulus and the safety of primary resection: Experience with 827 cases. *Dis Colon Rectum.* 2007;50(4):489–497.
43. Agaoglu N, Yucel Y, Turkyilmaz S. Surgical treatment of the sigmoid volvulus. *Acta Chir Belg.* 2005;105(4):365–368.
44. Bhuiyan MM, Machowski ZA, Linyama BS et al. Management of sigmoid volvulus in Polokwane-Mankweng Hospital. *S Afr J Surg.* 2005;43(1):17–19.
45. Raveenthiran V. Restorative resection of unprepared left-colon in gangrenous vs viable sigmoid volvulus. *Int J Colorectal Dis.* 2004;19(3):258–263.
46. De U, Ghosh S. Single stage primary anastomosis without colonic lavage for left-sided colonic obstruction due to acute sigmoid volvulus: A prospective study of one hundred and ninety-seven cases. *ANZ J Surg.* 2003;73(6):390–392.
47. Toure CT, Dieng M, Mbaye M et al. Results of emergency colectomy in the management of the colon volvulus in Dakar hospital. *Ann Chir.* 2003;128(2):98–101; discussion 102.
48. Kuzu MA, Aslar AK, Soran A et al. Emergent resection for acute sigmoid volvulus: Results of 106 consecutive cases. *Dis Colon Rectum.* 2002;45(8):1085–1090.
49. Madiba TE, Thomson SR. The management of sigmoid volvulus. *J R Coll Surg Edinb.* 2000;45(2):74–80.
50. Ballantyne GH. Review of sigmoid volvulus: History and results of treatment. *Dis Colon Rectum.* 1982;25(5):494–501.

## Commentary on Ogilvie's Syndrome and Colonic Volvulus

*Michael E. Lekawa*

Surgeons will commonly see Ogilvie's syndrome or acute colonic pseudo-obstruction (ACPO) either in consultation or for their own patients. Conservative therapies will have a 4%–20% failure rate, but pharmacologic and colonoscopic intervention is usually successful. As such, Ogilvie's syndrome now rarely requires surgical intervention. The author has presented an excellent data-supported review including a concise approach to diagnose a practical management strategy. The pathophysiology was not described, as it is not clearly understood.

As the author notes, the suspicion of ACPO often begins with impressive dilation of the cecum on plain radiograph. It is imperative that this be further evaluated, as a colonic closed loop obstruction is highly morbid. WSE has the potential advantage of therapeutic benefit. It is however work intensive, uncomfortable for the patient, and often difficult to obtain on nights and weekends. As noted earlier, it has been mostly replaced by the more readily available CT scan.

Our treatment approach mirrors that described by the author. We attempt conservative measures for 48 h. If there is no improvement, the patient is transferred to a monitored bed for Neostigmine IV push. If this is incomplete or unsuccessful, we follow with a Neostigmine infusion. This has largely replaced colonoscopic decompression, which we now reserve for pharmacologic failures or evaluation of suspected ischemia.

I have not routinely used PEG after treatment to prevent recurrence, though I likely will in response to this chapter! We do normally leave a colonic decompression tube as described.

Surgical intervention is reserved for persistent failure of medical therapy, perforation, or bowel necrosis. Cecostomy is a viable option for persistent dilation in a poor surgical candidate. While subtotal or total colectomy is described, it is often safe to simply resect the grossly abnormal colon.

Regarding the brief synopsis of colonic volvulus, we no longer use colostomy in the acute setting, but will usually protect an at risk colorectal anastomosis with a loop ileostomy. We take this down through a local incision in 6–12 weeks.

# 54

# *Hemorrhoids*

**Clarence E. Clark III and Jacquelyn Turner**

**CONTENTS**



## 54.1 Introduction

In the United States, the prevalence of symptomatic hemorrhoids has ranged from a rate of 4.4% (or 10 million people) up to a rate of 40% [1–3]. Nearly 3.2 million ambulatory care visits and over 300,000 hospitalizations are reported per year for hemorrhoids in the United States making this condition a significant health care issue [4].

Hemorrhoids are classified as internal, external, or mixed. Internal hemorrhoids (IH) are vascular cushions found above the dentate line, and external hemorrhoids (EH) are found below the dentate line [5]. IHs are further classified based on their symptoms: Grade I hemorrhoids are those that cause bleeding but do not prolapse; Grade II hemorrhoids prolapse out of the anal canal during defecation and spontaneously return to their anatomical position; Grade III hemorrhoids prolapse and require digital replacement; and Grade IV hemorrhoids are prolapsed and cannot be reduced [5].

Evaluation starts with history and physical exam paying close attention to complaints of anal bleeding, itching, discharge, discomfort, pain, or prolapse. Anoscopy is included to help classify the type of hemorrhoids in question.

Because this disease is commonly seen in general and colorectal surgical practices, evidence-based data are essential for guiding nonoperative and operative treatment decisions. Conservative measures (topical agents, stool softeners, and dietary/lifestyle modifications) are effective first-line treatments, but the focus of this chapter will be recent evidence-based data on the treatment of hemorrhoids after the failure of conservative management. Details of techniques for the listed interventions will not be discussed in this chapter and can be found in their original articles.

## 54.2 Management of Internal Hemorrhoids

### 54.2.1 Is Observation Alone a Viable Option for Symptomatic Internal Hemorrhoids?

The potential impact of doing nothing for symptomatic hemorrhoids should be discussed with the patient along with described nonoperative and operative treatment options. In a prospective randomized trial examining the natural history of first episode symptomatic Grade II hemorrhoids, Jensen et al. showed that treatment with rubber band ligation (RBL) had a better prognosis over observation alone over a median follow-up of 48 months. This trend includes the need to treat with hemorrhoidectomy for recurrent symptoms (29.6% versus 40.2%, respectively) and relief of symptoms after initial therapy (48% versus 19.8%, respectively) [6]. The authors further noted a significant difference in actuarial recurrence rates at 48 months favoring RBL over observation (33% versus 61%, $p < 0.05$).

*Recommendation*: This study shows observation significantly increases the risk of developing symptomatic hemorrhoids requiring surgery. Intervention should be considered early in these patients in light of the clear benefit of symptom relief. *Early intervention with RBL is superior to observation of Grade II internal hemorrhoids:*

*Level of evidence*: Ib

*Grade of recommendation*: A

### 54.2.2 Is There a Clear Advantage of One Nonexcisional Management Strategy for the Treatment of Symptomatic Hemorrhoids Over Others?

Anal dilation, injection sclerotherapy (IS), cryotherapy, infrared coagulation, laser therapy, diathermy coagulation, and RBL have been described as outpatient, nonexcisional options for treating symptomatic IHs [7–14]. Here, we will discuss the evidence-based data of these treatment modalities.

#### *54.2.2.1 Anal Dilation versus Hemorrhoidectomy*

A randomized prospective study in Europe with a 17-year follow-up compared anal dilation to surgical hemorrhoidectomy for Grades II–III hemorrhoids [7]. Three groups were assigned: Group A underwent Milligan hemorrhoidectomy (41 patients) alone, Group B underwent the original Lord's six-finger dilation with a dilator (46 patients), and Group C underwent anal dilation as described previously without a dilator (51 patients). More patients were symptom-free in Group A (52%) versus Group B (23%) and Group C (27%) after treatment. Recurrence of hemorrhoids was lower for the hemorrhoidectomy group. Fecal incontinence was the major complication found during follow-up for Groups B and C (52% of the total patients).

#### *54.2.2.2 Hemorrhoidectomy versus Rubber Band Ligation, Sclerotherapy, and Infrared Photocoagulation*

A meta-analysis by MacRae et al. compared several of the nonoperative treatment methods to surgical hemorrhoidectomy [8]. Overall, patients undergoing hemorrhoidectomy had a significantly better response to treatment than did patients treated with RBL ($p = 0.001$), although this was at a cost of a significantly greater risk of complications ($p = 0.02$) and pain ($p < 0.0001$). For Grade III hemorrhoids alone, no difference was shown. RBL was shown to be significantly better than IS in response to treatment ($p = 0.005$). This difference was shown for both Grades I and II hemorrhoids ($p = 0.007$) and Grade III hemorrhoids ($p = 0.042$), with no significant difference in the complication rate. Patients treated with RBL were less likely to require further therapy than those treated with either sclerotherapy ($p = 0.031$) or infrared photocoagulation ($p = 0.0014$). Despite this trend, pain was significantly more likely to occur following RBL. No difference was found between sclerotherapy and infrared photocoagulation for any of the outcomes. Therefore, the authors concluded RBL is the therapy of choice for Grades I–II hemorrhoids and the first-line treatment for Grade III prolapsing hemorrhoids, reserving hemorrhoidectomy for patients whose symptoms are not relieved with this modality.

#### *54.2.2.3 Rubber Band Ligation versus Laser Therapy*

Giamundo et al. randomized 60 patients with Grades II and III hemorrhoids to either RBL or Doppler-guided laser therapy (also known as hemorrhoidal laser procedure or HeLP) [9]. Immediate postprocedural pain and reduction of postprocedural analgesics were improved in the HeLP group ($p < 0.001$ and $p = 0.038$, respectively). In addition, downgrading of IHs by at least one grade ($p < 0.001$) and resolution of symptoms at 6 months ($p < 0.001$) was noticed in the HeLP group. The authors concluded both RBL and the HeLP procedure are effective for Grades II and III hemorrhoids, but favors the HeLP procedure over RBL in treating symptomatic hemorrhoids due to overall improvement of immediate postprocedural pain [9].

#### *54.2.2.4 Rubber Band Ligation versus Excisional Hemorrhoidectomy*

A meta-analysis of randomized controlled trials (RCTs) comparing RBL to excisional hemorrhoidectomy (closed or open) [10] found RBL to be as effective for Grade II hemorrhoids. For Grade III hemorrhoids, recurrence rate was improved with hemorrhoidectomy. Symptoms (incontinence, anal stenosis, sepsis, and significant bleeding), time from intervention to return to work, and complications were higher for excisional hemorrhoidectomy.

*Recommendation*: RBL is the therapy of choice for Grades I and II IHs. RBL should be the first-line treatment for Grade III prolapsing hemorrhoids, reserving hemorrhoidectomy for patients whose symptoms are not relieved. Laser therapy is another viable nonoperative option for Grades II and III IHs. Anal dilation should be abandoned due to significant morbidity associated with this treatment modality. RBL is preferred over anal dilation, sclerotherapy, and infrared photocoagulation for Grades I and II IHs. Doppler-guided laser therapy is as effective for Grades II and III hemorrhoids compared to RBL with likely improvement in immediate postprocedural pain:

*Level of evidence*: Ib

*Grade of recommendation*: A

### 54.2.3 What Are the More Recent Advances in Nonoperative Management of Internal Hemorrhoids?

Injectable sclerosing agents are currently being used as a less invasive approach to treating IHs. Sclerosants are irritants that produce inflammation and ultimately fibrosis that interrupt blood supply to the hemorrhoid and cause fibrotic fixation of the hemorrhoid, preventing prolapse [11–13]. Several agents have been used as a sclerosing medium such as hypertonic saline and phenol with varying degrees of success and effects. There have been several studies demonstrating that injectable sclerosing agents are a useful alternative to traditional hemorrhoidectomy [11,12]. Recently, a newer agent developed in Japan, aluminum potassium sulfate and tannic acid (ALTA), also known as OC-108, is being used for the treatment of hemorrhoids [11,13]. Hachiro et al. studied 1210 patients with Grades III and IV hemorrhoids and divided them into three cohorts: ALTA therapy alone (448 patients), ALTA therapy with excision (706 patients), and excision alone (56 patients) [13]. Recurrence rate was 3.6% in patients treated with ALTA alone compared to 0.3% in patient treated with both ALTA and excision. Reported complications include postoperative bleeding, rectal ulcer, and postoperative fever. Advantages of ALTA include avoidance of general anesthesia and overall morbidity is reduced such as postoperative pain and anal stenosis [13].

In addition, ALTA is being used in combination with other hemorrhoid treatment modalities such as RBL and with external hemorrhoidectomy. Abe et al. report their experience using both ALTA and distal hemorrhoidectomy in a cohort of 72 patients with Grades II–IV IHs with an external component [14]. With a median follow-up of 6 months, no recurrences of prolapse were noted. In addition, only 2.8% of the patients undergoing this novel approach experienced pain during defecation and constipation after 28 days.

*Recommendation*: The use of sclerosing agents for Grades II and IV hemorrhoids, specifically ALTA, is an alternative modality with favorable short-term outcomes. Postoperative complications such as bleeding, fever, and rectal ulcers have been reported without the need of any secondary procedures in most cases. *Sclerosing agents can effectively be used to treat Grades II–IV IHS:*

*Level of evidence*: 2b

*Strength of recommendation*: B

### 54.2.4 Which Invasive Operative Strategies Have More Favorable Outcomes When Managing Symptomatic Hemorrhoids?

If nonoperative management fails, surgery may be required. Specific technical aspects of various hemorrhoid procedures have been prospectively analyzed, including open versus closed hemorrhoidectomy (CH), stapled hemorrhoidectomy or hemorrhoidopexy, and hemorrhoidectomy with bipolar diathermy (BSH) or harmonic scalpel (HSH) [15–25]. In addition to these well-studied surgical modalities, transanal hemorrhoidal dearterialization (THD) has recently emerged as an alternative approach in the surgical armamentarium [26–34].

#### *54.2.4.1 Open versus Closed Hemorrhoidectomy*

Many RCT have compared open versus CH with no clear advantage of one technique over another. Recent RCTs have shown CH offers faster healing time. Arbman et al. found that at 3 weeks, 86% of patients in the Ferguson group (closed, $n = 38$) had completely healed wounds compared with 18% in the Milligan–Morgan (open, $n = 39$) group ($p < 0.001$) [15]. Arroyo et al. also found healing during the first postoperative month was faster in the CH group ($n = 100$) compared to open ($n = 100$; 90% versus 40% respectively; $p < 0.05$) [16]. Another RCT of 80 patients (40 open, 40 closed) showed the mean operating time in the open group ($35 \pm 7$ min) was significantly shorter than in the closed group ($45 \pm 8$ min; $p < 0.001$) [17]. No significant differences were observed, however, in the duration of hospital stay or the mean duration of inability to work. In addition, they also found mean healing time was significantly shorter in the closed group ($2.8 \pm 0.5$ weeks) than in the open group ($3.5 \pm 0.6$ weeks; $p < 0.001$).

The data for open versus CH do not favor one procedure over another. CH appears to offer faster wound healing but open hemorrhoidectomy offers shorter operative time and possibly improved morbidity [17].

It is important to note that most of these studies did include both IHs and EHs.

#### 54.2.4.2 Harmonic Scalpel versus Bipolar Diathermy

The original description of a Milligan–Morgan hemorrhoidectomy (MMH) used scissors for excision [18]. HSH™ and BSH are alternative modalities for hemorrhoid excision. Recently, a prospective double-blind randomized trial of 86 patients with prolapsing hemorrhoids compared MMH to BSH and HSH [19]. There were no significant differences in the complication rates among the three groups. Complete hemostasis was achieved in both BSH and HSH groups. HSH and BSH were found to be associated with less operative blood loss when compared with MMH ($p$ = 0.036, $p$ = 0.028, respectively). Cheung et al. note HSH™ is as safe and effective with similar complication and recurrence rates as diathermy or scissor excisional hemorrhoidectomy. In addition, the authors note patients who underwent HSH had less postoperative pain.

#### 54.2.4.3 Stapled Hemorrhoidopexy versus Hemorrhoidectomy

A more recent, novel approach to symptomatic hemorrhoids is stapled hemorrhoidopexy also known as procedure for prolapse and hemorrhoids (PPHs). Longo's hemorrhoidopexy, as described in 1998, does not involve removing mucosa or hemorrhoidal tissue [20,21]. The purpose of the hemorrhoidopexy procedure is to remove the feeding vessels to the symptomatic hemorrhoids. Jayaraman et al. performed a meta-analysis of 12 RCTs comparing stapled circular hemorrhoidopexy versus conventional open or CH for the treatment of Grades III and IV hemorrhoids [22]. Follow-up periods in the studies analyzed ranged from 6 to 39 months with a median follow-up period of 7–14 months.

In this meta-analysis, patients who underwent PPH were more likely to have recurrent hemorrhoids (7 trials, 537 patients, OR 3.85, CI 1.47–10.07, $p$ = 0.006), bleeding (9 trials, 699 patients, OR 1.33, CI 0.84–2.08), and prolapse (8 studies, 798 patients, OR 2.96, CI 1.33–6.58, $p$ = 0.008) in long-term follow-up at all time points than those patients treated with CH. In addition, soiling, maintenance of hygiene, presence of anal skin tags, and incontinence occurred more frequently in patients in the PPH groups as compared to CH groups at all time points. Conversely, patients treated with PPH were less likely to complain of pruritus ani at final follow-up for all time points than those treated with CH (4 studies, 273 patients, OR 0.66, CI 0.29–1.50). Last, the authors reported an increased reoperation rate, for any nature, in the PPH cohorts in long-term follow-up.

In a RCT comparing HSH hemorrhoidectomy to PPH, Chung et al. analyzed 88 patients with Grade III hemorrhoids (HSH = 45, PPH= 43) with median follow-up period of 15 months (range, 6–30) [23]. Comparing the two groups, the authors found no significant difference in operation time, blood loss, or time to first bowel movement. Despite the short follow-up and small sample size, they were able to conclude PPH derived greater short-term benefits including a reduction in pain, length of hospital stay, and time to return to work.

#### 54.2.4.4 Computer-Guided Bipolar Diathermy versus Stapled Hemorrhoidopexy

Recently, a meta-analysis of five RCTs comparing computer-guided BSH (LigaSure™) to PPH examined a total of 397 patients with symptomatic hemorrhoids ($n$ = 199 in the PPH arm and $n$ = 198 in the LigaSure arm) [24]. When comparing the two cohorts, there were no differences in postoperative complications such as bleeding, anal fissure, anal stenosis, or urinary retention. In addition, there was no difference in postoperative pain, return to normal activities, and hospital stay. The LigaSure™ technique had a significant reduction in recurrence rates ($p$= 0.01).

*Recommendation*: Conventional excisional surgery is the gold standard in the surgical treatment of Grades III and IV IHs. The data for open versus CH do not favor one procedure over the other. PPH has no clear advantage over conventional hemorrhoidectomy for Grade IV IHs. BSH is favored over stapled hemorrhoidopexy in terms of recurrence rate. Both LigaSure™ and stapled hemorrhoidopexy, however, are comparable in regards to postoperative complications, postoperative pain, and return to normal activities. Recommendations could not be made favoring BSH or HSH over traditional MMH. Trends of intraoperative bleeding, however, do favor the use of these advanced technologies over scissors for excision. *Conventional excisional hemorrhoidectomy, regardless of the technique, is preferred over PPH:*

*Level of evidence*: Ib

*Strength of recommendation*: A

### 54.2.5 What Are the More Recent Advances in Operative Management of Internal Hemorrhoids?

Hemorrhoid artery ligation (HAL) with Doppler guidance is an emerging treatment modality for hemorrhoids. HAL was popularized by Moringa et al. in 1995 [25–28]. The aim of this technique is to identify and ligate the terminal branches of the hemorrhoids arteries using a Doppler transducer. By ligating these terminal branches, the blood supply to the anal cushions is reduced [25]. This technique is commonly known as trandanal hemorrhoidal dearterialization (THD), Doppler-guided hemorrhoidal artery ligation, as well as HAL [27,29].

Moringa et al. noted a 96% improvement in pain, a 78% improvement with prolapse, and a 95% improvement with bleeding after THD was performed in 116 patients who underwent the procedure [26]. One hundred twelve patients were prospectively studied by Infantino et al. using THD with a mucopexy for prolapsed tissue. The authors noted pain, bleeding, dyschezia, and soiling improved postoperatively in patients with both Grades II and III hemorrhoids. Sohn et al. had similar results in regards to pain and bleeding after prospectively evaluating 60 patients with symptomatic hemorrhoids [28]. More than seven ligations was a predictor for treatment failure ($p$ = 0.002) in this study. Patients who failed THD were successfully retreated with RBL or hemorrhoidectomy. Furthermore, Tempel et al., in a survey of patient satisfaction following THD, reported 91.5% of the patients had an improvement of hemorrhoidal symptoms [30].

Schuurman et al. performed a randomized trial investigating the utility of Doppler-guided ligation versus non-Doppler-guided ligation for Grades II and III hemorrhoids [27]. One hundred five patients that were included in the study completed a written questionnaire was dictating their self-reported clinical parameters (pain, bleeding, prolapse, discomfort in daily life, and problems with defecation) before, 6 weeks, and 6 months after their operation. Both groups significantly improved all clinical parameters. However, recurrent prolapse at 6 months was most likely to occur with the Doppler group ($p$ = 0.047). Pain was better improved in the Doppler group, but not significant ($p$ = 0.702). Complications included postoperative pain or bleeding in the Doppler group. No complications were noted in the non-Doppler group. In the Doppler group, 13.2% of the patients needed an additional procedure such as banding or hemorrhoidectomy.

The utility of THD with Grade IV hemorrhoids is less studied. Ratto et al. prospectively studied 35 patients with Grade IV hemorrhoids [31]. Significant postoperative pain more than 3 days occurred in 14.3% of the patients. Postoperative complications included hemorrhoid thrombosis (8.6%), postoperative bleeding (5.7%), and urinary retention (14.3%). With a median follow-up of 10 months (range 6–28 months), the majority of patients (94%) had complete resolution or significant improvement of their symptoms. Residual prolapse was noted in 28.6% of which 5.7% needed further surgery. There was no report of anal stenosis or fecal incontinence.

To date there are few studies comparing THD with mucopexy to the gold standard of excisional hemorrhoidectomy. Denoya et al. conducted a double-blinded RCT comparing the two modalities [32]. Forty patients with symptomatic Grades III and IV hemorrhoids were randomized equally between the THD with mucopexy ($n$ = 20) and hemorrhoidectomy ($n$ = 20) treatments. Pain intensity was also lower in the THD/mucopexy group (2.9 ± 3.5) compared to the hemorrhoidectomy group (7.6 ± 2.9) on a scale of 0–10. The overall use of narcotics was less in the THD/mucopexy group ($p$ = 0.001). The hemorrhoidectomy group was more likely to experience urinary retention. Although not significant, the hemorrhoidectomy group was also more likely to experience postoperative constipation and the THD/mucopexy group was more likely to experience fecal urgency. Both groups equally experienced incontinence to flatus and stool. By postoperative day 7, the THD/mucopexy group reported better scores in general activity, mood, ability to sleep, and ability to return to work. Similar conclusion about postoperative pain was seen in a randomize trial performed by Bursics et al. [33] Sixty patients were randomized to THD ($n$ = 30) or hemorrhoidectomy ($n$ = 30) with a 1-year follow-up. In the hemorrhoidectomy group, one patient failed treatment for hemorrhoidal bleeding and underwent successful banding. In the THD group, one patient had recurrent bleeding which was treated with repeat THD.

*Recommendation*: THD with mucopexy is a viable option for treatment for Grades II and III hemorrhoids and select Grade IV hemorrhoids. THD with mucopexy has similar recurrence rates compared to hemorrhoidectomy. Pain, patient satisfaction, and return to work are significantly improved in patients undergoing THD with mucopexy. Reported postoperative complications include hemorrhoid thrombosis, postoperative bleeding requiring hospitalization, dysuria, urinary retention, and treatment failure requiring further treatment such as banding or hemorrhoidectomy. *THD with mucopexy is an acceptable alternative to conventional hemorrhoidectomy:*

*Level of evidence*: 1b

*Strength of recommendation*: A

## 54.3 Management of Thrombosed External Hemorrhoids

### 54.3.1 What Is the Best Management Strategy for Symptomatic External Hemorrhoids?

The most common findings with EHs are pain and/or ulceration of a thrombus through the skin [5]. Conservative measures are often utilized which include a combination of localize hygiene, tub baths, dietary changes, stool softeners, and oral and topical analgesics. There are very few quality studies looking at the management of EHs exclusively.

A prospective randomized trial examined conservative therapy versus surgery for the treatment of thrombosed EHs [34]. Three arms each had 50 patients: the first group was treated conservatively with 0.2% glyceryl trinitrate (GTN) ointment, the second group by incision, and the third group by excision of the thrombosed EH. At 4 days, there was a significantly less pain in patients treated by excision as compared to those treated with GTN or incision ($p < 0.001$). At 1 year all clinical outcomes significantly favored excision of thrombosed hemorrhoids. Based on their data, the authors recommend excision of perianal thrombosis under local anesthesia as the method of choice since it prevents recurrence of perianal thrombosis and development of anal skin tags [34].

Greenspon et al. retrospectively reviewed outcomes of 231 patients with thrombosed EHs [35]. One hundred nineteen patients (51.5%) were initially treated conservatively and 112 patients (48.5%) were treated surgically with a mean follow-up of 7.6 months (up to 7 years). The majority (97.3%) of the surgical patients had an excision of their EHs while only 2.7% had an incision. Time to symptom resolution was 24 days for conservatively managed patients versus 3.9 days for surgical patients ($p < 0.0001$). The frequency of recurrence was significantly higher for the conservative group (25.4%) than for the surgical group (6.3%; $p < 0.0001$). These data favor excision of thrombosed EHs over conservative therapy.

Jongen et al. reported the clinical outcomes of the 340 patients who underwent outpatient office excision of symptomatic EHs under local anesthesia alone [36]. All wounds were left open and office follow-up was achieved in 70% of the patients. Thrombosis recurrence was seen in 6.5% of patients more than 2 months from treatment. In addition, 16.5% of patients required subsequent RBL after complete wound healing. Anal stenosis, urinary retention, and fecal retention were not seen in this series. Based on their analysis, the authors recommend excision under local anesthesia in the office for thrombosed EHs.

Chan and Arthur systematically reviewed two prospective studies and two retrospective studies evaluating the management of thrombosed EHs with a total of 571 patients [37]. Excision of thrombosed EHs provided the best initial pain control compared to topical agents such as 0.2% GTN. There were no differences in pain relief after 1 month follow-up comparing conservative management to surgical management. In addition, 1 year recurrence rate was less in patients undergoing surgical treatment (6.1%) compared to those treated conservatively (25.4%; Tables 54.1 and 54.2).

*Recommendation*: Excision of EHs under local anesthesia is the method of choice for symptomatic EHs due to improved symptom relief. Practitioners can safely perform this procedure in the outpatient office setting. *Excision of symptomatic EHs is preferred over observation with medical management:*

*Level of evidence*: Ib

*Strength of recommendation*: A

**TABLE 54.1**

Clinical Questions

| Question | Answer | Grade of Recommendation | References |
|---|---|---|---|
| Is observation alone a viable option for symptomatic internal hemorrhoids (IHs)? | No. Clear benefit with intervention for Grade II and greater hemorrhoids | A | [6] |
| Is there a clear advantage of one nonexcisional management strategy over the others for the treatment of symptomatic hemorrhoids over others? | Yes. Rubber band ligation (RBL) is superior to anal dilation, sclerotherapy, and infrared photocoagulation. RBL is just as effective as Doppler-guided laser therapy for Grades II and III hemorrhoids | A | [7–9] |
| What are the more recent advances in nonoperative management of IHs? | Sclerosing agent can effectively be used to treat Grades II–IV IHs | B | [11–14] |
| Which invasive operative strategies have more favorable outcomes when managing symptomatic hemorrhoids? | Conventional hemorrhoidectomy, regardless of energy source or means of excision, is superior to procedure for prolapse and hemorrhoids (PPHs). There was no significant difference between Milligan–Morgan (open) hemorrhoidectomy and Ferguson hemorrhoidectomy (closed) | B | [15–23] |
| What are the more recent advances in operative management of IHs? | Hemorrhoid artery ligation (HAL) with Doppler guidance is as effective as conventional hemorrhoidectomy for Grades II and III hemorrhoids | A | [25–33] |
| What is the best management strategy for symptomatic external hemorrhoids (EHs)? | Excision of acutely thrombosis EHs is preferred over conservative treatment, topical agents, and incision | A | [34–37] |

**TABLE 54.2**
Levels of Evidence

| Subject | Year | Reference | Level of Evidence | Strength of Recommendation | Findings |
|---|---|---|---|---|---|
| First-line treatment of IHs | 2005 | [10] | Ib | A | RBL is the first-line therapy followed by hemorrhoidectomy if symptoms persist or Grade IV |
| Open or closed technique | 2002 | [17] | IIb | B | Both are acceptable operative strategies with no significant difference in outcomes |
| Conventional hemorrhoidectomy or PPHs | 2006 | [22] | Ia | A | Conventional hemorrhoidectomy is superior to PPHs |
| Conventional hemorrhoidectomy or HAL with Doppler guidance (THD) | 2013 | [32] | Ib | A | THD has similar outcomes to conventional hemorrhoidectomy with less pain and narcotic use |
| Management of symptomatic EHs | 2004 | [37] | IIb | B | Excision is superior to topical agents and incision of EHs |

## References


1. Johanson JF, Sonnenber A. The prevalence of hemorrhoids and chronic constipation: An epidemiologic study. *Gastroenterology*. 1990;98.
2. Janicke DM, Pundt MR. Anorectal disorders. *Emerg Med Clin North Am*. 1996;14.
3. Ohning GV, Machicado GA, Jensen DM. Definitive therapy for internal hemorrhoids; new opportunities and options. *Rev Gastrenterol Disord*. 2009;9.
4. Everhart JE. 2008. *The Burden of Digestive Diseases in the United States*. National Institute of Diabetes and Digestive and Kidney Diseases, U.S. Department of Health and Human Services: Bethesda, MD.
5. Kaidar-Person O, Person B, Wexner S. Hemorrhoidal disease: A comprehensive review. *J Am Coll Surg*. Jan 2007;204(1):102–117.
6. Jensen S, Harling H, Arseth-hansen P et al. The natural history of symptomatic hemorrhoids. *Int J Colorectal Dis*. 1989;4(1):41–44.
7. Konsten J, Baeten C. Hemorrhoidectomy vs Lord's method: 17-year follow-up of a prospective, randomized trial. *Dis Colon Rectum*. Apr 2000;43(4):503–206.
8. MacRae H, McLeod R. Comparison of hemorrhoidal treatment modalities: A meta-analysis. *Dis Colon Rectum*. 1995;38(7):687–694.
9. Giamundo P, Salfi R, Geraci M et al. The hemorrhoid laser procedure technique vs rubber band ligation: A randomized trial comparing 2 mini-invasive treatments for second- and third-degree hemorrhoids. *Dis Colon Rectum*. 2011;34:693–698.
10. Shanmugam V, Thaha M, Rabindranath K et al. Rubber band ligation versus excisional haemorrhoidectomy for haemorrhoids. *Cochrane Database Syst Rev*. 2005;Issue 1: Art. No.: CD005034.
11. Ono T, Goto K, Takagi S. Sclerosing effect of OC-108, a novel agent for hemorrhoids, is associated with granulomatous inflammation induced by aluminum. *J Pharmacol Sci*. 2005;99:353–363.
12. Ponsky J, Mellinger J, Simon I. Endoscopic retrograde hemorrhoidal sclerotherapy using 23.4% saline, a preliminary report. *Surg Today*. 2011;41:806–809.
13. Hachiro Y, Kunimoto M, Abe T et al. Aluminum potassium sulfate and tannic acid (ALTA) injection as the mainstay of treatment for internal hemorrhoids. *Surg Today*. 2011;41:806–809.
14. Abe T. Distal hemorrhoidectomy with ALTA injection: A new method for hemorrhoid surgery. *Int Surg*. 2014;99:295–298.
15. Arbman G, Krook H, Haapaniemi S. Closed vs open hemorrhoidectomy—Is there any difference? *Dis Colon Rectum*. Jan 2000;43(1):31–34.
16. Arroyo A, Perez F, Miranda E et al. Open versus closed day-case haemorrhoidectomy: Is there any difference? Results of a prospective randomized study. *Int J Colorectal Dis*. Jul 2004;19(4):370–373.
17. Gencosmanoglu R, Sad O, Koc D et al. Hemorrhoidectomy: Open or closed technique? A prospective, randomized clinical trial. *Dis Colon Rectum*. Jan 2002;45(1): 70–75.
18. Milligan E, Morgan C, Jones L et al. Surgical anatomy of the anal canal, and the operative treatment of haemorrhoids. *Lancet*. Nov 1937; ii:1120–1124.
19. Chung C, Ha J, Tai Y et al. Double-blind, randomized trial comparing Harmonic Scalpel™ hemorrhoidectomy, bipolar scissors hemorrhoidectomy and scissors excision: Ligation technique. *Dis Colon Rectum*. 2002;45:789–794.
20. Longo A. 1998. Treatment of hemorrhoids disease by reduction of mucosa and hemorrhoidal prolapse with a circular suturing device: A new procedure. *Proceedings of the 6th World Congress of Endoscopic Surgery*.
21. Corman M, Gravié T, Hager M et al. Longo Stapled haemorrhoidopexy: A consensus position paper by an international working party-indications, contra-indications and technique. *Colorectal Dis*. 5(4):304–310.
22. Jayaraman S, Colquhoun P, Malthaner R. Stapled versus conventional surgery for hemorrhoids. *Cochrane Database Syst Rev*. 2006;Issue 4.

23. Chung C, Cheung H, Chan E et al. Stapled hemorrhoidopexy vs. Harmonic Scalpel hemorrhoidectomy: A randomized trial. *Dis Colon Rectum*. Jun 2005;48(6):1213–1219.
24. Chen H, Woo X, Cui J et al. Ligasure versus stapled hemorrhoidectomy in the treatment of hemorrhoids: A meta-analysis of randomized control trials. *Surg Laparosc Endosc Percutan Tech*. 2014;1–5.
25. Infantino A, Bellomo R, Dal Monte P et al. Transanal haemorrhoidal artery echodoppler ligation and anopexy (THD) is effective for II and III degree haemorrhoids: A prospective multicentric study. *Colorectal Dis*. 2010;12:804–809.
26. Morinaga K, Hasuda K, Ikeda T. A novel therapy for internal hemorrhoids: Ligation of the hemorrhoidal artery with a newly devised instrument (Moricorn) in conjunction with a Doppler flowmeter. *Am J Gastroenterol*. 1995;90:610–613.
27. Schuurman J, Rinkes I, Go P. Hemorrhoidal artery ligation procedure with or without Doppler transducer in grade II and grade III hemorrhoidal disease: A blinded randomized clinical trial. *Ann Surg*. 2012;225:840–845.
28. Sohn N, Aronoff J, Cohen F, Weinstein M. Transanal hemorrhoidal dearterialization is an alternative to operative hemorrhoidectomy. *Am J Surg*. 2001;182:515–519.
29. Giordano P, Nastro P, Davies A, Gravante G. Prospective evaluation of stapled haemorrhoidopexy versus transanal haemorrhoidal dearterialization for stage II and III haemorrhoids: Three year outcomes. *Tech Coloproctol*. 2011;15:67–73.
30. Tempel M, Pearson E, Page M et al. Survey of patient satisfaction after Doppler-guided transanal hemorrhoidal dearterialization performed in ambulatory settings. *Tech Coloproctol*. 2014;18:607–610.
31. Ratto C, Giordano P, Donisi et al. Transanal haemorrhoidal dearterialization (THD) for selected fourth-degree haemorrhoids. *Tech Coloproctol*. 2011;15:191–197.
32. Denoya P, Fakhoury M, Chang K et al. Dearterialization with mucopexy versus haemorrhoidectomy for grade III or IV haemorrhoids: Short-term results of a double-blinded randomized controlled trial. *Colorectal Dis*. 2013; 15:1281–1288.
33. Bursics M, Kupcsulic F. Comparison of early and 1-year follow-up results of conventional hemorrhoidectomy and hemorrhoid artery ligation: A randomized study. *Int J Colorectal Dis*. 2004;19:178–180.
34. Cavcic J, Turcic J, Martinac P et al. Comparison of topically applied 0.2% glyceryl trinitrate ointment, incision and excision in the treatment of perianal thrombosis. *Dig Liver Dis*. 2001;33:335–340.
35. Greenspon J, Williams S, Young H et al. Thrombosed external hemorrhoids: Outcome after conservative or surgical management. *Dis Colon Rectum*. Sep 2004;47(9): 1493–1498.
36. Jongen J, Bach S, Stubinger S et al. Excision of thrombosed external hemorrhoid under local anesthesia: A retrospective evaluation of 340 patients. *Dis Colon Rectum*. Sep 2003;46(9):1226–1231.
37. Chan K, Arthur J. External haemorrhoidal thrombosis: Evidence for current management. *Tech Coloproctol*. 2013;17:21–25.

## Commentary on Hemorrhoids

*Michael J. Stamos*

The best treatment for hemorrhoidal disease has long been debated, but unfortunately, we are no closer to a definitive answer to that question now than we were 10 or even 20 years ago. We have learned a good bit over the past decade, but we have also failed to learn a few lessons. A point made early in this chapter highlights this issue but may be lost on the superficial reader, namely, that conservative measures are effective first-line therapy. Indeed, this first-line therapy (increased dietary fiber, avoidance of straining and prolonged squatting, topical agents) is pretty effective, and even when an operation is entertained or conducted, this therapy should be encouraged as it is complementary.

To address the specific questions asked and addressed in this manuscript.

### Is Observation Alone a Viable Option for Symptomatic Internal Hemorrhoids?

Rubber band ligation (RBL) has stood the test of time. It remains the standard of care for office-based therapy.

### Is There a Clear Advantage of One Nonexcisional Management Strategy for the Treatment of Symptomatic Hemorrhoids over Others?

It is important to separate truly office-based treatments from outpatient surgical procedures. RBL is the clearly preferred approach for Grade I and II hemorrhoids from the perspective of evidence-based data in the office setting. For Grade III hemorrhoids, the question needs to be framed properly. If the patient wants a "quick fix" with one treatment session, excisional hemorrhoidectomy is a clear winner, with the new modality of Doppler-guided laser therapy an intriguing option, which needs more study to become entrenched in our armamentarium. For a patient with more patience, willing to delay gratification, a series of RBLs remain a good option.

### What Are the More Recent Advances in Nonoperative Management of Internal Hemorrhoids?

Newer sclerosing agents are not readily available in the United States. Can their success overseas translate into success in an American population? Time will tell.

### Which Invasive Operative Strategies Have More Favorable Outcomes When Managing Symptomatic Hemorrhoids?

Conventional excisional hemorrhoidectomy is the current standard of care when operation is required. Using a scalpel, monopolar cautery, bipolar energy, and harmonic scalpel are all equivalent in terms of clinically meaningful outcomes. Stapled hemorrhoidopexy has faded in popularity for a good reason, it has potential for devastating complications rarely if ever seen with more traditional techniques and it has a higher rate of long-term pain in a minority of patients.

### What Are the Most Recent Advances in Operative Management of Internal Hemorrhoids?

Underpowered but promising studies of transanal hemorrhoidal dearterialization (THD) reflect attempts to decrease the pain experienced with a standard excisional hemorrhoidectomy. A noble goal but as yet not convincingly proven to me.

### What Is the Best Management Strategy for Symptomatic External Hemorrhoids?

The answer to this question really hinges on the presentation of the patient. For a patient who manages to get seen before the acute pain begins receding (typically 72–96 h) or with ischemic necrosis of the overlying skin, excision is the clearly preferred approach. For the other patients, the pain of excision often exceeds the benefit.

# 55

# *Anal Fissure, Fistula, and Abscess*

**W. Brian Perry**

**CONTENTS**



## 55.1 Introduction

Anorectal complaints are common, but often poorly understood—most physicians seem to have missed "Anus Day" in medical school. More often than not, a referral for "hemorrhoids" can mean any number of perineal maladies. Proper treatment absolutely depends on proper diagnosis. Once an accurate assessment is made, therapy can be based on evidence-based guidelines for the treatment of anorectal abscess, fistula, and fissure. Hemorrhoids and pilonidal disease are covered in other chapters (Table 55.1).

## 55.2 How Do Nonoperative Medical Therapies (Nitroglycerin, Calcium Channel Blockers, and Botulinum Toxin) Compare with Placebo and Lateral Internal Sphincterotomy in the Treatment of Anal Fissures?

Multiple randomized prospective trials have examined the role of various nonoperative therapies in the treatment of anal fissures. All effective modalities are aimed at decreasing the hypertonicity found in the internal anal sphincter of fissure patients. Therapies that do not lower sphincter pressures have been uniformly found to be no better than placebo. Most studies focus on chronic fissures [1].

Glyceryl trinitrate (GTN) and its derivatives are smooth muscle relaxants that have been shown to decrease internal anal sphincter pressures. In controlled trials, application of these nitric oxide donors is associated with a greater than 50% fissure healing rate, compared with only 30%–35% for placebo. A recent Cochrane review combining 15 studies showed a statistically better healing rate with GTN (49% vs. 37%). Headache is the principal adverse event with GTN use, causing about a quarter of patients to stop therapy; incontinence was not observed in any study. Interestingly, one small study showed no difference between anal application and distant transdermal delivery. In studies with follow-up periods of more than 1 year, recurrence after cessation of therapy approached 50% [2].

Calcium channel blockers, given either topically or orally, have been shown to heal fissures in 65%–95% of patients. Comparisons to GTN show similar results. Headache is less frequently reported with topical use, but oral administration has more side-effects and less efficacy [2].

Botulinum toxin (Botox) induces a temporary "chemical sphincterotomy" that initially heals approximately two-thirds of fissures with a single application. There is little consensus on dosing, injection sites, or repeated use. Transient incontinence to flatus and minor stool leakage is reported in up to 10% of patients. At 1 year, fissure recurrence rates are 40%–50% [2]. Adding topical GTN to patients treated with Botox does not improve healing rates but does have significant side-effects, primarily headache [4].

Surgical sphincterotomy outperforms all medical therapies in numerous randomized, controlled trials with an overall healing rate greater than 90%. A minor incontinence rate of less than 10% compares favorably with topical therapy [4–6].

*Recommendation*: Nonsurgical therapies are superior to placebo but inferior to lateral internal sphincterotomy for healing anal fissures.

*Level of evidence*: 1a

*Grade of recommendation*: A

## 55.3 What Is the Impact of Technique on the Outcomes of Patients Undergoing Surgery for Anal Fissure?

Surgical options for the treatment of anal fissure include anal stretch, open or closed lateral internal sphincterotomy (LIS), and posterior sphincterotomy, with or without papillae excision or dermal flap coverage [1]. Meta-analysis of stretch versus LIS clearly favors LIS for both recurrence (OR = 3.08, 95% CI 1.26–7.54) and incontinence (OR = 4.22, 95% CI 1.89–9.42). Randomized trials of surgical technique may suffer from performance variations. Nevertheless, multiple trials comparing open LIS to closed LIS show no difference in either recurrence or incontinence. Posterior sphincterotomy has been shown to be inferior to LIS for both persistence of the fissure and incontinence [7]. Additional procedures such as papillae excision and dermal flap coverage show a trend toward increased patient satisfaction in small trials [8,9]. Overall, the risk of incontinence is low and patient satisfaction following LIS is high, even in those patients with minor continence disturbances [10]. Sphincter-sparing fissurectomy, combined with either concomitant Botox injection [11] or anoplasty [12], shows promise in small observational series.

*Recommendation:* Lateral internal sphincterotomy (open or closed) is the surgical treatment of choice for chronic anal fissures.

*Level of evidence*: 1a

*Grade of recommendation*: A.

## 55.4 What Is the Healing and Incontinence Rate for Fistulotomy for Simple Fistula-in-Ano?

Anal fistulas vary in complexity from short, straight tracts involving primarily internal sphincter to branching complexes through a large amount of the external sphincter. With proper identification of the internal opening, fistulotomy is effective for simple fistulas, with recurrence rates less than 10% and minor incontinence rates of 0%–17%. While recurrence rates are similar, fistulectomy has shown to be inferior to fistulotomy due to longer healing times and a greater risk of incontinence. Marsupialization of the wound edges following fistulotomy has been shown in a small study to speed final healing and decrease bleeding. Most functional problems following surgery for simple fistulas improve in 1–2 years [13,14].

*Recommendation*: Fistulotomy is appropriate for simple fistula-in-ano with high rates of healing and low rates of incontinence.

*Level of evidence*: 2b

*Grade of recommendation*: B

## 55.5 What Is the Healing and Incontinence Rate for More Complex Fistulas Treated with Fibrin Glue, Fistula Plug, or a Seton?

Fistulotomy alone is contraindicated when division of a significant amount of external sphincter is divided, due to an increased risk of permanent incontinence [13]. Several surgical treatment modalities have been developed to increase the likelihood of durable fistula closure while reducing the risk of postoperative functional problems.

Utilizing fibrin glue to obliterate fistula tracts was initially considered an attractive option as no sphincter muscle is divided. Early series with short follow-up reported fistula closure rates of 60%–70% [14]. However, this has not been borne out in subsequent trials with longer periods of evaluation. In a prospective study, Singer randomized patients to fibrin sealant plus closure of the internal opening, fibrin sealant plus antibiotics, or fibrin sealant plus both; failures were offered retreatment. At 1 year, the rates of durable fistula closure were only 44%, 25%, and 35%, respectively, with no significant difference between groups [15].

In response to these findings, a bioabsorbable xenograft fistula plug made from lyophilized porcine intestinal submucosa (Surgisis®, Cook Surgical, Inc., Bloomington, IN) was developed. Initially, Champagne et al. demonstrated an overall success rate of 83% with a median follow-up of 12 months [16]. The results of subsequent studies have been highly variable, with success rates of 25%–81%, dependent on length of follow-up and fistula complexity, with simple fistulas faring better [17–20].

A seton is a flexible foreign body placed through a fistula and secured to itself to keep the tract open, preventing subsequent abscess formation, It may be placeholding or cutting, depending on how it is used. The fibrosis induced is thought to lessen subsequent incontinence. Overall recurrence rates are low—less than 10% in most series—but the rates of incontinence can be significant, up to 60% for minor disturbances in some cases [21].

*Recommendation*: Complex fistulas-in-ano may be successfully treated with fibrin glue, fistula plug, or a seton. Success and incontinence rates vary widely.

*Levels of evidence*: 2b–4

*Grade of recommendation*: C

## 55.6 What Is the Healing and Incontinence Rate for More Complex Fistulas Treated with an Endorectal Advancement Flap?

An endorectal advancement flap treats fistula-in-ano by obliterating the internal opening with a sliding "patch" of healthy tissue; no sphincter muscle need be divided. Numerous small case series demonstrate successful fistula closure in 55%–98% of patients, with low rates of major continence disturbance (<10%). Durable cure rates decrease with increasing fistula complexity—Crohn's radiation, large rectovaginal, and multiply recurrent fistulas fare worse than simpler ones [14,21]. Perez found little difference in patients with complex fistulae between flap repair and fistulotomy with immediate sphincter reconstruction, noting similar healing times, recurrences (10%), and incontinence rates (32%) [22]. Ellis found that adding fibrin glue as an adjunct for an endorectal advancement flap is actually detrimental, as recurrence rates were 46% in the fibrin glue group, compared with 20% in the flap alone group [23]. In one small series, Gottgens showed that the addition of platelet-rich plasma may improve healing, with 83% fistula closure success at 2 years [24].

*Recommendation*: Complex fistulas-in-ano may be successfully treated with an endorectal advancement flap. Success rates vary widely but incontinence is infrequent.

*Level of evidence*: 3

*Grade of recommendation*: C.

## 55.7 What Is the Role of Ligation of the Intersphincteric Fistula Tract in the Treatment of Fistula-in-Ano?

Ligation of the intersphincteric fistula tract (LIFT) is a sphincter-sparing procedure that may prove useful in the management of high transsphincteric anal fistulas [14]. Rojanasakul [25] after 3 months of follow-up showed a 94% healing rate. Subsequent reports of LIFT have shown success rates from 57% to 89%, with variable follow-up durations [26]. Adjuncts such as an interposed piece of a biologic sheet [27] or a fistula plug [28] have been investigated in small trials with modest improvements in healing rates.

*Recommendation*: Complex fistulas-in-ano may be successfully treated with ligation of the intersphincteric fistula tract. Success rates vary widely but incontinence is infrequent.

*Level of evidence*: 3

*Grade of recommendation*: C.

## 55.8 What Are the Results of Trials Comparing Different Surgical Techniques in the Management of Fistula-in-Ano?

There is a paucity of well-done randomized controlled trials addressing fistula-in-ano, especially comparing different techniques. In a randomized, prospective trial, Altomare compared cutting setons with fibrin glue; at 1 year, healing was much better in the seton group (88% vs. 39%, $p = 0.0007$), but incontinence was significantly worse [29]. A double-blinded multicenter randomized trial of advancement flap versus fistula plug showed equally disappointing results for each in the treatment of high transsphincteric fistulae, with healing rates of only 48% and 29% respectively [30]. One moderate-sized trial (70 total patients) comparing LIFT with mucosal advancement flap showed similar fistula closure rates at 1 year (74% vs. 66%, $p = 0.58$) [31].

*Recommendation*: No recommendation due to the paucity of trials.

**TABLE 55.1**
Overall Evidence Table

| Question | Answer | Levels of Evidence | Grade of Recommendation | References |
|---|---|---|---|---|
| How do nonoperative medical therapies (nitroglycerin, calcium channel blockers, and botulinum toxin) compare with placebo and lateral internal sphincterotomy in the treatment of anal fissures? | Nonsurgical therapies are superior to placebo but inferior to lateral internal sphincterotomy for healing anal fissures. | 1a | A | [1–6] |
| What is the impact of technique on the outcomes of patients undergoing surgery for anal fissure? | Lateral internal sphincterotomy (open or closed) is the surgical treatment of choice for chronic anal fissures. | 1a | A | [1,7–12] |
| What is the healing and incontinence rate for fistulotomy for simple fistula-in-ano? | Fistulotomy is appropriate for simple fistula-in-ano with high rates of healing and low rates of incontinence. | 2b | B | [13–14] |
| What is the healing and incontinence rate for more complex fistulas treated with fibrin glue, fistula plug, or a seton? | Complex fistulas-in-ano may be successfully treated with fibrin glue, fistula plug, or a seton. Success and incontinence rates vary widely. | 2b–4 | C | [13–21] |
| What is the healing and incontinence rate for more complex fistulas treated with an endorectal advancement flap? | Complex fistulas-in-ano may be successfully treated with an endorectal advancement flap. Success rates vary widely but incontinence is infrequent. | 3 | C | [14,21–24] |
| What is the role of ligation of the intersphincteric fistula tract (LIFT) in the treatment of fistula-in-ano? | Complex fistulas-in-ano may be successfully treated with ligation of the intersphincteric fistula tract. Success rates vary widely but incontinence is infrequent. | 3 | C | [14,25–28] |
| Are antibiotics unnecessary for most patients undergoing routine incision and drainage of perirectal abscesses? | Antibiotics are unnecessary for most patients following adequate abscess drainage. | 2c | B | [14,31] |

## 55.9 Are Antibiotics Unnecessary for Most Patients Undergoing Routine Incision and Drainage of Perirectal Abscesses?

Neither time to complete healing nor recurrence rates are improved by treating patients with antibiotics following incision and drainage of uncomplicated perirectal abscesses. These studies specifically excluded patients considered higher risk—those with diabetes, immunosuppression, or extensive cellulitis. While there are no large trials in these patients, antibiotics should be considered for this subset on a case-by-case basis [14]. According to American Heart Association guidelines, patients identified as high risk for the development of endocarditis should receive antibiotics prior to perirectal abscess incision and drainage [31].

*Recommendation*: Antibiotics are unnecessary for most patients following adequate abscess drainage.

*Level of evidence*: 2c

*Grade of recommendation*: B

## References


1. Perry WB, Dykes SL, Buie WD et al. Practice parameters for the management of anal fissures (3rd Revision). *Dis Colon Rectum.* 2010;53(8):1110–1115.
2. Nelson R. Non surgical therapy for anal fissure. *Cochrane Database Syst Rev.* 2006;4:Art No. CD003431.
3. Asim M, Lowrie N, Stewart J et al. Botulinum toxin versus botulinum toxin with low-dose glyceryltrinitrate for healing of chronic anal fissure. *N Z Med J.* 2014;127(1393):80–86.
4. Arsian K, Erenoglu B, Dogru O et al. Lateral Internal Sphincterotomy versus 0.25% isosorbide dinitrate ointment for chronic anal fissures: A prospective randomized controlled trial. *Surg Today.* 2013;43(5):500–505.
5. Nicholls J. Anal fissure; surgery is the best treatment. *Colorectal Dis.* 2008;10(5):529–530.
6. Nasr M, Ezzat H, Elsbae M. Botulinum toxin injection versus lateral internal sphincterotomy in the treatment of chronic anal fissure: A randomized controlled trial. *World J Surg.* 2010;34(11):2730–2734.
7. Nelson R. Operative procedures for fissure in ano. *Cochrane Database Syst Rev.* 2005;2:Art No. CD002199.

8. Gupta PJ, Kalaskar S. Removal of hypertrophied anal papillae and fibrous anal polyps increases patient satisfaction after anal fissure surgery. *Tech Coloproctol.* 2003;7(2):155–158.
9. Leong AF, Seow-Choen F. Lateral internal sphincterotomy compared with anal advancement flap for chronic anal fissure. *Dis Colon Rectum.* 1995;38(1):69–71.
10. Hyman N. Incontinence after lateral internal sphincterotomy: A prospective study and quality of life assessment. *Dis Colon Rectum.* 2004;47(1):35–38.
11. Witte ME, Klaase JM, Koop R. Fissurectomy combined with botulinum toxin A injection for medically resistant chronic anal fissures. *Colorectal Dis.* 2010;12(7 online):e163–e169.
12. Abramowitz L, Bouchard D, Souffran M et al. Sphincter-sparing anal-fissure surgery: A 1-year prospective, observational, multicenter study of fissurectomy with anoplasty. *Colorectal Dis.* 2013;15(3):359–367.
13. Bokhari S, Lindsey I. Incontinence following sphincter division for treatment of anal fistula. *Colorectal Dis.* 2010;12(7 online):e135–e139.
14. Steele SR, Kumar R, Feingold DL et al. Practice parameters for the management of perianal abscess and fistula-in-ano. *Dis Colon Rectum.* 2011;54(12):1465–1474.
15. Singer M, Cintron J, Nelson R et al. Treatment of fistulas-in-ano with fibrin sealant in combination with intra-adhesive antibiotics and/or surgical closure of the internal fistula opening. *Dis Colon Rectum.* 2005;48(6):799–808.
16. Champagne BJ, O'Connor LM, Ferguson M et al. Efficacy of anal fistula plug in closure of cryptoglandular fistulas: long term follow-up. *Dis Colon Rectum.* 2006;49(10):1817–1821.
17. van Koperen PJ, D'Hoore A, Wolthuis AM et al. Anal Fistula Plug for Closure of difficult anorectal fistula: A prospective study. *Dis Colon Rectum* 2007;50(12):2168–2172.
18. Ky AJ, Sylla P, Steinhagan R et al. Collagen fistula plug for the treatment of anal fistulas. *Dis Colon Rectum.* 2008;51(6):838–843.
19. El-Gazzaz G, Zutshi M, Hull T. A retrospective review of chronic anal fistulae treated by anal fistulae plug. *Colorectal Dis.* 2010;12(5):442–447.
20. Ellis CH, Rostas JW, Greiner FG. Long-term outcomes with the use of bioprosthetic plugs for the management of complex anal fistulas. *Dis Colon Rectum.* 2010;53(5):798–802.
21. Malik AI, Nelson RL. Surgical management of anal fistulae: a systematic review. *Colorectal Dis.* 2008;10(4): 420–430.
22. Perez F, Arroyo A, Serrano P et al. Randomized clinical and manometric study of advancement flap versus fistulotomy with sphincter reconstruction in the management of complex fistula-in-ano. *Am J Surg.* 2006;192(1): 34–40.
23. Ellis CN, Clark S. Fibrin glue as an adjunct to flap repair of anal fistulas: A randomized, controlled study. *Dis Colon Rectum.* 2006;49(10):1736–1740.
24. Gottgens KW, Vening W, van der Hagen SJ et al. Long-term results of mucosal advancement flap combined with platelet-rich plasma for high cryptoglandular perianal fistula. *Dis Colon Rectum.* 2014;57(2):223–227.
25. Rojansakul A, Pattanaarun J, Sahakitrungruang C et al. Total anal sphincter saving technique for fistula-in-ano: The ligation of the intersphincteric fistula tract. *J Med Assoc Thai.* 2007;90(8):581–586.
26. Vegara-Fernandez O, Espino-Urbina LA. Ligation of the intersphincteric fistula tract: What is the evidence in a review? *World J Gastroenterol.* 2013;19(40):6805–6813.
27. Ellis CN. Outcomes with the use of bioprosthetic grafts to reinforce the ligation of the intersphincteric fistula tract (BioLIFT procedure) for the management of complex anal fistulas. *Dis Colon Rectum.* 2010;53(10):1361–1364.
28. Han JG, Yi BQ, Wang ZJ. Ligation of the intersphincteric fistula tract plus a bioprosthetic anal fistula plug (LIFT-Plug): A new technique for fistula-in-ano. *Colorectal Dis.* 2013;15(5):582–586.
29. Altomare DF, Greco VJ, Tricomi N et al. Seton or glue for trans-sphincteric anal fistulae; a prospective randomized crossover clinical trial. *Colorectal Dis.* 2011;13(1):82–86.
30. Madbouly KM, El Shazly W, Abbas KS et al. Ligation of intersphincteric fistula tract versus mucosal advancement flap in patients with high transsphincteric fistula-in-ano, a prospective randomized trial. *Dis Colon Rectum.* 2014;57(10):1202–1208.
31. Dajani AS, Taubert KA, Wilson W et al. Prevention of bacterial endocarditis. Recommendations by the American Heart Association. *Circulation.* 1997;96(3):358–366.

## Commentary on Anal Fissure, Fistula, and Abscess

*Michael J. Stamos*

Over the past 25 years of my practice since completing my surgical training, much has changed. Treatment of the very common maladies of anal abscess/fistula disease and of anal fissures is no exception. The majority of the changes in the treatment of these diseases are based primarily on the observation that occasionally (or more often!), we fail to "do no harm," rendering the patient with some degree of anal incontinence as a direct consequence of our treatment. For many patients, concern for any degree of anal incontinence or even the threat of same will lead them to decline an operation, which carries *any* risk of this outcome. Indeed, the informed consent process and the education of our patients (either from us or the internet) has led to a surge in alternative treatments for these diseases, which are broadly termed sphincter sparing. The problem, of course, is that all these treatments suffer from lower success rates than the tried and true anal fistulotomy for anal fistula and lateral internal anal sphincterotomy (LIAS) for a chronic anal fissure. This is not meant to imply that the concerns over incontinence are unfounded, but rather that the pendulum may have swung a bit far, and to recognize that there is a price to pay for utilizing alternatives with less efficacy but greater safety. This price is not just in healthcare dollars but also in patient suffering, as many patients will choose to live with symptoms of an anal fissure and/or endure multiple operations before (hopefully) success is reached in the case of anal fistulae.

To address the specific questions asked and addressed in this manuscript.

### How Do Nonoperative Medical Therapies Compare to Placebo and LIAS in the Treatment of Anal Fissures?

The conclusion that nonoperative therapies that work by relaxing the anal sphincter are superior to placebo but inferior to LIAS is accurate, but with a binary endpoint of healing versus not, the studies may be missing the point, namely, that symptom relief is what patients care about. Indeed, many patients in my own practice prefer to use topical ointments and even repeat botulinum toxin injections rather than take a risk of even minor incontinence. Healing is less important to them than symptom relief. We also need to consider the long-term rate of incontinence from an LIAS, which might increase as patients age. No reliable data exists to guide us however.

### What Is the Impact of Technique on the Outcomes of Patients Undergoing Operation for Anal Fissure?

Not much controversy here, as LIAS is the clear choice when operating on an anal fissure. Decisions to excise the associated sentinel pile or hypertrophied anal papillae generally center around the current or likely symptomatology attributed to them. Anoplasty is a reasonable option for patients with pre-existing incontinence, but of course, those patients are rare, as a classic fissure requires sphincter hypertonicity.

### What Is the Healing and Incontinence Rate for Fistulotomy for Simple Fistula-in-Ano?

The devil is in the details for this question. What is the definition of a simple fistula? A simple answer is "Someone else's. " I would consider an intersphincteric fistula or a low transphincteric fistula simple, when it was located in the posterior aspect of the anal canal in a male patient. However, even in this scenario, the operation is at least as sphincter ablative as a LIAS, so can be expected to carry some risk of minor anal incontinence. When this is relayed to a patient, there still can be reluctance to consent.

### What Is the Healing and Incontinence Rate for More Complex Fistulae Treated with Fibrin Glue, Fistula Plug, or a Seton?

A mixed bag here, with glue being largely abandoned at least in its current form due to low success rates, while fistula plugs enjoying a modest surge in popularity until the ligation of intersphincteric tract (LIFT) procedure began to generate more enthusiasm. A 50% chance of healing with a plug (either of the two currently available) is a reasonable estimate based on recent prospective data, and incontinence risks seem to be nonexistent as one would expect. Setons are typically used to eradicate infection (draining or loose seton) in preparation for another procedure (plug or LIFT), or as definitive therapy (cutting seton). As noted by Dr Perry, cutting setons do not preserve continence reliably, so they should be used with utmost caution.

### What Is the Healing and Incontinence Rate for More Complex Fistulae Treated with an Endorectal Advancement Flap?

As noted, there is a paucity of high-quality studies to answer this question. However, this has become accepted as the most effective, time proven, sphincter-sparing operation for anal fistula. There is, however, a small risk of incontinence, and it is unclear if this is due to the anal stretch required to perform the operation or due to inadvertent or intentional internal sphincter injury during the operation. Intentional internal sphincter injury occurs when a flap deep to the submucosa is utilized, a preference of some surgeons.

### What Is the Role of LIFT in the Treatment of Fistula-in-Ano?

Like seemingly every new innovative approach to healing an anal fistula (see fibrin glue, fistula plugs), this operation was introduced with a bang in 2006 with the promise to be the holy grail of fistula treatment, a simple operation with a greater than 90% success, without incontinence. Alas, another relative disappointment. While arguably the best sphincter-sparing operation to use for most transphincteric fistula, success rates are settling out in the 60%–70% range. If history repeats itself, we will find that the lower end of that range is where it will settle.

### What Are the Results of Trials Comparing Different Surgical Techniques in the Management of Fistula-in-Ano?

A paucity of quality studies precludes definitive conclusions, but the simple observation that one of the reported RCTs had a success rate of 48% for an advancement flap while another had a success rate of 66%, which lends credence to the belief that patient selection and technical proficiency impact results.

### Are Antibiotics Necessary for Most Patients Undergoing Routine Incision and Drainage of Perirectal Abscesses?

Immunosuppression and extensive cellulitis with a concern for a necrotizing infection and high risk for heart valve infection are the only legitimate reasons to consider antibiotics. Most abscesses can be drained in the office or at the bedside, and unnecessary probing or breaking up of loculations is generally meddlesome.

# 56

# *Evidence-Based Practice: Acute Cholecystitis*

**Lane L. Frasier and Suresh K. Agarwal**

**CONTENTS**



## 56.1 Acute Cholecystitis

### 56.1.1 History and Epidemiology

Cholecystitis is not a new disease. Langenbuch is credited with the first cholecystectomy in history in 1882 [1]. In 1985, a German surgeon named Erich Muhe performed the first laparoscopic cholecystectomy. His approach was met with skepticism and disbelief, and it was not until French surgeon Mouret published his case series that the laparoscopic approach was recognized as a feasible alternative to open cholecystectomy [1]. Today, between 10% and 20% of Americans have gallstones, and up to a third of them will ultimately become symptomatic. A thorough understanding of the management of gallbladder disease remains essential for the practicing surgeon.

### 56.1.2 Anatomy and Physiology

Retrospective cohort studies delineate the frequency of anatomic variations in the extrahepatic biliary tree. Ectopic gallbladders (1/1600 autopsies), duplication or triplication of the gallbladder (1/4000 autopsies) and even gallbladder agenesis with biliary symptoms (<1 in 6000 live births) can all contribute to the therapeutic difficulty in a patient with acute cholecystitis [2]. Furthermore, textbook-like lateral cystic duct drainage in patients undergoing cholecystectomy was only encountered in 17% of several thousand cholangiograms reviewed [3]. Premature or delayed developmental separation or duplication or malrotation of the cystic duct can lead to significant variations in biliary anatomy. A prospective study of 186 consecutive laparoscopic cholecystectomies found that when dissection was limited to the neck of the gallbladder and Calot's triangle, variations in ductal anatomy were rarely visualized, although variations in arterial anatomy were more readily apparent [4]. There is increasing evidence that the visual perceptions and "biased confirmation" of anatomic patterns contribute significantly to bile duct injury mechanisms [5,6].

Obstruction of the cystic duct by a calculus is most often the cause of acute cholecystitis, but it can also be caused by blood clots or infectious organisms in immunosuppressed patients. Calculus obstruction is thought to be correlated with sterile bile in >50% of patients.

Stewart et al. have demonstrated a subset of patients with slime-forming bacteria imbedded into the gallstones [7].

### 56.1.3 Initial Evaluation and Diagnosis

#### 56.1.3.1 *What Are the Clinical Criteria Required for the Diagnosis of Acute Cholecystitis?*

A group in Japan has created and subsequently revised criteria for the diagnosis of acute cholecystitis (Tokyo Guidelines 2013 or TG13) [8]. They include local signs of inflammation (Murphy's sign, right upper quadrant pain, mass, or tenderness), systemic signs of inflammation (fever, elevated C-reactive protein, and elevated white blood cell count), and imaging findings characteristic of cholecystitis. Diagnosis can be suspected with one local and one systemic sign. Diagnosis is considered definite with the addition of imaging findings. In a retrospective review of 227 patients with pathology-confirmed acute cholecystitis, these updated criteria had a sensitivity and specificity of 91.2% and 96.9%, respectively [8].

*Recommendation*: No one clinical criterion is sufficient to predict or rule out acute cholecystitis; however, in the presence of one local and systemic sign of inflammation the diagnosis should be strongly suspected (Grade B recommendation).

#### 56.1.3.2 *What Is the Value of Imaging Studies for the Diagnosis of Acute Cholecystitis?*

Ultrasound remains the initial study of choice for most patients [9]. It is noninvasive, relatively easy to obtain, inexpensive, confers no radiation, and is moderately sensitive. Although it also provides the ability to assess for a sonographic Murphy's sign, this is a relatively low-specificity finding [10], and its absence does not exclude acute cholecystitis, especially if the patient has recently received narcotics for analgesia.

Several meta-analyses have confirmed the higher sensitivity and specificity of cholescintigraphy compared to abdominal ultrasound. A recent meta-analysis by Kiewiet et al. updated the findings of a previous study [11], estimating cholescintigraphy's sensitivity and specificity to be 96% and 90%, respectively, while abdominal ultrasound was estimated to have 81% sensitivity and 83% specificity [12].

Patients presenting with nonspecific abdominal pain or those who have negative ultrasound and/or cholescintigraphy may undergo computed tomography of the abdomen. While this study is not the ideal first test for evaluating the biliary system, it may nevertheless provide the diagnosis by identifying gallbladder wall enhancement, peri-cholecystic fluid, or complications like gangrene or gallbladder hemorrhage, as well as evaluating or ruling out competing alternative diagnoses [9].

*Recommendation*: Ultrasound remains the preferred initial study and will correctly diagnose most patients. If ultrasound is equivocal or does not correlate with the medical history, cholescintigraphy is an appropriate next step. Abdominal CT should be reserved for patients in whom the entire abdomen requires evaluation (Grade B recommendation).

### 56.1.4 Management

#### 56.1.4.1 *Should Laparoscopic or Open Cholecystectomy Be Performed in Acute and Complicated Acute Cholecystitis?*

Laparoscopy was originally contraindicated in the setting of acute cholecystitis and reserved for purely elective procedures in the setting of biliary colic. This is no longer the case. In 2009, the Society of American Gastrointestinal and Endoscopic Surgeons published its guidelines on indications, operative techniques, and management of complications for laparoscopic cholecystectomy based on a literature review. Of 219 abstracts reviewed, 38 articles were evaluated as pertinent, and the Society concluded that laparoscopy should be the preferred approach for acute cholecystitis [13].

Additionally, Boo et al. [14] studied inflammatory markers in patients randomized to open versus laparoscopic cholecystectomy in acute cholecystitis. Using blood samples obtained preoperatively and 24 and 72 h postoperatively, they found that laparoscopy patients had a faster normalization of C-reactive protein, and a less marked reduction in postoperative monocyte count and production of TNF-$\alpha$, suggesting reduced immunosuppression with the laparoscopic approach.

In 2008, Borzellino et al. completed a meta-analysis of outcomes for patients undergoing laparoscopic cholecystectomy for severe acute cholecystitis, defined by the presence of empyema or emphysematous gallbladder. Seven studies totaling 1408 patients were analyzed comparing surgery for severe versus nonsevere acute cholecystitis, and found a higher risk of conversion and overall complications (RR 3.2, CI 2.5–4.2 and RR 1.6, CI 1.2–2.2, respectively) [15]. However, the authors were unable to find any studies comparing outcomes after urgent laparoscopy with urgent open cholecystectomy and concluded that one should have a lower threshold for conversion when operating on patients with severe cholecystitis; no peer-reviewed articles appear to have been published in the interim.

The approach in a patient with Mirizzi syndrome, where a large stone impacted in the neck of the gallbladder causes extrinsic compression or fistula of the common bile duct, remains a controversial topic. The current literature suggests that the laparoscopic approach has a significantly higher rate of conversion [16–18] and the standard of care has not been definitively established.

*Recommendation*: Laparoscopic cholecystectomy should be the initial approach of choice in the vast majority of cases (Grade B recommendation). The best approach in Mirizzi syndrome is unknown (Grade D recommendation).

#### 56.1.4.2 What Should the Timing of Surgical Intervention Be?

In 2014, de Mestral et al. published a retrospective cohort study of Canadian patients presenting with acute cholecystitis. In a matched cohort of 14,220 patients, those undergoing early cholecystectomy (within 7 days) had, on average, hospital stays 1.9 days shorter and a relative risk of major biliary injury of 0.53 (CI 0.31–0.9) compared to patients undergoing later cholecystectomy, with nonsignificant differences in 30-day mortality or conversion [19].

In 2013, the Cochrane group updated its review on the timing of cholecystectomy for acute cholecystitis, summarizing the results of six trials [20]. Early cholecystectomy was defined as within 7 days of symptoms onset ($n = 244$), while delayed cholecystectomy occurred at least 6 weeks after symptom onset ($n = 244$). In the five trials reporting mortality data, there were no deaths in either group. There were no significant differences in conversion rates, bile duct injuries, or surgical complications in early versus late cholecystectomy. Patients undergoing early cholecystectomy had, on average, shorter hospital stay by 4 days (CI 3.03–5.22 days). In data summed from five of these trials, 18% of patients awaiting interval cholecystectomy had either persistent/recurrent symptoms necessitating emergent laparoscopic cholecystectomy, with a 45% conversion rate (Table 56.1). The authors noted that all studies were underpowered; nevertheless, they concluded that in the setting of equivalent rates of complications, early cholecystectomy was preferable as it conferred a shorter hospital stay and reduced the risk of interval symptoms and emergency surgery [20].

*Recommendation*: Early cholecystectomy is the preferred approach (Grade B recommendation).

#### 56.1.4.3 What Are the Indications and Outcomes for Nonsurgical Intervention?

Some patients with acute cholecystitis are severely ill and have a high perioperative risk due to comorbid illness. Cholecystostomy and gallbladder aspiration have both been reported as temporizing measures or definitive treatment for those patients. However, high-level evidence for these treatment modalities is scarce. Retrospective, nonrandomized case series remain a common source of outcome evaluations for cholecystostomy [21–23] as descriptive studies or comparing outcomes to emergency cholecystectomy in the absence of randomization. A large national retrospective analysis via the Nationwide Inpatient Sample from 1998 to 2010 found higher adjusted mortality rates for patients undergoing cholecystostomy versus cholecystectomy ($p < 0.001$) in patients with both calculous and acalculous cholecystitis [24].

Hatzidakis et al. [25] randomized 123 patients with acute cholecystitis and APACHE score >12 to conservative therapy (IV fluids, broad-spectrum antibiotics, and nonsteroidal anti-inflammatory drugs accompanied by proton pump inhibitors for stomach protection) versus percutaneous cholecystostomy followed by emergency surgery if there was no clinical improvement after 3 days.

**TABLE 56.1**

Summarized Results of a Systematic Review of Early versus Delayed Cholecystectomy for Acute Cholecystitis

| | Number of Trials | Number of Patients | Favors | Effect Size of Early Cholecystectomy |
|---|---|---|---|---|
| Mortality | 5 | 438 | Neither—there were no deaths in any studies | Not applicable |
| Biliary injury | 5 | 438 | Early cholecystectomy | Odds ratio 0.49<br>95% CI [0.05–4.72]<br>$p = 0.54$ |
| Other serious complication | 5 | 438 | Delayed cholecystectomy | Risk ratio 1.29<br>95% CI [0.61–2.72]<br>$p = 0.50$ |
| Conversion to open cholecystectomy | 6 | 488 | Early cholecystectomy | Risk ratio 0.89<br>95% CI [0.63–1.25]<br>$p = 0.50$ |
| Hospital length of stay | 4 | 373 | Early cholecystectomy | Mean difference (days): −4.12<br>95% CI [−5.22 to −3.03]<br>$p < 0.0001$ |
| Operative time | 6 | 488 | Early cholecystectomy | Mean difference (min): −1.22<br>95% CI: [−3.07 to −0.64]<br>$p = 0.20$ |

*Source:* Gurusamy, K et al., *Cochrane Database Syst Rev*, Issue 6, Art. No. CD005440, 2013.

They reported similar rates of symptom resolution (87% vs. 86%) and 30-day mortality (13% vs. 17.5%) in the conservative versus interventional groups, respectively, noting that more patients in the interventional group were initially admitted to the ICU. The authors concluded by recommending that this patient cohort be treated with initial conservative management, followed by percutaneous cholecystostomy if no clinical improvement was seen in 3 days [25]. Another trial randomized 70 high-risk patients (ASA grades II–IV, APACHE II score ≥12) to percutaneous cholecystostomy within 8 h of admission followed by immediate cholecystectomy if APACHE II scores decreased within 96 h, versus medical management followed by delayed cholecystectomy 8 weeks after recovery [26]. Patients who underwent cholecystostomy experienced faster symptom relief (mean time, 15 vs. 55 h, $p = 0.0001$). Patients who improved enough to undergo early laparoscopy had a conversion rate of 6.5%, while patients receiving conservative therapy and delayed cholecystectomy had a conversion rate of 13.4%. Patients randomized to cholecystostomy also had shorter mean hospital stay (5.3 vs. 15.2 days, $p = 0.0001$) and lower costs (mean $2612 vs. $3735, $p = 0.0001$) compared to those treated with delayed cholecystectomy. The authors concluded that patients treated with cholecystostomy and early cholecystectomy had a shorter time to resolution of symptoms and were able to safely undergo laparoscopic surgery, while avoiding the risks of recurrent cholecystitis and/or gallstone-induced pancreatitis [26].

*Recommendation*: The best approach remains unclear though conservative management with or without percutaneous cholecystostomy may be considered in high-risk patients (Grade D recommendation).

#### *56.1.4.4 What Are the Indications for Intraoperative Cholangiogram?*

Surgeons must determine which, if any, of their patients should undergo intraoperative cholangiography (IOC) with cholecystectomy. In 2012, Ford et al. [27] published a systematic review of randomized controlled trials published in the literature between 1980 and 2011 comparing routine, selective, or no IOC, ultimately evaluating eight trials with 1715 patients (Table 56.2). Six trials evaluated patients at "low-risk" for common bile duct stones, while two included any patient without frank jaundice or evidence of choledocholithiasis on preoperative imaging. Successful completion of cholangiography ranged from 66% to 98.9%, and added an average of 16 min additional operative time. There were 24 false-positive cholangiograms, two-thirds of which came from a single study, all of which prompted trans-cystic or common bile duct exploration.

In patients at low risk for choledocholithiasis, five patients had retained stones on follow-up; four had been randomized to no cholangiogram, while the last received IOC which was deemed normal. In the two nonselective IOC studies, a total of eight patients had retained stones, including three for whom IOC was attempted but unsuccessful. Two common bile duct injuries occurred, both in patients who did not receive IOC.

Given the low rates of retained stones and bile duct injury, the authors concluded that the studies were underpowered to evaluate the outcomes of interest and that neither routine nor selective IOC could be supported [27].

*Recommendation*: The best approach remains unclear (Grade D recommendation).

**TABLE 56.2**

Summarized Results of a Systematic Review of Routine versus No and Routine versus Selective Intraoperative Cholangiogram

| | Routine versus No Cholangiogram | | | Routine versus Selective Cholangiogram | | |
|---|---|---|---|---|---|---|
| **Outcome Assessed** | **Number of Trials** | **Number of Patients** | **Outcome** | **Number of Trials** | **Number of Patients** | **Outcome** |
| Common bile duct injury | 4 | 860 | 0 CBD injuries with routine IOC<br>2 CBD injuries with no IOC | 1 | 303 | 1 CBD injury with routine IOC<br>1 CBD injury with selective IOC |
| Intraoperative stones identified (true positives) | 6 | 1245 | 27 patients | 2 | 470 | 22 patients |
| Intraoperative stones identified (false positives) | 6 | 1245 | 23 patients with routine | 2 | 470 | 1 patients |
| Retained stones at follow-up | 6 | 1245 | 1 patient with routine IOC<br>4 patients with no IOC | 2 | 470 | 3 with routine IOC<br>5 patients with selective IOC |

*Source:* Ford, JA et al., *Br J Surg*, 99, 160, 2012.
*Abbreviations:* CBD, common bile duct; IOC, intraoperative cholangiogram.

#### *56.1.4.5 What Are the Indications for Drain Placement?*

Gurusamy et al. assessed the use of routine abdominal drainage for uncomplicated open cholecystectomy in a systematic review for the Cochrane database in 2007 [28]. Included were 28 open cholecystectomy trials (3659 patients) of which 20 trials evaluated the comparison of "no drain placement" vs. "drain placement" and 12 trials evaluated one drainage method versus another (closed suction vs. Penrose). No significant differences were encountered for intra-abdominal fluid collections; however, wound and chest infections were more frequent with drain placement [28].

In 2013, the same authors updated a separate review focusing on laparoscopic cholecystectomy (Table 56.3) [29]. In a meta-analysis of 12 randomized clinical trials totaling 1831 patients, consisting largely of patients undergoing elective cholecystectomy, there were no significant differences in serious adverse events, short-term mortality, hospital length of stay, or quality of life between patients who did and did not receive a drain. Drain recipients had a mean operative time, where reported, 5 min longer than nondrain patients (CI 2.6–7.3 min) [29].

A separate meta-analysis by Antoniou et al. of six randomized trials found higher pain scores 6–12 h (mean difference in pain score of 1.12 units, CI 1.01–1.24) postoperatively in patients receiving prophylactic drain placement, with no differences in 30-day morbidity or wound infections [30].

*Recommendation*: Routine drain placement does not appear to provide any benefit and may be associated with increased frequency of infections (Grade B recommendation).

#### *56.1.4.6 Which Antibiotic Therapy Is Warranted?*

The American Society of Health System Pharmacists' (ASHP) 2013 Therapeutic Guidelines recommends that for patients undergoing cholecystectomy electively or for mild–moderate, community-acquired cholecystitis, no antibiotic prophylaxis is needed for low-risk patients. Features placing a patient at higher risk of surgical site infection include: an episode of biliary colic within 30 days of surgery, emergent surgery, surgery lasting >120 min, intraoperative gallbladder rupture or bile spillage, age >70 years, pregnancy, a nonfunctioning gallbladder, American Society of Anesthesiologists classification ≥3, and diabetes. Because of the intraoperative nature of some of these risk factors and the higher rate of surgical site infection in patients undergoing open cholecystectomy, the authors state it may be reasonable to provide a single prophylactic dose of antibiotics to all patients undergoing laparoscopic cholecystectomy [31].

These guidelines include a meta-analysis comparing various antibiotic regimens in which no notable difference in outcomes between first-, second-, and third-degree cephalosporin was found. The guidelines therefore recommend cefazolin, cefoxitin, cefotetan, or ampicillin–sulbactam for noninfected biliary conditions, and ceftriaxone in patients suspected of acute cholecystitis or acute biliary infection with intraoperative redosing if case duration is longer than 4 h (cephalosporin) or 2 h (ampicillin–sulbactam) [31]. Broad-spectrum antibiotic

**TABLE 56.3**

Summarized Results of a Systematic Review of Routine Drainage During Laparoscopic Cholecystectomy

| | Number of Trials | Number of Patients | Favors | Effect Size of Drain |
|---|---|---|---|---|
| Mortality | 10 | 1681 | Drain | Risk ratio 0.41<br>95% CI [0.04–4.37]<br>$p = 0.46$ |
| Serious adverse events (proportion of patients) | 7 | 1143 | No drain | Risk ratio 2.12<br>95% CI [0.61–7.40]<br>$p = 0.24$ |
| Serious adverse events (total number) | 8 | 1286 | No drain | Risk ratio 1.60<br>95% CI [0.66–3.87]<br>$p = 0.30$ |
| Quality of life | 1 | 93 | Drain | Standard mean difference: 0.22<br>95% CI [−0.19 to 0.63] |
| Hospital length of stay | 5 | 449 | No drain | Mean difference (days): 0.22<br>95% CI [−0.06 to 0.50]<br>$p = 0.31$ |
| Operative time | 7 | 775 | No drain | Mean difference (minutes): 4.97<br>95% CI: [2.70–7.25]<br>$p < 0.0001$ |

*Source:* Gurusamy, KS et al., *Cochrane Database Syst Rev*, Issue 9, Art. No. CD006004, 2013.

coverage provides no benefit unless the patient has a known history of pseudomonal infection or drug-resistant colonization or infection and increases the risk of later drug resistance.

Currently, no randomized controlled trials or cohort studies are available evaluating the duration of antibiotic therapy for patients with acute cholecystitis. No randomized studies have been published examining the efficacy of 24 h of antibiotics versus greater than 24 h for acute cholecystitis. Based on evidence from studies on other procedures, the ASHP states that there is minimal evidence to support prophylactic postoperative antibiotics for most procedures, and should not be given for more than 24 h in the absence of systemic infection [31].

*Recommendation*: A single dose of prophylactic antibiotics is likely appropriate for all patients with acute cholecystitis (Grade B recommendation). A first-, second-, or third-generation cephalosporin or ampicillin-sulbactam is appropriate (Grade A recommendation). Antibiotic therapy greater than 24 h is not indicated (Grade B recommendation).

### *56.1.4.7 Which Perioperative Pain Therapy Is Effective?*

Kehlet et al. [32] published a procedure-specific systematic review and consensus recommendations for postoperative analgesia following laparoscopic cholecystectomy in 2005. Based on meta-analysis of 69 randomized trials, their recommendations for anesthesia providers included: use of dexamethasone and total IV anesthesia or partially IV anesthesia to prevent postoperative nausea and vomiting; and use of systemic nonsteroidal anti-inflammatory drugs, acetaminophen, and, when necessary, stepwise progression to weak opioids. Patients with severe pain or requiring conversion should receive strong opioids and consideration for epidural anesthesia. For surgeons, they recommend use of low-pressure $CO_2$ insufflation and combined use of intraperitoneal and incisional local anesthetic.

**TABLE 56.4**

Summary of Recommendations and Level of Evidence for Management of Acute Cholecystitis

| Question | Answer | Level of Evidence | Grade of Recommendation | References |
|---|---|---|---|---|
| What are the clinical criteria required for the diagnosis of acute cholecystitis? | No one clinical criterion is sufficient to predict or rule out acute cholecystitis; however, in the presence of one local and systemic sign of inflammation the diagnosis should be strongly suspected. | 3 | B | [8] |
| What is the value of imaging studies for the diagnosis of acute cholecystitis? | Ultrasound remains the preferred initial study and will correctly diagnose most patients. If ultrasound is equivocal or does not correlate with the medical history, cholescintigraphy is an appropriate next step. Abdominal CT should be reserved for patients in which the entire abdomen requires evaluation. | 4 | B | [9–12] |
| Should laparoscopic or open cholecystectomy be performed in acute and complicated acute cholecystitis? | Laparoscopic cholecystectomy should be the initial approach of choice in the vast majority of cases. | 2 | B | [13–18] |
| | The best approach in Mirizzi syndrome is unknown. | 7 | D | |
| What should the timing of surgical intervention be? | Early cholecystectomy is the preferred approach. | 1 | B | [19,20] |
| What are the indications and outcomes for nonsurgical intervention? | The best approach remains unclear though conservative management with or without percutaneous cholecystostomy may be considered in high-risk patients. | 2 | B | [21–26] |
| What are the indications for intraoperative cholangiogram? | The best approach remains unclear. | 2 | D | [27] |
| What are the indications for drain placement? | Routine drain placement does not appear to provide any benefit and may be associated with increased frequency of infections. | 1 | B | [28–30] |
| Which antibiotic therapy is warranted? | A single dose of prophylactic antibiotics is likely appropriate for all patients with acute cholecystitis. | 1 | B | [31] |
| | A first-, second-, or third-generation cephalosporin or ampicillin-sulbactam is appropriate. | 1 | A | |
| | Antibiotic therapy greater than 24 h is not indicated. | 7 | B | |
| Which perioperative pain therapy is effective? | A stepwise, multimodal approach is indicated. | 1 | A | [32–35] |

Mitra et al [33]. summarize more than 40 randomized trials comparing various regimens of intraperitoneal and incisional local anesthetic; most were found to be effective in reducing patient-reported pain severity but had mixed results relating to reduction of opioid use.

Since that time, transversus abdominis plane (TAP) block has been suggested as an additional method of analgesia. The higher dermatome distribution of post-cholecystectomy pain presented some question as to its effectiveness in cholecystectomy as compared to lower abdominal procedures. In 2013, Keir et al. [34] evaluated the four available randomized controlled trials of this technique and concluded that standard TAP was effective in reducing postoperative pain (either at rest and/or with coughing) but did not appear to be superior to infiltration of local anesthetic of the incision sites. They did identify one study [35] in which an alternative approach of subcostal TAP produced improved pain scores when compared to local anesthesia at incision sites. Keir et al. concluded that the costs of TAP and the risks associated with an invasive procedure must be weighed against the potential benefits, but that if TAP were to be performed for cholecystectomy, the subcostal approach should be performed [34]. Given the many approaches which could potentially utilize local anesthetic, coordination between anesthesia and surgery is vital to ensure that total doses of local anesthesia between the combined approaches remain within safe limits.

*Recommendation*: A stepwise, multimodal approach is indicated (Grade A recommendation).

## 56.2 Discussion

Biliary disease remains a common problem in general surgical practice. Many aspects of diagnosis, management, and postoperative care have not been rigorously evaluated with the gold standard of randomized controlled trials. Table 56.4 summarizes the current evidence and recommendations for the questions discussed in this chapter. Comparative effectiveness research, combined with ongoing randomized trials and meta-analyses and sound clinical judgment, will be necessary to provide the best possible care to our patients.

## References

1. Polychronidis A, Laftsidis P, Bounovas A, Simopoulos C. Twenty years of laparoscopic cholecystectomy: Phillip Mouret--March 17, 1987. *J Soc Laparoendosc Surg.* 2008;12(1):109–111.
2. Lamah M, Karanjia ND, Dickson GH. Anatomical variations of the extrahepatic biliary tree: Review of the world literature. *Clin Anat.* 2001;14(3):167–172.
3. Berci G. Biliary ductal anatomy and anomalies. The role of intraoperative cholangiography during laparoscopic cholecystectomy. *Surg Clin N Am.* 1992;72(5):1069–1075.
4. Larobina M, Nottle PD. Extrahepatic biliary anatomy at laparoscopic cholecystectomy: Is aberrant anatomy important? *Aust N Z J Surg.* 2005;75:392–395.
5. Way LW, Stewart L, Gantert W et al. Causes and prevention of laparoscopic bile duct injuries: Analysis of 252 cases from a human factors and cognitive psychology perspective. *Ann Surg.* 2003;237(4):460–469.
6. Hugh TB. New strategies to prevent laparoscopic bile duct injury—Surgeons can learn from pilots. *Surgery.* 2002;132(5):826–835.
7. Stewart L, Griffiss JM, Jarvis GA, Way LW. Gallstones containing bacteria are biofilms: Bacterial slime production and ability to form pigment solids determines infection severity and bacteremia. *J Gastrointest Surg.* 2007;11(8):977–983.
8. Yokoe M, Takada T, Strasberg SM et al. New diagnostic criteria and severity assessment of acute cholecystitis in revised Tokyo guidelines. *J Hepato-Biliary-Pancreatic Sci.* 2012;19:578–585.
9. Yarmish GM, Smith MP, Rosen MP et al. ACR appropriateness criteria right upper quadrant pain. *J Am Coll Radiol.* 2014;11(3):316–322.
10. Bree RL. Further observations on the usefulness of the sonographic Murphy sign in the evaluation of suspected acute cholecystitis. *J Clin Ultrasound.* 1995;23(3):169–172.
11. Shea JA, Berlin JA, Escarce JJ et al. Revised estimates of diagnostic test sensitivity and specificity in suspected biliary tract disease. *JAMA Intern Med.* 1994;154(22):2573–2581.
12. Kiewiet JJS, Leeuwenbrugh MMN, Bipat S, MBossuyt PMM, Stoker J, Boermeester MA. A systematic review and meta-analysis of diagnostic performance of imaging in acute cholecystitits. *Radiology.* 2012;264(3):708–720.
13. Overby DW, Awad Z, Haggerty S et al. 2010. Guidelines for the clinical application of laparoscopic biliary tract surgery. http://www.sages.org/publications/guidelines/guidelines-for-the-clinical-application-of-laparoscopic-biliary-tract-surgery. (accessed September 1, 2014.)
14. Boo Y-J, Kim W-B, Kim J et al. Systemic immune response after open versus laparoscopic cholecystectomy in acute cholecystitis: A prospective randomized study. *Scand J Clin Lab Invest.* 2007;67:207–214.
15. Borzellino G, Sauerland S, Minicozzi AM et al. Laparoscopic cholecystectomy for severe acute cholecystitis. A meta-analysis of results. *Surg Endosc.* 2008;22(1):8–15.
16. Antoniou SA, Antoniou GA, Makridis C. Laparoscopic treatment of Mirizzi syndrome: A systematic review. *Surg Endosc.* 2010;24(1):33–39.
17. Liedo JB, Barber SM, Ibanez JC, Torregrosa AG, Lopez-Andujar R. Update on the diagnosis and treatment of Mirizzi syndrome in laparoscopic era: Our experience in 7 years. *Surg Laparosc Endosc Percutan Tech.* 2014;24(6):495–501.

18. Erben Y, Benavente-Chenhalls LA, Donohue JM et al. Diagnosis and treatment of Mirizzi syndrome: 23-year Mayo Clinic experience. *J Am Coll Surg*. 2011;213(1):114–119.
19. de Mestral C, Rotstein OD, Laupacis A et al. Comparative operative outcomes of early and delayed cholecystectomy for acute cholecystitis: A population-based propensity score analysis. *Ann Surg*. 2014;259:10–15.
20. Gurusamy K, Davidson C, Gluud C, Davidson BR. Early versus delayed laparoscopic cholecystectomy for people with acute cholecystitis. *Cochrane Database Syst Rev*. 2013; Issue 6, Art. No. CD005440.
21. Flexer SM, Peter MB, Durham-Hall AC, Ausobsky JR. Patient outcomes after treatment with percutaneous choelcystostomy for biliary sepsis. *Ann R Coll Surg Engl*. 2014;96:229–233.
22. McKay A, Abulfaraj M, Lipschitz J. Short- and long-term outcomes following percutaneous cholecystostomy for acute cholecystitis in high-risk patients. *Surg Endosc*. 2012;26:1343–1351.
23. Karakayali FY, Akdur A, Kirnap M, Harman A, Ekici Y, Moray G. Emergency cholecystectomy vs percutaneous cholecystostomy plus delayed cholecystectomy for patients with acute cholecystitis. *Hepatobiliary Pancreat Dis Int*. 2014;13:316–322.
24. Anderson JE, Change DC, Talamini MA. A nationwide examination of outcomes of percutaneous cholecysteostomy compared with cholecystectomy for acute cholecystitis, 1998–2010. *Surg Endosc*. 2013;27:3406–3411.
25. Hatzidakis AA, Prassopoulos P, Petinarakis I et al. Acute cholecystitis in high-risk patients: Percutaneous cholecystostomy vs conservative treatment. *Eur Radiol*. 2002;12:1778–1784.
26. Akyurek N, Salman B, Yuksel O et al. Management of acute calculous cholecystitis in high-risk patients. Percutaneous cholecystostomy followed by early laparoscopic cholecystectomy. *Surg Laparosc Endosc Percutan Tech*. 2005;15(6):315–320.
27. Ford JA, Soop M, Du J, Loveday BPT, Rodgers M. Systematic review of intraoperative cholangiography in cholecystectomy. *Br J Surg*. 2012;99:160–167.
28. Gurusamy KS, Samraj K. Routine abdominal drainage for uncomplicated open cholecystectomy. *Cochrane Database Syst Rev*. 2007;Issue 2, Art. No. CD006003.
29. Gurusamy KS, Koti R, Davidson BR. Routine abdominal drainage versus no abdominal drainage for uncomplicated laparoscopic cholecystectomy. *Cochrane Database Syst Rev*. 2013; Issue 9, Art. No. CD006004.
30. Antoniou S, Koch O, Antoniou G et al. Routine versus on drain placement after elective laparoscopic cholecystectomy: Meta-analysis of randomized controlled trials. *Minerva Chir*. 2014;69(3):184–194.
31. Bratzler DW, Dellinger EP, Olsen KM et al. Clinical practice guidelines for antimicrobial prophylaxis in surgery. *Am J Health-Syst Pharm*. 2013;70:195–283.
32. Kehlet H, Gray AW, Bonnet F et al. A procedure-specific systematic review and consensus recommendations for postoperative analgesia following laparoscopic cholecystectomy. *Surg Endosc*. 2005;19:1396–1415.
33. Mitra S, Khandelwal P, Roberts K, Kumar S, Vadivelu N. Pain relief in laparoscopic cholecystectomy—A review of the current options. *Pain Pract*. 2012;12(6):485–496.
34. Keir A, Rhodes L, Kayal A, Khan OA. Does a transversus abdominis plane (TAP) local anaesthetic block improve pain control in patients undergoing laparoscopic cholecystectomy? A best evidence topic. *Int J Surg*. 2013;11:792–794.
35. Tolchard S, Davies R, Martindale S. Efficacy of the subcostal transversus abdominis plane block in laparoscopic cholecystectomy: Comparison with conventional port-site infiltration. *J Anaesthesiol Clin Pharmacol*. 2012;28(3):339–343.

## Commentary on Evidence-Based Practice: Acute Cholecystitis

*David H. Livingston*

The management of acute biliary tract disease is the mainstay of general and acute care surgery and one of the most common reasons for surgical consultation. As a surgeon who trained prior to the introduction of minimally invasive surgery, no single operation has been changed more than cholecystectomy. However with the exception of laparoscopic technique itself, the overall approach to the patient with symptomatic biliary tract disease has not changed drastically and still requires one to adhere to standard principles in treating organ space infection. The chapter clearly outlines the current issues in the overall management of acute cholecystitis although unfortunately the area of most concern, how best to manage those patients with difficult or complicated biliary tract infections, has much less evidence-based data on which to based firm therapeutic options than those symptomatic cholelithiasis or simple acute cholecystitis. So what does the modern acute care and general surgeon need to know about acute cholecystitis?

Simple acute cholecystitis versus symptomatic cholelithiasis: While the subtle difference is something that is asked of all trainees and medical students, in reality, it does not affect patient management to any great degree. The diagnosis is almost always made by history and physical examination accompanied by ultrasound evidence of cholelithiasis. When seeing a patient who presents to the emergency department with abdominal pain, the absence of any documented gallstones should make the diagnosis of biliary tract pathology very questionable and the surgeon should look for another source of the abdominal pain and infection. Patients with true acalculous cholecystitis and sepsis are almost always confined to the intensive care unit and are best treated by percutaneous drainage of the gallbladder. In contrast and as outlined in the chapter, patients with simple acute cholecystitis and symptomatic biliary cholelithiasis should undergo early laparoscopic cholecystectomy as this approach provides the most cost-effective treatment with respect to length of stay, morbidity, and mortality. These are level A recommendations.

Complicated cholecystitis: "Complicated" or "complex" cholecystitis can be thought of to occur in two groups of patients. In one group, the diagnosis is relatively simple and usually made or suggested preoperatively. Longstanding (greater than 5–7 days) duration of symptoms, CT, or ultrasound imaging suggesting an abscess, phlegmon or extension of the infection, systemic signs of sepsis, or cholecystitis in patients that are poor or prohibitive operative risks such as those early after an acute MI. In this group, control of infection by minimally invasive techniques (e.g., cholecystostomy) with appropriately dosed and chosen antibiotics is likely a better first-line therapy. The goal is to temporize, control the acute infection, which will allow the patient to recover and then address the gallbladder at a later date. Emergent operative intervention should be reserved for the subgroup of patients that do not improve and is most often done open. As well outlined in the chapter, there are no randomized prospective data to guide the decision making; however, it falls into the tried and true concept of risk to benefit ratio: the risk of intraoperative complications and perioperative morbidity versus the risk of failing to control the infection or early recurrence of the disease.

The more difficult and insidious group are those patients where complicated cholecystitis is only found or only appreciated during their attempted laparoscopic cholecystectomy. It is these cases where surgical judgment is most tested. Patients with Mirizzi's gallbladder, and those with markedly thickened gall bladder walls or impacted stones are just some examples of complex pathology. At this point, the number one goals should be to address the biliary pathology without injuring the common duct or other structures. Despite over two decades experience with laparoscopic cholecystectomy, the rate of common duct injuries remains at ~1%, which is still significantly higher than that reported during the open cholecystectomy era. In the event of a common bile duct injury, the ability to perform and biliary enteric reconstruction in patients with complicated cholecystitis with an inflamed porta hepatis is far more difficult. Thus, the acute care and general surgeon should not hesitate to open a patient where the critical view cannot be obtained. Familiarity with open and laparoscopic techniques to maximize exposure and minimize risk such as needle decompression, "top–down" dissection, opening the gall bladder with stone extraction, and hemicholecystectomy are necessary to achieve good outcomes. What has been made clear in the laparoscopic era is that there is no need to get close to the common duct but transection of the cystic duct high up on the gallbladder and even leaving a small remnant in the markedly inflamed patient is more than adequate.

Drains and antibiotics: The hardest thing to change in surgery and medicine is long held dogma. As well described, the use of perioperative antibiotics in simple cholecystitis is probably not warranted. This is different from older data in the open cholecystectomy era where antibiotic administration did decrease the superficial wound infection rate and it is likely that the lack of an open incision is the difference. However, if the decision is made to open or the patient's symptoms warrant it, a single dose of an appropriate antibiotic is supported by the data. Similarly, even in patients with more complicated disease who undergo cholecystectomy, there is no need for prolonged antibiotic administration. These are mostly Level A recommendations.

While it will likely take another generation or two, routine drainage in almost all surgical situations is not supported by data. In the case of cholecystectomy (Level B recommendations), if one is so concerned that there may be a ductal injury, one should not leave the operating room until it is proven one way of the other. Relying on postoperative drainage to guide this decision is likely to lead to increased morbidity and delayed recognition and treatment.

# 57

# *Acute Cholangitis*

**Adrian W. Ong and Shannon M. Foster**

**CONTENTS**



## 57.1 History and Epidemiology

Characterization of the features of acute cholangitis (AC) is attributed to Dr. Jean-Martin Charcot, a French neurologist, in 1877. Acute bacterial cholangitis remains a common surgical emergency. A study based on the Nationwide Inpatient Sample, a U.S. database comprising data from >1,000 hospitals estimated that there were 248,000 cases of acute cholangitis over a 10-year period in the United States with an overall mortality rate of about 6% [1]. Of the benign diseases, the most important cause is choledocholithiasis, with other less common causes being benign stricture, chronic pancreatitis, and primary sclerosing cholangitis. The scope of this chapter will be limited to a discussion of acute cholangitis related to choledocholithiasis.

## 57.2 Pathophysiology

An increase in intrabiliary pressure due to obstruction is postulated to play an important role in the pathogenesis of acute cholangitis [2]. In animal studies, the increased intrabiliary pressure leads to disruption of the tight junctions of the bile canalicular cells, and also impairment in the phagocytic function of the Kupffer cell. It is also thought that diversion of bile from the gastrointestinal tract due to obstruction could lead to altered endogenous gut flora and loss of gut mucosal integrity, thereby promoting bacterial translocation [2–4].

## 57.3 Initial Evaluation and Diagnosis

Recently, comprehensive guidelines establishing diagnostic criteria and a severity classification scheme were developed by expert consensus ("Tokyo Guidelines"). First developed and published in 2007 ("TG07") [5], the guidelines have recently been revised ("TG13") [6]. The challenges of establishing objective diagnostic criteria for AC were noted. A set of three standards were proposed (presence of purulent biliary drainage, clinical remission with biliary drainage, and improvement with antimicrobial agents alone when the biliary tree was the only infectious source) and applied to 1432 patients from several centers, to classify patients as those with or without acute cholangitis. Plausible variables were then refined iteratively. The revised TG13 diagnostic criteria (Table 57.1) were found to have a sensitivity of 92% and a specificity of 78% when applied against the aforementioned "gold standards." Of note, based on the TG13 guidelines, Charcot's triad had a low sensitivity but high specificity for diagnosis of acute cholangitis [6,7].

**TABLE 57.1**

Diagnostic Criteria for Acute Cholangitis Based on the Updated Tokyo Guidelines (TG13)

| | |
|---|---|
| A. Systemic inflammation | |
| A-1. Fever and/or shaking chills | |
| A-2. Laboratory data: evidence of inflammatory response | |
| B. Cholestasis | |
| B-1. Jaundice | |
| B-2. Laboratory data: abnormal liver function tests | |
| C. Imaging | |
| C-1. Biliary dilatation | |
| C-2. Evidence of the etiology on imaging (stricture, stone, stent, etc.) | |
| Suspected diagnosis: one item in A + one item in either B or C | |
| Definite diagnosis: one item in A, one item in B, and one item in C | |
| Thresholds | |
| A-1 Fever | >38°C |
| A-2 Evidence of inflammatory response | WBC (×10,000/μL) <4, or >10<br>CRP (mg/dL) ≥1 |
| B-1 Jaundice T-Bil ≥2 (mg/dL) | T-Bil ≥2 (mg/dL) |
| B-2 Abnormal liver function tests | ALP (IU) [1.5 × STD]<br>γGTP (IU) [1.5 × STD]<br>AST (IU) [1.5 × STD]<br>ALT (IU) [1.5 × STD] |

*Source:* Kiriyama, S et al., *J Hepatobiliary Pancreat Sci*, 19, 548, 2012.
*Abbreviations:* WBC, white blood count; T Bil, total bilirubin; ALP, alkaline phosphatase; γGTP, γ-glutamyl transpeptidase; AST, aspartate aminotransferase; ALT, alanine aminotransferase; CRP, C-reactive protein; STD, upper limit of normal value.

**TABLE 57.2**

Severity Assessment for Acute Cholangitis Based on the TG13 Guidelines

| | |
|---|---|
| Grade III (severe) acute cholangitis | |
| "Grade III" acute cholangitis is defined as acute cholangitis that is associated with the onset of dysfunction at least in any one of the following organs/systems: | |
| 1. Cardiovascular dysfunction | Hypotension requiring dopamine ≥5 mcg/kg/min, or any dose of norepinephrine |
| 2. Neurological dysfunction | Disturbance of consciousness |
| 3. Respiratory dysfunction | $PaO_2/FiO_2$ ratio <300 |
| 4. Renal dysfunction | Oliguria, serum creatinine >2.0 mg/dL |
| 5. Hepatic dysfunction | PT-INR >1.5 |
| 6. Hematological dysfunction | Platelet count <100,000/$mm^3$ |
| Grade II (moderate) acute cholangitis | |
| "Grade II" acute cholangitis is associated with any two of the following conditions: | |
| 1. Abnormal WBC count (>12,000/$mm^3$ or <4,000/$mm^3$) | |
| 2. High fever (≥39°C) | |
| 3. Age (≥75 years) | |
| 4. Hyperbilirubinemia (total bilirubin ≥5 mg/dL) | |
| 5. Hypoalbuminemia (<STD × 0.7) | |
| Grade I (mild) acute cholangitis | |
| "Grade I" acute cholangitis does not meet the criteria of "Grade III (severe)" or "Grade II (moderate)" acute cholangitis at initial diagnosis. | |

*Source:* Kiriyama, S et al., *J Hepatobiliary Pancreat Sci*, 19, 548, 2012.
*Abbreviations:* STD, upper limit of normal value.

Similarly, the TG13 severity classification attempted to address the inadequacies of TG07. The revised classification (Table 57.2) was based on the presence of organ dysfunction and several other criteria demonstrated to be associated with poor prognosis. The criterion of "responsiveness to medical management" was removed since this was not possible to determine on presentation. It is noted that the investigators also found that Charcot's triad was not associated with disease severity [6]. Using the TG13 diagnostic criteria, Grade III cholangitis (associated with organ dysfunction) (Table 57.2) was seen in 11%–20% of all cases [6,7].

## 57.4 Management

Essential elements of the initial management are: early recognition, risk stratification, prompt initiation of appropriate antibiotics, and consideration for urgent decompression of the obstructed biliary system.

## 57.5 Should the Initial Empiric Antibiotic Regimen Provide Coverage for Multidrug-Resistant Organisms?

In a retrospective study of patients with community acquired severe acute cholangitis, blood cultures were positive in 160 of 676 (24%) patients [8]. Another retrospective study of 65 patients with acute cholangitis where bile cultures were taken after biliary drainage found that only 22 of 65 (34%) had positive bile cultures [9]. In recent studies of bacteremic patients thought to be related to the biliary tract, the most common organisms were *Escherichia coli* (26%–62%), *Klebsiella* spp. (17%–28%), and *Enterococcus* spp. (1%–25%), *Pseudomonas aeruginosa* (3%–16%), *Enterobacter* spp. (2%–10%), and anaerobic bacteria (0%–7%) [10–14]. The spectrum of bacterial flora in bile cultures is fairly similar to that of blood cultures in the above studies. Of the *E. coli* and *Klebsiella* isolates in the blood, approximately 3%–44% were extended spectrum beta-lactamase (ESBL) positive [8,10,11,14,15]. The clinical impact of ESBL-positive strains is not well studied in acute cholangitis but one retrospective study noted that patients with ESBL-positive strains isolated from blood or bile (21 of 159) had a significantly higher 30-day mortality rate compared to those with ESBL-negative strains (3/21, 14.3% vs. 4/138, 2.9%). Inadequate antimicrobial therapy and septic shock were the other two factors associated with increased 30-day mortality [15]. It was noted that more than half of the patients with ESBL-positive strains had inadequate antimicrobial therapy in that study. This is supported by other studies showing that patients with bloodstream infections with ESBL-producing organisms had a higher mortality rate with inappropriate antibiotics for definitive therapy [16] but not necessarily inadequate initial antimicrobial therapy [16–18].

Evidence-based guidelines by the Infectious Diseases Society of America on complicated intra-abdominal infections suggest that routine coverage for enterococcus in these infections is not required since the pathogenicity of enterococcus is not established [19]. In addition, these guidelines also recommend that routine anti-pseudomonal coverage for mild to moderate (not severe) community-acquired intra-abdominal infections is not necessary. This is supported by a recent meta-analysis of randomized trials of ertapenem versus piperacillin/tazobactam which showed similar treatment success between the two arms [20]. Ertapenem has limited efficacy against *Enterococcus* spp. and is not efficacious against *Pseudomonas*. Other factors may play an equally important role in determining antibiotic coverage. In one study of intra-abdominal infections [21], health care-acquired infection, corticosteroid use, organ transplantation, liver disease, pulmonary disease, and a duodenal source were associated with resistant organisms. The vast majority (78%–90%) of ESBL-related bacteremias in other retrospective studies were also related health care related [16–18].

*Recommendation*: Local antimicrobial susceptibilities, comorbid conditions, and association with health care should be considered in the initial selection of antimicrobial therapy. Initial empiric coverage for multidrug-resistant organisms may not be necessary (level 3, Grade B).

## 57.6 Should Antibiotics Be Given for a Fixed Duration or Be Tailored to Response in Patients with Acute Cholangitis?

There is no high level evidence recommending a fixed duration of antibiotic treatment as opposed to a duration tailored to response to therapy. Kogure et al. [22] studied 18 patients prospectively where cefmetazole and meropenem were used as initial antibiotic therapy for patients with moderate and severe acute cholangitis, respectively. Patients underwent endoscopic biliary drainage within 24 h of diagnosis. When patients had a body temperature of 37°C maintained for 24 h, the antibiotics were stopped. The primary endpoint was the recurrence of acute cholangitis within 3 days after the withdrawal of antibiotic therapy. The median durations of antibiotic therapy were 3 days in patients with moderate cholangitis and 3.5 days for severe cholangitis. No patient developed recurrent cholangitis. There was no difference in the antibiotic duration between the bacteremic and nonbacteremic patients. Antibiotics were discontinued after 4 days in 14 of the 18 patients. Similarly, Van Lent et al. [23] studied 80 patients who received varying durations of different antibiotic regimens before or after ERCP. Forty-one patients received antibiotic therapy for 3 days or less, 19 for 4–5 days, and 20 patients longer than 5 days. The median period of follow-up was 6 months. The proportion of patients with recurrent cholangitis (24%) was not statistically different for the three groups. Death occurred in 6 of 41 (15%) patients with ≤3 days of antibiotics versus 1 of 20 (5%) with >5 days of antibiotics but this was not statistically significant. The authors concluded that short-term antibiotics (≤3 days) was adequate provided that endoscopic drainage was successful and that clinical improvement was seen.

Current guidelines recommend a duration limited to 4–7 days for complicated intra-abdominal infections "unless it is difficult to achieve adequate source control" [19]. The level of evidence of this recommendation was III (based on expert opinion).

*Recommendation*: There is insufficient evidence to recommend a specific duration of antimicrobial therapy. Antimicrobial therapy should be used in conjunction with drainage of the obstructed biliary system. Once the source control is achieved, the duration of antibiotic therapy may be guided by clinical response (level 3, Grade B).

## 57.7 How and When Should Biliary Drainage Be Performed in Acute Cholangitis due to Common Duct Stones?

After the diagnosis of acute bacterial cholangitis is made and antibiotics are started, expeditious biliary drainage should be considered. The TG13 guidelines advocate initial antibiotic therapy only for Grade I acute cholangitis, with biliary drainage for nonresponders. For Grade II diseases, "early" drainage should be performed and for Grade III diseases, "urgent" drainage should be performed, based on a consensus of experts [24]. However, the published literature has been vague as to what "early" or "urgent" means in terms of timing of biliary drainage in hours after presentation. A retrospective study of 250 patients [25] with moderate or severe cholangitis as defined by the TG07 guidelines divided the timing of biliary drainage into quartiles (0–11, 12–21, 22–42, and >42 h) and found that the risk of mortality was significantly lower for the 0–11 h group compared to the >42 h group, and that hospital readmission was significantly less for the 0–11 h group compared to those who had drainage after 22 h. There was no difference in mortality when ERCP was done <12 h versus 22–42 h.

Naveenathan et al. [26] in another retrospective study found that for all patients with acute cholangitis who underwent ERCP, 16% had a door-to-ERCP time of >72 h and this factor was independently associated with a composite adverse outcome (persistent organ failure or mortality) (odds ratio 3.36; 95% confidence interval, 1.12–10.2) as well as length of stay >10 days. The other risk factors were an American Society of Anesthesiologists classification of >3 and the presence of systemic inflammatory response syndrome.

Khashab et al. [27] found that in 90 patients who underwent ERCP for acute cholangitis that a delay of >72 h to ERCP (in 14.4% of the patients) was associated with an adverse composite outcome (mortality, organ failure) (odds ratio 5.5).

For acute cholangitis without organ failure, a retrospective study [28] found that patients who underwent ERCP within 24 h of presentation had similar mortality rates (0% vs. 0%) but shorter length of stay (6.8 ± 2.5 vs. 9.2 ± 4.5 days) and shorter intervention to discharge time (6.1 ± 2.5 vs. 7.2 ± 4.5 days) than patients who underwent ERCP after 24 h of presentation.

While it is clear that a delay of >72 h to ERCP is associated with a poorer outcome, expeditious drainage within 12 h of presentation may be beneficial.

The optimal method of drainage was addressed by Lai et al. [29] in a randomized trial: 82 patients were randomized after urgent ERCP was done: one group received papillotomy and nasobiliary catheter drainage and the other surgical intervention (with a mean of 2 h to anesthesia). The median time to randomization was 27 h in the surgical group versus 23 h in the endoscopic group. Mortality was 13/41 in the surgery group versus 4/41 in the endoscopic group ($p$ = 0.03). Other factors such as serum albumin, creatinine, leukocyte count, platelet count, age, serum urea nitrogen, and concomitant medical problems were also significant predictive factors for mortality. In another prospective randomized study, Javid et al. [30] allocated 84 patients to endoscopic biliary drainage versus surgery after emergency ERCP. The endoscopic group had a nasobiliary drain placed with or without sphincterotomy, and no attempt was made to extract stones during the initial biliary drainage. Subsequently, 24 of 42 underwent stone extraction after the sepsis resolved and the remainder underwent surgical intervention during the same admission. All surgical arm patients underwent choledochotomy. There was a significantly lower incidence of need for ventilator support (7/42 vs. 22/42), shorter time of ventilator support (38 vs. 74 h), and lower mortality (3/42 vs. 12/42) in the endoscopic arm.

In both these randomized studies, approximately half of the patients had shock or hypotension on presentation but there was no subgroup analysis based on disease severity at presentation in either of the two studies.

*Recommendations*: Endoscopic biliary decompression is preferred over surgery (level 2, Grade B).

Patients should undergo endoscopic drainage within 72 h of presentation (level 3, Grade B). Expeditious drainage within 12 h of presentation may be beneficial (level 3, Grade C).

## 57.8 When Should Cholecystectomy Be Done after Endoscopic Clearance of Common Duct Stones in the Setting of Acute Cholangitis?

A systematic review of several randomized trials [31] studied whether elective cholecystectomy should be performed in patients with gallbladders in situ who had endoscopic clearance of common duct stones. Overall mortality in the wait-and-see group was 47 out of 334 (14%) compared to 26 out of 328 (9%) in the prophylactic cholecystectomy group for a relative risk of 1.78 (95% confidence interval 1.15–2.75). Patients in the wait-and-see group had higher rates of recurrent biliary pain (relative risk 14.56) and jaundice or cholangitis (relative risk 2.53). Cholecystectomy was eventually performed in 35% of patients in the wait-and-see group. Williams et al. [32] reached a similar conclusion in another systematic review, recommending cholecystectomy for "all patients with CBDS and 'symptomatic gallbladder stones unless there are specific reasons for considering surgery inappropriate.'" In a retrospective study focusing only on patients with acute cholangitis who underwent ERCP, the incidence of recurrent biliary complications was 25% without cholecystectomy versus 5% with cholecystectomy with a median time to follow-up of 2 years [33].

The aforementioned studies advocate cholecystectomy after endoscopic clearance of common duct stones. However, the optimal timing of cholecystectomy after an episode of acute cholangitis is not clear. The TG13 guidelines could not recommend an optimal time period to perform cholecystectomy after common duct stone clearance [34]. Schiphorst et al. [35] examined 167 patients retrospectively and found that 20% developed biliary complications. The median time until the development of recurrent biliary complaints was 22 days (range 3–225 days), and 76% of the complications occurred after 1 week after sphincterotomy. The authors hence recommended surgery within a week of clearance of common duct stones. In this study, however, only 11% had cholangitis. Li et al. [36] studied patients treated for acute cholangitis who underwent early (within 6 weeks) versus late (after 6 weeks) laparoscopic cholecystectomy after clearance of the common duct. The two groups were fairly well matched for age, gender, and ASA class. The early surgery group had significantly fewer intraoperative complications (3/32 vs. 23/80) and postoperative complications (5/32 vs. 34/80) compared to the late surgery group. In a multivariate analysis of risk factors for postoperative complications, only late surgery (odds ratio 7.1) and endoscopic sphincterotomy (odds ratio 4.3) were independent risk factors. The authors therefore recommended surgery within 6 weeks of the episode of cholangitis especially if endoscopic sphincterotomy had been done during clearance of the common duct (Table 57.3).

*Recommendations*: Cholecystectomy should generally be done after endoscopic clearance of common duct stones

**TABLE 57.3**
Evidentiary Table

| Question | Answer | Level of Evidence | Grade of Recommendation | References |
|---|---|---|---|---|
| 1. Should the initial empiric antibiotic regimen provide coverage for multidrug-resistant organisms? | Local antimicrobial susceptibilities, comorbid conditions, and association with health care should be considered in the initial selection of antimicrobial therapy. Initial empiric coverage for multidrug-resistant organisms may not be necessary. | 3 | B | [8,10,11,14–21] |
| 2. Should antibiotics be given for a fixed duration or be tailored to response in patients with acute cholangitis? | There is insufficient evidence to recommend a specific duration of antimicrobial therapy. Antimicrobial therapy should be used in conjunction with drainage of the obstructed biliary system. Once the source control is achieved, the duration of antibiotic therapy may be guided by clinical response. | 3 | B | [22,23] |
| 3. How and when should biliary drainage be performed in acute cholangitis due to common duct stones? | Endoscopic biliary drainage is preferred over surgery. | 2 | B | [29,30] |
| | Patients should undergo endoscopic drainage within 72 h of presentation. | 3 | B | [25–28] |
| | Expeditious drainage within 12 h of presentation may be beneficial. | 3 | C | [25] |
| 4. When should cholecystectomy be done after endoscopic clearance of common duct stones in the setting of acute cholangitis? | Cholecystectomy should generally be done after endoscopic clearance of common duct stones after an episode of acute cholangitis unless the surgical risk is significant. | 1 | A | [31,32] |
| | It should be performed within 6 weeks following an episode of acute cholangitis. | 3 | C | [36] |

after an episode of acute cholangitis unless the surgical risk is significant (level 1, Grade A). It should be performed within 6 weeks following an episode of acute cholangitis (level 3, Grade C).

## References


1. McNabb-Baltar J, Trinh QD, Barkun AN. Biliary drainage method and temporal trends in patients admitted with cholangitis: A national audit. *Can J Gastroenterol.* 2013;27:513–518.
2. Huang T, Bass JA, Williams RD. The significance of biliary pressure in cholangitis. *Arch Surg.* 1969;98:629–632.
3. Sheen-Chen SM, Chau P, Harris HW. Obstructive jaundice alters Kupffer cell function independent of bacterial translocation. *J Surg Res.* 1998;80:205–209.
4. Diamond T, Dolan S, Thompson RL, Rowlands BJ. Development and reversal of endotoxemia and endotoxin-related death in obstructive jaundice. *Surg.* 1990; 108:370–374.
5. Wada K, Takadu T, Kawarada K et al. Diagnostic criteria and severity assessment of acute cholangitis: Tokyo guidelines. *J Hepatobiliary Pancreat Surg.* 2007;14:52–58.
6. Kiriyama S, Takada T, Strasberg SM et al. New diagnostic criteria and severity assessment of acute cholangitis in revised Tokyo guidelines. *J Hepatobiliary Pancreat Sci.* 2012;19:548–556.
7. Sun G, Han L, Yang Y et al. Comparison of two editions of Tokyo guidelines for the management of acute cholangitis. *J Hepatobiliary Pancreat Sci.* 2012;19:548–556.
8. Lee JK, Park CW, Lee SH et al. Updates in bacteriological epidemiology of community-acquired severe acute cholangitis and the effectiveness of metronidazole added routinely to the first-line antimicrobial regimen. *J Infect Chemother.* 2013;19:1029–1034.
9. Weber A, Huber W, Kamereck K et al. In vitro activity of moxifloxacin and piperacillin/sulbactam against pathogens of acute cholangitis. *World J Gastroenterol.* 2008;14:3174–3178.
10. Ortega M, Marco F, Soriano A et al. Epidemiology and prognostic determinants of bacteraemic biliary tract infection. *J Antimicrob Chemother.* 2012;67:1508–1513.
11. Sung YK, Lee JK, Lee KH et al. The clinical epidemiology and outcomes of bacteremic biliary tract infections caused by antimicrobial-resistant pathogens. *Am J Gastroenterol.* 2012;107:473–483.
12. Lee CC, Chang IJ, Lai YC et al. Epidemiology and prognostic determinants of patients with bacteremic cholecystitis or cholangitis. *Am J Gastroenterol.* 2007;102:563–569.
13. Weber A, Schneider J, Wagenpfeil S et al. Spectrum of pathogens in acute cholangitis in patients with and without biliary endoprosthesis. *J Infect.* 2013;67:111–121.
14. Melzer M, Toner R, Lacey S et al. Biliary tract infection and bacteraemia: Presentation, structural abnormalities, causative organisms and clinical outcomes. *Postgrad Med J.* 2007;83:773–776.
15. Kim HJ, Park JH, Park DI et al. Clinical impact of extended-spectrum β-lactamase-producing Enterobacteriaceae in patients with biliary tract infection. *Dig Dis Sci.* 2013;58:841–849.
16. Kang CI, Kim SH, Park WB et al. Bloodstream infections due to extended-spectrum β-lactamase-producing *Escherichia coli* and *Klebsiella pneumoniae*: Risk factors for mortality and treatment outcome, with special emphasis on antimicrobial therapy. *Antimicrob Agents Chemother.* 2004;48:4574–4581.
17. Frakking FNJ, Rottier WC, Dorigo-Zetsma JW et al. Appropriateness of empirical treatment and outcome in bacteremia caused by extended-spectrum β-lactamase-producing bacteria. *Antimicrob Agents Chemother.* 2013;57:3092–3099.
18. Tumbarello M, Sanguinetti M, Montuori E et al. Predictors of mortality in patients with bloodstream infections caused by extended-spectrum β-lactamase-producing Enterobacteriaceae: Importance of inadequate initial antimicrobial treatment. *Antimicrob Agents Chemother.* 2007;51:1987–1994.
19. Solomkin JS, Mazuski JE, Bradley JS et al. Diagnosis and management of complicated intra-abdominal infection in adults and children: Guidelines by the Surgical Infection Society and the Infectious Diseases Society of America. *Clin Infect Dis.* 2010;50:133–164.
20. An MM, Zou Z, Shen H et al. Ertapenem versus piperacillin/tazobactam for the treatment of complicated infections: A meta-analysis of randomized controlled trials. *BMC Infect Dis.* 2009;9:193.
21. Swenson BR, Metzger R, Hedrick TL et al. Choosing antibiotics for intra-abdominal infections: What do we mean by "high risk"? *Surg Infect.* 2009;10:29–39.
22. Kogure H, Tsujino T, Yamamoto K et al. Fever-based antibiotic therapy for acute cholangitis following successful endoscopic biliary drainage. *J Gastroenterol.* 2011;46:1411–1417.
23. Van Lent A, Bartelsman J, Tytgat G et al. Duration of antibiotic therapy for acute cholangitis after successful endoscopic drainage of the biliary tract. *Gastrointest Endosc.* 2002;55:518–522.
24. Miura F, Takada T, Strasberg SM et al. TG13 flowchart for the management of acute cholangitis and cholecystitis. *J Hepatobiliary Pancreat Sci.* 2013;20:47–54.
25. Mok SRS, Mannino CL, Malin J et al. Does the urgency of endoscopic retrograde cholangiopancreatography (ercp)/percutaneous biliary drainage (pbd) impact mortality and disease related complications in ascending cholangitis? (deim-i study). *J Interv Gastroenterol.* 2012;2(4):161–167.
26. Navaneethan U, Gutierrez NG, Jegadeesan R et al. Factors predicting adverse short-term outcomes in patients with acute cholangitis undergoing ERCP: A single center experience. *World J Gastrointest Endosc.* 2014;6(3):74–81.
27. Khashab MA, Tariq A, Tariq U et al. Delayed and unsuccessful endoscopic retrograde cholangiopancreatography are associated with worse outcomes in patients with acute cholangitis. *Clin Gastroenterol Hepatol.* 2012;10:1157–1161.

28. Jang SE, Park SW, Lee BS et al. Management for CBD stone-related mild to moderate acute cholangitis: Urgent versus elective ERCP. *Dig Dis Sci*. 2013;58:2082–2087.
29. Lai ES, Mok FPT, Tan ESY et al. Endoscopic biliary drainage for severe acute cholangitis. *N Engl J Med.* 1992;326:1582–1586.
30. Javid G, Zarger SA, Khateeb S et al. Surgery vs endoscopic biliary drainage for acute obstructive suppurative cholangitis due to cholelithiasis—A randomized trial. *J Dig Endosc.* 2009;1:6–11.
31. McAlister VC, Davenport E, Renouf E. Cholecystectomy deferral in patients with endoscopic sphincterotomy. *Cochrane Database Syst Rev.* 2007;4:CD006233.
32. Williams EJ, Green J, Beckingham I et al. Guidelines on the management of common bile duct stones (CBDS). *Gut*. 2008;57:1004–1021.
33. Poon RT, Liu CL, Lo CM et al. Management of gallstone cholangitis in the era of laparoscopic cholecystectomy. *Arch Surg.* 2001;136:11–16.
34. Yamashita Y, Takada T, Strasberg SM et al. TG13 surgical management of acute cholecystitis. *J Hepatobiliary Pancreat Sci.* 2013;20:89–96.
35. Schiphorst AH, Besselink MG, Boerma D et al. Timing of cholecystectomy after endoscopic sphincterotomy for common bile duct stones. *Surg Endosc.* 2008;22:2046–2050.
36. Li VK, Yum JL, Yeung YP. Optimal timing of elective laparoscopic cholecystectomy after acute cholangitis and subsequent clearance of choledocholithiasis. *Am J Surg.* 2010;200:483–488.

## Commentary on Acute Cholangitis

*Hemn Qader and David K. Imagawa*

The chapter by Ong outlines the role of empiric antibiotic and biliary drainage in the management of acute cholangitis (AC). The discussion includes (1) initial empiric antibiotic coverage for multidrug resistant organisms, (2) the duration of antibiotic therapy, (3) the timing of biliary drainage in AC secondary to choledocholithiasis, and (4) when should cholecystectomy be done after clearance of common bile duct stones in the setting of AC?

So what does a surgeon really need to know about AC?

### What Is AC and the Mechanism Leading to It

AC is the clinical condition of a bacterial infection that is superimposed on bile duct obstruction. In most cases, it is associated with choledocholithiasis. Cholangitis results from bile that has been obstructed, hence leading to increased intraductal pressure. This inevitably leads to cholangiolymphatic and cholangiovenous reflux. This will accelerate the spread of bacteria through the bloodstream and lymphatic tissues. Although bile is usually sterile, obstruction of the common bile duct reduces the flow of bile, increasing the chances of bacterial growth[*†‡]. More than one bacterial organism may be involved: *Klebsiella* species, *Streptococci*, and *Escherichia coli*, among others. Biliary procedures may lead to increase the risk of infections with *Pseudomonas* and anaerobes[‡].

### Other Causes of AC

Although the most common cause of AC is gallstones and choledocholithiasis, there are other factors including the following.

### Oriental Cholangiohepatitis (Recurrent Pyogenic Cholangiohepatitis)

This is a condition mostly found in southeast Asia and it is caused by hepatobiliary parasitic infestation (e.g., *Clonorchis sinensis*, *Ascaris lumbricoides*, and *Opisthorchis viverrini*). It is associated with intrahepatic brown pigment stone formation. The condition leads to obstructive jaundice with proximal stasis, intrahepatic ductal inflammation, and cholangitis. Associated with rural areas and poverty, the incidence is decreasing in southeast Asia, but increasing in the immigrant population of the United States[§].

### Primary Sclerosing Cholangitis (PSC)

This disorder of the bile duct is believed to be of autoimmune origin leading to inflammation and fibrosis of the intrahepatic and extrahepatic bile ducts. This may subsequently result in ascending cholangitis, cirrhosis, and liver cancer. Liver transplantation is definitive treatment in some patients.

### Autoimmune Cholangitis (AIC)

This condition is differentiated from PSC by its relation to IgG4-related disease. Autoimmune pancreatitis (IgG4 related) may often present with autoimmune cholangitis. Although it may be hard to differentiate between AIC and PSC, the following are characteristic features of AIC:

1. Biopsies using endoscopic retrograde cholangiopancreatography (ERCP) will demonstrate IgG4 plasma cells' infiltration and interstitial fibrosis.
2. Increase in serum levels of IgG4.
3. Involvement of extrabiliary organs especially autoimmune pancreatitis.
4. Disease response to glucocorticoid treatments[¶**].

### Tumors

Mechanical obstruction through internal or external compression (e.g., pancreatic cancer, cholangiocarcinoma, ampullary cancer, porta hepatitis tumors, or metastasis) may lead to obstruction of the bile duct and subsequent risk of cholangitis.

* Kimura Y, Takada T, Kawarada Y et al. Definitions, pathophysiology, and epidemiology of acute cholangitis and cholecystitis: Tokyo guidelines. *J Hepatobiliary Pancreat Surg.* 2007;14:15–26.

† Scott M and Brenner E. Acute cholangitis. Emedicine. Medscape. 2014. http://emedicine.medscape.com/article/774245-overview.

‡ Yusoff F, Bakun S, Barkun N. Diagnosis and management of acute cholecystitis and acute cholangitis. *Gastroenterol Clin North Am.* 2003;32:1145–1168.

§ Parry FQ, Wani A, Wani NA. Oriental cholangitis—Is our surgery appropriate? Int J Surg. 2014;12:789–793.

¶ Smit W, Barnes E. The emerging mysteries of IgG4-related disease. *Clin Med J.* 2014;14(6):S56–S60.

** Ghazale A, Chari ST, Zhang L et al. Immunoglobulin G4-associated cholangitis: Clinical profile and response to therapy. *Gastroenterology.* 2008;134:706–715.

### Other Benign Strictures

Most patients with benign biliary stricture remain asymptomatic until narrowing causes resistance to bile flow. The most common cause of benign stricture is iatrogenic due to injury of bile duct during cholecystectomy. Other even less common causes included anastomotic stricture following orthrotopic liver transplantation, Lemmel syndrome, Mirizzi syndrome, radiation, blunt abdominal trauma, and chemotherapeutic drugs.

### AIDS-Related Cholangiopathy

It is a condition characterized by biliary obstruction due to opportunistic infections in AIDS patients. The most common infections are *Cryptosporidium parvum*, cytomegalovirus, and microsporidia[*].

### Clinical Presentation and Diagnosis of AC

Patients may present with classic Charcot's triad of fever, right upper quadrant pain, and jaundice. In Reynold's pentad, confusion and hypotension are also present. However, the more recent Tokyo guidelines have attempted to provide more objective analysis[†‡]. Laboratory analysis will often show an increase in white blood cell count, elevated bilirubin, moderate elevated transaminase, elevated alkaline phosphatase, and elevated amylase. Right upper quadrant ultrasound should be performed to assess for cholelithiasis, gallbladder wall thickness as well as pericholecystic fluid. However, ultrasound has a low sensitivity to detect common bile duct (CBD) stones[§]. CT scan and magnetic resonance cholangiopancreatography (MRCP) are sensitive and give additional information about the anatomy of the bile duct[**]. ERCP is both a diagnostic and therapeutic tool for AC. It helps to identify the underlying cause as well as relieving the biliary compression[**].

### Initial Management of AC

The mortality of AC has reduced drastically due to advanced technology and better treatment methods[¶]. The treatment of AC is based upon two major factors of the disease: biliary obstruction and infection. Initial therapy may involve correction of body fluid and electrolyte deficits and empirical intravenous antibiotic therapy. There is no question that early institution of antibiotics should be part of initial treatment. Routine blood cultures may not be useful, as only a minority are positive[**]. Infectious disease guidelines do not recommend empiric coverage for *Enterococcus* and *Pseudomonas*[††‡‡]. Whether initial coverage for extended spectrum beta-lactamase stain should be utilized is less well defined[§§]. The choice of antibiotics needs to be individualized, based on the clinical situation and the known pathogens specific to the individual hospital.

### Approaches for Biliary Drainage

These approaches include percutaneous transhepatic biliary drainage (PTHC) by interventional radiology, endoscopic biliary drainage by gastroenterology as well as surgical biliary drainage. Surgical biliary drainage has a very high motility and morbidity rate as compared to other procedures; therefore, it is seldom utilized as first-line therapy. However, the surgeon still needs to know how to perform a laparoscopic or open bile duct exploration. Endoscopic biliary drainage is the preferred initial option, since it is characterized with shorter periods of hospitalizations, 90%–98% of success rate, and lower morbidity and mortality rates[¶¶***].

---

* Ali, A. Choledocholithiasis and cholangitis. Merck Manuals. 2013. http://www.merckmanuals.com/professional/hepatic_and_biliary_disorders/gallbladder_and_bile_duct_disorders/choledocholithiasis_and_cholangitis.html.

† Kiriyama S, Takada T, Strasberg SM et al. New diagnostic criteria and severity assessment of acute cholangitis in revised Tokyo guidelines. *J Hepatobiliary Pancreat Sci.* 2012;19:548–556.

‡ Sun G, Han L, Yang Y et al. Comparison of two editions of Tokyo guidelines for the management of acute cholangitis. *J Hepatobiliary Pancreat Sci.* 2012;19:548–556.

§ Yusoff F, Bakun S, Barkun N. Diagnosis and management of acute cholecystitis and acute cholangitis. *Gastroenterol Clin North Am.* 2003;32:1145–1168.

¶ Scott M and Brenner E. Acute cholangitis. Emedicine. Medscape. 2014. http://emedicine.medscape.com/article/774245-overview.

** Lee JK, Park CW, Lee SH et al. Updates in bacteriological epidemiology of community-acquired severe acute cholangitis and the effectiveness of metronidazole added routinely to the first-line antimicrobial regimen. *J Infect Chemother.* 2013;19:1029–1034.

†† Solomkin JS, Mazuski JE, Bradley JS et al. Diagnosis and management of complicated intra-abdominal infection in adults and children: Guidelines by the Surgical Infection Society and the Infectious Diseases Society of America. *Clin Infect Dis.* 2010;50:133–164.

‡‡ An MM, Zou Z, Shen H et al. Ertapenem versus piperacillin/tazobactam for the treatment of complicated infections: A meta-analysis of randomized controlled trials. *BMC Infect Dis.* 2009;9:193.

§§ Kang CI, Kim SH, Park WB et al. Bloodstream infections due to extended-spectrum β-lactamase-producing *Escherichia coli* and *Klebsiella pneumoniae*: Risk factors for mortality and treatment outcome, with special emphasis on antimicrobial therapy. *Antimicrob Agents Chemother.* 2004;48:4574–4581.

¶¶ Lai ES, Mok FPT, Tan ESY et al. Endoscopic biliary drainage for severe acute cholangitis. *New Engl J Med.* 1992;326:1582–1586.

*** Javid G, Zarger SA, Khateeb S et al. Surgery vs endoscopic biliary drainage for acute obtructive suppurative cholangitis due to cholelithiasis—A randomized trial. *J Dig Endosc.* 2009;1:6–11.

Complications may include perforation, stone impaction, bleeding, and pancreatitis. On other hand, PTHC may be preferable in conditions such as intrasegmental cholangitis and hepatolithiasis. Studies have shown that poor outcomes occur if ERCP is delayed over 72 h; best outcomes may occur if ERCP is performed within 12 h of presentation[*,†].

### Management of the Gallbladder and the Timing of Laparoscopic Cholecystectomy (LC) after Bile Duct Clearance in Patients with AC from Stones

It is recommended that patients with AC undergo cholecystectomy to avoid recurrence. Recent studies advocate for elective LC within 6 weeks after AC especially in patients who have undergone endoscopic sphincterotomy. The goal of early LC is to decrease the incidence of recurrent biliary complications, but caution should be considered, because the inflammation around the biliary tract may still be problematic. Conversion to an open cholecystectomy is mandatory if the anatomy cannot be definitively identified[‡].

### Management of AC in Patients with Previous History of Roux-en-Y Gastric Bypass by Doing "Laparoscopic Assisted ERCP"

A more problematic situation occurs when cholangitis occurs in a patient who has undergone a previous Roux-en-Y gastric bypass. The altered anatomy makes traditional ERCP extremely difficult, since the endoscope would need to be passed through the entire Roux limb and through the jejunojejunostomy to reach the common bile duct. Some centers have advocated the use of "laparoscopic-assisted ERCP": laparoscopic placement of a trocar into the gastric remnant followed by ERCP through the trocar[§]. However, this is typically a "one-shot" opportunity, since the gastric access is removed at the completion of surgery. We therefore recommend placement of a percutaneous transhepatic tube (PTHC) by interventional radiology in these patients. This allows for a more long-term biliary access in these patients[¶].

### Conclusion

AC is a condition that requires prompt attention with a multidisciplinary approach. Stabilization of the septic patients includes fluid resuscitation, intravenous antibiotics, and relieving the biliary obstruction. Surgical intervention is usually reserved for elective removal of the gallbladder within 6 weeks.

* Navaneethan U, Gutierrez NG, Jegadeesan R et al. Factors predicting adverse short-term outcomes in patients with acute cholangitis undergoing ERCP: A single center experience. *World J Gastrointest Endosc*. 2014;16:74–81.

† Khashab MA, Tariq A, Tariq U et al. Delayed and unsuccessful endoscopic retrograde cholangiopancreatography are associated with worse outcomes in patients with acute cholangitis. *Clin Gastroenterol Hepatol*. 2012;10:1157–1161.

‡ Li VK, Yum JL, Yeung YP. Optimal timing of elective laparoscopic cholecystectomy after acute cholangitis and subsequent clearance of choledocholithiasis. *Am J Surg*. 2010;200:483–488.

§ Samarasena JB, Nguyen NT, Lee JG. Endoscopic retrograde cholangiopancreatography in patients with roux-en-Y anatomy. *J Intervent Gastroenterol*. 2012;2:78–83.

¶ Sato KT. Percutanous management of biliary emergencies. *Semin Intervent Radiol*. 2006;23:249–257.

# 58

# Acute Pancreatitis

**Stephen W. Behrman**

**CONTENTS**



Acute pancreatitis (AP) is responsible for approximately one-quarter of a million hospital admissions in the United States annually [1]. While most cases are self-limiting, about 10%–20% of patients develop severe inflammation of the pancreas requiring intensive diagnostic and therapeutic intervention. While the basic algorithms for treatment of AP have not changed, new concepts in patient care have been proposed that represent, in many instances, a significant deviation from traditional management schemes. These evolving paradigm shifts in the treatment of those with AP represent an opportunity to enhance outcome by reducing infection-related morbidity while delivering care in a more cost-effective manner and with a reduction in hospital length of stay (LOS) (Table 58.1).

## 58.1 What is the Role (if Any) of Magnetic Resonance Cholangiopancreatography (MRCP) in Suspected Choledocholithiasis in Those with Acute Biliary Pancreatitis?

MRCP is a noninvasive technique that is more sensitive than ultrasound and CT scan as a modality to diagnose choledocholithiasis [2]. This advantage, however, is encumbered by higher financial costs and a potential delay in therapeutic intervention. Furthermore, the role of MRCP as a "screening" tool to identify candidates for preoperative endoscopic retrograde cholangiopancreatography (ERCP) has not been well defined. Finally, with respect to acute biliary pancreatitis (ABP), the need for MRCP or any other diagnostic testing in the absence of cholestasis has not been well delineated that is important since the vast majority of stones will pass spontaneously in this cohort. Given the high cost of this diagnostic test, it would be important that it be utilized only if there is a reasonable risk of choledocholithiasis and if it can be proven to have acceptable sensitivity and specificity. If so, it could prove to be advantageous toward reducing the need for ERCP with its inherent risks of bleeding, perforation, and pancreatitis.

Prediction of choledocholithiasis based on routine preoperative laboratory analysis and ultrasonography would be a first step toward deciding the need for further noninvasive and invasive diagnostic testing in ABP. Makary et al. [2] reported on 64 consecutive patients admitted with a presumed diagnosis of mild to moderate ABP that had routine performance of MRCP. A diagnosis of ABP was made based on a presentation of acute epigastric pain with a serum amylase twice the upper limit of normal. Only 48 had ultrasound and 36 CT imaging during the course of hospitalization, an unusual sequence of radiologic examinations. The time interval from presentation to MRCP was not reported. However, if choledocholithiasis was recognized, there was an orderly progression to ERCP and surgery at a median of 2 and 3 days, respectively. Seventeen patients had documented common bile duct (CBD) stones. MRCP resulted in one false-positive and one false-negative examination. Only *admission* liver chemistries were assessed relative to the final diagnosis of CBD stones. Any trend in laboratory data was not reported. Similarly, the combination of an abnormal liver profile with ultrasound diagnosed biliary dilation (>8 mm) as a means to predict choledocholithiasis by MRCP was not analyzed. The authors recommend that MRCP should be utilized as the initial imaging modality in those presenting with suspected ABP. However, their screening definition of gallstone pancreatitis would undoubtedly lead to overutilization at a great cost.

Barlow et al. [3] analyzed 173 patients admitted with ABP (diagnosed as amylase >300 U/L) that received an MRCP at a median of 4 days following admission. Unfortunately, this was *not* a consecutive series as all patients presenting with ABP ($n$ = 265) that *did not* receive an MRCP were *not* included. The presence of choledocholithiasis was correlated with liver chemistries and ultrasound. Biliary dilation was defined as a CBD ≥8 mm. Approximately two-thirds of the study population had increased liver chemistries and 25% had biliary dilation on ultrasound interrogation. CBD stones were noted on MRCP in 52 (30%) but stones were not confirmed by ERCP or at the time of surgery in at least eight patients. Furthermore, the timing of MRCP following admission relative to when it demonstrated choledocholithiasis was not reported. This study noted a poor sensitivity and specificity of increased liver chemistries and bile duct dilation to identify patients likely to have CBD stones. The authors conclude that neither biliary dilation nor abnormal liver chemistries predict CBD stones with enough sensitivity or specificity to allow selective use of MRCP and they support its routine use in all patients presenting with ABP. Given the limitations of this study as noted earlier this conclusion is certainly open to interpretation.

Mofidi et al. [4] retrospectively reviewed the clinical course of 249 patients admitted with ABP (diagnosis not defined) before and after the introduction of MRCP at their institution. Ninety-six patients with a nondilated CBD (<10 mm) and normal or resolving liver function tests within 48 h went directly to cholecystectomy (CCY) with IOC. Eight of ninety-six had CBD stones—the timing of cholangiography in this cohort was not reported. Preoperative diagnostic testing was utilized for nonresolving cholestasis or evidence of a dilated CBD by ultrasound examination in 106 patients. MRCP ($n$ = 49) was used to identify candidates for ERCP after its introduction. The incidence of choledocholithiasis in upfront ERCP versus MRCP was 17.5% and 14.2% respectively ($p$ = NS). Three of fifty-seven patients having ERCP suffered procedure-related complications. Those having MRCP had a significantly shorter LOS and the sensitivity and specificity of MRCP for CBD stones was 100% and 96%, respectively. The authors conclude that MRCP should be used selectively, preferential to ERCP, in those with clinical suggestion of retained CBD stones.

Liu et al. [5] assessed 440 patients eligible for laparoscopic cholecystectomy and analyzed results of a selective approach toward upfront ERCP and the need for preoperative MRCP based on risk stratification developed utilizing clinical presentation along with preoperative chemistry and ultrasound criteria. Patients ($n$ = 27) with a CBD >5 mm and elevated liver function tests in the absence of acute cholecystitis or ABP were triaged to upfront ERCP—93% of whom had choledocholithiasis. Patients ($n$ = 37) with similar criteria but *also* with either acute cholecystitis or pancreatitis had screening MRCP and if positive, underwent preoperative ERCP. Thirty-two percent had CBD stones and there was excellent correlation between MRCP and ERCP. Twenty-six patients in this group that had a negative MRC had intraoperative cholangiography only one of whom had a CBD stone. A third group ($n$ = 52) with cholecystitis or pancreatitis, a CBD <5 mm, and elevated liver function tests had upfront laparoscopic CCY with attempted cholangiography that was completed in 48 patients. Two (3.8%) had choledocholithiasis. The last group ($n$ = 324) had biliary colic or cholecystitis but not pancreatitis, a CBD <5 mm, and normal liver chemistries. Cholangiography was utilized in <1% and only three (0.9%) were found to have CBD stones on follow-up evaluation. This study suggests that MRCP can be avoided in those without pancreatitis or cholecystitis but with radiographic and chemical aberrations suggesting choledocholithiasis allowing more a more efficient progression to early ERCP. MRCP can be helpful in predicting CBD stones in those with cholecystitis and pancreatitis with hard signs by ultrasound and chemistries but can be avoided in those with discordant radiographic and laboratory studies.

In conclusion, there are contradictory findings in the literature regarding the use of MRCP in gallstone pancreatitis. Studies promoting its routine use have failed to report the critical timing of the procedure as MRCP delayed beyond the first 48 h may be more suggestive of choledocholithiasis whereas those performed earlier in the patient's clinical course might identify stones that may pass spontaneously. A selective approach that combines abnormal liver function tests and screening ultrasound criteria along with disease diagnosis seems prudent to identify a population appropriate for MRCP. When utilized under these circumstances, MRCP eliminates the need for invasive preoperative ERCP or the need for intraoperative IOC in two-thirds to three-fourths of patients studied while allowing an orderly progression to cholecystectomy. In the absence of serologic or radiographic abnormalities beyond the initial 24–48 h of presentation, MRCP and its cost can most often be avoided (Grade B recommendation).

## 58.2 What is the Role of Early Endoscopic Retrograde Cholangiopancreatography (ERCP) in Acute Biliary Pancreatitis?

The need for, and timing of ERCP in biliary pancreatitis has been a controversial subject in both the gastroenterology and surgical literature. The vast majority of stones will pass spontaneously into the duodenum and thus will neither aggravate the ensuing pancreatitis nor present a risk for the development of concurrent cholangitis. Indeed, early ERCP may exacerbate pancreatitis. However, the development of cholangitis in the face of severe acute pancreatitis (SAP) would most certainly contribute substantially to morbidity and mortality favoring early endoscopic evaluation. Perhaps more controversial is the role of early ERCP in ameliorating the degree of pancreatitis and the ensuing inflammatory cascade. Several randomized controlled studies and meta-analyses have addressed these issues.

In an early study, Neoptolemos et al. [6] prospectively randomized 121 patients with presumed biliary pancreatitis to early (<72 h from admission) ERCP with sphincterotomy and stone extraction if necessary versus conservative management alone with selective ERCP "if it was indicated." The severity of pancreatitis was assessed via the modified Glasgow criteria with severe disease defined as a score of three or higher [7]. Interpretation of the data in this study is somewhat clouded by the fact that gallstones could not be confirmed in 18 patients despite the availability of ultrasound and computed tomography. With this limitation in mind, early ERCP was successful in 52 of 59 (88%) patients and choledocholithiasis was confirmed in 19 (32%) (versus 3 of 14 [21%] in the conservative group) and successful stone extraction was accomplished in all. Early ERCP was associated with a statistically significant decrease in disease-related complications (pseudocyst, organ failure) and a reduction (not significant) in mortality in those with severe, but not mild, pancreatitis.

Fan et al. [8] studied the role of ERCP in AP of all causes (predominantly biliary in this oriental population) in a prospective randomized trial of 197 patients in an early study. The purpose of this study was to compare the efficacy of early (<24 h) ERCP with papillotomy if stones were identified versus initial conservative treatment with ERCP ± papillotomy reserved for those with clinical deterioration. Indications of clinical deterioration included rising fever, tachycardia, worsening leukocytosis, and/or an increase in bilirubin. Outcome was assessed on the basis of local and systemic complications as well as death. Severe pancreatitis was defined as a Ranson score of four or more. Impacted stones were found in 37 of 97 (38%) patients having early ERCP. In contrast, 27 of 98 patients initially followed conservatively required ERCP for deterioration, with stones found in the CBD or ampulla in only 12 (12%) confirming that the vast majority of stones pass spontaneously. Complications were higher in those with initial conservative treatment (29% versus 18%) but this difference was not significant ($p = 0.07$). With the exception of those developing cholangitis in the conservative group (eight versus zero patients), other complications did not differ dramatically. Mortality was higher in those treated conservatively (nine versus five patients) but did not reach statistical significance. All deaths occurred in those with severe pancreatitis—the vast majority of who had no stone found on endoscopic evaluation. Early ERCP did not seem to either worsen or improve the progression of pancreatitis. The authors, surprisingly, conclude that emergency ERCP is indicated in all patients with AP although their data seem to suggest otherwise.

Folsch et al. [9] conducted a prospective, randomized, multicenter study comparing early ERCP (<72 h) versus conservative management in those ABP *without* evidence of obstructive jaundice. Disease severity was measured by the modified Glasgow criteria (>3 severe). Indications for ERCP in the conservatively managed group were similar to those described by Fan et al. [8]. Out of 126 patients undergoing early ERCP, 58 had documented bile duct stones versus 13 of 112 in the conservative group. Of note, 22 of 112 patients in the conservatively managed group developed indications for ERCP and the incidence of choledocholithiasis in this group was 60%. Overall, morbidity and mortality did not differ between groups including the risk of developing pancreatic-related complications such as pseudocyst and necrosis. The authors conclude that early ERCP is not indicated in those with acute biliary pancreatitis in the absence of clinical evidence of biliary obstruction or sepsis.

In a more recent study, Oria et al. [10] examined the role of early (<48–72 h) ERCP in those presenting with acute gallstone pancreatitis *and* evidence of biliopancreatic obstruction defined as a CBD >8 mm or serum bilirubin >1.2 mg/dL. Importantly, patients with clinical evidence of cholangitis (Charcot's triad) were excluded as this condition was felt to mandate early ERCP in this randomized, prospective study. Severe pancreatitis was defined as an APACHE-II score >6. The specific aims of this study were to determine if early ERCP could reduce the severity of pancreatitis and thereby limit organ failure and complications of pancreatitis. The safety of early endoscopy was also assessed. Of 103 patients, 51 were randomized to early ERCP with choledocholithiasis noted on 47 (72%) successful cannulations with minimal complications. When comparing the two groups, early clearance of the common duct did not reduce organ failure, local complications of the pancreas, or mortality in either mild or severe pancreatitis. The authors concluded that early ERCP did not alter the course of acute gallstone pancreatitis and was not indicated in the absence of cholangitis.

In a prospective *observational* multicenter study from the Netherlands, the role of early ERCP in predicted severe ABP was examined in 153 patients [11]. Those with cholangitis were excluded but those with cholestasis or radiographic suggestion of choledocholithiasis ($n = 78$) were not. Severe pancreatitis was defined as an APACHE-II score ≥8, or Imrie score ≥3 or a C-reactive protein >150 mg/dL within 72 h of admission. A similar time frame defined "early" ERCP that was performed at the discretion of the treating physician. Early ERCP was successful in 70/91 patients in whom it was attempted and stones were found in 41 (29/52 in those with cholestasis). Overall complications (but not mortality) were reduced in those patients with cholestasis that received early ERCP ($n = 52$) primarily by a reduction in the extent of pancreatic necrosis. However, the incidence of multiorgan failure and/or the need for pancreas-related therapeutic intervention was not different between treatment groups. Those without cholestasis did not derive the same benefit from early ERCP ($n = 29$). The authors concluded that early ERCP did not alter the course of acute gallstone pancreatitis and was not indicated in the absence of cholangitis.

Three recent meta-analyses have yielded the same conclusions while recognizing the heterogeneity of patient populations, enrollment criteria, the arbitrary assignment of mild and severe pancreatitis, and the definition of "early" ERCP [12–14].

In conclusion, ERCP has proven to be safe when performed in the face of ABP. If performed early, the incidence of choledocholithiasis is substantially higher than if ERCP is performed selectively when there is evidence of persistent biliary obstruction based on routine radiologic and chemical analysis. However, in the studies to date, early clearance of the CBD has not correlated with a reduction in organ failure, pancreas-related complications, or mortality. For these reasons, in the absence of cholangitis or radiographic or laboratory evidence of biliary obstruction, early ERCP in gallstone pancreatitis is not recommended (Grade A recommendation).

## 58.3 Should Patients have Early or Delayed Cholecystectomy Following Acute Biliary Pancreatitis?

Acute biliary pancreatitis (ABP) is the most common etiology of AP worldwide and can vary from a mild self-limited disease to severe pancreatitis that may lead to pancreatic necrosis and death [15]. Within this spectrum includes patients that may require prolonged hospitalization and/or are at risk for delayed pancreatic pathology such as pseudocyst formation. Practically, it would be advantageous to perform cholecystectomy early and with minimally invasive techniques if anticipation of AP complications is limited *and* if the inflammatory response is minimized to the extent that one could predict a successful laparoscopic approach. Further, it would be helpful to avoid the need for more than one surgical intervention—i.e., performing gallbladder surgery when it might be anticipated that future surgery for pancreas-related disease would be necessary. Determining optimal timing of cholecystectomy in order to prevent disease recurrence is therefore not clear-cut. What is clear, however, is that prolonged delay in cholecystectomy is associated with a significant recidivism rate for not only gallstone-related diseases but also recurrent pancreatitis. Burch et al. compared outcomes of patients with similar degrees of pancreatitis that had CCY during their index admission for ABP versus those discharged and scheduled for elective surgery [16]. Morbidity and mortality was similar between these two groups. However, 29 of the 65 (44%) patients followed after discharge represented with either recurrent pancreatitis or biliary tract disease prior to definitive CCY—most within 3 months. Cameron and Goodman [17] noted a 25% incidence of hospital readmission when CCY was delayed beyond 4 weeks versus 6% when surgery occurred within that period following presentation for biliary pancreatitis. Complications resulting in readmission included cholecystitis, biliary colic, and recurrent pancreatitis. Similar outcomes have been reported by others and endoscopic sphincterotomy has not been found to be protective in terms of eliminating gallstone related complications if CCY is delayed [15,18].

Studies have examined the results of early versus delayed CCY most often in those mild to moderate pancreatitis. Rosing et al. [19] evaluated the impact of delayed versus early-lap CCY in those with mild to moderate AP defined as three or fewer Ranson criteria in a study comparing a retrospective review ($n = 177$) with a prospectively accumulated policy of mandated CCY within 48 h of admission ($n = 43$). A similar proportion of patients underwent ERCP in both treatment arms. There was only one conversion to open CCY that occurred in the early group. Length of stay (LOS) was significantly longer in the retrospective group (7 vs. 4 days) but there was no difference in morbidity and no mortality. A follow-up retrospective study by the same authors sought to confirm their original conclusion by combining data with a second university-affiliated urban medical center with a similar number of accrued patients during a 5-year period [20]. Exclusion criteria included >3 Ranson criteria, cholangitis, or high suspicion of a retained CBD stone. Approximately 40%

(117/303) of patients had early CCY and groups were well matched. CCY was accomplished laparoscopically in all with no procedure-related mortality. Median LOS was significantly decreased in the early cohort (3 vs. 6 days). Morbidity and readmission rates did not differ between treatment groups. The need for postoperative ERCP was equivalent (~10%).

A randomized prospective trial from yet this same institution was subsequently performed with mild pancreatitis defined similarly [21]. Forty-nine well-matched patients were randomized to laparoscopic CCY within 48 h ($n$ = 25) of admission or a delayed procedure until clinical and laboratory evidence of pancreatitis had resolved. Exclusion criteria were similar to their prior study. Patients in the delayed group had surgery performed at a mean of 77.8 vs. 35.1 h in those having early surgery. Laparoscopic CCY was successfully completed in all and there was no difference in the number requiring postoperative ERCP. LOS was significantly reduced in those with early surgery (median 3 vs. 4 days) and no procedure-related morbidity occurred in either group. The need for postoperative ERCP was equivalent and there were no readmissions in either study arm. Two meta-analyses have supported the role of early CCY in those with mild biliary pancreatitis at the index admission [22,23].

In contradistinction to those presenting with mild disease, patients with severe ABP are not uncommonly hemodynamically unstable, may develop multiple organ failure and are at risk for necrotizing pancreatitis or pseudocyst formation. Surgeons have been reluctant to proceed with early CCY under these circumstances due to patient instability, difficulty with successful laparoscopic removal, and the potential need for a second operation to address pancreas-specific complications arising from the inflammatory insult. Furthermore, early CCY might contaminate an otherwise sterile pancreatic fluid collection if one exists. There has been a paucity of literature examining early versus delayed CCY in SAP. Nealon et al. [24] reported on 187 patients with moderate to severe pancreatitis as defined by five or more Ranson criteria—151 of who had peripancreatic fluid collections equally distributed between those that had early and delayed CCY (defined as surgery deferred until a fluid collection resolved or required surgical intervention). Seventy-eight patients had "early" CCY that unfortunately was *not* defined in this study. The number of patients having attempted laparoscopic removal in the early group was not reported. Forty-four percent suffered postoperative complications and 49 patients in this group required reoperation following CCY for definitive management of a pancreatic pseudocyst. Of the 109 patients having delayed CCY, all required only one operation for definitive management including 56 that had successful laparoscopic CCY as their sole procedure, and 53 of whom had combined CCY and internal pseudocyst drainage. Postoperative morbidity was 5%. Similar results have been reported previously [25].

In summary, early cholecystectomy in mild to moderate ABP can be safely performed within 48 h, and can most often be accomplished laparoscopically, even if clinical symptoms have not completely abated and/or laboratory examinations normalized. Such a strategy results in decreased LOS with a low risk of procedure or disease-related morbidity or the need for hospital readmission. In contrast, a lower level of evidence suggests that CCY should be delayed in those with severe pancreatitis to allow sepsis and multiorgan failure to resolve, and to assess for pancreas-related complications that may require surgical intervention. Prophylactic endoscopic sphincterotomy is not recommended in this cohort unless hard evidence of choledocholithiasis exists [10] (Grade B recommendation).

## 58.4 What is the Role of Prophylactic Antibiotics in Severe Acute Pancreatitis?

Severe pancreatitis, defined by any grading system, is associated with a substantial risk for the development of pancreatic fluid collections and/or pancreatic necrosis as defined by the Atlanta Classification [26]. If these processes remain sterile, there is a good probability that patients will recover without the need for operative intervention. In contrast, secondary pancreatic infections mandate the need for operative drainage and debridement, markedly increase hospital LOS, and are associated with significant morbidity and mortality [27]. In theory, prophylactic antibiotics in those with severe AP might prevent the progression of a sterile process into an infected milieu. Questions remain if this mode of therapy is chosen. When should antimicrobial therapy be initiated and for how long? What antibiotic best penetrates pancreatic tissue? Finally, there may be a price to pay for such a strategy including antibiotic-associated colitis and the potential selection of resistant or fungal organisms given prolonged therapy that may augment, rather than protect against, the risk for mortality [28].

A review of antimicrobial agents with satisfactory tissue concentrations in the pancreatic bed is appropriate. In a classic study, Buchler et al. [29] measured the tissue (not serum) concentrations of 10 different antibiotics in 89 patients having *elective* pancreatic surgery. Antimicrobial agents with the highest tissue concentrations, as well as bactericidal activity included ciprofloxacin, ofloxacin, and imipenem. Further work from Bassi et al. examined the utility of these favored antibiotics in the face of human-necrotizing pancreatitis.

Tissue (not serum) levels of antimicrobials were obtained by needle biopsy, samples obtained at the time of surgery or from surgically placed drains in 12 patients [30]. In this study, fluoroquinolones and metronidazole had concentrations in pancreatic tissue higher than the minimal inhibitory concentration (MIC) for the most commonly cultured organisms. Carbapenem concentrations in necrotic tissue did not always exceed the MIC for common pathogens. The liposolubility of these agents proved to be a common trait and repeated administration enhanced their penetration in necrotic pancreatic tissue. In common with the study by Buchler, aminoglycosides proved inadequate presumably due to their limited liposolubility. Thus, the fluoroquinolones and the carbapenems have formed the basis of clinical studies investigating the role of antimicrobial prophylaxis in severe pancreatitis.

In an early, small multicenter, nonblinded trial, Penderzoli et al. [31] randomized 74 patients with evidence of pancreatic necrosis noted on CT scan within 72 h of admission to medical management alone versus the addition of prophylactic imipenem–cilastatin for 14 days (41 patients). Mean Ranson criteria for all patients was 3.7 and about one-half had pancreatitis on the basis of biliary disease. More patients receiving prophylaxis had >50% necrosis (14 versus 2). Only five patients receiving antimicrobial prophylaxis developed pancreatic sepsis (confirmed by culture) statistically different than those medically managed. However, mortality and the need for surgical debridement of the pancreas did not differ. Curiously, in addition to the five septic patients in the prophylaxis group, seven additional patients had laparotomy for reasons not stated. Culture data on those with pancreatic sepsis suggest that prophylaxis did not select out resistant organisms.

A study also supporting antibiotic prophylaxis was reported from seven Norwegian hospitals on 73 antibiotic-naive patients with SAP defined as a CRP >120 mg/L and evidence of necrosis by CT imaging [32]. Patients were randomized to imipenem for 5–7 days or control in a nonblinded fashion. While overall and infectious complications were significantly reduced in those that received prophylaxis, the incidence of organ failure, peripancreatic infection, need for pancreas specific therapeutic intervention, and death were not different between treatment groups. While admitting the study was underpowered, the authors surprisingly conclude that the utilization of antimicrobial prophylaxis in SAP is recommended.

In a study from Lithuania, the impact of antibiotic prophylaxis instituted within 72 h of presentation on the clinical course of 210 well-matched patients with SAP defined as CRP >120 mg/L, APACHE II score >7, and evidence of >30% pancreatic necrosis by CT imaging was assessed [33]. Results were analyzed based on two time periods: 2 years during which prophylaxis was employed (ciprofloxacin 800 mg/day, metronidazole 1500 mg/day for 14 days) and 1 subsequent year when it was withdrawn (103 and 107 patients, respectively). There was no difference in the incidence of infected necrosis, the need for necrosectomy, organ failure, LOS, or mortality between treatment groups.

Isenmann et al. [34] performed a multicenter, randomized, placebo-controlled, double-blind study on the effect of ciprofloxacin and flagyl, administered for a minimum of 14 days, in preventing infected pancreatic necrosis and thereby reducing mortality. One hundred and fourteen patients with SAP defined as a C-reactive protein level (CRP) >150 mg/L and/or the presence of pancreatic necrosis on contrast-enhanced CT and entering within 72 h of admission were studied. Study patients were converted to open antibiotic therapy if extra or de novo pancreatic sepsis was documented, multiple organ failure developed or CRP levels increased. The etiology of pancreatitis was predominantly biliary and alcohol related. Of the 58 patients randomized to treatment, only 16 required conversion to open antimicrobial administration versus 26 in the placebo group—a significant difference. However, the incidence of secondary and extrapancreatic infections was not different nor was the mortality rate. Approximately one-half of the isolates in both groups with infected necrosis were gram-positive organisms. However, it was not noted how these isolates were obtained—open versus percutaneous. Thus, while empiric antibiotic treatment did not lead to development of resistant or fungal organisms, it failed to prevent pancreatic and systemic infections and it did not reduce mortality in this study. It should be noted, however, that the initial power analysis called for a study population of 200 patients assuming an incidence of pancreatic infection of 40%. Surprisingly, this study was terminated after an interim analysis because, the authors state, infected pancreatic necrosis occurred in 7/53 treated patients versus 5/52 receiving placebo and this was a reverse trend. Certainly, it could be argued that study recruitment should have continued.

Dellinger and colleagues reported a multicenter similarly designed study and patient population to that of Isenmann comparing prophylactic meropenem infusion to placebo in 40 patients each within 5 days of onset of SAP and delivered for 7–21 days [35]. In contrast to the study by Isenmann, most patients in this study had documented pancreatic necrosis >30% consistent with severe disease. The incidence of developing pancreatic infection, the number of operative interventions on the pancreas, and the mortality rate were not different between groups. The utilization of prophylaxis did not increase the incidence of resistant organisms with gram-positive and negative flora predominating. The authors concluded the antibiotic prophylaxis did not reduce septic pancreatic infections in those with SAP as was confirmed in two recent meta-analyses [36,37]. This study again did not reach its desired power analysis assuming an incidence of pancreatic infection of 40% and it was not continued to reach the desired number of patients due to a "restriction of resources."

To summarize, the utilization of prophylactic antibiotics in severe necrotizing pancreatitis is well tolerated and may alter the flora recovered if infection ensues but is not associated with the development of resistant organisms. Randomized, double-blinded, placebo-controlled studies to date have failed to recruit enough patients to establish a statistically significant difference, if it exists, between prophylaxis and placebo. It is unlikely that given the low incidence of severe pancreatitis as well as the heterogeneity of patients and the treatment they receive that future studies might improve on those reported to date. Although not an absolute contraindication, the routine use of antibiotic prophylaxis in those with severe pancreatitis *and* significant necrosis should be discouraged (Grade B recommendation).

## 58.5 Is Enteral Nutrition (EN) Safe and Superior to Total Parenteral Nutrition (TPN) in Acute Pancreatitis?

Nutritional support in severe acute pancreatitis is vital due to the local and systemic inflammatory response that increases metabolic demands resulting in hypercatabolism [38]. In an attempt to "rest" the pancreas and not worsen its severity, hyperalimentation has traditionally provided the backbone of therapy to meet nutritional needs. In addition, severe pancreatitis is often associated with gastric stasis and/or intestinal ileus limiting enteral feeding and many patients are simply too ill to consume adequate calories. It has long been recognized that EN is superior to the parenteral route in terms of immune competence, metabolic homeostasis, reducing catheter-related sepsis and the overall cost of support and its utilization in other areas of surgical care has been well established [39]. Most recently, the paradigm that EN in severe pancreatitis exacerbates the disease or will not be tolerated has been challenged. The utilization of this mode of nutritional support, however, must not present its own set of complications *and* it must prove superior outcomes to standard therapy with TPN.

In the setting of SAP, the utilization of jejunal nutrition has its own inherent limitations and potential associated complications beyond just intolerance secondary to disease-associated ileus. Naso-jejunal (NJ) tube placement typically requires either radiologic or endoscopic advancement either of which can be problematic in an unstable intensive care unit patient. Bedside placement can be utilized but is cumbersome and time-consuming [40]. In addition, jejunal feedings in hypotensive patients, those with large volume fluid requirements and patients with clinical evidence of an ileus, have been associated with the development of catastrophic small bowel necrosis [41]. With these caveats in mind, jejunal feedings have been successfully implemented in AP in several comparison studies with TPN.

Windsor et al. investigated the impact of EN on decreasing the acute phase response and thereby the disease severity of AP when compared with TPN in a randomized trial of 34 patients [42]. Severe pancreatitis was defined as an Imrie score >3 and NJ tubes were placed under radiographic guidance. Enrollment was within 48 h of admission and the influence of nutritional support was assessed after 7 days of implementation. Patients were followed clinically for the development of the systemic inflammatory response syndrome, intra-abdominal sepsis, multiple organ failure, the need for operative intervention, and mortality. Four of sixteen patients in the EN group required a temporary reduction in their goal rate due to intolerance. The EN group had a significant reduction in CRP levels and APACHE II scores—a trend *not* found in the TPN group. EN significantly reduced measured inflammatory mediators versus TPN. The clinical parameters assessed demonstrated a superior trend favoring EN. The authors conclude that EN is superior to TPN in attenuating the acute-phase response of pancreatitis that may translate to an improved clinical course.

McClave et al. randomized 32 well-matched patients to EN via an NJ tube placed endoscopically or TPN within 48 h [43]. Ranson scores were only modestly elevated suggesting these patients did not have severe pancreatitis. The vast majority of patients in both groups reached goal calories by day 4 of implementation. There was no mortality and no difference between groups with respect to pain scores, serum albumin level, hospital LOS, and the incidence of nosocomial infection. Serial Ranson and APACHE III scores were reduced in the EN group and increased in the TPN group but this difference reached significance on only one occasion and it is unclear how to interpret "serial" Ranson criteria. EN was significantly less expensive. One patient had an exacerbation of pancreatitis when the NJ tube migrated back into the stomach and three patients in the EN group had recurrent pancreatitis on initiation of an oral diet. LOS was not improved. The authors tenuously conclude that EN may promote more rapid resolution of the toxicity and stress response of pancreatitis and that this should be the preferred method of caloric delivery.

The issue was reexamined in those with *severe* pancreatitis in a well-performed randomized study of 38 patients by Kalfarentzos et al. [44]. Severe pancreatitis was defined as three or more Imrie criteria or an APACHE II score >8 combined with a CRP concentration >120 mg/L within 48 h of admission and Grade D or E findings by Balthazar CT criteria. All patients received antibiotic prophylaxis with imipenem. The 18 patients randomized to EN had a naso-enteric tube placed fluoroscopically within 48 h of admission (two patients had unsuccessful placement and were excluded from analysis). Feedings were initiated immediately thereafter in resuscitated, "stable" patients. There was no difference in the clinical course of either group with respect to the need for operation, LOS, and mortality. Target nutritional goals were reached and nitrogen balance improved progressively and equally in both groups. The mean number of infections per patient as well as the overall complication rate was significantly less in those receiving EN; however, a few pancreatic infections were noted. EN was significantly less expensive. The authors conclude that early EN in those with severe pancreatitis is safe and preferential to TPN.

Petrov et al. [45] examined the impact of EN on reducing secondary pancreatic infections and mortality in a randomized trial of 69 well-matched patients presenting with SAP defined as an APACHE II score >8 and/or a CRP concentration >150 mg/dL. Nutritional support was initiated within 72 h of presentation with enteral catheters positioned radiologically. The hemodynamic stability, or lack thereof, of patients receiving EN was not reported. Prophylactic antibiotics were routinely utilized in both groups. When compared with TPN, EN was associated with a statistically significant reduction in pancreatic and extrapancreatic septic morbidity. Since pancreatic infection mandated operative intervention the need for surgery was significantly reduced in those receiving EN as well. Mortality from pancreatic sepsis and/or multiple organ failure was significantly worse in those receiving TPN. The need for additional feeding-tube positioning, abdominal bloating, diarrhea, and a reduction in the rate of administration of support were all more common in those receiving EN. The authors conclude that EN could be an important adjunct in reducing pancreatic infectious complications and thereby mortality in those with SAP.

A study from Poland assessed the impact of early (<48 h) versus delayed ($n = 100$) EN (3–7 days after admission) on infectious complications and clinical outcome in 197 well-matched patients with predicted SAP [46]. The diagnosis of SAP was similar to that in other studies. Exclusion criteria included those admitted after 72 h of onset of symptoms. The authors make no mention of withholding feedings in the hemodynamically unstable patient. NJ tube placement was made by a "medical staff" while endoscopy was reserved for those that had failure of bedside placement. The need for surgical intervention for pancreas-related complications was not different between treatment groups (7 early, 11 delayed). The incidence of infected peripancreatic collections and mortality was higher in those with delayed EN. With the exception of respiratory failure, systemic complications were not different between treatment groups. The authors conclude that early EN should be instituted following admission for SAP. Caution, however, needs to be utilized in those with hemodynamic instability to reduce the risk of bowel infarction.

In conclusion, when compared with TPN, careful utilization of early EN is well tolerated, reduces the inflammatory response of AP, reduces infectious morbidity, and is less expensive. Data demonstrating a *clinical* improvement with respect to the need for operative intervention, a shorter hospital LOS, and disease-related mortality when EN is utilized remain sparse but promising due to the small number of patients reported in comparative studies to date. While further study is needed and with the acknowledged difficulty in feeding-tube placement, EN in the hemodynamically stable patient with severe pancreatitis is favored with close monitoring of tolerance (Grade B recommendation). In those undergoing surgical debridement, a surgically placed jejunostomy tube is strongly recommended [47]. If jejunal feeding is not tolerated due to hemodynamic instability or ileus, TPN remains an important therapy.

## 58.6 Is Gastric Feeding Safe and Equivalent to Jejunal Feeding in Acute Pancreatitis?

With the aforementioned benefits of jejunal feedings, a reasonable extrapolation would be to simplify the limitations of tube placement by feeding directly into the stomach. As previously noted, such a management scheme may be associated with its own inherent complications—specifically intolerance due to gastric stasis, the possibility of aspiration in those without airway protection, and an exacerbation of pancreatitis due to stimulation of the pancreas. Several clinical trials have compared these routes of administration.

Eatock et al. [48] randomized 49 well-matched patients with SAP defined as an Imrie score >3, and APACHE II score >6 or a CRP >150 mg/dL to nasogastric (NG) versus endoscopically placed NJ feedings beginning within 72 h of onset of symptoms. All but one patient tolerated the enteral route and the majority of patients in both groups were receiving at least 75% of goal calories within 48 h of initiation of feedings. Groups did not differ with respect to follow-up APACHE II scores, CRP levels, or pain analog scales and mortality was not statistically different (24.5% of study population). Gastrointestinal complications were equivalent between groups. One patient required to repeat endoscopy to replace an NJ tube. The authors conclude that NG feeding is simpler, less expensive, and equivalent to the NJ route.

Kumar et al. [49] randomized 31 evenly matched patients with SAP defined as organ failure and an APACHE II score >8 or Balthazar score >7 to NG ($n$ = 15) or NJ (placed endoscopically) feedings. Importantly, patients in shock (systolic blood pressure <90 mmHg) were appropriately excluded and feedings were gradually increased over a 7-day period. Patients were assessed for study accrual up to 4 weeks after onset of symptoms—a delay in initiation that might allow better tolerance of feedings. No patient required TPN once the goal rate of feeding was achieved (day 7). When compared with the NJ route, NG feedings were associated with similar rates of pancreatic infection and operative intervention and the LOS and mortality were not different between groups. Anthropometric and nutritional parameters declined regardless of the route of administration and complications were similar. Neither modality exacerbated pancreatitis. The authors conclude that both routes of administration, when gradually delivered are well tolerated but fail to reverse the catabolism associated with the disease.

Eckerwall et al. [50] compared NG feedings to TPN in 48 well-matched patients with SAP defined as an APACHE II score >8 and/or a CRP level >150 mg/dL. The goal of the study was to assess the impact of nutrient delivery on the inflammatory response of AP during the first 10 days of illness. Nutritional support was started within 24 h of admission with a target goal reached in 66% of the entire population with no difference between groups. No patient receiving NG feeds had aspiration. A measure of inflammation decreased equally in both groups during the study period. Only one patient in the entire series required operative pancreatic surgery. The authors concluded that NG feedings were tolerated well in those with predicted SAP but did not attenuate the inflammatory response associated with the disease when compared with TPN.

Finally, Singh et al. [51] randomized 78 well-matched patients with SAP defined as organ failure, APACHE II score >8 or a CT Balthazar score >7 to NG or NJ feedings. Patients in shock were excluded. The NJ tube was placed endoscopically and feedings were initiated within 48 h aimed at achieving nutrient goal within 3–4 days that was successful in all study patients. Diarrhea occurred in three and four patients with NJ and NG feedings, respectively. There were less overall infectious complications including those within the pancreatic bed in those having NG feeds. However, four and two patients in the NG and NJ pathways, respectively, required surgery for infected necrosis. The author's claim that some with infected necrosis were treated with antibiotics alone, however, this would seem exceptional in terms of definitive treatment. In addition, the total number of patients with infected necrosis was not clearly stated. Measures of intestinal permeability and endotoxemia were not different between groups. Given these limitations their data would support their conclusion that NG feeding was not inferior to that provided by the NJ route.

In summary, these preliminary studies suggest that NG feeding seems to be tolerated as well as NJ feeding in those with SAP *in the hemodynamically stable patient*

**TABLE 58.1**

Controversies in Pancreatitis, Recommendations, Level of Evidence, and References

| Question | Answer | Levels of Evidence | Grade of Recommendation | References |
|---|---|---|---|---|
| What is the role (if any) of MRCP in suspected choledocholithiasis in those with ABP? | Routine use discouraged. Selective approach is based on ultrasound and liver profile to identify candidates for preoperative ERCP. | IIc | B | [2–5] |
| What is the role of ERCP in ABP? | Only if evidence of cholangitis or biliary obstruction exists. | Ia | A | [6,8–14] |
| Should patients have early or delayed cholecystectomy following ABP? | Early in mild to moderate disease. Delay in those with SAP. | IIb | B | [18–25] |
| What is the role of prophylactic antibiotics in SAP? | Studies do not show a routine benefit. Reasonable in those with multiorgan failure. | Ib | B | [31–37] |
| Is EN safe and superior to TPN in AP? | Safe and less expensive but clinical benefit is unclear. | IIb | B | [42–44] |
| Is gastric feeding safe and equivalent to jejunal feeding in AP? | Safe in hemodynamically stable patients if tolerated. | IIb | B | [48–51] |

*Abbreviations:* MRCP, magnetic resonance cholangiopancreatography; ERCP, endoscopic cholangiopancreatography; SAP, severe acute pancreatitis; AP, acute pancreatitis; EN, enteral nutrition; TPN, total parenteral nutrition.

without exacerbating the disease process provided close assessment of tolerance is made (Grade B recommendation). Tube placement is easier and less costly. The relationship of NG feedings to a decline in secondary pancreatic infections and disease-related mortality has yet to be ascertained.

## References


1. Whitcomb DC. Acute pancreatitis. *N Engl J Med.* 2006;354(20):2142–2150.
2. Makary MA, Duncan MD, Harmon JW et al. The role of magnetic resonance cholangiopancreatography in the management of patients with gallstone pancreatitis. *Ann Surg.* 2005;241:119–124.
3. Barlow AD, Haqq J, McCormack D et al. The role of magnetic resonance cholangiopancreatography in the management of acute gallstone pancreatitis. *Ann R Coll Engl.* 2013;95:503–506.
4. Mofidi R, Lee AC, Madhavan KK et al. The selective use of magnetic resonance cholangiopancreatography in the imaging of the axial biliary tree in patients with acute gallstone pancreatitis. *Pancreatology.* 2008;8:55–60.
5. Liu TH, Consorti ET, Kawahima A et al. Patient evaluation and management with selective use of magnetic resonance cholangiography and endoscopic retrograde cholangiopancreatography before laparoscopic cholecystectomy. *Ann Surg.* 2001;234:33–40.
6. Neoptolemos JP, Carr-Locke DL, London NJ et al. Controlled trial of urgent endoscopic cholangiopancreatography and endoscopic sphincterotomy versus conservative treatment for acute pancreatitis due to gallstones. *Lancet.* 1988;2(8618):979–983.
7. Blamey S, Imrie C, O'Neill J et al. Prognostic factors in acute pancreatitis. *Gut.* 1984;25(12):1340–1346.
8. Fan S, Lai E, Mok F et al. Early treatment of acute biliary pancreatitis by endoscopic papillotomy. *N Engl J Med.* 1993;328(4):228–232.
9. Folsch UR, Nitsche R, Ludtle R et al. Early ERCP and papillostomy compared with conservative treatment for acute biliary pancreatitis. The German Study Group on acute biliary pancreatitis. *N Engl J Med.* 1997;336(4):237–242.
10. Oria A, Cimmino D, Ocampo C et al. Early endoscopic intervention versus early conservative management in patients with acute gallstone pancreatitis and biliopancreatic obstruction: A randomized clinical trial. *Ann Surg.* 2007;245(1):10–17.
11. Van Santvoort HC, Besselink MG, de Vries AC et al. Early endoscopic retrograde cholangiopancreatography in predicted severe acute biliary pancreatitis. *Ann Surg.* 2009;250:68–75.
12. Behrns KE, Ashley SW, Hunter JG et al. Early ERCP for gallstone pancreatitis: For whom and when? *J Gastrointest Surg.* 2008;12(4):629–633.
13. Petrov MS, van Santvoort HC, van der Heijden GJ et al. Early endoscopic retrograde cholangiopancreatography versus conservative management in acute biliary pancreatitis: A meta-analysis of randomized trials. *Ann Surg.* 2008;247(2):250–257.
14. Uy MC, Daez ML, Sy PP et al. Early ERCP in acute gallstone pancreatitis without cholangitis: A meta-analysis. *JOP.* 2009;10:299–305.
15. Ito K, Ito H, Whang EE. Timing of cholecystectomy for biliary pancreatitis: Do the data support current guidelines? *J Gastrointest Surg.* 2008;12:2164–2170.
16. Burch JM, Feliciano DV, Mattox KL et al. Gallstone pancreatitis. *Arch Surg.* 1990;125:853–860.
17. Cameron DR, Goodman AJ. Delayed cholecystectomy for gallstone pancreatitis: Re-admissions and outcomes. *Ann R Coll Engl.* 2004;86:358–362.
18. Nebiker CA, Frey DM, Hamel CT et al. Early versus delayed cholecystectomy in patients with biliary acute pancreatitis. *Surgery.* 2009;145:260–264.
19. Rosing DK, de Virgilio C, Yaghoubian A et al. Early cholecystectomy for mild to moderate gallstone pancreatitis shortens hospital stay. *J Am Coll Surg.* 2007;205:762–766.
20. Falor AE, de Virgilio C, Stabile BE et al. Early laparoscopic cholecystectomy for mild gallstone pancreatitis. *Arch Surg.* 2012;147:1031–1035.
21. Aboulian A, Chan T, Yaghoubian A et al. Early cholecystectomy safely decreases hospital stay in patients with mild gallstone pancreatitis. *Ann Surg.* 2010;251:615–619.
22. van Baal MC, Besselink MG, Bakker OJ et al. Timing of cholecystectomy after mild biliary pancreatitits. *Ann Surg.* 2012;255:860–866.
23. Perez LJR, Parra JF, Dimas GA. The safety of early laparoscopic cholecystectomy (<48 h) for patients with mild gallstone pancreatitis: A systematic review of the literature and meta-analysis. *Cir Esp.* 2014;92: 107–113.
24. Nealon WH, Bawduniak J, Walser EM. Appropriate timing of cholecystetomy in patients who present with moderate to severe gallstone-associated acute pancreatitis with perpancreatic fluid collections. *Ann Surg.* 2004;239:741–751.
25. Tang E, Stain SC, Tang G et al. Timing of laparoscopic surgery in gallstone pancreatitis. *Arch Surg.* 1995;130:496–500.
26. Bradley EL. A clinically based classification system for acute pancreatitis. Summary of the *International Symposium on Acute Pancreatitis*, Atlanta, GA, September 11 through 13, 1992. *Arch Surg.* 1993;128(5):586–590.
27. Rodriguez JR, Razo AO, Targarona J et al. Debridement and closed packing for sterile or infected necrotizing pancreatitis: Insights into indications and outcomes in 167 patients. *Ann Surg.* 2008;247(2):294–299.
28. Hoerauf A, Hammer S, Muller Myhsok B et al. Intra-abdominal *Candida* infection during acute necrotizing pancreatitis has a high prevalence and is associated with increased mortality. *Crit Care Med.* 1998;26(12):2010–2015.

29. Buchler M, Malfertheiner P, Friess, H et al. Human pancreatic tissue concentration of bactericidal antibiotics. *Gastroenterology.* 1992;103(6):1902–1908.
30. Bassi C, Pederzoli P, Vesentini S et al. Behavior of antibiotics during human necrotizing pancreatitis. *Antimicrob Agents Chemother.* 1994;38(4):830–836.
31. Penderzoli P, Bassi C, Vesentini S et al. A randomized multicenter clinical trial of antibiotic prophylaxis of septic complications in acute necrotizing pancreatitis with imipenim. *Surg Gynecol Obstet.* 1993;176(5):480–483.
32. Rokke O, Harbitz TB, Liljedal J et al. Early treatment of severe pancreatitis with imipenem: A prospective randomized clinical trial. *Scan J Gastroenterol.* 2007;42: 771–776.
33. Ignatavicius P, Vitkauskiene A, Pundzius J et al. Effects of prophylactic antibiotics in acute pancreatitis. *HPB.* 2012;14:396–402.
34. Isenmann R, Runzi M, Kron M et al. Prophylactic antibiotic treatment in patients with predicted severe acute pancreatitis: A placebo-controlled, double-blind trial. *Gastroenterology.* 2004;126(4):997–1004.
35. Dellinger EP, Tellado JM, Soto NE et al. Early antibiotic treatment for severe necrotizing pancreatitis: A randomized, double-blind, placebo-controlled study. *Ann Surg.* 2007;245(5):674–683.
36. Bai Y, Gao J, Zou D et al. Prophylactic antibiotics cannot reduce infected pancreatic necrosis and mortality in acute necrotizing pancreatitis: Evidence from a meta-analysis of randomized controlled trials. *Am J Gastroenterol.* 2008; 103(1):104–110.
37. Jafri NS, Mahid SS, Idstein SR et al. Antibiotic prophylaxis is not protective in severe acute pancreatitis: A systematic review and meta-analysis. *Am J Surg.* 2009;197: 806–813.
38. Dickerson RN, Vehe KL, Mullen JL et al. Resting energy expenditure in patients with pancreatitis. *Crit Care Med.* 1991;19(4):484–490.
39. Kudsk KA. Beneficial effect of enteral nutrition. *Gastrointest Endosc Clin N Am.* 2007;17(4):647–662.
40. Zaloga GP. Bedside method for placing small bowel feeding tubes in critically ill patients. A prospective study. *Chest.* 1991;100(6):1643–1646.
41. Schunn CD, Daly JM. Small bowel necrosis associated with postoperative jejunal tube feeding. *J Am Coll Surg.* 1995;180(4):410–416.
42. Windsor A, Kanwar S, Li A et al. Compared with parenteral nutrition, enteral feeding attenuates the acute-phase response and improves disease severity in acute pancreatitis. *Gut.* 1998;42(3):431–435.
43. McClave SA, Greene LM, Snider HL et al. Comparison of the safety of early enteral vs parenteral nutrition in mild acute pancreatitis. *J Parenter Enter Nutr.* 1997;21(1):14–20.
44. Kalfarentzos F, Kehagias J, Mead N et al. Enteral nutrition is superior to parenteral nutrition in severe acute pancreatitis: Results of a randomized prospective trial. *Br J Surg.* 1997;84(12):1665–1669.
45. Petrov MS, Kukosh MV, Emelyanov NV. A randomized controlled trial of enteral versus parenteral feeding in patients with predicted severe acute pancreatitis shows a significant reduction in mortality and in infected pancreatic complications with total enteral nutrition. *Dig Surg.* 2006;23(5–6):336–345.
46. Wereszczynska-Siemiatkowska U, Swidnicka-Siergiejko A, Siemiatkowski A et al. Early enteral nutrition is superior to delayed enteral nutrition for the prevention of infected necrosis and mortality in acute pancreatitis. *Pancreas.* 2013;42:640–646.
47. Kudsk K, Campbell S, O'Brien T et al. Postoperative jejunal feedings following complicated pancreatitis. *Nutr Clin Pract.* 1990;5(1):14–17.
48. Eatock F, Chong P, Menezes N et al. A randomized study of early nasogastric versus nasojejunal feeding in severe acute pancreatitis. *Am J Gastroenterol.* 2005;100(2):432–439.
49. Kumar A, Singh N, Prakash S et al. Early enteral nutrition in severe acute pancreatitis: A prospective randomized controlled trial comparing nasojejunal and nasogastric routes. *J Clin Gastroenterol.* 2006;40(5):431–434.
50. Eckerwall G, Axelsson J, Andersson R. Early nasogastric feeding in predicted severe acute pancreatitis: A clinical randomized study. *Ann Surg.* 2006;244(6):959–967.
51. Singh N, Sharma B, Sharma M et al. Evaluation of early enteral feeding through nasogastric and nasojejunal tube in severe acute pancreatitis. *Pancreas.* 2012;41:153–159.

## Commentary on Acute Pancreatitis

*Samir M. Fakhry*

Many surgical services no longer admit or primarily manage acute pancreatitis (AP). Most do manage AP in the setting of cholelithiasis, or are consulted to help with the care of patients who have complicated AP. In a recent report, hepaticopancreaticobiliary disease was the most common category of admissions for emergency general surgery in the United States over the past decade*. Acute care surgeons are likely to continue to see increasing numbers of these patients as the population ages given the higher frequency of complicated disease in that population. This (aging) reminds me that medicine in general and surgery in particular have changed significantly in my approximately quarter-century career. Although the changes in surgical technologies have perhaps been the most prominent, the scientific advances that affect our clinical decision making and patient care practices have also been dramatic. There are many things we did routinely or took for granted that have now been shown to be unnecessary, useless or (worse yet) harmful. The primary driver for these ongoing changes has been the improvement in the quality of the research produced and the emphasis on evidence-based medicine. If I practiced today the way I was trained, there are many things I would be doing that would be unacceptable or even wrong. For that reason, staying abreast of quality scientific advances in our field is vital to remaining relevant as a surgeon. Separating the wheat from the chaff is especially critical, but for most of us clinicians, that may be easier said than done†. Credible guidance as to what is a valuable manuscript whose findings we should incorporate into our practice and what is a weak study we should ignore can be quite helpful. The questions addressed in this chapter are commonly encountered by surgeons in the care of patients with AP.

### What Is the Role (If Any) of Magnetic Resonance Cholangiopancreatography (MRCP) in Suspected Choledocholithiasis in Those with Acute Biliary Pancreatitis?

The use of MRCP as a precursor to ERCP has increased tremendously in recent years. For some endoscopists, it is a prerequisite to ERCP. My main conclusion in this context is that the data are few and generally of poor quality. I agree with the author that the methodological flaws of many of the available studies make it hard to draw conclusions. The reports by Mofidi et al. and Lim et al. provide some direction: use MRCP selectively in patients with persistent signs and symptoms of common bile duct (CBD) obstruction or gallstone pancreatitis prior to ERCP and many patients can be spared the invasive procedure. Note that the timing of the decision to "work up" the CBD is important, since most CBD stones will pass on their own. Early use of MRCP will result in a higher number of patients referred for stone extraction by ERCP. It appears prudent to follow the clinical, ultrasound, and biochemical variables and if they and the patient are improving, neither MRCP nor ERCP is likely needed.

### What Is the Role of Early Endoscopic Retrograde Cholangiopancreatography (ERCP) in Acute Biliary Pancreatitis?

The data in support of reserving ERCP in patients with acute biliary pancreatitis for those with evidence of likely CBD obstruction or those with cholangitis are reasonably good and I would therefore not recommend ERCP in a patient with uncomplicated acute biliary pancreatitis. One additional conclusion was also drawn from this dataset: early ERCP in patients with AP has relatively little detrimental impact on the course of the pancreatitis. This represents a departure from the older mindset that manipulation of the CBD in AP will result in progression of the pancreatitis. This is another example of something that made a lot of sense intuitively but has been shown to be a relatively unfounded concern.

### Should Patients Have Early or Delayed Cholecystectomy Following Acute Biliary Pancreatitis?

The author's conclusions regarding the data for this question are consistent with the practice of most surgeons in that we perform laparoscopic cholecystectomy early on patients with mild to moderate acute biliary pancreatitis while delaying surgery for those with severe pancreatitis. The data are not conclusive, however, and I wonder if further studies may yet reveal that early cholecystectomy combined with early ECRP for duct clearance may benefit some patients with severe acute biliary pancreatitis.

### What Is the Role of Prophylactic Antibiotics in Severe AP?

Prophylactic antibiotics for patients with severe AP became popular when Penderzoli et al published their

* Gale SC, Shafi S, Dombrovski AY, Arumugam D, Crystal JS. The public health burden of emergency general surgery in the United States: A 10 year analysis of the Nationwide Inpatient Sample—2001 to 2010. *J Trauma Acute Care Surg.* 2014;77(2):202–208.

† Ioannidis, JPA. Why most published research findings are false. *PLOS Med.* 2005;2(8):696–701.

study in 1993 showing a lower incidence of pancreatic sepsis in the group receiving antibiotics. The study had a number of methodological weaknesses and, in addition, the rates of surgical intervention on the pancreas and the hospital mortality were not different. In spite of these issues, the use of prophylactic antibiotics in severe AP became commonplace. Several studies and meta-analyses have been conducted since that time with no clear evidence showing benefit with prophylactic antibiotic use. Not all physicians are convinced however, and the use of prophylaxis continues underlining the challenge of changing ingrained practices. Based on the available evidence, the recommendation in this chapter is the correct one: "... the routine use of antibiotic prophylaxis in those with severe pancreatitis *and* significant necrosis should be discouraged."

### Is Enteral Nutrition (EN) Safe and Superior to Total Parenteral Nutrition (TPN) in AP?

Enteral nutrition has displaced parenteral nutrition in most clinical scenarios in surgery. Broad consensus exists regarding many of the issues related to enteral nutrition in acutely ill patients as outlined in a recent consensus document*. The evidence in favor of enteral nutrition is substantial and consistent across many disease entities. The use of enteral nutrition in AP should therefore be standard with the exception of patients with hemodynamic instability.

### Is Gastric Feeding Safe and Equivalent to Jejunal Feeding in AP?

Another long-held assumption was that gastric feedings would worsen pancreatitis, because it would stimulate pancreatic secretions. The available evidence indicates that gastric feedings are acceptable in many patients with AP provided the feedings are tolerated and there is no hemodynamic instability. This is another example of progressively accumulating evidence challenging established dogma. I am not aware of data on the percentage of physicians who have adopted this practice and used gastric feedings in AP but suspect that there are many clinicians who remain reluctant to do so. This underlines the often relatively slow progression from published data to dissemination to physicians and then adoption into clinical practice.

---

* McClave SA, Martindale RG, Vanek VW et al. Guidelines for the provision and assessment of nutrition support therapy in the adult critically ill patient. *J Parenter Enteral Nutr.* 2009;33(3):277–316.

# 59

## *Pancreatic Pseudocysts*

**Olga N. Tucker, Raul J. Rosenthal, Conrad H. Simpfendorfer, and Marcelo J. Lacayo Baez**

**CONTENTS**



### 59.1 Introduction

Pancreatic pseudocysts (PPs) comprise ≥75% of all cystic lesions of the pancreas. They generally arise as a complication of acute or chronic pancreatitis, however, other causes exist. Acute pancreatitis is usually a mild and self-limiting disorder, but approximately 20% of patients develop a severe form with local and systemic complications. Fluid collections representing an exudative or serous reaction to injury of the pancreas occur in approximately 50% of patients with moderate to severe pancreatitis. Approximately 50% of these collections resolve spontaneously within 6 weeks. However, 5%–15% progress to pseudocyst formation [1,2]. Approximately 20%–40% of PPs develop in patients with chronic pancreatitis, due to chronic and progressive ductal obstruction, dilation, and disruption [1,2]. Other causes include trauma, iatrogenic surgical pancreatic injury, pancreatic ductal adenocarcinoma, and very rarely hemorrhagic PPs associated with autoimmune pancreatitis [3–6].

Important issues to consider in the management of these lesions are the exclusion of other causes of peri- or intrapancreatic fluid collections that may complicate acute pancreatitis requiring alternative approaches of therapeutic intervention, determination of optimal time for intervention once the diagnosis of PP has been confirmed, and consideration of the optimal management approach.

#### 59.1.1 What is the Definition of a Pancreatic Pseudocyst?

To understand the definition of PP, it is important to review the 2012 Atlanta classification from the Acute Pancreatitis Classification Working Group, which was developed through virtual web-based consensus and evidence-based literature [7]. The new classification focuses on two phases of acute pancreatitis: the early phase (1–2 weeks) and the late phase (beyond the 1–2 weeks mark) [8] (Level IV evidence). Two types of acute pancreatitis are described: interstitial edematous pancreatitis, which corresponds to 80%–90% of cases, is the milder form and lacks the presence of necrosis, and necrotizing pancreatitis, which corresponds to 10% of cases, is the more severe form and is characterized by the presence of necrosis [8].

With regards to severity, the new classification bases severity on the presence or absence of local complications, systemic complications and persistent versus transient organ failure, and the way these affect timing. Local complications are defined based on the type of acute pancreatitis and are all a form of pancreatic or peripancreatic collections [8]. Local complications of interstitial edematous pancreatitis are characterized by the lack of necrotic tissue (lack of heterogeneity) and lack of infection. An acute peripancreatic fluid collection (APFC) is present within 4 weeks from the onset of acute pancreatitis. It corresponds to a fluid-only (homogeneous) collection confined by the fascial planes of the peripancreatic retroperitoneum (not intrapancreatic). A PP is present beyond 4 weeks from the onset of acute pancreatitis. It, like its counterpart, is a fluid-only collection, but in this case walled off and well-circumscribed. The definition of PP is particularly relevant given the fact that the term has been misused repeatedly in the published literature. The pathogenesis of the PP has been currently defined as the focal disruption of pancreatic ducts with subsequent outflow of pancreatic fluid and inflammatory formation of a walled-off homogeneous collection but the absence of necrosis. A PP is commonly found to be peripancreatic and rarely intrapancreatic. An APFC may develop into a PP [8]. Local complications of necrotizing pancreatitis are characterized by the presence of necrotic tissue (heterogeneous collections) and the possible presence of infection. An acute necrotic collection (ANC) is a peripancreatic or intrapancreatic heterogeneous (fluid and solid components—the solid component corresponding to necrotic tissue) collection that is not well circumscribed (has no definitive wall). Beyond 4 weeks the ANC will usually develop into a walled-off necrosis, which will likewise be an intrapancreatic or peripancreatic heterogeneous collection but with a well-defined wall. These local complications of necrotizing pancreatitis may be infectious or not infectious [8].

Systemic complications are defined as being directly related to the systemic inflammatory response syndrome (SIRS) product of the acute pancreatic insult. SIRS would lead to respiratory, circulatory or renal disease, or the exacerbation of an already present comorbid condition. Cited examples include exacerbation of chronic obstructive pulmonary disease, liver disease, or congestive heart failure [8]. Organ failure is defined according to the Modified Marshall Scoring System that uses respiratory ($PaO_2/FiO_2$), cardiac (systolic blood pressure in mmHg), and renal (serum creatinine, μmol/L) parameters to define organ failure. Organ failure is present if a patient scores 2 or more points in one or more systems. Organ failure is considered transient if it lasts <48 h or persistent if it lasts >48 h [8]. Mild acute pancreatitis is defined as lasting approximately 7 days (confined to early phase acute pancreatitis), not requiring any form of intervention and not presenting with local complications, systemic complication, or organ failure of any sort. Moderate acute pancreatitis is defined as lasting beyond 7 days and often related to local complications ± systemic complications and only transient (<48 h) organ failure. Severe acute pancreatitis is characterized particularly by persistent organ failure, but it usually is accompanied by one or more local ± systemic complications. Moderate and severe acute pancreatitis are both usually confined to late phase acute pancreatitis. Severe acute pancreatitis that develops within the early phase of acute pancreatitis is related to a 36%–50% mortality rate [8]. Infected necrotizing pancreatitis is accompanied by clinical manifestations such as fevers and chills as well as leukocytosis and tachycardia. It is also manifest in extraluminal gas and/or gas fluid levels on computed tomography (CT) [8].

*Recommendation*: The 2012 revision of the Atlanta classification of acute pancreatitis provides well-developed evidence-based definitions for intrapancreatic or peripancreatic homogeneous (fluid) or heterogeneous (fluid- and solid-necrotic) collections. It also reclassifies the severity of disease based on three aspects: local complications, systemic complications, and organ failure. Following this new classification, the PP described in much of the literature would have to be redefined based on a more categorical system: an intrapancreatic or peripancreatic collection would be defined by timing (early-versus late-phase acute pancreatitis), the presence or absence of necrosis, the presence or absence of a well-circumscribed wall, the presence or absence of infection. This would be in counter to a continuum, where a patient with a PP develops a necrotic collection and/or an infected collection. This new classification system is promising but requires further validation since it was recently published in January of 2013 (Level IV evidence; Grade C recommendation).

### 59.1.2 What is the Incidence of Pancreatic Pseudocysts?

The true incidence of PPs is unknown due to inconsistencies in the application of a uniform definition, the timing of diagnosis, differing techniques of clinical monitoring, the use of varying diagnostic modalities, the use of varying clinical and radiological severity grading systems, the complexity and variety of the underlying pathology, and the wide use of multiple interventional techniques with poor reporting of treatment outcomes. Incidence rates of pseudocyst formation after acute pancreatitis, trauma, iatrogenic injury, and autoimmune pancreatitis have been reported in case reports, multiple case series, and review articles (Level IV evidence). Many reported case series on the incidence and management of pseudocysts are limited by population heterogeneity, small patient numbers, and mixed data on patients with mild acute nonnecrotizing and severe acute pancreatitis, and/or the inclusion of patients with varying etiology including acute and chronic pancreatitis. Mild acute and severe acute pancreatitis represent contrasting ends of a wide spectrum of disease severity with significant differences in complication and survival rates. The majority of acute fluid collections complicating acute nonnecrotizing pancreatitis will resolve spontaneously with pseudocyst formation in a minority [9]. The incidence of acute PPs is higher after severe acute pancreatitis, with higher morbidity and mortality rates related to a higher incidence of complications [10]. The use of inaccurate and imprecise definitions of acute PPs has resulted in inaccurate representation of data. One of the most common difficulties is the differentiation of organized pancreatic and peripancreatic necrosis with associated fluid sequestration from an acute PP with pancreatic necrosis [11]. These clinical entities are very different in terms of treatment approach, and prognosis.

*Recommendation*: The true incidence of PP is unknown, due to the heterogeneity of published reports and inconsistencies in the published literature (Level IV evidence; Grade C recommendation).

### 59.1.3 What is the Incidence of Complicated Pancreatic Pseudocysts?

In the presence of a PP complications can arise including pseudocyst infection with abscess formation, intracystic hemorrhage, rapid expansion with increasing abdominal pain, obstruction of adjacent organs including esophagus, stomach, duodenum, jejunum, colon, biliary tree, or retroperitoneal structures, and/or rupture into an adjacent viscus such as the stomach, duodenum, colon or body cavity including the peritoneal cavity causing ascites, pleural space resulting in an effusion, bronchus, or pericardium with fistula formation [10,12–15]. Pseudocysts may erode into an adjacent major artery, more commonly the splenic artery, resulting in a pseudoaneurysm and/or hemorrhage. A massive gastrointestinal bleed can occur if the pseudoaneurysm communicates with the main pancreatic duct, a condition known as hemosuccus pancreaticus. Portal and splenic vein thrombosis have been reported in patients with PPs with persistent inflammatory response.

Although the occurrence of complications is uncommon, no accurate figures are available from the published literature on the true incidence of morbidity associated with pancreatic pseudocysts. Available data have been extracted from multiple case series, case reports, and review articles (Level IV evidence) [10,15–18]. The incidence of complicated pseudocysts is higher in patients following severe acute pancreatitis, as the majority of acute fluid collections in patients with mild acute nonnecrotizing pancreatitis resolve without pseudocyst formation [9]. In a recent study by Ocampo et al. [10], 43 (59%) of 73 patients over a 10 year period with an acute PP following severe acute pancreatitis developed complications including infection in 74%, perforation in 21%, and bleeding in 4.6%.

*Recommendation*: Complications of PPs are uncommon, however, no accurate figures of the true incidence are available in the published literature (Level IV evidence; Grade C recommendation).

### 59.1.4 What is the Optimal Time for Intervention Once the Diagnosis of Pancreatic Pseudocyst Has Been Confirmed?

Once identified, the timing of intervention for PPs remains controversial [9,17–23]. Experimental studies by Warren et al. [24] suggested a minimum period of 6 weeks to allow cyst wall maturation. As it is not always possible to date the onset of pseudocyst formation, a wait period of 6 weeks from the time of diagnosis has been recommended [18,26]. Some authors advocate elective intervention in all patients with uncomplicated acute pancreatic pseudocysts greater than 6 cm in size that persist for greater than 6 weeks regardless of symptoms due to reduction in the possibility of spontaneous resolution and a reported increase in complications (rupture, abscess, jaundice, and hemorrhage) during extended periods of observation [10,18,22]. In a series by Bradley et al. [18], a 41% complication rate and a 14% mortality rate were observed during an expectant period of observation, with 23% of the complications developing in the first 6 weeks. Others advocate a nonoperative, noninterventional approach in selected patients [15,20,23]. In a series by Vitas and Sarr [23], spontaneous resolution was seen in 48% of patients with asymptomatic PPs treated conservatively, while only 19 of 68 patients required elective surgery over a 5 year period. Severe life-threatening complications developed in six patients (9%) over a mean period of 46 months. Operative intervention was more common in large PPs ≥6.9 cm diameter, however, no serious complications occurred in seven patients with pseudocysts ≥10 cm diameter treated expectantly [23]. Cooperman [20] also advocated expectant management of asymptomatic pseudocysts due to the natural history of spontaneous resolution. Yeo et al. [15] also support a conservative approach in asymptomatic patients able to tolerate oral intake, with a reported spontaneous resolution rate of 60% at 1 year with stability or size reduction in 40% treated nonoperatively in the absence of pseudocyst-related mortality. Again, large pseudocyst size predicted the need for surgical intervention, with operative drainage required in 67% of those greater than 6 cm diameter while only 40% less than 6 cm diameter required operative intervention [15]. Warshaw and Rattner [22] defined clinical and biochemical criteria in a series of 42 patients, of whom 28 had underlying chronic pancreatitis, to guide the time of optimal drainage in patients with PP. They observed differences in the natural history and treatment requirements dictated by etiology. Spontaneous resolution occurred in only three patients following antecedent acute pancreatitis, while it was not seen in any patient with chronic pancreatitis. They suggested that a pseudocyst is unlikely to resolve when persistent for greater than 6 weeks, in the presence of chronic pancreatitis, a thick cyst wall on ultrasound, and a pancreatic duct abnormality other than communication with the pseudocyst [22]. In the setting of chronic pancreatitis, the authors concluded that internal drainage procedures should be performed at the time of diagnosis to avoid unnecessary additional expense and potential increased complications [22]. Serum levels of old amylase may help guide the optimal drainage time indicating a mature pseudocyst [22].

*Recommendation*: There are no published randomized controlled trials in the literature that define the optimal time of intervention for PPs. Evidence from highly selected multiple case series, case reports, and review articles support an expectant approach in patients with asymptomatic pseudocysts following acute pancreatitis regardless of size for a minimum of 6 weeks after diagnosis. In the setting of chronic pancreatitis immediate intervention is feasible, and may reduce the incidence of potential complications (Level III evidence; Grade C recommendation).

### 59.1.5 What are the Optimal Imaging Modalities for the Diagnosis of a Pancreatic Pseudocyst?

A variety of radiological techniques are utilized in diagnosis, monitoring, and planning of therapeutic intervention for PPs including transabdominal ultrasonography, contrast-enhanced abdominal CT (CECT), magnetic resonance imaging (MRI), and magnetic resonance cholangiopancreatography. Combined radiological and endoscopic modalities include endoscopic retrograde cholangiopancreatography (ERCP) and endoscopic ultrasound (EUS). Upper gastrointestinal endoscopy can be performed to plan endoscopic or surgical drainage. However, prospective data from randomized controlled trials and large patient series comparing currently available imaging modalities are lacking. CECT is the preferred and most commonly utilized modality to facilitate the accurate diagnosis, define extent of disease, and plan percutaneous intervention if appropriate [27]. Balthazar's CT severity index, based on combined assessments of peripancreatic inflammatory collections and degree of pancreatic necrosis, can be used to predict morbidity and mortality in patients with severe acute pancreatitis [27]. However, the CT appearances cannot characterize the local complications of acute pancreatitis, and in the acute phase cannot predict the development or extent of pseudocyst formation. Controversies exist regarding interobserver variability in interpretation of CECT, and the varying definitions used to define APFCs including PPs. A recent study performed to assess the interobserver agreement of categorizing peripancreatic collections on CECT using the Atlanta classification in patients with acute necrotizing pancreatitis, who underwent surgery from 2000 to 2003, involving five radiologists from 11 hospitals demonstrated poor concordance despite the radiologists' awareness of the clinical condition of the patient and the timing of the scan. All five radiologists agreed in only 4% of 70 cases, four of five agreed in 19%, and three agreed in 60% using terminology defined by the Atlanta criteria to define CECT findings [28]. In most published series the differentiation between an acute fluid collection and a pseudocyst was determined 4 weeks from onset of disease, however, different time periods have been described from 3 to 8 weeks [29–31]. In further publications, pseudocysts have been defined as collections containing fluid and necrotic debris [32–34]. As previously stated pseudocysts should be devoid of solid necrotic debris. Controversy also exists in correctly differentiating pseudocysts and pancreatic abscesses as CECT has a low sensitivity in the detection of necrotic debris in collections predominantly containing fluid, and poor discriminatory ability between sterile and infected collections [11,26,35]. Misinterpretation of CECT findings may result in instrumentation of sterile collections causing infection, or a delay in appropriate intervention. MRI and EUS can more accurately detect the presence of necrotic debris, and may be of additional benefit in guiding appropriate intervention [26,35].

*Recommendation*: There are no published randomized controlled trials in the literature to define the optimal imaging modality in the diagnosis and management of PPs. Evidence from multiple case series, case reports, and review articles support CECT as the imaging modality of choice. Prior to anticipated intervention, an MRI scan or EUS should be performed to exclude necrotic debris in the collection (Level III evidence; Grade C recommendation).

### 59.1.6 What is the Optimal Method of Therapeutic Intervention?

Indications for intervention include symptomatic, large (>6 cm diameter), enlarging, and complicated pseudocysts, and where there is a suspicion of an underlying malignancy [2,18,22]. Options include percutaneous external drainage, ERCP with transpapillary pancreatic duct stenting, endoscopic internal drainage, laparoscopic, laparoscopic-assisted, or open surgical internal drainage and/or resection [33,36–39]. Factors that determine the approach and timing of intervention include etiology, maturity of the cyst wall, cyst location, the presence or absence of complications, and the availability of local expertise [18,22,24,25,37]. Percutaneous drainage is generally performed under CT guidance to diagnose and/or drain septic foci in infected PPs, or in patients with symptomatic or complicated pseudocysts that are medically unfit to undergo a more definitive procedure [10,39]. In a recent series by Ocampo et al., CT guided percutaneous and endoscopic drainage were successful in controlling sepsis in 11 of 13 patients (85%)

with severe organ failure and facilitated subsequent definitive surgical management [10,39].

Open surgical drainage as an initial therapeutic option has been largely replaced by minimally invasive techniques including endoscopic and laparoscopic approaches [36]. Endoscopic drainage can be performed transmurally through the wall of the stomach or duodenum, or transpapillary via the pancreatic duct [33,36,41]. Transpapillary drainage is performed when the PP is demonstrated to communicate with the main pancreatic duct at ERCP, or in the presence of a distal pancreatic duct stricture. Laparoscopic techniques include endogastric, transgastric, or exogastric cystgastrostomy, roux en Y or loop cystjejunostomy [36].

In Aljarabah et al.'s [36] review of the published literature on laparoscopic and endoscopic approaches to internal drainage of PPs from 1974 to 2005, the mean cyst diameter was significantly smaller in the endoscopic group with a mean cyst diameter of 7 cm compared to 13 cm in the laparoscopic group. The success rate in achieving pseudocyst drainage and resolution was higher after the laparoscopic (98.3%) compared to the endoscopic (80.8%) approach. Postprocedural complications were observed in 4.2% of patients after laparoscopic versus 12% after endoscopic drainage. Two patients died after endoscopic drainage (mortality rate 0.35%) with no deaths after laparoscopic drainage. The mean follow-up period was longer at 24 months (range 0.5–70) after endoscopic than laparoscopic drainage at 13 months (range 1–59) with reported recurrence in 14.4% and 2.5%, respectively [36].

Seifert et al.'s study [44] focused on transluminal retroperitoneal endoscopy for debridement of solid infected necrosis in the setting of severe necrotizing pancreatitis. This was a retrospective multicenter study with long-term prospective follow-up involving six different medical centers (Level III evidence). Fifty-four of the 93 patients had previously undergone percutaneous radiologic drainage and/or transgastric stent drainage. All 93 patients underwent an initial session with transgastric (80 patients) or transduodenal (12 patients) access to the retroperitoneum via endoscopic or endosonographic guidance, followed by stent(s) insertion. The following session consisted of balloon dilation for the introduction of a gastroscope into the retroperitoneum for subsequent "forceful" irrigation and suction as well as endoscopic removal of necrotic tissue and debris. Patients underwent further endoscopic sessions at 1–4 days until vital structures were visible at the walls of the collection (this represents a mean of 6.2 sessions with a range of 1–35 sessions per patient). Finally, stent drainage of the empty cavity continued for 6–12 weeks and was reassessed afterward using CT or US.

The primary end point for this study was long-term clinical success of endoscopic necrosectomy defined as a symptom-free state requiring no further interventions, with a mean long-term follow-up of 44 months (range 4–96 months). Clinical failure was defined as a persistent collection, need for other interventions, failure to significantly improve symptoms, the presence of complications requiring the use of a different treatment modality (such as surgery), and death. Initial clinical success was based on the initial 30 days of follow-up. Seventy-five of 86 patients (87%) underwent endotherapy and were clinically successful initially, 57 of 86 endotherapy patients (66%) were clinically successful long-term, 14 of 93 patients (15%) were converted to surgery, 14 of 93 patients (15%) died during the study period. This study is limited by the fact that it is a retrospective review, albeit with prospective follow-up. It lacks a formal comparison group: the surgical group was composed of patients who had failed endotherapy, required emergent management, or suffered a complication. Finally, more than half of the patients had previously undergone endoscopic or percutaneous drainage procedures for management of necrotic pancreatic or peripancreatic collections [44].

The only known randomized controlled trial evaluating the management of necrotizing pancreatitis is the minimally invasive step-up approach versus maximal necrosectomy in patients with acute necrotizing pancreatitis, published in 2010 (Level I evidence). The PANTER trial [45] prospectively followed patients from 2005 to 2008 in 7 university hospital medical centers and 12 large teaching hospitals from the Dutch Pancreatitis Study Group. Patients with infected pancreatic or peripancreatic necrosis either confirmed (by fine-needle aspiration, open drainage, or presence of gas within the fluid collection) or suspected (progressive clinical deterioration despite maximal intensive care unit support or persistent sepsis) were randomly allocated to the minimally invasive "step-up approach" or to open necrosectomy followed by post operative lavage (traditional approach). The "step-up approach" consists of retroperitoneal percutaneous drainage of pancreatic or peripancreatic collections, with preference for left retroperitoneal access due to seamless transition to video-assisted retroperitoneal debridement (VARD). From 43 patients managed with the "step-up approach," 35% of patients were successfully managed with percutaneous drainage alone, whereas in 60% of patients percutaneous drainage was followed by VARD. In 33% of these patients, additional interventions were necessary for either further necrosectomy or for management of complications. In 27% of these patients, additional percutaneous drainage was warranted. In the 44 patients undergoing open necrosectomy followed by postoperative lavage, 19 patients (42%) required further management. This included open laparotomy surgery for sepsis

(8 of 44 patients), complications (5 of 44 patients), or both (6 of 44 patients). Of note, 15 patients (33%) ultimately required percutaneous drainage.

The primary end point of the PANTER trial was death during admission or within 3 months after discharge or a composite of major complications including new-onset multiple organ failure, systemic complications, enterocutaneous fistula, perforation of a visceral organ, or intra-abdominal bleeding requiring intervention. The primary end point was reached in 31 of 45 patients (69%) in the open necrosectomy group. It was reached in 17 of 43 patients (40%) in the "step-up approach" group. The risk ratio with the "step-up approach" was 0.57 with a 95% confidence interval, 0.38–0.87, $p = 0.006$. New-onset multiple organ failure and multiple systemic complications were significantly ($p = 0.001$) more common in the open necrosectomy group. Death rate between groups was not significantly different (8 of 43 patients [19%] in the "step-up approach" group and 7 of 45 patients [16% in the open necrosectomy group, $p = 0.70$]). At 6 months of follow-up the open necrosectomy group demonstrated significantly higher rate of incisional hernias (24% versus 7%, $p = 0.03$), new-onset diabetes (38% versus 16%, $p = 0.02$) and use of pancreatic enzymes (33% versus 7%, $p = 0.002$). With regards to healthcare costs, the "step-up approach" represented a 12% cost reduction with a mean difference of $15,963 per patient. The difference in mean total cost between groups was statistically significant with a $p$ value of 0.004 [45].

*Recommendation*: Minimally invasive internal drainage techniques by endoscopic and laparoscopic approaches are commonly employed. These two approaches are safe with minimal morbidity and mortality. Although laparoscopic drainage has a higher success rate in achieving pseudocyst drainage and resolution, a lower postprocedural complication rate, and a lower recurrence rate, reported follow-up periods are significantly shorter. The heterogeneity of the published reports and the lack of consistency of reported data limit direct comparison between endoscopic and laparoscopic techniques. Endotherapy via transmural endoscopic or endosonographic stent placement initially, followed by balloon dilation and serial endoscopic irrigation/suction and debris removal and final 6–12-week stent drainage yields a 66% success rate but these data are retrospective and limited by a lack of comparison group. Randomized controlled trials are warranted to further elucidate outcome superiority between endoscopic and laparoscopic techniques. However, the only known randomized controlled trial is based on the laparoscopic approach and demonstrates that the minimally invasive "step-up approach" is clinically and economically superior to the traditional open necrosectomy with lavage (Levels I–II evidence; Grade A recommendation).

### 59.1.7 Do Delays in Surgical Intervention Affect Outcome?

Initial interventions in the management of PPs are increasingly directed toward nonsurgical therapies including percutaneous external drainage or endoscopic approaches due to the perceived benefits of reduced invasiveness, and lower morbidity and mortality rates. However, these techniques can be associated with significant failure rates and complications [35,41,42]. Subsequent surgical intervention is often required as a salvage procedure to treat persistent or recurrent pseudocysts, or complications such as infection following percutaneous drainage [35,41,43]. Some authors have suggested that primary nonoperative intervention with delayed surgery is associated with a higher incidence of postoperative complications, readmission, morbidity, and mortality [41,44]. Rao et al. retrospectively reviewed outcome in 52 patients who underwent early surgical intervention compared to 18 who underwent delayed surgery after failed CT and endoscopic drainage [41]. Perioperative morbidity was twice as frequent in the delayed surgery group (33% versus 14%), with increased time to PP resolution from the initial drainage attempt [41]. In a study by Ito et al., 284 consecutive patients admitted with PPs over a 15 and a half year period were identified retrospectively, of which 46 underwent initial operative intervention [44]. Percutaneous drainage was performed in 89 patients of whom 42 required subsequent surgical intervention for failure, while endoscopic drainage was performed in 73 patients of whom 33 required subsequent surgical intervention for failure. There was no significant difference in patient demographics, etiology of pancreatitis, location, number, and diameter of pseudocysts, or morphology of the main pancreatic duct in patients treated with initial surgery versus those undergoing delayed surgery. However, the median time from diagnosis to surgery was three times longer in the delayed surgery group. The main indication for intervention in the delayed group was pseudocyst infection in 43% versus 13% in the early group. The delayed surgery group had a significantly higher incidence of postoperative pancreatic complications, infectious complications, perioperative morbidity, and readmission rates. Five patients died in the postoperative period due to sepsis in two and organ failure secondary to necrotizing pancreatitis in the remainder. On univariate analysis failure of nonsurgical intervention was associated with pseudocyst diameter ≥6 cm, main pancreatic duct stricture, ≥2 nonsurgical interventional procedures, and pseudocyst infection [44].

*Recommendation*: Surgical intervention after failed nonoperative drainage procedures is associated with higher incidences of postoperative infection, pancreatic complications, morbidity, mortality, and readmission rates (Level III evidence; Grade C recommendation; Table 59.1).

**TABLE 59.1**

Summary of Evidence and Recommendations

| No. | Question | Answer | Grade of Recommendation | Level of Evidence | References |
|---|---|---|---|---|---|
| 1. | What is the definition of a pancreatic pseudocyst (PP)? | The 2013 Atlanta classification system defines a PP as a walled-off and well-circumscribed fluid-only peripancreatic collection with no associated necrosis or infection | C | 2 | [7,8] |
| 2. | What is the incidence of PPs? | The true incidence of PP is unknown | C | 4 | [9–11] |
| 3. | What is the incidence of complicated PPs? | The true incidence of complicated PP is unknown | C | 4 | [9,10,12–18] |
| 4. | What is the optimal time for intervention once the diagnosis of PP has been confirmed? | The optimal time of intervention for PPs is unknown, but timing of intervention is determined by etiology, symptoms, and complications | C | 3 | [9,15,17–24,26] |
| 5. | What are the optimal imaging modalities for diagnosis of a PP? | CECT is the imaging modality of choice. Prior to intervention, an MRI or EUS should be performed to exclude necrotic debris | C | 3 | [26–35] |
| 6. | What is the optimal method of therapeutic intervention? | The optimal approach to PP drainage is the "step-up approach" which is clinically safe and economic | A | 1 | [44,45] |
| 7. | Do delays in surgical intervention affect outcome? | Surgical intervention after failed nonoperative drainage is associated with a worse outcome | C | 3 | [40,41,44] |

## References


1. Whitcomb DC. Clinical practice. Acute pancreatitis. *N Engl J Med.* May 18, 2006;354(20):2142–2150.
2. Rosao EL, Sonnenday CJ, Lillemoe KD, Yeo CJ. 2007. Pseudocysts and other complications of pancreatitis. In: Yeo CJ, ed. *Shackelford' Surgery of the Alimentary Tract*, 6th edn. Saunders: Philadelphia, PA, pp. 1329–1357.
3. Kawakami H, Kuwatani M, Shinada K, Yamato H, Hirano S, Kondo S, Yonemori A, Itoh T, Matsuno Y, Asaka M. Autoimmune pancreatitis associated with hemorrhagic pseudocysts: A case report and literature review. *Intern Med.* 2008;47(7):603–608.
4. Welsch T, Kleeff J, Esposito I, Buchler MW, Friess H. Autoimmune pancreatitis associated with a large pancreatic pseudocyst. *World J Gastroenterol.* September 28, 2006;12(36):5904–5906.
5. Lin BC, Fang JF, Wong YC, Liu NJ. Blunt pancreatic trauma and pseudocyst: Management of major pancreatic duct injury. *Injury.* May 2007;38(5):588–593.
6. Yamaguchi T, Takahashi H, Kagawa R, Takeda R, Sakata S, Yamamoto M, Nishizaki D. Huge pseudocyst of the pancreas caused by poorly differentiated invasive ductal adenocarcinoma with osteoclast-like giant cells: Report of a case. *Hepatogastroenterology.* March 2007;54(74):599–601.
7. Banks PA, Bollen TL, Dervenis C, Gooszen HG, Johnson CD, Sarr MG, Tsiotos GG, Vege SS. Acute Pancreatitis Classification Working Group. Classification of acute pancreatitis—2012: Revision of the Atlanta classification and definitions by international consensus. *Gut.* January 2013;62(1):102–111.
8. Sarr MG. 2012 revision of the Atlanta classification of acute pancreatitis. *Pol Arch Med Wewn.* 2013;123(3):118–124.
9. Lenhart DK, Balthazar EJ. MDCT of acute mild (non-necrotizing) pancreatitis: Abdominal complications and fate of fluid collections. *AJR Am J Roentgenol.* March 2008;190(3):643–649.
10. Ocampo C, Oria A, Zandalazini H, Silva W, Kohan G, Chiapetta L, Alvarez J. Treatment of acute pancreatic pseudocysts after severe acute pancreatitis. *J Gastrointest Surg.* March 2007;11(3):357–363.
11. Baron TH, Morgan DE, Vickers SM, Lazenby AJ. Organized pancreatic necrosis: Endoscopic, radiologic, and pathologic features of a distinct clinical entity. *Pancreas.* July 1999;19(1):105–108.
12. Boudaya MS, Alifano M, Baccari S, Regnard JF. Hemothorax as the clinical presentation of a pancreaticopleural fistula: Report of a case. *Surg Today.* 2007;37(6):518–520.
13. Rigaux J, Poreddy V, Al-Kawas F. Intraperitoneal and retroperitoneal hemorrhage associated with coumadin-induced bleeding into a pancreatic pseudocyst. *Clin Gastroenterol Hepatol.* June 2007;5(6):A32.
14. Yoon SE, Lee YH, Yoon KH, Choi CS, Kim HC, Chae KM. Spontaneous pancreatic pseudocyst-portal vein fistula presenting with pancreatic ascites: Strength of MR cholangiopancreatography. *Br J Radiol.* January 2008;81(961):e13–e16.

15. Yeo CJ, Bastidas JA, Lynch-Nyhan A, Fishman EK, Zinner MJ, Cameron JL. The natural history of pancreatic pseudocysts documented by computed tomography. *Surg Gynecol Obstet.* May 1990;170(5):411–417.
16. Beger HG, Rau B, Isenmann R. Prevention of severe change in acute pancreatitis: Prediction and prevention. *J Hepatobiliary Pancreat Surg.* 2001;8(2):140–147.
17. Kourtesis G, Wilson SE, Williams RA. The clinical significance of fluid collections in acute pancreatitis. *Am Surg.* December 1990;56(12):796–799.
18. Bradley EL, Clements JL, Jr., Gonzalez AC. The natural history of pancreatic pseudocysts: A unified concept of management. *Am J Surg.* January 1979;137(1):135–141.
19. Aghdassi AA, Mayerle J, Kraft M, Sielenkamper AW, Heidecke CD, Lerch MM. Pancreatic pseudocysts—When and how to treat? *HPB (Oxford).* 2006;8(6):432–441.
20. Cooperman AM. An overview of pancreatic pseudocysts: The emperor's new clothes revisited. *Surg Clin North Am.* April 2001;81(2):391–397, xii.
21. Andren-Sandberg A, Dervenis C. Pancreatic pseudocysts in the 21st century. Part I: Classification, pathophysiology, anatomic considerations and treatment. *JOP.* January 2004;5(1):8–24.
22. Warshaw AL, Rattner DW. Timing of surgical drainage for pancreatic pseudocyst. Clinical and chemical criteria. *Ann Surg.* December 1985;202(6):720–724.
23. Vitas GJ, Sarr MG. Selected management of pancreatic pseudocysts: Operative versus expectant management. *Surgery.* February 1992;111(2):123–130.
24. Warren WD, Marsh WM, Mullen WH, Jr. Experimental production of pseudocysts of the pancreas with preliminary observations on internal drainage. *Surg Gynaecol Obstet.* 1957;105:385.
25. Frey CF. Pancreatic pseudocyst—Operative strategy. *Ann Surg.* November 1978;188(5):652–662.
26. Bollen TL, van Santvoort HC, Besselink MG, van Es WH, Gooszen HG, van Leeuwen MS. Update on acute pancreatitis: Ultrasound, computed tomography, and magnetic resonance imaging features. *Semin Ultrasound CT MR.* October 2007;28(5):371–383.
27. Balthazar EJ, Robinson DL, Megibow AJ, Ranson JH. Acute pancreatitis: Value of CT in establishing prognosis. *Radiology.* February 1990;174(2):331–336.
28. Besselink MG, van Santvoort HC, Bollen TL, van Leeuwen MS, Lameris JS, van der Jagt EJ, Strijk SP, Buskens E, Freeny PC, Gooszen HG. Describing computed tomography findings in acute necrotizing pancreatitis with the Atlanta classification: An interobserver agreement study. *Pancreas.* November 2006;33(4):331–335.
29. De WJ, Vogelaers D, Decruyenaere J, De VM, Colardyn F. Infectious complications of acute pancreatitis. *Acta Clin Belg.* March 2004;59(2):90–96.
30. Soliani P, Franzini C, Ziegler S, Del RP, Dell'Abate P, Piccolo D, Japichino GG, Cavestro GM, Di MF, Sianesi M. Pancreatic pseudocysts following acute pancreatitis: Risk factors influencing therapeutic outcomes. *JOP.* September 2004;5(5):338–347.
31. Zhou ZG, Zheng YC, Shu Y, Hu WM, Tian BL, Li QS, Zhang ZD. Laparoscopic management of severe acute pancreatitis. *Pancreas.* October 2003;27(3):e46–e50.
32. Andren-Sandberg A, Ansorge C, Eiriksson K, Glomsaker T, Maleckas A. Treatment of pancreatic pseudocysts. *Scand J Surg.* 2005;94(2):165–175.
33. Kruger M, Schneider AS, Manns MP, Meier PN. Endoscopic management of pancreatic pseudocysts or abscesses after an EUS-guided 1-step procedure for initial access. *Gastrointest Endosc.* March 2006;63(3):409–416.
34. Nealon WH, Walser E. Surgical management of complications associated with percutaneous and/or endoscopic management of pseudocyst of the pancreas. *Ann Surg.* June 2005;241(6):948–957.
35. Merkle EM, Gorich J. Imaging of acute pancreatitis. *Eur Radiol.* August 2002;12(8):1979–1992.
36. Aljarabah M, Ammori BJ. Laparoscopic and endoscopic approaches for drainage of pancreatic pseudocysts: A systematic review of published series. *Surg Endosc.* November 2007;21(11):1936–1944.
37. Palanivelu C, Senthilkumar K, Madhankumar MV, Rajan PS, Shetty AR, Jani K, Rangarajan M, Maheshkumaar GS. Management of pancreatic pseudocyst in the era of laparoscopic surgery–Experience from a tertiary centre. *Surg Endosc.* December 2007;21(12):2262–2267.
38. Pryor A, Means JR, Pappas TN. Laparoscopic distal pancreatectomy with splenic preservation. *Surg Endosc.* December 2007;21(12):2326–2330.
39. Stiles GM, Berne TV, Thommen VD, Molgaard CP, Boswell WD. Fine needle aspiration of pancreatic fluid collections. *Am Surg.* December 1990;56(12):764–768.
40. Rao R, Fedorak I, Prinz RA. Effect of failed computed tomography-guided and endoscopic drainage on pancreatic pseudocyst management. *Surgery.* October 1993;114(4):843–847.
41. Bartoli E, Delcenserie R, Yzet T, Brazier F, Geslin G, Regimbeau JM, Dupas JL. Endoscopic treatment of chronic pancreatitis. *Gastroenterol Clin Biol.* May 2005;29(5):515–521.
42. Jacobson BC, Baron TH, Adler DG et al. ASGE guideline: The role of endoscopy in the diagnosis and the management of cystic lesions and inflammatory fluid collections of the pancreas. *Gastrointest Endosc.* March 2005;61(3):363–370.
43. Ito K, Perez A, Ito H, Whang EE. Pancreatic pseudocysts: Is delayed surgical intervention associated with adverse outcomes? *J Gastrointest Surg.* October 2007;11(10):1317–1321.
44. Seifert H, Biermer M, Schmitt W. Transluminal endoscopic necrosectomy after acute pancreatitis: A multicentre study with long-term follow-up (the GEPARD Study). *Gut.* April 2009;58:1260–1266.
45. Van Santvoort HC, Besselink MG, Bakker OJ. A step-up approach or open necrosectomy for necrotizing pancreatitis. *N Engl J Med.* April 2010;362:1491–1502.

## Commentary on Pancreatic Pseudocysts

*Lewis Flint*

Reading the very thorough review of the clinical problem of pancreatic pseudocysts by Tucker et al. gave me the opportunity to reflect on the changes that have occurred over my surgical career (which now spans more than four decades) in our understanding of the natural history of pancreatic pseudocysts, the impact of precise diagnosis, and carefully thought-out treatment strategies on clinical outcomes, and the trend toward less invasive approaches to management.

I spent my clinical years practicing in public, safety net hospitals. The lesson learned about pancreatic pseudocysts that seems important, upon reflection, is that published clinical results differ largely because of differences in the patient population that is being reported. The peripancreatic fluid collections that I encountered arose mostly in patients with alcoholic pancreatitis and this meant that outcomes were impacted significantly by the severity of the complications of alcoholism (primarily hepatic cirrhosis and malnutrition) as well as the comorbid conditions that commonly accompanied long-standing alcohol abuse such as lung and cardiovascular disease in large part due to tobacco use. The chapter authors note that there is significant heterogeneity in the published literature about pancreatic pseudocysts and I am fairly certain that much of this is due to differing proportions of patients with alcoholic, biliary, and "idiopathic" pancreatitis in the patient cohorts in published reports.

We have learned much about the natural history of peripancreatic fluid collections and pancreatic pseudocysts. Pancreatic and peripancreatic necrosis due to severe inflammation was, in the early part of my career, assumed to be destined to become infected and stimulate the systemic inflammatory response syndrome leading to multiple organ failure. We used the same approach to this condition as we did to severe burns and performed early debridement. We learned, probably after too much delay, that necrosis was not uniformly destined to become infected and could be treated expectantly if evidence of infection or progression of organ failure was not present. As the authors note, the Atlanta classification system* for pancreatitis has assisted us in determining disease severity and monitoring the course of the disease and this information has informed clinical decision-making. What has been learned about the natural history of peripancreatic fluid collections and pancreatic pseudocysts has been translated into clinical practice guidelines. The guidelines promulgated by the American College of Gastroenterology† provide a strong recommendation that an expectant approach be used in stable patients without organ failure or evidence of infection. We have also learned that peripancreatic fluid collections due to acute pancreatitis almost always resolve and do not need to be drained unless symptomatic tense ascites or pleural effusion occurs. Our belief that complications of pseudocysts increase with increasing size of the cyst has also been challenged and the clinical practice guidelines† recommend, based on "strong" evidence, that asymptomatic pseudocysts be managed nonoperatively regardless of pseudocyst size.

Obviously, other factors need to be considered when deciding about the need for a surgical approach to patients with pancreatic pseudocysts. Cyst location may be important; we know that cysts adjacent to major visceral arteries carry a risk of pseudoaneurysm formation and bleeding. Cysts adjacent to mesenteric veins may cause venous thrombosis that results in left-sided portal hypertension and a risk of variceal bleeding‡§.

Pseudocysts that are associated with pancreatic ductal strictures or ductal disruption require careful definition of ductal anatomy. As the authors point out, ductal anatomy is a key factor in determining the need for and technique of pseudocyst management. What is the take-home message from these lessons learned? Successful management of patients with pancreatic pseudocysts will probably require a multidisciplinary team to facilitate diagnosis and management. Such a team would probably need participation by gastroenterologists and/or surgeons with endoscopic expertise so that cyst anatomy could be carefully defined (using endoscopic ultrasound, for example). The presence of debris and septations in the cyst demonstrated on endoscopic ultrasound suggests the diagnosis of cystic pancreatic neoplasm rather than pseudocyst.

* Banks PA, Bollen TL, Dervenis C et al. Classification of acute pancreatitis—2012: Revision of the Atlanta classification and definitions by international consensus. *Gut*. 2013;62(1):102–111.

† Tenner S, Baillie J, DeWitt J et al. American College of Gastroenterology guideline: Management of acute pancreatitis. *Am J Gastroenterol*. 2013;108(9):1400–1416.

‡ Nadkarni NA, Khanna S, Vege SS. Splanchnic venous thrombosis and pancreatitis. *Pancreas*. 2013;42(6):924–931.

§ Easler J, Muddana V, Furlan A et al. Portosplenomesenteric venous thrombosis in patients with acute pancreatitis is associated with pancreatic necrosis and usually has a benign course. *Clin Gastroenterol Hepatol*. 2014;12(5):854–862.

Ductal anatomy can be defined using magnetic resonance imaging. Because of this, the team needs to have a radiologist to provide accurate interpretation of imaging. Endoscopic retrograde cholangiopancreatography (ERCP) will serve diagnostic and therapeutic functions. Surgeons and/or gastroenterologists with endoscopic expertise will be needed to perform these procedures. We know that patients who are diagnosed with "idiopathic" pancreatitis often have sphincter of Oddi dysfunction and can be treated with endoscopic sphincterotomy. Patients with pseudocysts or chronic pancreatitis with ductal strictures can have these defined and, sometimes, treated using ERCP; for patients requiring operation for management of pseudocysts or ductal obstruction, ERCP is performed shortly before the operative procedure to carefully define ductal anatomy. Chronic pancreatitis with multiple ductal strictures will occasionally produce intrapancreatic pseudocysts that will need to be treated using ductal decompression procedures such as the Frey procedure or the Beger procedure*. Patients with pancreatic ductal disruption present a specific array of challenges. Precise definition of the ductal anatomy is necessary to determine the proper approach and preoperative angioembolization can be used to reduce the risk of severe intraoperative hemorrhage†. The team will, therefore, need to have access to an interventional radiologist. The value of a team approach to patients with pancreatic pseudocysts was suggested in the Swedish national study reported by Andersson and coauthors‡ and the importance of the multidisciplinary team approach is further supported by the success of the team review of therapeutic strategies in the prospective, randomized study of the "step-up" approach to treatment of infected pancreatic necrosis§.

The final important trend I would like to comment on is the increasing use of minimally invasive approaches for management of pancreatic necrosis and pancreatic pseudocysts. Available research supports the usefulness of laparoscopic cystogastrostomy or cyst enterostomy¶**. There is also evidence of the value of endoscopic cyst gastrostomy†† accomplished by placing a stent through the gastric wall into a pseudocyst that is located adjacent to the stomach. The main disadvantage of the endoscopic approaches is the need for multiple procedures; the mean number of procedures needed averages four. An alternative approach that places a large diameter stent through the gastric wall into the pseudocyst or area of infected necrosis using a laparoscopic, transgastric approach may have value as a means of reducing the number of procedures needed and this approach should be evaluated further‡‡.

I enjoyed reading the chapter by Tucker et al and I recommend it to the surgeons at all career levels who need carefully evaluated information regarding the management of pancreatic pseudocysts. The trends that interested me, and other trends as well, need to be followed carefully by surgeons so that the outcomes of our patients with acute and chronic pancreatitis can continue to improve.

* Andersen DK, Frey CF. The evolution of the surgical treatment of chronic pancreatitis. *Ann Surg.* 2010;251(1):18–32.

† Fischer TD, Gutman DS, Hughes SJ et al. Disconnected pancreatic duct syndrome: Disease classification and management strategies. *J Am Coll Surg* 2014 October;219(4):704–712.

‡ Andersson B, Andren-Sandberg A, Andersson R. Survey of the management of pancreatic pseudocysts in Sweden. *Scand J Gastroenterol.* 2009;44(10):1252–1258.

§ van Santvoort HC, Besselink MG, Bakker OJ et al. A step-up approach or open necrosectomy for necrotizing pancreatitis. *N Engl J Med.* 2010;362(16):1491–1502.

¶ Khaled YS, Malde DJ, Packer J et al. Laparoscopic versus open cystgastrostomy for pancreatic pseudocysts: A case-matched comparative study. *J Hepatobiliary Pancreat Sci.* 2014 November;21(11):818–823.

** Gibson SC, Robertson BF, Dickson EJ et al. 'Step-port' laparoscopic cystgastrostomy for the management of organized solid predominant post-acute fluid collections after severe acute pancreatitis. *HPB (Oxford).* 2014;16(2):170–176.

†† Varadarajulu S, Bang JY, Sutton BS et al. Equal efficacy of endoscopic and surgical cystogastrostomy for pancreatic pseudocyst drainage in a randomized trial. *Gastroenterology.* 2013;145(3):583–590.e1.

‡‡ Worhunsky DJ, Qadan M, Dua MM et al. Laparoscopic transgastric necrosectomy for the management of pancreatic necrosis. *J Am Coll Surg.* 2014;219(4):735–743.

# 60

# Liver Abscess

**David M. Levi and Andreas G. Tzakis**

**CONTENTS**



## 60.1 Introduction

Among the various infectious diseases that affect the liver, pyogenic abscess and amebic abscess have classically been the concern of the surgeon. The fundamentals of our understanding of pyogenic and amebic abscesses can be traced to two seminal publications by Ochsner and DeBakey in the 1930s [1,2]. Yet, from the critical perspective of evidence-based practice, these papers present level 4 data. Liver abscesses result from varied etiologies, may be isolated to the liver or occur in the context of multiorgan involvement, and occur in a heterogeneous patient population, making rigorous, high-level clinical studies difficult to perform. The high morbidity and mortality associated with liver abscess is proof that clinically relevant questions regarding its diagnosis and management remain inadequately answered. Recently, trials that address specific aspects of the treatment of liver abscess have emerged that meet the high standards of evidence-based practice and will be noted in this chapter.

## 60.2 Epidemiology

Pyogenic liver abscesses are relatively uncommon; their incidence varies by geographic region and patient population. In 1938, Ochsner et al. reported an incidence of 8 per 100,000 admissions at New Orleans' Charity Hospital [2]. A large series from the Johns Hopkins Hospital in Baltimore reported that from 1973 to 1993 the incidence rose from 13 to 20 per 100,000 hospital admissions and that the increase was attributed to the increase in patients seen during that time interval with malignant disease, especially hepatobiliary and pancreatic cancer [3]. Does this change reflect a true increase in incidence or simply the experience of the authors? The inherent limitation of case series limits a high-level, evidence-based answer. A group from Alberta, Canada reported an incidence of 2.3 per 100,000 hospital admissions, the majority of patients being male and older [4]. In most large case series, the average patient age is the fifth and sixth decades of life, with a slight predominance of men [3–5]. Pyogenic liver abscesses are more common in Asia; a retrospective series from Taiwan reported an incidence of 17.6 per 100,000 population [6]. The authors speculate that different bacteriology and patient factors accounts for this variation. In a large, population-based study of U.S. data involving over 17,000 patients from 1994 to 2005, the overall incidence of pyogenic liver abscess was 3.6 per 100,000 population with an inhospital mortality of 5.6% [7].

Amebic abscesses result from infection with the protozoan parasite *Entamoeba histolytica*. The liver is the most common extraintestinal site of ameba infection. The organism is found throughout the world and infection is common in places with inadequate sanitation. In the United States, the amebic liver disease is seen predominantly in individuals who have traveled to or have emigrated from endemic areas [8]. In adults, men are more commonly affected than women, while among children, boys and girls are equally affected. Possibly, the higher rate of alcohol use by men contributes to this difference.

Conditions that affect cell-mediated immunity, such as extremes of age, pregnancy, corticosteroid therapy, malignancy, and malnutrition, may also increase the chances that *E. histolytica* infection results in invasive disease with liver involvement [8].

## 60.3 Pathophysiology/Microbiology

Most pyogenic liver abscesses arise secondary to an infection that originates elsewhere in the body. They can be categorized by the mode of spread to the liver. Knowledge of these routes and mechanisms aids in diagnosis and often dictates treatment. The liver can become the site of abscess formation via (1) the biliary tree, from ascending cholangitis; (2) the portal vein, as in pylephlebitis resulting from appendicitis or diverticulitis; (3) the hepatic artery, as in bacteremia from endocarditis or an oral cavity abscess; (4) direct extension, from a contiguous disease process; and (5) post-traumatic, from penetrating injuries or iatrogenic events. Rarely no source is found.

In the past, the most common underlying etiology was acute appendicitis [2]. However, biliary tract pathology is now the most common cause of pyogenic liver abscess, accounting for 40%–60% of cases [9,10]. Malignant biliary obstruction has been noted to be a more frequent cause than in the past [3,11]. Pyogenic abscess formation as a procedure-related complication is being reported anecdotally in recent years. These iatrogenic events include abscess formation after biliary intervention, percutaneous liver biopsy, hepatic tumor ablation or embolization, hepatic artery thrombosis after liver transplantation, and hepatic artery or biliary injury during laparoscopic cholecystectomy [10,12–15].

The microbiology of pyogenic liver abscesses varies and often reflects the underlying etiology and route of liver involvement. Many liver abscesses are polymicrobial and include anaerobes. *Klebsiella pneumoniae, Escherichia coli,* and *Enterococcus* species predominate in series where biliary tract pathology is the common etiology [9]. In case series from New York and San Diego, *K. pneumoniae* was the most common cause of pyogenic liver abscess and was noted to be particularly virulent [9,11,16]. In Asia, especially Taiwan, *K. pneumoniae* is by far the most common pathogen and can be associated with bacteremia, meningitis, endophthalmitis, and necrotizing fasciitis especially in the diabetic or immunosuppressed host [17]. In the United States, a specific organism, is identified in nearly half of patients, and about half of those are bacteremic. The most common organisms cultured are *Enterococcus* species and *E. coli.* [7] *S. aureus, Streptococcus* species, *Pseudomonas aeruginosa* and *Candida* species are important but less common causative organisms [18,19]. Because the causative organism is unpredictable and may possess antibiotic resistance, cultures from the abscess (including those for anaerobic bacteria) and blood cultures are important for determining the optimal antimicrobial therapy.

Liver abscesses due to *E. histolytica* infection occur most commonly in patients that have spent time in an endemic area. Infection occurs when individuals ingest food or water contaminated with feces containing *E. histolytica*; sexual transmission is uncommon. While *E. histolytica* infection occurs in men and women equally, invasive amebic diseases, such as abscess formation, predominates in men at a ratio of about 3:1 [20]. Once ingested, the organism penetrates the intestinal mucosa eventually reaching the portal venous system. In the liver, *E. histolytica* has membrane-based molecules that shield it from complement-mediated lysis and releases proteases that destroy host IgA and IgG allowing abscess formation [8].

## 60.4 Clinical Presentation

Many of the clinical characteristics of pyogenic abscess and amebic abscess are similar, nonspecific, and are inconsistently present making their respective diagnosis dependent on adjunct testing and imaging. Pain, localized to the right upper quadrant and epigastrium, is common. Pain radiating to the right scapular region suggests right hemidiaphragm irritation. Fever is common; nausea and vomiting, weight loss, malaise, anorexia, chills are less common, and equally nonspecific [21–23]. Patients with amebiasis can have diarrhea from colitis and symptoms from a simultaneous liver abscess [8]. Elderly patients may present with only fever of unknown origin.

The physical examination findings of fever, upper abdominal tenderness, and hepatomegaly may suggest the diagnosis of a hepatic infection. These coupled with relevant historical clues may suggest the diagnosis. A history of travel to an endemic area may suggest amebic abscess while a recent biliary procedure or history of diverticulitis suggests pyogenic abscess. In a large series of adults in Pakistan, distinguishing between patients with pyogenic and amebic abscess was studied. The authors found that patients with pyogenic abscess were usually older with a history of diabetes, more likely to present with jaundice, and pulmonary findings. Patients with amebic abscess were younger with epigastric pain, lower serum albumin levels, and positive amebic titres [24]. It is unlikely that their conclusions hold true for patients in nonendemic areas.

## 60.5 What is the Optimal Diagnostic Strategy for Liver Abscess?

Diagnosis of and differentiation between pyogenic abscess and amebic abscess on clinical grounds may be impossible. As already mentioned, the clinical presentation varies and is usually nonspecific. Laboratory examinations may suggest an infection or inflammatory process. In a series of 63 patients with pyogenic liver abscesses reviewed at a single center in Australia, most patients had an elevated white blood cell count with neutrophils dominating. One-quarter of the patients were anemic and, in the 47 patients in whom it was measured, C-reactive protein level was elevated. Most patients had mild amino transaminase elevation and hyperbilirubinemia [25].

Modern abdominal imaging studies that exploit the nuanced radiographic characteristics of liver abscesses have become imperative for an accurate diagnosis. Computerized tomography (CT) is slightly superior to ultrasound (US) for detecting small liver abscesses; both have made radionucleotide scans second-line studies [4]. Magnetic resonance imaging (MRI) can occasionally be useful but does not add greatly to CT imaging. The literature provides little high-level evidence supporting the superiority of either CT or MRI. CT offers the potential for guided, diagnostic aspiration and therapeutic drainage; a distinct, practical advantage over MRI. Once a cystic liver lesion is identified to be a pyogenic abscess, CT- or US-guided aspiration of the cyst fluid is important for isolating the causative organism(s) and tailoring antimicrobial therapy. Image-guided aspiration/biopsy of a hepatic lesion may be essential to distinguish between liver abscess and benign and malignant neoplasms.

Pyogenic liver abscesses are solitary or multifocal discrete masses, usually round or lobulated. In the same series from Australia, two of three patients had solitary lesions with a median diameter of 6.3 cm [25]. Contrast-enhanced CT demonstrates peripheral rim enhancement with central low attenuation. Abscesses can be complex with loculations and may have an air-fluid level. In another recent series of 58 patients with pyogenic abscess, CT was the imaging study used for making the diagnosis in 56 cases, or 97% of the time [11].

CT and US are the imaging modalities of choice for diagnosing amebic liver abscess. Both are very sensitive but lack needed specificity. Imaging may reveal solitary or multiple lesions, usually less complex than pyogenic abscesses. Ultrasonographic features include a smooth wall, hypoechoic center with internal echoes. Because many amebic abscesses are treated nonoperatively, serial US examinations are useful for tracking the progress of medical therapy.

Serologic testing and analysis of aspirated cyst fluid are important for discerning amebic liver abscess from pyogenic liver abscess and other mass lesions of the liver. Patients with amebic abscess usually do not have concomitant intestinal involvement; thus *E. histolytica* antigen or DNA is usually not detected in the stool of affected patients. The detection of serum antibodies *E. histolytica* may be due to amebiasis in the past, limiting the tests' utility. Real-time DNA PCR assay of urine and saliva are important tests for making the diagnosis. When either urine or saliva are positive, *E. histolytica* DNA is detectable in the liver abscess 97% of the time [26].

*Answer:* Patients with liver abscess present with nonspecific symptoms and complaints, physical findings, and laboratory abnormalities. US, CT, and MRI are very sensitive studies but can be nonspecific. Definitive diagnosis may require image-guided aspiration and culture of the cyst fluid. The use of serologic testing for amebic abscess, while useful, has been supplanted by PCR testing for the causative organisms DNA. Recommendation: Grade B (Table 60.1).

## 60.6 What is the Treatment for Liver Abscess?

In recent years, evidenced-based studies have emerged that address controversies regarding the treatment of pyogenic and amebic liver abscess. The fundamental precepts guiding the treatment of pyogenic liver abscess are the administration of appropriate antibiotics and/or antifungal agents, drainage of the abscess, and treatment of the root cause. When the abscess is secondary to biliary obstruction, biliary drainage via the transhepatic or endoscopic retrograde route may be required.

Historically, open surgery with either abscess drainage or hepatic resection was regarded as the treatment of choice [4]. Percutaneous catheter drainage has developed with the emergence of interventional radiology, and has almost replaced open surgical drainage [11]. Correspondingly, there has been a significant decrease in mortality related to pyogenic abscess [9]. There are still proponents of open surgical drainage as more effective for patients with large, multifocal, and multiloculated abscesses, but the trend toward percutaneous drainage is clear [27]. In a nonrandomized series comparing open to percutaneous drainage, Ferraioli and colleagues reported no percutaneous drainage failures while open surgical drainage was associated with longer hospitalization and greater morbidity [28]. Contrastingly, in a series from China of 44 patients with pyogenic liver abscess complicating hepatobiliary or

**TABLE 60.1**

Evidence-Based Surgery Table

| Question | Answer | Levels of Evidence | Grade of Recommendation | References |
|---|---|---|---|---|
| What is the optimal diagnostic strategy for liver abscess? | Patients with liver abscess present with nonspecific symptoms and complaints, physical findings, and laboratory abnormalities. US, CT, and MRI are very sensitive studies but can be nonspecific. Definitive diagnosis may require image (CT or US)-guided aspiration and culture of the cyst fluid. The use of serologic testing for amebic abscess, while useful, has been supplanted by PCR testing for the causative organisms DNA. | 2–3 | B | [4,11,25,26] |
| What is the treatment for liver abscess? | The treatment of pyogenic liver abscess has become less invasive over the years, with percutaneous drainage and antibiotics supplanting surgery in most cases. An open or laparoscopic approach may be useful in selected cases, such as for multiloculated abscesses or when biliary pathology can be simultaneously addressed. Surgery should be considered early if percutaneous drainage is failing. Amebic liver abscess responds to medical treatment with metronidazole, although there is occasionally a role for percutaneous drainage or aspiration. | 2–3 | B | [4,8,9,11,27–33] |

pancreatic cancer, 15% or 34% of patients failed percutaneous catheter drainage; 12 required open surgery; 8 of whom experienced abscess resolution [29]. The authors concluded that patients with multiloculated abscesses or with abscesses that directly connect with the biliary tree were more likely to fail percutaneous catheter drainage and should be considered for early surgical intervention.

Small abscesses, defined as less than 3 cm may be treated with antibiotics alone in selected patients [30]. In a randomized trial of 64 patients, Yu and colleagues demonstrated that percutaneous aspiration without catheter placement was as effective as percutaneous drainage, with no difference in length of hospitalization or mortality [31].

Recently, the role of laparoscopic surgery for treating pyogenic liver abscess has been examined. In a series from Singapore of 85 patients, laparoscopic drainage was compared to percutaneous drainage. No difference in hospital length of stay or duration of antibiotic use was noted. The authors reported a lower failure rate with the laparoscopic approach but acknowledged their study is limited by its nonrandomized design and small sample size; there were just 18 patients in the laparoscopy group [32]. In another small, nonrandomized series, from China, 31 patients with biliary tract pathology and pyogenic liver abscess were treated with either open or laparoscopic surgery. A variety of procedures were performed including liver resection or abscess drainage and concomitant cholecystectomy with or without common bile duct exploration. Both approaches were equally safe and effective in treating the abscess and the underlying biliary tract pathology but the laparoscopic approach was associated with a quicker postoperative recovery of gastrointestinal function and a shorter postoperative hospital stay [33].

The mainstay of treatment for amebic liver abscess is metronidazole. The majority of patients will respond needing no drainage. There is controversy regarding the role of percutaneous drainage in the management of amebic liver abscess. It has been suggested that aspiration or drainage of large abscesses may shorten the time to resolution. In one detailed review, the author suggests that intervention beyond medical management should be reserved for patients for whom the diagnosis is uncertain, seriously ill patients that may benefit from more rapid treatment, and patients that have not responded as expected with resolution of fever and decreased abdominal pain within 4 days [8].

*Answer*: The treatment of pyogenic liver abscess has become less invasive over the years, with percutaneous drainage and antibiotics supplanting surgery in most cases. An open or laparoscopic approach may be useful in selected cases, such as for multiloculated abscesses or when biliary pathology can be simultaneously addressed. Surgery should be considered early if percutaneous drainage is failing. Amebic liver abscess responds to medical treatment with metronidazole, although there is occasionally a role for percutaneous drainage or aspiration. Recommendation: Grade B (Table 60.1).

## References

1. Ochsner A, DeBakey M. Liver abscess part I: Amebic abscess analysis of 73 cases. *Am J Surg.* 1935;29:173–194.
2. Ochsner A, DeBakey M, Murray S. Pyogenic abscess of the liver: II. An analysis of 47 cases with review of the literature. *Am J Surg.* 1938;40:292–319.

3. Huang CJ, Pitt HA, Lipsett PA et al. Pyogenic hepatic abscess. *Ann Surg.* 1996;223:600–607.
4. Kaplan GG, Gregson DB, Laupland KB. Population-based study of the epidemiology of and risk factors for pyogenic liver abscess. *Clin Gastroenterol Hepatol.* 2004;2:1032–1038.
5. Alvarez Perez JA, Gonzalez JJ, Baldonedo RF et al. Clinical course, treatment, and multivariate analysis of risk factors for pyogenic liver abscess. *Am J Surg.* 2001;181:177–186.
6. Tsai FC, Huang YT, Chang LY et al. Pyogenic liver abscess as endemic disease, Taiwan. *Emerg Infect Dis.* 2008;14:1592–1600.
7. Meddings L, Myers RP, Hubbard J et al. A population-based study of pyogenic liver abscesses in the United States: Incidence, mortality, and temporal trends. *Am J Gastroenterol.* 2010;105:117–124.
8. Stanley SL. Amoebiasis. *Lancet.* 2003;361:1025–1034.
9. Rahimian J, Wilson T, Oram V et al. Pyogenic liver abscess: Recent trends in etiology and mortality. *Clin Infect Dis.* 2004;39:1654–1659.
10. Lam YH, Wong SK, Lee DW et al. ERCP and pyogenic liver abscess. *Gastrointest Endosc.* 1999;50:340–344.
11. Mezhir JJ, Fong Y, Jacks LM et al. Current management of pyogenic liver abscess: Surgery is now second-line treatment. *J Am Coll Surg.* 2010;210:975–983.
12. Mezhir JJ, Fong Y, Fleischer D et al. Pyogenic Abscess after hepatic artery embolization: A rare but potentially lethal complication. *J Vasc Interv Radiol.* 2011;22:177–182.
13. Kong WT, Zhang WW, Qiu YD et al. Major complications after radiofrequency ablation for liver tumors: Analysis of 255 patients. *World J Gastroenterol.* 2009;15:2651–2656.
14. Nikeghbalian S, Salahi R, Salahi H et al. Hepatic abscesses after liver transplant: 1997–2008. *Exp Clin Transplant.* 2009;7:256–260.
15. Stewart L, Robinson TN, Lee CM et al. Right hepatic artery injury associated with laparoscopic bile duct injury: Incidence, mechanism, and consequences. *J Gastrointest Surg.* 2004;8:523–530.
16. Lederman ER, Crum NF. Pyogenic liver abscess with a focus on *Klebsiella pneumoniae* as a primary pathogen: An emerging disease with unique clinical characteristics. *Am J Gastroenterol.* 2005;100:322–331.
17. Siu LK, Yeh KM, Lin JC, Fung CP, Chang FY. Klebsiella pneumonia liver abscess: A new invasive syndrome. *Lancet Inf Dis.* 2012;12:881–887.
18. Smith BM, Zyromski NJ, Allison DC. Community-acquired methicillin-resistant *Staphylococcus aureus* liver abscess requiring resection. *Surgery.* 2007;141:110–111.
19. Ulug M, Gedik E, Girgin S et al. Pyogenic liver abscess caused by community acquired multidrug resistance Pseudomonas aeruginosa. *Braz J Infect Dis.* 2010;14:218.
20. Acuna-Soto R, Maguire JH, Wirth DF. Gender distribution in asymptomatic and invasive amebiasis. *Am J Gastroenterol.* 2000;95:1277–1283.
21. Conter RL, Pitt HA, Tompkins RK et al. Differentiation of pyogenic from hepatic abscess. *Surg Gynecol Obstet.* 1986;162:114–120.
22. Akgun Y, Tacyildiz IH, Celik Y. Amebic liver abscess: Changing trends over 20 years. *World J Surg.* 1999;23:102–106.
23. Hoffner JR, Kilaghbian T, Esekogwu VI et al. Common presentations of amebic liver abscess. *Ann Emerg Med.* 1999;34:351–355.
24. Lodhi S, Sarwari AR, Muzammil, M et al. Features distinguishing amebic from pyogenic liver abscess: A review of 577 adult cases. *Trop Med Inter Health.* 2004;9: 718–723.
25. Pang T, Fung T, Samra J et al. Pyogenic liver abscess: An audit of 10 years' experience. *World J Gastroenterol.* 2011;17:1622–1630.
26. Haque R, Kabir M, Noor Z et al. Diagnosis of amebic liver abscess and amebic colitis by detection of *E histolytica* DNA in blood, urine, and saliva by a real-time PCR assay. *J Clin Microbiol.* 2010;48:2798–2801.
27. Tan YM, Chung AY, Chow PK et al. An appraisal of surgical and percutaneous drainage for pyogenic liver abscesses greater than 5 cm. *Ann Surg.* 2005;241:485–490.
28. Ferraioli G, Garlaschelli A, Zanaboni D et al. Percutaneous and surgical treatment of pyogenic liver abscesses: Observation over a 21-year period in 148 patients. *Dig Liver Dis.* 2008;40:690–696.
29. Lai KC, Cheng KS, Jeng LB et al. Factors associated with treatment failure of percutaneous catheter drainage of pyogenic liver abscess in patients with hepatobiliary-pancreatic cancer. *Am J Surg.* 2013;205:52–57.
30. Hope WW, Vrochides DV, Newcomb WL et al. Optimal treatment of hepatic abscess. *Am Surg.* 2008;74:178–182.
31. Yu SC, Ho SS, Lau WY et al. Treatment of pyogenic liver abscess: Prospective randomized comparison of catheter drainage and needle aspiration. *Hepatology.* 2004;39:932–938.
32. Tan L, Zhou HJ, Hartman M et al. Laparoscopic drainage of cryptogenic liver abscess. *Surg Endosc.* 2013;27:3308–3314.
33. Tu JF, Huang XF, Hu RY et al. Comparison of laparoscopic and open surgery for pyogenic liver abscess and biliary pathology. *World J Gastroenterol.* 2011;17:4339–4343.

## Commentary on Liver Abscess

*Ali Salim*

I must admit that despite training at a safety net hospital in Southern California, liver abscesses were not very common. This was encountered following severe liver trauma or sometimes as a complication of an intra-abdominal infection with subsequent pylephlebitis as patients would often seek treatment very late in their course. We would occasionally see patients with amoebic liver abscess, as we frequently saw patients that had immigrated to the United States. Nevertheless, it was fascinating to watch the evolution of treatment even in the short time period during my residency. Open surgical drainage was often the treatment of choice. Although not a very satisfying operation, it did provide adequate treatment. Then we started with this new tool of laparoscopic surgery to unroof and drain the abscess. Though it was less satisfying than the open surgical approach, the patients seemed to recover much quicker. Then our radiology colleagues got into the game and were involved in aspiration and drainage with the deployment of their various sizes of pigtail catheters. It became clearly evident that this noninvasive modality was the best tolerated of all the treatment options. As an acute care surgeon today, we were rarely invited to solve this interesting problem anymore. Patients are managed conservatively with antibiotics, with or without percutaneous pigtail drainage.

This chapter provides a nice summary regarding the epidemiology, pathophysiology, and diagnostic and therapeutic options of a fairly uncommon clinical problem. It is presented in an excellent evidence-based practice approach. Two major questions were raised that I will briefly comment on.

### What Is the Optimal Diagnostic Strategy for Liver Abscess?

As the authors noted, since the clinical symptoms are variable and not pathognomonic, there needs to be a high index of suspicion. There is no gold standard for diagnostic imaging, but the two most widely used modalities are computed tomography and ultrasound. Ultrasound has the advantage of being widely accessible, noninvasive, and lower cost, but the disadvantage is that it is operator dependent. This may explain the fairly high false-negative rate (especially for smaller abscesses). Computed tomography appears to be a better choice and, in addition, appears to have a higher sensitivity rate for smaller lesions. Diagnostic percutaneous aspiration is then performed to ensure treatment with appropriate antibiotics.

### What Is the Treatment for Liver Abscess?

As the authors carefully noted, a distinction must first be made between a pyogenic liver abscess and an amoebic liver abscess as the treatment algorithms are usually different. Antibiotics alone are effective for smaller pyogenic abscesses and most amoebic abscesses. The majority of abscess can be successfully treated with percutaneous drainage. Surgical drainage is reserved for large abscesses, those with multiloculations ruptured, difficult anatomy that precludes aspiration or those that fail percutaneous drainage. The preferred method for surgery is laparoscopic drainage. Open surgical drainage may be reserved for patients with clinical deterioration, those who require extensive debridement (i.e., hepatic lobectomy), or in patients who have failed laparoscopic drainage. With appropriate antimicrobial therapy and appropriate drainage when necessary, outcomes have improved dramatically over time.

# 61

# *Diagnosis and Treatment of Variceal Hemorrhage Due to Cirrhosis*

**Robert M. Esterl, Jr., Aaron Lewis, Juan Marcano, Abdul Alarhayem, Gregory A. Abrahamian, and K. Vincent Speeg**

**CONTENTS**

Cirrhosis is a histological description of end-stage liver disease characterized by nodular regeneration and bridging fibrosis in the liver. Portal hypertension (PH) is defined as a hepatic vein pressure gradient (HVPG) (gradient between portal and central venous pressure) of >12 mmHg [1]. Variceal hemorrhage is a common and serious complication of PH, with mortality rates as high as 50% with the initial episode [2]. This chapter will review the pathophysiology, diagnosis, and treatment of variceal hemorrhage, including primary and secondary prophylaxis and control of active hemorrhage. We present practice guidelines that have been developed and endorsed by the American Association for the Study of Liver Disease and the American College of Gastroenterology and reviewed at the most recent international Baveno V consensus conference [1,3].

## 61.1 Pathophysiology

PH develops as a consequence of both increased resistance to portal blood flow and increased portal blood flow. Increased resistance to portal blood flow is due not only to architectural fibrotic distortion but also to vasoconstriction in the liver. This is mediated by contractile stellate cells responding both to decreased production of nitric oxide by adjacent hepatic endothelial cells and increased response to several endogenous vasoconstrictors, including endothelin, norepinephrine, angiotensin II, vasopressin, leukotrienes, and thromboxane A2. PH also occurs as a consequence of increased splanchnic arterial flow from decreased systemic vascular resistance, increased cardiac output, and direct splanchnic arteriolar vasodilatation mediated by multiple vasoactive agents [4].

## 61.2 What is the Most Reliable Predictor of Variceal Development in Cirrhotics?

### 61.2.1 Measurement of the Hepatic Vein Pressure Gradient

The HVPG is the preferred method to assess portal venous pressure and the most reliable predictor of variceal development [1]. This technique involves advancing a balloon catheter into the hepatic vein to measure the wedge hepatic vein pressure (WHVP) (balloon inflated) and the free hepatic vein pressure (FHVP) (balloon deflated). The HVPG is WHVP–FHVP. Normal HVPG is 3–5 mmHg, and in PH, the HVPG is >12 mmHg. The HVPG is elevated in sinusoidal causes of PH, but is normal in presinusoidal causes of PH [1].

There is strong evidence that reduction in HVPG with pharmacological intervention reduces the risk of variceal hemorrhage. Reduction in HVPG ("responders") can include HVPG ≤12 mmHg or HVPG ≥20% from baseline, regardless of final HVPG. Variceal hemorrhage does not occur when HPVG ≤12 mmHg, and the risk of recurrent variceal hemorrhage decreases significantly when HPVG ≥20% from baseline. Two large meta-analyses determined that the risk of variceal hemorrhage and liver-related mortality were lower in patients who achieved HVPG reduction [5]. Another study involving 71 cirrhotics confirmed that propranolol ± isosorbide mononitrate significantly reduced the 8-year cumulative probability of no variceal hemorrhage to 90% in responders vs. 45% in nonresponders, but there were no significant differences in liver-related mortality [6]. Patients with HVPG ≥20 mmHg had greater failure to control variceal hemorrhage (29% vs. 83%), earlier recurrent hemorrhage, longer intensive care unit and hospital stays, more transfusion requirements, and worse 1-year mortality (20% vs. 64%) [7].

*Recommendation*: Although invasive, measurement of the HVPG is the preferred method to assess portal pressure and is predictive of variceal development (1b/A).

## 61.3 What is the Best Diagnostic Test to Detect the Presence of Esophageal Varices?

### 61.3.1 Role of Upper Endoscopy in Diagnosis of Varices

Upper endoscopy is the gold standard to detect the presence of esophageal varices [1]. Consensus guidelines recommend that all patients with a new diagnosis of cirrhosis undergo screening upper endoscopy [1,3]. Additionally, upper endoscopy is a primary technique for initial control of variceal hemorrhage [1].

*Recommendation*: Upper endoscopy remains the best diagnostic test to detect the presence of esophageal varices (2a/C to 5/D).

## 61.4 What is the Best Treatment to Prevent the Development of Varices in Cirrhotics Who Have No Varices by Upper Endoscopy?

### 61.4.1 Preprimary Prophylaxis

Without prior assessment of the presence of varices with screening upper endoscopy, there is no evidence to support treating all cirrhotics with β-blockers [3]. If upper endoscopy demonstrates no varices, treating patients with empiric β-blockers does not prevent the formation of varices [1,3]. In a study of 213 patients without varices at screening endoscopy who were randomized to timolol (108 patients) vs. placebo (105 patients), the development of varices did not differ (39% vs. 40%, respectively) at a mean follow-up of 54.9 months. Furthermore, timolol had more serious adverse events including bradycardia, severe fatigue, wheezing, and syncope (timolol 18% vs. placebo 6%) [8]. Instead of β-blocker therapy, consensus guidelines suggest that compensated cirrhotics with no varices should undergo surveillance upper endoscopy every 2–3 years; cirrhotics who develop hepatic decompensation should undergo surveillance endoscopy at that time and then annually in order to document new varices [1].

*Recommendation*: When upper endoscopy reveals no varices, data suggest that β-blockers are not helpful to prevent the formation of varices (1b/A). These patients should undergo regular surveillance upper endoscopy (1/C). Treatment should be directed at the underlying liver disease to reduce PH and prevent the development of varices (1b/A).

## 61.5 What is the Best Treatment to Prevent First Variceal Hemorrhage in Cirrhotics Who Have Small Varices?

### 61.5.1 Primary Prophylaxis

#### *61.5.1.1 Small Varices*

##### *61.5.1.1.1 Nonselective β-Blockers*

Several studies suggest that compensated cirrhotics who have small varices on screening upper endoscopy should receive nonselective β-blockers to prevent growth to large varices and first variceal hemorrhage. In a study of 161 cirrhotics with small varices on screening endoscopy randomized to the nonselective β-blocker nadolol vs. placebo, annual surveillance upper endoscopy was performed for 5 years to document growth from small to large varices. Nine (11%) patients on nadolol and 29 (37%) patients on placebo had growth from small to large varices, but there were no differences in survival. Freedom from first variceal hemorrhage was significantly higher in the nadolol group vs. the placebo group (88% vs. 78%), but more patients on nadolol (11%) vs. placebo (1%) were removed from the trial because of adverse side effects [9].

Consensus guidelines suggest that compensated cirrhotics with small varices that have not bled should probably receive nonselective β-blockers, although survival benefit is unclear [1,3]. Patients with small varices who have red wale marks by upper endoscopy or Child-Pugh Class C have increased risk of hemorrhage and should receive nonselective β-blockers to prevent growth to larger varices [1,3]. Compensated cirrhotics with small varices who receive β-blockers do not require repeat screening upper endoscopy. Compensated cirrhotics with small varices that have not bled and choose not to receive nonselective β-blockers should undergo surveillance upper endoscopy every 2 years [1].

*Recommendation*: Compensated cirrhotics with small varices may receive nonselective β-blockers to prevent growth to large varices (1b/A to 3/B). Patients with small varices who have increased risk of hemorrhage (1b/A) should receive nonselective β-blockers (2a/C to 5/D).

## 61.6 What is the Best Treatment to Prevent First Variceal Hemorrhage in Cirrhotics Who Have Large Varices?

### 61.6.1 Medium to Large Varices

#### *61.6.1.1 β-Blockers*

A meta-analysis of 11 trials with 1189 cirrhotics with medium or large varices reported that β-blockers significantly reduced the risk of first variceal hemorrhage vs. placebo (14% vs. 30%) [10]. In a trial of 105 cirrhotics with large varices who received intravenous propranolol followed by oral nadolol, responders had significantly lower risk of first variceal hemorrhage, fewer hospitalizations for decompensated cirrhosis, and lower mortality [11]. A randomized controlled trial of 104 cirrhotics with varices and elevated HVPG evaluated propranolol vs. carvedilol for primary prophylaxis. In a substantial number of nonresponders to propranolol, carvedilol achieved a hemodynamic response, resulting in improved prevention of variceal hemorrhage. Both carvedilol and propranolol demonstrated fewer episodes of hepatic decompensation and death, as compared to endoscopic variceal ligation (EVL) [12]. Abraczinskas et al. noted that prophylactic β-blockers in patients with medium to large varices should be used indefinitely because removal of prophylactic β-blockers leads to an equal risk of first variceal hemorrhage with an increased mortality compared to an untreated population [13].

#### *61.6.1.2 EVL versus No Therapy*

A meta-analysis of five trials with 601 patients who had medium or large varices reported that prophylactic EVL vs. no therapy significantly reduced the relative risk of first variceal hemorrhage, hemorrhage-related mortality, and all-cause mortality [14]. A cohort study of 76 cirrhotics with contraindications, intolerance, or unresponsiveness to β-blockers showed that EVL had similar episodes of variceal hemorrhage compared to cirrhotics with good hemodynamic response to β-blockers [15]. Another abstract comparing EVL to no therapy in cirrhotics with contraindications or intolerance to β-blockers was discontinued prematurely after patients had more variceal hemorrhage than expected in the EVL group. This was the first study to suggest that EVL was no better than no therapy, and should be used cautiously for primary prophylaxis [16].

#### 61.6.1.3 Nonselective β-Blockers versus EVL

A meta-analysis of 19 trials involving 1504 patients with medium- to high-risk varices receiving EVL (731 patients) or β-blockers (773 patients) showed EVL to be slightly better than β-blockers for the prevention of variceal hemorrhage (14% vs. 20% incidence of hemorrhage); however, the benefit of EVL was not confirmed when comparing adequately randomized trials, and there was no difference in hemorrhage-related mortality between the two groups [17]. A meta-analysis of eight trials (596 patients) demonstrated that EVL (285 patients) compared to β-blockers (311 patients) reduced rates of first variceal hemorrhage in cirrhotics with medium and large varices by 43%, but hemorrhage-related mortality and all-cause mortality were similar. Adverse events were significantly less frequent with EVL than β-blockers (4% vs. 13%); however, side effects with β-blockers (hypotension, fatigue, and shortness of breath) resolved soon after cessation and did not require hospitalization. Although less frequent, the side effects of EVL were much more severe, including esophageal ulcers (10 patients) and esophageal perforation (1 patient). Most of these side effects required hospitalization and blood transfusions, and resulted in two deaths [18].

Consensus guidelines recommend that, when β-blockers are used, they should be adjusted upward to the maximally tolerated dose and surveillance upper endoscopy is not necessary [1]. When EVL is used, it should be repeated every 1–2 weeks until variceal obliteration (usually 2–4 sessions). Surveillance endoscopy should occur 1–3 months after variceal obliteration and repeated every 6–12 months for recurrent varices which are again treated with EVL [1]. After EVL, shallow ulcers at the base are common and sometimes bleed, and a short course of intravenous pantoprazole significantly reduces the size of the ulcers [19]. Sclerotherapy or shunt therapy alone should not be used to prevent first variceal hemorrhage in patients with large varices [1,3].

#### 61.6.1.4 EVL Plus Nonselective β-Blocker versus EVL Alone

One trial of 144 cirrhotics with high-risk varices reported that EVL and propranolol (72 patients) compared to EVL alone (72 patients) were equally effective in the prevention of first variceal hemorrhage and hemorrhage-related death. The addition of propranolol, however, decreased recurrent variceal hemorrhage, although side effects were seen in 22% of patients, 34% of whom required drug removal [20]. Another trial of 140 cirrhotics with high-risk esophageal varices randomized to EVL and nadolol (70 patients) vs. nadolol alone showed no statistical difference in the rate of first variceal hemorrhage or hemorrhage-related mortality, and the addition of EVL to nadolol carried increased adverse events [21].

*Recommendation*: Nonselective β-blockers or EVL should be used to prevent initial hemorrhage in cirrhotics with large varices (1a/A). Nonselective β-blockers reduce the risk of first variceal hemorrhage in patients with large varices (1a/A). Propranolol is the drug of choice, but carvedilol is an attractive alternative, especially in patients who are nonresponders to propranolol (1b/A). EVL is probably more effective than nonselective β-blockers to reduce the risk of first variceal hemorrhage in these patients, but it may not improve survival and carries more severe adverse events (1a/A). EVL should be recommended when these patients have contraindications, intolerance, or unresponsiveness to β-blockers 1a/A). No data suggest that combined nonselective β-blockers and EVL, sclerotherapy, or shunt therapy should be used in primary prophylaxis of large varices (3/A to 1a/A).

## 61.7 What Specific Resuscitative Fluids Should be Given in Cirrhotics Who Have Acute Variceal Hemorrhage?

### 61.7.1 Acute Variceal Hemorrhage

Current treatment strategies for acute variceal hemorrhage have resulted in improved survival in the United States [1]. Initial management includes airway assessment/protection and placement of large peripheral venous catheters for blood volume resuscitation. Airway protection with a cuffed endotracheal tube prior to endoscopy is crucial to avoid aspiration. Replacement of blood loss should be done promptly but cautiously often with colloid infusion to maintain hemodynamic stability and with packed red cells to maintain Hg 7–8 g/dL [1,3].

Overzealous blood transfusion can lead to increased PH and persistent hemorrhage. A randomized controlled trial showed a lower rate of recurrent variceal hemorrhage and a survival advantage when restrictive transfusion strategies were employed [22]. Saline solutions should generally be avoided due to their potential to increase portal pressure and to cause extravascular fluid accumulation in cirrhotics [1]. Transfusions of fresh frozen plasma and platelets can be considered in patients with significant coagulopathy and thrombocytopenia, but data are limited [1,3]. A multicenter, randomized, controlled trial of recombinant factor VIIa in cirrhotics with gastrointestinal hemorrhage failed to show benefit over standard therapy [23].

*Recommendation*: Prompt but careful resuscitation of blood loss from variceal hemorrhage should occur with colloid to maintain hemodynamic stability and with packed cells to maintain Hg 7–8 g/dL (1b/B to 1b/A). Data regarding management of coagulopathy and thrombocytopenia are limited (5/D).

## 61.8 What is the Role of Prophylactic Antibiotics, if Any, in Cirrhotics Who Have Acute Variceal Hemorrhage?

Bacterial infections occur in many cirrhotics who are admitted to the hospital with gastrointestinal hemorrhage. Bacterial overgrowth and translocation from the gastrointestinal tract, combined with increased susceptibility to infection, mainly due to reticuloendothelial system dysfunction, predispose cirrhotics to spontaneous bacterial peritonitis and bacteremia—both of which can lead to septic shock, multiorgan dysfunction, and death [24].

Recent reports indicate that bacterial infections have also been directly associated with variceal hemorrhage. Endotoxin released during bacterial infections causes contraction of hepatic stellate cells, resulting in increased intrahepatic vascular resistance and portal pressure. Endotoxins also inhibit platelet aggregation through nitric oxide and prostaglandin I2 release, increasing bleeding tendency. In a meta-analysis of 12 trials examining cirrhotics with upper gastrointestinal hemorrhage, prophylactic antibiotics significantly reduced the number of bacterial infections, mortality from bacterial infections, recurrent hemorrhage, length of hospitalization, and all-cause mortality [25].

Consensus guidelines {Garcia-Tsao, 2007 #107} recommend short-term (≤7 days) antibiotic prophylaxis in any patient with cirrhosis and upper gastrointestinal hemorrhage [1,3]. Oral norfloxacin or intravenous ciprofloxacin (when oral administration is not possible) are the recommended antibiotics. A recent randomized trial of 100 patients with advanced cirrhosis and variceal hemorrhage found intravenous ceftriaxone to be superior to oral norfloxacin in preventing bacterial infections [26].

*Recommendation*: Short-term (≤7 days) prophylactic antibiotics should begin at hospital admission for all cirrhotics who present with acute variceal hemorrhage (1a/A). Oral norfloxacin (400 mg BID) or intravenous ciprofloxacin (when oral administration is contraindicated) are the recommended antibiotics (1b/A). Intravenous ceftriaxone can be considered in hospital settings with high rates of quinolone-resistant infections (1b/A).

## 61.9 What is the Best Treatment to Control Hemorrhage in Cirrhotics Who Have Acute Variceal Hemorrhage?

### 61.9.1 Pharmacological Intervention in Acute Variceal Hemorrhage

Pharmacological intervention should begin promptly, even before upper endoscopy confirms the diagnosis of acute variceal hemorrhage, and should continue for up to 5 days [1,3]. Pharmacological therapy alone controls acute variceal hemorrhage in most cases. A meta-analysis of 15 trials reported that pharmacological therapy (vasopressin and its analogs and somatostatin and its analogs) was equivalent to sclerotherapy but had much fewer severe side effects, suggesting that pharmacological intervention should be the first-line therapy in the control of acute variceal hemorrhage [27]. β-blockers should not be administered with active variceal hemorrhage because they drop systolic blood pressure and mask tachycardia that occurs as a normal response to blood loss. In a meta-analysis of 30 trials involving 3111 cirrhotics with acute variceal hemorrhage, the use of vasoactive agents in acute variceal hemorrhage was associated with significantly lower transfusion requirements, improved hemostasis, shorter hospitalization, and lower 7-day all-cause mortality [28].

*Vasopressin* is a potent splanchnic vasoconstrictor that decreases portal venous inflow, thus reducing portal pressure. Vasopressin is administered as a continuous infusion at 0.2–0.4 U/min and can be increased to a maximal rate of 0.8 U/min. Because vasopressin can cause cardiac, intestinal, and peripheral ischemia, it should not be used beyond 24 h; because of these ischemic consequences, its use has dropped out of favor for treatment of acute variceal hemorrhage. Nitroglycerin can be used as a continuous infusion to counteract these ischemic side effects [1]. Seven studies in a recent meta-analysis demonstrated that terlipressin, a synthetic analogue of vasopressin with longer biological activity and significantly fewer side effects, is useful in the control of variceal hemorrhage, but offers no survival benefit [28].

*Octreotide*, currently the only somatostatin analog available in the United States, causes splanchnic vasoconstriction by suppressing the release of vasodilatory gastrointestinal hormones such as glucagon. Octreotide is administered as an initial 50 mcg bolus followed by a continuous 50 mcg/h infusion. This agent is relatively safe compared to vasopressin and can be used for five continuous days or more, allowing treatment during a period when the risk of recurrent hemorrhage is greatest. Because of its rare risk of tachyphylaxis, octreotide should not be used alone, but appears to be most beneficial when administered in conjunction with endoscopic therapy [1]. A Cochrane review of 21 trials involving 2588 cirrhotics with acute variceal hemorrhage noted that octreotide decreased the number of patients who failed initial control of hemorrhage and the number of blood transfusions, but did not reduce the number of patients with recurrent variceal hemorrhage or mortality rates [29].

### 61.9.2 Endoscopic Intervention in Acute Variceal Hemorrhage

Consensus guidelines recommend a combination of initial pharmacological intervention followed by prompt upper endoscopy (within 12 h). When variceal hemorrhage is confirmed by upper endoscopy, EVL should be employed for hemorrhage control [1,3]. In a meta-analysis of eight trials in 939 cirrhotics with acute variceal hemorrhage, this combined approach vs. endoscopic therapy alone improved initial control of variceal hemorrhage and continuous 5-day hemostasis, although severe adverse side effects and 5-day mortality rates were equal [30]. A meta-analysis of 10 trials in 404 cirrhotics with acute variceal hemorrhage reported better initial control of variceal hemorrhage with EVL vs. sclerotherapy [31]. Consensus guidelines recommend EVL as the preferred endoscopic technique for hemorrhage control, and sclerotherapy is used only when EVL is technically difficult or not feasible [1,3]. Early failure of control of acute variceal hemorrhage with this combined approach is best managed with a second attempt of endoscopic therapy before considering rescue therapy [3].

### 61.9.3 Rescue Therapy for Acute Variceal Hemorrhage

#### *61.9.3.1 Sengstaken–Blakemore Tube*

Balloon tamponade with a Sengstaken–Blakemore tube should only be used as a bridge to definitive therapy, whether transjugular intrahepatic portosystemic shunt (TIPSS) or surgical shunt. Although effective in controlling hemorrhage in >80% of patients, its usefulness is limited by a prohibitive side-effect profile (aspiration, tube migration, esophageal necrosis, and perforation), which carries a 20% mortality rate [1,3].

#### *61.9.3.2 Shunt Therapy*

Ten to twenty percent of patients with acute variceal hemorrhage fail combined pharmacological and endoscopic treatment [1]. Because a surgical shunt reduces HVPG promptly, it has proven efficacy in limited retrospective trials of patients who fail combined therapy [1]. TIPSS is also very effective in controlling hemorrhage in these patients by reducing HVPG, but may worsen hepatic encephalopathy and offers no survival benefit due to further decompensated liver failure. In a randomized controlled trial of advanced cirrhotics with active hemorrhage, the use of early TIPSS (within 72 h) was associated with significant reductions in treatment failure and mortality compared to standard pharmacological and endoscopic therapy followed by rescue TIPSS when necessary [32].

#### *61.9.3.3 Liver Transplantation*

Liver transplantation is not a feasible rescue therapy for acute variceal hemorrhage due to lack of regular donor organs. Liver transplantation might be feasible for patients who develop hepatic decompensation after TIPSS or surgical shunt.

*Recommendation*: Pharmacological therapy should be initiated as soon as variceal hemorrhage is suspected, even before endoscopic confirmation (1b/A to 1a/A). Vasoactive drugs should be used in conjunction with upper endoscopy (1a/A). Upper endoscopy should be performed promptly to confirm the diagnosis and to control variceal hemorrhage, preferably with EVL. Sclerotherapy is used only when EVL is technically difficult or not feasible (1b/A). Early re-hemorrhage should prompt a second endoscopic attempt before considering rescue therapy with TIPSS or surgical shunt (2b/B). Persistent or severe recurrent hemorrhage despite combined pharmacological and endoscopic therapy is best treated by TIPSS (1/C to 2b/B). Early use of TIPSS may be warranted (1b/A). Balloon tamponade should only be used as a temporizing measure to definitive therapy

(TIPSS/surgical shunt) (1b/B to 5/D). There is no role for liver transplantation in acute variceal hemorrhage due to lack of regular donor organs.

## 61.10 What is the Best Treatment to Prevent Recurrence in Cirrhotics Who Recover from Acute Variceal Hemorrhage?

### 61.10.1 Secondary Prophylaxis

Patients who survive the first variceal episode carry a high risk of recurrent hemorrhage and mortality. Therefore, patients who recover from variceal hemorrhage should receive secondary prophylaxis soon after the first variceal episode to prevent recurrent hemorrhage. Patients who required rescue therapy with TIPSS or surgical shunt do not need secondary prophylaxis. If suitable candidates otherwise, all of these patients should be referred to liver transplant centers early [1].

### 61.10.2 β-Blockers

Historically, nonselective β-blockade with propranolol or nadolol has been shown to significantly reduce rates of recurrent variceal hemorrhage and mortality. The addition of isosorbide mononitrate to β-blockade may improve the efficacy of therapy in hemodynamic nonresponders, which, in turn, may be more effective in the prevention of recurrent variceal hemorrhage, but the combination carries greater side effects and has no survival benefit [3].

### 61.10.3 β-Blockers Plus EVL

Consensus guidelines recommend a combination of β-blockers and EVL to prevent recurrent hemorrhage [1,3]. A meta-analysis comparing β-blockers and EVL to either modality alone reported that combination therapy significantly reduced the risk of recurrent variceal hemorrhage but not overall mortality [33]. Patients who are unable or unwilling to have EVL should have combination therapy with β-blockers and isosorbide mononitrate [3]. Patients who have contraindications or intolerance to β-blockers should have EVL as the preferred therapy [3].

### 61.10.4 TIPSS

Patients who fail β-blockers, EVL, or a combination of β-blockers and EVL as secondary prophylaxis should be considered for TIPSS as the preferred therapy. If TIPSS is unavailable, an alternative option is a surgical shunt for lower-risk Child-Pugh Class A or B patients. TIPSS can be used as a bridge to liver transplantation; transplantation provides excellent long-term outcomes in appropriate candidates and should be seriously considered [3].

### 61.10.5 Sclerotherapy

Sclerotherapy is no longer recommended in the secondary prophylaxis of variceal hemorrhage. Compared to sclerotherapy, EVL shows superior results in relation to rates of recurrent variceal hemorrhage, mortality, and esophageal stricture [1].

*Recommendation*: For cirrhotics who recover from acute variceal hemorrhage, data support a combination of β-blockers and EVL for secondary prophylaxis (1a/A). Patients who fail combined therapy should be considered for TIPSS or surgical shunt (2b/B to 1a/A). TIPSS can be used as a bridge to transplantation (4/C), and suitable candidates should be referred to liver transplant centers early (2b/B). Sclerotherapy is no longer recommended for secondary prophylaxis of variceal hemorrhage.

## 61.11 Conclusion

Results from evidenced-based protocols have clearly changed the treatment of variceal hemorrhage. HVPG measurement has become the most reliable predictor of variceal development, and screening upper endoscopy remains the best tool to detect varices. No medical therapy is available to prevent the formation of varices, but nonselective β-blockers and EVL are equivalent therapies to prevent first variceal hemorrhage in patients with medium or large varices. Acute variceal hemorrhage requires prompt but careful resuscitation, and overzealous resuscitation can lead to persistent variceal hemorrhage. Prophylactic antibiotic therapy is critical to prevent bacterial infections associated with acute variceal hemorrhage. A combination of immediate pharmacological therapy followed by prompt endoscopic therapy appears to be the most reasonable approach for acute variceal hemorrhage. For patients who fail optimal medical therapy for acute variceal hemorrhage, rescue techniques (Sengstaken–Blakemore tube placement, TIPSS, and surgical shunts) should be carefully considered. A combination of β-blockers and EVL appears to be the most effective approach in the prevention of recurrent variceal hemorrhage, and TIPSS and operative shunts are reserved for patients who fail secondary prophylaxis. TIPSS can be used as a bridge to liver transplantation, and suitable patients should be referred to specialized liver transplant centers early (Table 61.1).

**TABLE 61.1**

Evidence-Based Diagnosis and Treatment of Variceal Hemorrhage

| Question | Answer | Level of Evidence | References |
|---|---|---|---|
| In cirrhotics, what is the most reliable predictor of variceal development? | Measurement of the HVPG is the preferred method to assess portal pressure and is predictive of variceal development. | 1b/A | [1,3,5–7] |
| What is the best diagnostic test to identify esophageal varices? | Upper endoscopy remains the best diagnostic test to detect the presence of esophageal varices. All patients with a new diagnosis of cirrhosis should undergo screening upper endoscopy at diagnosis. | 2a/C to 5/D | [1,3] |
| In cirrhotics who have no varices by upper endoscopy, what is the best treatment to prevent the development of varices? | When screening upper endoscopy reveals no varices, β-blockers are not helpful to prevent formation of varices.[1] Instead, these patients should undergo regular surveillance upper endoscopy.[2] Treatment should be directed at the underlying liver disease to reduce PH.[3] | 1b/A1[1], 1/C[2], 1b/A[3] | [1,3,8] |
| In cirrhotics who have small varices, what is the best treatment to prevent first variceal hemorrhage? | Patients with small varices but no hemorrhage may receive nonselective β-blockers to prevent growth to larger varices.[1] Patients with small varices but increased risk of hemorrhage should receive nonselective β-blockers to prevent growth to larger varices.[2] | 1b/A to 3/B[1], 2a/C to 5/D[2] | [1,3,9] |
| In cirrhotics who have large varices, what is the best treatment to prevent first variceal hemorrhage? | Nonselective β-blockers or EVL reduce the risk of first variceal hemorrhage in patients with large varices. | 1a/A | [1,3,10–21] |
| In cirrhotics who have acute variceal hemorrhage, what specific resuscitative fluids should be given? | Prompt but careful resuscitation of blood loss due to acute variceal hemorrhage should occur with colloid solution to maintain hemodynamic stability and with packed red cells to maintain Hg 7–8 g/dL. | 1b/B to 1b/A | [1,3,22,23] |
| In cirrhotics who have acute variceal hemorrhage, what is the role of prophylactic antibiotics, if any? | Prophylactic antibiotics should begin at hospital admission for all patients who present with acute variceal hemorrhage because they decrease bacterial infections, recurrent variceal hemorrhage, length of hospitalization, and mortality. | 1a/A | [1,3,24–26] |
| In cirrhotics who have acute variceal hemorrhage, what is the best treatment to control hemorrhage? Upper endoscopy should be performed promptly to confirm the diagnosis and to control hemorrhage, preferably with EVL.[3] | When acute variceal hemorrhage is suspected, pharmacological intervention should begin immediately, even before endoscopic confirmation.[1] Vasoactive drugs should be used in conjunction with upper endoscopy.[2] Early re-hemorrhage should prompt a second endoscopic attempt before considering rescue therapy with TIPSS (or surgical shunt).[4] Persistent or severe recurrent hemorrhage is best treated by TIPSS.[5] Balloon tamponade should be considered as a temporizing measure to definitive therapy.[6] | 1b/A to 1a/A[1], 1a/A[2], 1a/A[3], 2b/B[4], 1/C to 2b/C[5], 1b/B to 5/D[6] | [1,3,27–32] |
| In cirrhotics who recover from acute variceal hemorrhage, what is the best treatment to prevent recurrence? | Data support a combination of β-blockers and EVL for secondary prophylaxis.[1] Patients who fail combined therapy should be considered for TIPSS or surgical shunt.[2] TIPSS can be used as a bridge to transplantation,[3] and suitable candidates should be referred to liver transplant centers early.[4] | 1a/A[1], 2b/B to 1a/A[2], 4/C[3], 2b/B[4] | [1,3,33] |

## References


1. Garcia-Tsao G, Sanyal AJ, Grace ND, Carey W, Practice Guidelines Committee of the American Association for the Study of Liver Diseases, Practice Parameters Committee of the American College of Gastroenterology. Prevention and management of gastroesophageal varices and variceal hemorrhage in cirrhosis. *Hepatology*. 2007;46(3):922–938.
2. Qureshi W, Adler DG, Davila R et al. ASGE guideline: The role of endoscopy in the management of variceal hemorrhage, updated July 2005. *Gastrointest Endosc*. 2005;62(5):651–655.
3. de Franchis R, Baveno V, Faculty. Revising consensus in portal hypertension: Report of the baveno V consensus workshop on methodology of diagnosis and therapy in portal hypertension. *J Hepatol*. 2010;53(4):762–768.

4. Garcia-Pagan JC, Gracia-Sancho J, Bosch J. Functional aspects on the pathophysiology of portal hypertension in cirrhosis. *J Hepatol.* 2012;57(2):458–461.
5. D'Amico G, Garcia-Pagan JC, Luca A, Bosch J. Hepatic vein pressure gradient reduction and prevention of variceal bleeding in cirrhosis: A systematic review. *Gastroenterology.* 2006;131(5):1611–1624.
6. Turnes J, Garcia-Pagan JC, Abraldes JG, Hernandez-Guerra M, Dell'Era A, Bosch J. Pharmacological reduction of portal pressure and long-term risk of first variceal bleeding in patients with cirrhosis. *Am J Gastroenterol.* 2006;101(3):506–512.
7. Moitinho E, Escorsell A, Bandi JC et al. Prognostic value of early measurements of portal pressure in acute variceal bleeding. *Gastroenterology.* 1999;117(3):626–631.
8. Groszmann RJ, Garcia-Tsao G, Bosch J et al. Beta-blockers to prevent gastroesophageal varices in patients with cirrhosis. *N Engl J Med.* 2005;353(21):2254–2261.
9. Merkel C, Marin R, Angeli P et al. A placebo-controlled clinical trial of nadolol in the prophylaxis of growth of small esophageal varices in cirrhosis. *Gastroenterology.* 2004;127(2):476–484.
10. D'Amico G, Pagliaro L, Bosch J. Pharmacological treatment of portal hypertension: An evidence-based approach. *Semin Liver Dis.* 1999;19(4):475–505.
11. Villanueva C, Aracil C, Colomo A et al. Acute hemodynamic response to beta-blockers and prediction of long-term outcome in primary prophylaxis of variceal bleeding. *Gastroenterology.* 2009;137(1):119–128.
12. Reiberger T, Ulbrich G, Ferlitsch A et al. Carvedilol for primary prophylaxis of variceal bleeding in cirrhotic patients with haemodynamic non-response to propranolol. *Gut.* 2013;62(11):1634–1641.
13. Abraczinskas DR, Ookubo R, Grace ND et al. Propranolol for the prevention of first esophageal variceal hemorrhage: A lifetime commitment? *Hepatology.* 2001;34(6):1096–1102.
14. Imperiale TF, Chalasani N. A meta-analysis of endoscopic variceal ligation for primary prophylaxis of esophageal variceal bleeding. *Hepatology.* 2001;33(4):802–807.
15. Dellera A, Sotela JC, Fabris FM et al. Primary prophylaxis of variceal bleeding in cirrhotic patients: A cohort study. *Dig Liver Dis.* 2008;40(12):936–943.
16. Triantos C, Vlachogiannakos J, Armonis A et al. Primary prophylaxis of variceal bleeding in cirrhotics unable to take beta-blockers: A randomized trial of ligation. *Aliment Pharmacol Ther.* 2005;21(12):1435–1443.
17. Gluud LL, Krag A. Banding ligation versus beta-blockers for primary prevention in oesophageal varices in adults. *Cochrane Database Syst Rev.* 2012;8:CD004544.
18. Khuroo MS, Khuroo NS, Farahat KL, Khuroo YS, Sofi AA, Dahab ST. Meta-analysis: Endoscopic variceal ligation for primary prophylaxis of oesophageal variceal bleeding. *Aliment Pharmacol Ther.* 2005;21(4):347–361.
19. Shaheen NJ, Stuart E, Schmitz SM et al. Pantoprazole reduces the size of postbanding ulcers after variceal band ligation: A randomized, controlled trial. *Hepatology.* 2005;41(3):588–594.
20. Sarin SK, Wadhawan M, Agarwal SR, Tyagi P, Sharma BC. Endoscopic variceal ligation plus propranolol versus endoscopic variceal ligation alone in primary prophylaxis of variceal bleeding. *Am J Gastroenterol.* 2005;100(4):797–804.
21. Lo GH, Chen WC, Wang HM, Lee CC. Controlled trial of ligation plus nadolol versus nadolol alone for the prevention of first variceal bleeding. *Hepatology.* 2010;52(1):230–237.
22. Villanueva C, Colomo A, Bosch A et al. Transfusion strategies for acute upper gastrointestinal bleeding. *N Engl J Med.* 2013;368(1):11–21.
23. Bosch J, Thabut D, Bendtsen F et al. Recombinant factor VIIa for upper gastrointestinal bleeding in patients with cirrhosis: A randomized, double-blind trial. *Gastroenterology.* 2004;127(4):1123–1130.
24. Garcia-Tsao G, Wiest R. Gut microflora in the pathogenesis of the complications of cirrhosis. *Best Pract Res Clin Gastroenterol.* 2004;18(2):353–372.
25. Chavez-Tapia NC, Barrientos-Gutierrez T, Tellez-Avila F et al. Meta-analysis: Antibiotic prophylaxis for cirrhotic patients with upper gastrointestinal bleeding—An updated cochrane review. *Aliment Pharmacol Ther.* 2011;34(5):509–518.
26. Fernandez J, Ruiz del Arbol L, Gomez C et al. Norfloxacin vs ceftriaxone in the prophylaxis of infections in patients with advanced cirrhosis and hemorrhage. *Gastroenterology.* 2006;131(4):1049–1056; quiz 1285.
27. D'Amico G, Pietrosi G, Tarantino I, Pagliaro L. Emergency sclerotherapy versus vasoactive drugs for variceal bleeding in cirrhosis: A Cochrane meta-analysis. *Gastroenterology.* 2003;124(5):1277–1291.
28. Wells M, Chande N, Adams P et al. Meta-analysis: Vasoactive medications for the management of acute variceal bleeds. *Aliment Pharmacol Ther.* 2012;35(11):1267–1278.
29. Gotzsche PC, Hrobjartsson A. Somatostatin analogues for acute bleeding oesophageal varices. *Cochrane Database Syst Rev.* 2008;(3):CD000193.
30. Banares R, Albillos A, Rincon D et al. Endoscopic treatment versus endoscopic plus pharmacologic treatment for acute variceal bleeding: A meta-analysis. *Hepatology.* 2002;35(3):609–615.
31. Garcia-Pagan JC, Bosch J. Endoscopic band ligation in the treatment of portal hypertension. *Nat Clin Pract Gastroenterol Hepatol.* 2005;2(11):526–535.
32. Garcia-Pagan JC, Caca K, Bureau C et al. Early use of TIPS in patients with cirrhosis and variceal bleeding. *N Engl J Med.* 2010;362(25):2370–2379.
33. Thiele M, Krag A, Rohde U, Gluud LL. Meta-analysis: Banding ligation and medical interventions for the prevention of rebleeding from oesophageal varices. *Aliment Pharmacol Ther.* 2012;35(10):1155–1165.

## Commentary on Diagnosis and Treatment of Variceal Hemorrhage due to Cirrhosis

*Todd W. Costantini and Raul Coimbra*

Cirrhosis is the most common cause of portal hypertension in the United States and frequently leads to the formation of varices when low resistance venous collaterals become dilated by elevated hepatic venous pressure gradient. Portal hypertension is associated with a high risk of esophageal varices that are a common cause of significant upper GI hemorrhage. In fact, patients with cirrhosis have an annual risk of variceal bleeding of 10%–20% based on patient characteristics such as Child–Pugh class and the size of varices present*. This chapter nicely reviews the importance of screening and primary prophylaxis to prevent the development of esophageal varices in patients with cirrhosis. While important to review, this is rarely the responsibility of the acute care surgeon. Instead, the acute care surgeon or surgical intensivist is more frequently called to the emergency department or intensive care unit to manage the unstable cirrhotic patient with acute, and often massive, upper GI bleeding.

Acute variceal bleeding in patients with cirrhosis is associated with a mortality rate of 20%–30% at 6 weeks after the bleeding episode†. While rarely treated with surgical intervention, these patients require prompt, aggressive management to provide resuscitation and control of hemorrhage. The following are critical elements in the management of cirrhotic patients with upper GI bleeding from esophageal varices:

1. *A, B, C's*: As with any acute illness associated with blood loss, the initial assessment of upper GI bleeding should include evaluation of airway, breathing, and circulation. The patient should be admitted to the intensive care unit for frequent monitoring of vital signs, resuscitation, and treatment. An airway should be secured by orotracheal intubation due to the high risk for aspiration. Patients should have two large bore IVs placed for transfusion of blood or IV fluids as needed. Patients should be transfused packed red blood cells with goal hemoglobin of 7–8 g/dL. Transfusion to higher hemoglobin targets may result in increased portal hypertension and increased risk of rebleeding and should be avoided‡.
2. *Correct coagulopathy*: Coagulopathy is common in cirrhotics and should be corrected promptly. Transfusion of fresh frozen plasma to correct the INR and platelet transfusion to address the thrombocytopenia, common findings in cirrhotics. The use of recombinant factor VIIa has been considered as a treatment to correct coagulopathy in patients with variceal hemorrhage; however, a randomized, double-blind trial failed to demonstrate any advantage compared to standard therapy§.
3. *Pharmacologic* treatment: Vasoactive medications should be administered as soon as bleeding from esophageal varices is diagnosed and prior to endoscopic intervention. Vasopressin is a potent splanchnic vasoconstrictor that decreases blood flow through the varices and can aid in hemorrhage control. Its administration is limited by systemic side effects including myocardial ischemia, hypertension, and ischemic abdominal pain. Octreotide, a somatostatin analogue, is another splanchnic vasoconstrictor that can provide bleeding control prior to definitive endoscopic therapy. A proton pump inhibitor should be added to suppress gastric acid secretion.
4. *Endoscopic therapy*: Emergent esophagogastroduodenoscopy (EGD) can confirm the diagnosis of variceal bleeding and provide hemorrhage control using either variceal band ligation or sclerotherapy, with variceal band ligation considered first-line endoscopic therapy due to a lower complication rate. Rebleeding from esophageal varies occurs in approximately 60% of patients within 2 years of the initial bleeding episode¶.
5. *Balloon tamponade*: Failure of both medical and endoscopic maneuvers to control hemorrhage from variceal bleeding is life-threatening. Balloon luminal tamponade using either a Minnesota or Sengstaken–Blakemore tube can

* Garcia-Tsao G, Bosch J. Management of varices and variceal hemorrhage in cirrhosis. *N Engl J Med*. 2010;362:823–832.

† Chalasani N, Kahi C, Francois F, Pinto A, Marathe A, Bini EJ, Pandya P, Sitaraman S, Shen J. Improved patient survival after acute variceal bleeding: A multicenter, cohort study. *Am J Gastroenterol*. 2003;98:653–659.

‡ Garcia-Tsao G, Sanyal AJ, Grace ND, Carey W. Prevention and management of gastroesophageal varices and variceal hemorrhage in cirrhosis. *Hepatology*. 2007;46:922–938.

§ Bosch J, Thabut D, Bendtsen F, D'Amico G, Albillos A, Gonzalez Abraldes J, Fabricius S, Erhardtsen E, de Franchis R. Recombinant factor VIIa for upper gastrointestinal bleeding in patients with cirrhosis: A randomized, double-blind trial. *Gastroenterology*. 2004;127:1123–1130.

¶ O'Brien J, Triantos C, Burroughs AK. Management of varices in patients with cirrhosis. *Nat Rev Gastroenterol Hepatol*. 2013;10:402–412.

provide temporary hemorrhage control, while more definitive interventions are planned. These tubes are equipped with large balloons that can compress the gastroesophageal junction and decrease blood flow through the esophageal varices. While these tubes are usually successful in controlling hemorrhage initially, a majority will rebleed once the balloon is deflated.

6. *Antibiotic prophylaxis*: Antibiotics should be administered at the time of admission and can decrease infectious complications and have actually been shown to decrease the risk of early rebleeding*. Fluoroquinolones have traditionally been considered the antibiotic of choice; however, third-generation cephalosporins are now part of the first-line therapy due to the increased incidence of quinolone-resistant bacteria.

Transjugular intrahepatic portosystemic shunts (TIPSs) are placed percutaneously, where a stent is deployed to create a portocaval shunt within the liver. TIPS can be used in patients after pharmacologic and endoscopic treatment failure for acute variceal hemorrhage. Surgical shunts, while performed less frequently since the advent of TIPS, are still an option for patients with preserved liver function. These shunts divert portal blood flow away from the liver, resulting in decompression of the esophageal varices, but are reserved for patients with preserved synthetic function in cases where TIPS is unavailable†.

* Hou MC, Lin HC, Liu TT, Kuo BI, Lee FY, Chang FY, Lee SD. Antibiotic prophylaxis after endoscopic therapy prevents rebleeding in acute variceal hemorrhage: A randomized trial. *Hepatology*. 2004;39:746–753.

† Thabut D, D'Amico G, Tan P, De Franchis R, Fabricius S, Lebrec D, Bosch J, Bendtsen F. Diagnostic performance of Baveno IV criteria in cirrhotic patients with upper gastrointestinal bleeding: Analysis of the F7 liver-1288 study population. *J Hepatol*. 2010;53:1029–1034.

# 62

# *Acute Arterial Embolus*

**Christopher J. Busken, Georges Haidar, Ryan Hagino, and Boulos Toursarkissian**

**CONTENTS**



Peripheral artery embolus is associated with a high risk of limb loss and death—ranging from 5% to 40% for limb loss [1–5]. A mortality rate of up to 25% is reported [3]. Patients with acute peripheral embolus are often a medically disadvantaged population. Frequently they have a cardiogenic nidus for the embolus, often a clot from the left atrium due to atrial fibrillation. The next most common cause is a myocardial thrombus that occurs within several weeks of a myocardial infarction.

The five "Ps" of acute limb ischemia—pain, paresthesia, pallor, paralysis, and pulselessness—characterize acute arterial embolus. Not all of these signs and symptoms necessarily must be present; however, the added findings typically relate an increasingly dire clinical scenario. Ischemia will initially affect the sensory nerves, which will lead to pain, paresthesia, and loss of proprioception. More prolonged or intense ischemia will cause loss of gross sensation and motor function. Impaired motor function is an immediate precursor to irreversible tissue loss, and paralysis indicates severe, likely irreversible, muscle death and compartment swelling. Evaluation of function is more important than the absolute elapsed time following the development of the inciting embolus [4]. Prevention of thrombus propagation by initiation of anticoagulation and revascularization of the ischemic, but still salvageable, limb is strongly recommended [6,7]. Categories of viability include "viable," "threatened," and "irreversible" [8]. Articles report 45% of limbs present as viable, 45% present as threatened, and 10% of limbs present with irreversible ischemia [6].

History and physical examination aid in diagnosing the nidus of the event. Complaints of claudication or an abnormal examination on the opposite leg suggest thrombosis instead of an embolus. Differentiating between acute thrombosis due to atherosclerotic disease or a peripheral aneurysm and an acute embolus can be difficult [5]. The difference is important as it does impact diagnostic testing and treatment.

Treatment options for acute arterial embolus include observation, primary amputation, surgical revascularization, intra-arterial thrombolysis, or a combined approach with thrombolysis and open revascularization. Anticoagulation is of primary importance in any treatment regimen [6,7]. Three questions are of importance in this situation—embolic versus thrombotic etiology, anticoagulation strategy, and choice of revascularization approach.

## 62.1 Is It Possible to Diagnose an Embolic versus Thrombotic Etiology for Acute Limb Ischemia Based on History and Physical Examination?

Retrospective reviews of consecutive patient cohorts and one prospective study do provide information on the subject. A retrospective review[3] examined patients treated with surgical embolectomy for acute limb ischemia. The patients had a preoperative diagnosis of acute arterial embolism. The group looked to define a group of patients misdiagnosed with arterial embolism instead of acute thrombosis. A diagnosis of arterial embolus was made if an embolic source was discovered (atrial fibrillation and/or myocardial infarction), the event was acute, and the patient had no history of chronic arterial insufficiency (intermittent claudication). The main criteria for diagnosis of arterial thrombosis were an absence of a cardiovascular source for the embolus, a rapid (not sudden) onset of symptoms with less than 7 days duration, and a history of symptomatic peripheral arterial disease. Twenty-five percent of the patients were misdiagnosed with an embolic etiology for their ischemia (Level 4). Twenty-six percent of patients had an etiology of acute limb ischemia that was not identifiable in a more recent cohort (Level 3b) [2]. Cambria and Abbott in 1984 established that the diagnosis of embolus was wrong in 17% of their patients [9]. The presence of atrial fibrillation was the only distinguishing feature between the two groups. Forty percent of thrombotic patients had preceding symptoms of arterial insufficiency (Level 3b). A 1-year prospective study of patients treated for acute limb ischemia based on examination alone demonstrated an incorrect diagnosis in 9% of patients. However, no impact on the outcome was seen due to misdiagnosis [1] (Level 2b).

In conclusion, it is possible to distinguish between embolic versus thrombotic etiology on examination. However, there is a substantial subset of patients that will need further testing and/or exploration (Grade C recommendation).

## 62.2 Is Perioperative Anticoagulation Necessary in the Treatment of Acute Limb Ischemia?

Anticoagulation is an important treatment for prevention of propagation of thrombus. Stasis created by the initial occlusive event leads to thrombosis and loss of collateral flow via secondary occlusion from propagation of thrombus [6,7] (Level 5). Surgical embolectomy can be delayed if anticoagulation alone is administered and if there is no evidence of impending muscle loss [1,2,4,5,9]. However, this is not always an acceptable measure as up to 50% of patients require immediate revascularization [2].

Patients undergoing revascularization without anticoagulants and patients receiving anticoagulants before surgery, during, and after revascularization were reviewed at one center [10]. Patients with temporary anticoagulation and those with incomplete records were omitted. Patients receiving anticoagulation were twice as likely to have a "good result" defined as amputation-free survival at 4 months. No difference in hospital deaths was found, but patients receiving anticoagulation had significantly more bleeding complications. Recurrence rates at 36 months were not different (Level 4). One hundred and eighteen patients with acute limb ischemia randomized to anticoagulation or no anticoagulation along with thromboembolectomy were prospectively studied at multiple centers. Anticoagulation with heparin was then transitioned to Coumadin. Results were evaluated at 30 days. No significant difference was found in amputation-free survival, mortality, or reoperation [11] (Level 2b).

In conclusion, consensus panels recommend perioperative anticoagulation in the absence of definitive evidence (Grade C).

## 62.3 Is Percutaneous Catheter-Directed Intra-Arterial Thrombolysis the Preferred Initial Treatment over Surgical Revascularization?

Catheter-directed intra-arterial therapy has fewer bleeding complications and improved clot resolution compared with systemic thrombolysis [12]. It is believed that thrombolytic therapy allows for improved clearance of thrombus from vessels too small for traditional embolectomy catheters, a more gradual reperfusion of the ischemic limb, and the ability to diagnose underlying pathology in the angiography suite or operating room. This does come at the cost of increased time to reperfusion, cost, and hospital resource use, hemorrhage, and distal embolization.

A systematic review found 27 patients treated with thrombolytic therapy taken from larger cohorts [13]. Limb salvage was 100% at 6–12 months. Mortality was 0. However, selection bias played a large role in the choice of therapy. Current thinking follows that cardiogenic embolic material is more organized and is more resistant to thrombolysis than in situ thrombosis [6]. Surgical therapy has been compared with percutaneous thrombolysis in several prospective randomized trials. Unfortunately, the end points of the studies vary as does the patient populations. Patients with embolic sources were excluded from randomization [14]. No differences in limb salvage were found in several single center trials [15,16] (Level 2b). The Thrombolysis Or Peripheral Arterial Surgery (TOPAS) trial was a randomized, multicenter prospective trial comparing thrombolysis or surgery in patients with <2 weeks of acute ischemia. There was no difference in 1-year mortality or amputation-free survival. Forty-six percent of patients needed no further surgical revascularization following thrombolysis (Level 2b) [17]. And 548 patients were evaluated in phase 2. The primary end point was amputation-free survival, and there was no difference between the two groups. Bleeding complications were significantly higher in the thrombolysis group. There was no demonstrable difference between limbs treated for thrombotic etiology versus embolic etiology. The major conclusion is that there is a decreased need for open surgical revascularization, but there is a higher rate of bleeding with thrombolytic therapy (Level 2b).

**TABLE 62.1**

Clinical Questions

| Question | Answer | Levels of Evidence | Grade of Recommendation | References |
|---|---|---|---|---|
| Is it possible to diagnose embolus versus thrombus by history and physical? | Yes, but many patients will require further testing. | 2b, 3b, 4 | C | [1,2,3,9] |
| Is preoperative anticoagulation indicated? | Yes, consensus panels support this. | 5, 4, 2b | C | [1,2,4,5,9,10] |
| Is percutaneous thrombectomy preferred over surgical revascularization? | No, they are equivalent in obtaining limb salvage and mortality. | 2b, 1a | B | [6,12–14, 17,18] |

A Cochrane Database meta-analysis examined five randomized trials including 1283 patients. The primary end point of amputation-free survival at 1, 6, and 12 months after thrombolysis versus open surgery was found to be no different. There was no difference in mortality as the secondary end point. Initial thrombolysis had an increased risk of major hemorrhage at 30 days (OR 2.8; 95% CI 1.7–4.6), stroke at 30 days (OR 6.41; 95% CI 1.57–26.2), and distal embolization (OR 8.35; 95% CI 4.47–15.58) [19] (Level 1a).

Intra-arterial catheter-directed thrombolysis as initial therapy for acute limb ischemia is equivalent to surgical therapy in obtaining limb salvage and reducing mortality. It may decrease further need for surgical revascularization. However, there is an increased risk of major hemorrhage, stroke, and distal embolization. The treatment of acute embolic ischemia is extrapolated from broader patient cohorts (Grade B) (Table 62.1).

## References


1. McPhail N, Fratesi SJ, Barger GG, Scobie TK. Management of acute thromboembolic limb ischemia. *Surgery.* 1983;93:381–385.
2. Jivegard L, Arfvidsson B, Holm J, Schersten T. Selective conservative and routine early operative treatment in acute limb ischemia. *Br J Surg.* 1987;74:798–801.
3. Jivegard L, Holm J, Schersten T. The outcome in arterial thrombosis misdiagnosed as arterial embolism. *Acta Chir Scand.* 1986;152:251–256.
4. Dale W. Differential management of acute peripheral arterial ischemia. *J Vasc Surg.* 1984;1:269–278.
5. Blaisdell F, Steele M, Allen RE. Management of acute lower extremity arterial ischemia due to embolism and thrombosis. *Surgery.* 1978;84:822–834.
6. Norgren LHW, Dormandy JA, Nehler MR, Harris KA, Fowkes FGR. Inter-societal consensus for the management of peripheral arterial disease (TASC II). *J Vasc Surg.* 2007;45:S1–S67.
7. Clagett GPSM, Jackson MR, Lip GYH, Tangelder M, Verhaeghe R. Antithrombotic therapy in peripheral arterial occlusive disease: The Seventh ACCP Conference on antithrombotic and thrombolytic therapy. *Chest* 2004;126:609–626.
8. Rutherford R, Baker JD, Ernst C et al. Recommended standards for reports dealing with lower extremity ischemia: Revised version. *J Vasc Surg.* 1997;26:517–538.
9. Cambria R, Abbott WM. Acute arterial thrombosis of the lower extremity. *Arch Surg.* 1984;119:784–787.
10. Jivegard LHJ, Schersten T. Arterial thromboembolectomy—Should anticoagulants be administered? *Acta Chir Scand.* 1986;152:493–497.
11. Jivegard L, Holm J, Bergqvist D et al. Acute lower limb ischemia: Failure of anticoagulant treatment to improve one-month results of arterial thromboembolectomy. A prospective randomized multi-center study. *Surgery.* 1991;109:610–616.
12. Berridge D, Gregson RHS, Hopkinson BR et al. Randomized trial of intra-arterial recombinant tissue plasminogen activator, intravenous recombinant tissue plasminogen activator and intra-arterial streptokinase in peripheral arterial thrombolysis. *Br J Surg.* 1991;78:988–995.
13. Diffin D, Kandarpa K. Assessment of peripheral intraarterial thrombolysis versus surgical revascularization in acute lower-limb ischemia: A review of limb-salvage and mortality statistics. *J Vasc Inv Rad.* 1996;7:57–63.
14. The STILE Investigators. Results of a prospective randomized trial evaluating surgery versus thrombolysis for ischemia of the lower extremity. The STILE trial. *Ann Surg.* 1994;220:251–268.
15. Ouriel K, Shortell CK, DeWeese JA et al. A comparison of thrombolytic therapy with operative revascularization in the initial treatment of acute peripheral arterial ischemia. *J Vasc Surg.* 1994;19:1021–1030.
16. Nilsson L, Albrechtsson U, Jonung T et al. Surgical treatment versus thrombolysis in acute arterial occlusion: a randomised controlled study. *Eur J Vasc Surg.* 1992;6:189–193.
17. Ouriel K, Veith FJ, Sasahara AA et al. Thrombolysis or peripheral arterial surgery: Phase I results. *J Vasc Surg.* 1996;23:64–73.
18. Ouriel K, Veith FJ, Sasahara AA et al. A comparison of recombinant urokinase with vascular surgery as initial treatment for acute arterial occlusion of the legs. *N Engl J Med.* 1998;338:1105–1111.
19. Berridge DC, Kessel D, Robertson I. The Cochrane Database of Systematic Reviews: Surgery versus thrombolysis for initial management of acute limb ischemia. *Cochrane Database Syst Rev.* 2013;6:CD002784.

## Commentary on Acute Arterial Embolus

*Todd W. Costantini and Raul Coimbra*

Acute limb ischemia (ALI) is one of the most common problems that a vascular surgeon is called upon to manage. The underlying etiologies are varied, but the most frequent ones include thrombosis superimposed upon pre-existing atherosclerosis, iatrogenic and noniatrogenic trauma, and peripheral arterial embolization, most commonly from a cardiac source. The authors have addressed the diagnosis and treatment of peripheral artery embolus. The spectrum of disease and degree of ischemia can be quite variable, and thus, the options for and timing of treatment are also wide-ranging. Each case taxes the judgment of a vascular surgeon.

### Is It Possible to Diagnosis Embolic versus Thrombotic Etiology for Acute Limb Ischemia Based on History and Physical Examination?

History, in this day of rampant medical imaging remains of major importance. Physical examination is likewise extremely important and is unfortunately often neglected, given the widespread prompt access to CTA, MRA, and duplex imaging. In most cases, it is possible to distinguish a thrombotic source from an embolic source. Nearly 90% of peripheral emboli originate from the heart, so most commonly, such patients will present with ALI either in the setting of atrial fibrillation or after a recent myocardial infarction. ALI developing in either of these settings should be presumed to be embolic in origin until proven otherwise.

Most active patients who have pre-existing atherosclerosis will report having had symptoms of claudication and will also have evidence on physical examination and basic noninvasive testing of peripheral arterial occlusive disease, often bilaterally. In these patients, pre-existing collaterals often make the situation less urgent. Many of these patients, if their degree of ischemia is not profound, can be managed with an initial course of systemic heparinization, followed by urgent, rather than emergent, thrombolysis to uncover the culprit lesion and angioplasty with or without stenting to treat it. There are a small number of patients in whom the differential diagnosis is difficult to make and some patients who have a combination of an embolic source and pre-existing atherosclerotic occlusive disease in whom the diagnosis may not be totally clear even after treatment. Nonetheless, a complete history and physical examination with attention to underlying risk factors and previous lower extremity vascular symptoms will most often point the diagnostician in the proper direction. The distinction is important, since the treatment approach may well differ.

### Is Perioperative Anticoagulation Necessary in the Treatment of Acute Limb Ischemia?

Perioperative anticoagulation to prevent propagation of thrombus is the standard treatment for patients with acute arterial occlusion in the absence of absolute contraindications to anticoagulation therapy, such as recent major GI hemorrhage or recent intracranial hemorrhage. In addition, in patients who are treated for embolic ALI, maintenance of perioperative and postoperative anticoagulation is extremely important as one of the major causes of subsequent morbidity and mortality in these patients is either recurrent embolization or recurrent thrombosis of the treated arterial segment, presumably due to the combined effects of residual thrombus and underlying endothelial damage from the treatment pathway chosen. Although there are no randomized prospective trials, abundant long-term clinical experience suggests that perioperative and long-term anticoagulation in patients with cardiogenic emboli is indicated.

### Is Percutaneous Catheter-Directed Intra-Arterial Thrombolysis the Preferred Initial Treatment over Surgical Revascularization?

Nearly all prospective randomized trials have focused on a mix of patients who have either thrombosis of a preexisting arterial atherosclerotic stenosis or embolic limb ischemia. In addition, most of the randomized trials have included a broad spectrum of ischemia. It is extremely important to stratify the patient's degree of ischemia preoperatively using the standard Rutherford ALI classification system.* Category I patients have viable limbs that are not immediately threatened and they can be treated with anticoagulation and subsequent urgent or semielective revascularization if the degree of ischemia warrants it. These patients have no sensory loss, no muscle weakness, and audible arterial and venous Doppler signals. Threatened limbs, which include Category IIA and IIB, are salvageable with immediate revascularization, but revascularization cannot usually be delayed. In Category IIA patients, there may be minimal or no sensory findings or sensory disturbances are confined to the distal forefoot, and these patients can be treated somewhat less aggressively than those who have more severe sensory loss or those with motor dysfunction.

* Rutherford RB, Baker JD, Ernst C et al. Recommended standards for reports dealing with lower extremity ischemia: Revised version. *J Vasc Surg*. 1997;26(3):517–538.

Patients with irreversible ischemia are best treated with anticoagulation and subsequent amputation, but in some of these cases, one is still forced to do some sort of revascularization in order to allow even an amputation to heal.

ALI management depends on the underlying cause, location, ease of accessibility and details of presentation.* The modern treatment of ALI for patients with acute thrombosis superimposed upon previous atherosclerotic disease, especially for category I and IIA patients, generally involves an initial endovascular approach with thrombolysis to identify the culprit lesion, which can then be treated appropriately. Many Category IIA and most Category IIB and III patients are best treated in the operating room with a combination of open and endovascular techniques, or so-called hybrid approaches. Nearly all high level vascular care centers have access to advanced imaging in the operating room setting, which would be utilized in these cases. Catheter-directed thrombolysis should not be performed in patients for whom lysis for 12–48 h would not be safe and in those with absolute contraindications to thrombolysis such as recent major surgery, intracranial hemorrhage or vascular brain neoplasm, or recent active bleeding. In addition, thrombolysis should not be performed in a nonviable limb. There are newly available mechanical thrombectomy devices that can speed the process, but they often prove unsatisfactory for the effective removal of large cardiac emboli. Major emboli at surgically accessible sites (saddle emboli, common femoral artery, and brachial artery) are still most often and expeditiously treated by surgical cut-down and Fogarty catheter embolectomy, with fasciotomy, if indicated, due to duration and or severity of ischemia. A contemporary study based on the U.S. National Inpatient Sample reported that (1) embolectomy was associated with decreased mortality and amputation risk and that (2) fasciotomy was done in 4.3% of limbs coded for acute embolism and thrombosis of the lower extremities.† Fasciotomy was more common (25%) in a concomitant, retrospective experience at a major academic institution. Those patients requiring fasciotomy were also at greater risk of amputation and death, presumably reflecting more advanced ischemia, and perhaps a selection bias based on the tertiary referral pattern.†

The onus on the surgeon treating ALI is to rapidly establish the diagnosis, base treatment on a logical algorithm considering the most likely cause, severity, and duration of ischemia, and patient comorbidities. Diagnosis and treatment delays and failure to perform fasciotomy can lead to severe morbidity and even mortality.

* Branco BC, Montero-Baker MF, Mills JL. The pros and cons of endovascular and open surgical treatments for patients with acute limb ischemia. *J Cardiovasc Surg.* 2015 June;56(3):401–407.

† Eliason JL, Wainess RM, Proctor MC, Dimick JB, Cowan JA Jr., Upchurch GR Jr., Stanley JC, Henke PK. A national and single institutional experience in the contemporary treatment of acute lower extremity ischemia. *Arch Surg.* 2003;238(3):383–389.

# 63

## *Ruptured Abdominal Aortic Aneurysm*

**Boulos Toursarkissian**

CONTENTS



A ruptured abdominal aortic aneurysm (rAAA) is a serious life-threatening surgical emergency. It ranks among the 15 leading causes of death in the United States, despite many advances in anesthesia and critical care medicine.

Important considerations in the care of a patient with a rAAA include preoperative resuscitation goals and methods, criteria used to select patients for surgery (i.e., survival prediction), the nature of imaging studies needed before surgical intervention and the delay impact this can cause, the type of intervention to be performed, the use of anticoagulants intraoperatively, and the need to monitor patients for frequent postoperative complications. Patients with rAAA are prone to the development of complications including ischemic colitis (IC), paraplegia from spinal cord ischemia, renal failure, peripheral atheroembolic complications, and abdominal compartment syndrome (ACS) (Tables 63.1 and 63.2).

### 63.1 What are the Optimal Resuscitation Goals and Methods to Be Used in Patients with Ruptured Aneurysms?

As far as resuscitation goals, measures, and fluids, only expert opinions and some prospective cohort studies are available in the literature (level IV and V evidence). The suggestions are based on extrapolations from the trauma literature. One of the main limitations to be kept in mind, however, is that trauma patients are usually younger and healthier as a group compared to patients with rAAA.

One prospective trial evaluated 90 patients requiring emergency surgery for trauma; patients were randomized to either intraoperative hypotensive resuscitation (mean arterial pressure of 50 mmHg) or standard fluid resuscitation (target mean arterial pressure of 65 mmHg). Patients in the low pressure arm required less fluids and blood, had less coagulopathy and had a lower mortality in the early postoperative period [1] (level I evidence).

Many experts suggest that it is acceptable to tolerate a systolic blood pressure under 100 mmHg or even lower (down to 70 mmHg) in patients with rAAA as long as adequate mentation is maintained (Grade C recommendation). The rationale presented is that a higher pressure may exacerbate the tendency for retroperitoneal hemorrhage and convert what was otherwise a contained rupture into a free one. The added fluids required may also exacerbate postoperative coagulopathy. A retrospective study of 248 patients with rAAA over a 10-year period suggested that aggressive volume resuscitation before proximal aortic control predicted an increased perioperative risk of death, which was independent of systolic blood pressure [2] (level IIb evidence). On the other hand, retrospective analysis of data from the British IMPROVE trial [3; see below] suggests that a systolic pressure under 70 mmHg was independently associated with increased mortality (51% vs. 34%).

Although there are no definitive studies in patients with rAAA, it seems intuitive to recommend avoiding overt hypertension [4].

**TABLE 63.1**

Clinical Questions

| Question | Answer | Grade of Recommendation | References |
|---|---|---|---|
| What are the optimal resuscitation goals? | Low-grade hypotension is acceptable | C | [1,2] |
| What are the preferred resuscitation fluids? | Blood products are preferred | B | [5,6] |
| Should a CT scan be obtained in patients with suspected rAAA? | Yes, except in most extreme cases | B | [20] |
| Can EVAR be used in patients with rAAA? | Yes | A, B | [3,24] |
| What can be done to avoid paraplegia and/or ischemic colitis? | Try to maintain flow to at least one hypogastric artery | B | [35] |

**TABLE 63.2**

Levels of Evidence

| Subject | Year | References | Level of Evidence | Strength of Recommendation | Findings |
|---|---|---|---|---|---|
| Choice of fluids for resuscitation | 2010 | [5,6] | IIb | B | Early administration of blood products may be beneficial |
| Imaging prior to treatment | 2014 | [20] | IIb | B | Spiral CT scanning is a reasonable test in most patients |
| Repair technique | 2013–2014 | [3,24] | I | A | EVAR is an acceptable alternative to open repair |
| Ischemic colitis post rAAA repair | 2013 | [37] | IIb | B | Ischemic colitis is frequent and vigilance is required for early detection |

The nature of fluids to be used for resuscitation purposes in the perioperative period in patients with rAAA has been the subject of at least one prospective cohort study (level IIa evidence). In this Danish study, 55 patients with rAAA were proactively administered fresh frozen plasma and platelet concentrates immediately when the diagnosis of rAAA was suspected [5]. Thirty days survival improved to 66% as compared to a 44% survival for the 93 patients treated by conventional means in the preceding 2-year period. All patients in the study group were treated with an open aneurysm surgery. Another prospective cohort study from Denmark used a "transfusion package" of red cells (five units), plasma (five units), and platelets (two units) combined with thromboelastography to guide transfusion, resulting in a decrease in mortality at 30 days from 56% in historic controls to 34% in treated patients [6]. From these studies as well as other data on massively injured patients [7], an aggressive approach toward the use of blood products appears justified (Grade B recommendation).

*Recommendation*: Moderate hypotension is acceptable and blood products should be used early (Grades B and C recommendations).

## 63.2 Can Mortality from rAAA be Predicted?

Mortality after repair of rAAA remains high. One of the factors that has been associated with increasing mortality in a number of studies is advanced age, especially when comparing patients over the age of 80 years to younger individuals (level IIIb evidence). However, an age cutoff beyond which survival is unlikely has never been identified, and survival rates over 50% have been reported by some in octogenarians [8]. Therefore, age alone cannot be used as a contraindication to attempting surgical repair of a rAAA (Grade B recommendation).

There is no single preoperative parameter to indicate whether or not a patient with a rAAA will survive a surgical attempt to repair the rAAA. Many models have been developed to help predict mortality and survival. The Glasgow aneurysms score is equal to the age in years, plus 17 points for the presence of shock, plus 7 points for a prior myocardial infarction or ongoing angina, plus 10 points for any prior stroke or transient ischemic attacks (TIA), plus 14 points for renal insufficiency [9]. A retrospective nationwide survey in Finland [10] found the Glasgow score to be predictive of mortality, with a score greater than 98 to be associated with an 80% postoperative mortality (level IIIb evidence). The Hardman index is another such model and gives one point for each of age greater than 76 years, creatinine over 190 μmol/L, hemoglobin less than 9 g/dL, myocardial ischemia on EKG, and a history of loss of consciousness after arrival in hospital [11]. The presence of over three or more points was reported as uniformly fatal in one study [12]. Both the Glasgow score and the Hardman index have been reported as poor predictors of survival in at least one retrospective study from Scotland [13]. It appears therefore that there are currently no scores to allow reliable prediction of mortality (Grade B recommendation).

While preoperative predictors of survival may be poor, there are formulas which use postoperative data to predict short-term mortality. For instance, in patients who are alive after 48 h from surgery, the sequential organ failure assessment (SOFA) score has been shown to be predictive of mortality. The SOFA score evaluates respiratory, coagulation, hepatic, cardiovascular, renal, and neurologic function, with each a sign value from 0 to 4 [14]. In one retrospective study [15], a 48 h SOFA score greater than 11 predicted mortality with 93% specificity (level IIIb evidence).

*Recommendation*: Neither age nor any of the available formulas are accurate enough to allow mortality prediction (Grade B recommendation).

## 63.3 Do Delays in Reaching an Operating Room Affect Outcomes?

Controversy continues as to whether delays in reaching an operating room affect the ultimate mortality of patients with rAAA. Studies have been published with completely conflicting results [16–18]. All these studies however are retrospective cohort studies (level III evidence). Many but not all exclude patients who do not survive till hospital arrival, thereby creating a clear selection bias. It appears rather intuitive to try to minimize any delays in accessing an operating room, given the overall risks and benefit ratios (Grade B recommendation).

The question of delay in getting to surgery has become particularly relevant with the increasing use of endovascular repair (EVAR) for treating rAAA (see below). In order to allow proper EVAR planning, a CT scan of the abdomen and pelvis is usually needed. With spiral CT units, the time needed for an abdomen scan has diminished. In a study of time-to-death in patients with rAAA not operated upon, 87.5% of patients admitted to hospital with rAAA died after more than 2 h of admission [19], with most of those not being treated aggressively. Data from the British IMPROVE trial (see the following text) suggests that for most patients there is sufficient time to obtain a CT scan and that the resulting delay is very minimal [20]. It appears therefore reasonable to consider a CT angiogram of the abdomen and pelvis in all except the most unstable patients (Grade B recommendation).

The other reason why delays may be important has to do with the possible need to regionalize the care of patients with rAAAs. Increasing data are showing that high volume surgeons in high volume facilities with subspecialty training may produce better results for patients with rAAAs (level IIb evidence) [21,22]. Other data suggest that large centers that are able to more rapidly mobilize large resources may produce better outcomes for rAAA [23]. Transfer may be time-consuming although data from both the British IMPROVE trial and the Amsterdam trial [24] (see below) suggest that such transfers do not affect outcomes. A selection bias may however be present in that only more robust patients may survive a transfer.

*Recommendation*: The data are controversial. However, getting a CT scan is reasonable in the majority of cases (Grade B recommendation).

## 63.4 Is Endovascular Repair Preferred in Patients with rAAA?

A rAAA is usually a fatal condition unless treated surgically. There are two major choices of surgical intervention: open repair and stent graft placement or EVAR. The EVAR1 trial compared open repair to EVAR in patients undergoing elective repair of a nonruptured AAA [25]. The group undergoing EVAR had a lower early mortality and fewer complications. Given this finding, and given the fact that open repair for rAAA has continued to have a high mortality, the question has arisen as to whether EVAR should be preferred over open repair for patients presenting with rAAA.

Numerous retrospective studies have suggested that EVAR for rAAA may be beneficial over open repair. The largest retrospective review published was a study of 283 cases over a 10 year period at Albany Medical Center and showed a decreased 30 days and 5 year mortality in patients treated with EVAR as opposed to open repair (24% vs. 44% at 30 days). They did note an increased reintervention rate for EVAR patient group [26]. A meta-analysis of 41 studies (all retrospective except for one prospective small trial) published in 2013 showed less mortality with EVAR as well as less respiratory and renal complications [27]. All such studies suffer from an inherent selection bias, in that more stable patients with less complicated anatomy may be selected for EVAR as opposed to open repair.

Two randomized prospective trials have tried to address the question of EVAR vs. OR for rAAAs [3,24].

The Amsterdam trial [24] randomized 116 patients with rAAA, who had anatomy suitable for both EVAR and OR. EVAR used an aorto-uniliac graft configuration with a crossover femoro-femoral bypass. All rAAA care in the Amsterdam area was centralized to three participating centers. Overall, 20% of patients presented with systolic pressures under 90 mmHg. The greatest reason for exclusion among the 520 potential patients was unsuitable anatomy for EVAR. The 30-day mortality was 21% in patients assigned to EVAR vs. 25% in those assigned to OR (no difference; intention to treat). Crossover from EVAR to OR was 14%. Hospital stay, ICU stay, and estimated blood loss were all less in patients assigned to EVAR. Mortality in the nonrandomized cohort that was treated was 30%, a number lower than seen in other studies; this may be explained by the centralization of care and protocols.

The British IMPROVE trial [3] had a different design, in that it randomized patients with suspected rAAA to either an endovascular strategy (CT scan followed by EVAR if anatomically suitable) or an immediate open surgery (with CT scan optional). Six hundred twenty-three patients were randomized out of 1275 possible at 30 centers. One-half of the patients had systolic blood pressure less than 90 mmHg. Of the 316 patients randomized to an endovascular approach, 87% had ruptures confirmed and 36% of those were not suitable for EVAR. EVAR was attempted in 154 patients and open repair in 112 cases in the endovascular strategy group. Of the 297 randomized to an open approach, 88% had rupture confirmed and open repair was attempted in 220. The 30-day mortality in patients with confirmed rAAA was the same in both groups (36.4% and 40.6%). In women, the endovascular strategy seemed beneficial in terms of 30-day mortality (37% vs. 57%). ICU and hospital lengths of stay were shorter in the endovascular strategy group. When looking at treatment actually received, the mortality, however, was lower with EVAR than open repair (25% vs. 38%).

A number of points can be made from reviewing all these studies.

Even with versatile devices and the use of aorto-mono-iliac configurations (with crossover femoro-femoral bypass), there is still a very significant proportion of patients with rAAA who have anatomy not suitable for EVAR [28]. The proportion of ineligible patients is higher than seen in patients presenting for elective repair. There is also a trend toward accepting less than optimal anatomy for EVAR in patients with rAAA [29]. In those patients who can undergo EVAR, the morbidity, blood loss, and ICU length of stay are decreased. Emergency EVAR is also likely to be more technically challenging and requires the use of adjunctive techniques such as placement of temporary aortic occlusion balloons for instance.

The use of local anesthesia may be beneficial in patients undergoing EVAR for rAAA. The British IMPROVE trial showed that patients treated under local anesthesia had a fourfold survival advantage compared to those treated with EVAR under general anesthesia [20]; this has also been suggested in retrospective reviews [30].

We conclude that EVAR for rAAA is a viable therapeutic option when offered by an experienced surgeon in a center familiar with elective EVAR therapy and with quick access to a variety of stent graft sizes.

*Recommendation*: EVAR is an acceptable treatment method (Grade A recommendation).

## 63.5 Should Anticoagulation Be Used Intraoperatively?

Heparin anticoagulation prior to aortic clamping is routinely done in elective rAAA surgery. Patients with rAAA have already lost large volumes of blood and may be coagulopathic and hypothermic. It seems therefore reasonable in those cases to avoid full anticoagulation. There are no good studies on the subject and only expert opinion is available (level V evidence). The data from Albany [26] recommend avoidance of anticoagulation in EVAR for rAAA. The decision to use anticoagulants must be individualized.

In patients who develop coagulopathy intraoperatively, the use of abdominal packing is an option. A retrospective series of 23 patients identified from a prospective surgical database (level III evidence) had a 48% survival, but a high 22% incidence of early or late infectious complications [31]. Even the use of vacuum-assisted closure and mesh-mediated fascial traction is still associated with a risk of infectious issues and fistulas [32]. Use of packing should therefore be very selective (Grade C recommendation).

Intraoperative hypothermia has been shown to be correlated with increased mortality in a retrospective review of 100 consecutive patients treated for rAAA at one institution [33] (level IIb evidence). Therefore, every effort should be made to avoid hypothermia starting in the preoperative period (Grade B recommendation). The room should be warmed, blankets used, and fluids and gas administered should be heated.

The final issue relates to the level of aortic clamping for cases done via an open approach. Again, no prospective or retrospective data on the subject have been published and only expert opinion is available (level V evidence). Infrarenal clamping appears desirable when possible, as it avoids renal and mesenteric ischemia. However, this is often not possible as a large hematoma with a large rAAA may obscure the planes and mandate a supraceliac clamp.

*Recommendation*: No data are available regarding intraoperative anticoagulation and decision must be individualized. Hypothermia should be avoided (Grade C recommendation).

## 63.6 Can Paraplegia Be Avoided?

Spinal cord ischemia can be caused by shock, massive atheroembolization, interruption of flow to the artery of Adakiewicz, and interruption of flow to the hypogastric arteries.

The incidence with open repair of rAAA is between 1% and 2% [34].

One retrospective review of 35 patients with rAAA treated with EVAR noted an 11.5% incidence [35]; a statistical association was noted with occlusion of one or more hypogastric arteries with the stent graft (level III evidence). Other reports have not suggested as high an incidence.

Prevention should focus on maintenance of spinal cord perfusion pressure by maintenance of blood pressure and avoiding collateral disruption. It seems prudent to try to maintain flow to at least one hypogastric artery during stent graft placement for rAAA (Grade B recommendation).

Cerebrospinal fluid drainage in elective settings is useful but not practical for emergencies. However, it can be placed postoperatively if symptoms develop and may result in reversal of symptoms.

*Recommendation*: Paraplegia cannot always be avoided. Try to maintain flow to at least one hypogastric artery (Grade B recommendation).

## 63.7 Should Sigmoidoscopy Be Performed Routinely in the Postop Period?

IC after repair of rAAA is a common occurrence. It may be related to hypotension, embolization or interruption of flow to the inferior mesenteric, and hypogastric arteries. Earlier studies showed that endoscopically verified IC after open repair of rAAA may be present in as many as 42% of cases [36] (level I evidence). More recent studies have shown a lesser incidence of 22%, and most cases are mild [37]. This is similar to the incidence reported after EVAR for rAAA [38]. Unfortunately, there are no predictive parameters and even patients with transmural ischemia may fail to show early laboratory anomalies. Retrospective data do suggest that early detection of IC may be associated with decreased mortality (level III evidence). As a consequence, many surgeons advocate routine flexible sigmoidoscopy at 24 h after surgery for rAAA (Grade C recommendation).

*Recommendation*: IC is frequent enough that sigmoidoscopy should be performed with any clinical suspicion (Grade C recommendation).

## 63.8 Should Patients Be Monitored for Abdominal Compartment Syndrome?

ACS can affect 4%–12% of patients following open repair of rAAA, while the incidence after EVAR may be higher, up to 20% [39]. In one retrospective series from Albany, ACS was responsible for 31% of deaths [26].

In retrospective series, a number of risk factors for ACS have been identified to include coagulopathy, massive transfusion, and the need for an aortic occlusion balloon for hypotension [39] (level IIb evidence). Early recognition of ACS via bladder pressure monitoring and aggressive management appears to result in decreased mortality, and appears therefore reasonable (Grade B recommendation).

*Recommendation*: The ACS is frequent enough that bladder monitoring should be performed (Grade B recommendation).

## References

1. Morrison CA, Carrick MM, Norman MA et al. Hypotensive resuscitation strategy reduces transfusion requirements and severe postoperative coagulopathy in trauma patients with hemorrhagic shock: Preliminary results of a randomized controlled trial. *J Trauma Injury Infect Crit Care.* 2011;70(3):652–663.
2. Dick F, Erdoes G, Opfermann P et al. Delayed volume resuscitation during initial management of ruptured abdominal aortic aneurysm. *J Vasc Surg.* 2013;57:943–950.
3. Improve Trial Investigators. Endovascular or open repair strategy for ruptured abdominal aortic aneuryms: 30 day outcomes from IMPROVE randomized trial. *Br Med J.* 2014;348:7661.
4. Piffaretti G, Caronno R, Tozzi M et al. Endovascular versus open repair of ruptured abdominal aortic aneurysms. *Expert Rev Cardiovasc Ther.* 2006;4(6):839–852.
5. Johansson PI, Stensballe J, Rosenberg I et al. Proactive administration of platelets and plasma for patients with a ruptured abdominal aortic aneurysm: Evaluating a change in transfusion practice. *Transfusion.* 2007;47:593–598.
6. Johansson PI. Goal directed hemostatic resuscitation for massively being patients: The Copenhagen concept. *Transfusion Apheresis Sci.* 2010:43:401–405.
7. Cinat ME, Wallace WC, Nastanski F et al. Improved survival following massive transfusion in patients who have undergone trauma. *Arch Surg.* 1999;134:964–970.
8. Chiesa R, Setacci C, Tshomba Y et al. Ruptured abdominal aortic aneurysm in the elderly patient. *Acta Chir Belg.* 2006;106:508–516.
9. Samy AK, Murray G, MacBain G. Glasgow Aneurysm score. *Cardiovasc Surg.* 1994;2:41–44.

10. Korhonen SJ, Ylonen K, Biancari F et al. Glasgow aneurysm score as a predictor of immediate outcome after surgery for ruptured abdominal aortic aneurysm. *Br J Surg.* 2004;91:1449–1452.
11. Hardman DT, Fisher CM, Patel MI et al. Ruptured abdominal aortic aneurysms: Who should be offered surgery? *J Vasc Surg.* 1996;23:123–129.
12. Prance SE, Wilson YG, Cosgrove CM et al. Ruptured abdominal aortic aneurysms: Selecting patients for surgery. *Eur J Vasc Endovasc Surg.* 1999;17:129–132.
13. Tambyraja AL, Fraser SCA, Murie JA et al. Validity of the Glasgow aneurysm store and the Hardman Index in predicting outcome alter ruptured abdominal aortic aneurysm repair. *Br J Surg.* 2005;92:570–573.
14. Kniemayer HW, Kessler T, Reber PU et al. Treatment of ruptured abdominal aortic aneurysm, a permanent challenge or a waste of resources? Prediction of outcome using a multi-organ-dysfunction score. *Eur J Vasc Endovasc Surg.* 2000;19:190–196.
15. Laukontaus SJ, Lepantalo M, Hynninen M et al. Prediction of survival after 48 hours of intensive care following open surgical repair of ruptured abdominal aortic aneurysm. *Eur J Vasc Endovasc Surg.* 2005;30:509–515.
16. DeSouza VC, Strachan DP. Relationship between travel time to the nearest hospital and survival from ruptured abdominal aortic aneurysms: Record linkage study. *J Public Health.* 2005;27(2):165–170.
17. Hames H, Forbes TL, Harris JR et al. The effect of patient transfer on outcomes after rupture of an abdominal aortic aneurysm. *Can J Surg.* 2007;50(1):43–47.
18. Salhab M, Farmer J, Osman I. Impact of delay on survival the patient's with a ruptured abdominal aortic aneurysm. *Vascular.* 2006;14(1):38–42.
19. Lloyd GM, Bown MJ, Norwood MGA et al. Feasibility of preoperative computer tomography in patients with ruptured abdominal aortic aneurysm: A time-to-death study in patients without operation. *J Vasc Surg.* 2004;39:788–791.
20. Powell JT and the Improve Trial Investigators. Observations from the IMPROVE trial concerning the clinical care of patients with ruptured abdominal aortic aneurysm. *Br J Surg.* 2014;101(3):216–224.
21. Dueck AD, Kucey DS, Johnston KW et al. Survival after ruptured abdominal aortic aneurysm: Effect of patient, surgeon and hospital factors. *J Vasc Surg.* 2004;39:1253–1260.
22. Holt PJ, Poloniecki JD, Gerrard D et al. Meta-analysis and systematic review of the relationship between volume and outcome in abdominal aortic aneurysm surgery. *Br J Surg.* 2007;94:395–403.
23. Utter GH, Maier RV, Rivara FP et al. Outcomes after ruptured abdominal aortic aneurysms: The halo effect of trauma center designation. *J Am Coll Surg.* 2006;203:498–505.
24. Reimerink JJ, Hoornweg LL, Vahl AC et al. Endovascular repair versus open repair of ruptured abdominal aortic aneurysms: A multicenter randomized controlled trail. *Ann Surg.* 2013;258(2):248–256.
25. EVAR Trial Participants. Endovascular aneurysm repair versus open repair in patients with abdominal aortic aneurysm (EVAR trial 1): Randomized controlled trial. *Lancet.* 2005;365:2187–2192.
26. Mehta M, Byrne J, Darling RC et al. Endovascular repair of ruptured infrarenal abdominal aortic aneurysm is associated with lower 30-day mortality and better 5-year survival rates than open surgical repair. *J Vasc Surg.* 2013;57:368–375.
27. Antoniou GA, Georgiadis GS, Antoniou SA et al. Endovascular repair for ruptured abdominal aortic aneurysm confers an early survival benefit over open repair. *J Vasc Surg.* 2013;58:1091–1105.
28. Hoornweg LL, Wisselink W, Vahl A et al. The Amsterdam Acute Aneurysm trial: Suitability and application rate for endovascular repair of ruptured abdominal aortic aneurysms. *Eur J Vasc Endovasc Surg.* 2007;33:679–683.
29. Dillon M, Cardwell C, Blair PH et al. Endovascular treatment for ruptured abdominal aortic aneurysm. *Cochrane Database Syst Rev.* 2014;7:CD0005261.
30. Mayer D, Pfammatter T, Rancic Z et al. Ten years of emergency endovascular aneurysm repair fro ruptured abdominal aortoiliac aneurysms: Lessons learned. *Ann Surg.* 2009;249:510–515.
31. Adam DJ, Fitridge RA, Raptis S. Intra-abdominal packing for uncontrollable haemorrhage during ruptured abdominal aortic aneurysm repair. *Eur J Vasc Endovasc Surg.* 2005;30:516–519.
32. Sorelius K, Wanhainen A, Acosta S. et al. Open abdomen treatment after aortic aneurysm repair with vacuum-assisted wound closure and mesh mediated fascial traction. *Eur J Vasc Endovasc Surg.* 2013;45(6):588–594.
33. Janczyk RJ, Howells GA, Blar HA et al. Hypothermia is an independent predictor of mortality in ruptured abdominal aortic aneurysms. *Vasc Endovasc Surg.* 2004;38:37–42.
34. Peppelenbosch AG, Vermulen Windsant IC, Jacobs MJ et al. Open repair for ruptured abdominal aortic aneurysm and the risk of spinal cord ischemia: Review of the literature and risk factor analysis. *Eur J Vasc Endovasc Surg.* 2010:40(5):589–595.
35. Peppelenbosch N, Cuypers PWM, Vahl AC et al. Emergency endovascular treatment for ruptured abdominal aortic aneurysm and the risk of spinal cord ischemia. *J Vasc Surg.* 2005;42:608–614.
36. Champagne BJ, Darling RC, Daneshmand M et al. Outcome of aggressive surveillance colonoscopy in ruptured abdominal aortic aneurysm. *J Vasc Surg.* 2004;39:792–796.
37. Tottrup M, Fedder AM, Jensen RH et al. The value of routine flexible sigmoidoscopy within 48 hours after surgical repair of ruptured abdominal aortic aneurysms. *Ann Vasc Surg.* 2013;27(6):714–718.
38. Champagne BJ, Lee EC, Valerian B et al. Incidence of colonic ischemia after repair of ruptured abdominal aortic aneurysm with endograft. *J Am Coll Surg.* 2007;204:597–602.
39. Mehta M, Darling RC, Roddy SP et al. Factors associated with abdominal compartment syndrome complicating endovascular repair of ruptured abdominal aortic aneurysms. *J Vasc Surg.* 2005;42:1047–1051.

## Commentary on Ruptured Abdominal Aortic Aneurysm

*Roy M. Fujitani*

Ruptured abdominal aortic aneurysms (rAAAs) are intra-abdominal vascular catastrophes that can lead to rapid hemorrhagic shock and death, if not treated in timely fashion at the time of presentation. As is often the case, the diagnosis of the presence of an abdominal aortic aneurysm (AAA) that rupture is often unknown to the patient until the day of the rupture. This fact inherently would make early preemptive detection through screening for AAAs an appealing idea. Although several screening methods exist, ultrasonography is accepted as the standard screening imaging method for AAA, because it has a high sensitivity (94%–100%) and specificity (98%–100%). It is also readily accepted by patients, since it is very quick, safe, noninvasive, and inexpensive. Very recently, the U.S. Preventive Services Task Force (USPSTF) has issued recommendations for AAA screening.* The task force recommends one-time AAA screening for men aged 65–75, who have ever smoked (B recommendation). For men aged 65–75 who have never smoked, the task force recommends discussion with one's health care provider about whether one-time AAA screening is appropriate based on health history and potential benefits/harms of screening (C recommendation). Task force determined that current evidence is insufficient to weigh benefits and harms of screening for AAA in women aged 65–75 years who have ever smoked (I statement) and recommends against routine screening for AAA in women who have never smoked (D recommendation). These proposals form the basis of a draft recommendation statement as published at the time of this commentary preparation. However, despite more aggressive attempts at widespread screening programs, AAAs still remains the 15th leading cause of death in the United States.

Many patients may not survive an acutely ruptured AAA and succumb in our communities prior to receiving emergent surgical care upon arrival at an acute healthcare facility. When they do present however, surgeons must be in a position to offer the best care possible in expedient, expert fashion. This chapter authored by Dr. Toursarkissian very nicely outlines the current evidence-based practices to optimize caring for these critically ill patients at death's threshold.

During the entire stretch of my career, I have had ample opportunity to emergently treat many patients presenting with rAAAs and have seen a substantial evolution in their management. Endovascular therapies have significantly changed the paradigm in which many of these patients are managed. Experience with ruptured endovascular aortic aneurysm repair (REVAR) has gained much ground and is currently our primary choice in managing patients presenting with rAAAs having favorable anatomic characteristics. For selected patients with rAAA, national datasets and single center series suggest that endovascular repair is associated with a lower operative mortality than open surgical repair. The option of open rAAA repair is still however an important and necessary alternative treatment modality reserved for patients with unfavorable anatomy for endovascular repair. Additionally, from a realistic more global health-care system standpoint, not all acute hospital facilities can offer endovascular therapies at all times due to limitation in resources and support personnel.

To comment on specific evidence-based answers to queries addressed in this chapter.

### What Are the Optimal Resuscitation Goals and Methods to Be Used in Patients with rAAAs?

Consistent with the stated available evidence, our current practice allows patients diagnosed with rAAAs to be managed with "permissive hypotension," provided there is clinical evidence of adequate perfusion allowing for adequate mentation. This management is even requested of paramedics when transferring patients from outside facilities, when being transferred for higher level of care to our tertiary center. This, of course, requires very critical monitoring with judicious adjustments in resuscitation until the proximal suprarenal aorta is controlled, usually using percutaneous endovascular balloon occlusion under local anesthesia. Once the proximal aorta is controlled, our preferred resuscitation is use of blood products as noted in the Danish study.

### Can Mortality from rAAA Be Predicted?

There is no argument that mortality from a rAAA is very high, with an estimated 50% of patients never making it to the hospital when rupturing at home. Patients who survive more protracted times from the sentinel rupture event have, in essence, selected themselves as "survivors." As noted, advanced age alone is not predictive of mortality and should not preclude aggressive management. The bottom line is that nearly all patients will not survive a rAAA without expedient surgical intervention. The implementation of structured rAAA protocols streamlining the treatment of these otherwise moribund patients with rapid aortic control is essential to optimize chances for survival.

* LeFevre, ML, on behalf of the U.S. Preventive Services Task Force. Screening for abdominal aortic aneurysm: U.S. Preventive Services Task Force recommendation statement. *Ann Intern Med.* 2014;161(4):281–290.

### Do Delays in Reaching an Operating Room Affect Outcomes?

The goal in optimizing patient outcomes is to have the afflicted patient with a rAAA be treated as quickly and efficiently as possible, which in turn, translates to getting the patient to the operating room emergently. However, having stated this, there is almost always enough time to quickly obtain a CTA en route to the operating suite. The ready availability and close proximity of the CT scanner to the emergency receiving center is important as one wants to avoid taking a patient to a remote part of the hospital when in critical condition. As noted by the author, a preoperative CTA is particularly helpful to allow for deciding between REVAR and open rAAA repair. If REVAR is determined to be feasible, the CTA will facilitate determining choice of endograft device, configuration, and operative approach including potential need for ancillary procedures. This thorough, but expedient preoperative planning, in turn, will lead to more favorable surgical outcomes regardless of REVAR or open rAAA repair.

### Is Endovascular Repair Preferred in Patients with rAAA?

Published national databases and large single center series suggest that REVAR is associated with a lower operative mortality than open rAAA repair. However, it remains controversial with two European randomized trials (Amsterdam Trial and British IMPROVE Trial), noted in the chapter, having failed to show any difference in operative mortality between the two types of repair.[*†] A recent publication, performing a very comprehensive meta-analysis of outcome data of treatment modalities for rAAAs compared perioperative outcomes between REVAR and open rAAA repair in 59,941 patients across 41 studies.[‡] The in-hospital mortality occurred in 30% of patients treated with REVAR and in 42% of patients who underwent open rAAA repair (odds ratio 0.56; 95% confidence interval; 0.50–0.64; $P < 0.01$). The very narrow confidence intervals make the conclusion that REVAR is favorable to open rAAA repair very convincing.

From personal experience, I am absolutely convinced that REVAR is not only acceptable treatment, but favorable to open rAAA repair. The ability to perform the operation using only local anesthesia in REVAR is a significant advantage. Local anesthesia avoids need for general anesthesia and the inherent adverse hemodynamic manifestations it may produce, particularly upon induction in a patient presenting in hemorrhagic shock.

Rapid aortic control is essential for anyone who tries to treat a patient presenting with a rAAA. In our experience, the ability to rapidly percutaneously insert a suprarenal aortic occlusion balloon under local anesthesia to gain proximal aortic control has supplanted need for open aortic cross-clamping. This offers immediate vascular control, allowing for more immediate resuscitation, if the clinical situation requires it. The mortality rate for patients presenting with rAAA has fallen with use of endovascular techniques, partly which may be based on the rapid insertion of an aortic occlusion balloon. Additionally, this proximal aortic control can be used whether subsequently managing with REVAR or open rAAA repair.

### Should Anticoagulation Be Used Intraoperatively?

As alluded to by the lack of evidence-based recommendations, we individualize our decision to administer full systemic anticoagulation based upon the clinical presentation of the patient with a rAAA. In those patients presenting with advanced hemorrhagic shock and significant hemorrhage, we avoid heparin anticoagulation during the conduct of the operation to avoid exacerbating uncontrolled bleeding. When performing REVAR in unstable patients with preexisting, large retroperitoneal hematomas, systemic anticoagulation may only exacerbate the development of subsequent abdominal compartment syndrome postoperatively. Whenever possible, expedient performance of the operation will avoid thrombotic complications. We are liberal in flushing the access sheaths in REVAR cases perioperatively with low concentration heparinized saline to avoid thrombotic complications in the access arteries.

In hemodynamically normal patients presenting with symptomatic but contained rAAAs, we use the same emergency protocols, whether REVAR or open rAAA repair. However, we will generally systemically anticoagulate the patient in this situation, as if performing the procedure in an elective case. This minimizes undesired thrombotic worries while having minimal hemorrhagic difficulties.

Avoidance of hypothermia is essential to minimize risk of the development of coagulopathy and other undesirable physiologic consequences. Having an environmentally toasty operating suite and using perioperative ancillary warming techniques, including heating blankets, warmed intravenous fluids is of paramount importance.

[*] IMPROVE trial investigators. Endovascular or open repair strategy for ruptured abdominal aortic aneurysms: 30 day outcomes from IMPROVE randomized trial. *Br Med J.* 2014;348:7661

[†] Reimerink JJ, Hoornweg LL, Vahl AC et al. Endovascular repair versus open repair of ruptured abdominal aortic aneurysms: A multicenter randomized controlled trial. *Ann Surg.* 2013;258(2):248–256.

[‡] Antoniou GA, Georgiadis GS, Antoniou SA et al. Endovascular repair for ruptured abdominal aortic aneurysm confers an early survival benefit over open repair. *J Vasc Surg.* 2013;58:1091–1110

### Can Paraplegia Be Avoided?

Paraplegia is a known, devastating potential complication of thoracic and thoracoabdominal aortic aneurysm repair. The development of paraplegia following the repair of infrarenal rAAAs occurs much less frequently. Generally, interference with the pelvic blood supply, prolonged aortic cross-clamping, prolonged suprarenal clamping, intraoperative hypotension, thromboembolic phenomena, and interference with a low-origin of the great radicular artery of Adamkiewicz (arteria radicularis magna) have all been suggested as possible causes of spinal cord ischemia.

### Should Sigmoidoscopy Be Performed Routinely in the Post-Op Period?

The treatment of rAAAs is a known risk factor for the development of postoperative ischemic colitis. In a recent review of this topic, we searched the American College of Surgeons National Surgical Quality Improvement Program (ACS NSQIP®) database to examine clinical data of patients undergoing AAA repair during 2011–2012 developing postoperative ischemic colitis.* When analyzing the cohort of 3486 patients who underwent AAA repair (11.6% open repair and 88.4% EVAR), the incidence of postoperative ischemic colitis was 2.2% (5.2% for open repair and 1.8% for EVAR). However, the diagnosis was associated with a 38.7% mortality rate. Of note, ruptured aneurysms, need for perioperative transfusion, juxtarenal aneurysms, renal failure needing dialysis, diabetes, and female gender were predictors for ischemic colitis. Patients who developed ischemic colitis had a four times higher mortality compared to those without the diagnosis. Surgical treatment was needed in nearly half of these patients and was associated with a higher mortality.* With this in mind, liberal performance of flexible sigmoidoscopy postoperatively following rAAA repair (REVAR or open rAAA repair) is prudent in this high-risk group.

### Should Patients Be Monitored for Abdominal Compartment Syndrome?

The careful clinical observation for the development of abdominal compartment syndrome following rAAA repair, particularly following REVAR, is prudent. This recognized syndrome of intra-abdominal hypertension resulting from aortic hemorrhage and generalized physiological dysfunction in these critically ill patients should be aggressively treated with abdominal decompression surgery. Postoperative bladder pressure monitoring is an easy, reliable method for monitoring for abdominal compartment syndrome and should be routinely performed in this cohort of rAAA patients.

* Moghadamyeghaneh Z, Sgroi MD, Fujitani RM. Risk factors and outcomes of post-operative ischemic colitis in contemporary open and endovascular abdominal aortic aneurysm repair. *J Vasc Surg.* 2015.

# 64

## *Acute Aortic Dissection*

**Chad N. Stasik and Edward Y. Sako**

**CONTENTS**



### 64.1 Introduction

An aortic dissection occurs when a tear in the intima permits blood to flow into and separate the layers of the media, resulting in a "false" lumen that is divided from the true aortic lumen by a thin dissection flap. The incidence is reported at approximately 2–3.5/100,000 persons annually in the United States, though this is likely an underestimate due to the catastrophic nature of the initial event. Two-thirds of those affected are men, with a peak incidence in the sixth and seventh decades of life. Over 60% of aortic dissections involve the ascending aorta, while the remainder of cases involve primarily the descending thoracic and abdominal aorta. The pathophysiology often involves episodes of extreme hypertension, which increases shearing forces on the aortic wall. Those with aortic disease, either acquired or congenital, are also at increased risk. Although treatment has evolved over the past several decades, numerous controversies remain (Table 64.1).

### 64.2 How are Aortic Dissections Classified?

Aortic dissections are classified according to their chronicity as well as anatomic features. An acute aortic dissection (AAD) is one that is detected within 14 days from the onset of pain. Between 2 weeks and 2 months they are considered subacute, and after 2 months from the onset of symptoms they are referred to as chronic.

The two widely accepted classification systems are the DeBakey and the Stanford systems. The DeBakey classification divides AADs into three categories based on the origin of the intimal tear and the extent of the dissection [1]. DeBakey type I dissections originate in the ascending aorta and extend distally to at least the aortic arch and usually into the descending thoracic aorta and beyond. Type II dissections originate in and are confined to the ascending aorta. DeBakey type III dissections originate distal to the left subclavian artery and are subdivided into type IIIa dissections that are confined to the descending thoracic aorta and type IIIb dissections that extend beyond the diaphragm.

The Stanford classification simply divides aortic dissections into two groups, those that involve the ascending aorta (type A) and those that do not (type B) [2]. Therefore, Stanford type A encompasses DeBakey types I and II, while Stanford type B includes DeBakey types IIIa and IIIb. The Stanford system is commonly used clinically because, as discussed subsequently, it separates those dissections that are typically treated with emergency surgery (type A) from those that are most commonly managed medically (type B). For that reason, the Stanford system will be used throughout this chapter.

Stanford type B aortic dissections (TBADs) are further classified as complicated (cTBAD) or uncomplicated (uTBAD), as defined in a recent consensus statement [3]. This distinction is important because the approximately 25% of patients who present with complicating features are at increased risk of morbidity and mortality during medical management. These complicating features include malperfusion syndrome and rupture or impending rupture, which may be indicated by persistent hypertension and/or pain despite full medical therapy, or by an increase in the size of a periaortic hematoma or hemorrhagic pleural effusion. Malperfusion syndrome refers to compromised end-organ perfusion as a result of a dynamic or static obstruction of the renal, mesenteric, spinal, or iliac arteries [4]. This may occur secondary to true lumen collapse or from branch vessel obstruction from extension of the dissection.

Two related conditions worth mentioning are intramural hematoma (IMH) and penetrating aortic ulcer (PAU) [5]. IMH is believed to be caused by ruptured vasa vasorum or a microscopic intimal tear. It is characterized by crescentic or circumferential aortic wall thickening in the absence of a discernible dissection flap or blood flow into a false lumen [6]. Two-thirds of IMH will evolve to become classic dissections, aneurysms, or pseudoaneurysms, leading some authors to believe that IMH is the precursor to all AAD. In general, IMH is treated the same way as AAD based on anatomy and complicating features [7,8]. PAU is the result of the erosion of an atherosclerotic lesion through the internal elastic lamina into the media, forming a false aneurysm. They occur more frequently in the descending aorta (type B). Treatment of PAU is more individualized and less data driven. Ulcers in the ascending aorta are more prone to aneurysmal expansion and surgery should be considered early. Some also advocate early surgical intervention for asymptomatic type B PAU when the ulcer neck is >10 mm or diameter is >20 mm at diagnosis, but this is controversial [9].

*Recommendation*: Aortic dissections are classified based on their chronicity and anatomic features. They may be acute, subacute, or chronic. The two most common classification schemes are the DeBakey and the Stanford system. IMH and PAU are related diagnoses that fall along the spectrum of acute aortic syndromes with AAD.

## 64.3 What is the Best Imaging Modality for the Diagnosis of Acute Aortic Dissection?

Early and accurate diagnosis of AAD is critical. A careful history and physical examination, along with a high degree of clinical suspicion, should suggest the diagnosis. The most common symptoms for patients presenting with AAD are chest, back, and/or abdominal pain. Pain is almost invariably present and may be sharp or tearing in nature. Many patients also have a history of hypertension, and a personal or family history of aneurysm or connective tissue disorder should raise suspicion. Possible physical examination abnormalities include a murmur of aortic regurgitation and an abnormal pulse exam. A plain chest radiogram may show a widened mediastinum, irregular aortic contour, deviated trachea, enlarged cardiac silhouette, or pleural effusion, but is not diagnostic of AAD. An electrocardiogram should be obtained to evaluate for acute coronary syndrome. Be aware that as an ascending dissection may involve the coronary ostia, myocardial ischemia may be present. Therefore both entities, myocardial infarction and aortic dissection, may need to be evaluated if clinically indicated.

Aortic imaging may be performed with computed tomographic angiography (CTA), magnetic resonance angiography (MRA), or transthoracic or transesophageal echocardiography (TTE or TEE, respectively). In a systematic review and meta-analysis of CT, MR, and TEE for the diagnosis of AAD, all three modalities were equally reliable, with pooled sensitivity of 98%–100% and specificity of 95%–98% [10]. Due largely to practical reasons, CTA has become the mainstay of diagnosis in most centers. It is widely available, relatively operator independent, and can provide detailed imaging of the entire aorta from the aortic valve to the femoral arteries in less than a minute. In addition to demonstrating the true and false aortic lumens and the dissection flap, it may also reveal the primary entry tear, distal fenestrations, coronary artery and branch vessel involvement, and the presence of aneurysmal or atherosclerotic disease. Furthermore, CTA provides anatomic information critical for operative planning in the case of thoracic endovascular aortic repair (TEVAR). However, some unstable patients may not be suitable for transfer to the CT scanner, and it does require ionizing radiation and nephrotoxic contrast. CTA has a 100% sensitivity and 98% specificity for detecting AAD.

MRA is extremely sensitive (98%) and specific (98%) for the diagnosis of AAD [10]. However, it is not often used as the initial imaging modality due to lack of availability, longer acquisition times (up to 30 min), and clinician unfamiliarity. The scanners are generally not as accessible as CT scanners and not suitable for unstable patients. In addition, the most commonly used contrast agent, gadolinium, has been implicated in a many-fold increase in nephrogenic systemic fibrosis and should be avoided in patients with chronic renal insufficiency.

TTE is commonly used as a screening test for cardiovascular disease because it is widely available, portable, fast, noninvasive, and does not require ionizing radiation or contrast. It is especially useful for diagnosing myocardial or valvular dysfunction or pericardial effusion, but it has limited utility in visualizing the distal ascending aorta, aortic arch, and descending aorta. It has a reported sensitivity of only 59%–85% and specificity of 63%–96% for the diagnosis of AAD [11]. TEE, on the other hand, has a sensitivity of 98% and specificity of 95% for the diagnosis of AAD [10]. It is often used as a confirmatory test if there is any doubt or equivocation on the CTA images. It is also extremely useful when there is a high index of suspicion for AAD in a hemodynamically unstable patient. Such a patient can be transported to the operating room and TEE performed while the patient is being stabilized. If an ascending aortic dissection is confirmed then repair is immediately undertaken. Disadvantages of TEE are that it provides limited visualization of the distal thoracic aorta and that it is more operator dependent than CTA or MRA.

Invasive imaging such as contrast aortography, while once the gold standard, is nearly obsolete for the diagnosis of AAD. Likewise, intravascular ultrasound has a limited role in diagnosis but may be a useful adjunct for intraoperative imaging of the aorta and its branch vessels, including defining the true and false lumens.

*Recommendation*: CTA, MRA, and TEE are equally sensitive and specific for the diagnosis of AAD. The most common first test is CTA and this is considered the mainstay of diagnosis (Grade B recommendation).

## 64.4 What is the Role of Medical Management in the Treatment of Acute Aortic Dissection?

The initial management of both Stanford types A and B AAD is to decrease aortic wall stress by controlling heart rate and blood pressure [8]. Appropriate, early, and judicious regulation of blood pressure in the patient with an AAD can decrease early mortality and ameliorate symptoms of both pain and malperfusion. The importance of early initiation of beta blockade cannot be overemphasized. Intravenous beta blockade, usually with an esmolol infusion, should be initiated and titrated to a goal heart rate of 60 beats/min or less. By reducing both the absolute pressure as well as diminishing the change in pressure over time (dP/dT), beta blockade plays a crucial role in the prevention of extension or rupture of the dissection. If blood pressure remains above 120 mmHg despite achieving the goal heart rate, then an angiotensin-converting enzyme inhibitor, calcium channel blocker, or vasodilator such as sodium nitroprusside should be added. If there is a contraindication to beta blockade then an intravenous calcium channel blocker such as nicardipine should be used. In addition to heart rate and blood pressure control, intravenous opiates should be used to achieve adequate pain control.

*Recommendation*: In the acute setting, beta blockade is the mainstay of therapy with additional vasoactive agents used as needed. Pain control with intravenous opiates is also required (Grade D recommendation).

## 64.5 When is Surgery Indicated for Acute Aortic Dissection?

Acute Stanford type A aortic dissection is a true surgical emergency. Without operation it carries an extremely high risk of mortality from rupture and tamponade, myocardial ischemia from coronary artery dissection, acute heart failure from aortic valve insufficiency, stroke from carotid artery dissection, or malperfusion of the viscera or lower extremities. Together this leads to an overall mortality rate of about 1% *per hour* [12]. Therefore, the presence of a dissection in the ascending aorta is an indication for emergency surgical repair in all but the highest risk patients. Surgical repair may include one, some, or all of the following: ascending aorta replacement, arch replacement with implantation or bypass of the brachiocephalic vessels, aortic root or valve replacement, and coronary artery bypass grafting. Even in contemporary series in experienced referral centers, the overall in-hospital mortality following surgery for acute type A dissection has not changed significantly in the past 20 years and is still 25% [13]. For patients surviving to hospital discharge, the 5 year survival rate is excellent at 88% [14].

Hospital survival for acute uncomplicated Stanford TBAD is above 90% with medical therapy, and early open surgery for these patients does not lead to improved survival [15]. Guidelines from American and European task forces recommend medical management including control of heart rate, blood pressure, and pain for acute uTBAD [7,8]. For cTBAD, TEVAR is recommended as the first-line therapy when feasible [3]. The goal of treatment is to cover the primary entry tear, stent open the true lumen, and completely occlude the false lumen if possible. Others have advocated a "complication-specific" approach, whereby a rupture or impending rupture is treated with TEVAR (or open tube graft replacement), and end-organ ischemia from malperfusion is treated with endovascular or open fenestration [16]. Either way, endovascular therapy has largely supplanted open surgery for cTBAD and has led to improved outcomes.

*Recommendation*: Type A AADs are true surgical emergencies and mandate immediate operative repair. Acute uTBADs are generally treated medically, while acute cTBADs require operative intervention (Grade B recommendation).

## 64.6 What is the Role of TEVAR for Acute Type B Dissection?

As stated earlier, TEVAR has nearly replaced open aortic repair for cTBAD. The authors of a recent meta-analysis found a pooled rate for 30-day mortality of 7.3% for

TEVAR vs. 19.0% for open repair [17]. The pooled estimates for stroke, spinal cord ischemia, and total neurologic events were also lower for TEVAR, at 3.9%, 3.1%, and 7.3%, respectively; compared to 6.8%, 3.3%, and 9.8% for open repair.

With the greater than 90% hospital survival achieved with medical management for acute uTBAD, TEVAR will only challenge the established treatment paradigm if it leads to fewer complications, reinterventions, and deaths during long-term follow-up. A report out of the International Registry of AAD (IRAD) evaluated long-term survival in patients who underwent TEVAR ($n = 276$) for acute TBAD vs. those who underwent medical management alone ($n = 853$) [18]. As expected, patients treated with TEVAR were more likely to have presented with complicated dissection (61.7%) than those in the medical management group (37.2%). Despite this difference, in-hospital mortality was similar at 10.9% in the TEVAR group and 8.7% in the medical group. At 5 years, patients in the TEVAR group had a lower death rate than those treated medically (15.5% vs. 29.0%). The diameter of the descending aorta was also smaller in the TEVAR group after 5 years in comparison to the medical therapy group.

In the Investigation of Stent Grafts in Aortic Dissection (INSTEAD) trial, 140 patients with subacute *uncomplicated* TBAD were randomized to receive optimal medical therapy (OMT) alone vs. OMT plus TEVAR in seven European centers [19]. There were two periprocedural deaths, one retrograde type A dissection, two cases of spinal cord ischemia, and one stroke after TEVAR. Based on intention-to-treat analysis, there was no significant difference in survival between the OMT group (95.6%) and the TEVAR group (88.9%) after 2 years. There was also no difference in aorta-specific survival. There was, however, expansion of the true aortic lumen, regression of the false lumen, and a higher incidence of false lumen thrombosis in the thoracic aorta in the TEVAR group compared with the OMT group. To see if this aortic remodeling would lead to improved long-term survival, the trial follow-up was extended and 5-year results were recently reported [20]. In this INSTEAD-XL trial, there was a trend toward decreased all-cause mortality with TEVAR (11.1%) vs. OMT (19.3%) at 5 years and there was a significant reduction in aorta-specific mortality and disease progression. Some have used this data to justify routine TEVAR in acute uTBAD but caution must be exercised until further data become available to support this practice.

Another small randomized trial, the Acute Dissection Stentgraft OR Best Medical Treatment (ADSORB) trial followed 61 patients with acute uTBAD in 17 European centers. One-year results have been published [21]. The trial was not powered for mortality and instead used a composite primary end point of freedom from false lumen thrombosis, aortic dilation, or rupture. The result was, not surprisingly, that TEVAR was more effective than OMT at inducing false lumen thrombosis. Similar to the INSTEAD trial, it also showed an increase in true lumen size and concomitant decrease in false lumen size. However, it did not help to answer the question of whether TEVAR should replace medical management as the first-line therapy for acute uTBAD.

In general, stent grafting should be avoided in patients with Marfan's syndrome or other connective tissue disorders [22,23]. Connective tissue disorders have consistently been an exclusion criterion in clinical trials of endovascular stent grafts. That being said, TEVAR may be considered when there is a clear indication for aortic repair, suitable anatomy, and contraindication to open surgery. In addition, given the unknown long-term results with TEVAR, stent grafting in younger patients should be guided by careful risk stratification and extensive discussion with the patient and family, including counseling with regards to the need for lifetime follow-up.

**TABLE 64.1**

Levels of Evidence

| Question | Answer | Level of Evidence | Grade of Recommendation | References |
|---|---|---|---|---|
| How are aortic dissections classified? | By chronicity: acute, subacute, and chronic. By anatomy: the DeBakey and Stanford classification systems | N/A | N/A | [1–3] |
| What is the best imaging modality for the diagnosis of acute aortic dissection (AAD)? | CTA is considered the mainstay of diagnosis, though CTA, MRA, and TEE are equally sensitive and specific | Level II | Grade B | [10,11] |
| What is the role of medical management in the treatment of AAD? | Beta blockade is the mainstay of therapy with additional vasoactive agents used as needed. Pain control is also required | Level V | Grade D | [8] |
| When is surgery indicated for AAD? | Type A AADs mandate immediate operative repair. Acute uTBADs are generally treated medically, while cTBADs require operative intervention | Level II | Grade B | [3,7,8,12–16] |
| What is the role of TEVAR for acute type B dissection? | TEVAR is the first-line therapy for acute cTBAD. Medical management is recommended for acute uTBAD, though TEVAR may play an increasing role in the future | Level II | Grade B | [15–21] |

*Recommendation*: When feasible, TEVAR is the first-line therapy for acute cTBAD. Medical management is recommended for acute uTBAD, though TEVAR shows promise in aortic remodeling and may play an increasing role in the future (Grade B recommendation).

## References

1. Debakey ME, Henly WS, Cooley DA, Morris GC, Jr., Crawford ES, Beall AC, Jr. Surgical management of dissecting aneurysms of the aorta. *J Thorac Cardiovasc Surg.* 1965;49:130–149.
2. Daily PO, Trueblood HW, Stinson EB, Wuerflein RD, Shumway NE. Management of acute aortic dissections. *Ann Thorac Surg.* 1970;10(3):237–47.
3. Fattori R, Cao P, De Rango P et al. Interdisciplinary expert consensus document on management of type B aortic dissection. *J Am Coll Cardiol.* 2013;61(16):1661–1678.
4. Ryan C, Vargas L, Mastracci T et al. Progress in management of malperfusion syndrome from type B dissections. *J Vasc Surg.* 2013;57(5):1283–1290; discussion 90.
5. Bonaca MP, O'Gara PT. Diagnosis and management of acute aortic syndromes: Dissection, intramural hematoma, and penetrating aortic ulcer. *Curr Cardiol Rep.* 2014;16(10):536.
6. Bossone E, Suzuki T, Eagle KA, Weinsaft JW. Diagnosis of acute aortic syndromes: Imaging and beyond. *Herz.* 2013;38(3):269–276.
7. Authors/Task Force Members, Erbel R, Aboyans V et al. ESC Guidelines on the diagnosis and treatment of aortic diseases: Document covering acute and chronic aortic diseases of the thoracic and abdominal aorta of the adultThe Task Force for the Diagnosis and Treatment of Aortic Diseases of the European Society of Cardiology (ESC). *Eur Heart J.* 2014;35(41):2873–2926.
8. Hiratzka LF, Bakris GL, Beckman JA et al. ACCF/AHA/AATS/ACR/ASA/SCA/SCAI/SIR/STS/SVM guidelines for the diagnosis and management of patients with Thoracic Aortic Disease: A report of the American College of Cardiology Foundation/American Heart Association Task Force on Practice Guidelines, American Association for Thoracic Surgery, American College of Radiology, American Stroke Association, Society of Cardiovascular Anesthesiologists, Society for Cardiovascular Angiography and Interventions, Society of Interventional Radiology, Society of Thoracic Surgeons, and Society for Vascular Medicine. *Circulation.* 2010;121(13):e266–e369.
9. Ganaha F. Prognosis of aortic intramural hematoma with and without penetrating atherosclerotic ulcer: A clinical and radiological analysis. *Circulation.* 2002; 106(3):342–348.
10. Shiga T, Wajima Z, Apfel CC, Inoue T, Ohe Y. Diagnostic accuracy of transesophageal echocardiography, helical computed tomography, and magnetic resonance imaging for suspected thoracic aortic dissection: Systematic review and meta-analysis. *Arch Intern Med.* 2006;166(13):1350–1356.
11. Kamalakannan D, Rosman HS, Eagle KA. Acute aortic dissection. *Crit Care Clin.* 2007;23(4):779–800, vi.
12. Hirst AE, Jr., Johns VJ, Jr., Kime SW, Jr. Dissecting aneurysm of the aorta: A review of 505 cases. *Medicine* 1958;37(3):217–279.
13. Trimarchi S, Nienaber CA, Rampoldi V et al. Contemporary results of surgery in acute type A aortic dissection: The International Registry of Acute Aortic Dissection experience. *J Thorac Cardiovasc Surg.* 2005;129(1):112–122.
14. Chiappini B, Schepens M, Tan E et al. Early and late outcomes of acute type A aortic dissection: Analysis of risk factors in 487 consecutive patients. *Eur Heart J.* 2005;26(2):180–186.
15. Tolenaar JL, Froehlich W, Jonker FH et al. Predicting in-hospital mortality in acute type B aortic dissection: Evidence from International Registry of Acute Aortic Dissection. *Circulation* 2014;130(11 Suppl 1):S45–S50.
16. Ziganshin BA, Dumfarth J, Elefteriades JA. Natural history of Type B aortic dissection: Ten tips. *Ann Cardiothorac Surg.* 2014;3(3):247–254.
17. Moulakakis KG, Mylonas SN, Dalainas I, Kakisis J, Kotsis T, Liapis CD. Management of complicated and uncomplicated acute type B dissection. A systematic review and meta-analysis. *Ann Cardiothorac Surg.* 2014;3(3):234–246.
18. Fattori R, Montgomery D, Lovato L et al. Survival after endovascular therapy in patients with type B aortic dissection: A report from the International Registry of Acute Aortic Dissection (IRAD). *JACC Cardiovasc Interv.* 2013;6(8):876–882.
19. Nienaber CA, Rousseau H, Eggebrecht H et al. Randomized comparison of strategies for type B aortic dissection: The INvestigation of STEnt Grafts in Aortic Dissection (INSTEAD) trial. *Circulation.* 2009;120(25):2519–2528.
20. Nienaber CA, Kische S, Rousseau H et al. Endovascular repair of type B aortic dissection: Long-term results of the randomized investigation of stent grafts in aortic dissection trial. *Cir Cardiovasc Interv.* 2013;6(4):407–416.
21. Brunkwall J, Kasprzak P, Verhoeven E et al. Endovascular repair of acute uncomplicated aortic type B dissection promotes aortic remodelling: 1 year results of the ADSORB trial. *Eur J Vasc Endovasc Surg Offic J Eur Soc Vasc Surg.* 2014;48(3):285–291.
22. Grabenwoger M, Alfonso F, Bachet J et al. Thoracic Endovascular Aortic Repair (TEVAR) for the treatment of aortic diseases: A position statement from the European Association for Cardio-Thoracic Surgery (EACTS) and the European Society of Cardiology (ESC), in collaboration with the European Association of Percutaneous Cardiovascular Interventions (EAPCI). *Eur Heart J.* 2012;33(13):1558–1563.
23. Svensson LG, Kouchoukos NT, Miller DC et al. Expert consensus document on the treatment of descending thoracic aortic disease using endovascular stent-grafts. *Ann Thorac Surg.* 2008;85(1 Suppl):S1–S41.

## Commentary on Acute Aortic Dissection

*Jeffrey H. Lawson*

Acute aortic dissection is one of major arterial catastrophes that can challenge even the most experienced acute care and cardiovascular surgeons. Understanding the correct classification terminology, appropriate imaging modalities, and the role of medical, surgical, and endovascular treatments are critical for the management of this potentially devastating cardiovascular problem. The chapter on aortic dissection highlights these issues with an appropriate and up-to-date perspective. With wide-spread advancement of endovascular techniques, the treatment of both acute and chronic dissection has evolved quite rapidly where the sealing of entry site tears, covering of penetrating ulcers, and the fenestration of false lumens are now common place. While treatment of acute aortic dissection has made significant progress in the past decade with the development of aortic care centers of excellence, improved medical management, and advanced endovascular techniques, little progress has been made in the basic understanding of the pathophysiology and prevention of the cardiovascular process. One might ask the simple question "what makes the most robust vascular structure in the body unravel?" Unfortunately, to date the question remains unanswered. We currently react to aortic dissection and have limited insight into the prevention of the process. The chapter outlined in the text presents a comprehensive approach to current issues in treating this problem.

To comment briefly on the questions addressed in this chapter.

### How Are Aortic Dissections Classified?

Both the duration of the dissection (acute, subacute, and chronic) and the two most widely used classification systems, the DeBakey and Stanford systems, are discussed in the chapter. While describing the duration of the dissections is relevant for classification, the distinction among acute, subacute, and chronic is somewhat arbitrary and may merely highlight the difference of those individuals who, for unclear reasons, survive when their aorta unravels. It is quite likely that this arbitrary temporal classification creates some element of selection bias in our understanding of the pathology. A significant and unknown number of acute aortic dissections are never counted, because they do not survive for medical evaluation and are dismissed as an unexplained acute death of unknown cause. Further, many of the chronic dissections have already demonstrated the capacity to survive this process and will likely continue to do so as long as our interventions do not induce an associated iatrogenic catastrophe. Thus, while timing of dissection may be important as a mode of classification, it is unclear if it changes what we do. If the patient is alive at the time of diagnosis, the algorithm is relatively simple: formal imaging, acute blood pressure and heart rate control, and anatomic treatment based on the identified pathology.

While both the DeBakey and Stanford classification systems have been used for many years, the Stanford system has become more widely accepted for academic utility, comparing clinical outcomes and treating the problem and thus is appropriately used in this text. Stanford type A dissections most often require emergent surgical repair to prevent rupture, coronary ischemia, or aortic valve failure. This in contrast to Stanford type B dissections that require a more measured combination of medical and surgical judgment. One confounder in comparing clinical outcomes using the Stanford system is distinction between complicated type B dissections (cTBADs) and uncomplicated type B dissections (uTBADs). This assumes an all or none response to complications when it truly represents a spectrum of pathology. There is no doubt that cTBAD involving the visceral segment of the aorta with associated intestinal/renal ischemia is a much more catastrophic and different complication than an aortic dissection flap at the common iliac artery with modest limb perfusion symptoms. With many innovative technologies used to treat this problem and many more on the horizon, it seems like a more granular classification system of cTBAD distinction would be useful.

### What Is the Best Imaging Modality for the Diagnosis of Acute Aortic Dissection?

Imaging technology had evolved dramatically over the past 20 years. There was a time when an abnormal aortic silhouette on a chest x-ray led to an angiogram and a hopeful surgical procedure. In 2015, there is no question that CTA of the chest, abdomen, and pelvis (and runoff vessels if needed) is the most rapid and appropriate test for both the evaluation and treatment of acute aortic dissection. High-quality cross-sectional imaging is essential for any interventional strategy that may preserve both life and limb. CTA with rapid and appropriate three-dimensional reconstruction has revolutionized the care of patients with both acute and chronic aortic dissection and been instrumental in the application of endovascular techniques for treatment. Even in the setting of renal impairment, it is likely that the benefit of a single strategically timed CT angiogram will outweigh the risk and morbidity of contrast-induced renal failure. The only role for formal angiography is in the hybrid operating room if endovascular treatments are planned based on the CT scan. There is almost no logistical utility of obtaining an MRI or MRA of the chest and great vessels in the setting of aortic dissection. The only imaging modality other than a CT angiography, which may impact the planning and treatment of aortic dissection, is cardiac echo where both trans-thoracic (TTE) and trans-esophageal (TEE) echo have been utilized. Cardiac echo allows for immediate analysis of aortic valve and left ventricular wall motion to aid in both critical care management and the surgical requirement to address aortic valve or coronary artery function.

### What Is the Role of Medical Management in the Treatment of Acute Aortic Dissection?

Medical management still has a very important role in the treatment of aortic dissection. Even in the setting of a surgical emergency for an unstable Stanford type A dissection, blood pressure, heart rate, and pain control are essential even while proceeding to the operating room. Medical management of uTBAD has long been the mainstay of treatment. It is clear that many patients with a moderate tear in intimal layer of their aortic arch will require no future intervention if both heart rate and blood pressure are controlled. Beta-blockade has provided longstanding and durable medical treatment. For those patients treated medically, serial imaging of the aorta is important with a minimum of an annual CT scan. For those patients who show changes of aortic sac geometry while on optimal medical treatment, endovascular relining of that portion of the aorta is now recommended. With the advance of endovascular techniques some even recommend earlier and aggressive treatment and longitudinal studies of best medical care versus early endovascular treatment are ongoing.

### When Is Surgery Indicated for Acute Aortic Dissection?

Surgery has always been the mainstay of treatment for acute Stanford Type A dissection. Proximal aortic arch reconstruction is critical to prevent rupture, maintain coronary and cerebral perfusion, and secure aortic valve function. For cTBAD, a hybrid or endovascular approach has become the mainstay of treatment. Challenges in managing the descending aorta primarily involve preventing visceral and spinal cord ischemia where branched endovascular devices and/or formal aortic debranching with visceral reconstruction may be required. Controversy exists in the ability to cover the origin of the left subclavian artery with an endograft to obtain a proximal seal zone. If left arm ischemia is noted, a carotid to subclavian bypass may be required. As noted earlier, for uTBAD, medical management is still the mainstay of early treatment with endovascular treatment reserved for those patients who show progressive signs of aortic deterioration.

### What Is the Role of TEVAR for Acute Type Dissection?

Endovascular techniques to manage all aspects of aortic pathology have evolved rapidly in the past 15 years. It is now inconceivable to not have endovascular options available for the treatment of acute aortic dissection. TEVAR has now become the standard of care for managing nearly all descending aortic dissection pathology with adjuvant surgical techniques reserved to maintain limb and solid organ perfusion. With innovative branched devices now entering clinical testing, it is likely that many ascending aortic arch tears will be amenable to endovascular techniques in the future. This highlights the essential need for acute care and cardiovascular surgeons to continue to obtain the essential wire and imaging skills required for advanced endovascular treatments.

# 65

# *Deep Venous Thrombosis*

**Casey J. Allen, Evan J. Valle, Shevonne S. Satahoo, and Enrique Ginzburg**

**CONTENTS**



Deep venous thrombosis (DVT) is a major health problem with an annual incidence of 0.5–1 per 1000 [1]. The main short-term complication of DVT is pulmonary embolism (PE) while the long-term complication is postthrombotic syndrome [2]. Multiple evidence-based reviews of the diagnosis and treatment of DVT [3–5] and practice guidelines [6–8] have been published. This chapter reviews several aspects of DVT treatment. Some of the questions address the broader topics of both DVT and PE, that is, venous thromboembolism (VTE).

## 65.1 What Are the Optimal Preventative Strategies for DVT?

Heparin binds to antithrombin III, which inhibits a cascade of procoagulation factors. Low-molecular-weight heparin (LMWH) is a fractionated heparin with fewer pentasaccharide chains. LMWH is more expensive than heparin, although its advantages include once-daily dosing. Current recommendations are that major trauma patients receive either heparin or LMWH [9].

Direct thrombin inhibitors are the newest agents for prophylaxis. In contrast to other agents, they do not require a plasma cofactor; rather, they bind to thrombin and block its enzymatic activity. Their main role is for prophylaxis in patients with heparin-induced thrombocytopenia, and their use is limited because no specific antidote is available for reversal.

Lower-extremity compression devices minimize the effect of immobilization and circulatory stasis. Mechanical prophylaxis is only recommended for patients who are at low risk for DVT or for those in whom pharmacologic prophylaxis is contraindicated (risk for bleeding, traumatic brain injury, etc.). Intermittent pneumatic compression (IPC) devices are the preferred mechanical prophylaxis devices [9].

There are several ongoing areas of research in DVT prophylaxis, and recommendations are often changing. There is evidence of decreased VTE rates when LMWH is titrated based upon antifactor Xa levels [10]. Clinical trials are underway to examine the utility of using thromboelastography [11] to guide prophylaxis regimens. Improved prophylaxis regimens may decrease VTE rates in high-risk patients; however, more studies are needed.

*Recommendation*: Current optimal prophylaxis is with low-dose unfractionated heparin (LMWH, Grade 1B) over no prophylaxis.

*Level of evidence*: 1b

*Grade of recommendation*: A

Adding mechanical prophylaxis with elastic stockings or IPC to pharmacologic prophylaxis is suggested.

*Level of evidence*: 2c

*Grade of recommendation*: B

## 65.2 How Is DVT Diagnosed?

Duplex ultrasonography (US) is the most widely used method for diagnosing DVT and has the same sensitivity and specificity value of 98% [12]. The advantages of US include the following: being rapid, cost-effective, and noninvasive. The US probe is used to compress the lumen of a vein, and the presence of a thrombus prevents compression and is diagnostic for a DVT. However, the compression technique is not sensitive in diagnosing DVT below the knee [13]. The sensitivity of US is also lower in patients with asymptomatic DVT, largely due to a higher distribution of DVT in the calf veins in these asymptomatic patients [14]. US screening has been effective in high-risk trauma patients [15]; however, controversy remains and routine US screening is not currently recommended [16].

*Recommendation*: Duplex US for diagnosis of DVT, yet surveillance in high-risk patients, is not currently recommended.

*Level of evidence*: 2c

*Grade of recommendation*: B

## 65.3 What Is the Best Initial Treatment for Venous Thromboembolism?

Traditionally, DVT was treated with intravenous, unfractionated heparin until a therapeutic level of oral anticoagulation was achieved with vitamin K antagonists (VKAs). However, frequent lab tests with the adjustment of the unfractionated heparin dose are necessary due to variable clinical effects. On the other hand, the effects of LMWH are more predictable and do not require routine lab testing [17]. Multiple randomized controlled trials have been performed comparing the efficacy and safety of unfractionated heparin versus LMWH and have been summarized in evidence-based reviews [3,4,7,17,18] and society-sponsored practice guidelines [6,7].

A Cochrane review [18] performed an analysis of 22 randomized trials with a total of 8867 patients. The primary outcome of recurrence of symptomatic VTE using the pooled data revealed a significant reduction using LMWH during the initial treatment (odds ratio [OR] 0.68; 95% confidence interval [CI] 0.48–0.97) and at the end of follow-up (OR 0.68; 95% CI 0.55–0.84) compared to unfractionated heparin. Secondary outcomes of reduction in major hemorrhage during the initial treatment (OR 0.57; 95% CI 0.39–0.83) and lower overall mortality at the end of follow-up (OR 0.76; 95% CI 0.62–0.92) also favored the LMWH group.

LMWH has the advantages of providing predictable anticoagulation levels in patients using weight-adjusted dosing without laboratory monitoring in most patients. However, clinical situations such as renal failure or pregnancy may require dose adjustment using plasma anti-Xa levels [7]. Furthermore, LMWH use provides the convenience of once-daily administration.

Another Cochrane review [19] examined five studies with a total of 1508 participants. The pooled data showed no significant difference in recurrent VTE between the two treatment regimens (OR 0.82; 95% CI 0.49–1.39; $p$ = 0.47). A comparison of major hemorrhagic events (OR 0.77; 95% CI 0.40–1.45; $p$ = 0.41), improvement of thrombus size (OR 1.41; 95% CI 0.66–3.01; $p$ = 0.38), and mortality (OR 1.14; 95% CI 0.62–2.08; $p$ = 0.68) also showed no significant differences between the two treatment regimens. The review concluded that once-daily treatment with LMWH is as effective and safe as twice-daily treatment with LMWH.

For DVT of the upper extremity, treatment is similar as for DVT of the leg [20]. For DVT of the distal lower extremity, treatment with anticoagulants is only indicated if severely symptomatic [20].

*Recommendation*: LMWH is the preferred initial treatment for DVT compared to unfractionated heparin in most patients.

*Level of evidence*: 1a

*Grade of recommendation*: A

## 65.4 Is Home Therapy for Venous Thromboembolism Safe and Effective Compared to Inpatient Care?

Multiple trials have been performed comparing the safety of DVT treatment at home with LMWH with the safety of hospitalization and treatment with unfractionated heparin or LMWH; these trials have been summarized in several evidence-based reviews [4,7,21,22]. A Cochrane review [22] performed an analysis of six randomized trials containing 1708 participants. VTE recurrence was significantly lower in the LMWH patients treated at home (relative risk [RR, fixed] 0.6; 95% CI 0.42–0.90) compared to hospitalized patients. In addition, patients treated at home exhibited a lower mortality and fewer major bleeding complications but were more likely to have minor bleeding complications compared to patients treated in the hospital; however, these differences were not significant. Home therapy was also deemed to be cost-effective and preferred by patients.

Study limitations to home versus inpatient treatment of DVT include differences in the treatments studied, such as using unfractionated heparin in the hospital but LMWH for home treatment [4,21,22]. Furthermore, strict criteria for patients considered for home treatment were used and may affect the generalizability of the studies to patients seen in clinical practice [21,22].

More recently, the viability of home therapy has been extended to PE in consensus studies [23]. Randomized trials, as well as other studies, have supported outpatient management of PE in selected patients and circumstances [24,25].

*Recommendation*: Home therapy for DVT with LMWH is safe and cost-effective in carefully chosen patients. PE can be treated on an outpatient basis in select patients.

*Level of evidence*: 1b

*Grade of recommendation*: A

## 65.5 What Is the Optimal Oral Starting Dose of VKA Therapy?

Vitamin K–dependent clotting factors have circulating half-lives ranging from 6 to 60 h. Because factor II has the longest circulating half-life of 60 h, the full anticoagulant effect of VKA, such as warfarin, may be delayed by a week or more. Furthermore, initiation of VKA therapy can result in a transient hypercoagulable state due to the circulating half-lives of 6 and 42 h for the anticoagulant protein C and protein S, respectively. Thus, unfractionated heparin or LMWH therapy is initiated and maintained for several days until oral VKA therapy is therapeutic, as measured by an international normalized ratio (INR) with values generally between 2 and 3 [26]. Achieving a therapeutic INR with warfarin as soon as possible is important because this minimizes the duration of parenteral medication necessary to attain immediate anticoagulation, and it potentially decreases the cost and inconvenience of treatment. Although a 5 mg loading-dose nomogram tends to prevent excessive anticoagulation, a 10 mg loading-dose nomogram may achieve a therapeutic INR more quickly.

Six prospective, randomized trials [27–32] compared starting doses of 5 or 10 mg of warfarin therapy. These trials have been previously reviewed [7,26,33], and guidelines for the initial dosing of VKA have been published by several societies [7,33,34]. Two small trials randomized 49 patients [29] and 53 patients [28] to receive an initial dose of 5 or 10 mg of warfarin and measured the time necessary to attain therapeutic INR. Harrison et al. [29] determined that at 36 h, significantly more patients were therapeutic in the 10 mg group (44% versus 8%, $p = 0.005$) compared to the 5 mg group. In contrast, Crowther et al. [28] determined that significantly more patients in the 5 mg group exhibited a therapeutic INR on days 1–5 of therapy (66% versus 24%, $p < 0.003$) compared to the 10 mg group. The 10 mg group in both studies exhibited an increased risk of excessive anticoagulation [28,29], and there was a faster rate of decrease in protein C levels in the first 36 h of treatment with the 10 mg group [29], leading the authors to speculate that the 5 mg warfarin dose maybe less likely to induce a hypercoagulable state. Both studies recommended using a 5 mg dose for initiation of warfarin therapy.

Kovacs et al. [27] randomized 210 patients to receive 5 or 10 mg initial doses of warfarin; the study was powered to detect a 0.5 day difference in time necessary to reach a therapeutic INR. Patients receiving 10 mg of warfarin achieved a therapeutic INR 1.4 days faster that patients receiving 5 mg ($4.2 \pm 1.1$ vs. $5.6 \pm 1.4$ days, $p < 0.001$) with no significant increase in excessive anticoagulation. However, this study excluded patients at high risk for bleeding.

A recent Cochrane review [33] involving four of these trials [27,30–32] found that no difference was observed in recurrent VTE (RVTE) at 90 days when the warfarin nomogram of 10 mg was compared with the warfarin nomogram of 5 mg (RR 1.48; 95% CI 0.39–5.56); no difference was observed in major bleeding at 14 days (RR 1.69; 95% CI 0.22–13.04) and at 90 days (RR 0.62; 95% CI 0.10–3.78). No difference was observed in minor bleeding at 14–90 days (RR 0.32; 95% CI 0.15–1.83) or in length of hospital stay (mean difference 2.30 days; 95% CI 7.96–3.36).

*Recommendation*: In patients with acute VTE (DVT or PE), considerable uncertainty surrounds the use of a 10 mg or a 5 mg loading dose for initiation of VKA, and there is currently no consensus on the optimal starting dose of VKA. Clinicians should consider patient-specific factors for determining the optimal starting dose. Patients at low risk for bleeding may safely tolerate a 10 mg loading dose if appropriate nomograms are strictly followed.

*Level of evidence*: 2b

*Grade of recommendation*: B

## 65.6 What Is the Optimal Length of Oral VKA Treatment for DVT?

Currently, the most frequently used secondary treatment for patients with VTE consists of VKA targeted at an INR of 2.5 (range 2.0–3.0). However, based on the continuing risk of bleeding and uncertainty regarding the risk of recurrent VTE, the discussion on the proper duration of treatment with VKA for these patients is ongoing. Multiple trials have evaluated the duration of therapy with VKA on VTE; these trials have been summarized in several evidence-based reviews [4,7,35,36] and society-sponsored practice guidelines [6,7]. A recent Cochrane review [36] performed an analysis of 11 randomized trials with a total of 3716 patients. A consistent and strong reduction in the risk of recurrent VTE events was observed during prolonged treatment with VKA (RR 0.20; 95% CI 0.11–0.38) independent of the period elapsed since the index thrombotic event. A statistically significant "rebound" phenomenon (i.e., an excess of recurrences shortly after cessation of prolonged treatment) was not found (RR 1.28; 95% CI 0.97–1.70). In addition, a substantial increase in bleeding complications was observed for patients receiving prolonged treatment during the entire period after randomization (RR 2.60; 95% CI 1.51–4.49). No reduction in mortality was noted during the entire study period (RR 0.89; 95% CI 0.66–1.21, $p$ = 0.46). Thus, the authors concluded that the efficacy of VKA therapy decreased over time and that the optimal duration of therapy would vary between different groups of patients dependent upon balancing risk/benefit profiles [36].

Segal et al. [4] identified 10 trials that included 4240 patients that utilized objective radiologic documentation of VTE and used INR to monitor VKA therapy. Durations of VKA therapy were evaluated in multiple trials. Only one randomized blinded trial [37] compared 1 versus 3 months of therapy for DVT associated with a transient event, such as surgery. Treatment for 1 month resulted in increased rates of RVTE with similar bleeding complications compared to 3 months of therapy. The trial was stopped for slow patient accrual and was only able to randomize 165 patients of the estimated 390 patients needed to provide conclusive results.

*Recommendation*: Extended therapy with VKA is warranted to prevent RVTE. Risks of bleeding versus recurrence of VTE for individual patients may alter the optimal duration of therapy.

*Level of evidence*: 1a

*Grade of recommendation*: A

*DVT associated with a* transient event maybe effectively treated with 3 months of VKA.

*Level of evidence*: 2b

*Grade of recommendation*: B

## 65.7 Does Catheter-Directed Thrombolysis Decrease DVT Recurrences and Incidence of Postthrombotic Syndrome?

The goal of catheter-directed thrombolysis is to rapidly remove thrombus, thereby potentially preserving venous valvular function and reducing the incidence and severity of postthrombotic syndrome. A recent Cochrane review evaluated catheter-directed thrombolysis and anticoagulation compared to anticoagulation alone for acute DVT [38]. It consisted of 17 studies with 1103 participants. Complete lysis of clot was more often achieved in those with catheter-directed thrombolysis in both early (up to 1 month) and intermediate (after 6 months) follow-ups (RR 4.91, 95% CI 1.66–14.53, and $p$ = 0.004 and RR 2.37, 95% CI 1.48–3.80, and $p$ = 0.0004, respectively). Similarly, postthrombotic syndrome occurred less in the catheter-directed thrombolysis group (RR 0.64; 95% CI 0.52–0.79, $p$ < 0.001). However, catheter-directed thrombolysis was associated with significantly more bleeding complications than anticoagulation alone (RR 2.23, 95% CI 1.41–3.52, $p$ = 0.0006). No significant difference was shown in regard to mortality at early or intermediate follow-ups. In regard to PE and recurrent DVT, the data were inconclusive.

A randomized, controlled trial by Enden et al. evaluated 103 participants aged 18–75 years with iliofemoral DVT to assess if additional catheter-directed thrombolysis versus anticoagulation alone improved iliofemoral patency after 6 months [39]. Patency in the catheter-directed thrombolysis group was 64% compared to 35.8% in the anticoagulation group, equivalent to an absolute risk reduction of 28.2%, 95% CI 9.7–46.7, and $p$ = 0.004. Venous obstruction was seen in 20.0% with catheter-directed thrombolysis compared to 49.1% (absolute risk reduction of 29.1%, 95% CI 20.0–38.0, and $p$ = 0.004). There was no difference in femoral vein insufficiency. Enden et al. [40] performed another analysis using iliofemoral DVT treated with catheter-directed thrombolysis and anticoagulation versus anticoagulation alone. After 24-month follow-up, 189 participants were assessed. Postthrombotic syndrome was observed in 41.1% of the catheter-directed thrombolysis group compared to 55.6% in the anticoagulation alone group, $p$ = 0.047 (which corresponded to an absolute risk reduction of 14.4%, 95% CI 0.2–27.9). Patency after 6 months was higher in the catheter-directed thrombolysis group (65.9% versus 47.4%, $p$ = 0.012). However, 20 bleeding complications were noted in the catheter-directed thrombolysis group.

Strict eligibility criteria to reduce the risk of bleeding complications are needed and these limit the general use of catheter-directed thrombolysis [38]. Other interventions that combine chemical lysis with mechanical or ultrasound energy clot removal have been reviewed [41]. There is a randomized trial that is ongoing with promising midterm results (TORPEDO Trial) [42]. Thus far, the authors have shown that these percutaneous endovenous interventions with anticoagulation are superior to anticoagulation alone in regard to the reduction of VTE and postthrombotic syndrome.

*Recommendation*: While catheter-directed thrombolysis results in increased venous patency and decreased incidence of postthrombotic syndrome, bleeding complications limit the routine use of this technology.

*Level of evidence*: 1a

*Grade of recommendation*: A

## 65.8 Do Compression Stockings Reduce the Long-Term Complication of Postthrombotic Syndrome?

There have been historical data supporting the use of compression stockings to reduce the incidence of postthrombotic syndrome. A Cochrane review in 2004 included three randomized controlled trials to evaluate the role of compression therapy versus no intervention [43]. At 2 years, compression therapy was associated with a significantly decreased incidence of postthrombotic syndrome (OR, 0.31, 95% CI 0.20–0.48). In regard to severe postthrombotic syndrome, the OR was 0.39 (95% CI 0.20–0.76). There was also reduction in regard to swelling, pain, and clinical scores observed in those undergoing compression therapy ($p < 0.05$), with no serious adverse events.

A subsequent meta-analysis expanded on these results [44] by including five randomized controlled trials. Similarly, there was a reduction in the incidence of postthrombotic syndrome. Overall, compression therapy was associated with postthrombotic syndrome incidence of 26% compared to 46% in the control group (RR 0.54). Mild-to-moderate postthrombotic syndrome occurred in 22% in the compression stocking group versus 37% in the control group (RR 0.52). When evaluating severe postthrombotic syndrome, the incidence was 5% with compression therapy, while it was 12% without compression therapy (RR 0.38).

However, there has been a recent shift in paradigm. Kahn et al. [45] performed the first multicenter, randomized, placebo-controlled trial assessing compression stockings (30–40 mm Hg) compared to placebo (<5 mm Hg at the ankle) for 2 years. Stockings were initiated within 2 weeks of DVT diagnosis and were replaced every 6 months or sooner if they were torn or leg size changed. With 806 participants, this serves as the largest trial to date. The authors found that the incidence of postthrombotic syndrome was not significantly different between treatment and control groups (14.2% versus 12.7%, respectively, with center-adjusted hazard ratio of 1.13, 95% CI 0.73–1.76, and $p = 0.58$). There was no difference in rates of RVTE, ipsilateral DVT, ipsilateral venous valvular reflux at 12 months, or death. There were also similar generic and disease-specific quality of life scores between the two groups. No differences were observed on subgroup analyses by age, body mass index, or extent of DVT, though sex showed marginal benefit for women ($p = 0.047$). There were no serious adverse events.

*Recommendation*: Routine use of compression stockings to reduce postthrombotic syndrome is not supported.

*Level of evidence*: 1b

*Grade of recommendation*: A (Table 65.1)

**TABLE 65.1**
Summary of Clinical Questions

| Question | Answer | Grade | References |
|---|---|---|---|
| 1. What are the optimal preventative strategies for DVT? | LMWH over no prophylaxis. | A | [9] |
| | Adding mechanical prophylaxis to pharmacologic prophylaxis is suggested. | B | |
| 2. How is DVT diagnosed? | Duplex US for diagnosis, yet surveillance in high-risk patients, is not currently recommended. | B | [12] |
| 3. What is the best initial treatment for VTE? | LMWH is the preferred initial treatment for DVT compared to unfractionated heparin in most patients. | A | [3,4,6,7,17–20] |
| 4. Is home therapy for VTE safe and effective compared to inpatient care? | Home therapy for DVT with LMWH is safe and cost-effective in carefully chosen patients. | A | [4,7,21,22] |
| 5. What is the optimal oral starting dose of VKA? | There is no consensus on the optimal starting dose of warfarin. Clinicians should consider patient-specific factors for determining a warfarin dose. Patients at low risk for bleeding may safely tolerate a 10 mg loading dose. | B | [7,33,34] |
| 6. What is the optimal length of oral VKA treatment for DVT? | Extended therapy with VKA is warranted to prevent RVTE. Risks of bleeding versus recurrence of VTE for individual patients may alter the optimal duration of therapy. | A | [4,6,7,35,36] |
| | DVT associated with a transient event maybe effectively treated with 3 months of VKA. | B | [4,37] |
| 7. Does catheter-directed thrombolysis decrease DVT recurrences and incidence of postthrombotic syndrome? | While catheter-directed thrombolysis results in increased venous patency and decreased incidence of postthrombotic syndrome, bleeding complications limit the routine use of this technology. | A | [38–40] |
| 8. Do compression stockings reduce the long-term complication of postthrombotic syndrome? | Graded compression stockings do not reduce the incidence of postthrombotic syndrome. | A | [43–45] |

*Abbreviations:* LMWH, low-molecular-weight heparin; DVT, deep venous thrombosis; US, ultrasound; VKA, vitamin K antagonist.

## References

1. Fowkes FJ, Price JF, Fowkes FG. Incidence of diagnosed deep vein thrombosis in the general population: Systematic review. *Eur J Vasc Endovasc Surg.* 2003;25(1):1–5.
2. Brandjes DP, Buller HR, Heijboer H et al. Randomised trial of effect of compression stockings in patients with symptomatic proximal-vein thrombosis. *Lancet.* 1997;349(9054):759–762.
3. Segal JB, Eng J, Jenckes MW et al. Diagnosis and treatment of deep venous thrombosis and pulmonary embolism. *Evid Rep Technol Assess (Summ).* 2003(68):1–6.
4. Segal JB, Streiff MB, Hofmann LV, Thornton K, Bass EB. Management of venous thromboembolism: A systematic review for a practice guideline. *Ann Intern Med.* 2007;146(3):211–222.
5. Segal JB, Eng J, Tamariz LJ, Bass EB. Review of the evidence on diagnosis of deep venous thrombosis and pulmonary embolism. *Ann Fam Med.* 2007;5(1):63–73.
6. Snow V, Qaseem A, Barry P et al. Management of venous thromboembolism: A clinical practice guideline from the American College of Physicians and the American Academy of Family Physicians. *Ann Intern Med.* 2007;146(3):204–210.
7. Buller HR, Agnelli G, Hull RD, Hyers TM, Prins MH, Raskob GE. Antithrombotic therapy for venous thromboembolic disease: The Seventh ACCP Conference on Antithrombotic and Thrombolytic Therapy. *Chest.* 2004;126(3 Suppl):401S–428S.
8. Qaseem A, Snow V, Barry P et al. Current diagnosis of venous thromboembolism in primary care: A clinical practice guideline from the American Academy of Family Physicians and the American College of Physicians. *Ann Intern Med.* 2007;146(6):454–458.
9. Gould MK, Garcia DA, Wren SM et al. Prevention of VTE in nonorthopedic surgical patients: Antithrombotic Therapy and Prevention of Thrombosis, 9th ed: American College of Chest Physicians Evidence-Based Clinical Practice Guidelines. *Chest.* 2012;141(2 Suppl):e227S–e277S.
10. Lin H, Faraklas I, Saffle J, Cochran A. Enoxaparin dose adjustment is associated with low incidence of venous thromboembolic events in acute burn patients. *J Trauma.* 2011;71(6):1557–1561.
11. Harrington RA, Becker RC, Cannon CP et al. Antithrombotic therapy for non-ST-segment elevation acute coronary syndromes: American College of Chest Physicians Evidence-Based Clinical Practice Guidelines (8th Edition). *Chest.* 2008;133(6 Suppl):670S–707S.
12. Kearon C, Julian JA, Newman TE, Ginsberg JS. Noninvasive diagnosis of deep venous thrombosis. McMaster Diagnostic Imaging Practice Guidelines Initiative. *Ann Intern Med.* 1998;128(8):663–677.
13. Wicky J, Bongard O, Peter R, Simonovska S, Bounameaux H. Screening for proximal deep venous thrombosis using B-mode venous ultrasonography following major hip surgery: Implications for clinical management. *VASA Zeitschrift fur Gefasskrankheiten.* 1994;23(4):330–336.
14. Kearon C. Noninvasive diagnosis of deep vein thrombosis in postoperative patients. *Semin Thromb Hemost.* 2001;27(1):3–8.
15. Thorson CM, Ryan ML, Van Haren RM et al. Venous thromboembolism after trauma: A never event?. *Crit Care Med.* 2012;40(11):2967–2973.
16. Bates SM, Jaeschke R, Stevens SM et al. Diagnosis of DVT Antithrombotic Therapy and Prevention of Thrombosis, 9th ed: American College of Chest Physicians Evidence-Based Clinical Practice Guidelines. *Chest.* 2012;141(2):E351s–E418s.
17. Krishnan JA, Segal JB, Streiff MB et al. Treatment of venous thromboembolism with low-molecular-weight heparin: A synthesis of the evidence published in systematic literature reviews. *Respir Med.* 2004;98(5):376–386.
18. van Dongen CJ, van den Belt AG, Prins MH, Lensing AW. Fixed dose subcutaneous low molecular weight heparins versus adjusted dose unfractionated heparin for venous thromboembolism. *Cochrane Database Syst Rev.* 2004(4):CD001100.
19. Bhutia S, Wong PF. Once versus twice daily low molecular weight heparin for the initial treatment of venous thromboembolism. *Cochrane Database Syst Rev.* 2013;7:CD003074.
20. Kearon C, Akl EA, Comerota AJ et al. Antithrombotic therapy for VTE disease: Antithrombotic Therapy and Prevention of Thrombosis, 9th ed: American College of Chest Physicians Evidence-Based Clinical Practice Guidelines. *Chest.* 2012;141(2 Suppl):e419S–e494S.
21. Segal JB, Bolger DT, Jenckes MW et al. Outpatient therapy with low molecular weight heparin for the treatment of venous thromboembolism: A review of efficacy, safety, and costs. *Am J Med.* 2003;115(4):298–308.
22. Othieno R, Abu Affan M, Okpo E. Home versus inpatient treatment for deep vein thrombosis. *Cochrane Database Syst Rev.* 2007(3):CD003076.
23. Wells PS, Forgie MA, Rodger MA. Treatment of venous thromboembolism. *JAMA.* 2014;311(7):717–728.
24. Aujesky D, Roy PM, Verschuren F et al. Outpatient versus inpatient treatment for patients with acute pulmonary embolism: An international, open-label, randomised, non-inferiority trial. *Lancet.* 2011;378(9785):41–48.
25. Erkens PM, Gandara E, Wells P et al. Safety of outpatient treatment in acute pulmonary embolism. *J Thromb Haemost: JTH.* 2010;8(11):2412–2417.
26. Eckhoff CD, Didomenico RJ, Shapiro NL. Initiating warfarin therapy: 5 mg versus 10 mg. *Ann Pharmacother.* 2004;38(12):2115–2121.
27. Kovacs MJ, Rodger M, Anderson DR et al. Comparison of 10-mg and 5-mg warfarin initiation nomograms together with low-molecular-weight heparin for outpatient treatment of acute venous thromboembolism. A randomized, double-blind, controlled trial. *Ann Intern Med.* 2003;138(9):714–719.
28. Crowther MA, Ginsberg JB, Kearon C et al. A randomized trial comparing 5-mg and 10-mg warfarin loading doses. *Arch Intern Med.* 1999;159(1):46–48.

29. Harrison L, Johnston M, Massicotte MP, Crowther M, Moffat K, Hirsh J. Comparison of 5-mg and 10-mg loading doses in initiation of warfarin therapy. *Ann Intern Med.* 1997;126(2):133–136.
30. Farahmand S, Saeedi M, Seyed Javadi HH, Khashayar P. High doses of warfarin are more beneficial than its low doses in patients with deep vein thrombosis. *Am J Emerg Med.* 2011;29(9):1222–1226.
31. Kovacs MJ, Cruickshank M, Wells PS et al. Randomized assessment of a warfarin nomogram for initial oral anticoagulation after venous thromboembolic disease. *Haemostasis.* 1998;28(2):62–69.
32. Quiroz R, Gerhard-Herman M, Kosowsky JM et al. Comparison of a single end point to determine optimal initial warfarin dosing (5 mg versus 10 mg) for venous thromboembolism. *Am J Cardiol.* 2006;98(4):535–537.
33. Garcia P, Ruiz W, Loza Munarriz C. Warfarin initiation nomograms for venous thromboembolism. *Cochrane Database Syst Rev.* 2013;7:CD007699.
34. Hirsh J, Fuster V, Ansell J, Halperin JL. American Heart Association/American College of Cardiology Foundation guide to warfarin therapy. *J Am Coll Cardiol.* 2003;41(9):1633–1652.
35. Hutten BA, Prins MH. Duration of treatment with vitamin K antagonists in symptomatic venous thromboembolism. *Cochrane Database Syst Rev.* 2006;(1):CD001367.
36. Middeldorp S, Prins MH, Hutten BA. Duration of treatment with vitamin K antagonists in symptomatic venous thromboembolism. *Cochrane Database Syst Rev.* 2014;8:CD001367.
37. Kearon C, Ginsberg JS, Anderson DR et al. Comparison of 1 month with 3 months of anticoagulation for a first episode of venous thromboembolism associated with a transient risk factor. *J Thromb Haemost: JTH.* 2004;2(5):743–749.
38. Watson L, Broderick C, Armon MP. Thrombolysis for acute deep vein thrombosis. *Cochrane Database Syst Rev.* 2014;1:CD002783.
39. Enden T, Klow NE, Sandvik L et al. Catheter-directed thrombolysis vs. anticoagulant therapy alone in deep vein thrombosis: Results of an open randomized, controlled trial reporting on short-term patency. *J Thromb Haemost: JTH.* 2009;7(8):1268–1275.
40. Enden T, Haig Y, Klow NE et al. Long-term outcome after additional catheter-directed thrombolysis versus standard treatment for acute iliofemoral deep vein thrombosis (the CaVenT study): A randomised controlled trial. *Lancet.* 2012;379(9810):31–38.
41. McLafferty RB. Endovascular management of deep venous thrombosis. *Perspect Vasc Surg Endovasc Ther.* 2008;20(1):87–91.
42. Sharifi M, Bay C, Mehdipour M, Sharifi J, Investigators T. Thrombus Obliteration by Rapid Percutaneous Endovenous Intervention in Deep Venous Occlusion (TORPEDO) trial: Midterm results. *J Endovasc Ther Offic J Int Soc Endovasc Spec.* 2012;19(2):273–280.
43. Kolbach DN, Sandbrink MW, Hamulyak K, Neumann HA, Prins MH. Non-pharmaceutical measures for prevention of post-thrombotic syndrome. *Cochrane Database Syst Rev.* 2004;(1):CD004174.
44. Musani MH, Matta F, Yaekoub AY, Liang J, Hull RD, Stein PD. Venous compression for prevention of post-thrombotic syndrome: A meta-analysis. *Am J Med.* 2010;123(8):735–740.
45. Kahn SR, Shapiro S, Wells PS et al. Compression stockings to prevent post-thrombotic syndrome: A randomised placebo-controlled trial. *Lancet.* 2014;383(9920):880–888.

## Commentary on Deep Venous Thrombosis

*M. Margaret Knudson*

Venous thromboembolic disease (VTE), which includes deep venous thrombosis (DVT) and pulmonary embolism (PE), has long been recognized as a source of morbidity and mortality after surgical procedures. This association was first described in autopsy studies performed over 80 years ago in patients who had a sudden (and obviously fatal) cardiac arrest postoperatively. These findings prompted the widespread use of low doses of subcutaneous unfractionated heparin administered in the perioperative period aimed at prevention of DVT and subsequent PE. Despite these efforts, *symptomatic* VTE still occurs in at least 1% of surgical patients undergoing elective procedures. However, since most VTE events are silent, hospitals that routinely scan high-risk patients with duplex ultrasound examination (surveillance) will report much higher rates of DVT. Additionally, liberal use of CT angiography in surgical patients has facilitated the detection of nonfatal PE. In trauma patients, PE is recognized as the third leading cause of death. Thus, while we continue to search for more effective methods of *prevention* of VTE events after surgery and trauma, the chapter by Ginzberg et al on the *treatment* of established VTE remains relevant for the acute care surgeon.

The authors of this chapter first explore the use of the low-molecular-weight heparin (LMWH) enoxaparin in the treatment of VTE. Initially introduced in the United States by orthopedic surgeons, enoxaparin has been shown to be more effective in preventing DVT when compared to unfractionated heparin due to its improved bioavailability and its higher affinity for antithrombin. Most studies also report a lower risk of bleeding with the use of LMWH in postoperative patients. An additional benefit, when compared to traditional treatment with the vitamin K antagonist Coumadin, is that LMWH can be administered in a standard dose without the need for expensive and inconvenient laboratory monitoring. However, as we gain more experience with LMWH, we have learned that the recommended full anticoagulant dose of 1mg/kg administered subcutaneously twice daily may not be adequate for all patients. The effect of LMWH can be estimated by measuring anti-Xa activity, but this laboratory test is expensive and not routinely performed in most centers. Another method of measuring the activity of LMWH is with TEG (thromboelastography), but this is not yet considered standard of care. Additional challenges in the field of anticoagulation include the increasing use of anti-Xa agents that can be given orally as well as novel direct thrombin inhibitors. Like LMWH, these new oral agents cannot be easily monitored nor can they be easily reversed should bleeding occur. Certainly, these new medications will be a topic for future chapters in this textbook.

Should patients with established VTE be treated at home with LMWH as opposed to in-hospital treatment? The authors present some data on the safety of this practice, but there are several factors to be considered prior to embarking on this course of action, including the proximity to the surgical procedure (i.e., concern for postoperative hemorrhage induced by the anticoagulant), the estimated compliance of the patient (is he/she willing to continue twice daily self-injections?), and the cost (does the patient have insurance that will cover this out of hospital treatment?). An additional concern is that should the patient be inadequately protected due to ineffective dosing or missed injections and develop a PE at home, there is no chance for a medical response team to intervene and potentially provide life-saving measures ("failure to rescue"). In my mind, this practice is perhaps more suited for medical patients rather than those treated by the acute care surgeon and who have undergone emergency surgical procedures.

Regarding the optimal starting dose of vitamin K antagonist therapy, I agree with the authors that we should be cautious with administering doses larger than the traditional 5 mg in our trauma/acute care surgical patients. This concern comes from the unique changes in the coagulation system that have been elucidated from research into the acute coagulopathy of trauma. Of particular interest is the role of protein C, levels of which may drop off quickly in the trauma patient and potentially render the patient hypercoagulable early after injury. Further decreasing this protein with high doses of Coumadin may have significant consequences.

Patients who develop VTE following surgery or trauma are typically treated with anticoagulation for 3–6 months after the event, but we have no solid data on which to make this recommendation. Most surgical patients do not have a permanent "hypercoagulable" state and thus are at relatively low risk for subsequent VTE events. In addition to the bleeding risk and other side effects of the anticoagulants that we prescribe (such as interaction with other medications and induced dietary changes), some patients report psychological consequences such as fear of falling while on anticoagulation, reluctance to return to exercise routines, and other life-style changes that have significantly affected their sense of well-being. A more reasonable approach would be to bring patients back for serial venous ultrasound scans and discontinue anticoagulants when the DVT has resolved by imaging. Using DVT as a surrogate marker for PE, a more informed time-frame for the course of treatment for postoperative/posttraumatic VTE could be developed.

One frequently overlooked consequence of DVT is the postthrombotic syndrome. Most acute care surgeons will not treat such patients, but our vascular surgical colleagues will attest to the seriousness of this chronic condition, including leg pain, persistent leg swelling, ulceration, inability to resume previous work and athletic pursuits, and occasionally even amputation. While catheter-based infusion of thrombolytics is indicated in life-threatening cases of pulmonary embolism, this therapy is rarely indicated in the routine treatment of DVT especially in the postoperative patient. One exception might be in the unfortunate patient with iliac vein thrombosis with severe leg swelling (cerulea dolens). Not surprisingly, compression stockings have been demonstrated to be ineffective in preventing the long-term sequelae associated with the postthrombotic syndrome. Another area of research that might prove fruitful is a study of venous insufficiency using plethysmography in patients with a history of DVT to identify patients with subclinical venous insufficiency who might benefit from therapy.

Postsurgical VTE is considered by the Centers for Medicare and Medicaid as a complication that is preventable ("a never event"). In emergency general surgery and trauma patients, this is an unreasonable goal as currently there is no method of VTE prophylaxis that is both safe and 100% effective in this heterogeneous group of patients. Thus, the advice provided by Ginzberg and colleagues on the current state of the art regarding treatment of VTE has implications for our everyday practice as we focus on quality, patient safety, and patient-centered care.

# 66

## *Pulmonary Embolism*

**George C. Velmahos**

**CONTENTS**



### 66.1 Introduction

Pulmonary embolism (PE) is a national health problem, claiming over 50,000 lives in the United States. PE has been found in 32% of surgical patients who had autopsy, and in about half of these cases, PE was thought to be the causing or contributing factor for death [1]. Although the sample of patients in that study was not representative of the entire surgical population and was subject to variable thromboprophylactic practices, the high figures indicate the importance of the problem. Currently, the PE rates are estimated to be overall lower but vary significantly (0.3%–30%) due to the inconsistent screening and diagnosis among centers. The exact percentage of fatal PE is unknown for the same reasons.

The pathogenesis of PE is based on the theory of clot dislodgment from a lower extremity or pelvic deep venous thrombosis (DVT). Neck and upper extremity veins contribute on occasions. However, there is a consistent disconnect in the literature between DVT and PE. Although one would expect that a lower extremity or pelvic DVT would be found on patients with PE, this is only infrequently the case. In the past, this discrepancy was explained by the inaccuracy of available diagnostic methods to detect DVT, particularly of pelvic origin. With the development of CT venography and high-definition ultrasonography, this is no longer the case. These tests evaluate accurately the pelvic and proximal extremity veins and frequently fail to discover DVT associated with an existing PE. Therefore, the original theory of PE pathogenesis may be incorrect. It is possible that PE does not always originate from peripheral veins but may be formed de novo in the pulmonary circulation [2].

There are more unknowns than standards in PE. The optimal diagnosis, prevention, and treatment are under constant debate.

### 66.2 Risk Factors

#### 66.2.1 Who is at Risk for PE?

The classic Virchow's triad places the surgical patient at risk for PE, but the exact level of risk that allows intelligent risk-to-benefit calculations and decisions about the administration of potentially harmful thromboprophylaxis is unknown. Multiple risk factors have been suggested: obesity, immobility, cancer, major abdominal or pelvic operations, trauma, oral contraceptives, increasing age, previous thromboembolism, pregnancy and postpartum period, smoking, coagulation abnormalities, and acute medical illness, including heart, renal, and respiratory failure. There is poor evidence documenting the impact of each one of these risk factors on the pathogenesis of PE, and contradictory studies are common. For example, it is unknown which exact level of obesity, exact duration, and level of immobility; exact age, type and stage of cancer, or severity of medical illness predisposes the patient for PE. A systematic review and meta-analysis of the existing literature among trauma patients underscore precisely this inconsistency [3]. Although gender, head injuries, spinal fractures, spinal cord injuries, long-bone fractures, and pelvic fractures were examined as possible risk factors among studies of trauma patients, only spinal fractures and spinal cord injuries were found on pooled analysis to affect the incidence of venous thromboembolism (Level 2b evidence). The study also found that the likelihood of venous thromboembolism increases with older age and higher Injury Severity Score, and the threshold at which the rate of the outcome increases significantly could not be determined by the available literature.

The seventh ACCP conference created a stratification of risk according to the presence of risk factors [4]. This stratification makes clinical sense but is based on variable levels of evidence (typically Level 3) and, therefore, should be considered with caution. Patients younger than 40 years, no other risk factors, and minor surgery are at low risk for PE. Patients at moderate risk have only one of the following: age 40–60 years, major surgery, or a major preexisting risk factor. Patients at high risk are those who are either older than 60 years or older than 40 years but with major surgery and a major preexisting risk factor present. At the highest risk are patients who are older than 40 years of age and have major surgery *and* one of the following: previous thromboembolic event, cancer, or hypercoagulable condition; major trauma; spinal injury; hip/knee arthroplasty; and hip surgery. Major surgery was considered as a thoracic or abdominal operation under general anesthesia lasting over 30 min. The authors calculated a risk of 2%–4% for PE and 0.4%–1% for fatal PE in patients at high risk and 4%–10% for PE and 0.5%–5% for fatal PE in patients at the highest risk.

*Recommendation*: There is inconsistent evidence about the exact risk factors that predispose to PE. It seems that major trauma—and particularly spinal injuries—older age, major surgery, previous history of thromboembolism, and cancer increase the risk of PE. The effect of other factors, such as immobility, obesity, and medical illness, is ill-defined (Grade B recommendation).

## 66.3 Diagnosis

### 66.3.1 What is the Optimal Diagnostic Test for PE?

The ventilation-perfusion (V-P) scan and pulmonary angiography (PA) have been the main tests for diagnosis of PE for more than 20 years. The prospective investigation of pulmonary embolism diagnosis study [5] showed that V-P scan is 96% sensitive when the index of clinical suspicion is high. However, 75% of the patients belong to the intermediate category in which V-P scan is less sensitive. PA may still remain the standard of reference but is invasive and requires significant time spent in the angiography suite, a major setback for critically ill patients.

Over the past 10 years, computed tomographic pulmonary angiography (CTPA) has evolved to become the preferred diagnostic method for PE in surgical patients. In a meta-analysis of the diagnostic performance of CTPA and V-P scan, Hayashino et al. [6] examined 12 studies from 1985 to 2003, which were selected according to the following three criteria: the tests were performed for the diagnosis of acute PE; PA was used as the standard of reference; and absolute numbers of true-positive, true-negative, false-positive, and false-negative findings were given. Based on these studies, a random effects model found CTPA to have 86% sensitivity (95% confidence interval [CI]: 80.2%, 92.1%) and 93.7% specificity (95% CI: 91.1%, 96.3%). V-P scan was found to have low sensitivity (39%) and high specificity (97.1%) with high probability threshold but high sensitivity (98.3%) and low specificity (4.8%) with normal threshold. The authors concluded that, although V-P scan and CTPA have similar diagnostic ability for patients with a high probability for PE, CTPA has higher discriminatory power than V-P scan for patients with normal and near-normal probability (Level 1b evidence).

In another systematic review of the literature, Quiroz et al. [7] examined the clinical validity of a negative CTPA for suspected PE. Of particular concern was the alleged low sensitivity of CTPA for peripheral PE. To calculate the overall negative likelihood ratio of PE after a negative or inconclusive CTPA, the authors included PE, which was confirmed by another diagnostic test within 3 months of CTPA. Fifteen studies with a total population of 3500 patients were included from 1994 to 2002. Single-slice, multidetector, and electron-beam scanners were used in the different studies. The negative predictive value of a normal CTPA was 99.7% (95% CI: 98.7%, 99.5%), and the negative likelihood ratio of a PE after a normal CTPA was 0.7 (95% CI: 0.05, 011). There was no difference in the risk of PE based on the different types of computed tomographic scanner. The authors concluded that the clinical validity of CTPA to rule out PE is similar to that reported for conventional PA (Level 1b evidence). This study shows that even if the diagnosis of peripheral PE is the principal limitation of CTPA, undiagnosed peripheral PE (which can exist in as many as 30% of "normal" CTPA) is usually not clinically significant and does not cause subsequent clinically detectable PE or death from PE.

Finally, a meta-analysis of different diagnostic strategies for PE by Roy et al. [8] included 48 of the 1012 articles examined from 1990 to 2003. The study attempted to determine the clinical application of each test according to pretest clinical probability. In patients with a high pretest probability, a high-probability V-P scan, a positive CTPA, and a positive lower extremity venous ultrasound was associated with a higher than 85% posttest probability of PE. In patients with an intermediate or low pretest probability, a normal or near-normal V-P scan, a normal CTPA in combination with normal lower extremity venous ultrasound, and a D-dimer concentration of less than 500 μg/L measured by quantitative enzyme-linked immunosorbent assay was associated with a less than 5% posttest probability of PE. CTPA, magnetic resonance angiography, a low-probability V-P scan, and a quantitative latex or hemoagglutination D-dimer test could only exclude PE in patients with low pretest probability. The authors concluded that the accuracy of the different tests vary significantly and according to the pretest clinical probability for PE (Level 2 evidence).

*Recommendation*: CTPA is convenient, safe, and accurate for the diagnosis of clinically significant PE. It is the preferred diagnostic method for most emergency surgery and trauma patients (Grade A recommendation).

## 66.4 Prevention

### 66.4.1 Is Heparin and Compression Devices Adequate for PE Prophylaxis?

The use of low-dose unfractionated heparin (UFH), usually administered subcutaneously, for prevention of PE was established in the mid-1970s by the seminal study of Kakkar et al. [9]. That study included only elective surgery patients; emergency surgery and trauma patients were excluded. Despite this fact, thromboprophylaxis by UFH became common practice for all surgical patients. An overview of randomized trials of general, orthopedic, and urologic surgery patients concluded that UFH reduced symptomatic PE rates from 2% to 1.3% and fatal PE rates from 0.8% to 0.3%, but the risk of perioperative bleeding increased from 3.8% to 5.9% [10]. However, the evidence about UFH in trauma is controversial, and the evidence about UFH in emergency non-traumatic general surgery patients simply does not exist. Low-molecular-weight heparin (LMWH), also administered subcutaneously, has shown increased stability and bioavailability compared to UFH, benefits possibly associated with improved effectiveness and safety. There are multiple randomized studies and meta-analyses in general surgery patients documenting equivalence or superiority of LMWH over UFH [11,12], but again, this evidence is only modestly applicable to the emergency surgery population because the majority of included patients had elective operations.

Sequential compression devices (SCDs) have been used extensively based on the assumption that they promote blood flow, simulating muscle function, and trigger the release of fibrinolytic agents from the vascular endothelium. The evidence on their effectiveness is also questionable, and at least two studies document poor compliance [13,14]. This could be the ultimate drawback for their use, as it gives the physician a false sense of security, while the patient receives no benefit from the prescribed treatment.

There are a number of noncontrolled studies and a few prospective randomized trials in trauma patients. Knudson et al. [15] produced three randomized trials (Level 1c evidence). In 1992, the authors randomized 113 trauma patients to UFH or SCD and found no significant difference in thromboembolic complications (five patients with DVT, four with PE, and three with DVT and PE) between the two groups. In 1994, the authors compared patients receiving UFH, SCD, or no treatment and found similar VT rates in the three groups, except for a mild advantage of SCD over no treatment in neurosurgical patients [16]. There were only two documented PEs, one in a SCD patient and one in a patient who received no thromboprophylaxis. In 1996, they randomized 181 patients to LMWH or SCD and failed to find any significant difference in DVT [17]. There were no documented cases of PE in any of the randomized groups.

In a study of LMWH against SCD in head and spinal trauma, 60 patients were randomized to LMWH and 60 to SCD [18]. The incidence of PE was not different between the two groups, with 7% in the LMWH group and 3% in the SCD group. This high incidence of PE could indicate a poor thromboprophylactic effect of LWMH and SCD (Level 1c evidence). In another randomized study, spinal cord injury patients received either UFH with SCD or LMWH and showed no difference in proximal DVT or PE rates [19]. The total number of thromboembolic events was very high and almost identical in the two groups (65.5% for LMWH and 63.3% for UFH with SCD, $p = 0.81$), placing again in doubt the effectiveness of these regimens (Level 1c evidence).

Probably, the two best-designed randomized trials in trauma patients examined LMWH vs. SCD [20] or LMWH vs. UFH [21]. In both, DVT and not PE (or total thromboembolic events) was the principal outcome. In the study by Ginzburg et al. [20], the DVT rates were similar between LMWH and SCD. There was one PE in each group. There was no difference in thromboembolic events when a sub-analysis of patients with

Injury Severity Score higher than 19 was undertaken. The rate of bleeding was not different either (Level 1b evidence). In the study by Geerts et al. [21], LMWH was associated with lower DVT rates compared to UFH. There was only one patient with documented PE (a high-probability V-P scan), and he belonged to the LMWH group. The rate of major bleeding was not different (0.6% vs. 2.9%, $p = 0.12$), but of the six documented episodes, one was in the UFH group and five in the LMWH group (Level 1b evidence). Two systematic reviews of the existing evidence in trauma confirmed the low level of evidence that exists about UFH, SCD, and LMWH, and the uncertainty about their exact profile of effectiveness and safety [22,23] (Level 1b evidence).

*Recommendation*: Although general surgery patients with elective operations seem to benefit from the current thromboprophylactic methods, the effectiveness of UFH, LMWH, and SCD in emergency surgery and trauma patients remains uncertain. An individual risk-to-benefit assessment should be made for each such patient at risk of PE. LMWH is probably more effective than UFH or SCD (Grade B recommendation).

### 66.4.2 Are PE and Mortality from PE Reduced by IVC Filters?

The effectiveness of inferior vena cava (IVC) filters relies on their ability to capture clot originating from lower extremity or pelvic veins. Three scenarios may hamper this ability. First, a misplaced or tilted filter may not function adequately. A tilt of as little as 10° in relationship with the IVC axis has been reported to compromise optimal function [24]. Second, the capture of a primary clot at the apex of the filter may force blood circulation toward the periphery of the vessel and recurrent clots to escape in this way. Third, clots may originate from upper extremity or neck veins [25] or, even possibly, form de novo in the pulmonary circulation [2], in which case, a device in the IVC is obviously of no use. One can argue that a filter is never used therapeutically, as its effect never involves a PE that has already occurred but only the embolus that may follow. The use of IVC filters in patients with "breakthrough" PE (occurring while the patient is fully anticoagulated) or with primary PE and inability to anticoagulate is well-accepted. Other criteria are more controversial and include a contraindication for prophylactic anticoagulation in the presence of high risk for PE, added prophylaxis in patients at very high risk for PE even if prophylactic anticoagulation is feasible, and added prophylaxis in patients who have already sustained a significant PE and are therapeutically anticoagulated but would be at risk of death, if a breakthrough PE occurred [26] (Level 3b evidence).

Currently, retrievable filters have replaced temporary filters for most indications. Unless it is deemed that a filter needs to remain in place for life, as it may happen with spinal cord injury patients or very old patients with significant co-morbidities, most trauma and emergency surgery patients have only a finite period of risk and, therefore, do not need a permanent device. Unfortunately, a multicenter study [27] has shown that only 19% of these filters are being removed, and therefore, most are left permanently, even if not designed for this purpose (Level 3a evidence).

There is not a single prospective randomized study on the use of IVC filters in trauma and emergency surgery patients. Decousous et al. [28] randomized a mixed population of 200 predominantly medical patients with DVT into IVC filter versus no filter. After a 2-year follow-up, those with filters had a significant decrease in PE but a significant increase in DVT. There was no difference in mortality. When this population was followed-up for 8 years [29], the results remained unchanged: the IVC filter group had a lower incidence of PE (6.2% vs. 15.1%, $p = 0.008$), higher incidence of DVT (35.7% vs. 27.5%, $p = 0.042$), and no difference in mortality, compared to the no filter group (Level 1b evidence). Studies of trauma patients have failed to consistently prove that the insertion of vena cava filters resulted in a decrease of PE or death from PE [30–32] (Level 3b evidence).

IVC filters are not complication free. Morbidity related to access (bleeding, thrombosis, arterial damage), catheter advancement (vessel damage), contrast material (anaphylaxis, renal failure), and the filter itself (vessel wall perforation, migration, IVC thrombosis, DVT, misplacement) is detected in approximately 4%–7% of the cases, although the variability in rates among studies is great [26] (Level 3a evidence). A new class of complications is now related to the removal of retrievable filters, including all of the aforementioned problems as well as dislodgement of clot captured by the filter, damage of the IVC wall, and inability to retrieve.

Most importantly, the theory of "de novo" formation of clots in the pulmonary circulation, which contradicts the traditional theory of clot embolization from the deep venous system of the extremities, may in large part defy the logic behind IVC filter use. If clots form directly into the pulmonary arteries and do not travel from the legs, then the placement of an IVC filter to interrupt the course of such travel is obsolete. In an elegant study of 99 patients with proven PE, Van Langevelde et al. [33] performed a total-body magnetic resonance imaging to identify venous clots. No thrombus was found in 55 patients, and of the 44 patients who had venous thrombi, 12 had isolated calf thrombosis and 5 had isolated superficial vein thrombosis. At the end, only 44% were presumed to have a peripheral venous origin of PE, and only slightly over 27% had it at the major deep venous system. In other words, an IVC filter could be unable to prevent the PE in more than half of the patients.

*Recommendation*: There is no convincing evidence that in emergency surgery and trauma patients, IVC filters reduce the incidence of PE and mortality from PE. Use of IVC filters should be made based on an individual patient-by-patient risk-to-benefit analysis (Grade C recommendation).

## 66.5 Treatment

### 66.5.1 Is LMWH as Safe and Effective as UFH for the Treatment of PE?

Dose-adjusted intravenous UFH is used for the treatment of PE. However, subcutaneous LMWH at therapeutic doses presents significant benefits over UFH, as monitoring is not required and treatment can be self-administered at home. There are multiple randomized

**TABLE 66.1**

Clinical Questions

| Question | Answer | Grade of Recommendation | References |
|---|---|---|---|
| Who is at risk for PE? | Patients with spinal injuries, older age, major surgery or trauma, previous history of thromboembolism, and cancer. | B | [3,4] |
| What is the optimal diagnostic test for PE? | CTPA | A | [6–8] |
| Are heparin and compression devices adequate for PE prophylaxis? | The effectiveness of heparin and compression devices in trauma and emergency surgery patients is unclear. LMWH seems to perform better than UFH. | B | [11–23] |
| Are PE and mortality from PE reduced by IVC filters? | The effectiveness of IVC filters in reducing PE and mortality from PE in trauma and emergency surgery patients is unclear. | C | [28–32] |
| Is LMWH as safe and effective as UFH for the treatment of PE? | Yes | A | [33] |

**TABLE 66.2**

Evidence-Based Table

| Study | Design | Intervention | Description | Results |
|---|---|---|---|---|
| #15 | RCT | Duplex within 24 h of admission and every 5 days. Prophylaxis by SCD or UFH or nothing | 113 patients included. 76 randomized to SCD and 37 to UFH | VT developed in 12 (5 DVT, 4 PE, 3 both); 9 SCD and 3 UFH. Risk factor for DVT was spinal trauma. |
| #16 | RCT | Duplex within 24 h of admission and then every 5–7 days. Prophylaxis by SCD or UFH or nothing | Division in three groups and randomization within each group. Group I: UFH or SCD or nothing; Group II: UFH or nothing; Group III: SCD or nothing | 255 patients—15 developed DVT—unclear PE. No difference in Group I (2.3% UFH, 14.2% SCD, 3.2% nothing) and Group II (5.5% UFH, 8% nothing). Lower DVT in Group III (0% SCD, 14.7% nothing). |
| #17 | RCT | Duplex on admission and every 5–7 days. Prophylaxis by LMWH, SCD, AVF. | 487 patients included, 372 analyzed. 202 stratified to the heparin group and randomized to LMWH (120) or SCD (61)/AVF (21). 170 stratified to the no heparin group and received SCD/AVF. | DVT in nine (2.4%) and PE in one. In randomized patients, one LMWH and two SCD patients had DVT. The other six DVT were in the nonrandomized group. |
| #20 | RCT | Duplex within 24 h of admission and weekly after that | 294 moderately and 148 severely injured patients randomized separately into LMWH and SCD. | DVT in 2.7% of SCD and 0.5% of LMWH ($p = 0.12$). PE in one patient per group. |
| #21 | RCT | Venography 10–14 days after admission. Prophylaxis by UFH or LMWH | 265 included; 136 randomized to UFH and 129 to LMWH | DVT (44% UFH, 31% LMWH, $p = 0.014$). Proximal DVT (15% UFH, 6% LMWH, $p = 0.012$). One PE in LMWH. |
| #28 | RCT | V-P scan, and if necessary PA | 400 randomized: 200 to filter and 200 to no filter | At day 12, PE developed in 1.1% of filters and 4.8% of no filters ($p = 0.03$). At 2 years, 20.8% filter and 11.6% no filter patients had recurrent DVT ($p = 0.02$). |

*Abbreviations:* RCT, randomized controlled trial; SCD, sequential compression device; UFH, unfractionated heparin; LMWH, low-molecular-weight heparin; AVF, arteriovenous foot pumps; DVT, deep venous thrombosis; PE, pulmonary embolism; V-P scan, ventilation-perfusion scan.
*Note:* The intervention described refers to DVT. No study except #28 had a protocolized routine intervention for PE.

studies in the literature, and all of them include either exclusively or predominantly medical patients. Therefore, the evidence on emergency surgery and trauma patients is poor. A meta-analysis of 12 randomized studies [34] found that LMWH was associated with a non-significant decrease of symptomatic PE (1.7% vs. 2.3%) and asymptomatic PE (1.2% vs. 3.2%), while offering a non-significant advantage in decreasing bleeding (1.3% vs. 2.1%), compared to UFH (Level 1a evidence). The authors concluded that LMWH was at least as safe and effective as UFH for the initial treatment of PE. It is expected that in emergency surgery and trauma patients, the rates of the aforementioned outcomes—and specifically of bleeding—may be different, but there is little reason to believe that the equivalence between the two groups will not be maintained. However, concerns about the inability to reverse LMWH effectively by protamin if a high-risk patient were to bleed may still create discomfort in consistently using LMWH over UFH.

*Recommendation*: LMWH is as safe and effective as UFH for the treatment of PE. It may be the preferred treatment in patients at lower risk of bleeding, based on the convenience of outpatient self-administration, and there is no need for monitoring (Grade A recommendation) (Tables 66.1 and 66.2).

## References


1. Lindblad B, Eriksson A, Bergqvist D. Autopsy-verified pulmonary embolism in a surgical department. Analysis of the period from 1951 to 1988. *Br J Surg.* 1991;78:849–852.
2. Velmahos GC, Spaniolas K, Tabbara M et al. The relationship of pulmonary embolism and deep venous thrombosis in trauma. Are they really related? *Arch Surg.* October 2009;144(10):928–932.
3. Velmahos GC, Kern J, Chan LS, Oder D, Murray JA, Shekelle P. Prevention of venous thromboembolism after injury: An evidence-based report--part II: Analysis of risk factors and evaluation of the role of vena caval filters. *J Trauma.* 2000;49(1):140–144.
4. Geerts WH, Pineo GF, Heit HA et al. Prevention of venous thromboembolism: The seventh ACCP conference on antithrombotic and thrombolytic therapy. *Chest.* 2004;126(3 Suppl):338S–400S.
5. The PIOPED Investigators. Value of the ventilation/perfusion scan in the diagnosis of pulmonary embolism: Results of the prospective investigation for pulmonary embolism diagnosis (PIOPED). *JAMA.* 1990;263;2753–2759.
6. Hayashino Y, Goto M, Noguchi Y, Fugul T. Ventilation-perfusion scanning and helical CT in suspected pulmonary embolism: Meta-analysis of diagnostic performance. *Radiology.* 2005;234:740–748.
7. Quiroz R, Kucher N, Zou KH et al. Clinical validity of a negative computed tomography scan in patients with suspected pulmonary embolism. A systematic review. *JAMA.* 2005;293:2012–2017.
8. Roy PM, Colombet I, Durieux P, Chatellier G, Sors H, Meyer G. Systematic review and meta-analysis of strategies for the diagnosis of suspected pulmonary embolism. *Br Med J.* 2005;331:1–9.
9. Kakkar VV, Corrigan TP, Fossard DP et al. Prevention of fatal postoperative pulmonary embolism by low doses of heparin. An international multicentre trial. *Lancet.* 1975;2(7924):45–51.
10. Collins R, Scrimgeour A, Yusuf S, Peto R. Reduction in fatal pulmonary embolism and venous thrombosis by perioperative administration of subcutaneous heparin. Overview of results of randomized trials in general, orthopedic, and urologic surgery. *N Engl J Med.* 1988;318:1162–1173.
11. Koch A, Bouges S, Ziegler S et al. Low molecular weight heparin and unfractionated heparin in thrombosis prophylaxis after major surgical intervention: Update of previous meta-analyses. *Br J Surg.* 1997;84:750–759.
12. Mismetti P, Laporte S, Darmon JY et al. Meta-analysis of low molecular weight heparin for the prevention of venous thromboembolism in general surgery. *Br J Surg.* 2001;88:913–930.
13. Cornwell EE, Chang D, Velmahos G et al. Compliance with sequential compression device prophylaxis in at-risk trauma patients: A prospective analysis. *Am Surg.* 2002;68:470–473.
14. Comerota AJ, Katz ML, White JV. Why does prophylaxis with external pneumatic compression for deep vein thrombosis fail? *Am J Surg.* 1994;164:265–268.
15. Knudson MM, Collins JA, Goodman SB, McCrory DW. Thromboembolism following multiple trauma. *J Trauma.* 1992;32:2–11.
16. Knudson MM, Lewis FR, Clinton A, Atkinson K, Megerman J. Prevention of venous thromboembolism in trauma patients. *J Trauma.* 1994;37:480–487.
17. Knudson MM, Morabito D, Paiement GD, Schackleford S. Use of low molecular weight heparin in preventing thromboembolism in trauma patients. *J Trauma.* 1996;41:446–459.
18. Kurtoglou M, Yanar H, Bilsel Y et al. Venous thromboembolism prophylaxis after head and spinal trauma: Intermittent pneumatic compression devices versus low molecular weight heparin. *World J Surg.* 2004;28:807–811.
19. Merli G and the Spinal Cord Injury Thromboprophylaxis Investigators. Prevention of venous thromboembolism in the acute treatment phase after spinal cord injury: A randomized, multicenter trial comparing low-dose heparin plus intermittent pneumatic compression with enoxaparin. *J Trauma.* 2003;54:1116–1126.

20. Ginzburg E, Cohn SM, Lopez K et al. Randomized clinical trial of intermittent pneumatic compression and low molecular weight heparin in trauma. *Br J Surg.* 2003;90:1338–1344.
21. Geerts WH, Jay RM, Code KI et al. A comparison of low-dose heparin with low-molecular-weight heparin as prophylaxis against venous thromboembolism after major trauma. *N Engl J Med.* 1996;335:701–707.
22. Velmahos GC, Kern J, Chan LS, Oder D, Murray JA, Shekelle P. Prevention of venous thromboembolism after injury: An evidence-based report—part I: Analysis of risk factors and evaluation of the role of vena caval filters. *J Trauma.* 2000;49(1):132–138.
23. Rogers FB, Cipolle MD, Velmahos GC, Rozycki G, Luchette FA. Practice management guidelines for the prevention of venous thromboembolism in trauma patients: The EAST practice management guidelines work group. *J Trauma.* 2002;53:142–164.
24. Rogers FB, Stringberg G, Schackford GR et al. Five-year follow-up of prophylactic vena cava filters in high-risk trauma patients. *Arch Surg.* 1998;133:406–411.
25. Hingorani A, Ascher E, Lorenson E et al. Upper extremity deep venous thrombosis and its impact on morbidity and mortality rates in a hospital-based population. *J Vasc Surg.* 1997;26(5):853–860.
26. Martin MJ, Salim A. Vena cava filters in surgery and trauma. *Surg Clin N Am.* 2007;87:1229–1252.
27. Karmy-Jones R, Jurkovich G, Velmahos GC et al. Practice patterns and outcomes after retrievable vena cava filters in trauma patients: A AAST multicenter study. *J Trauma.* 2007;62:17–25.
28. Decousous A, Leizorovicz S, Parent F et al. for the PREPIC study group. A clinical trial of vena cava filters in the prevention of pulmonary embolism in patients with deep vein thrombosis. *N Engl J Med.* 1998;338:409–415.
29. The PREPIC study group. Eight year follow-up of patients with permanent vena cava filters in the prevention of pulmonary embolism. *Circulation.* 2005;112:416–422.
30. Antevil JL, Sise MJ, Sack DI et al. Retrievable vena cava filters for preventing pulmonary embolism in trauma patients: A cautionary tale. *J Trauma.* 2006;60:35–40.
31. Rogers FB, Shackford SR, Ricci MA, Wilson JT, Parsons S. Routine prophylactic vena cava filter insertion in severely injured trauma patients decreases the incidence of pulmonary embolism. *J Am Coll Surg.* 1995;180:641–647.
32. McMurtry AL, Owings JT, Anderson JT, Battistella FD, Gosselin R. Increased use of prophylactic vena cava filters in trauma patients failed to decrease overall incidence of pulmonary embolism. *J Am Coll Surg.* 1999;189:314–320.
33. Van Langevelde K, Sramek A, Vincken PWJ, van Rooden JK, Rosendaal FR, Cannegieter SC. Finding the origin of pulmonary emboli with a total-body magnetic resonance direct thrombus imaging technique. *Haematologica.* 2013;98:309–315.
34. Quinlan DJ, McQuillan AM, Eikelbloom JW. Low-molecular-weight heparin compared with intravenous unfractionated heparin for treatment of pulmonary embolism. *Ann Intern Med.* 2004;140:175–183.

## Commentary on Pulmonary Embolism

*Kenneth L. Mattox*

"There are more unknowns than standards in PE. The optimal diagnosis, prevention, and treatment are under constant debate," states Dr. George Velmahos in his well-written chapter on, "Pulmonary Embolism." And, truer words were never spoken. With this chapter, Dr. Velmahos confirms my frustrations with textbook chapters, journal articles, lectures, and "best practice guidelines" on the subject. The writings, recommendations, and repeated opinions have been confusing since major venous clot formation, embolization of these clots, fatal pulmonary embolism, and vascular thrombosis/clot formation were first reported. Dr. Velmahos underscores my own belief that the diagnosis and management of *pulmonary embolism* is one of the most confusing areas in medical science, especially for the surgeon.

### Definitions/Terminology (Words)

The very phrase "pulmonary embolism" creates different images and definitions in the mind of the beholder, be that person an internist, vascular physician, surgeon, radiologist, pathologist, lawyer, emergency physician, thoracic surgeon, billing coder, electronic medical record computer programmer, or insurance company adjuster. "Venous thromboembolism" might actually be more descriptive, but this term, likewise, presumes both a site for formation of a blood clot and that it traveled to another location. From a coding standpoint, neither term is specific in defining the etiology, the pathology producing process, or the exact location where the clot is found by whatever means. The modifying words, "acute" and "chronic," may be added to both pulmonary embolism and deep venous thrombosis (DVT). The ICD-10 classifications for pulmonary continue due to the lack of specificity as to etiology, site of origin, and the ultimate location of a clot in the pulmonary arteries that is slightly better, but there is still room for confusion.

### Etiology of Clot in the Pulmonary Arteries

The definition of pulmonary embolism is a clot located in the pulmonary arteries, either central or in the terminal pulmonary arterioles. Following a clinical diagnosis of a possible pulmonary, confirmation is made by pulmonary arteriography, CT scanning (using a defined PE protocol), operation, or autopsy. Some laboratory tests are supportive but not diagnostic of PE. The etiology of the clots found in these locations continues to be debated—thromboembolic versus primarily forming in the pulmonary arteries or arterioles. Even the time of the clot formation is not known in the majority of patients. When the etiology is considered to be thromboembolic, the exact location of origin is almost always speculative, and in most instances of larger central occluding thromboemboli, the source is most likely either the iliac veins and/or the infrarenal venal cava. It is believed by many physicians (including this author) that thromboemboli originating from the veins of the leg or arm rarely are the etiology for the central large fatal thromboemboli. It is also believed by many physicians that the small clots seen in the peripheral pulmonary arterioles on CT scan or at autopsy are virtually never embolic, but most likely are secondary to low flow states, either at time of injury, early in the course of an illness, or late in the course of a terminal illness. Should such a peripheral clot develop in the distal pulmonary arterioles near the time of death, it should be so described. The patient is then appropriately described as a patient that dies with pulmonary emboli being present, rather than a patient dying secondary to pulmonary emboli. The finding of different kinds of clot in different locations and at different times in a patient's course of disease becomes very confusing in attempting to establish both etiologies and reasonable, scientific, standard treatment best practices. Dr. Velmahos, in his chapter, has made reference to this confusion.

### Confusion

A major cause of confusion relates to the *classification* and *coding* of pulmonary embolism cited earlier in this section. Both the ICD-9 and CD-10 codes have *no* qualifier as to the *location* of the pulmonary artery clots (central vs. peripheral), timing of clot formation, or origin of clot formation (nontruncal veins, iliac veins, a IVC, upper extremity veins, intracardiac, etc.). This lack of specificity carries through the hospital record and, often, the autopsy report. In that autopsy and operation are infrequently performed, a detailed description of the characteristics of the clot gives no clues as to the origin of the clot or even that it was, indeed, thromboembolic in origin. Finally, a chart reviewer might assume that the mere presence of a pulmonary artery clot (with an ICD-9 or ICD-10 diagnosis of pulmonary embolism) is a very serious and near-fatal condition, but such is certainly not always the case, especially for tiny peripheral pulmonary artery clots most likely caused by low flow states during terminal events. Thus, confusion continues, in that a person may die or have a major complication because of a thromboembolic central pulmonary artery clot *or* a person may develop a clot in the pulmonary artery distribution as a complication of injury, illness, or low flow state.

## Conclusion

This disease needs *major* reconsideration relating to etiology, definition, classification, causation, location of initial clot formation, association of the presence of the type of pulmonary artery clot to other conditions (such as DVT), and the type and timing of treatment.

This commentary has not included the additional complicating and confusing issues when pulmonary embolism is due to amniotic fluid, decidua tissue from a pregnancy, air, bone marrow, tumors, or fat (all of which have been described as being a source of pulmonary emboli). I have also not addressed the specifics of surgical or medical therapy, as this has been addressed in the parent chapter.

Doctor Velmahos repeatedly points out the lack of convincing evidence for current approaches to risk factors, treatment, use of filters, and prevention. I totally concur with his general conclusion that more evidence-based answers on this condition need to be sought.

# 67

# *Necrotizing Soft Tissue Infections*

**Mark D. Sawyer**

**CONTENTS**



## 67.1 Introduction and Definitions

Necrotizing soft tissue infections (NSTIs) are a subject that would seem to lend itself poorly to a textbook of evidence-based surgery. Such uncommon and highly lethal disease processes make quality large, prospective, randomized trials extremely difficult to design and implement. Further complicating the picture is that a large proportion of current practice is by necessity based upon individual observations and deductions concerning the disease, which as one might expect can engender strong biases, which at times seem to be in inverse proportion to available evidence. Thus, an evidence-based discussion of questions concerning NSTIs may have more the appearance of a photographic negative—deciding which tentative conclusions are likely not justified because there is no quality evidence to support them, rather than raising to the fore those conclusions best supported by solid statistical evidence. This also points out the need for a larger, cooperative effort to glean more substantial evidence from the 3800 to 5800 cases per year that occur [11].

While NSTIs comprise a wide variety of clinical scenarios as reflected by the bewildering array of terms utilized in the literature, a simple division—predominantly fascial versus predominantly muscular involvement—categorizes these infections reasonably well both in terms of their behavior and a pragmatic approach to empiric treatment [6,7]. Although anyone may be affected, the immunocompromised and debilitated—most commonly those with advancing age and diabetes mellitus—are disproportionately represented both in terms of acquiring the disease, and in suffering poorer outcomes.

## 67.2 Necrotizing Fasciitis

### 67.2.1 The Disease

Necrotizing fasciitis is an infection involving the investing fascia of muscle, primarily the superficial layer, and may secondarily involve a modest amount of juxtaposed fat and muscle. It has a predilection for the immunocompromised, in which it is more morbid and lethal as well. Originally described as a streptococcal or streptococcal-predominant infectious process [1,2] it is usually a polymicrobial infection, although monomicrobial forms of the disease (*Vibrio, Pseudomonas, Klebsiella*, and others) exist as well. Studies carefully culturing the tissues may show a mix of Gram-positive, Gram-negative, and anaerobic bacteria, as well as candidal species in some.

Necrotizing fasciitis has been described as a rapidly progressive process, but at least some patients may describe a relatively indolent period prior to seeking medical attention, with subsequent decompensation giving the outward appearance of rapid progression [3,4]. These patients are primarily those with the polymicrobial form of the disease. The monomicrobial forms of the disease—group A *Streptococcus*, Clostridial species, and marine gram negatives such as *Vibrio vulnificans*—are rapidly progressive, extraordinarily lethal disease processes.

### 67.2.2 Diagnosis

Incision and exploration with open biopsy of suspected tissues has been the standard of care for diagnosis, although radiographic studies such as CT scans can provide useful data regarding the location and extent of disease.

## 67.3 Mainstay Therapy

There are two cornerstones of initial therapy: expeditious and complete debridement, and broad-spectrum antimicrobial therapy. Immediate initiation of empiric broad-spectrum antimicrobial therapy based on an anti-Streptococcal component is key; awaiting culture or even Gram stain data to guide therapy would constitute an unnecessary and potentially dangerous delay. With one study utilizing careful culture techniques showing Candida species in a majority of patients and the dangers of superinfection following potent broad-spectrum antimicrobial therapy, many would advocate empiric therapy with an antifungal agent as well, although this is not considered standard of care. The Infectious Disease Societies of America have recently published an update to their evidence-based recommendations for antimicrobial choices in skin and soft tissue infections, including necrotizing fasciitis and myositis (Table 67.1). As with other evidence-based recommendations for NSTIs, the recommendations are strong, but with weak evidence.

The other unequivocal cornerstone of therapy is expeditious and complete excision of the infected and necrotic fascia to prevent further progression and begin the healing process. Although some have advocated staged resections in the past, it would seem more logical to remove as much of the involved fascia as the patient will tolerate at the first resection. Regardless of initial philosophy, returning to the operating room for "second-look" procedures to at least assess if not complete the resection process is ubiquitous. Necrotizing fasciitis is a progressive disease, and assuring that progression has been halted is mandatory. Though excision and debridement can be debilitating and disfiguring, completeness is essential to halt the progression of disease and maximize survival. Following the initial phase, a prolonged healing convalescent phase is usual in survivors, with care of open wounds that may constitute a large percentage of the patient's body surface area. In addition to standard techniques for dressing and closing such wounds, newer technologies such as vacuum-assisted wound closure devices may be helpful.

## 67.4 Supplemental Therapy

There are a number of therapies that have been utilized in NSTIs to try and improve outcome, such as hyperbaric oxygen and antistreptococcal immunoglobulin administration. The rationale for the former had its genesis in the treatment of anaerobic NSTIs such as clostridial necrotizing myositis, and the latter as an attempt to improve treatment of aggressive group A streptococcal infections and their complications such as streptococcal toxic shock syndrome. While theoretically attractive, neither has definitively proven itself as a mainstay of treatment in NSTIs. Unfortunately, these therapies have not been shown to improve outcomes.

## 67.5 Necrotizing Myositis

The most common eponyms for necrotizing muscle infections are gas gangrene, clostridial/streptococcal myonecrosis, and necrotizing myositis. The latter most term is simple, descriptive, and alliteratively associates the disease process with its fascial counterpart. The infection infects, spreads, and necroses entire muscle compartments with celerity; it is rapidly progressive and in contradistinction to necrotizing fasciitis has no recognized indolent variants. Pragmatically, this means that exceptionally aggressive surgery such as proximal amputation may be required to gain control of the disease process before the patient succumbs, which may occur within hours of presentation. In further contradistinction to necrotizing fasciitis, necrotizing myositis is usually a monomicrobial infection, most commonly a toxin-producing *Clostridium* or *Streptococcus* species.

**TABLE 67.1**

Treatment of Necrotizing Infections of the Skin, Fascia, and Muscle

| Type of Infection | First-Line Antimicrobial Agent | Adult Dosage | Pediatric Dosage Beyond the Neonatal Period | Antimicrobial Agent for Patients with Severe Penicillin Hypersensitivity |
|---|---|---|---|---|
| Mixed infections | Piperacillin-tazobactam plus vancomycin | 3.375 g every 6–8 h IV | 60–75 mg/kg/dose of the piperacillin component every 6 h IV | Clindamycin or metronidazole[a] with an aminoglycoside or fluoroquinolone |
| | Imipenem-cilastatin | 30 mg/kg/dose in 2 divided doses | 10–13 mg/kg/dose every 8 h IV | N/A |
| | Meropenem | 1 g every 6–8 h IV | N/A | N/A |
| | Ertapenem | 1 g every 8 h IV | 20 mg/kg/dose every 8 h IV | |
| | Cefotaxime plus metronidazole or clindamycin | 1 g daily IV | 15 mg/kg/dose every 12 h IV for children | |
| | | 2 g every 6 h IV | 3 months-12 year | |
| | | 500 mg every 6 h IV | 50 mg/kg/dose every 6 h IV | |
| | | 600–900 mg every 8 h IV | 7.5 mg/kg/dose every 6 h IV | |
| | | | 10–13 mg/kg/dose every 8 h IV | |
| *Streptococcus* | Penicillin plus clindamycin | 2–4 million units every 4–6 h IV (adult) | 60,000–100,000 units/kg/dose every 6 h IV | Vancomycin, linezolid, quinupristin/dalfopristin, daptomycin |
| | | 600–900 mg/every 8 h IV | 10–13 mg/kg/dose every 8 h IV | |
| *Staphylococcus aureus* | Nafcillin | 1–2 g every 4 h IV | 50 mg/kg/dose every 6 h IV | Vancomycin, linezolid, quinupristin/dalfopristin, daptomycin |
| | Oxacillin | 1–2 g every 4 h IV | 50 mg/kg/dose/every 6 h IV | Bacteriostatic; potential cross-resistance and emergence of resistance in erythromycin-resistant strains; inducible resistance in MRSA[b] |
| | Cefazolin | 1 g every 8 h IV | 33 mg/kg/dose every 8 h IV | |
| | Vancomycin (for resistant strains) | 30 mg/kg/dose in 2 divided doses IV | 15 mg/kg/dose every 6 h IV | |
| | Clindamycin | 600–900 mg every 8 h IV | 10–13 mg/kg/dose every 8 h IV | |
| *Clostridium* species | Clindamycin plus penicillin | 600–900 mg every 8 h IV<br>2–4 million units every 4–6 h IV (adult) | 10–13 mg/kg/dose every 8 h IV<br>60,000–100,000 units/kg/dose every 6 h IV | N/A |
| *Aeromonas hydrophila* | Doxycycline plus ciprofloxacin or ceftriaxone | 100 mg every 12 h IV<br>500 mg every 12 h IV<br>1–2 g every 24 h IV | Not recommended for children but may need to use in life-threatening situations | N/A |
| *Vibrio vulnificus* | Doxycycline plus ceftriaxone or cefotaxime | 100 mg every 12 h IV<br>1 g qid IV<br>2 g tid IV | Not recommended for children but may need to use in life-threatening situations | N/A |

*Abbreviations:* IV, intravenous; MRSA, methicillin-resistant *Staphylococcus aureus*; N/A, not applicable; qid, four times daily; tid, three times daily.

[a] If *Staphylococcus* present or suspected, add an appropriate agent.

[b] If MRSA is present or suspected; add vancomycin not to exceed the maximum adult daily dose.

## 67.6 Diagnosis: Is Open Fascial Exploration and Biopsy Still the Standard for Diagnosis of NSTI, or Has it Been Supplanted by Radiographic Studies?

The standard of diagnosis in NSTIs is clinical diagnosis, confirmed by open incision, examination of the tissues, and optionally to obtain a biopsy with frozen section [12–14]. In order for imaging modalities to confer a benefit beyond this clinical standard, they would need to provide some additional benefit, either in providing more timely positive support of the diagnosis and thus shorten the time to definitive surgical therapy, or definitively ruling out the diagnosis, obviating the need for diagnostic surgery. This second benefit would be more difficult to provide, as the negative predictive value would need to approach perfection; a missed diagnosis due to an imperfect prediction would delay surgery and increase mortality.

Imaging modalities—CT, MRI, and ultrasound—have all developed increasingly finer resolution, software sophistication, and in the case of ultrasound portability allowing for point of care use. The CT characteristics of NSTIs are well delineated, but are not terribly specific, as exemplified by elements such as fascial thickening and edema without asymmetry. Other more specific findings, such as gas within soft tissues, are not ubiquitous, and therefore, their absence does not rule out the disease [13,14]. If it does not delay definitive surgical therapy, computed tomography may help in planning a thorough surgical intervention by showing the extent of disease, but should not be relied upon to rule in or out the diagnosis of NSTI.

MRI would be thought to be an ideal instrument in the circumstance of NSTIs, as its strength is in delineation of soft tissue pathology, and it has been propounded as such by some authors [22,23]. However, findings have been found to be any more specific than computed tomography; one author found the MRI findings similar between necrotizing fasciitis, dermatomyositis, and posttraumatic muscle injury [15]. While it has been shown that necrotizing infectious fasciitis can at times be differentiated from noninfectious necrotizing fasciitis, there remains some diagnostic uncertainty and interobserver variation—and therefore imperfect negative predictive value. MRI is not as rapidly obtained as CT scan, and does not seem to convey any significant additional diagnostic advantage over CT. Its role in NSTIs is therefore very limited.

Point of care ultrasound is a rapidly expanding field, especially in the field of emergency medicine. There have been recent interesting reports and limited case series utilizing point of care ultrasound to assess soft tissue infections [19–21]. While interesting, these do not as yet provide compelling evidence for their routine use, nor should they be relied upon as a substitute for a surgical consultation. It may be that they could shorten the time to surgical consultation by virtue of being able to be used at point of care, but predictive values have yet to be established.

*Recommendation*: The standard for diagnosis in NSTI is clinical; confirmation by open exploration and inspection of the tissues with biopsy and frozen section if the diagnosis is still uncertain. Recommendation Grade: C.

## 67.7 Mainstay Therapy: Which Is a Better Approach to Initial Resection in NSTI, Staged, or "Complete"?

There has been little in the literature to suggest a standardized approach to NSTI. Certainly, the objective is to remove all necrotic and infected tissue as quickly as possible. Whether or not this may be achieved in one operative intervention, however, depends heavily upon the patient's ability to tolerate extended, aggressive resection. Regardless of whether the first procedure is considered complete, nearly all patients will require at least 1 s look procedure to ensure a lack of disease progression. Recently, Wong et al. have advocated a standardized approach to resection, involving a complete resection in the first procedure, with second look operations to follow [33]. While the approach seems sensible in those who will tolerate their complete approach to the initial procedure, it is not on the basis of prospective randomized data, but the authors considered approach to the problem. It is, as noted above, a logical approach to the disease process, with the caveat that it would seem prudent to halt the procedure once the patient's tolerance for operative intervention is reached and return when they have been further resuscitated and stabilized.

*Recommendation*: As complete an initial resection as the patient will tolerate. Recommendation Grade: C.

## 67.8 Supplemental Therapy: Is There Convincing Evidence for the Use of Hyperbaric Oxygen Therapy in the Treatment of Necrotizing Soft Tissue Infections?

Hyperbaric oxygen (HBO) therapy was originally devised as a way to treat decompression sickness after deep underwater diving ("the bends"). At many atmospheres of depth, more nitrogen is solubilized in the bloodstream, and too-rapid ascent results in nitrogen desolubilizing out of the bloodstream as bubbles, which then cause gas emboli. The use of hyperbaric oxygen is currently unregulated, and usage ranges from legitimate and proven (treating decompression sickness), to therapeutic and experimental use in medicine such as carbon monoxide poisoning and NSTIs, to "oxygen bar" like operations hawking sessions for their purported general health benefits.

Hyperbaric oxygen therapy is a theoretically attractive potential therapy for NSTIs, utilizing oxygen as a direct toxin to combat anaerobic bacterial [29]. What comparative studies exist generally are not randomized, and controls may be historical. One recent comparative but nonrandomized study in a small number of patients showed a shorter length of treatment when utilizing HBO [27]. Most studies of NSTIs are observational in nature [25,26,28,30]; there are synergistic factors that make randomized controlled trials in NSTIs difficult to complete. The first is the rarity of the infections; it can take a single center decades to accrue a few dozen cases, making adequate statistical analysis difficult as well as weakening any conclusions by virtue of the rapid general advances made in medicine over such a long period of time—the longer the study, the less comparable the first patients entered into such a study are to the last. The second factor is the zeal with which proponents of hyperbaric oxygen therapy for NSTIs maintain despite any solid statistical evidence to support its use in these infections. Some have gone so far as to say that randomized controlled trials of its use are "unethical" because they believe it is so clearly beneficial. This attitude may be compounded by the long time between patients, and in fact, there are studies spanning decades that use the "prehyperbaric chamber" era as a historical control for the "posthyperbaric chamber" era. A further potential bias is inherent in the purchase of these expensive chambers; having spent millions of dollars for one such, two questions must be asked: (1) would such an expensive piece of equipment have been purchased if it was not thought to be efficacious *a priori* and (2) having made the investment, how objective can one be regarding its supposed benefits in the absence of the objective evidence of a randomized controlled trial? Two recent studies bear mention. In the first, the authors queried the University Health Consortium database from 2008 to 2010 for NSTIs in centers with hyperbaric oxygen capabilities. They found that the most direly ill patients with necrotizing fasciitis who underwent hyperbaric oxygen therapy had significantly improved mortality (4% vs. 26%, $p < 0.01$) and fewer complications (45% vs. 66%, $p < 0.01$) with NSTIs [32]. However, only 7% of patients actually received HBO, and these 117 patients were stratified into four small groups based on severity of illness, increasing the risk of a type I error. The nature of the database did not allow for a more granular analysis, such as which patients were selected for HBO therapy, a critical element for comparison. While the results are promising, confirmation with other studies would be important in that particular group of patients; to date, the extant literature has not shown a preponderance of evidence for HBO being of benefit for the population of NSTIs as a whole. In another database study, the Nationwide Inpatient Sample was queried for NSTIs from 1998 to 2010 and found that the use of hyperbaric oxygen therapy had decreased from 1.6% to 0.8% over the epoch studied ($p < 0.0001$), while overall survival of patients with NTSIs improved from 9.0% to 4.9% ($p < 0.0001$) [31]. These findings were in the face of worsening patient acuity and increasing complication rates. While no direct correlation between the HBO and mortality trends in this study can be made, it does suggest that the overall gestalt of current treatment has increased patient survival and that survival is not correlated with the use of HBO.

*Recommendation*: No, hyperbolic oxygen should not be part of the standard treatment for NSTIs. More rigorous trials are needed. Recommendation Grade: C.

## 67.9 Supplemental Therapy: Is Immunoglobulin Therapy Part of Standard Care for Necrotizing Soft Tissue Infections?

As streptococcal species have been strongly implicated in NSTIs since their initial description, and immunoglobulin has been utilized in the treatment of *Streptococcus pyogenes* (Group A streptococcus) and streptococcal toxic shock syndrome, it is reasonable to examine whether or not immunoglobulin therapy has any salutary effect on NSTIs [24]. The use of immunoglobulin therapy has been utilized in an attempt to improve survival in cases of streptococcal toxic shock syndrome [25,26]. While case reports and observational studies have been encouraging, the efficacy of gamma globulin in streptococcal toxic shock syndrome has not been confirmed by randomized studies.

*Recommendation*: No, intravenous immunoglobulin treatment has not been convincingly proven to improve outcomes. Recommendation grade: C.

## 67.10 Conclusions

NSTIs are uncommon, highly lethal diseases requiring rapid diagnosis and treatment in order to achieve optimal outcomes. With only a thousand or so cases a year across the United States, however, prospective randomized trials are difficult, and in the case of a single institution near impossible. With agreement on the basics of therapy—aggressive surgical debridement and broad-spectrum antimicrobials—the important questions at present involve secondary therapies that remain unproven at best. In order to obtain quality data for questions such as the use of hyperbaric oxygen and polyclonal immunoglobulin administration, multicenter studies and databases will almost certainly be required to obtain a level of evidence sufficient to recommend their use with confidence. The recent study utilizing a multicenter database to gather data is encouraging and is a novel manner with which to address the

**TABLE 67.2**
Evidence

| Question | Answer | Grade | References |
|---|---|---|---|
| What is the standard for diagnosis in NSTIs? | Clinical; confirmation by open biopsy | C | [5–10] |
| What is the best approach to initial resection? | As complete as the patient will tolerate | C | [21] |
| Should hyperbaric oxygen be part of the standard treatment for NSTIs? | No. More rigorous trials are needed. | C | [14–20] |
| Should intravenous immunoglobulin be part of the standard treatment for NSTIs? | No, it has not been proven to improve outcomes. | C | [11–13] |

difficulties of researching a rare disease. The success in caring for patients with these difficult infections has improved, but secondary therapies for now remain unproven (Table 67.2).

## References

### General


1. Meleny FL. Hemolytic streptococcus gangrene. *Arch Surg.* 1924;9:317–364.
2. Wilson B. Necrotizing fasciitis. *Am Surg.* 1952;18:416.
3. Wong CH, Tan SH. Subacute necrotizing fasciitis. *Lancet.* 2004;364:1376.
4. Wong CH, Wang YS. What is subacute necrotizing fasciitis? A proposed clinical diagnostic criteria. *J Infection.* 2006;52:415–419.
5. Cainzos M, Gonzalez-Rodriguez FJ. Necrotizing soft tissue infections. *Curr Opin Crit Care.* 2007;13:433–439.
6. Sawyer MD, Dunn DL. Deep soft tissue infections. *Curr Opin Infect Dis.* 1991;4:649–654.
7. Dunn DL, Sawyer MD. Deep soft-tissue infections. *Curr Opin Infect Dis.* 1990;3:691–696.
8. Hakkarainen T. Necrotizing soft tissue infections: Review and current concepts in treatment, systems of care, and outcomes. *Curr Prob Surg.* 2014;51:344–362.
9. Stevens D, Bisno A, Chambers H, Dellinger E, Goldstein E, Gorbach S, Hirschmann J, Kaplan S, Montoya J, Wade J. Practice guidelines for the diagnosis and management of skin and soft tissue infections: 2014 update by the infectious diseases Society of America. *CID.* 2014;59: 47–159.
10. Ustin J, Malangoni M. Necrotizing soft-tissue infections. *Crit Care Med.* 2011;39(9):2156–2162.
11. Psoinos C, Flahive J, Shaw J, YouFu L, Sing Chau N, Tseng J, Santry H. Contemporary trends in necrotizing soft tissue infections in the United States. *Surgery.* 2013;153:819–827.


### Diagnosis: Imaging and Open Biopsy


12. Stamenkovic I, Lew PD. Early recognition of potentially fatal necrotizing fasciitis: The use of frozen section biopsy. *N Engl J Med.* 1984;310:1689–1693.
13. Majeski JA, Majeski E. Necrotizing fasciitis: Improved survival with early recognition by tissue biopsy and aggressive surgical treatment. *South Med J.* 1997;90:1065–1068.
14. Wong CH, Wang YS. The diagnosis of necrotizing fasciitis. *Curr Opin Infect Dis.* 2005;18:101–106.
15. Levenson RB, Singh AK, Novelline RA. Fournier gangrene: Role of imaging. *Radiographics.* 2008;28:519–528.
16. Wysoki MG, Santora TA, Sha RM, Friedman AC. Necrotizing fasciitis: CT characteristics. *Radiology.* 1997;203:859–863.
17. Arslan A, Pierre-Jerome C, Borthne A. Necrotizing fasciitis: Unreliable MRI findings in the preoperative diagnosis. *Eur J Radiol.* 2000;36:139–143.
18. Malghem J, Lecouvet FE, Omoumi P et al. Necrotizing fasciitis: Contribution and limitations of diagnostic imaging. *Joint Bone Spine.* March 2013;80(2):146–154.
19. Oelze L, Wu S, Carnell J. Emergency ultrasonography for the early diagnosis of necrotizing fasciitis: A case series from the ED. *Am J Emerg Med.* 2013;31:632, e5–e7.
20. Kehrl T. Point-of-care ultrasound diagnosis of necrotizing fasciitis missed by computed tomography and magnetic resonance imaging. *J Emerg Med.* 2014;47(2):172–175.
21. Castleberg E, Jenson N, Dinh VA. Diagnosis of necrotizing faciitis with bedside ultrasound: The STAFF exam. *Western J Emerg Med.* 2014;15(1):111–113.
22. Rahmouni A, Chosidow O, Mathieu D, Gueroguieva E, Jazaerli N, Radier C, Faivre J, Roujeau J, Vasile N. MR Imaging in acute infectious cellulitis. *Radiology* 1994;192:493–496.
23. Kim K, Yeo J, Lee J, Kim Y, Park S, Lim M, Suh C. Can necrotizing infectious fasciitis be differentiated from nonnecrotizing infectious fasciitis with MR Imaging? *Radiology.* 2011;259(3):816–824.


### Use of Immunoglobulin/Streptococcal Toxic Shock


24. Stevens DL. Streptococcal toxic shock syndrome associated with necrotizing fasciitis. *Annu Rev Med.* 2000;51:271–288.
25. Barry W, Hudgins L, Donta S, Pesanti E. Intravenous immunoglobulin therapy for toxic shock syndrome. *JAMA.* 1992;267:3315–3316.
26. Kaul R, McGeer A, Norrby-Teglund A et al. Intravenous immunoglobulin therapy for streptococcal toxic shock syndrome—A comparative observational study. *Clin Infect Dis.* 1999;28:800–807.

## Hyperbaric Oxygen


27. Jallali N, Withey MS, Butler PE. Hyperbaric oxygen as adjuvant therapy in the management of necrotizing fasciitis. *Am J Surg.* 2005;189:462–466.
28. Sugihara A, Watanabe H, Oohashi M, Kato N, Murakami H, Tsukazaki S, Fujikawa K. The effect of hyperbaric oxygen therapy on the bout of treatment for soft tissue infections. *J Infect.* 2004;48:330–333.
29. Kornonen K. Hyperbaric oxygen therapy in acute necrotizing infections with special reference to the effects on tissue gas tensions. A clinical and experimental study. *Ann Chirurg Gynaecol Suppl.* 2000;214:3–36.
30. Kornonen K, Klossner J, Hirn M, Niinkoski J. Management of Clostridial gas gangrene and the role of hyperbaric oxygen. *Ann Chirurg Gynaec.* 1999;88:139–142.
31. Massey P, Sakran J, Mills A, Sarani B, Aufhauser D, Sims C, Pascual J, Kelz R, Holena D. Hyperbaric oxygen therapy in necrotizing soft tissue infections. *J Surg Res.* 2012;177:146–151.
32. Shaw JJ, Psoinos C, Emhoff TA, Shah SA, Santry HP. Not just full of hot air: Hyperbaric oxygen therapy increases survival in cases of necrotizing soft tissue infections. *Surg Infect (Larchmt).* June 2014;15(3):328–335.


## Operative Approach


33. Wong CH, Yam AKT, Tan ABH, Song C. Approach to debridement in necrotizing fasciitis. *Am J Surg.* September 2008;196(3):e19–e24.

## Commentary on Necrotizing Soft Tissue Infections

*E. Patchen Dellinger*

This chapter nicely summarizes the clinical situation in necrotizing soft tissue infections (NSTIs) and the poor quality of data available to draw conclusions about the management of this uncommon but devastating disease. NSTI occurs uncommonly enough that few physicians or surgeons outside of specialty referral centers ever see enough cases to become comfortable managing the disease and frequently enough that most surgeons will encounter at least one or two cases during a professional career. Dr. Sawyer correctly notes that the grades of evidence for all of his recommendations are due to the absence of any prospective trials in the diagnosis or treatment of this condition. All the information that we have comes from case series.

Early on Dr. Sawyer refers to "the monomicrobial forms of the disease—Group A *Streptococcus*, Clostridial species, and marine gram negatives such as *Vibrio vulnificans*." We should now also include methicillin-resistant *Staphylococcus aureus* (MRSA), especially with the Panton–Valentine leucocidin as an important consideration for monomicrobial NSTI.*

The chapter recommends open incision and examination of affected tissue for diagnosis of the disease and correctly notes that radiological studies (CT and MRI) lack specificity although sensitivity is rather good. Mention is made of frozen section examination of biopsy, and while this is not harmful, in my experience, it is rarely needed. The greatest risk to a patient with NSTI is failure of the medical and surgical team to recognize the necrotizing nature of the condition and then to treat expectantly for cellulitis without necrosis. Some case series demonstrate a significant increase in mortality associated with delay between onset of symptoms and definitive operation and between hospitalization and operation.† What is needed is a high index of suspicion for the diagnosis of NSTI. Once the suspicion is raised, a small incision for biopsy usually reveals to the naked eye the nature of the process and adequate debridement can be undertaken without waiting for a frozen section. Regarding the recommendation that initial debridement be as complete as the patient will tolerate, there are no useful data, but the clinical experience of surgeons who have managed this disease suggests that this is the correct approach.

Dr. Sawyer correctly notes that there is an absence of data supporting the use of hyperbaric oxygen for NSTI. One potential harm that can come from efforts to use hyperbaric oxygen occurs when attempts to get a patient to a hyperbaric chamber delay the mandatory aggressive debridement of the infection, which is the most important initial step along with antibiotic administration and aggressive support of vital signs. The initial debridement should never be postponed in order to get a patient to a chamber. On the other hand, if a chamber is close by or if the opportunity is readily available for transfer after the first operation and prior to the second look procedure that Dr. Sawyer correctly recommends, there is no harm in transfer. Because of the widespread though unproven belief in the possible value of hyperbaric oxygen, the surgeons and physicians in some hyperbaric centers may have a greater experience with the disease than the average practitioner. Thus, any benefit may stem from experience with the disease rather than use of the hyperbaric chamber.

The data on immunoglobulin therapy are correctly noted to be quite weak, but they are probably not harmful except to the medical budget. New, adjunctive therapies would be nice, but I am not aware of any on the horizon. It may be worth mentioning that although there are not good human data, in animal studies, clindamycin appears to reduce the severity of response to NSTI, especially Clostridial, *Streptococcal*, and MRSA infections due to the action of clindamycin in inhibiting protein synthesis, specifically synthesis of bacterial toxins.‡§¶ Table 4 of the chapter recommends using clindamycin with penicillin for *Streptococcal* and Clostridial infections and might consider adding the recommendation for clindamycin to be combined with the first-line antibiotics also in the Staphylococcal section.

* Miller LG, Perdreau-Remington F, Rieg G et al. Necrotizing fasciitis caused by community-associated methicillin-resistant *Staphylococcus aureus* in Los Angeles. *N Engl J Med*. 2005;352:1445–1453.

† Wong CH, Chang HC, Pasupathy S, Khin LW, Tan JL, Low CO. Necrotizing fasciitis: Clinical presentation, microbiology, and determinants of mortality. *J Bone Joint Surg Am*. 2003;85(A):1454–1460.

‡ Stevens DL, Bryant AE, Hackett SP. Antibiotic effects on bacterial viability, toxin production, and host response. *Clin Infect Dis*. 1995;2:S154–S157.

§ Stevens DL, Ma Y, Salmi DB, McIndoo E, Wallace RJ, Bryant AE. Impact of antibiotics on expression of virulence-associated exotoxin genes in methicillin-sensitive and methicillin-resistant *Staphylococcus aureus*. *J Infect Dis*. 2007;195:202–211.

¶ Wong CJ, Stevens DL. Serious group a streptococcal infections. *Med Clin North Am*. 2013;97:721–736, xi–xii.

# 68

# *Incarcerated Hernias*

**Rachel E. Beard and Steven D. Schwaitzberg**

**CONTENTS**



## 68.1 Introduction

Incarcerated hernia is one of the more common emergencies for the general surgeon. There are several important questions to consider when dealing with this entity. Emergent imaging has become ubiquitous and seems to replace physical examination in an increasing number of settings. In addition, hernia repair has evolved over the last decade with several new options and paradigms to consider. Certain dilemmas remain unchanged such as determining the viability of incarcerated intestine. Finally, the age-old dilemma of what to do when the incarcerated hernia turns out to be the strangulated hernia with contamination remains a formidable challenge.

### 68.1.1 What are the Appropriate Physical Examination and Imaging Evaluations Necessary to Diagnose Incarcerated Hernias?

There are no randomized trials in the literature comparing physical examination alone to imaging in securing the diagnosis of incarcerated abdominal wall hernia. However, there are numerous case reports and short retrospective series that offered testimonial benefit to the use of computed tomography (CT) or ultrasound (US) in the diagnosis of abdominal wall incarcerated hernia [1,2] (Level 4 evidence). Imaging appeared to be of the greatest benefit in three categories: obese patients, spigelian hernias, and obturator hernias [3–9] (Level 4 and 5 evidence) (Grade C Recommendation). The literature also describes an unusual case of small bowel obstruction (SBO) following open repair of an incarcerated inguinal hernia caused by intestine trapped in a hernia sac that was protruding into the preperitoneal space and ultimately required laparotomy for repair. The authors pointed out the diagnostic difficulty and the need for CT scan in this case [10] (Level 5 evidence). Aside from these unusual circumstances, the vast majority of inguinal and ventral hernias appear to be diagnosed clinically. In fact, one large nationwide retrospective study from Sweden, which included more than 100,000 patients, demonstrated that patients who lacked a well-documented physical examination of the groin (37%) were more likely to undergo preoperative imaging ($p < 0.001$), resulting in an unnecessary delay in surgery [11] (Level 2B evidence). A thorough physical examination is mandatory, and there is no evidence that a diagnosis made on physical examination requires imaging confirmation (Grade B Recommendation).

*Recommendation*: A thorough physical examination is mandatory and, except in rare cases, is acceptable for the diagnosis of most incarcerated hernias. Adjunctive imaging, usually CT or US, is acceptable in specific clinical scenarios where diagnosis is difficulty, such as spigelian or obturator hernias or if obesity limits physical examination, but routine imaging can lead to delay in surgical management (Grade B Recommendation).

### 68.1.2 What are the Technical Considerations for Treating Incarcerated Hernia that Influence Choice of Repair?

Prior to the mid-1980s, the choices for elective and emergent hernia repairs were simple. Primary tissue repairs were exclusively performed. The introduction of the first polypropylene mesh then expanded polytetrafluoroethylene (PTFE) change the face of elective hernia repairs almost completely by the mid-1990s. The use of mesh for elective hernia repairs is well established now [12–15] (Level 4 evidence). Laparoscopic repairs were added to the elective hernia repair options in the early 1990s, and all utilize some form of prosthesis. It was inevitable that these options would be considered for urgent/emergent repairs as well.

There are a few small prospective trials performed in order to determine optimal repair of incarcerated hernias with cohort sizes ranging from 40 to 54 patients [16,17,20] (Level 2B evidence), as well as a few retrospective studies [18,19] (Level 4 evidence). Karatepe concludes that preperitoneal repair with mesh for strangulated hernias is superior to Lichtenstein mesh-only repair because it allows for bowel resection if needed and avoids the need for an additional incision, which was significantly associated with increased morbidity ($p = 0.003$) in their patient population [16]. Elsebae concluded that Lichtenstein mesh repair also decreased recurrence when compared to repair with Bassini technique, without increasing complication rates. This study, however, excluded patients with peritonitis and who underwent bowel resection from mesh repair [17]. Derici's retrospective study included 113 patients and suggests that Lichtenstein repair with mesh is preferred in incarcerated inguinal hernias because it significantly lowers recurrence rates when compared to primary repair ($p = 0.036$) without increasing complications [18]. Papziogas included 75 patients in his comparative study and concluded that a tension-free mesh repair did not increase complication rates or lead to mesh removal when compared to a modified Bassini repair, even in the setting of bowel resection [19]. Lastly, Abdel-Baki randomized patients with incarcerated paraumbilical hernias to either prosthetic repair with a polypropylene mesh-only or tissue repair and concluded that prosthetic repair significantly reduced recurrence rates ($p < 0.05$) without increasing complications [20]. The studies indicate that mesh repair is not contraindicated for strangulated hernias even if bowel resection is needed. For inguinal hernias, Lichtenstein repair reduces recurrence rates as compared to tissue repairs, though there is some suggestion that a preperitoneal approach may better allow for bowel resection if needed.

Laparoscopic repair as an option for the repair of incarcerated hernia continues to be studied. It is well established that operator experience will influence outcome in laparoscopic repairs, though the breadth of laparoscopic experience among surgeons is likely narrowing, as it is increasingly an integral part of surgical training [21] (Level 2B evidence). There are a number of retrospective series and case reports indicating success repairing inguinal, femoral, and ventral hernias with Lichtenstein repairs, transabdominal laparoscopic repairs (TAP), and totally extraperitoneal laparoscopic repairs (TEP) [22–26] (Level 4 evidence). As with the aforementioned studies that examined open mesh repairs, these studies conclude that laparoscopic repair with mesh is not contraindicated for incarcerated and strangulated hernias and also suggest that the TAP approach is preferable for strangulated inguinal hernias as it allows for good visualization of abdominal contents and bowel resection if needed.

*Recommendation*: Repair with mesh is not contraindicated for strangulated hernias (Grade B Recommendation). For inguinal hernias, Lichtenstein repair reduces recurrence rates as compared to tissue repairs, though there is some suggestion that a preperitoneal approach may better allow for bowel resection if needed (Grade B Recommendation). Laparoscopic repair with mesh is not contraindicated for incarcerated and strangulated hernias and also suggest that the TAP approach is preferable for strangulated inguinal hernias as it allows for good visualization of abdominal contents and bowel resection if needed (Grade C Recommendation).

### 68.1.3 What are the Repair Options in the Face of GI Contamination or Infection?

The challenge of repairing and abdominal wall defects in the face of significant gastrointestinal (GI) contamination or infection is formidable. Primary tissue repair avoids foreign body-based infections; however, subsequent recurrences are common [17,18,20] (Level 2B and 4 evidence). Retrospective studies support the use of polypropylene mesh in selected settings, including patients who are immunosuppressed following solid organ transplantation, cases categorized as clean-contaminated or even contaminated, and in the setting of bowel resection without frank peritonitis [19,29–33] (Level 3B and 4 evidence). These studies do not demonstrate any increased morbidity, morality, or need for mesh removal in such cases. The use of biologic prosthesis has become popular despite the fact that there are no long-term or randomized outcome studies concerning the use of biologic prosthesis such as acellular dermis or reconstituted collagen in the contaminated or infected setting. Retrospective reviews suggest clearly imperfect but acceptable results in grossly contaminated fields with modest complication rates (infection, hernia, and reoperation) considering the magnitude of the clinical problem [34–40] (Level 3B and 4 evidence).

*Recommendation*: Primary repair is discouraged, as subsequent recurrence rates are clearly higher. The use of synthetic prostheses for use in contaminated cases has been shown to be safe and superior for reducing long-term recurrence (Grade B Recommendation). The use of biologic prostheses is well described and is acceptable for use in high-risk and contaminated repairs (Grade B Recommendation).

### 68.1.4 What are the Characteristics of Incarceration/Strangulation that Impact Mortality/Morbidity?

General features of risk stratification have been well worked out for emergency surgery. Apache classification assigns increasing risk for derangements of physiology, laboratory parameters, age greater than 55, and emergent surgery [41] (Level 2B evidence). The increased mortality noted in the large Swedish prospectively recorded database of nearly 108,000 hernia repairs clearly highlight the increased risk of emergent surgery [42] (Level 2B evidence). A more recent large retrospective study by the same group, analyzing over 107,000 patients, confirms that emergency surgery increases mortality and additionally suggest that femoral hernias increase morality by 7-fold when compared to inguinal hernias and that mortality is increased 20-fold if bowel resection is undertaken. They also found that women overall had a higher mortality risk than men even when accounting for the higher proportion of femoral hernias and emergency surgery among women [43] (Level 2B evidence). Other retrospective series also generally suggest that increased mortality is most significantly influenced by the need for bowel resection, long duration of symptoms, delay to hospitalization, concomitant illness, and high American Society of Anesthesiologists (ASA) scores [44–48] (Level 4 evidence). Retrospective studies by other groups also confirm the suggestion of worsened outcomes associated with femoral hernias, which are more common in women and are attributable to a higher risk of bowel resection in these patients [49,50] (Level 2B and 3B evidence).

*Recommendation*: Emergent surgery for incarcerated hernias is clearly associated with increased complications as compared to elective hernia repairs (Grade B Recommendation). Specific risk factors associated with increased morbidity and mortality include long duration of symptoms, bowel resection, concomitant illness, high ASA scores, femoral hernia, and female gender (Grade B Recommendation).

### 68.1.5 What are the Most Effective Intra-Op Evaluation Tools to Assess Bowel Viability?

Every abdominal surgeon has been faced with the need to evaluate abnormally appearing bowel in order to determine its viability. In addition, there are circumstances where the reduction of an incarcerated hernia leaves a question of bowel viability unanswered. The surgical myth that "strangulated bowel will not reduce" has been disproven on many occasions. A number of techniques have been offered to assess intestinal viability in trial currently. Most comparative studies were performed in preclinical settings. The most commonly evaluated modalities were clinical assessment, Doppler ultrasound, fluorescein dye administration, myoelectric activity, surface pulse oximetry, and non-contact laser Doppler blood flow assessment [51–61] (Level 2B and 3B evidence). Preclinical comparative assessments show mixed results when comparing pulse oximetry, Doppler ultrasound, and fluorescein that are superior to clinical judgment alone. Laser Doppler may be superior when compared to fluorescein, and pulse oximetry, and nonrandomized prospective evaluation demonstrated excellent predictive assessment when compared to clinical assessment [53,62,63] (Level 3B evidence). Multiple accounts of the utility of laparoscopy or hernioscopy report clinical utility when assessing bowel liability in those cases where intestinal reduction occurs prior to clinical evaluation of intestinal viability [64–68] (Level 4 evidence).

*Recommendation*: Objective techniques are superior to clinical evaluation alone when assessing intestinal ischemia. Laser Doppler flowmetry may be the most sensitive technique; however, Doppler ultrasound and/or fluorescein dye are likely to be more readily available (Grade B Recommendation). Laparoscopy transabdominally or through the hernia sac is a useful technique for assessing intestinal viability in selected cases (Grade C Recommendation).

### 68.1.6 Should Hernias be Repaired in Order to Prevent Incarceration and Strangulation?

Many authors recommend elective repair of inguinal hernia as a strategy to prevent complications and poorer outcomes associated with emergent repairs for incarcerated or strangulated hernias particularly in elderly patients [11,50,69,70] (Level 2B, 3B, and 44 evidence). These studies show that approximately 5% of the hernia repairs reviewed were performed emergently. These cases were the source of most of the significant morbidity and mortality in the population studied. Comorbidities contributed significantly to poor outcome in the emergent setting [11,71]. Elective hernia repairs even in the very elderly population are safe, particularly when performed under local anesthesia [70,72] (Level 3B evidence).

Previously, the recommendation was to repair inguinal hernias as they were discovered in order to prevent complications; however, this practice has been challenged. The prospective Veterans Administration

**TABLE 68.1**

Evidence-Based Issues Concerning Incarcerated Hernia

| Question | Answer | Grade of Recommendation | Level of Evidence | References |
|---|---|---|---|---|
| What are the appropriate physical examination and imaging evaluations necessary to diagnose and incarcerated hernia? | A thorough physical examination is mandatory and, except in rare cases, is acceptable for diagnosis of most incarcerated hernias. Adjunctive imaging, usually CT or US, is acceptable in specific clinical scenarios where diagnosis is difficulty, such as spigelian or obturator hernias or if obesity limits physical examination, but routine imaging can lead to delay in surgical management. | B | 2B, 4, 5 | [3–11] |
| What are the technical considerations for treating incarcerated hernia that influence choice of repair? | Repair with mesh is not contraindicated for strangulated hernias. | B | 2B | [17–20] |
| | For inguinal hernias, Lichtenstein repair reduces recurrence rates as compared to tissue repairs, though there is some suggestion that a preperitoneal approach may better allow for bowel resection if needed. | B | 2B | [16–19] |
| | Laparoscopic repair with mesh is not contraindicated for incarcerated and strangulated hernias, and also suggest that the TAP approach is preferable for strangulated inguinal hernias as it allows for good visualization of abdominal contents and bowel resection if needed. | C | 4 | [22–26] |
| What are the repair options in the face of GI contamination or infection? | Primary repair is discouraged, as subsequent recurrence rates are clearly higher. The use of synthetic prostheses in contaminated cases has been shown to be safe and superior for reducing long-term recurrence | B | 2B, 3B, 4 | [17–20,29–33] |
| | The use of biologic prostheses is well described and is acceptable for use in high-risk and contaminated repairs. | B | 3B, 4 | [34–40] |
| What are the characteristics of incarceration/strangulation that impact mortality/morbidity? | Emergent surgery for incarcerated hernias clearly is clearly associated with increased complications as compared to elective hernia repairs. | B | 2B | [41,42] |
| | Specific risk factors associated with increased morbidity and mortality include long duration of symptoms, bowel resection, concomitant illness, high ASA scores, femoral hernia, and female gender. | B | 2B, 3B, 4 | [43–50] |
| What are the most effective intraoperative evaluation tools to assess bowel viability? | Objective techniques are superior to clinical evaluation alone when assessing intestinal ischemia. Laser Doppler flowmetry may be the most sensitive technique; however, Doppler ultrasound and/or fluorescein dye are more likely to be readily available. | B | 2B, 3B | [51–63] |
| | Laparoscopy transabdominally or through the hernia sac is a useful technique for assessing intestinal viability in selected cases. | C | 4 | [27,28,64–68] |
| Should hernias be repaired in order to prevent incarceration and strangulation? | Authors continue to cite the need for elective hernia repair to avoid morbidity and mortality; however, watchful waiting appears safe for healthy patients with minimally symptomatic hernias, though patients should be counseled that symptoms will likely progress and require eventual repair. | B | 1B, 2B, 3B, 4 | [11,50,69,70,73,74] |

multicenter trial of immediate tension-free repair versus "watchful waiting" demonstrated a less than 1% risk of catastrophic event related to observation and study population [73] (Level 1B evidence). The limitations of this initial study include a 30% rate of nonparticipation of the patients screened, a follow-up time of only 2 years, the exclusion of sicker patients, and that about only half the patients' hernias were detectable on cough impulse examination. This latter finding indicates a large proportion of very small, if actually real, hernias were included in the study. Nonetheless, this remains one of the best attempts to understand the natural history of modern hernias within the context of the severe limitations. A long-term follow-up to this study was published in 2013 which published findings after Fitzgibbons and colleagues continued to follow the men in the "watchful waiting" group for an additional 7 years [74] (Level 2B evidence). At the end of the initial study period, 32% of patients had crossed over and had their hernias repaired, and at the end of the additional follow-up period, this number had risen to 68%. The most common reason for repair was pain (54%) and men over 65 crossed over at a higher rate than those who were younger (79% vs. 62%). Only three patients required an emergency operation, and there were no mortalities. Thus, watchful waiting appears safe for healthy patients with minimally symptomatic hernias; however, patients should be counseled that symptoms will likely progress and require eventual repair (Grade B Recommendation).

*Recommendation*: Authors continue to cite the need for elective hernia repair to avoid morbidity and mortality; however, watchful waiting appears safe for healthy patients with minimally symptomatic hernias, though patients should be counseled that symptoms will likely progress and require eventual repair (Grade B Recommendation) (Table 68.1).

## References


1. Chen SC, Lee CC, Liu YP et al. Ultrasound may decrease the emergency surgery rate of incarcerated inguinal hernia. *Scand J Gastroenterol.* 2005;40:721–724.
2. Ramseyer L, Abernethy EA, 3rd, McCune EA, Steffen HL. The role of CT in the diagnosis of small bowel obstruction: A case and literature review. *J Okla State Med Assoc.* 1998;91:103–106.
3. Buljevac M, Grgurevic I, Lackovic Z, Kujundzic M, Banic M. Duplex ultrasonography in diagnosis of spigelian hernia with incarcerated jejunal loop. *Acta Med Croat.* 2001;55:225–227.
4. van der Linden FM, Puylaert JB, De Vries BC. Ultrasound diagnosis of incarcerated obturator hernia. *Eur J Surg.* 1995;161:531–532.
5. Losanoff JE, Kjossev KT. Incarcerated Spigelian hernia in morbidly obese patients: The role of intraoperative ultrasonography for hernia localization. *Obes Surg.* 1997;7:211–214.
6. Avaro JP, Biance N, Savoie PH et al. Incarcerated obturator hernia: Early diagnostic using helical computed tomography. *Hernia.* 2008;12:199–200.
7. Rodriguez-Hermosa JI, Codina-Cazador A, Maroto-Genover A et al. Obturator hernia: Clinical analysis of 16 cases and algorithm for its diagnosis and treatment. *Hernia.* 2008;12:289–297.
8. Engin O, Cicek E, Oner SR, Yidirim M. Incarcerated femoral hernia containing the right uterine tube. A preoperative diagnosis is possible. *Ann Ital Chir.* 2011; 82(5):409–412.
9. Larson DW, Farley DR. Spigelian hernias: Repair and outcome for 81 patients. *World J Surg.* 2002;26:1277–1281.
10. Berney CR. Beware of spontaneous reduction "en masse" of inguinal hernia. *Hernia.* 2014.
11. Nilsson H, Nilsson E, Angeras U, Nordin P. Mortality after groin hernia surgery: Delay of treatment and cause of death. *Hernia.* 2011;15:301–307.
12. Mathes SJ, Steinwald PM, Foster RD, Hoffman WY, Anthony JP. Complex abdominal wall reconstruction: A comparison of flap and mesh closure. *Ann Surg.* 2000;232:586–596.
13. Luijendijk RW, Hop WC, van den Tol MP et al. A comparison of suture repair with mesh repair for incisional hernia. *N Engl J Med.* 2000;343:392–398.
14. Amid PK, Shulman AG, Lichtenstein IL. An analytic comparison of laparoscopic hernia repair with open "tension-free" hernioplasty. *Int Surg.* 1995;80:9–17.
15. Klaristenfeld DD, Mahoney E, Iannitti DA. Minimally invasive tension-free inguinal hernia repair. *Surg Technol Int.* 2005;14:157–163.
16. Karatepe O, Adas G, Battal M et al. The comparison of preperitoneal and Lichtenstein repair for incarcerated groin hernias: A prospective randomized study. *Int J Surg.* 2008;6:189–192.
17. Elsebae MM, Nasr M, Said M. Tension-free repair versus Bassini technique for strangulated inguinal hernia: A controlled randomized study. *Int J Surg.* 2008;6:302–305.
18. Derici H, Unalp HR, Nazli O et al. Prosthetic repair of incarcerated inguinal hernias: Is it a reliable method? *Langenbecks Arch Surg.* 2008;395:575–579.
19. Papaziogas B, Lazaridis Ch, Makris J, Koutelidakis J, Patsas A, Grigoriou M, Chatzimavroudis G, Psaralexis K, Atmatzidis K. Tenstion-free repair versus modified Bassini technique (Andrews technique for strangulated inguinal hernia: A comparative study. *Hernia.* 2005;9:156–159.
20. Abdel-Baki NA, Bessa SS, Abdel-Razek AH. Comparison of prosthetic mesh repair and tissue repair in the emergency management of incarcerated para-umbilical hernia: A prospective randomized study. *Hernia.* 2007;11:163–167.
21. Neumayer L, Giobbie-Hurder A, Jonasson O et al. Open mesh versus laparoscopic mesh repair of inguinal hernia. *N Engl J Med.* 2004;350:1819–1827.

22. Landau O, Kyzer S. Emergent laparoscopic repair of incarcerated incisional and ventral hernia. *Surg Endosc.* 2004;18:1374–1376.
23. Shah RH, Sharma A, Khullar R, Soni V, Baijai M, Chowbey PK. Laparoscopic repair of incarcerated ventral abdominal wall hernias. *Hernia.* 2008;12:457–463.
24. Ferzli G, Shapiro K, Chaudry G, Patel S. Laparoscopic extraperitoneal approach to acutely incarcerated inguinal hernia. *Surg Endosc.* 2004;18:228–231.
25. Wysocki A, Pozniczek M, Krzywon J, Strzalka M. Lichtenstein repair for incarcerated groin hernias. *Eur J Surg.* 2002;168:452–454.
26. Yau KK, Siu WT, Cheung YS, Wong CH, Chung CC, Li KW. Laparoscopic management of acutely incarcerated femoral hernia. *J Laparoendosc Adv Surg Tech A.* 2007;17:759–762.
27. Legnani GL, Rasini M, Pastori S, Sarli D. Laparoscopic trans-peritoneal hernioplasty (TAPP) for the acute management of strangulated inguino-crural hernias: A report of nine cases. *Hernia.* 2008;12:185–188.
28. Rebuffat C, Galli A, Scalambra MS, Balsamo F. Laparoscopic repair of strangulated hernias. *Surg Endosc.* 2006;20:131–134.
29. Antonopoulos IM, Nahas WC, Mazzucchi E, Piovesan AC, Birolini C, Lucon AM. Is polypropylene mesh safe and effective for repairing infected incisional hernia in renal transplant recipients? *Urology.* 2005;66:874–877.
30. Muller V, Lehner M, Klein P, Hohenberger W, Ott A. Incisional hernia repair after orthotopic liver transplantation: A technique employing an inlay/onlay polypropylene mesh. *Langenbecks Arch Surg.* 2003;388:167–173.
31. Kelly ME, Behrman SW. The safety and efficacy of prosthetic hernia repair in clean-contaminated and contaminated wounds. *Am Surg.* 2002;68:524–528; discussion 8–9.
32. Catena F, La Donna M, Gagliardi S et al. Use of prosthetic mesh in complicated incisional hernias. *Minerva Chir.* 2002;57:363–369.
33. Geisler DJ, Reilly JC, Vaughan SG, Glennon EJ, Kondylis PD. Safety and outcome of use of nonabsorbable mesh for repair of fascial defects in the presence of open bowel. *Dis Colon Rectum.* 2003;46:1118–1123.
34. Bellows CF, Albo D, Berger DH, Awad SS. Abdominal wall repair using human acellular dermis. *Am J Surg.* 2007;194:192–198.
35. Bachman S, Ramshaw B. Prosthetic material in ventral hernia repair: How do I choose? *Surg Clin North Am.* 2008;88:101–112, ix.
36. Franklin ME, Jr., Trevino JM, Portillo G, Vela I, Glass JL, Gonzalez JJ. The use of porcine small intestinal submucosa as a prosthetic material for laparoscopic hernia repair in infected and potentially contaminated fields: Long-term follow-up. *Surg Endosc.* 2008;22:1941–1946.
37. Diaz JJ, Jr., Guy J, Berkes MB, Guillamondegui O, Miller RS. Acellular dermal allograft for ventral hernia repair in the compromised surgical field. *Am Surg.* 2006;72:1181–1187; discussion 7–8.
38. Gupta A, Zahriya K, Mullens PL, Salmassi S, Keshishian A. Ventral herniorrhaphy: Experience with two different biosynthetic mesh materials, Surgisis and Alloderm. *Hernia.* 2006;10:419–425.
39. Kim H, Bruen K, Vargo D. Acellular dermal matrix in the management of high-risk abdominal wall defects. *Am J Surg.* 2006;192:705–709.
40. Patton JH, Jr., Berry S, Kralovich KA. Use of human acellular dermal matrix in complex and contaminated abdominal wall reconstructions. *Am J Surg.* 2007;193:360–363; discussion 3.
41. Knaus WA, Wagner DP, Draper EA et al. The APACHE III prognostic system. Risk prediction of hospital mortality for critically ill hospitalized adults. *Chest.* 1991;100:1619–1636.
42. Nilsson E, Haapaniemi S, Gruber G, Sandblom G. Methods of repair and risk for reoperation in Swedish hernia surgery from 1992 to 1996. *Br J Surg.* 1998;85:1686–1691.
43. Nilsson H, Stylianidis G, Haapamaki M, Milsson E, Nordin P. Mortality after groin hernia surgery. *Ann Surg.* 2007;245:656–660.
44. Kulah B, Kulacoglu IH, Oruc MT et al. Presentation and outcome of incarcerated external hernias in adults. *Am J Surg.* 2001;181:101–104.
45. Alvarez JA, Baldonedo RF, Bear IG, Solis JA, Alvarez P, Jorge JI. Incarcerated groin hernias in adults: Presentation and outcome. *Hernia.* 2004;8:121–126.
46. Kurt N, Oncel M, Ozkan Z, Bingul S. Risk and outcome of bowel resection in patients with incarcerated groin hernias: Retrospective study. *World J Surg.* 2003;27:741–743.
47. Alvarez-Perez JA, Baldonedo-Cernuda RF, Garcia-Bear I, Suarez-Solis JA, Alvarez-Martinez P, Jorge-Barreiro JI. [Presentation and outcome of incarcerated external hernias in adults]. *Cir Esp.* 2005;77:40–45.
48. Heydorn WH, Velanovich V. A five-year U.S. Army experience with 36,250 abdominal hernia repairs. *Am Surg.* 1990;56:596–600.
49. Corder AP. The diagnosis of femoral hernia. *Postgrad Med J.* 1992;68:26–28.
50. Koch A, Edwards A, Haapaniemi S, Nordin P, Kald A. Prospective evaluation of 6895 groin hernia repairs in women. *Br J Surg.* 2005;92:1553–1558.
51. Johansson K, Ahn H, Kjellstrom C, Lindhagen J. Laser Doppler flowmetry in experimental mesenteric vascular occlusion. *Int J Microcirc Clin Exp.* 1989;8:183–190.
52. Orland PJ, Cazi GA, Semmlow JL, Reddell MT, Brolin RE. Determination of small bowel viability using quantitative myoelectric and color analysis. *J Surg Res.* 1993;55:581–587.
53. Ando M, Ito M, Nihei Z, Sugihara K. Assessment of intestinal viability using a non-contact laser tissue blood flowmeter. *Am J Surg.* 2000;180:176–180.
54. Holmes NJ, Cazi G, Reddell MT et al. Intraoperative assessment of bowel viability. *J Invest Surg.* 1993;6:211–221.
55. Horgan PG, Gorey TF. Operative assessment of intestinal viability. *Surg Clin North Am.* 1992;72:143–155.
56. Shah SD, Andersen CA. Prediction of small bowel viability using Doppler ultrasound. Clinical and experimental evaluation. *Ann Surg.* 1981;194:97–99.
57. Bergman RT, Gloviczki P, Welch TJ et al. The role of intravenous fluorescein in the detection of colon ischemia during aortic reconstruction. *Ann Vasc Surg.* 1992;6:74–79.

58. Erikoglu M, Kaynak A, Beyatli EA, Toy H. Intraoperative determination of intestinal viability: A comparison with transserosal pulse oximetry and histopathological examination. *J Surg Res.* 2005;128:66–69.
59. Freeman DE, Gentile DG, Richardson DW et al. Comparison of clinical judgment, Doppler ultrasound, and fluorescein fluorescence as methods for predicting intestinal viability in the pony. *Am J Vet Res.* 1988;49:895–900.
60. Tollefson DF, Wright DJ, Reddy DJ, Kintanar EB. Intraoperative determination of intestinal viability by pulse oximetry. *Ann Vasc Surg.* 1995;9:357–360.
61. Wright CB, Hobson RW, 2nd. Prediction of intestinal viability using Doppler ultrasound techniques. *Am J Surg.* 1975;129:642–645.
62. Redaelli CA, Schilling MK, Carrel TP. Intraoperative assessment of intestinal viability by laser Doppler flowmetry for surgery of ruptured abdominal aortic aneurysms. *World J Surg.* 1998;22:283–289.
63. Redaelli CA, Schilling MK, Buchler MW. Intraoperative laser Doppler flowmetry: A predictor of ischemic injury in acute mesenteric infarction. *Dig Surg.* 1998;15:55–59.
64. Lavonius MI, Ovaska J. Laparoscopy in the evaluation of the incarcerated mass in groin hernia. *Surg Endosc.* 2000;14:488–489.
65. Al-Naami MY, Al-Shawi JS. The use of laparoscopy to assess viability of slipped content in incarcerated inguinal hernia: A case report. *Surg Laparosc Endosc Percutan Tech.* 2003;13:292–294.
66. Guvenc BH, Tugay M. Laparoscopic evaluation in incarcerated groin hernia following spontaneous reduction. *Ulus Travma Acil Cerrahi Derg.* 2003;9:143–144.
67. Lin E, Wear K, Tiszenkel HI. Planned reduction of incarcerated groin hernias with hernia sac laparoscopy. *Surg Endosc.* 2002;16:936–938.
68. Morris-Stiff G, Hassn A. Hernioscopy: A useful technique for the evaluation of incarcerated hernias that retract under anaesthesia. *Hernia.* 2008;12:133–135.
69. Nehme AE. Groin hernias in elderly patients. Management and prognosis. *Am J Surg.* 1983;146:257–260.
70. Alvarez Perez JA, Baldonedo RF, Bear IG, Solis JA, Alvarez P, Jorge JI. Emergency hernia repairs in elderly patients. *Int Surg.* 2003;88:231–237.
71. Kulah B, Duzgun AP, Moran M, Kulacoglu IH, Ozmen MM, Coskun F. Emergency hernia repairs in elderly patients. *Am J Surg.* 2001;182:455–459.
72. Rigberg D, Cole M, Hiyama D, McFadden D. Surgery in the nineties. *Am Surg.* 2000;66:813–816.
73. Fitzgibbons RJ, Jr., Giobbie-Hurder A, Gibbs JO et al. Watchful waiting vs repair of inguinal hernia in minimally symptomatic men: A randomized clinical trial. *JAMA.* 2006;295:285–292.
74. Fizgibbons RJ, Jr., Ramanan B, Arya S et al. Long-term results of a randomized controlled trial of a nonoperative strategy (watchful waiting) for men with minimally symptomatic inguinal hernias. *Ann Surg.* 2013;258:508–515.

## Commentary on Incarcerated Hernias

*Michael E. Lekawa*

The authors have presented an excellent data supported synopsis on the optimal management of an incarcerated hernia, an issue that continues to be both a controversial and entertaining component of M & M conference. This is partly because, as the authors point out, there is a paucity of Level I or II evidence to support one management strategy over another. It has been my experience that older surgeons tend to be more dogmatic in their management, i.e., "all hernias should be repaired" or "mesh should never be placed in a potentially compromised wound." If a complication occurs when these dogmas are compromised, the junior surgeon is exposed to various levels of... let us say constructive criticism. Many older surgeons would never implant mesh into a contaminated field. This may be the case regardless of data that support that mesh appears safe and lowers recurrence. On the other hand, younger surgeons were trained after laparoscopic hernia repair was commonplace and the use of mesh became universal. I queried a few of my chief residents who noted they had never done an inguinal hernia repair without mesh. Thus, their own experience and comfort level would have them push the envelope toward using mesh in a contaminated field.

To better analyze the broad range of questions, I would like to comment on each of the questions addressed by the authors.

### What Are the Appropriate Physical Examination and Imaging Evaluations Necessary to Diagnose Incarcerated Hernia?

I completely agree with the authors' conclusions as they relate to groin hernias. I think it is important to differentiate between inguinal and ventral/obturator hernias. I cannot think of an indication to routinely obtain a CT or ultrasound on a groin hernia. The study noted by the author related an inadequate groin exam to an increased use of confirmatory studies perfectly illustrates the negative unintended consequences of our newer technology. Incarcerated hernias should be repaired. Surgeons must push their emergency medicine associates to not order CT scans for suspected groin hernias. Incarcerated groin hernia is a clinical diagnosis based on history and exam and should be managed in the OR with expedience. It is a perfect procedure for an acute care service, where the presence of an in-house surgeon and a prompt surgical evaluation would decrease unnecessary radiologic studies, decrease dwell time in the emergency department, and improving patient outcomes by intervening earlier. Radiographic work-up for groin hernias does not maintain any tangible benefit over surgical clinical evaluation. Whether it is used as a delay tactic, fodder for ultrasound trained EM physicians, or as a habit by well-meaning clinicians, it should be discarded. For ventral hernias, the higher risk of wound complications in very obese patients does, however, make it a reasonable option if the initial surgical evaluation is not reasonably certain of the diagnosis. The difficulty in making certain clinical diagnosis for suspected obturator or spigelian hernia makes CT not only an option, but likely the standard of care. The unusual case the author noted illustrates a "reduction en mass or en bloc." Patients with signs or symptoms of an small bowel obstruction (SBO) after hernia reduction should undergo prompt CT scanning.

### What Are the Technical Considerations for Treating Incarcerated Hernia That Influence Choice of Repair?

The authors present an excellent review of what is possible for repair of incarcerated and even strangulated hernia. The lack of high-quality evidence, however, continues to leave many options and the choice of repair will likely be determined by the surgeons experience with routine hernia repair. Again, it is critical to differentiate between groin and ventral hernias. For groin hernia repair, most surgeons have narrowed their elective repair to one approach, usually some variation of a Lichtenstein repair. Regardless, the approach used for elective repair will likely be used for an incarcerated repair. The authors note the evidence that mesh is safe to use, an important point, as many young surgeons have no experience with tissue repair of groin hernias. While there is evidence that an incarcerated groin hernia can be repaired laparoscopically, most elective hernia repairs are still done open. This experience will make it even more unlikely that an incarcerated groin hernia would be approached laparoscopically. This is in contradistinction to ventral hernias, where most elective repairs are performed laparoscopically. As such, the evidence that it is safe to repair an incarcerated ventral hernia laparoscopically is much more useful. My own experience is to consider if the abdomen will be too hostile for a laparoscopic approach and proceed accordingly. Most important in this chapter is the data supporting the use of mesh for incarcerated and even strangulated hernias.

### What Are the Repair Options in the Face of GI Contamination or Infection?

Hernia repair in the face of gross contamination will likely integrate surgical judgment more than any other circumstance. It is encouraging to see the evidence presented by the authors indicated the safety of mesh. As I stated earlier, the lack of experience with tissue repair for groin hernias makes the safety of mesh I contaminated wounds quite appealing. For ventral hernias though, smaller defects are still likely to be repaired without mesh. With larger ventral defects, many surgeons would still avoid the use of mesh. This would be the most common situation where biological mesh will be considered. The initial enthusiasm for biological mesh has been mitigated by high costs and questionable long-term efficacy. The potential safety of mesh onlays described by the author will likely evolve as a treatment paradigm. Our service has managed several mesh infections recently. These are difficult, painful, and morbid procedures and should give thoughtful pause to the casual use of permanent mesh in contaminated or infected hernias. More complex abdominal reconstructions such as component separation are highly effective but should generally be deployed in an elective setting without existing infection.

### What Are the Characteristics of Incarceration/Strangulation That Impact Mortality/Morbidity?

The authors illustrate the evidence that supports the common sense answer to this question; Emergent operations have higher risks for death or complications. Again, this is a where we could find an opportunity to produce better outcomes with an acute care service. Careful preoperative optimization, collaboration with out anesthesia colleagues, timely repair, and comprehensive detail-oriented postoperative management are all part and parcel to a quality acute care surgery team. The increased operative risks described for femoral hernia repair and for women are noteworthy though difficult to understand.

### What Are the Most Effective Intra-Op Evaluation Tools to Assess Bowel Viability?

While the author concludes that objective techniques are superior to clinical evaluation alone to assess bowel viability, I feel this is not always practical. Much of the literature presented was dated and not necessarily directed at incarcerated hernias. It is our group's practice to use clinical assessment alone as an initial tool for assessment of bowel viability. If the bowel is pink and healthy with palpable pulses, no other assessment is done. If the clinical evaluation is unclear, then objective methods may be appropriate. Once the bowel is freed up and warmed with wet laparotomy pads, Doppler pulses are evaluated. Laser flow angiography has replaced standard fluorescein in our practice. All said, if the bowel does not appear viable on subjective evaluation, no objective finding would prevent me from performing a bowel resection.

### Should Hernias Be Repaired in Order to Prevent Incarceration and Strangulation?

The authors nicely summarize the current data and thoughts on elective groin hernia repair in elderly patients. We offer repair to elderly patients with symptomatic hernia or with clinically present hernia and patient request for repair. We do not normally offer repair for groin hernias that are not clinically apparent.

# 69

# *Surgical Endocrine Emergencies*

**Sara B. Edwards, Steven Brower, and Jennifer L. Marti**

**CONTENTS**

## 69.1 Endocrine Surgical Emergencies

Although endocrine surgical emergencies are uncommon, a surgeon should have a basic knowledge of the pathophysiology of these crises in order to properly diagnose, evaluate, and treat affected patients. Such disorders include central diabetes insipidus, carcinoid crisis, thyroid storm, hypercalcemic crisis, adrenal crisis, and hypertensive crisis secondary to pheochromocytoma.

## 69.2 Central Diabetes Insipidus

### 69.2.1 Introduction

Central diabetes insipidus (CDI) results from inadequate secretion of the hypothalamic polypeptide antidiuretic hormone (ADH). ADH originates in the supraoptic and paraventricular nuclei of the hypothalamus and is excreted by the posterior pituitary gland [1]. Hypovolemia or increased serum osmolality stimulates ADH secretion, which increases renal water reabsorption. Insufficient ADH secretion results in polyuria that can lead to severe hypovolemia, hypotension, and hypernatremia if unrecognized.

With CDI, urine output exceeds 30 mL/kg in 24 h, despite fluid restriction [2]. The urine is dilute, with specific gravity below 1.005, and urine osmolality below 200 mOsm/kg. Plasma osmolality and serum sodium are increased as a result. Other causes of polyuria in the differential diagnosis include osmotic diuresis of diabetes mellitus (DM), psychogenic polydipsia, primary polydipsia from excessive water intake, and diuretic use. The osmotic diuresis of DM may be distinguished from CDI by the presence of glucosuria. With polydipsia, specific gravity and osmolality will increase with fluid restriction, and plasma vasopressin levels will increase with decreased water intake. This is in contrast to CDI, where the vasopressin levels remain low [1–3].

#### *69.2.1.1 What are the Causes of CDI?*

CDI most commonly occurs in the setting of traumatic brain injury (TBI), brain tumors, or following neurosurgery [2–4]. CDI has also been identified in thoracic spinal injury [5]. Injury to the hypothalamic osmoreceptors, supraoptic or paraventricular nuclei, or the supraopticohypophyseal tract halts ADH production and release, resulting in CDI [1–4]. Injury to the posterior pituitary gland, the site of storage and secretion of ADH, will often result with transient CDI. In the setting of such injury, the hypothalamus may directly release ADH [1,4].

*Recommendation*: CDI is most commonly seen in traumatic brain injury (TBI), brain tumors, or following neurosurgery.

*Recommendation Grade*: C

#### *69.2.1.2 What is the Optimal Treatment of CDI?*

*Recommendation*: Initial treatment of CDI involves replacement of fluids with hypotonic solution to match urine output, and replacement of ADH with a synthetic analog, d-DAVP or desmopressin [3,6]. This medication can be delivered orally, intravenously, or as a nasal spray. The doses are titrated using urine and blood osmolality and sodium levels. Patients must be monitored closely as overcorrection can lead to hemodilution and hyponatremia [6,7].

*Recommendation Grade*: B

## 69.3 Carcinoid Crisis

### 69.3.1 Introduction

Carcinoid tumors are of neuroendocrine origin and are derived from enterochromaffin, or Kultschitzky cells. They may occur in sites of the developmental foregut, midgut or hindgut, including the lungs, thymus, gastrointestinal tract, liver, pancreas, or genitourinary system. Primary tumors most commonly present in the small intestine, and 30% of small intestinal tumors will metastasize [8]. Fifteen percent of patients present with metastatic disease to the liver [9].

Carcinoid tumors are rare, occurring in 2 of 100,000 people. Distribution is bimodal, with peak incidences in adolescence and in the elderly. Although most carcinoid tumors occur spontaneously, 1% may be familial [9].

Carcinoid syndrome is caused by tumor secretion and systemic action of polypeptides, biogenic amines, and prostaglandins. The most significant carcinoid secretions are serotonin, histamine, tachykinins, kallikrein, and prostaglandins. These hormones are hepatically cleared. Tumor secretions must overwhelm or bypass the hepatic metabolism to produce symptoms. Therefore, carcinoid syndrome is limited to patients with metastatic disease to the liver, primary lung tumors, high tumor burden, or direct tumor manipulation [9,10].

Carcinoid crisis is a severe sequela of carcinoid syndrome, characterized by excessive diarrhea and flushing. Fluid losses may result in dehydration, electrolyte abnormalities, arrhythmias, and hypovolemic or cardiogenic shock. Chronic exposure to serotonin and other tumor secretions may contribute to carcinoid heart disease (CHD), a severe fibrosis of the endocardium with resultant valvular and wall motion abnormalities [10]. Venous telangiectasia, bronchospasm, pellagra, and muscle wasting may also be present [9].

#### *69.3.1.1 How is a Carcinoid Tumor Diagnosed?*

Patients with carcinoid tumors are definitively diagnosed with tissue biopsy. With carcinoid syndrome, serum platelet serotonin and urinary 5-HIAA, a metabolite of serotonin, will be elevated. Chromogranin A (CgA), a protein found on neuroendocrine cells, is not limited to serotonin-secreting tumors and can help identify the presence of inactive tumors. Imaging to localize the carcinoid primary and to evaluate the extent of disease includes CT, video enterography, endoscopy and MIBG scans. FDG PET scans have poor utility, as carcinoid tumors display limited metabolic activity and are consequently not FDG avid. Octreotide scintigraphy scans may also aid in tumor localization [9,11].

*Recommendation*: Carcinoid tumors are definitively diagnosed with tissue biopsy. Tumors may be difficult to identify on imaging and multiple modalities may be needed for localization. Serum platelet serotonin, urinary 5-HIAA, and CgA levels are commonly elevated.
*Recommendation Grade*: B

#### *69.3.1.2 What is the Optimal Treatment of Carcinoid Crisis?*

Carcinoid crisis is treated with octreotide, a somatostatin analog with a prolonged half-life of 100 h. Octreotide binds to somatostatin tumor receptors, limiting hormone, and neurotransmitter release. An initial bolus of 25–500 mcg is administered, followed by a continuous infusion of 50–150 mcg/h. Higher doses of octreotide may be required in patients with CHD or those previously treated with octreotide. Interferon-α has been used as an adjunct to octreotide, though efficacy has varied and the mechanism of action is poorly understood [9,11,12].

The hypotension of carcinoid crisis results from diarrhea-induced hypovolemia and from vasoactive peptide-induced vasodilatation. Vasopressors are often ineffective and may be deleterious as they may exacerbate bronchospasm [12,13]. To prevent carcinoid crisis, patients with carcinoid syndrome should receive aggressive fluid resuscitation to prevent hypovolemia, with close monitoring of electrolytes. They may also benefit from antidiarrheals, such as loperamide [9–11,14].

*Recommendation*: Carcinoid crisis is treated with intravenous fluids, electrolyte supplementation, and octreotide.

*Recommendation Grade*: C

## 69.4 Thyroid Storm

### 69.4.1 Introduction

Thyroid storm (TS) is characterized by severe thyrotoxicosis and may result in multiorgan system failure [15]. TS is rare, occurring in only 1%–2% of patients with thyrotoxicosis. TS occurs primarily in the setting of Graves disease; rarely, it may be due a solitary toxic adenoma, toxic multinodular goiter, subacute thyroiditis, TSH-secreting pituitary tumors, or amiodarone. Thyroid storm may occur in patients with poorly controlled hyperthyroidism or be precipitated by stressors and such inciting events include trauma, surgery, infection, cerebral vascular accidents, diabetic ketoacidosis, myocardial infarction, radioactive iodine, or pregnancy. Nonsteroidal anti-inflammatory drugs, antidepressants, steroids, insulin, and thiazide diuretics may exacerbate thyrotoxicosis [16,17]. As mortality approaches 15%, timely intervention is critical [15–17].

#### *69.4.1.1 What are the Symptoms and Signs of Thyroid Storm?*

Thyroid hormones, prohormone thyroxine ($T_4$) and triiodothyronine ($T_3$), alter gene expression by systemically binding to mitochondrial and nuclear deoxyribo nucleic acid (DNA)-binding proteins, promoting metabolism and growth. Symptoms and signs of thyroid storm include fever, palpitations, atrial fibrillation, tachypnea, congestive heart failure (CHF), diarrhea, vomiting, jaundice, delirium, seizures, and coma [16]. Serum $T_4$ and $T_3$ levels are markedly elevated. Thyroid-stimulating hormone (TSH) is suppressed, unless the source of hyperthyroidism is due to a TSH-secreting pituitary tumor [15]. Additional laboratory abnormalities may include leukocytosis, elevated liver enzymes, elevation in lactate dehydrogenase, metabolic acidosis, and hyperglycemia [16].

To aid in the differentiation of TS from simple thyrotoxicosis, Burch and Wartofsky, in 1993, developed a point system based on a history of hyperthyroidism, the presence of fever, altered mental status, gastrointestinal and hepatic manifestations (nausea, vomiting, diarrhea, lactic acidosis, liver failure), atrial fibrillation, and heart failure [18]. In a Japanese sampling modeled after Burch and Wartofsky, nausea, vomiting, and diarrhea were found to be nearly exclusive to TS. Atrial fibrillation and CHF were noted common complications and were associated with increased mortality [17].

*Recommendation*: Thyroid storm presents in the setting of thyrotoxicosis and physiologic stress. Diagnostic criteria for TS require the presence of thyrotoxicosis (low TSH and elevated free thyroxine) and symptoms and signs, including fever, altered mental status, gastrointestinal and hepatic manifestations, atrial fibrillation, and CHF.

*Recommendation Grade*: C

### 69.4.1.2 What is the Appropriate Management of Thyroid Storm?

The management of TS is primarily pharmacologic. Medical treatment includes antithyroid agents, antihypertensive agents, glucocorticoids, anticoagulants, and antipyretic agents.

β-Adrenergic blockade is given to treat hypertension and tachycardia associated with TS [15]. Propranolol is preferred over other β-blockers, for its dual effect of β-blockade and the prevention of peripheral conversion of T4 to T3 [15,16,19]. Propranolol should not be administered in the setting of decompensated heart failure, as suppression of sympathetic stimulation may precipitate cardiovascular collapse [16].

The antithyroid medications propylthiouracil (PTU) and methimazole (MMI) are used in the treatment of thyrotoxicosis. Both inhibit formation of thyroid hormone by reducing iodine organification. PTU also reduces peripheral deiodination of T4 to T3 and should be used preferentially in the setting of a life-threatening thyrotoxicosis [15,16,20].

The indications for antithyroid agents are informed by side-effect profiles. MMI should be avoided in the first trimester of pregnancy as severe congenital abnormalities may occur. Hepatotoxicity, necessitating liver transplant, has occurred with the administration of PTU, and therefore, MMI is preferentially used for the initial treatment of non-TS hyperthyroidism. Monitoring of hepatic function has not been shown to improve outcomes in fulminant PTU-induced hepatotoxicity [19,20].

Iodine, administered as sodium iodide or Lugol's solution (a mixture of elemental iodine and potassium iodide), can be used to treat TS by temporarily preventing synthesis and release of thyroid hormone. Iodine solutions should be administered no sooner than 1 h prior to antithyroid medications, to avoid stimulation of hormone production. Lithium carbonate ($Li_2CO_3$) prevents proteolysis of colloid and may also be used in the treatment of TS [15].

Glucocorticoids are used as adjuncts in the treatment of TS. Glucocorticoid stores are depleted in the hypermetabolic state of TS. Exogenous administration of glucocorticoids helps to stabilize blood pressure and inhibit peripheral deiodination of T4 to T3. They also serve as an antipyretic and promote vasomotor stability [15,16,21].

Circulating pro-coagulation factors are increased in TS while inhibitors, such as plasminogen and proteins C and S, are transiently reduced. Consequently, thromboembolic events may occur in TS and are responsible for up to 18% of thyrotoxic-related deaths [21]. Prophylactic anticoagulation should be administered. Patients with pre-existing coagulation disorders or atrial fibrillation, present in 40% of TS cases, should be considered for therapeutic anticoagulation [15,17].

In thyroid storm refractory to standard treatment, other agents may be considered. Reserpine, an inhibitor of norepinephrine transport, may successfully treat hypertension in patients who are refractory to β-blockade. Guanethidine, a norepinephrine antagonist, is a useful alternative to β-blockers or reserpine in the setting of asthma or bronchospasm. Cholestyramine can be used as a binding agent to lower thyroid hormone levels by facilitating intestinal excretion. L-carnitine inhibits cellular uptake of thyroid hormone. As a last resort, plasmapheresis, dialysis, or charcoal hemoperfusion may be used to temporarily reduce circulating T3 and T4 [15–17,21].

Fever in thyrotoxicosis may exceed 38°C, resulting in increased cardiac output, vasodilation, tachyarrhythmias, lactic acidosis, tachypnea, coma, and even death. Salicylates should be avoided in TS, as they increase free T3 and T4 by inhibiting binding in serum to thyroxine-binding globulin (TBG). Therefore, acetaminophen is the preferred agent for fever. External cooling measures include alcohol sponges, ice packs, and cooling blankets may be necessary [15–17].

Insensible fluid losses in TS may lead to profound hypovolemia. Therefore, fluid resuscitation should begin early. Given the risk in TS for cardiac complications and CHF, administration of IVF should be performed with close monitoring of intravascular volume status to avoid hypervolemia.

*Recommendation*: The management of thyroid storm is primarily treated with β-blockers, antithyroid agents, and glucocorticoids. Fluid resuscitation and thermoregulation are crucial. Underlying stressors leading to TS should be aggressively treated.

*Recommendation Grade*: B

### 69.4.1.3 When, in the Setting of Thyroid Storm, is Thyroidectomy Indicated?

Thyroidectomy may be required for cases refractory to medical management. Surgery has been recommended for patients who fail to improve after 12–24 h of treatment, as mortality approaches 75% without surgery (vs. 10% with surgery) [19,22–25]. Plasmapheresis or dialysis may be attempted to achieve temporary euthyroidism prior to surgery [23].

*Recommendation*: Surgical management during thyroid storm may be urgently required in patients who are refractory to medical management.

*Recommendation Grade*: C

## 69.5 Hypercalcemic Crisis

### 69.5.1 Introduction

Hypercalcemic crisis most commonly arises as a consequence of primary hyperparathyroidism or malignancy; rarely, it can be due to parathyroid carcinoma or sarcoidosis. Hypercalcemic crisis generally occurs at levels above 14 mg/dL. Gastrointestinal symptoms are common and include nausea, vomiting, abdominal pain, and constipation. Changes in cognitive function range from fatigue to confusion, seizures, and coma. Hypovolemia, tetany, arrhythmias, heart block, cardiac arrest, pancreatitis, nephrolithiasis, nephrogenic diabetes insipidus, and renal failure may also occur [26].

#### *69.5.1.1 What are the Causes of Hypercalcemic Crisis?*

Primary hyperparathyroidism and malignancy are the most common causes of hypercalcemic crisis. If due to primary hyperparathyroidism, a single parathyroid adenoma is the most common pathology [26]. Hypercalcemic crisis may also occur in the setting of malignancy, from either direct osteolysis by bony metastases, or osteolysis from osteoclastic activity stimulated by PTHrP or proinflammatory mediators release by the tumor. Hypercalemia due to malignancy most commonly occurs with breast, lung, and hematologic malignancies. The prognosis for patients with hypercalcemic crisis of malignancy is often dismal, with a median survival of 30 days [27].

Secondary hyperparathyroidism (SHPT) from end-stage renal disease (ESRD) results from inadequate renal activation of vitamin D, inadequate phosphate excretion, and low calcium levels, resulting in parathyroid gland hypertrophy. Although calcium levels typically do not exceed 11 mg/dL, hypercalcemia has been shown to correlate with increased mortality in dialysis patients [28]. The treatment of SHPT initially includes active vitamin D and phosphate binders. Cinacalcet, a calcimimetic, may be added if initial medical management fails to lower PTH and calcium levels. Patients with SHPT due to ESRD who fail medical management or who have persistent disease after renal transplant can be treated with subtotal parathyroidectomy [29].

*Recommendation*: Hypercalcemic crisis is most commonly caused by primary hyperparathyroidism or malignancy.

*Recommendation Grade*: B

#### *69.5.1.2 How is Hypercalcemic Crisis Evaluated and Treated?*

In the evaluation of patients with hypercalcemia, laboratory tests to be ordered include calcium, intact PTH, creatinine, 25-OH vitamin D, and PTHrP levels. In the setting of primary hyperparathyroidism, calcium and PTH will be elevated, while PTHrP is normal [27]. PTH levels will be suppressed in hypercalcemia of malignancy.

Initial treatment of hypercalcemia involves administration of intravenous fluids, to restore intravascular volume and promote diuresis. A one-liter bolus is given, followed by a continuous infusion, titrated to a urine output of 1–2 mL/kg/h [27]. Loop diuretics may then be initiated to increase the renal excretion of calcium. Bisphosphonates may be administered to limit osteoclastic activity and prevent release of calcium from bone [27]. Calcitonin, cinacalcet, and glucocorticoids may be given to patients refractory to initial medical therapy. In life-threatening hypercalcemia, as with arrhythmias or coma, hemodialysis may be used for rapid calcium clearance.

The underlying etiology of hypercalcemia should be identified. Once the patient is medically optimized and calcium has decreased with medical management to less than 12 mg/dL, primary hyperparathyroidism may be definitively treated with parathyroidectomy. When preoperative localization suggests a single adenoma, a focused surgical approach can be performed.

*Recommendation*: Treatment of hypercalcemia includes aggressive fluid resuscitation, loop diuretics, and bisphosphonates. Calcitonin, glucocorticoids, and cinacalcet may be added for refractory cases. Hypercalcemia due to hyperparathyroidism is definitively treated with surgery.

*Recommendation Grade*: C

## 69.6 Adrenal Crisis

### 69.6.1 Introduction

The adrenal gland is composed of the cortex, which produces steroid hormones, and the medulla, responsible for the secretion of catecholamines. Adrenal crisis occurs with disruption of the hypothalamic–pituitary–adrenal axis, primarily resulting in acute mineralocorticoid deficiency. Common causes include Addison disease, discontinuation of exogenous corticosteroids, hemorrhagic adrenalitis, adrenal infarct, or severe physiologic stress [30]. Adrenal crisis in the critically ill is likely caused by an exaggerated inflammatory response, tissue resistance to corticosteroids, and intrinsic adrenal gland deficiency [31].

#### *69.6.1.1 What Signs and Symptoms are Found in Patients with Adrenal Crisis?*

Adrenal crisis presents with hypovolemic shock, refractory to fluid resuscitation and vasopressors. A delay in diagnosis and treatment can be fatal. Other symptoms include nausea, vomiting, abdominal pain, fever, confusion, and lethargy. Close monitoring of electrolytes is required, as patients may develop hyponatremia and hyperkalemia. Adrenal insufficiency should be suspected in all septic patients unresponsive to fluids and vasopressors.

*Recommendation*: Symptoms of adrenal insufficiency include nausea, vomiting, abdominal pain, fever, and lethargy. Adrenal crisis is characterized by hypotension unresponsive to fluid resuscitation or vasopressors.

*Recommendation Grade*: B

#### 69.6.1.2 *What is the Appropriate Workup When Adrenal Insufficiency is Suspected?*

Adrenal insufficiency is defined by low serum cortisol levels (<10 mcg/dL) or failure of cortisol to rise (<9 mcg/dL) after attempted stimulation with corticotropin (ACTH) 250 mcg [31,32]. Low-dose (1 mcg) corticotropin stimulation testing is more sensitive than high-dose testing [33]. In the septic patient, empiric treatment is recommended if adrenal insufficiency is suspected, and therefore, testing is not necessary.

*Recommendation*: Patients with adrenal insufficiency will commonly have decreased serum cortisol levels, and will often fail low-dose corticotropin stimulation testing. However, as these tests are not 100% sensitive, critically ill patients unresponsive to intravenous fluids and vasopressors should be empirically treated for adrenal insufficiency.

*Recommendation Grade*: B

#### 69.6.1.3 *What is the Optimal Treatment for Patients in Adrenal Crisis?*

Patients suspected of having adrenal crisis should be treated empirically, as mortality is considerable if left untreated. Hydrocortisone is the mainstay of treatment, for its dual mineralocorticoid and glucocorticoid action. Patients require close hemodynamic monitoring during treatment. Fluid resuscitation and electrolyte repletion are essential. Patients with hypothalamic–pituitary–adrenal (HPA) axis disruption may have concurrent hypothyroidism. Precipitating factors, such as infection or myocardial ischemia, should be identified and treated [30,34].

Empiric treatment of adrenal insufficiency with hydrocortisone should be considered in patients with septic shock who are unresponsive to fluid resuscitation and vasopressors [35]. Given the variability of corticosteroid levels during periods of septic shock, corticotropin-stimulation testing may not accurately identify patients who require supplementation [35,36].

*Recommendation*: A trial of corticosteroids should be instituted in patients in septic shock refractory to fluid resuscitation and vasopressors.

*Recommendation Grade*: B

## 69.7 Hypertensive Crisis due to Pheochromocytoma

### 69.7.1 Introduction

Paragangliomas (PGL) occur within the adrenal gland (pheochromocytoma) or in an extra-adrenal location, such as the neck, mediastinum, abdomen, pelvis, or the organ of Zuckerkandl. Nearly, half of all pheochromocytomas are identified incidentally, and most are sporadic [37]. They may also be associated with familial disorders, such as MEN2A and MEN2B, neurofibromatosis type 1, Von Hippel–Lindau syndrome, or succinate dehydrogenase B and D (SDHB, SDHD) gene mutations [37,38].

#### 69.7.1.1 *What are the Signs and Symptoms of Pheochromocytoma?*

Pheochromocytomas are classically associated with a triad of headaches, palpitations, and diaphoresis. Other symptoms such as anxiety, dizziness, syncope, or flushing may occur [37]. Pheochromocytomas are responsible for 1% of all cases of hypertension and may result in hypertensive emergency. As hypertension is often episodic, up to 50% of patients with pheochromocytomas may be normotensive at presentation [38].

In pregnancy, the hypertension of pheochromoctyoma may be mistaken for preeclampsia. Mortality may be as high as 50% for mother and fetus. Hypertension of pheochromocytoma may be distinguished from preeclampsia by the absence of proteinuria, and an early trimester presentation [38].

*Recommendation*: Pheochromocytomas are associated with a triad of headaches, palpitations, and diaphoresis. Other symptoms may include anxiety, dizziness, syncope, or flushing.

*Evidence Grade*: B

#### 69.7.1.2 *How are Pheochromocytomas Diagnosed?*

Evaluation begins with measurement of plasma or urinary metanephrines in symptomatic patients, or those with an adrenal mass. The diagnosis is made biochemically. Metanephrine levels are typically elevated fourfold [39,40]. CT or MRI is the initial imaging modalities of choice to localize tumors. Pheochromocytomas will often appear hyperintense on a T2-weighted MRI, and hypointense on T1-weighted images [41]. On CT, pheochromocytomas may be homogenous, heterogeneous or cystic, and typically have attenuation greater than 10 Hounsfield units (HU) on noncontrast CT. Functional imaging with $^{131}$I-radiolabeled MIBG may be performed, in the setting of a negative CT or MRI, or in cases of suspected bilateral tumors or metastatic disease [42]. FDG-PET CT may also be used to assess extent of disease in the setting of known malignant pheochromocytoma, or when $^{131}$I MIBG is negative.

*Recommendation*: Pheochromocytoma is diagnosed biochemically, with elevated plasma or urinary metanephrines. CT or MRI is the initial imaging modality of choice.

*Recommendation Grade*: B

#### 69.7.1.3 How Does a Pheochromocytoma Cause Hypertensive Crisis?

Hypertensive crisis in patients with pheochromoctyoma is due to high levels of catecholamine production and release. Commonly, it occurs in cases of locally advanced or metastatic disease, or it may be precipitated by anesthesia induction or direct tumor manipulation. The release of catecholamines leads to vasoconstriction and tachycardia, resulting in hypertension. Complications of hypertensive crisis include myocardial infarction, cerebrovascular accidents, seizures, cardiovascular collapse, and shock. Pheochromocytoma multisystem crisis (PMC) is characterized by hyperthermia, encephalopathy, and multiorgan system failure. Mortality rates may exceed 85% [30,43].

*Recommendation*: Hypertensive crisis results from excess catecholamine release. Uncontrolled hypertension may lead to significant morbidity, including multiorgan failure and death.

*Evidence Grade*: B

#### 69.7.1.4 What is the Recommended Treatment for Hypertensive Crisis due to Pheochromocytoma?

Treatment begins with an α-blocker; the agent of choice is phenoxybenzamine, a nonselective α-blocker. In all patients with pheochromocytoma, α-blockade should be administered for 10–14 days prior to operative intervention [38]. Dosing is titrated to orthostatic hypotension and to a blood pressure below 160/90 [43].

Alternatives to phenoxybenzamine include selective α-1 receptor blockers such as terazosin, prazosin, and doxazosin. Due to shorter half-lives, the incidence of postoperative reflex tachycardia and hypotension may be reduced with these agents.

β-Blockers are added to treat reflex tachycardia arising from α-blockade. Administration of β-blockers should occur only after α-blockade is initiated; otherwise, the patient will develop hypertensive crisis through unopposed α-stimulation.

During α-blockade, the patient is encouraged to liberally consume salt and fluids to replenish intravascular volume. This is critical in preparation for adrenalectomy, as immediate loss of α-stimulation and vasoconstriction with tumor extirpation can result in significant hypotension if the patient is hypovolemic. Calcium-channel antagonists (e.g., nicardipine) may also be used in the treatment of pheochromocytoma [30,43]. In refractory cases, α-methyl tyrosine (metyrosine) may be administered to decrease catecholamine biosynthesis [30,38,43].

Intraoperative management of pheochromocytomas requires careful hemodynamic monitoring, with prompt treatment of hemodynamic instability. Nitroglycerine or nitroprusside may be delivered as a continuous infusion for hypertension. Magnesium sulfate may be administered to lower blood pressure, stabilize hyperdynamic myocardium, and prevent arrhythmias. Nicardipine, clevidipine, esmolol, and phentolamine are also used to lower blood pressure intraoperatively.

*Recommendation*: Initial management of patients with hypertensive crisis from a pheochromocytoma includes α-blockade, subsequent β-blockade, and intravascular volume repletion. Other agents, including calcium-channel blockers or α-methyl tyrosine, may be required. Nitroglycerine or nitroprusside may be required intraoperatively for refractory cases.

*Recommendation Grade*: A

#### 69.7.1.5 How are Pheochromocytomas Approached Surgically?

Definitive treatment for pheochromocytomas is adrenalectomy, after medical optimization with α-blockade, intravascular volume repletion, and hemodynamic stabilization. Most adrenalectomies can be performed with a minimally invasive approach, either laparoscopically or retroperitoneoscopically. When compared to an open approach, the minimally invasive approach results in decreased blood loss and shorter recovery time, with no difference in intraoperative hemodynamics or operative length [44,45]. Contraindications to a minimally invasive approach include suspected malignancy and large tumors (>8–10 cm), due to the risk of incomplete resection or seeding of the tumor bed [45,46].

Emergency adrenalectomy for patients in PMC carries significant morbidity and mortality. However, surgery may be the only option for patients with multiorgan failure refractory to medical management [47,48].

*Recommendation*: A minimally invasive approach is preferred to open adrenalectomy. Contraindications to minimally invasive surgery include suspected malignant disease or very large tumors. In patients with PMC, patients refractory to medical management may require emergency adrenalectomy (Tables 69.1 and 69.2)

*Recommendation Grade*: B

**TABLE 69.1**
Question and Answer Summaries and Recommendations

| Question | Answer | Levels of Evidence | Grade of Recommendation | References |
|---|---|---|---|---|
| What are the causes of CDI? | CDI is most commonly observed in traumatic brain injury (TBI), brain tumors, or following neurosurgery. | 2a, 3a | C | [1–4] |
| What is the optimal treatment of CDI? | Initial treatment of CDI involves replacement of fluids with hypotonic solution to match urine output, and replacement of ADH with a synthetic analog, d-DAVP or desmopressin. This medication can be delivered orally, intravenously, or as a nasal spray. The doses are titrated using urine and blood osmolality and sodium levels. Patients must be monitored closely as overcorrection can lead to hemodilution and hyponatremia. | 2a, 3 | B | [3–7] |
| How is a carcinoid tumor diagnosed? | Carcinoid tumors are definitively diagnosed with tissue biopsy. Tumors may be difficult to identify on imaging and multiple modalities may be needed for localization. Serum platelet serotonin, urinary 5-HIAA, and CgA levels are commonly elevated. | 2a, 3b | B | [9,11] |
| What is the optimal treatment of carcinoid crisis? | Carcinoid crisis is treated with intravenous fluids, electrolyte supplementation, and octreotide. | 2a, 3 | C | [9–14] |
| What are the symptoms and signs of thyroid storm? | Thyroid storm presents in the setting of thyrotoxicosis and physiologic stress. Diagnostic criteria for TS require the presence of thyrotoxicosis (low TSH and elevated free thyroxine) and symptoms and signs, including fever, altered mental status-gastrointestinal and hepatic manifestations, atrial fibrillation, and congestive heart failure. | 3a | C | [16–18] |
| What is the appropriate management of thyroid storm? | The management of thyroid storm is primarily treated with β-blockers, antithyroid agents, and glucocorticoids. Fluid resuscitation and thermoregulation are crucial. Underlying stressors leading to thyroid storm should be aggressively treated. | 2a, 3a | B | [15–21] |
| When, in the setting of thyroid storm, is thyroidectomy indicated? | Surgical management during thyroid storm may be urgently required in patients who are refractory to medical management. | 2a, 3 | C | [19,22–25] |
| What are the causes of hypercalcemic crisis? | Hypercalcemic crisis is most commonly caused by primary hyperparathyroidism or malignancy. | 2a, 3a | B | [26–29] |
| How is hypercalcemic crisis evaluated and treated? | Treatment of hypercalcemia includes aggressive fluid resuscitation, loop diuretics, and bisphosphonates. Calcitonin, glucocorticoids, and cinacalcet may be added for refractory cases. Hypercalcemia due to hyperparathyroidism is definitively treated with surgery. | 3a | C | [27] |
| What signs and symptoms are found in patients with adrenal crisis? | Symptoms of adrenal insufficiency include nausea, vomiting, abdominal pain, fever, and lethargy. Adrenal crisis is characterized by hypotension unresponsive to fluid resuscitation or vasopressors. | 3 | B | [30–31] |

(Continued)

**TABLE 69.1 (*Continued*)**

Question and Answer Summaries and Recommendations

| Question | Answer | Levels of Evidence | Grade of Recommendation | References |
|---|---|---|---|---|
| What is the appropriate workup when adrenal insufficiency is suspected? | Patients with adrenal insufficiency will commonly have decreased serum cortisol levels and will often fail low-dose corticotropin stimulation testing. However, as these tests are not 100% sensitive, critically ill patients unresponsive to intravenous fluids and vasopressors should be empirically treated for adrenal insufficiency. | 2a, 3a | B | [31–33] |
| What is the optimal treatment for patients in adrenal crisis? | A trial of corticosteroids should be instituted in patients in septic shock refractory to fluid resuscitation and vasopressors. | 2 | B | [30,34–36] |
| What are the signs and symptoms of pheochromocytoma? | Pheochromocytomas are associated with a triad of headaches, palpitations, and diaphoresis. Other symptoms may include anxiety, dizziness, syncope, or flushing. | 2a | B | [37,38] |
| How are pheochromocytomas diagnosed? | Pheochromocytoma is diagnosed biochemically, with elevated plasma or urinary metanephrines. CT or MRI is the initial imaging modality of choice. | 2, 3a | B | [39–41] |
| How does a pheochromocytoma cause hypertensive crisis? | Hypertensive crisis results from excess catecholamine release. Uncontrolled hypertension may lead to significant morbidity, including multiorgan failure and death. | 2 | B | [30,43] |
| What is the recommended treatment for hypertensive crisis due to pheochromocytoma? | Initial management of patients with hypertensive crisis from a pheochromocytoma includes α-blockade, subsequent β-blockade, and intravascular volume repletion. Other agents, including calcium-channel blockers or α-methyl tyrosine, may be required. Nitroglycerine or nitroprusside may be required intraoperatively for refractory cases. | 2 | A | [30,38,40] |
| How are pheochromocytomas approached surgically? | A minimally invasive approach is preferred to open adrenalectomy. Contraindications to minimally invasive surgery include suspected malignant disease or very large tumors. In patients with PMC, patients refractory to medical management may require emergency adrenalectomy. | 1b, 2a, 3b | B | [44–48] |

**TABLE 69.2**
Review of References

| Author (References) | Year | Level of Evidence | Groups | Design | Median Follow-up | Endpoint |
|---|---|---|---|---|---|---|
| Babey et al. [1] | 2011 | 2a | Patients with familial central diabetes insipidus | Review | N/A | Review of clinical presentation, treatment, and molecular characteristics |
| Schneider et al. [4] | 2007 | 2a | Patients with pituitary abnormalities due to traumatic brain injury or subarachnoid hemorrhage | Meta-analysis | 3 months–22 years (median not calculated) | Anterior hypopituitarism: insulin level, insulin tolerance, GHRH, GH, TSH, LH/FSH ACTH, arginine, and growth hormone releasing peptide 6 levels Posterior hypopituitarism: prevalence of DI |
| Vande Walle et al. [7] | 2007 | 2a | Patients treated with desmopressin for diabetes insipidus | Review of retrospective cohort studies and RCTs | NR | Resolution of symptoms or onset of complications |
| Zuetenhurst and Taal [9] | 2005 | 2C | Patients with carcinoid tumors | Review of retrospective cohort, RCTs, and outcomes research | NR | Examine the epidemiology, current diagnostic criteria, treatments, and prognosis |
| Seymour and Sawh [11] | 2013 | 2A | Patients treated with high-dose octreotide for carcinoid crisis | Review of retrospective cohort studies and consensus statements | NR | Resolution of symptoms, side effects, mortality |
| Castillo et al. [12] | 2012 | 3B | Carcinoid tumor-induced cardiac disease | Review of case series and retrospective cohort studies | NR | Patient optimization and octreotide dosing |
| Kinney et al. [14] | 2001 | 2B | Patients who underwent abdominal surgery for metastatic carcinoid tumors | Retrospective cohort study | 30 days | Perioperative morbidity and mortality |
| Akamizu et al. [17] | 2012 | 2C | Japanese patients with thyrotoxicosis, with and without thyroid storm (TS) | Outcomes research | NR | Onset of thyroid storm, irreversible complications, death, resolution of TS |
| Burch and Wartofsky [18] | 1993 | 2A | Patients with thyroid storm | Review of retrospective cohort studies | NR | Resolution of symptoms, death |
| Bahn et al. [19] | 2011 | Grade B | Recommendations for the management of hyperthyroidism | Consensus statement (national task force) | NA | NA |
| Stagnaro-Green et al. [20] | 2011 | Grade B | Recommendations for the diagnosis and management of thyroid disease in pregnancy and in the postpartum period | Consensus statement (national task force) | NA | NA |
| Klubo-Gwiezdzinska and Wartofsky [21] | 2012 | 2A | Recommendations for the management of hypothyroid and hyperthyroid emergencies | Review of retrospective cohort studies | N/A | N/A |
| Clines [27] | 2011 | 2A | Patients with hypercalcemia of malignancy | Retrospective cohort studies, RCTs | NA | NA |

*(Continued)*

**TABLE 69.2 (*Continued*)**

Review of References

| Author (References) | Year | Level of Evidence | Groups | Design | Median Follow-up | Endpoint |
|---|---|---|---|---|---|---|
| Fukagawa et al. [28] | 2014 | 2B | Patients with secondary hyperparathyroidism due to ESRD | Prospective case-cohort study | 3 years | All-cause mortality |
| Tucci and Sokari [30] | 2014 | 2A | Patients with adrenal emergencies | Review of retrospective cohorts, RCTs | NA | NA |
| Marik et al. [31] | 2008 | Grade B | Recommendations for corticosteroid insufficiency | Consensus statement (international task force) | NA | NA |
| Annane et al. [32] | 2006 | 2B | Septic and nonseptic patients | Consecutive cohort study | NR | Baseline cortisol level, free cortisol level, and delta cortisol level after stimulation |
| Siraux et al. [33] | 2005 | 2B | Patients administered low-dose (1 μg) corticotropin stimulation test vs. the standard (250 μg) test for the diagnosis of relative adrenal insufficiency | Consecutive cohort study | 28 days | Cortisol levels, maximum cortisol levels, hemodynamic stability, length of ICU stay, ICU mortality, 28-day survival |
| Dellinger et al. [35] | 2013 | Grade B | Recommendations for the management of severe sepsis and septic shock | Consensus statement (international task force) | NA | NA |
| Briegel et al. [36] | 2009 | 2B | Patients in septic shock | Retrospective cohort study | NR | Cortisol level, diagnosis of corticosteroid insufficiency |
| Wachtel et al. [37] | 2014 | 2B | Adrenalectomy in patients with incidental or symptomatic pheochromocytoma | Retrospective cohort study | NR | Histologic evidence of malignant or benign disease |
| Chen et al. [38] | 2010 | Grade B | Recommendations for the diagnosis and management of neuroendocrine tumors | Consensus statement (international task force) | NA | NA |
| Kirshtein et al. [39] | 2007 | 2C | Adrenalectomy for adrenal incidentaloma | Outcomes research | NR | NA |
| Lenders et al. [40] | 2002 | 2B | Patients evaluated for pheochromocytoma (1994–2001) | Retrospective cohort study | NR | Sensitivities and specificities of the biochemical markers of pheochromocytoma |
| Bhatia et al. [42] | 2005 | 2B | Patients who underwent both preoperative [(123)I]MIBG and cross-sectional imaging for confirmed pheochromocytoma and paraganglioma | Retrospective analysis | NR | Sensitivity of MIBG vs. CT/MRI scans for the detection of adrenal and extra-adrenal tumors |
| Tiberio et al. [44] | 2008 | 1B | Comparison of laparoscopic vs. open adrenalectomy for pheochromocytoma | Prospective randomized controlled trial | NR | Operative time, hypertensive episodes, and long-term follow-up |
| Bentrem et al. [45] | 2002 | 2B | Laparoscopic, laparoscopic-assisted, and open adrenalectomies | Retrospective cohort study | 6.5 days | Operative times, blood loss, length of stay |
| Phitayakom and McHenry [46] | 2008 | 2B | Comparison of laparoscopic adrenalectomy to laparoscopic adrenalectomy converted to open | Retrospective cohort study | NR | Conversion to open procedure |

## Acknowledgments

We gratefully acknowledge Christopher Busken, MD, Rebecca Coefield, MD, and Robert Kelly, MD, who contributed to a prior version of this chapter [49].

## References

1. Babey M, Kopp P, Robertson GL. Familial forms of diabetes insipidus: Clinical and molecular characteristics. *Nat Rev Endocrinol*. 2011;7(12):701–714.
2. Leroy C, Karrouz W, Douillard, C et al. Diabetes insipidus. *Ann Endocrinol* (*Paris*). 2013;74(5–6):496–507.
3. Devin JK. Hypopituitarism and central diabetes insipidus: Perioperative diagnosis and management. *Neurosurg Clin North Am*. 2012;23(4):679–689.
4. Schneider HJ, Kreitschmann-Andermahr I, Ghigo E et al. Hypothalamopituitary dysfunction following traumatic brain injury and aneurysmal subarachnoid hemorrhage: A systematic review. *JAMA*. 2007;298(12):1429–1438.
5. Kuzeyli K, Cakir E, Baykal S et al. Diabetes insipidus secondary to penetrating spinal cord trauma: Case report and literature review. *Spine* (Phila Pa 1976). 2001;26(21): E510–E511.
6. Chanson P, Salenave S. Treatment of neurogenic diabetes insipidus. *Ann Endocrinol* (*Paris*). 2011;72(6):496–499.
7. Vande Walle J, Stockner M, Raes A, Nørgaard JP. Desmopressin 30 years in clinical use: A safety review. *Curr Drug Safety*. 2007;2(3):232–238.
8. Modlin IM, Lye KD, Kidd M. A 5-decade analysis of 13,715 carcinoid tumors. *Cancer*. 2003;97(4):934–959.
9. Zuetenhorst JM, Taal BG. Metastatic carcinoid tumors: A clinical review. *Oncologist*. 2005;10(2):123–131.
10. Mehta AC, Rafanan AL, Bulkley R et al. Coronary spasm and cardiac arrest from carcinoid crisis during laser bronchoscopy. *Chest*. 1999;115(2):598–600.
11. Seymour N, Sawh SC. Mega-dose intravenous octreotide for the treatment of carcinoid crisis: A systematic review. *Can J Anaesth*. 2013;60(5):492–499.
12. Castillo JG, Silvay G, Solis J. Current concepts in diagnosis and perioperative management of carcinoid heart disease. *Semin Cardiothorac Vasc Anesth*. 2013;17(3):212–223.
13. Vaughan DJ, Brunner MD. Anesthesia for patients with carcinoid syndrome. *Int Anesthesiol Clin*. 1997;35(4):129–142.
14. Kinney MA, Warner ME, Nagorney DM et al. Perianaesthetic risks and outcomes of abdominal surgery for metastatic carcinoid tumours. *Br J Anaesth*. 2001;87(3):447–452.
15. Papi G, Corsello SM, Pontecorvi A. Clinical concepts on thyroid emergencies. *Front Endocrinol* (*Lausanne*). 2014;5:102.
16. Hampton J. Thyroid gland disorder emergencies: Thyroid storm and myxedema coma. *AACN Adv Crit Care*. 2013;24(3):325–332.
17. Akamizu T, Satoh T, Isozaki O et al. Diagnostic criteria, clinical features, and incidence of thyroid storm based on nationwide surveys. *Thyroid*. 2012;22(7):661–679.
18. Burch HB, Wartofsky L. Life-threatening thyrotoxicosis. Thyroid storm. *Endocrinol Metab Clin North Am*. 1993;22(2):263–277.
19. Bahn RS, Burch HB, Cooper DS et al. Hyperthyroidism and other causes of thyrotoxicosis: Management guidelines of the American Thyroid Association and American Association of Clinical Endocrinologists. *Endocr Pract*. 2011;17(3):456–520.
20. Stagnaro-Green A, Abalovich M, Alexander E et al. Guidelines of the American Thyroid Association for the diagnosis and management of thyroid disease during pregnancy and postpartum. *Thyroid*. 2011;21(10):1081–1125.
21. Klubo-Gwiezdzinska J, Wartofsky L. Thyroid emergencies. *Med Clin North Am*. 2012;96(2):385–403.
22. Uchida N, Suda T, Ishiguro K. Thyroidectomy in a patient with thyroid storm: Report of a case. *Surg Today*. 2013;45(1):110–114.
23. Yamamoto J, Dostmohamed H, Schacter I et al. Preoperative therapeutic apheresis for severe medically refractory amiodarone-induced thyrotoxicosis: A case report. *J Clin Apher*. 2014;29(3):168–170.
24. Scholz GHHE, Arkenau C, Engelmann L, Lamesch P, Schreiter D, Schoenfelder M, Olthoff D, Paschke R. Is there a place for thyroidectomy in older patients with thyrotoxic storm and cardiorespiratory failure? *Thyroid*. 2003;13(10):933–940.
25. Reichmann I, Frilling A, Hormann R et al. Early operation as a treatment measure in thyrotoxic crisis. *Chirurg*. 2001;72(4):402–407.
26. Khan MA, Rafiq S, Lanitis S et al. Surgical treatment of primary hyperparathyroidism: Description of techniques and advances in the field. *Indian J Surg*. 2014;76(4):308–315.
27. Clines GA. Mechanisms and treatment of hypercalcemia of malignancy. *Curr Opin Endocrinol Diabetes Obes*. 2011;18(6):339–346.
28. Fukagawa M, Kido R, Komaba H et al. Abnormal mineral metabolism and mortality in hemodialysis patients with secondary hyperparathyroidism: Evidence from marginal structural models used to adjust for time-dependent confounding. *Am J Kidney Dis*. 2014;63(6):979–987.
29. Dewberry LK, Weber C, Sharma J. Near total parathyroidectomy is effective therapy for tertiary hyperparathyroidism. *Am Surg*. 2014;80(7):646–651.
30. Tucci V, Sokari T. The clinical manifestations, diagnosis, and treatment of adrenal emergencies. *Emerg Med Clin North Am*. 2014;32(2):465–484.
31. Marik PE, Pastores SM, Annane D et al. Recommendations for the diagnosis and management of corticosteroid insufficiency in critically ill adult patients: Consensus statements from an international task force by the American College of Critical Care Medicine. *Crit Care Med*. 2008;36(6):1937–1949.
32. Annane D, Maxime V, Ibrahim F et al. Diagnosis of adrenal insufficiency in severe sepsis and septic shock. *Am J Respir Crit Care Med*. 2006;174(12):1319–1326.

33. Siraux V, De Backer D, Yalavatti G et al. Relative adrenal insufficiency in patients with septic shock: Comparison of low-dose and conventional corticotropin tests. *Crit Care Med.* 2005;33(11):2479–2486.
34. Bancos I, Hahner S, Tomlinson J et al. Diagnosis and management of adrenal insufficiency. *Lancet Diabetes Endocrinol.* March 2014;3(3):216–226.
35. Dellinger RP, Levy MM, Rhodes A et al. Surviving Sepsis Campaign: International guidelines for management of severe sepsis and septic shock, 2012. *Intensive Care Med.* 2013;39(2):165–228.
36. Briegel J, Sprung CL, Annane D et al. Multicenter comparison of cortisol as measured by different methods in samples of patients with septic shock. *Intensive Care Med.* 2009;35(12):2151–2156.
37. Wachtel H, Cerullo I, Bartlett EK et al. Characteristics of incidentally identified pheochromocytoma. *Ann Surg Oncol.* January 2015;22(1):132–138.
38. Chen H, Sippel RS, O'Dorisio MS et al. The North American Neuroendocrine Tumor Society consensus guideline for the diagnosis and management of neuroendocrine tumors: Pheochromocytoma, paraganglioma, and medullary thyroid cancer. *Pancreas.* 2010;39(6):775–783.
39. Kirshtein B, Ragliarello G, Yelle JD et al. Incidence of pheochromocytoma in trauma patients during the management of unrelated illness: A retrospective review. *Int J Surg.* 2007;5(5):332–335.
40. Lenders JW, Eisenhofer G, Mannelli M et al. Biochemical diagnosis of pheochromocytoma: Which test is best? *JAMA.* 2002;287(11):1427–1434.
41. Mayo-Smith WW, Boland GW, Noto RB et al. State-of-the-art adrenal imaging. *Radiographics.* 2001;21(4):995–1012.
42. Bhatia KS, Ismail MM, Sahdev A et al. 123I-metaiodobenzylguanidine (MIBG) scintigraphy for the detection of adrenal and extra-adrenal phaeochromocytomas: CT and MRI correlation. *Clin Endocrinol (Oxford).* 2008;69(2):181–188.
43. Kinney MA, Narr BJ, Warner MA. Perioperative management of pheochromocytoma. *J Cardiothorac Vasc Anesth.* 2002;16(3):359–369.
44. Tiberio GA, Baiocchi GL, Arru L et al. Prospective randomized comparison of laparoscopic versus open adrenalectomy for sporadic pheochromocytoma. *Surg Endosc.* 2008;22(6):1435–1439.
45. Bentrem DJ, Pappas SG, Ahuja Y et al. Contemporary surgical management of pheochromocytoma. *Am J Surg.* 2002;184(6):621–624; discussion 624–625.
46. Phitayakorn R, McHenry CR. Laparoscopic and selective open resection for adrenal and extraadrenal neuroendocrine tumors. *Am Surg.* 2008;74(1):37–42.
47. Bos JC, Toorians AWFT, van Mourik JC et al. Emergency resection of an extra-adrenal phaeochromocytoma: Wrong or right? A case report and a review of literature. *Neth J Med.* 2003;61(8):258–265.
48. Uchida N, Ishiguro K, Suda T et al. Pheochromocytoma multisystem crisis successfully treated by emergency surgery: Report of a case. *Surg Today.* 2010;40(10):990–996.
49. Busken C, Kelly B. 2009. *Acute Care Surgery and Trauma: Evidence Based Practice*, 1st edn. Surgical Endocrine Emergencies. Boca Raton, FL:CRC Press, pp. 451–456.

## Commentary on Surgical Endocrine Emergencies

*Amirhossein Razavi and Timothy G. Buchman*

The importance of endocrine surgical emergencies including central diabetes insipidus (CDI), carcinoid crisis, thyroid storm, hypercalcemic crisis, adrenal crisis, and hypertensive crisis secondary to pheochromocytoma cannot be stresses. Delay in treatment can be lethal. Recognition and urgent management of these states requires high clinical suspicion and vigilance. The chapter on "Surgical Endocrine Emergencies" is incisive and worth reading every few months to maintain mental preparedness.

The scope and depth of most endocrine emergencies discussed in this chapter will require ICU admission for close monitoring and medical management. Surgery is reserved for refractory cases and if contemplated ought to trigger multiple consultations from critical care, anesthesiology, surgery, and endocrinology to generate a master plan to minimize risk. The key point is that early recognition and aggressive medical management is important to reduce the need for urgent operation.

### Central Diabetes Insipidus

CDI results from decreased release of antidiuretic hormone (ADH), causing polyuria, nocturia, and polydipsia. Unfortunately, these patients are often confused with other causes of massive urinary water loss including nephrogenic diabetes insipidus, diabetes mellitus, adverse drug effects (we have seen patients with aminoglycoside toxicity void more than 1 L/h), and even psychogenic polydipsia. The most important step is to replace the fluid loss with intravenous hypotonic solutions, arrest the rise in serum sodium, and begin to slowly bring it—and with it the blood and urine osmolality—back into the normal range. The specific hypotonic fluid—5% glucose, 0.45% saline or together—is less important than the fact that the solution is hypotonic. Regardless, treatment will require hourly monitoring in an ICU setting. ADH treatments are done so commonly in a surgical ICU (vasopressin is another name for ADH, and DDAVP is used to address platelet dysfunction in renal failure) that it is important to remind staff that the medication is being used for a different purpose and hourly monitoring as described is crucial.

### Carcinoid Crisis

Carcinoid crisis is blessedly rare. One trap for the unwary is that patients with carcinoid problems lying just subclinical—that is, patients with carcinoid tumors that have just begun to spread and escape hepatic metabolism—can drop into full-blown serotonin syndrome when a well-meaning practitioner prescribes an SSRI-class antidepressant medication. While there are other more common causes for the serotonin syndrome upon SSRI administration, this one should be kept in mind.

### Thyroid Storm

Thyroid storm is also blessedly rare in an era where thyroid function is commonly measured. Unfortunately, it is seen periodically in patients who do not have regular medical care and therefore, the earlier manifestations of thyrotoxicosis have gone both unnoticed and untreated. If the diagnosis is even entertained, fluids should be initiated and consideration given to immediate propranolol treatment unless there is clinical evidence of heart failure. Use of intravenous propranolol is rare in the modern era. Those of us who grew up with that drug as the only beta-blocker available in intravenous form learned to administer it one (1) mg at a time watching the heart rate with great care for about 10 min after each dose. Once the diagnosis is confirmed, the other interventions come into play.

### Hypercalcemic Crisis

"Crisis" is fairly rare in hypercalcemia. The usual situation is that the lab reports a high calcium level following relatively nonspecific complaints as enumerated in the chapter. The goals are to stop the rise in calcium, get rid of excess calcium, make a diagnosis, and get to specific treatment. This is one of the few situations that a true "saline diuresis"—meaning the use of 0.9% saline—is indicated. We usually administer a liter to an adult and then follow with a loop diuretic such as furosemide, which will accelerate the excretion of calcium. If a sustained diuresis is required (more saline, more furosemide, often side by side as continuous infusions), then regular determinations of sodium, potassium, chloride, bicarbonate, magnesium, and phosphate should be made until the calcium level is near normal. Bear in mind that calcium stores are large and the condition can recur until a specific diagnosis is made and specific treatment is initiated.

### Adrenal Crisis

Adrenal crisis is potentially lethal. Fever, hyponatremia, hyperkalemia, and leukocytosis are common but of course can be masked by various treatments. Shock is fairly common, fluids are important, and making the diagnosis is even more important. Measurement of a random cortisol is usually diagnostic. If the patient is not terribly ill, then low-dose cosyntropin test is useful to verify the diagnosis. However, if the patient is at all unstable and the diagnosis, it is better to draw the random cortisol and immediately give a modest dose of hydrocortisone—the usual 100 mg is probably excessive, but no one will fault you—intravenously. Once that is done, the next step is a thorough review of prior medications—the most common cause of adrenal crisis th is unrecognized inadvertent interruption of pharmacologic glucocorticoid treatment sufficient to suppress the adrenal glands.

### Hypertensive Crisis Secondary to Pheochromocytoma

Pheochromocytoma is diagnosed either as incidental adrenal mass on imaging, based on clinical symptoms such as attacks of headache, palpitation, and sweating or based on positive family history. Generally, the first step in diagnosis where the diagnosis is suspected is to measure urinary and plasma fractionated metanephrines and catecholamines. The emergency aspect arises when the patient shows up with extremely high blood pressures. If nothing else is remembered, block alpha-adrenergic receptors first, and then beta-adrenergic receptors to suppress the reflex tachycardia and give fluids liberally. Once the blood pressure is controlled, it is well to reflect on whether one is dealing with an isolated pheochromocytoma, or alternatively with a multiple endocrine neoplasia, type 2a or 2b. Recall the different MEN syndromes:

MEN 1 = Parathyroid tumors, pancreatic tumors, and pituitary tumors

MEN 2a = Medullary thyroid cancers, pheochromocytoma, and parathyroid tumors

MEN 2b = Medullary thyroid cancers, pheochromocytoma, and neuromas

Appropriate testing should be done.

There are three other pearls that are worth mentioning in the context of surgical endocrine emergencies.

1. First, take a detailed medication history. Avoid precipitating an emergency such as adrenal insufficiency or symptomatic hypothyroidism, because there was an inadequate review of a medication list. Interrupt or discontinue such endocrine replacement therapies in surgical patients only with very good reason.
2. Second, endocrine emergencies in surgery are more commonly "medical" than "surgical." Avoid creating an emergency such as serotonin syndrome or hypoglycemia with casual administration of SSRIs (and the multiple drugs that interact with SSRIs to precipitate the serotonin syndrome) and hypoglycemic agents.
3. Third, recall that uncommon presentations of common problems are more common than common presentations of uncommon problems. Learn the myriad causes and presentations of hyperglycemic states, hypothyroidism, and the common electrolyte abnormalities in addition to the less common problems described in this chapter. All are important, but timely treatment of the less glamorous medical conditions will have a far greater impact on patients.

# Section III

# Surgical Critical Care

# 70

## *Bacteremia*

**Spyridon Fortis and Greg J. Beilman**

**CONTENTS**



### 70.1 Introduction

Bacteremia, the presence of bacteria in the bloodstream, was described more than a century ago by Libman, in 1897. Transient bacteremia can occur in daily activities such as tooth brushing with no clinical sequelae because the host immune system eliminates the bacteria. Bacteremia may occur after tooth brushing up to 50% depending on the intensity, while periodontal surgeries may be associated with an incidence rate of bacteremia as high as 90% [1]. Up to 16% of the patients may develop bacteremia after intubation or bronchoscopy, while bacteremia can occur in an average of 16% of patients in ICU after nasotracheal suctioning [1]. Gastrointestinal procedures may be associated with transient bacteremia in a rate that ranges from 0% to 17%, while the incidence of bacteremia after esophageal dilation can be as high as 45% [1]. Urinary tract interventions may be complicated with transient bacteremia in a rate of 11%–86% depending on the sterility of the urine and the intensity of the procedure [1]. The rate of transient bacteremia after a simple urinary catheterization is about 13%, while the incidence of bacteremia after a vaginal birth is about 3% [1]. When the host immune system fails to clear the bacteria, bacteremia can lead to blood stream infection (BSI) and sepsis. Since transient bacteremia is not associated with clinically significant conditions, the term bacteremia is reserved for bacteremia associated with clinical signs and is often used instead of BSI. Bacteremia and BSI can be further classified as primary or secondary. Primary BSI is a BSI without a known source [2]. In the presence of an indwelling catheter, a primary bacteremia is considered a catheter-related BSI [2]. The incidence of hospital-acquired BSI in United States is 189 per 100,000 person-years and BSI accounts for 2.2% of total admissions [3]. Half of the BSI take place in the ICU [4] and 5% of all ICU patients develop BSI [5]. BSI is a leading cause of death with a case fatality rate ranging from 10% to 60% [2]. In addition to being an important cause of death, BSIs lead to prolonged length of hospitalizations and higher cost of care [4,6].

In this chapter, we will review the literature concerning risk factors, the diagnosis, management, and prognosis of BSIs and provide recommendations as supported by the current level of evidence (Table 70.1).

#### 70.1.1 How Do We Identify Patients at Risk for Bacteremia?

A number of conditions and diseases that impair host immunity increase the risk for BSI. The incidence of BSI can be even 10 times greater in patients above 80 years of age compared to patients in their 40s and 50s [3,7]. Male sex increases the risk for BSI in the elder population but it is not a risk factor in younger ages [3,7]. Other risk factors for acquiring bacteremia (relative risk [RR], 95% confidence interval [95% CI]) are alcoholism (RR: 5.6; 95% CI: 3.8–8.0) chronic diseases and conditions such as diabetes mellitus (DM) (RR: 5.9; 95% CI: 4.4–7.8), heart disease (RR: 2.0; 95% CI: 1.4–3.0), hemodialysis (RR: 208.7, 95% CI: 142.9–296.3), HIV infection (RR: 7.8; 95% CI: 0.9–28.5), lung disease (RR: 3.8; 95% CI: 2.6–5.4), and malignancy (RR: 7.5; 95% CI: 5.3–10.3) [7]. Immunosuppressive medications, liver disease, obesity, and smoking are also risk factors for BSI [8].

Apart from host immunity, the risk of bacteremia depends on the location of the infection. The pretest probability of bacteremia in a patient with meningitis is 0.53, in a patient with pyelonephritis is 0.19–0.25 while in patients with community-acquired pneumonia is 0.07 and cellulitis is 0.02 [9]. Patients with septic shock have a pretest probability of bacteremia of 0.69, and patients with sepsis have a probability of 0.39 [9]. Patients from the community have a lower probability for BSI as opposed to patients from a health care facility [9].

A number of interventions and procedures increase patients at risk for bacteremia, particularly in ICU. The rate of bacteremia in ICU is higher than the rate in the general ward [4], but this is probably due to the increased number of interventions in the ICU such as central venous line, arterial lines, urinary catheters, mechanical ventilation, etc. Overall, the rate of BSI in patients with an intravascular catheter in ICU is about 0.6%–1% [10–12]. Central venous lines are one of the most common procedures and are associated with a 0.94% risk for BSI [11]. Arterial catheterization is an underrecognized cause of BSI with a rate between 0.68% and 0.96% [11,12]. Urinary catheters also carry a 0.4% risk for BSI [13]. Another very common intervention in the ICU that can result in bacteremia is invasive mechanical ventilation (MV). The rate of bacteremia in mechanically ventilated patient is about 8.7% [14]. Sorting out the rate of bacteremia from the ventilator alone is difficult as most patients also have additional lines. Red blood cell (RBC) transfusions in ICU are also associated with 1.65–5 times higher chance to acquire BSI [15] compared to patients that do not receive transfusions. Similarly, patients with gastrostomy and patients with parenteral nutrition are more likely to develop bacteremia [8,16].

Although patients in ICU are more likely to be complicated with bacteremia [4] due to more interventions, the distribution of most common isolated pathogens is similar in ICU and non-ICU patients [4]. Thirteen percent of all BSI are polymicrobial. Of monomicrobial cultures in ICU, coagulase-negative *Staphylococcus aureus* (*S. aureus*) (CoNS) is the most common isolate with 35.9% and *S. aureus* ranks second with 16.8%. *Candida* species (10.1%) come next and are followed by *Enterococci* (9.8%), *Enterobacter* species (4.7%), *Pseudomonas aeruginosa* (*P. aeruginosa*) (4.7%), *Klebsiella* species (4%), and *E. coli* (3.7%) [4]. As the age of population increases, the proportion of CoNS decreases to 27% in patients aged above 65 years, while *S. aureus* increases to 24% [4].

Is there any way to predict which patients have or will develop bacteremia? Which patients need blood cultures (BCs)? A recent meta-analysis of studies in ICU and non-ICU populations describes predictors of bacteremia [9]. The positive likelihood ratio (LR) of bacteremia in a patient with fever is 1.9 (95% CI: 1.4–2.4) while in a patient without fever, the negative LR is 0.54 (95% CI: 0.38–0.78) [9]. In patients with chills (shaking), the probability of bacteremia increases with a positive LR of 4.7 (95% CI: 3.0–7.2). Tachycardia is not a good predictor but absence of tachycardia decreases the chance for bacteremia with a negative LR of 0.67 (95% CI: 0.59–0.77). Elevated WBC has a positive LR for bacteremia between 1.3 and 1.7 depending on the cutoff, while leucopenia has LR of 2.5 (95% CI: 1.4–4.4). The absence of elevated WBC, however, is not helpful. The presence of SIRS increases the probability of bacteremia with a positive LR of 1.8 (95% CI: 1.6–2.0), while its absence has a negative LR of 0.09 (95% CI: 0.03–0.26) [9]. Septic shock or hypotension doubles the chance for bacteremia [9]. The clinician's impression is relatively reliable with a positive LR of 2.3 (95% CI: 1.4–3.6) when there is a high suspicion and a negative LR 0.48 (95% CI: 0.24–0.97) when there is a low suspicion [9]. A decision rule by Shapiro has similar accuracy with SIRS to predict bacteremia. According to Shapiro decision rule, the risk of bacteremia is low when none of the major criteria (suspicion of endocarditis, fever >39.4°C, indwelling catheter) and fewer than two minor criteria (fever >38.3°C, age >65 years, chills, vomiting, systolic blood pressure <90 mmHg, WBC >18,000 μL, creatinine >2 mg/dL) are present [9]. Both SIRS and Shapiro decision rule are very sensitive but not specific. From the rest of the few available scoring systems for the prediction of BSI, none of them provide superior accuracy to SIRS [9,17].

Procalcitonin is a promising biomarker for bacteremia. A procalcitonin level below 0.1 ng/mL can rule out bacteremia in patients with urosepsis with a sensitivity of 99% and negative predictive value of 98% [18]. However, according to a meta-analysis, its diagnostic ability for the detection of bacteremia in ambulatory patients is modest [19]. In a prospective study in patients with SIRS, a cutoff of 0.1 ng/mL failed to detect 7% of patients with bacteremia [20]. Although the utility of BC have been questioned [21,22], there are no available randomized clinical trial to assess whether affect the clinical outcome, because the mortality of critically ill patients with bacteremia is very high and can reach 60% [5,7], clinicians must be more proactive.

*Recommendation*: Because of the high mortality of patients in ICU with bacteremia, clinicians must be more vigilant. Based on one large meta-analysis and several prospective cohorts, BCs should be performed in patients with high clinical suspicion and pretest probability for bacteremia (Grade A recommendation). However, isolated fever or leukocytosis should not be considered sufficient to draw BCs in immunocompetent patients or those without suspicion of infectious endocarditis. SIRS or the Shapiro decision rule should be used to identify patients that do not need BCs (Grade A recommendation). Procalcitonin may be helpful to rule out the presence of bacteremia, but further studies are needed to determine the cutoff (Grade A recommendation).

### 70.1.2 What is the Protocol for Diagnosis of Bacteremia?

BCs are the current cornerstone for detection of BSIs [23]. A BC is defined as a specimen of blood obtained from a single venipuncture or intravascular access device. Peripheral blood draw is the preferred approach for obtaining BC. From a retrospective study in hospitalized patients, the false-positive ratio of peripheral BC was 2.6% versus 13% which is the false-positive ratio of catheter-drawn cultures [24]. The sensitivity, however, in both peripheral and catheter-drawn BCs of patients in ICU is low, with a range of 64.7%–65% for venipuncture, and 78%–82.4% for catheter-drawn BCs [25,26]. Obtaining BCs both from venipuncture and from catheters can increase the sensitivity [25–27]. Arterial catheter BCs have similar sensitivity with venipuncture or central venous line BC [24].

The yield of BCs to detect bacteremia also depends on the number of BCs. Cockerill and colleagues performed an observational study at the Mayo clinic and found that two BCs detected only 80% of blood stream infections, three detected 96% of blood stream infections and that four BCs were necessary to detect 100% of blood stream infections [28]. These findings were confirmed in another retrospective observational study performed by Lee et al. They analyzed their data to determine the cumulative sensitivity of BCs obtained sequentially during a 24 h time period. The results of their study demonstrated that two BCs in a 24 h period will detect approximately 90% of blood stream infections. They further concluded that to achieve a greater than 99% detection rate, as many as four BCs may be necessary. They further observed that *S. aureus* was the most likely microorganism to be detected with the initial BC and *Pseudomonas aeruginosa* and *Candida albicans* are the least likely blood stream pathogens to be detected with the initial BC [29].

The volume of BC should be at least 20 mL per draw [28]. A set of two 30 mL draws can detect more pathogens than a set of two 20 mL drawings and has similar sensitivity to a set of three 20 mL draws [30]. While volume of BC is crucial, drawing cultures at the time of fever does not affect the yield of BC to detect pathogens [31].

What is the relevance of the routine use of the anaerobic BC bottle? Classically, two bottles are collected routinely, an aerobic and an anaerobic bottle. However, Murray et al. conducted a retrospective review and demonstrated that the frequency of obligate anaerobic bacteremia has declined significantly and with the exception of obligate anaerobic bacteria, many organisms grow preferentially in aerobic bottles [32]. Based on these results, the routine use of two aerobic BCs with selective use of anaerobic bottles has been proposed in the literature. Grohs and colleagues performed a retrospective study on BCs focusing on the relevance of routine use of the anaerobic bottle and demonstrated that 13.5% of patients with a positive BC had a positive anaerobic bottle in the absence in any positive aerobic bottle and two-thirds of these grew with nonobligate anaerobes. Further, they demonstrated that in 64% of the BCs growing *Enterobacter,* the anaerobic bottles detected growth earlier than the corresponding aerobic bottle. They concluded that in their institution the use of anaerobic bottle is still relevant [23]. A recent study also showed that the addition of an anaerobic bottle increases the sensitivity [30].

From a technical aspect, the choice of skin disinfectant does not affect the contamination rate of BCs while delay of BC to be sent to the laboratory after collection may affect their accuracy [33].

Despite being the cornerstone for the diagnosis of bacteremia, BCs have certain limitations. These limitations are: delay in diagnosis, poor sensitivity for slow growing and fastidious organisms and decrease in sensitivity when blood samples are taken after the start of antimicrobial therapy [34,35]. New diagnostic techniques are necessary to increase the sensitivity and specificity, decrease turnaround time and reduce inhibitory effects of antibiotics on the detection of pathogens. One of the most promising developments is the direct detection of bacteria in whole blood with multiplex polymerase chain reaction (PCR) assays

Louie et al. performed a prospective cohort study to test multiplex PCR for simultaneous detection of multiple organisms in blood stream infections [34]. Two hundred adult patients at risk of blood stream infections had blood samples collected for PCR and BC. When PCR assay results were compared to BC results, PCR detected bacteria and fungi in 45 cases compared to 37 detected by BCs. More than 68% of PCR results were confirmed by blood, urine, and catheter cultures. PCR did not detect *Enterococcus faecalis* in five BC confirmed cases. In conclusion, multiplex PCR detected bacteria and fungi that were not found by BC, and BC identified organisms that were not detected by PCR. A major limitation of all molecular techniques is the lack of simultaneous provision of the antimicrobial susceptibility pattern [36,37]. Despite limitations of both methods, PCR may serve as an adjunct to BC to improve speed and sensitivity of detection of organisms in the case of bacteremia.

*Recommendation*: Despite the lack of level I evidence precluding grade A recommendations, BCs remain the gold standard for the diagnosis of blood stream infections. Until the advent of further microarray-based techniques, multiplex PCR methods may be used as an adjunct to BCs (Grade B Recommendation). Based on the currently available data, the number of BCs drawn and the use of anaerobic BC bottles should be left at the discretion of the clinician.

### 70.1.3 What is the Significance of Empiric Therapy in the Patient with Bacteremia?

Empiric therapy is defined as the initiation of an antimicrobial regimen in a patient with suspected infection before the type of infecting organism has been identified [38]. The administration of appropriate antibiotics in a timely manner is crucial to improving outcome. Failure of the empiric antimicrobial treatment in chronic ICU patients with high complexity may be related to the higher rate of infections from resistant microorganisms to the typical antibiotic coverage in this population. Appropriate empiric therapy has been shown to be a predictor of mortality in numerous analyses.

In a large prospective cohort study, Leibovici and colleagues reported mortality rates of 20% compared to 34% in patients receiving appropriate ($n$ = 2158) versus inappropriate ($n$ = 1255) antibiotic therapy ($p$ = 0.0001). Further, hospital stay of survivors who were given appropriate empirical treatment was shorter than in those given inappropriate treatment. They concluded that appropriate empirical antibiotic treatment was associated with a significant reduction in fatality in patients with BSIs [39].

Ibrahim et al. performed a prospective cohort study with 492 patients. They established that 29.9% of these patients received inadequate antimicrobial treatment for their bacteremia. The hospital mortality of these patients was statistically greater than the hospital mortality rate of patients with BSIs who received adequate treatment (62% vs. 28% respectively, $p$ = 0.001). Independent risk factors for inappropriate antimicrobial therapy were: BSIs with *Candida* species, prior antibiotic administration during the same hospitalization, low serum albumin concentration, and increasing central venous catheter duration [6]

A recent multinational prospective study in ICU population with 1156 patients showed that delay of appropriate treatment of BSI is associated with higher 28-day mortality. Among the patients with inadequate treatment the 28-day mortality was 48.7%, while in patients with adequate treatment, the 28-day mortality was 33.7% ($p$ < 0.0007) [40]. Timing to adequate treatment (before day 6 from blood collection) was also associated with higher mortality [40].

To decrease mortality, length of hospital stay and cost, appropriate empiric therapy should be initiated in a timely fashion. To achieve this goal, in the face of increasing antimicrobial resistance, it is necessary to follow hospital and if possible unit-specific pathogen type and sensitivity and resistance patterns of these pathogens causing BSIs. Another key to proper antibiotic selection is the patient's history of previous antibiotic therapy.

It is important to achieve a balance between the need for effective empiric antibiotic treatment and the potential risk of predisposing the patient to subsequent emergence of antibiotic-resistant infections. This goal may be achieved by early administration of effective antimicrobial treatment to patients with suspected BSI. With the availability of culture results, the antimicrobial regimen should then be rapidly tailored or discontinued.

*Recommendation*: The timely administration of effective empiric antimicrobial treatment in patients with suspected BSI leads to a decrease mortality rate (Grade B Recommendation). The choices in empiric antimicrobial agents should be based on knowledge of local distribution of pathogens and their resistance patterns, as well as the cause of BSI and recent administration of antimicrobial agents. This recommendation is based on the results of observational studies, as randomized control trials and withholding of treatment would not have been ethical (Grade B Recommendation).

### 70.1.4 When Can I Safely Stop Antibiotics for the Treatment of Bacteremia?

There have been no large randomized clinical trials in adults to guide us in our prescribing practices in treating patients with bacteremia. Great variability exists in the treatment duration for BSIs in the critically ill patient.

To have a better understanding of differences in current prescribing practices, Corona and colleagues performed a large-scale international survey by sending questionnaires to national and international intensive care societies. As expected, the responses from 254 ICUs in 34 countries revealed a wide variation in the duration of antibiotic treatment for bacteremia, ranging from short courses (≤5 days) of a restricted-spectrum antibiotic to long courses (≥10 days) of broad-spectrum antibiotics. The survey results further revealed that the greater the involvement of infectious disease specialists and/or microbiologists, the shorter was the duration of therapy ($p$ < 0.0001) [41].

Corona and colleagues' routine practice in their ICU at University College London Hospitals is to use short course monotherapy (5–6 days) for BSIs unless there was deep-seated infection present. The authors carried out a prospective observational study to assess their management policy by monitoring clinical response and relapse rate. From 84 bacteremic patients in the ICU, a total of 78 patients with BSIs were treated with short course monotherapy. The results demonstrated a death rate of 23.8% directly related to BSI and a satisfactory clinical response of 72%. The incidence of ICU-acquired resistant gram-negative bacteremias (6.5%) and fungemias (3%) were low. They further observed that none of the patients discharged from the ICU developed a bacteremic relapse. They concluded that a short-course antibiotic monotherapy strategy provides a satisfactory clinical response, low relapse rate, and no long-term infectious complications [38]. One of the limitations of this study was that only a small number of patients were involved.

In their guidelines for the management of intravascular catheter-related BSIs, Mermel and colleagues state that patients with catheter-related bacteremias are to be separated into those with complicated and uncomplicated infections. They describe complicated infections as those bacteremias associated with endocarditis, osteomyelitis, possible metastatic seeding, and septic thrombosis. They recommend 10–14 days of antimicrobial therapy in uncomplicated cases of bacteremia excluding BSIs with coagulase-negative staphylococci in which case they recommend only 5–7 days of antibiotic treatment. They further recommend 4–6 weeks of antibiotic therapy for complicated cases of bacteremia and in cases of persistent bacteremia or fungemia after catheter removal. In the presence of osteomyelitis, their recommendation is 6–8 weeks of antimicrobial therapy. The authors state that there are no compelling data to support their specific recommendations [42].

The only strong evidence for the duration of antimicrobial treatment comes from a recent meta-analysis that included small randomized clinical trial from both pediatric and adult populations with various severity and different types of infections. Only one study, included in the analysis, focused exclusively in bacteremia and this was in neonates. The rest of the treatment outcomes of bacteremic patients were derived from subgroup analysis of the different trials. The authors showed no difference between short (5–7 days) versus long (7–21 days) duration of antimicrobial treatment in terms of survival, clinical, and microbiological improvement [43].

*Recommendation*: Taking into consideration the cause of bacteremia and types of pathogens involved, clinicians should strive for the shortest course of antimicrobial treatment of BSIs, finding a balance between successful eradication of the infecting microorganism and low relapse rate and avoidance of drug toxicity, fungemia and development of antimicrobial resistance. Unless in the presence of complicated BSIs requiring a prolonged course of antimicrobial treatment, antibiotic therapy should be stopped with the resolution of bacteremia-related clinical findings and improvement in related organ dysfunction (Grade B). There is an urgent need for a large-scale randomized control trial to guide us in terms of optimal duration of antimicrobial treatment of BSIs.

### 70.1.5 What are Adjuvant Treatment for Bacteremia?

The treatment of bacteremia has traditionally focused around the control of the infectious source and the immunosuppressed status of the host. Immune status of the host is a main determinant of the outcome in BSI. A multinational prospective study in 132 ICUs from 26 different countries showed that increasing age (every decade) (OR: 1.14; 95% CI: 1.04–1.27), chronic liver failure (OR: 4.1; 95% CI: 1.44–11.67), and immunosuppression (OR: 1.64; 95% CI: 1.06–2.53) are associated with increased mortality [44]. Alcohol use, cancer, and pulmonary diseases also increase mortality in patients with bacteremia [40,45]. On the other side, trauma is associated with more favorable outcome [44], which may mean that bacteremia in this population result from transient loss of integrity of vascular compartmentalization and not from an infection. The medical (OR: 3.71; 95% CI: 2.01–6.95) and surgical patients (OR: 2.32; 95% CI: 1.10–4.97) are more likely to die if they are complicated with bacteremia compared to trauma patients [46]. Severity of the critical illness determines the prognosis of the bacteremic patients. Higher APACHE II [44,47] and SAPS II scores [44,46] are associated with increased mortality. Critically ill bacteremic patients with septic shock have about 3–12 times higher chance of death [44,47–49]. Acute kidney injury in bacteremic ICU patients with community-acquired pneumonia is associated with higher mortality (OR: 11.3; 95% CI: 6.6–19.4) [45,46].

Multidrug-resistant microorganism, Enterobacteriaceae other than *Escherichia coli, Pseudomonas, Candida* species are also associated with worse outcome [40,48].

Apart from the host- and pathogen-associated factors, interventions play an important role in the outcome of these patients. As we mentioned previously, early effective antimicrobial treatment is a major determinant of outcome [6,39,40]. Source control of the infection is another one [40]. The mortality can increase up to six times when infection source is uncontrolled [40].

Moreover, although traditionally the research about the outcome of infection and bacteremia has focused primarily on the pathogens (microorganism) and the immunosuppressed status of the host, excessive inflammatory response can also be deleterious. The hallmark of sepsis is an uncontrolled exaggerated pro-inflammatory response which mediates SIRS. Recently, compensatory anti-inflammatory response syndrome (CARS) has attracted more attention. CARS is the homeostatic mechanism of the host to deactivate the immune system and reduce the inflammatory response as opposed to SIRS. Both pro-inflammatory response (SIRS) and ant-inflammatory response (CARS) are present early in sepsis. Interventions to reduce the pro-inflammatory response and increase the anti-inflammatory response have been attempted with limited success. Glucocorticoids have

**TABLE 70.1**
Clinical Questions

| Question | Answer | Grade of Recommendation | References |
|---|---|---|---|
| How do we identify patients at risk for bacteremia? | Based on one large meta-analysis and several prospective cohorts, BCs should be ordered in patients with high clinical suspicion and pretest probability for bacteremia | A | [3,4,7–14,16–21] |
| What is the protocol for diagnosis of bacteremia? | BCs remain the gold standard. Multiple PCR methods can be used as an adjunct | B | [25,27–31,34,36,37] |
| What is the significance of empiric therapy in the patient with bacteremia? | Early administration of effective empiric antimicrobial treatment leads to a decrease in the mortality rate, duration of hospital stay, and hospital costs | B | [6,39,40] |
| When can I safely stop antibiotics for the treatment of bacteremia? | Unless in the presence of complicated BSIs requiring a prolonged course of antimicrobial treatment, antibiotic therapy should be stopped with the resolution of bacteremia-related clinical findings and improvement in related organ dysfunction. There is an urgent need for a large-scale randomized control trial to guide us in terms of optimal duration of antimicrobial treatment of BSIs | B | [43] |
| Are any adjuvant treatment for bacteremia? | Early recognition and early treatment with appropriate antimicrobial treatment and source control can reduce mortality. There are no available adjuvant treatment for bacteremia or sepsis | B | [40,50,51] |

not been shown to result in mortality benefit. However, the benefit of glucocorticoid administration is ambiguous as there is not a reliable diagnostic test to detect patients with overexaggerated inflammatory response [50]. Other anti-inflammatory agents like tifacogin, which is a recombinant tissue factor pathway inhibitor, or drotrecogin alfa, which is human recombinant–activated protein C have been tried with early positive results that failed to be sustained in following trials [51].

*Recommendation*: Mortality of critical ill patients with bacteremia increases in immunosuppressed patients. Certain pathogens like multidrug-resistant microorganism, pseudomonas, *Candida* species are associated with worse outcome. Patients with septic shock and high severity score have greater risk of death (Grade A). Early recognition and early treatment with appropriate antimicrobial treatment and source control can reduce mortality (Grade A). There are no currently adjuvant treatments for sepsis and bacteremia (Grade B).

## References


1. Durack DT. Prevention of infective endocarditis. *N Engl J Med.* 1995;332(1):38–44.
2. Juan-Torres A, Harbarth S. Prevention of primary bacteraemia. *Int J Antimicrob Agents.* 2007;30(Suppl 1):S80–S87.
3. Uslan DZ, Crane SJ, Steckelberg JM et al. Age- and sex-associated trends in bloodstream infection: A population-based study in Olmsted County, Minnesota. *Arch Intern Med.* 2007;167(8):834–839.
4. Wisplinghoff H, Bischoff T, Tallent SM, Seifert H, Wenzel RP, Edmond MB. Nosocomial bloodstream infections in US hospitals: Analysis of 24,179 cases from a prospective nationwide surveillance study. *Clin Infect Dis Offic Publ Infect Dis Soc Am.* 2004;39(3): 309–317.
5. Prowle JR, Echeverri JE, Ligabo EV et al. Acquired bloodstream infection in the intensive care unit: Incidence and attributable mortality. *Crit Care.* 2011;15(2):R100.
6. Ibrahim EH, Sherman G, Ward S, Fraser VJ, Kollef MH. The influence of inadequate antimicrobial treatment of bloodstream infections on patient outcomes in the ICU setting. *Chest.* 2000;118(1):146–155.
7. Laupland KB, Gregson DB, Zygun DA, Doig CJ, Mortis G, Church DL. Severe bloodstream infections: A population-based assessment. *Crit Care Med.* 2004;32(4): 992–997.
8. Kaye KS, Marchaim D, Chen TY et al. Predictors of nosocomial bloodstream infections in older adults. *J Am Geriatr Soc.* 2011;59(4):622–627.
9. Coburn B, Morris AM, Tomlinson G, Detsky AS. Does this adult patient with suspected bacteremia require blood cultures? *JAMA.* 2012;308(5):502–511.
10. Timsit JF, Schwebel C, Bouadma L et al. Chlorhexidine-impregnated sponges and less frequent dressing changes for prevention of catheter-related infections in critically ill adults: A randomized controlled trial. *JAMA.* 2009;301(12):1231–1241.

11. Lucet JC, Bouadma L, Zahar JR et al. Infectious risk associated with arterial catheters compared with central venous catheters. *Crit Care Med.* 2010;38(4): 1030–1035.
12. O'Horo JC, Maki DG, Krupp AE, Safdar N. Arterial catheters as a source of bloodstream infection: A systematic review and meta-analysis. *Crit Care Med.* 2014;42(6):1334–1339.
13. Srinivasan A, Karchmer T, Richards A, Song X, Perl TM. A prospective trial of a novel, silicone-based, silver-coated foley catheter for the prevention of nosocomial urinary tract infections. *Infect Control Hosp Epidemiol Offic J Soc Hosp Epidemiol Am.* 2006;27(1):38–43.
14. Ko HK, Yu WK, Lien TC et al. Intensive care unit-acquired bacteremia in mechanically ventilated patients: Clinical features and outcomes. *PLoS One.* 2013;8(12):e83298.
15. Michalia M, Kompoti M, Panagiotakopoulou A et al. Impact of red blood cells transfusion on ICU-acquired bloodstream infections: A case-control study. *J Crit Care.* 2012;27(6):655–661.
16. Pontes-Arruda A, Dos Santos MC, Martins LF et al. Influence of parenteral nutrition delivery system on the development of bloodstream infections in critically ill patients: An international, multicenter, prospective, open-label, controlled study—EPICOS study. *J Parenter Enteral Nutr.* 2012;36(5):574–586.
17. Paul M, Andreassen S, Nielsen AD et al. Prediction of bacteremia using TREAT, a computerized decision-support system. *Clin Infect Dis Offic Publ Infect Dis Soc Am.* 2006;42(9):1274–1282.
18. van Nieuwkoop C, Bonten TN, van't Wout JW et al. Procalcitonin reflects bacteremia and bacterial load in urosepsis syndrome: A prospective observational study. *Crit Care.* 2010;14(6):R206.
19. Jones AE, Fiechtl JF, Brown MD, Ballew JJ, Kline JA. Procalcitonin test in the diagnosis of bacteremia: A meta-analysis. *Ann Emerg Med.* 2007;50(1):34–41.
20. Hoenigl M, Raggam RB, Wagner J et al. Procalcitonin fails to predict bacteremia in SIRS patients: A cohort study. *Int J Clin Pract.* 2014;68(10):1278–1281.
21. Kennedy M, Bates DW, Wright SB, Ruiz R, Wolfe RE, Shapiro NI. Do emergency department blood cultures change practice in patients with pneumonia? *Ann Emerg Med.* 2005;46(5):393–400.
22. Chen Y, Nitzan O, Saliba W, Chazan B, Colodner R, Raz R. Are blood cultures necessary in the management of women with complicated pyelonephritis? *J Infect.* 2006;53(4):235–240.
23. Grohs P, Mainardi JL, Podglajen I et al. Relevance of routine use of the anaerobic blood culture bottle. *J Clin Microbiol.* 2007;45(8):2711–2715.
24. McBryde ES, Tilse M, McCormack J. Comparison of contamination rates of catheter-drawn and peripheral blood cultures. *J Hosp Infect.* 2005;60(2):118–121.
25. Beutz M, Sherman G, Mayfield J, Fraser VJ, Kollef MH. Clinical utility of blood cultures drawn from central vein catheters and peripheral venipuncture in critically ill medical patients. *Chest.* 2003;123(3):854–861.
26. Martinez JA, DesJardin JA, Aronoff M, Supran S, Nasraway SA, Snydman DR. Clinical utility of blood cultures drawn from central venous or arterial catheters in critically ill surgical patients. *Crit Care Med.* 2002;30(1):7–13.
27. Rodriguez L, Ethier MC, Phillips B, Lehrnbecher T, Doyle J, Sung L. Utility of peripheral blood cultures in patients with cancer and suspected blood stream infections: A systematic review. *Support Care Cancer Offic J Multinatl Assoc Support Care Cancer.* 2012;20(12): 3261–3267.
28. Cockerill FR, 3rd, Wilson JW, Vetter EA et al. Optimal testing parameters for blood cultures. *Clin Infect Dis Offic Publ Infect Dis Soc Am.* 2004;38(12):1724–1730.
29. Lee A, Mirrett S, Reller LB, Weinstein MP. Detection of bloodstream infections in adults: How many blood cultures are needed? *J Clin Microbiol.* 2007;45(11):3546–3548.
30. Patel R, Vetter EA, Harmsen WS, Schleck CD, Fadel HJ, Cockerill FR, 3rd. Optimized pathogen detection with 30- compared to 20-milliliter blood culture draws. *J Clin Microbiol.* 2011;49(12):4047–4051.
31. Riedel S, Bourbeau P, Swartz B et al. Timing of specimen collection for blood cultures from febrile patients with bacteremia. *J Clin Microbiol.* 2008;46(4):1381–1385.
32. Murray PR, Traynor P, Hopson D. Critical assessment of blood culture techniques: Analysis of recovery of obligate and facultative anaerobes, strict aerobic bacteria, and fungi in aerobic and anaerobic blood culture bottles. *J Clin Microbiol.* 1992;30(6):1462–1468.
33. Sautter RL, Bills AR, Lang DL, Ruschell G, Heiter BJ, Bourbeau PP. Effects of delayed-entry conditions on the recovery and detection of microorganisms from BacT/ALERT and BACTEC blood culture bottles. *J Clin Microbiol.* 2006;44(4):1245–1249.
34. Louie RF, Tang Z, Albertson TE, Cohen S, Tran NK, Kost GJ. Multiplex polymerase chain reaction detection enhancement of bacteremia and fungemia. *Crit Care Med.* 2008;36(5):1487–1492.
35. Peters RP, van Agtmael MA, Danner SA, Savelkoul PH, Vandenbroucke-Grauls CM. New developments in the diagnosis of bloodstream infections. *Lancet Infect Dis.* 2004;4(12):751–760.
36. Safdar N, Fine JP, Maki DG. Meta-analysis: Methods for diagnosing intravascular device-related bloodstream infection. *Ann Intern Med.* 2005;142(6):451–466.
37. DesJardin JA, Falagas ME, Ruthazer R et al. Clinical utility of blood cultures drawn from indwelling central venous catheters in hospitalized patients with cancer. *Ann Intern Med.* 1999;131(9):641–647.
38. Corona A, Wilson AP, Grassi M, Singer M. Short-course monotherapy strategy for treating bacteremia in the critically ill. *Minerva Anesthesiol.* 2006;72(10):841–857.
39. Leibovici L, Shraga I, Drucker M, Konigsberger H, Samra Z, Pitlik SD. The benefit of appropriate empirical antibiotic treatment in patients with bloodstream infection. *J Intern Med.* 1998;244(5):379–386.

40. Tabah A, Koulenti D, Laupland K et al. Characteristics and determinants of outcome of hospital-acquired bloodstream infections in intensive care units: The EUROBACT International Cohort Study. *Intens Care Med.* 2012;38(12):1930–1945.
41. Corona A, Bertolini G, Ricotta AM, Wilson A, Singer M. Variability of treatment duration for bacteraemia in the critically ill: A multinational survey. *J Antimicrob Chemother.* 2003;52(5):849–852.
42. Mermel LA, Farr BM, Sherertz RJ et al. Guidelines for the management of intravascular catheter-related infections. *J Intraven Nurs Offic Publ Intraven Nurs Soc.* 2001;24(3):180–205.
43. Havey TC, Fowler RA, Daneman N. Duration of antibiotic therapy for bacteremia: A systematic review and meta-analysis. *Crit Care.* 2011;15(6):R267.
44. Corona A, Bertolini G, Lipman J, Wilson AP, Singer M. Antibiotic use and impact on outcome from bacteraemic critical illness: The BActeraemia Study in Intensive Care (BASIC). *J Antimicrob Chemother.* 2010;65(6):1276–1285.
45. Lisboa T, Blot S, Waterer GW et al. Radiologic progression of pulmonary infiltrates predicts a worse prognosis in severe community-acquired pneumonia than bacteremia. *Chest.* 2009;135(1):165–172.
46. Magret M, Lisboa T, Martin-Loeches I et al. Bacteremia is an independent risk factor for mortality in nosocomial pneumonia: A prospective and observational multicenter study. *Crit Care.* 2011;15(1):R62.
47. Valles J, Palomar M, Alvarez-Lerma F et al. Evolution over a 15-year period of clinical characteristics and outcomes of critically ill patients with community-acquired bacteremia. *Crit Care Med.* 2013;41(1):76–83.
48. Sancho S, Artero A, Zaragoza R, Camarena JJ, Gonzalez R, Nogueira JM. Impact of nosocomial polymicrobial bloodstream infections on the outcome in critically ill patients. *Eur J Clin Microbiol Infect Dis Offic Publ Eur Soc Clin Microbiol.* 2012;31(8):1791–1796.
49. Ortega M, Marco F, Soriano A et al. Epidemiology and prognostic determinants of bacteraemic catheter-acquired urinary tract infection in a single institution from 1991 to 2010. *J Infect.* 2013;67(4):282–287.
50. Sprung CL, Annane D, Keh D et al. Hydrocortisone therapy for patients with septic shock. *N Engl J Med.* 2008;358(2):111–124.
51. Ranieri VM, Thompson BT, Barie PS et al. Drotrecogin alfa (activated) in adults with septic shock. *N Engl J Med.* 2012;366(22):2055–2064.

## Commentary on Bacteremia

*Donald H. Jenkins*

Described first more than a century ago, bacteremia is endemic in humans for actions as natural as childbirth and dental hygiene. It is quite common in the hospital setting from seemingly innocuous procedures (intubation, placement of a urinary catheter, endoscopy, etc.) with a fascinating regularity (1 in 6 such procedures may be associated with bacteremia despite the variability in these organ systems). The eventual outcome of transient, primary and secondary bacteremia depends on numerous factors that include: host defenses/weaknesses; virulence of the bacteria; source of the bacteria; presence of artificial devices and; urgency of diagnosis and action by the clinical team. Bacteremia is a serious condition, which can lead to significant complications, organ failure, prolonged hospitalization, and death. The authors have done a very nice job of answering all the questions posed and this is one of the most well-defined, studied, and reported topics in critical care literature, making many of their recommendations with the highest possible supporting evidence. In my personal experience and in the practice in which I have and currently work in, each recommendation presented is not only representative of that practice but also my personal approach to patients with bacteremia and appropriately based on the available evidence.

### How Do We Identify Patients at Risk for Bacteremia?

Nonmodifiable factors (age, gender, etc.) and chronic underlying conditions (lung/kidney disease, etc.), especially those related to immunocompromise, rise to the top of the factors placing patients at increased risk of bacteremia. Hospitalized patients, patients having undergone procedures, or placement of foreign bodies or who develop a hospital-acquired infection are more susceptible to development of bacteremia than outpatients without such risk factors. Patients requiring ICU are more susceptible than patients not requiring the level of invasive care (central venous catheters, endotracheal intubation, etc.) undertaken in the ICU. Even transfusion carries with it an increased risk of bacteremia. Patients receiving platelet transfusion are at a 10-fold increased risk of development of sepsis compared to patients receiving red blood cell transfusion (1:25,000 versus 1:250,000 incidence).*

* Blajchman MA, Beckers EAM, Dickmeiss E, Lin L, Moore G, Muylle L. Bacterial detection of platelets: Current problems and possible resolutions. *Transfus Med Rev.* 2005;19(4):259–272.

### What Is the Protocol for Diagnosis of Bacteremia?

The diagnosis involves establishing a level of suspicion that the patient has bacteremia and then acting on that suspicion. The presence of SIRS is likely the most sensitive marker of the presence of bacteremia. The authors provide a very nice summary of the components of SIRS and then describe the role of procalcitonin elevation in prediction/diagnosis of bacteremia. In many scenarios, the lack of elevation or presence of a given marker is more powerful in negative prediction than its presence is in the positive prediction of the presence of bacteremia. Blood cultures remain the hallmark test to diagnose bacteremia. Once a patient at risk is identified, diagnosis with multiple and possibly serial blood cultures are undertaken. Various protocols exist to direct the blood culture regimen. The more blood cultures drawn, the more cultures drawn peripherally, the more blood cultures drawn serially over time intervals, the more blood cultures drawn across the spectrum of types of microbes (aerobes, anaerobes, fungi, etc.) increase the likelihood of accurate diagnosis. Atleast 2–4 cultures, at least one including anaerobes and based upon patient risk factors and drawn peripherally, give the highest likelihood of accurate diagnosis. The location of the patient in the health care spectrum (home versus ICU) and underlying factors (immunocompromised transplant patient, abdominal abscess, etc.) will influence this process. PCR adds to this classic diagnostic regimen and has the potential to replace blood cultures in some of these clinical settings. Clinical areas caring for specific patient populations have well-established and frequently updated biograms elucidating the typical bacteria present in infections in that patient population as well as the susceptibilities of those microorganisms.

### What Is the Significance of Empiric Therapy in the Patient with Bacteremia?

Timing of initiation, selection of antimicrobial regimen, and duration of treatment have a significant role in eventual outcome for patients who develop bacteremia. Improved mortality, decreased ICU, and hospital length of stay and avoidance of other morbidities (e.g., organ failure) are the benefits of an aggressive and well-designed empiric antimicrobial regimen protocol based upon the patient population/unit location. A closely coordinated plan of care involving the primary clinical team, pharmacologists, microbiology, and infectious disease efforts are paramount to a successful treatment regimen.

### When Can I Safely Stop Antibiotics for Treatment of Bacteremia?

The duration of therapy remains one of the more controversial areas under the topic of bacteremia. Only half-jokingly do we often tell our team to treat the patient with antibiotics for a duration resembling a football score: 7–10, 10–14, 14–21, or 21–28 days. Microorganisms of low virulence and without an ongoing source (e.g., central line removed) can be treated with shorter duration regimens while those of a greater virulence and resistance profile without prompt source control (osteomyelitis, septic thrombi, etc.). Only ongoing study within the patient population and location can help to guide this regimen. The shortest, most accurate regimen would be best but must be monitored for recurrence/success. Microorganisms prone to rapid development of resistance should be treated with a broader regimen for a longer duration while monitoring potential side effects of the antimicrobial agents themselves.

### What Are Adjuvant Treatments for Bacteremia?

The adjuvant treatments for bacteremia are few and revolve mainly around source control. Draining infections, removing foreign bodies (pacemaker leads, arthroplasty hardware, central venous catheters), and optimizing patient condition (nutrition, oxygenation, prevention of organ dysfunction) where possible (you can't make the patient younger) are paramount to successful treatment of bacteremia. In today's electronic health care environment, rapid diagnosis may be more achievable than ever using the electronic medical record to inform the astute clinician to a constellation of signs and symptoms that indicates their patient is in the process of development of bacteremia or sepsis. Such "sniffers" have been developed and represent the future of surveillance for development of bacteremia, leading to even more rapid diagnosis and treatment. Logically, based upon the data presented by the authors, this would lead to decreased mortality and morbidity related to bacteremia. Development of even more rapid diagnostic tools would further this goal.

# 71

## *Prevention of Central Venous Catheter Infections*

**Antonio Aponte-Feliciano and Stephen O. Heard**

**CONTENTS**



Central venous catheter (CVC) infections are commonly known as catheter-related bloodstream infections (CRBSI) or central line-associated bloodstream infections (CLABSI). A CRBSI must satisfy specific laboratory criteria (e.g., catheter tip cultures and blood cultures growing the same organism, time to positivity of paired catheter blood and peripheral blood cultures) as to whether or not the catheter is the cause of the bacteremia [1]. A CLABSI is a surveillance definition: the presence of a primary bloodstream infection without any other obvious source in a patient who currently has or had a CVC 48 h prior to the positive blood cultures [1]. Either definition is reported as cases per 1000 catheter days. CRBSIs cause significant morbidity and result in an increased hospital length of stay (average of 12 days), increased health care costs by an average of $32,000 per episode, and, after adjusting for severity of illness, a 2.27-fold increased risk of death [2]. The Center for Disease Control and Prevention (CDC) has reported that ICU central line infections decreased by 58% from 2001 to 2009 resulting in about 6000 saved lives and an estimated savings of $414 million in excess health care costs for 2009 [3]. The most common pathogens causing CLABSIs are coagulase-negative *Staphylococci* spp., *Staphylococcus aureus*, *Enterococcus* spp., *Candida* spp., *Escherichia coli*, and *Klebsiella* spp. [4]. New data from participating ICUs in the CDC National Nosocomial Infections Surveillance System and the National Healthcare Safety Network [5] demonstrate that since 2006 adult ICU CLABSIs have decreased annually by 18% for *S. aureus*, 18% for *Enterococcus* species, 16% for gram-negative organisms, and 14% for *Candida* species. This reduction is the result of the adoption of evidence-based practices to reduce CLABSI. These practices will be reviewed in this chapter.

### 71.1 What Is the Best Site to Insert Intravascular Catheters?

In a randomized controlled trial of three different insertion sites in ICU patients, Merrer et al. found that the femoral site had a significantly higher rate of colonization when compared to the subclavian site, and a trend toward a higher rate of CRBSI [6]. Subsequent observational studies corroborated those findings with few exceptions. Evidence from multiple randomized and/or prospective trials designed to evaluate the effectiveness of anti-infective or multiple lumen catheters have shown that the subclavian insertion site is associated with the lowest rate of significant catheter colonization, followed by the internal jugular (IJ) and then the femoral site [7]. Recent meta-analyses of this issue give conflicting results. One concluded that the subclavian site was associated with the lowest risk of infection [8], whereas the other found no difference in infection rates among the three sites [9]. Differences in the studies that were included in each analysis, channeling, confounding bias, and heterogeneity likely explain the differences between the two meta-analyses.

*Recommendation*: The subclavian site is the preferred site for catheter insertion (Grade B).

## 71.2 What Is Needed to Prevent Contamination during Catheter Insertion?

Adherence to strict sterile technique during insertion of the catheter is considered important to prevent catheter and site contamination. The classic randomized, controlled trial by Raad et al. demonstrated that the use of maximum barrier precautions reduces the incidence of CRBSI [10]. However, one recent prospective randomized trial in general surgery patients failed to demonstrate that the use of maximum barrier precautions reduced the incidence of CRBSI [11]. Nonetheless, numerous studies continue to support maximum barrier precautions as part of an overall bundle to prevent CRBSI in the adult and pediatric populations [12,13].

*Recommendation*: Maximum barrier precautions (cap, mask, sterile gown and gloves, and a sterile drape that completely covers the patient) should be used during catheter insertion (Grade B).

## 71.3 What Is the Role of Chlorhexidine in Insertion and Management of Central Venous Catheters?

### 71.3.1 Insertion

Skin antisepsis is an important component in preparing for catheter insertion and postinsertion care. Several studies have evaluated and compared a variety of skin antiseptics. Chaiyukaunlapruk et al. demonstrated that chlorhexidine solutions were the best skin antiseptic agents to reduce catheter colonization and CRBSI in a meta-analysis of eight randomized controlled trials comparing the effectiveness of chlorhexidine to povidone-iodine solutions [14]. Other limited data demonstrated that the combination of alcoholic chlorhexidine (0.5%/70%) and 10% povidone-iodine was more effective than either alone in preventing catheter colonization. A cost analysis study showed that the use of a chlorhexidine skin prep resulted in a cost reduction of $113 per catheter [15].

### 71.3.2 Management

Timsit et al. performed a randomized prospective trial of chlorhexidine-impregnated sponges and found that the incidence of CBRSI was significantly lower in the chlorhexidine sponge group. Furthermore, the frequency of dressing change could be extended from 3 to 7 days without increasing the risk of catheter infection [16]. A recent meta-analysis of nine randomized controlled trials evaluating the effectiveness of chlorhexidine-impregnated dressings for the prevention of CRBSI also found that the use of chlorhexidine-impregnated dressings significantly reduced the incidence of catheter colonization and CRBSIs [17].

In an observational cohort study with historical controls, Dixon and Carver demonstrated that daily 2% chlorhexidine gluconate nonrinse cloth bathing significantly reduced the rate of CLABSI from 12.07 to 3.17 per 1000 catheter days [18]. Other data showed that chlorhexidine gluconate bathing of trauma patients decreased the rate of colonization by methicillin-resistant *S. aureus* and *Acinetobacter* species and decreased the rate of CLABSI from 8.4 to 2.1 per 1000 catheter days [19]. However, the salutatory effect of chlorhexidine may be due to the reduction of false-positive CLABSIs as several studies have shown that daily chlorhexidine bathing decreases skin bacterial colonization thereby leading to a lower contamination rate of blood cultures and as a consequence fewer false positives. Nonetheless, Climo et al., in a randomized, nonblinded, cluster trial evaluating the effect of chlorhexidine bathing on the rate of CLABSI, showed that chlorhexidine bathing decreased both skin colonization and CLABSI rates (gram-positive organisms and fungi) [20].

*Recommendation*: An aqueous or alcoholic chlorhexidine solution is the preferred skin antiseptic prior to catheter insertion and during catheter maintenance (Grade A). Chlorhexidine-impregnated dressings at the entry point of the central line have been shown to reduce catheter colonization and CLABSI (Grade A). Dressing changes can be performed between 3 and 7 days when chlorhexidine sponges are used. The dressings should be monitored closely for separation, soiling, or leaking to prevent contamination (Grade A). Chlorhexidine gluconate bathing helps reduce skin colonization with a further decrease in the rates of CLABSI and false-positive blood cultures (Grade B).

## 71.4 Is Education Useful in Preventing CRBSI?

Available evidence shows that catheterization by less experienced providers is associated with a higher risk of infection. Sherertz et al. showed that an educational didactic program and a "hands-on" demonstration of insertion of both arterial and CVCs offered to beginning PGY-1 physicians resulted in a steady and significant reduction in catheter-related infection over time [21]. Coopersmith et al. [22] used a focused educational initiative that consisted of a self-study module with a pretest and posttest that had to be completed by interns, ICU nurses, residents, and attending physicians. When the educational program was implemented, a sustained reduction in CLABSI was documented in both surgical and medical ICUs. Similar educational interventions have resulted in reductions in CRBSI in nonteaching, community hospitals. Simulation-based medical education has emerged as a frequent tool to aid medical schools and residency programs in the training of medical students and residents. Barsuk et al., in two observational cohort studies, used a simulation-based CVC placement learning program and showed a significant decrease in CLABSIs when compared to the presimulation period [23]. In a randomized, controlled single-blinded trial, Khouli et al. evaluated the sterile technique during simulated central vein catheterization by medical residents. They found subsequent to this intervention that the incidence of CLABSI decreased threefold [24].

*Recommendation*: An education program for all staff including nurses, physicians, and affiliate practitioners will reduce the risk of CLABSI (Grade B). A simulation-based education program in conjunction with video training will assist in decreasing CLABSI rates (Grade A).

## 71.5 How Frequently Should Catheters Be Changed?

The risk of significant catheter colonization and/or CLABSI does not increase with the length of catheterization, as shown in numerous studies summarized by Timsit [25]. Small underpowered studies using CVCs, peripheral arterial catheters, and pulmonary artery catheters demonstrated that routine changes irrespective of method did not result in a reduction of infection rates [26,27]. Furthermore, Cook et al. performed a meta-analysis of 12 prospective randomized trials and determined that scheduled guide wire changes were associated with a higher risk of catheter colonization and a trend toward a higher risk of CLABSI [28]. However, a decrease in the rate of mechanical complications was noted with scheduled guide wire changes compared to insertion at a new site. It is recommended that catheters should be removed as soon as they are not needed [29].

*Recommendation*: Catheters should not be routinely changed. If the catheter needs to be changed, a new insertion site should be used unless mechanical complications are expected; risk versus benefit evaluation should be exercised (Grade B).

## 71.6 Should Anti-Infective Catheters Be Utilized?

In the United States, three anti-infective catheters with different protective coatings or impregnated materials are currently commercially available: (1) second-generation chlorhexidine and silver sulfadiazine, (2) minocycline–rifampin, and (3) silver in a carbon/platinum matrix. Wang et al. showed in a recent network meta-analysis that most anti-infective-impregnated catheters are effective in reducing catheter colonization [30]. When compared to standard catheters, minocycline–rifampin catheters are the most efficacious in reducing CRBSI [30,31]. However, the use of anti-infective catheters is an ineffective way to reduce CRBSIs in ICUs where the baseline rates of infection are low [32].

*Recommendation*: Anti-infective catheters will reduce catheter colonization and CLABSI if the endemic rates are high (Grade A).

## 71.7 Do Anti-Infective Catheters Promote Antibiotic Resistance?

The increased use of antiseptic or antibiotic-impregnated catheters has raised fears about the development of antiseptic or antibiotic resistance. Several randomized, prospective controlled trials by Maki et al. [33], Brun-Buisson et al. [34], and Rupp et al. [35] suggest that the chlorhexidine–silver sulfadiazine catheters do not promote antiseptic nor antibiotic resistance. Rosato et al. did not observe antiseptic resistance in coagulase-negative *Staphylococcus* isolates exposed to silver sulfadiazine and chlorhexidine in vitro [36]. In a retrospective cohort study using the minocycline and rifampin-impregnated catheters, Chatzinikolaou et al.

demonstrated no change in the susceptibility of staphylococcal strains to minocycline or rifampin [37]. Furthermore, in vitro studies and randomized control trials evaluating the minocycline–rifampin-impregnated catheters suggest that bacterial resistance does not develop; however, small increases in the minimum inhibitory concentration of either antibiotic with *S. epidermidis* may occur [38–40]. In a retrospective clinical cohort study, Ramos et al. [41] evaluated catheters placed from 1999 to 2006 (8009 patients) at a tertiary university-based cancer center before and after switching to catheters impregnated with minocycline and rifampin. During the study period the incidence of CRBSIs gradually decreased from 8.3 to 1.2 per 1000 catheter days after the implementation of an infection control bundle and the use of the antibacterial-coated CVC. They found no evidence of change in the sensitivity of staphylococcal isolates from their ICU to tetracycline or rifampin.

*Recommendation*: The use of impregnated catheters with antibiotics or antiseptics does not promote antibiotic or antiseptic resistance (Grade B).

## 71.8 What Evidence Is Available on Peripherally Inserted Central Catheters?

Peripherally inserted central catheters (PICCs) are not immune to develop CLABSIs. Much of the literature available on these catheters is derived from oncology studies. Cotogni et al. performed a single-center prospective observational study, and found a total CLABSI rate of 0.05 cases/1000 catheter days [42]. In another prospective study, Bellesi et al. found a rate of 1.5 cases per 1000 catheter days [43]. In both studies, the PICCs were inserted and cared for by specialized teams. In addition, a meta-analysis by Chopra et al. determined that PICCs carry a lower risk of CLABSI when compared to CVCs in the outpatient population [44]. The data for hospitalized patients are conflicting. Two small single-center retrospective cohort studies showed a trend toward decreased infection rates with PICC lines in surgical and burn ICUs when compared to CVCs [45,46]. However, a retrospective analysis of prospective randomized studies of chlorhexidine sponge dressings showed no difference in the rate of CLABSI between standard CVCs and PICCs [47].

*Recommendation*: PICC lines are associated with lower incidence of CLABSI in the outpatient setting (Grade B). There is no difference in the incidence of PICC-related CLABSI in the inpatient setting when compared to standard central lines (Grade B).

## 71.9 What Is the Evidence Available if We Bundle the Aforementioned Techniques and Recommendations?

Berenholtz et al. [32] utilized and modified the existing behavioral and educational model to prevent CLABSI. Their intervention consisted of five parts:

1. An online education program (including the following recommendations: *preinsertion*, subclavian vein as preferred insertion site, hand hygiene, chlorhexidine skin preparation; *during insertion*, full barrier precautions, maintenance of sterile field; *postinsertion*, proper catheter care) and a test that all practitioners were required to take and pass before they could insert CVCs.
2. Creation of a central line insertion cart that included all necessary equipment and supplies.
3. Use of a check list during daily rounds where the need for CVC was reviewed.
4. Use of a checklist by the bedside nurse to insure adherence to best practices during insertion of a CVC.
5. Empowering nurses to stop the procedure as soon as the best practice guidelines were not met.

They found that bundle program resulted in sustained reductions in CLABSIs. Subsequently, Pronovost et al. [48] demonstrated that a similar educational and interventional program introduced into 108 ICUs in the state of Michigan resulted in a sustained reduction in CBSI for up to 18 months. Incidence-rate ratios of CLABSI were 2.7/1000 catheter days at baseline and decreased continuously from 0.62 at the 0–3-month time interval to 0.34 at the 16–18-month interval. A 36th-month follow-up revealed a sustained reduction on central line-related infections. Multiple recently published studies continue to support the notion that a bundled approach to catheter insertion and care will reduce the rate of CLABSI [13,49] (Table 71.1).

*Recommendation*: The use of catheter bundles or multimodal interventional programs reduces the incidence of CLABSI (Grade B).

**TABLE 71.1**

Summary of Evidence-Based Questions for the Prevention of Central Venous Catheter Infections

| Question | Answer | Levels of Evidence | Grade of Recommendation | References |
|---|---|---|---|---|
| What is the best site to insert intravascular catheters? | The subclavian site is the preferred site for catheter insertion. | 1B, 2A | B | [6–9] |
| What is needed to prevent contamination? | Maximum barrier precautions (cap, mask, sterile gown and gloves, and a sterile drape that completely covers the patient) should be used during catheter insertion. | 1B, 2A | B | [10–13] |
| What is the role of chlorhexidine in insertion and management of central venous catheters? | An aqueous or alcoholic chlorhexidine solution is the preferred skin antiseptic prior to catheter insertion and during catheter maintenance. | 1A | A | [14,15] |
| | Chlorhexidine-impregnated dressings at the entry point of the central line have been shown to reduce catheter colonization and CLABSI. | 1A | A | [16,17] |
| | Dressing changes can be performed between 3 and 7 days when chlorhexidine sponges are used. The dressings should be monitored closely for separation, soiling, or leaking to prevent contamination. | 1B | A | [16] |
| | Chlorhexidine gluconate bathing helps reduce skin colonization with a further decrease in the rates of CLABSI and false-positive blood cultures. | 2A | B | [18–20] |
| Is education useful in preventing CRBSI? | An education program for all staff including nurses, physicians, and affiliate practitioners will reduce the risk of CRBSI. | 2A | B | [21,22] |
| | A simulation-based education program in conjunction with video training will assist in decreasing CRBSI rates. | 2A | B | [23,24] |
| How frequent should catheters be changed? | Catheters should not be routinely changed. If the catheter needs to be changed, a new insertion site should be used unless mechanical complications are expected; risk versus benefit evaluation should be exercised. | 1B, 2A | B | [25–29] |
| Should anti-infective catheters be utilized? | Anti-infective catheters will reduce catheter colonization and CLABSI if the endemic rates are high. | 1A | A | [30–32] |
| Do anti-infective catheters promote antibiotic resistance? | The use of impregnated catheters with antibiotics or antiseptics does not change sensitivities to chlorhexidine, silver sulfadiazine, minocycline, or rifampin. | 2A | B | [33–41] |
| What evidence is available on peripherally inserted central catheters (PICC)? | PICC lines are associated with a lower incidence of CLABSI in the outpatient setting. | 2A | B | [42–44] |
| | There is no difference in the incidence of PICC-related CLABSI in the inpatient setting when compared to standard central lines. | 2A | B | [45–47] |
| What is the evidence available if we bundle the aforementioned techniques and recommendations? | The use of catheter bundles or multimodal interventional programs will reduce the incidence of CLABSI. | 2A | B | [13,32,48,49] |

## References


1. Chen XX, Lo YC, Su LH, Chang CL. Investigation of the case numbers of catheter-related bloodstream infection overestimated by the central line-associated bloodstream infection surveillance definition. *J Microbiol Immunol Infect.* 2014. http://dx.doi.org/10.1016/j.jmii.2014.03.006.
2. Steven V, Geiger K, Concannon C, Nelson RE, Brown J, Dumvati G. Inpatient costs, mortality and 30 day readmissions in patients with central-line-associated bloodstream infections. *Clin Microbiol Infect.* 2014;20:318–324.
3. Vital signs: Central line-associated blood stream infections—United States, 2001, 2008, and 2009. *MMWR Morb Mortal Wkly Rep.* March 4, 2011;60(8):243–248.
4. Wisplinghoff H, Bischoff T, Tallent SM, Seifert H, Wenzel RP, Edmond MB. Nosocomial bloodstream infections in US hospitals: Analysis of 24,179 cases from a prospective nationwide surveillance study. *Clin Infect Dis.* 2004;39(3):309–317.
5. Fagan RP, Edwards JR, Park BJ, Fridkin SK, Magill SS. Incidence trends in pathogen-specific central line-associated bloodstream infections in US intensive care units, 1990–2010. *Infect Control Hosp Epidemiol.* 2013;34(9):893–899.

6. Merrer J, De Jonghe B, Golliot F et al. French Catheter Study Group in Intensive Care. Complications of femoral and subclavian venous catheterization in critically ill patients: A randomized controlled trial. *JAMA.* 2001;286(6):700–707.
7. Heard SO, Wagle M, Vijayakumar E et al. Influence of triple-lumen central venous catheters coated with chlorhexidine and silver sulfadiazine on the incidence of catheter- related bacteremia. *Arch Intern Med.* 1998;158(1):81–87.
8. Parienti JJ, du Cheyron D, Timsit JF et al. Meta-analysis of subclavian insertion and nontunneled central venous catheter-associated infection risk reduction in critically ill adults. *Crit Care Med.* 2012;40(5):1627–1634.
9. Marik PE, Flemmer M, Harrison W. The risk of catheter-related bloodstream infection with femoral venous catheters as compared to subclavian and internal jugular venous catheters: A systematic review of the literature and meta-analysis. *Crit Care Med.* 201240(8):2479–2485.
10. Raad, II, Hohn DC, Gilbreath BJ et al. Prevention of central venous catheter-related infections by using maximal sterile barrier precautions during insertion. *Infect Control Hosp Epidemiol.* 1994;15(4 Pt 1):231–238.
11. Ishikawa Y, Kiyama T, Haga Y et al. Maximal sterile barrier precautions do not reduce catheter-related bloodstream infections in general surgery units: A multi-institutional randomized controlled trial. *Ann Surg.* 2010;251(4):620–623.
12. Tang HJ, Lin HL, Lin YH, Leung PO, Chuang YC, Lai CC. The impact of central line insertion bundle on central line-associated bloodstream infection. *BMC Infect Dis.* 2014;14:356.
13. Walz JM, Ellison RT, 3rd, Mack DA et al. The Bundle "Plus": The effect of a multidisciplinary team approach to eradicate central line-associated bloodstream infections. *Anesth Analg.* 2013.
14. Chaiyakunapruk N, Veenstra DL, Lipsky BA, Saint S. Chlorhexidine compared with povidone-iodine solution for vascular catheter-site care: A meta-analysis. *Ann Intern Med.* 2002;136(11):792–801.
15. Chaiyakunapruk N, Veenstra DL, Lipsky BA, Sullivan SD, Saint S. Vascular catheter site care: The clinical and economic benefits of chlorhexidine gluconate compared with povidone iodine. *Clin Infect Dis.* 2003;37(6):764–771.
16. Timsit JF, Schwebel C, Bouadma L et al. Chlorhexidine-impregnated sponges and less frequent dressing changes for prevention of catheter-related infections in critically ill adults: A randomized controlled trial. *JAMA.* 2009;301(12):1231–1241.
17. Safdar N, O'Horo JC, Ghufran A et al. Chlorhexidine-impregnated dressing for prevention of catheter-related bloodstream infection: A meta-analysis. *Crit Care Med.* 2014;42(7):1703–1713.
18. Dixon JM, Carver RL. Daily chlorhexidine gluconate bathing with impregnated cloths results in statistically significant reduction in central line-associated bloodstream infections. *Am J Infect Control.* 2010;38(10):817–821.
19. Evans HL, Dellit TH, Chan J, Nathens AB, Maier RV, Cuschieri J. Effect of chlorhexidine whole-body bathing on hospital-acquired infections among trauma patients. *Arch Surg.* 2010;145(3):240–246.
20. Climo MW, Yokoe DS, Warren DK et al. Effect of daily chlorhexidine bathing on hospital-acquired infection. *N Engl J Med.* 2013;368(6):533–542.
21. Sherertz RJ, Ely EW, Westbrook DM et al. Education of physicians-in-training can decrease the risk for vascular catheter infection. *Ann Intern Med.* 2000;132(8):641–648.
22. Coopersmith CM, Rebmann TL, Zack JE et al. Effect of an education program on decreasing catheter-related bloodstream infections in the surgical intensive care unit. *Crit Care Med.* 2002;30(1):59–64.
23. Barsuk JH, Cohen ER, Potts S et al. Dissemination of a simulation-based mastery learning intervention reduces central line-associated bloodstream infections. *BMJ Qual Safety.* 2014;23(9):749–756.
24. Khouli H, Jahnes K, Shapiro J et al. Performance of medical residents in sterile techniques during central vein catheterization: Randomized trial of efficacy of simulation-based training. *Chest.* 2011;139(1):80–87.
25. Timsit JF. Scheduled replacement of central venous catheters is not necessary. *Infect Control Hosp Epidemiol.* 2000;21(6):371–374.
26. Cobb DK, High KP, Sawyer RG et al. A controlled trial of scheduled replacement of central venous and pulmonary-artery catheters. *N Engl J Med.* 1992;327(15):1062–1068.
27. Eyer S, Brummitt C, Crossley K, Siegel R, Cerra F. Catheter-related sepsis: Prospective, randomized study of three methods of long-term catheter maintenance. *Crit Care Med.* 1990;18(10):1073–1079.
28. Cook D, Randolph A, Kernerman P et al. Central venous catheter replacement strategies: A systematic review of the literature. *Crit Care Med.* 1997;25(8):1417–1424.
29. O'Grady NP, Alexander M, Burns LA et al. Summary of recommendations: Guidelines for the Prevention of Intravascular Catheter-related Infections. *Clin Infect Dis.* 2011;52(9):1087–1099.
30. Wang H, Huang T, Jing J et al. Effectiveness of different central venous catheters for catheter-related infections: A network meta-analysis. *J Hosp Infect.* 2010;76(1):1–11.
31. Darouiche RO, Raad II, Heard SO et al. A comparison of two antimicrobial-impregnated central venous catheters. Catheter Study Group. *N Engl J Med.* 1999;340(1):1–8.
32. Berenholtz SM, Pronovost PJ, Lipsett PA et al. Eliminating catheter-related bloodstream infections in the intensive care unit. *Crit Care Med.* 2004;32(10):2014–2020.
33. Maki DG, Stolz SM, Wheeler S, Mermel LA. Prevention of central venous catheter-related bloodstream infection by use of an antiseptic-impregnated catheter. A randomized, controlled trial *Ann Intern Med.* 1997;127(4):257–266.
34. Brun-Buisson C, Doyon F, Sollet JP, Cochard JF, Cohen Y, Nitenberg G. Prevention of intravascular catheter-related infection with newer chlorhexidine-silver sulfadiazine-coated catheters: A randomized controlled trial. *Intensive Care Med.* 2004;30(5):837–843.

35. Rupp ME, Lisco SJ, Lipsett PA et al. Effect of a second-generation venous catheter impregnated with chlorhexidine and silver sulfadiazine on central catheter-related infections: A randomized, controlled trial. *Ann Intern Med.* 2005;143(8):570–580.
36. Rosato AE, Tallent SM, Edmond MB, Bearman GM. Susceptibility of coagulase-negative staphylococcal nosocomial bloodstream isolates to the chlorhexidine/silver sulfadiazine-impregnated central venous catheter. *Am J Infect Control.* 2004;32(8):486–488.
37. Chatzinikolaou I, Hanna H, Graviss L et al. Clinical experience with minocycline and rifampin-impregnated central venous catheters in bone marrow transplantation recipients: Efficacy and low risk of developing staphylococcal resistance. *Infect Control Hosp Epidemiol.* 2003;24(12):961–963.
38. Sampath LA, Tambe SM, Modak SM. In vitro and in vivo efficacy of catheters impregnated with antiseptics or antibiotics: Evaluation of the risk of bacterial resistance to the antimicrobials in the catheters. *Infect Control Hosp Epidemiol.* 2001;22:640–646.
39. Munson EL, Heard SO, Doern GV. In vitro exposure of bacteria to antimicrobial impregnated-central venous catheters does not directly lead to the emergence of antimicrobial resistance. *Chest.* 2004;126(5):1628–1635.
40. Aslam S, Darouiche RO. Prolonged bacterial exposure to minocycline/rifampicin-impregnated vascular catheters does not affect antimicrobial activity of catheters. *J Antimicrob Chemother.* 2007;60(1):148–151.
41. Ramos ER, Reitzel R, Jiang Y et al. Clinical effectiveness and risk of emerging resistance associated with prolonged use of antibiotic-impregnated catheters: More than 0.5 million catheter days and 7 years of clinical experience. *Crit Care Med.* 2011;39(2):245–251.
42. Cotogni P, Barbero C, Garrino C et al. Peripherally inserted central catheters in non-hospitalized cancer patients: 5-Year results of a prospective study. *Support Care Cancer.* 2014.
43. Bellesi S, Chiusolo P, De Pascale G et al. Peripherally inserted central catheters (PICCs) in the management of oncohematological patients submitted to autologous stem cell transplantation. *Support Care Cancer.* 2013;21(2):531–535.
44. Chopra V, O'Horo JC, Rogers MA, Maki DG, Safdar N. The risk of bloodstream infection associated with peripherally inserted central catheters compared with central venous catheters in adults: A systematic review and meta-analysis. *Infect Control Hosp Epidemiol.* 2013;34(9):908–918.
45. Gunst M, Matsushima K, Vanek S, Gunst R, Shafi S, Frankel H. Peripherally inserted central catheters may lower the incidence of catheter-related blood stream infections in patients in surgical intensive care units. *Surg Infect (Larchmt).* 2011;12(4):279–282.
46. Fearonce G, Faraklas I, Saffle JR, Cochran A. Peripherally inserted central venous catheters and central venous catheters in burn patients: A comparative review. *J Burn Care Res.* 2010;31(1):31–35.
47. Safdar N, Maki DG. Risk of catheter-related bloodstream infection with peripherally inserted central venous catheters used in hospitalized patients. *Chest.* 2005;128(2):489–495.
48. Pronovost P, Needham D, Berenholtz S et al. An intervention to decrease catheter-related bloodstream infections in the ICU. *N Engl J Med.* 2006;355(26):2725–2732.
49. DePalo VA, McNicoll L, Cornell M, Rocha JM, Adams L, Pronovost PJ. The Rhode Island ICU collaborative: A model for reducing central line-associated bloodstream infection and ventilator-associated pneumonia statewide. *Qual Safety Health Care.* 2010;19(6):555–561.

## Commentary on the Prevention of Central Venous Catheter Infections

*Addison K. May*

While your spouse may not appreciate compulsivity much in the home, compulsivity in the delivery of health care nearly always leads to higher quality. Sweat the small stuff; attention to detail matters in health care quality. Humans, however, are poor at maintaining high compliance with simple routine tasks without appropriate systems in place to support performance. These truisms are well demonstrated in the literature regarding the prevention of central venous catheter infections. This chapter successfully and succinctly outlines the current recommendations regarding the prevention of central venous catheter infections. Somewhat implied, but not explicitly stated, are the vagaries of the quality and safety medical literature, where the success of any one intervention may be dependent on the presence or absence of a set of conditions or other interventions. These may be unknown and unmeasured. Change a single condition or intervention and the results from quality efforts may change.

Central line–associated blood stream infections (CLABSIs) have declined significantly in the past decade. The acceptance and application of a number of practices in central line insertion and maintenance likely has contributed significantly to this reduction. Whether or not this reduction in CLABSI translates linearly to a reduction in central line–related blood stream infections (CLRBSIs) remains unknown. As highlighted in this chapter, CLABSI is a term used for surveillance, alterable by interventions that do not change the actual infection rate. The most obvious—"no blood culture, no CLABSI." While public reporting appropriately creates pressure to lower CLABSI rates, this pressure encourages both preventive strategies and strategies to reduce reporting. As the CLABSI definition begins with a positive blood culture, a reduction in blood cultures will reduce the CLABSI rate, yet will not directly result in a true improvement in patient outcome. While a reduction in the frequency of obtaining blood cultures may actually be a laudable goal, reducing blood cultures as a method of reducing CLABSI rates highlights the complexity of implementing public policy to address health care quality.

Central venous catheters may become colonized or infected through three common routes: (1) contamination of the external surface by bacteria from the skin or contamination during insertion, (2) contamination of the intravascular portion of the external catheter surface by blood-borne bacteria, or (3) introduction of bacteria into the lumen of the catheter during infusions or catheter maintenance. Progression of catheter colonization to clinical infection is significantly dependent on the patient's susceptibility to infection and the pathogenicity of colonizing bacteria. Each specific recommendation for the prevention of CLABSI and CLRBSI predominately addresses one of the three routes. Elimination of CLRBSI requires that all three routes be addressed. Success or failure of any one particular intervention may be altered by host susceptibility, compliance with other interventions, and possibly unknown factors neither observed nor measured.

To comment briefly on the specific questions addressed in this chapter.

### What Is the Best Site to Insert Intravascular Catheters?

As outlined, the subclavian position is our site of choice when inserting central venous catheters. However, while the answer seems clear for the majority of patients, details may alter the answer for individual patients. As noted, the subclavian site has the lowest infection rate, followed by the internal jugular and femoral positions in most studies. This is predominately believed to be related to two factors: (1) the density of bacterial colonization at each site and (2) the ease of maintaining an intact sterile dressing. Certain circumstances that may alter these two factors may exist in individual patients and have not been inadequately studied. The presence of a tracheostomy likely significantly increases the degree of bacterial colonization and contamination of the subclavian site, and securing devices around the neck may limit the ability to appropriately apply dressings to an internal jugular catheter. At any site, conditions that alter skin integrity skin and the presence of hair may increase bacterial colonization or limit dressing integrity.

While infection risk is clearly part of the risk/benefit ratio for each insertion location, the risk of other complications should also be considered. The risk of pneumothorax may have markedly greater implications in certain patients. Venous stenosis risk in patients requiring long-term dialysis, coagulopathy, and carotid disease should be considered.

### What Is Needed to Prevent Contamination during Catheter Insertion?

As noted by the authors, although recommendations for the use of maximum barrier precautions during insertion, not all studies have consistently demonstrated a requirement for all components. Ishikawa and colleagues failed to demonstrate a difference between the use of gloves, prep, and a regional drape versus full barrier precautions in a multicenter, randomized study.* However, patients included were not critically ill, likely with a much lower susceptibility to infection from contamination during insertion. Whether or not catheters were antibiotic/antiseptic coated was not discussed in the reference, their use potentially having implications on the results.

### What Is the Role of Chlorhexidine in Insertion and Management of Central Venous Catheters?

More data exists that chlorhexidine is better than povidine-iodine for skin preparation than the data that exists for the effectiveness of povidine-iodine as a prep. However, attention to detail likely matters when applying chlorhexidine solution. Contact time is important, particularly with no alcoholic component and the application technique should allow the solution to dry on the skin for maximal effectiveness.

### Is Education Useful in Preventing CRBSI?

That a provider should be fully knowledgeable about the risks, contraindications, anatomy, and techniques required to minimize complications prior to undertaking a procedure that could result in severe disability and even death seems self-evident and requires little comment. Perhaps, to some, this is not self-evident. It is, however, the standard to which we should all hold ourselves.

### How Frequently Should Catheters Be Changed?

Every time a sterile catheter is manipulated, the risk of colonization and infection is increased. Each new central venous catheter placement has associated complication risks. That no routine exchange or replacement of indwelling central venous catheters be undertaken without signs of clinical infection is clear. If an existing indwelling central venous catheter has local signs of infection, then it should be removed and a new site selected if central access is still required. However, the best approach to catheter management for patients undergoing diagnostic evaluation for a suspected infection is much less straight forward. This chapter accepts the verbiage put forth by O'Grady et al., that central lines suspected of infections should have a new site rather than a catheter exchange.† Clearly, if the central venous catheter has erythema or purulence at the entry site, this approach is justified. However, in critically ill patients, a significant portion of catheter replacement occurs when central venous catheter infection is one of the several possible infection sites within a differential diagnosis, and local signs are absent. Limited data are available to guide recommendations in this setting. The risk of short- and long-term complications of repeated percutaneous central catheter placement must also be considered. Rewiring a catheter in this setting with culture of the indwelling portion of the replaced catheter may be recommended to limit complications and venous stenosis.‡

### Should Anti-Infective Catheters Be Utilized?

### Do Anti-Infective Catheters Promote Antibiotic Resistance?

Sections "Should Anti-Infective Catheters Be Utilized?" and "Do Anti-Infective Catheters Promote Antibiotic Resistance?" are discussed together. Only two significant arguments support using nonantibiotic-/antiseptic-coated catheters: (1) anti-infective catheters are more expensive, and (2) concerns regarding resistance. No significant data to date suggests that anti-infective catheters promote resistance. In theory, prevention of CLRBSI reduces systemic antibiotic use, the strongest single risk factor for acquiring a subsequent resistant hospital infection. Thus, the decision to utilize anti-infective catheters falls solely to complex cost/benefit analysis.

### What Evidence Is Available on Peripherally Inserted Central Catheters (PICCs)?

The lower risk profile for the insertion of PICCs and similar infection risks make PICCs an attractive alternative when rapid infusion and monitoring are not required.

### What Is the Evidence Available If We Bundle the Aforementioned Techniques and Recommendations?

And now we have completed the circle to beginning of the discussion. The impact of individual components of prevention bundles is difficult to test. Aspects of line maintenance not addressed by components of prevention bundles may also alter infection rates, as recently reported.§ Attention to detail matters.

---

* Ishikawa Y, Kiyama T, Haga Y et al. Maximal sterile barrier precautions do not reduce catheter-related bloodstream infections in general surgery units: A multi-institutional randomized controlled trial. *Ann Surg*. 2010;251(4):620–623.

† O'Grady NP, Alexander M, Burns LA et al. Guidelines for the prevention of intravascular catheter-related infections. *Am J Infect Control*. 2011;39(4 Suppl. 1):S1–S34.

‡ Cobb DK, High KP, Sawyer RG et al. A controlled trial of scheduled replacement of central venous and pulmonary-artery catheters. *N Engl J Med*. 1992;327(15):1062–1068.

§ Klintworth G, Stafford J, O'Connor M et al. Beyond the intensive care unit bundle: Implementation of a successful hospital-wide initiative to reduce central line-associated bloodstream infections. *Am J Infect Control*. 2014;42(6):685–687.

# 72

# *Ventilator-Associated Pneumonia*

**Aaron M. Fields**

**CONTENTS**



## 72.1 Are Invasive Methods Better for Diagnosing Ventilator-Associated Pneumonia (VAP)?

The concept that tracheal aspirate is as good as bronchoalveolar lavage (BAL) is not new. In 1998, Sanchez-Nieto et al. [1] performed a pilot study of 51 patients. They were randomized to invasive and noninvasive groups. The invasive group received a bronchoscopy with protected brush specimen collection and BAL plus tracheal aspirate. The noninvasive group received only tracheal aspirate. In this small, single-center study, the authors found no difference in mortality, length of mechanical ventilation, or stay in the intensive care unit (ICU). In their conclusion, they called for larger trials.

In 2000, three studies were published that responded to this call. Solé Violán et al. [2] randomized 91 patients at a single institution to either invasive or noninvasive diagnosis of VAP. The patients in the invasive group received bronchoscopy with either a protected brush or BAL. Tracheal aspiration was performed in the noninvasive group. Once again, they found no difference in mortality, length of mechanical ventilation, or length of stay in the ICU.

Ruiz et al. [3] randomized 76 patients at a single center to invasive and noninvasive groups. There was no difference in length of mechanical ventilation or ICU stay. They were also unable to show a difference in 30-day mortality. They were able to show a statistical difference in cost: ~$30 USD for noninvasive and ~$370 USD for invasive testing ($p < 0.0001$).

In 2006, The Canadian Critical Care Trials Group [4] performed a randomized controlled trial (RCT) in which they obtained samples for the diagnosis of VAP using either noninvasive tracheal aspirate or BAL. This large study of 740 patients was performed at 28 institutions. There were no differences in the primary outcome, which was a 28-day mortality. Additionally, there were no differences in targeted therapy, days alive without antibiotics, or length of ICU or hospital stay.

Finally, in a 2009 observational study of 2436 patients in Europe, 74.8% were diagnosed using noninvasive techniques.

*Recommendation*: Invasive methods of diagnosing VAP are no better than noninvasive methods and are much less expensive.

*Grade of recommendation*: A

## 72.2 What Are the Modifiable Risk Factors for VAP?

The use of closed versus open suctioning systems has been identified as a potentially modifiable risk factor for developing VAP. Several studies have examined their use. In 2005, Lorente et al. [6] randomized 443 patients to open suction versus closed suction changed daily. They showed no difference in incidence of VAP, but a higher cost associated with the closed system. The same group in 2006 [7] showed that in patients intubated longer than 4 days and their systems changed only when clinically indicated, the closed loop systems became less expensive, although they were still unable to change the incidence of VAP.

Topeli et al. [8] conducted an RCT examining the use of closed versus open systems in 78 patients. While they found increased rates of colonization of ventilator tubing in the closed suction group, there was no difference in mortality, rate of VAP, length of ICU stay, or length of hospital stay. Other smaller studies have reached the same conclusions [9,10].

*Recommendation*: Closed suction systems should be used in all intubated patients. Multiple smaller studies failed to find a difference in rates of VAP using a closed suction system. However, over time, these systems are less expensive and expose healthcare workers to fewer secretions. Closed loop systems should not be changed daily.

### 72.2.1 Endotracheal Tube Attributes

Continuous subglottic suctioning was shown to decrease the incidence of all types of VAP by Vallés et al. [11] in an RCT of 190 patients (RR 1.98; $p < 0.03$). Mahul et al. [12] conducted a 2 × 2 randomized study using endotracheal tubes (ETTs) with and without subglottic suctioning and patients were randomized to antacids or sucralfate. They were able to show a statistically significant reduction in pneumonia (29.1% versus 12.8%, $p < 0.05$). Additionally, the pneumonia that occurred in the subglottic suctioning group was much later than in the regular ETT group (8 versus 16 days). The use of sucralfate versus antacids failed to show any difference in rates of VAP. Kollef et al. [13] showed that using continuous subglottic secretions in cardiac patients did not change the rate of VAP, but did decrease the incidence of early VAP.

In a 2015 RCT, subglottic secretion suctioning resulted in a significant reduction of VAP prevalence [14] ($p = 0.018$). Mortality, length of ICU stay, were not statistically changed by the use of the subglottic suctioning device.

Metz et al. [15] investigated whether lavage of the pharynx and the subglottic area decreased the rates of VAP. They found that large volume pharyngeal lavage reduced the bacterial counts briefly in the subglottic area, but led to a slightly higher incidence in VAP. Lavage of the subglottic area offered no advantage over simple suctioning of the subglottic port.

Lorente et al. [16] randomized 280 patients to receive a standard ETT or a tube with both a polyurethane cuff (PUC) and a subglottic suctioning channel that was placed to suction intermittently. They showed a statistically significant decrease in the development of both early and late VAP (HR 3.3, $p < 0.001$.) Unfortunately, at the time of this writing, this type of tube is not available in the United States. However, standard ETT with a PUC is available and was used by Poelaert et al. [17] in a small randomized study of 134 patients. They were able to show a statistically significant protective effect using the PUC ETT.

Silver-coated ETT tubes were shown to reduce bacterial colonization and VAP rates in intubated patients in two small RCTs [18].

*Recommendation*: ETT with subglotting suctioning ports and silver coatings reduce the incidence of VAP and should be used in anyone anticipated needing invasive ventilation for more than 48 h.

### 72.2.2 Heat and Moisture-Inducing Devices

Gases entering the nose are warmed and humidified before reaching the lungs. Endotracheal intubation removes this protective barrier. Attempts to overcome the drying effects of the tubes have included heat and moisture exchangers (HME), and heated water baths that include a wire in the circuit to prevent condensation. Both are efficacious in preventing tracheal mucosa and desiccation. Multiple studies have examined if either are associated with an increased risk of VAP. Most recently, Boots et al. [19] showed that the rate of VAP was the same for both types of heater/moisturizer systems. Three hundred and eighty-one patients were randomized to either hot water bath with circuit wires, or HME with viral and bacterial filters. There was no difference in rates of VAP in the groups. HME were shown to have a higher resistance over time.

Other studies have failed to show a difference in VAP rates [20–24].

Lorente et al. [25] showed that a modern hot water bath was protective for VAP when compared to HME. They acknowledged the fact that their findings were contradictory to previous studies showing no difference in HME and the hot water bath. They attributed this to the fact that the hot water bath they used was able to deliver higher partial pressures of water and the ability to refill its reservoir without opening it.

*Recommendation*: Newer water bath humidifiers should be used whenever possible. However, HME are a suitable alternative.

### 72.2.3 Semirecumbent Position

The semirecumbent position received considerable attention after a study by Drakulovic [26] was stopped early due to an early clinically and statistically significant decrease in VAP rates among patients in the semirecumbent position. The rate decreased from 11/47 (23%) to 2/39 (5%) where $p = 0.018$. Some critics of this study felt that supine was not the standard of care at the time. In answer to these questions, van Nieuwenhoven [27] randomized 221 patients to standard of care (which turned out to be 10°) versus treatment, which was 45°. They were unable to achieve 45°, and succeeded in only reaching 28° in the treatment group. However, no differences were found between the groups.

*Recommendation*: Avoid the supine position in intubated patients. It may not be possible to achieve 45° elevation, but some elevation should be attempted.

*Recommendation*: The use of closed suction systems, ETT with subglottic suctioning ports, PUC and silver coating, new water bath type humidifiers, and the semirecumbent position all decrease the rates of VAP.

*Grade of recommendation*: A

## 72.3 How Should Antibiotics Be Used to Treat VAP?

Empiric coverage is defined as antibiotic coverage for VAP prior to having culture results. Only one randomized study was found regarding empiric versus late antibiotic coverage. The 2003 study by Baker et al. [28] randomized 98 trauma patients to empiric coverage or beginning antibiotic coverage after having invasively obtained samples (BAL). They found a trend toward decreased hospital costs associated with late antibiotic usage.

Alvarez-Lerma [29] conducted a prospective nonrandomized observational study of 16,872 ICU patients. They found that mortality was 24.7% in those whose initial coverage was inadequate, but only 16.2% in those who received adequate empiric antibiotic coverage for VAP ($p = 0.034$.)

Luna et al. [30] performed an observational study using BAL to diagnose VAP. When patients had received appropriate antibiotics early in their VAP course (i.e., before bronchoscopy), their mortality was 37%. However, if this therapy was inadequate, their mortality was 91% ($p < 0.001$).

Another nonrandomized trial examining the timing of antibiotics was performed by Iregui et al. [31]. They showed that mortality from VAP was significantly increased if appropriate antibiotics were given more than 24 h after diagnostic criteria were met (OR 7.68; $p < 0.001$).

Mortality benefit may be attributed to prescribing antibiotic coverage to which the pathogen is sensitive. Kollef and Ward [32] performed a cohort study using mini BAL. They showed that VAP due to a pathogen resistant to the empiric antibiotics led to an increased mortality (OR 3.28; $p < 0.006$).

Similar findings were demonstrated in trauma patients by Mueller et al. [33]. Many of their patients had multiple instances of VAP. They demonstrated that mortality increased as the number of times that each patient received inadequate empiric coverage. Mortality increased from 3.6% for no episodes, 8.8% for one episode, and 45% for more than one episode ($p < 0.001$).

In 2008, Heyland et al. [34] showed, in a subgroup of patients who had pseudomonas randomized to either monotherapy with meropenem or dual coverage with meropenem plus ciprofloxacin, that those with double empiric coverage had a higher rate of adequate initial coverage (18.8% versus 84.2%; $p < 0.001$).

*Recommendations*: When clinical diagnosis of VAP is met, broad spectrum antibiotics (multiple) should be given without delay. Attempts to elucidate speciation and sensitivity should be made as soon as possible.

### 72.3.1 Double Coverage

Damas et al. [35] showed that in patients diagnosed with pneumonia who were given adequate empiric coverage with a single agent, there was no benefit to other antibiotics for double coverage or synergy.

Rubinstein et al. [36] prospectively randomized patients with many types of infections, including pseudomonas, to either ceftazidime monotherapy or ceftriaxone/tobramycin. Those with pseudomonas had the same mortality despite monotherapy. There was no increased incidence of resistance or superinfection in those treated with a single agent.

*Recommendation*: After speciation and sensitivities are proven, antibiotics should be tailored and monotherapy should be continued.

### 72.3.2 Linezolid versus Vancomycin for Methicillin-Resistant *Staphylococcus aureus* (MRSA) Pneumonia

Rubinstein et al. [37] conducted a prospective RCT comparing linezolid and vancomycin for the treatment of MRSA pneumonia. While there was a trend toward linezolid causing increased cure rates, no statistically significant differences were found between the two groups.

Wunderink et al. [38] conducted an additional RCT using the same agents in patients with pneumonia. Again, no statistically significant differences were found in the two groups. There were also no differences in drug-related adverse events between the two groups.

Most recently, Niederman et al. [39] performed a post hoc analysis comparing these two agents for MRSA nosocomial pneumonia. They found no statistically significant differences in clinical outcomes. They did find that diagnosis of renal failure was greater on vancomycin, which resulted in higher health car resource sue.

*Recommendation*: Unless there is a concern for renal failure, vancomycin should be the empiric and treatment of choice for MRSA pneumonia.

### 72.3.3 Length of Treatment

A meta-analysis from 2013 looked at four RCTs comparing short (7–8 days) to long (10–15 days) antibiotic treatment and failed to show a difference in mortality. A trend toward significance was shown in decreasing relapses in the long treatment groups [40].

*Recommendation*: Empiric coverage should be broad and nearly always includes more than one drug. Studies have not demonstrated any advantage to double covering any microbe after speciation including pseudomonas. Vancomycin is as effective as linezolid. Antibiotics should be given for no more than 8 days.

*Grade of recommendation*: A

## 72.4 Does Timing of Tracheotomy Change Outcomes in PTS with VAP?

Rumbak et al. [41] conducted a prospective, randomized, multicenter, controlled trial evaluating the timing of percutaneous tracheotomy versus long-term endotracheal intubation in 120 patients. The patient population was limited to those anticipated needing longer than 14 days of mechanical ventilation. Patients randomized to early tracheotomy had the procedure performed during the first 48 h of their intubation. They found that mortality, pneumonia, and accidental extubation were all reduced in the early tracheotomy group. The length of ICU stay and mechanical ventilation was also reduced. Finally, damage to the mouth and larynx was significantly less in the early tracheotomy group. Lower mortality rates were attributed to fewer diagnoses of pneumonia and less need for sedation.

In contrast, Bouderka et al. [42] found no difference in frequency of pneumonia or mortality in head-injured patients. They did, however, find a shorter length of mechanical ventilation in the early tracheostomy group. This study included only 62 patients at a single center.

Several other studies were examined but were felt to offer little evidence in support or rebuttal of early tracheostomy. In 1990, Rodriguez et al. [43] showed that tracheostomy had a low morbidity and mortality. Sugerman et al. [44] designed an elegant multicenter trial assessing the effects of early versus late tracheostomy in ICU patients. However, of the 157 patients entered, only 14 late tracheostomy patients completed the study. It seems they were unable to eliminate physician bias. They were able to again show low morbidity and mortality associated with tracheostomy.

A recent meta-analysis suggested that early trachеotomy decreased mortality, reduced ICU stay hospital stay, and mechanical ventilation duration [45].

*Recommendation*: In centers that frequently perform percutaneous tracheostomies, patients expected to be intubated longer than 14 days should have early tracheostomy due to a possible decrease in mortality and low risk of the procedure.

*Recommendation*: Yes, early tracheostomy should be performed.

*Grade of recommendation*: B

## 72.5 What Is the Epidemiology of VAP?

Hedrick et al. [46] performed a retrospective analysis of rates of VAP in trauma and nontrauma ICU patients. They found VAP in 71% of trauma admissions and 29% in nontrauma admissions.

Quartin et al. [47] found a VAP mortality rate of 13.7 in contrast to previous studies demonstrating a much higher rate. This suggests that VAP mortality may be decreasing over time.

*Recommendation*: Rates of VAP are between 29% and 71% with wide variability based on patient population. Rates of VAP increase as time of intubation accumulates and may be decreasing when compared to historical rates.

*Grade of recommendation*: B

Q: What is the best method to assess and tailor treatment for VAP?

Raman et al. [48] conducted a retrospective observational cohort study in 89 patients. Those who had antibiotics stopped within 1 day of a negative bronchoscopy culture were classified as early discontinuation. Those who had antibiotics stopped later than 1 day were classified as late discontinuation. There was no difference in mortality and there was a lower frequency of multidrug-resistant superinfections in the early discontinuation group.

*Recommendation*: Antibiotics can be stopped when clinical signs of infection have resolved (Tables 72.1 and 72.2).

*Grade of recommendation*: B

**TABLE 72.1**

Clinical Questions

| Question | Answer | Grade of Recommendation | References |
|---|---|---|---|
| Are invasive methods better for diagnosing ventilator-associated pneumonia (VAP)? | Invasive methods of diagnosing VAP are no better than noninvasive methods and are much less expensive | A | [1–5] |
| What are the modifiable risk factors for VAP? | The use of closed suction systems, ETT with subglottic suctioning ports, PUC and silver coating, new water bath type humidifiers, and the semirecumbent position all decrease the rates of VAP | A | [6–27] |
| How should antibiotics be used to treat VAP? | Empiric coverage should be broad and nearly always includes more than one drug. Studies have not demonstrated any advantage to double covering any microbe after speciation including pseudomonas. Vancomycin is as effective as linezolid. Antibiotics should be given for no more than 8 days | A | [28–40] |
| Does timing of tracheotomy change outcomes in PTS with VAP? | Yes, early tracheostomy should be performed | B | [41–45] |
| What is the epidemiology of VAP? | Rates of VAP are between 29% and 71% with wide variability based on patient population. Rates of VAP increase as time of intubation accumulates and may be decreasing when compared to historical rates | B | [46–47] |
| What is the best method to assess and tailor treatment for VAP? | Antibiotics can be stopped when clinical signs of infection have resolved | B | [48] |

**TABLE 72.2**

Levels of Evidence

| Subject | Year | Reference | Level of Evidence | Strength of Recommendation | Findings |
|---|---|---|---|---|---|
| Invasive or noninvasive methods of VAP diagnosis | 2009 | [5] | Ib | A | Invasive methods of VAP diagnosis do not change outcomes |
| Closed circuit suctioning | 2004 | [8] | Ib | A | Closed circuit suctioning devises should be used and only changed on a clinical basis |
| ETT with subglottic suctioning | 1992 | [12] | Ia | A | ETT with subglottic suctioning decreases the rates of VAP |
| Double antibiotic coverage for VAP | 1995 | [36] | Ia | A | Monotherapy is as good as double coverage for VAP treatment |

## References


1. Sanchez-Nieto JM, Torres A, Garcia-Cordoba F et al. Impact of invasive and noninvasive quantitative culture sampling on outcome of ventilator-associated pneumonia: A pilot study. *Am J Respir Crit Care Med.* 1998;157(2):371–376.
2. Solé Violán J, Fernández JA, Benítez AB et al. Impact of quantitative invasive diagnostic techniques in the management and outcome of mechanically ventilated patients with suspected pneumonia. *Crit Care Med.* 2000;28(8):2737–2741.
3. Ruiz M, Torres A, Ewig S et al. Noninvasive versus invasive microbial investigation in ventilator-associated pneumonia: Evaluation of outcome. *Am J Respir Crit Care Med.* 2000;162(1):119–125.
4. Canadian Critical Care Trials Group. A randomized trial of diagnostic techniques for ventilator-associated pneumonia. *N Engl J Med.* 2006;355(25):2619–2630.
5. Koulenti D, Lisboa T, Brun-Buisson C et al. Spectrum of practice in the diagnosis of nosocomial pneumonia in patients requiring mechanical ventilation in European intensive care units. *Crit Care Med.* 2009;37(8):2360–2368.
6. Lorente L, Lecuona Ma, Martín MaM et al. Ventilator-associated pneumonia using a closed versus an open tracheal suction system. *Crit Care Med.* 2005;33(1):115–119.
7. Lorente L, Lecuona Ma, Jiménez A et al. Tracheal suction by closed system without daily change versus open system. *Intensive Care Med.* 2006;32(4):538–544.
8. Topeli A, Harmanci A, Cetinkaya Y et al. Comparison of the effect of closed versus open endotracheal suction systems on the development of ventilator-associated pneumonia. *J Hosp Infect.* 2004;58(1):14–19.
9. Deppe SA, Kelly JW, Thoi LL et al. Incidence of colonization, nosocomial pneumonia, and mortality in critically ill patients using a Trach Care closed-suction system versus an open-suction system: Prospective, randomized study. *Crit Care Med.* 1990;18(12):1389–1393.

10. David D, Samuel P, David T et al. An open-labelled randomized controlled trial comparing costs and clinical outcomes of open endotracheal suctioning with closed endotracheal suctioning in mechanically ventilated medical intensive care patients. *J Crit Care.* 2011;26(5):482–488.
11. Vallés J, Artigas A, Rello J et al. Continuous aspiration of subglottic secretions in preventing ventilator-associated pneumonia. *Ann Intern Med.* 1995;122(3):179–186.
12. Mahul P, Auboyer C, Jospe R et al. Prevention of nosocomial pneumonia in intubated patients: Respective role of mechanical subglottic secretions drainage and stress ulcer prophylaxis. *Intensive Care Med.* 1992;18(1):20–25.
13. Kollef MH, Skubas NJ, Sundt TM. A randomized clinical trial of continuous aspiration of subglottic secretions in cardiac surgery patients. *Chest.* 1999;116(5):1339–1346.
14. Damas P, Frippiat F, Ancion A. Prevention of ventilator-associated pneumonia and ventilator-associated conditions: A randomized controlled trial with subglottic secretion suctioning. *Crit Care Med.* January 2015;43(1):22–30.
15. Metz C, Linde H-J, Göbel L, Göbel F, Taeger K. Influence of intermittent subglottic lavage on subglottic colonisation and ventilator-associated pneumonia. *Clin Intensive Care.* 1998;9(1):20–25.
16. Lorente L, Lecuona Ma, Jiménez A et al. Influence of an endotracheal tube with polyurethane cuff and subglottic secretion drainage on pneumonia. *Am J Respir Crit Care Med.* 2007;176(11):1079–1083.
17. Poelaert J, Depuydt P, De Wolf A et al. Polyurethane cuffed endotracheal tubes to prevent early postoperative pneumonia after cardiac surgery: A pilot study. *J Thoracic Cardiovasc Surg.* 2008;135(4):771–776.
18. Li X1, Yuan Q, Wang L et al. Silver-coated endotracheal tube versus non-coated endotracheal tube for preventing ventilator-associated pneumonia among adults: A systematic review of randomized controlled trials. *J Evid Based Med.* 2012;5(1):25–30.
19. Boots RJ, George N, Faoagali JL et al. Double-heater-wire circuits and heat-and-moisture exchangers and the risk of ventilator-associated pneumonia. *Crit Care Med.* 2006;34(3):687–693.
20. Dreyfuss D, Djedaïni K, Gros I et al. Mechanical ventilation with heated humidifiers or heat and moisture exchangers: Effects on patient colonization and incidence of nosocomial pneumonia. *Am J Respir Crit Care Med.* 1995;151(4):986–992.
21. Kollef MH, Shapiro SD, Boyd V et al. A randomized clinical trial comparing an extended-use hygroscopic condenser humidifier with heated-water humidification in mechanically ventilated patients. *Chest.* 1998;113(3):759–767.
22. Boots RJ, Howe S, George N et al. Clinical utility of hygroscopic heat and moisture exchangers in intensive care patients. *Crit Care Med.* 1997;25(10):1707–1712.
23. Memish ZA, Oni GA, Djazmati W et al. A randomized clinical trial to compare the effects of a heat and moisture exchanger with a heated humidifying system on the occurrence rate of ventilator-associated pneumonia. *Am J Infect Contr.* 2001;29(5):301–305.
24. Lacherade J-C, Auburtin M, Cerf C et al. Impact of humidification systems on ventilator-associated pneumonia: A randomized multicenter trial. *Am J Respir Crit Care Med.* 2005;172(10):1276–1282.
25. Lorente L, Lecuona Ma, Jiménez A et al. Ventilator-associated pneumonia using a heated humidifier or a heat and moisture exchanger: A randomized controlled trial [ISRCTN88724583]. *Crit Care.* 2006;10(4):R116.
26. Drakulovic MB, Torres A, Bauer TT et al. Supine body position as a risk factor for nosocomial pneumonia in mechanically ventilated patients: A randomised trial. *Lancet.* 1999;354(9193):1851–1858.
27. van Nieuwenhoven CA, Vandenbroucke-Grauls C, van Tiel FH et al. Feasibility and effects of the semirecumbent position to prevent ventilator-associated pneumonia: A randomized study. *Crit Care Med.* 2006;34(2):396–402.
28. Baker AM, Meredith JW, Chang M. Bronchoscopically guided management of ventilator-associated pneumonia in trauma patients. *J Bronchol.* 2003;10(1):7–16.
29. Alvarez-Lerma F. Modification of empiric antibiotic treatment in patients with pneumonia acquired in the intensive care unit. ICU-Acquired Pneumonia Study Group. *Intensive Care Med.* 1996;22(5):387–394.
30. Luna CM, Vujacich P, Niederman MS et al. Impact of BAL data on the therapy and outcome of ventilator-associated pneumonia. *Chest.* 1997;111(3):676–685.
31. Iregui M, Ward S, Sherman G et al. Clinical importance of delays in the initiation of appropriate antibiotic treatment for ventilator-associated pneumonia. *Chest.* 2002;122(1):262–268.
32. Kollef MH, Ward S. The influence of mini-BAL cultures on patient outcomes: Implications for the antibiotic management of ventilator-associated pneumonia. *Chest.* 1998;113(2):412–420.
33. Mueller EW, Hanes SD, Croce MA et al. Effect from multiple episodes of inadequate empiric antibiotic therapy for ventilator-associated pneumonia on morbidity and mortality among critically ill trauma patients. *J Trauma.* 2005;58(1):94–101.
34. Heyland DK, Dodek P, Muscedere J et al. Randomized trial of combination versus monotherapy for the empiric treatment of suspected ventilator-associated pneumonia. *Crit Care Med.* 2008;36(3):737–744.
35. Damas P, Garweg C, Monchi M et al. Combination therapy versus monotherapy: A randomised pilot study on the evolution of inflammatory parameters after ventilator associated pneumonia. *Crit Care.* 2006;10(2):R52.
36. Rubinstein E, Lode H, Grassi C. Ceftazidime monotherapy vs. ceftriaxone/tobramycin for serious hospital-acquired gram-negative infections. Antibiotic Study Group. *Clin Infect Dis.* 1995;20(5):1217–1228.
37. Rubinstein E, Cammarata S, Oliphant T, Wunderink R. Linezolid (PNU-100766) versus vancomycin in the treatment of hospitalized patients with nosocomial pneumonia: A randomized, double-blind, multicenter study. *Clin Infect Dis.* 2001;32(3):402–412.

38. Wunderink RG, Cammarata SK, Oliphant TH, Kollef MH. Continuation of a randomized, double-blind, multicenter study of linezolid versus vancomycin in the treatment of patients with nosocomial pneumonia. *Clin Therap.* 2003;25(3):980–992.
39. Niederman MS, Chastre J, Solem CT et al. Health economic evaluation of patients treated for nosocomial pneumonia caused by methicillin-resistant *Staphylococcus aureus*: Secondary analysis of a multicenter randomized clinical trial of vancomycin and linezolid. *Clin Therapy.* 2014;36(9):1233–1243.
40. Dimopoulos G, Poulakou G, Pneumatikos IA et al. Short- vs long-duration antibiotic regimens for ventilator-associated pneumonia: A systematic review and meta-analysis. *Chest.* 2013;144(6):1759–1767.
41. Rumbak MJ, Newton M, Truncale T et al. A prospective, randomized, study comparing early percutaneous dilational tracheotomy to prolonged translaryngeal intubation (delayed tracheotomy) in critically ill medical patients. *Crit Care Med.* 2004;32(8):1689–1694.
42. Bouderka MA, Fakhir B, Bouaggad A et al. Early tracheostomy versus prolonged endotracheal intubation in severe head injury. *J Trauma.* 2004;57(2):251–254.
43. Rodriguez JL, Steinberg SM, Luchetti FA et al. Early tracheostomy for primary airway management in the surgical critical care setting. *Surgery.* 1990;108(4):655–659.
44. Sugerman HJ, Wolfe L, Pasquale MD et al. Multicenter, randomized, prospective trial of early tracheostomy. *J Trauma.* 1997;43(5):741–747.
45. Shan L, Hao P, Xu F et al. Benefits of early tracheotomy: A meta-analysis based on 6 observational studies. *Respir Care.* 2013;58(11):1856–1862.
46. Hedrick TL, Smith RL, McElearney ST et al. Differences in early- and late-onset ventilator-associated pneumonia between surgical and trauma patients in a combined surgical or trauma intensive care unit. *J Trauma.* 2008;64(3):714–720.
47. Quartin AA, Scerpella EG, Puttagunta S et al. A comparison of microbiology and demographics among patients with healthcare-associated, hospital-acquired, and ventilator-associated pneumonia: A retrospective analysis of 1184 patients from a large, international study. *BMC Infect Dis.* 2013;13:561.
48. Raman K, Nailor MD, Nicolau DP et al. Early antibiotic discontinuation in patients with clinically suspected ventilator-associated pneumonia and negative quantitative bronchoscopy cultures. *Crit Care Med.* 2013;41(7):1656–1663.

## Commentary on Ventilator-Associated Pneumonia

*Martin A. Croce*

Pneumonia is a surgical disease. The fact that operations are rarely required does not matter. Depending on the patient population, it is a disease that carries significant morbidity and mortality. Despite its impact on patients, it is a disease that is shrouded by baffling mysteries, including prevention, diagnosis, and therapy.

Nosocomial pneumonia, and especially ventilator-associated pneumonia, is probably the most significant of all hospital acquired infections and is the leading cause of death from nosocomial infection. Accurate diagnosis and prompt therapy are extremely important; however, the accurate diagnosis of ventilator-associated pneumonia is difficult. The conventional clinical criteria of fever, leukocytosis, and purulent sputum in the presence of a new or changing infiltrate on chest x-ray are not specific for the diagnosis of pneumonia—especially in the multiply injured trauma patient. Routine tracheal aspirates have been shown to be notoriously inaccurate and will not differentiate *colonization* from *infection*. The lack of diagnostic accuracy has led to more invasive techniques that are more specific for culturing the lower airways. Bronchoalveolar lavage (BAL) and protected specimen brushing have been studied extensively but are invasive and will significantly increase hospital costs. However, if these invasive procedures can distinguish between SIRS and pneumonia, then the additional costs may be more than offset by savings in unnecessary costs.

Now I have given my perspective on some of the questions addressed in this chapter.

### Are Invasive Methods Better for Diagnosing Ventilator-Associated Pneumonia?

In a word, yes.

As mentioned earlier, much depends on the patient population. There is a distinct difference between medical ICU patients (in whom the majority of the references describe) and patients cared for by acute care surgeons in surgical ICUs. The medical patients develop VAP in response to their chronic illnesses, while the surgical patients develop VAP in the setting of an acute insult causing a systemic inflammatory response, such as trauma or perforated viscus. Thus, it is imperative that the diagnostic method be able to differentiate between systemic inflammatory response due to the acute event and invasive infection. Quantitative cultures of the lower airway obtained via bronchoscopy with BAL are able to differentiate inflammation from infection. Interpretation of the references cited by the author must be taken with caution. Some of the studies involve only medical ICU patients, and all of them include only a minority of surgical patients. Most of the studies also allow for continued antibiotic therapy, even if the cultures are negative (including the Canadian study), which make meaningful interpretation impossible. A study from our institution demonstrated that in trauma patients, antibiotic therapy could be based *solely* on the quantitative BAL results, with a low rate of false-negative cultures. Earlier work also illustrated an actual cost reduction with quantitative BAL, with the true savings based on eliminating unnecessary antibiotics.

### What Are the Modifiable Risk Factors for VAP?

We all want things like fancy endotracheal tubes and the ventilator bundle to work. The endotracheal tubes that allow for subglottic suctioning are interesting, and may actually be of benefit in patients who have prolonged mechanical ventilation. However, these tubes are more expensive and may not be available in all areas where intubation occurs (such as prehospital). One must weigh the risks of changing out an established airway for a tube with marginal potential benefit. The ventilator bundle of DVT and stress ulcer prophylaxis, head of bed elevation, and sedation vacation with daily weaning assessment have been shown in a prospective multi-institutional study to be of no benefit in preventing VAP. Whether the addition of chlorhexidine mouth care will make the bundle more effective is unknown.

### How Should Antibiotics Be Used to Treat VAP?

Empiric antibiotic treatment can be based on the duration of time the patient has been in the ICU and the typical flora present in the individual ICU. Earlier VAP is typically caused by sensitive Gram-positive organisms and *H. influenza*. Later VAP is typically caused by nosocomial Gram negatives and MRSA. Careful interpretation of the ICU antibiograms will identify the best empiric regimen for that specific ICU.

Duration of therapy may also be based on the organism. Waiting for resolution of clinical signs of infection can lead to prolonged unnecessary antibiotic use, since the inflammatory response from the acute insult may persist and does not require antibiotics. Early VAP typically requires 7 days of antibiotics. Most late VAP may need 10 days of therapy. *P. aeruginosa* usually needs 14 days for eradication, and appropriate monotherapy is adequate. Basing therapy duration on the *organism* and not *resolution of clinical signs* is cost-effective.

Vancomycin may safely be used for treatment of VAP due to MRSA. It is important to follow serum levels to ensure adequate dosing. Some of the data comparing linezolid to vancomycin may be skewed, since some studies did not allow vancomycin dose adjustments.

### Does Timing of Tracheostomy Change Outcomes in Patients with VAP?[*†‡]

Regarding the timing of tracheostomy, it is difficult to separate evidence-based medicine from faith-based medicine. We are believers in early tracheostomy especially in patients with brain injuries. We also believe it is easier to provide pulmonary toilet in patients with tracheostomy. The procedure is well tolerated and will improve the patient's comfort level[§¶**††].

* Croce MA, Fabian TC, Shaw B et al. Analysis of charges associated with diagnosis of nosocomial pneumonia: Can routine bronchoscopy be justified? *J Trauma*. 1994 November;37:721–727.

† Croce MA, Fabian TC, Schurr MJ et al. Using bronchoalveolar lavage to distinguish nosocomial pneumonia from systemic inflammatory response syndrome: A prospective analysis. *J Trauma*. 1995 December;39:1134–1140.

‡ Croce MA, Fabian TC, Waddle-Smith L et al. Utility of Gram's stain and efficacy of quantitative cultures for post traumatic pneumonia: A prospective study. *Ann Surg*. 1998 May;227(5):743–756.

§ Mueller EW, Croce MA, Boucher BA et al. Repeat bronchoalveolar lavage to guide antibiotic duration for ventilator-associated pneumonia. *J Trauma*. 2007 December;64(6):1329–1337.

¶ Magnotti LJ, Croce MA, Zarzaur BL et al. Causative pathogen dictates optimal duration of antimicrobial therapy for ventilator-associated pneumonia in trauma patients. *J Am Coll Surg*. 2011 April;212(4):476–486.

** Magnotti LJ, Croce MA, Zarzaur BL et al. Causative pathogen dictates optimal duration of antimicrobial therapy for ventilator-associated pneumonia in trauma patients. *J Am Coll Surg*. 2011 April;212(4):476–486.

†† Sharpe JP, Magnotti LJ, Weinberg JA et al. Impact of pathogen-directed antimicrobial therapy for ventilator-associated pneumonia in trauma patients on charges and recurrence. *J Am Coll Surg*. 2015 April;220(4):489–495.

# 73

# *Management of Acute Myocardial Infarction and Cardiogenic Shock*

**Antonio Hernandez**

**CONTENTS**



## 73.1 Introduction

Cardiovascular disease remains to be the leading cause of death in the United States. In 2010, the overall rate of death attributed to cardiovascular disease was 235.5 per 100,000; however, there was a decline of 31% from 2000 to 2010 [1]. According to the Centers for Disease Control and Prevention, about 720,000 Americans have a myocardial infarction (MI) each year of which approximately 380,000 die [2]. Our focus in this chapter is related to the incidence of MI and consequent cardiogenic shock in perioperative patients. Although there is good evidence for the use of thrombolytic therapy in ST-elevation MI, based on the 2013 ACCF/AHA guidelines [3], thrombolytic therapy is often contraindicated in the postoperative population. Hence I review therapies suggested by the ACC/AHA for ST-elevation and non-ST-elevation MI [4] and how they apply to our postoperative population. In this chapter, I attempt to describe the evidence related to MI with respect to the etiology and pathophysiology, diagnosis, and management. At the conclusion of the chapter, I review current evidenced-based strategies for the management of cardiogenic shock.

## 73.2 Diagnosis

The typical presentation of an ECG for an acute MI includes ST segment elevation in two "consecutive" or "contiguous" leads that represent the same coronary artery territory, and not how they appear in sequence on the ECG. ST-elevation should be ≥1 mm or 0.1 mV. Other ECG findings include inversion of T waves and finally the development of a Q wave. The area that may be elusive on an ECG includes the inferior lateral wall. The presentation here would include increased voltage over the R waves, peaked T waves, and ST depression on leads $V_1$–$V_2$. Also, the development of a new left bundle branch block should be approached as an acute MI and managed as such, until biomarker data exclude the likelihood of an acute event.

The biomarkers listed here follow a pattern of progression that often makes it challenging to assess for reinfarction. Upon the onset of MI, creatine phosphokinase (CPK), and creatine kinase MB (CKMB), serum levels begin to rise at 4–8 h, peak at approximately 18 h, and return to baseline after 2–4 days. Troponin levels are more specific, and are the better biomarker to follow. Troponin serum levels rise at 6 h, and may remain elevated for a few days, particularly if the patient has coexisting renal insufficiency. Specific levels of biomarkers should be referenced with the specific institutional standards, as they may vary.

Due to improved accessibility and portability, the role of echocardiography is an excellent complement to the methods described. Echocardiography provides information about specific segments of each wall. Previously we used a 16-segment model for the interpretation of systolic function [5], but have recently adopted a 17-segment model for the left ventricle (LV), septum, and true apex. When taking the transthoracic approach, it is noninvasive and essentially harmless to the patient. In the hands of a skilled echocardiographer, hemodynamic parameters can be estimated, to include cardiac output, pulmonary artery (PA) systolic pressure and mean arterial pressure, valvular structural abnormalities to include endocarditis, and it also provides information about cardiomyopathy patterns and pericardial integrity and estimation of pericardial volume. Although the PA catheter was considered the gold standard in previous years, invasive monitoring is becoming less utilized. Use of a PA catheter may complement the techniques described above. Information that can be obtained from a PA catheter that is not offered from an ECG is oxygen saturation and oxygen tension of mixed venous blood as a measure of appropriate delivery of oxygen. In the next section, I discuss the management strategies of an acute MI.

Last, there are emerging techniques that are promising for the rapid detection of myocardial ischemia. I direct you to a recent review of these techniques, which include sestamibi myocardial perfusion single photon emission (SPECT), rubidium PET scan, ischemic memory imaging, cardiac MRI, and cardiac CT [6]. Of the techniques described, I will focus on SPECT as there is a substantial body of evidence supporting the use of this technique with inconsequential economic burden to payers or healthcare systems [7–11]. Briefly, SPECT has a negative predictive value of acute MI when used in the Emergency Department of greater than 99%, and in a study by Kontos in which 361 patients were evaluated within 6 h of initial symptoms, and only two received a negative SPECT test that progressed to a MI 5 days after admission [10]. The use of SPECT led to a reduction in hospitalization from 52% to 42% [11].

## 73.3 Management

### 73.3.1 Right versus Left Ventricular Infarction

One of the first steps in managing acute MI is to identify which chamber is being affected so that one can implement the appropriate strategy for achieving target hemodynamic goals. The primary method of improving delivery of oxygen to the myocardium is by improving blood flow, since the myocardium is already maximally extracting oxygen at a ratio of approximately 75%. The higher the coronary perfusion pressure (CPP), the better the blood flow. So, at this time we should define the determining variables for CPP. For the left ventricle, the CPP is diastolic blood pressure (DBP)—left ventricular end diastolic pressure (LVEDP). This is particularly unique to the left ventricle, since it primarily perfuses during diastole. The right ventricle perfuses during the entire cardiac cycle, which is understood to be represented by the following relationship: mean arterial pressure—mean pulmonary arterial pressure.

Generally, the goals for both LV and RV acute MI are to reduce the oxygen consumption and increase the delivery of oxygen to the myocardium. However, one of the strategies for the LV in reducing the oxygen consumption will affect the RV in a negative fashion. That is, afterload reduction or reducing LV work will aid in reducing the LV oxygen consumption. But, if the patient is experiencing RV infarction rather than LV infarction, decreasing the MAP will have a negative effect on the delivery of oxygen to the RV and exacerbate the oxygen demand/supply ratio. Therefore, it is imperative to identify what coronary artery territories are being affected, before proceeding with management. In the following two sections, I will describe the management for ST-elevation MI and non-ST-elevation MI independently as per the ACC/AHA guidelines. Overall, the goal is to establish revascularization.

### 73.3.2 Thrombolytic Therapy

There is good evidence for the use of thrombolytic therapy for revascularization during an acute MI [12]. However, in postoperative patients the use of thrombolytic therapy is often contraindicated due to recent surgery. Nevertheless, I have included a list of contraindications:

- Active internal bleeding
- Intracranial neoplasm, aneurysm, or A-V malformation
- Neurosurgery or cerebral vascular accident within 6 weeks
- Trauma or major surgery within 2 weeks
- Aortic dissection

### 73.3.3 ST-Elevation MI

The following strategies for management of an acute MI will be based on current guidelines forwarded by the ACC/AHA for ST-elevation MI [3].

The current recommendation is to establish reperfusion as quickly as possible. For patients experiencing a coronary event, the health system goal should be to have the patient receive an intervention within 90 min, from arrival to "balloon" time [13]. For our particular patient population, access to a percutaneous coronary intervention (PCI) laboratory should be quite easy. It has been demonstrated that outcomes are better when patients are cared for in centers of high volume PCI experience [14]. In their analysis of the National Registry of Myocardial Infarction, they compared in-hospital mortality and times to treatment in STEMI across different levels of hospital specialization with PCI. They divided 463 hospitals into quartiles of PCI specialization based on the relative proportion of reperfusion-treated patients who underwent a PCI. After adjusting for patient and hospital characteristics, including percutaneous intervention volume, they found that greater PCI specialization was associated with a lower relative risk of in-hospital mortality in patients treated with PCI (adjusted relative risk comparing the highest and lowest quartiles, 0.64; $p < 0.006$) but not in those treated with fibrinolytic therapy. Because this patient population is likely to have a contraindication to fibrinolytic therapy, prompt arrival to the PCI laboratory is very important.

#### *73.3.3.1 Beta-Blocker Therapy*

According to the updated guidelines by the ACC/AHA, oral beta-blocker therapy should be initiated in the first 24 h for patients that do not have the following: (1) signs of heart failure, (2) evidence of a low output state, (3) increased risk for cardiogenic shock, or (4) other relative contraindications to beta blockade such as heart block, asthma, or reactive airway disease [3]. In previous studies, intravenous (IV) beta-blocker therapy had not shown to be superior to the oral route of administration with the exception of IV atenolol [15]. In previous studies, IV beta-blocker therapy had not shown to be superior to the oral route of administration, with the exception of IV atenolol [15]. The GUSTO-I experience, aside from comparing one of four thrombolytic strategies, also compared IV versus oral atenolol. The atenolol protocol recommended that patients without hypotension, bradycardia, or signs of heart failure be given atenolol 5 mg IV over 5 min as soon as possible after enrollment, followed 10 min later by another 5 mg IV over 5 min. Oral atenolol (50 mg given 10 min after the last IV dose, followed by 50–100 mg daily) was to be given if no contraindications existed. They compared the 30-day mortality of patients given no atenolol ($n$ = 10,073), any atenolol ($n$ = 30,771), any IV atenolol ($n$ = 18,200), only oral atenolol ($n$ = 12,545), and both IV and oral drug ($n$ = 16,406), after controlling for baseline differences and for early deaths (before oral atenolol could be given). Patients given any atenolol had a lower baseline risk than those not given atenolol. Adjusted 30-day mortality was significantly lower in atenolol-treated patients, but patients treated with IV and oral atenolol treatment versus oral treatment alone were more likely to die (odds ratio, 1.3; 95% confidence interval, 1.0–1.5; $p < 0.02$). IV atenolol use was associated with more heart failure, shock, recurrent ischemia, and pacemaker use than oral atenolol use. The rates of stroke, intracranial hemorrhage, and reinfarction were similar among the IV and oral versus oral atenolol groups. This post hoc analysis of atenolol use identified no significant change in mortality [15,16]. Current class I level A recommendations include the initiation of oral beta-blocker (metoprolol) therapy unless contraindicated within 24 h of the acute event; this is beneficial for secondary prevention and related complications [17]. The oral dose can be titrated to achieve rate control, and vigilance must be maintained to monitor for plausible complications from beta-blocker therapy. It should be noted that oral doses of beta-blocker therapy can be harmful if not titrated carefully. The POISE trial demonstrated that administration of an extended release dose of metoprolol 100 mg preoperatively led to an increase risk of stroke and death, further stressing the strategy to begin with a low dose and titrate to effect [18].

#### *73.3.3.2 Antiplatelet Therapy*

Aspirin 162–325 mg should be initiated on all patients suspected of experiencing an acute MI unless contraindicated. The use of aspirin alone reduces the incidence of reinfarction and mortality by 23% without any other adjuncts [19].

The efficacy of thienopyridines in the management of ST-elevation MI, clopidogrel primarily, has been tested in two large trials since the 2004 ACC/AHA guidelines publication. The COMMIT-CCS-2 included 45,852 patients who received 75 mg of clopidogrel daily in addition to a daily dose of 162 mg of aspirin. This trial achieved an end point of all-cause mortality reduction from 8.1% in the placebo group to 7.5% in the clopidogrel group ($p$ = 0.03), and the rate of cerebral and major noncerebral bleeding was 0.55% in the placebo group and 0.58% in the clopidogrel group ($p$ = 0.59) [20]. The other trial was the CLARITY-TIMI 28 that included clopidogrel added to thrombolytic therapy. I will not elaborate on this study as it is not relevant to the postsurgical population, but I will comment that there was an improvement of the end point that was occluded infarct artery on angiography or death or recurrent

MI before angiography. This was reduced from 21.7% in the placebo group versus 15.0% in the clopidogrel group [21]. Suffice to say that clopidogrel is considered a class I level A recommendation for adjuvant therapy for ST-elevation MI. Nevertheless, in our postsurgical and trauma patient population, thienopyridines should be used with caution.

Glycoprotein IIb/IIIa receptor antagonists are used in conjunction with PCI, and have no role in independent use as an adjuvant, without the involvement of a PCI specialist.

#### *73.4.3.3 Anticoagulants*

Administration of unfractionated heparin is often administered on a weight-based protocol to include a bolus of 60 U/kg up to a maximum of 4000 U and an initial infusion rate of 12 U/kg/h with a goal to keep the partial thromboplastin time between 50 and 70 s. Unfractionated heparin currently holds a class IIa level B recommendation. Fondaparinux is beneficial when compared to LMWH in the absence of a PCI with respect to reducing the risk of bleeding [22]. However, in the setting of a PCI, there is no superiority of one agent over the other, nor is there a difference in risk of bleeding in nonsurgical patients [23]. Currently the 2013 ACCF/AHA guidelines for managing ST-elevation MI list Fondaparinux as a class III with B level of evidence [24]. Bivalirudin is attractive due to its shorter half-life when compared to unfractionated heparin with respect to risk of bleed, and there is recent evidence that bivalirudin increases the risk of MI and stent thrombosis while reducing the risk of bleeding [25]. However, according to the recent 2013 ACCF/AHA guidelines for managing ST-elevation MI lists bivalirudin (with or without heparin) as a class I with B level of evidence as an alternative to heparin [24] pending further studies.

#### *73.3.3.4 Nitrates*

Although not addressed by current guidelines, the use of nitrates continues to be the standard of practice. In particular, nitroglycerin (NTG) transdermal, sublingual or via infusion therapy is frequently initiated to aid in improving angina and perfusion to the injured myocardium until direct revascularization is implemented. It should be noted that there is a lack of evidence to demonstrate an improvement in mortality from nitrates. Recently, the GISSI-3 trial compared ACE-I versus transdermal NTG versus ACE-I with transdermal NTG versus placebo. All patients received aspirin, IV and oral beta-blocker therapy, and thrombolytic therapy. The result demonstrated a benefit from the use of lisinopril, regardless of whether transdermal NTG was added [26]. When used IV, the dose of NTG is either 0.25–0.5 mcg/kg/min or 10 mcg/min and titrated to effect as long as the patient is hemodynamically appropriate. Remember to use appropriate tubing to avoid chelating of NTG before entering the patient.

### 73.3.4 ACE-I

Several trials have demonstrated the benefit of initiating ACE-I therapy as soon as the patient tolerates its use. In the CONSENSUS II trail, 103 Scandinavian centers studied patients with an acute MI and blood pressure above 100/60 mmHg. Subjects were randomly assigned to treatment with either enalapril or placebo, in addition to conventional therapy. Therapy was initiated with an IV infusion of enalapril (enalaprilat) within 24 h after the onset of chest pain, followed by administration of oral enalapril. Of the 6090 patients enrolled, 3046 were assigned to placebo and 3044 to enalapril. The mortality rates in the two groups at 1 and 6 months were not significantly different (6.3% and 10.2% in the placebo group versus 7.2% and 11.0% in the enalapril group, $p = 0.26$). The relative risk of death in the enalapril group was 1.10 (95% confidence interval, 0.93–1.29). Death due to progressive heart failure occurred in 104 patients (3.4%) in the placebo group and 132 (4.3%) in the enalapril group ($p = 0.06$).

As for oral ACE-I therapy, data from the SAVE and later HOPE trials both support the use of oral ACE-I in the postacute MI setting if not contraindicated. In the SAVE trial, 2231 patients with left ventricular ejection fraction (LVEF) <40% were randomized to receive either placebo ($n = 1116$) or oral captopril ($n = 1115$) within 3–16 days postacute MI. The initial dose of captopril was 12.5 mg, but the dose was reduced to 6.25 mg for subjects with marked decreases in blood pressure. The target for the study was 25 mg three times a day with the maximum of 50 mg three times a day. Subjects were observed for 2 years, and the following data were obtained. All-cause mortality was 20% in the captopril group compared to 25% in the placebo group, with a relative risk reduction of 19% (95% confidence interval, 3%–32%; $p = 0.019$). In the HOPE trial, a total of 9297 high-risk patients who had evidence of vascular disease or diabetes plus one other cardiovascular risk factor and who were not known to have a low ejection fraction or heart failure were randomly assigned to receive ramipril (10 mg once per day orally) or matching placebo for a mean of 5 years. The primary outcome was a composite of MI, stroke, or death from cardiovascular causes as defined by the investigators. A total of 651 patients received ramipril (14.0%) and reached the primary end point, as compared with 826 patients who were assigned to receive placebo (17.8%). Treatment with ramipril reduced the rates of death from cardiovascular causes (6.1%, as compared with 8.1% in the placebo group; relative risk, 0.74; $p < 0.001$), MI (9.9% versus 12.3%; relative risk, 0.80; $p < 0.001$), stroke (3.4% versus 4.9%; relative risk, 0.68; $p < 0.001$), death from any cause (10.4% versus 12.2%; relative risk, 0.84; $p$ = 0.005), revascularization procedures (16.0% versus 18.3%; relative risk, 0.85; $p$ = 0.002), cardiac arrest (0.8% versus 1.3%; relative risk, 0.63; $p$ = 0.03), heart failure (9.0% versus 11.5%; relative risk, 0.77; $p$ < 0.001), and complications related to diabetes (6.4% versus 7.6%; relative risk, 0.84; $p$ = 0.03). In conclusion, for LVEF <40%, it is a class I level A recommendation; for low-risk patients that have >40% LVEF, it is class IIa level B recommendation.

The SAVE trial [27] demonstrated an improvement in mortality of just over 20%; the HOPE trial [28] improved survival related to cardiac events as well as a reduction in stroke. ACE-I should be initiated within 24 h if tolerated, and, like beta-blockers, the oral route of administration results in improved outcomes.

The recommendation is to initiate a low dose and titrate the dose as tolerated. For those patients that do not tolerate ACE-I due to the adverse reactions, similar benefits have been noted with angiotensin receptor blockers (ARBs). The VALIANT trial assessed the effect of captopril, valsartan, and the combination of both [29]. It was noted that both captopril and valsartan were as effective, but when used together the risks of an adverse effect outweighed the benefit to the patient.

### 73.3.5 Non-ST-Elevation MI

The key for non-ST-elevation MI is to establish reperfusion by thrombolytic therapy if PCI is not available.

#### *73.3.5.1 Beta-Blocker Therapy*

Like with ST-elevation MI, the use of oral beta-blockers is more advantageous than that of IV beta-blockers. The recommendation is a class I level B to initiate within 24 h of the acute coronary event, as long at the patient does not have any contraindications as listed in the ST-elevation section [30]. Initiate a low dose and titrate to achieve rate control.

#### *73.3.5.2 Antiplatelet Therapy*

As before, the use of aspirin is invaluable and should be initiated within 10 min of identifying signs and symptoms of an acute MI, unless contraindicated. The patient should continue to receive this therapy as it not only reduces mortality in the group by nearly 50%, but it also reduces reinfarction.

The addition of clopidogrel to the group of 12,562 patients in the CURE trial demonstrated a benefit in mortality, MI, and stroke with only a 1% risk of major nonlife threatening bleeds ($p$ = 0.001) [31]. The current guidelines recommend either/or clopidogrel 300 mg load or a GP IIb/IIIa load if an early intervention strategy is anticipated, and this is class I level A recommendation [30]. Again, clopidogrel should be used with caution in the postoperative population.

#### *73.3.5.3 Anticoagulants*

Unfractionated heparin as well as LMWH remains a class I level A recommendation. In this patient population, based on the ESSENCE trial that included 22,000 patients, they noted a statistically significant reduction in the combined end point of death or nonfatal MI at 30 days for enoxaparin versus unfractionated heparin in the overall trial populations (10.1% versus 11.0%; OR, 0.91; 95% CI, 0.83–0.99; number needed to treat, 107) [32]. In the TIMI 11B trial, LMWH was demonstrated to be superior to unfractionated heparin without increased risk of bleeding [33]. The dose for LMWH is 1 mg/kg every 12 h subcutaneously. The unfractionated heparin dose is the same as described in the ST-elevation section.

#### *73.3.5.4 Nitrates*

Like with ST-elevation MI, there is no evidence that nitrates will improve outcome, but are helpful in managing the patient's symptoms of angina. Initiate at the same doses described above, and titrate to effect as long as the patient tolerates its use. Avoid use in patients with a systolic blood pressure below 90 mmHg.

### 73.3.6 Cardiogenic Shock

Cardiogenic shock is one of the complications from an acute MI. Management strategies vary, and there is no evidence to clearly guide our choice in agents with improved outcome in a large, multicenter trial. However, both Dobutamine and Milrinone have demonstrated improved cardiac index with their use in left ventricular failure, but no conclusive evidence of improved outcome in the setting of acute MI. There is an increasing evidence for the use of sildenafil for right ventricular failure, but its role in right ventricular failure in the setting of acute MI is limited. There is limited evidence that support the efficacy of sildenafil as a good agent to reduce pulmonary vascular resistance, while decreasing LVEDP and improving cardiac index [34]. Right ventricular failure as a result of pulmonary hypertension will respond well to sildenafil and actually improves the quality of life after 12 weeks [35] and after 6 months [36]. Since nitrates are the standard of therapy in an acute MI, sildenafil should likely be avoided until more evidence is available.

Intra-aortic balloon counterpulsation (IABCP) in acute MI has been used for nearly 30 years. Unfortunately, there are limited data to determine if its use impacts mortality, even though a study in which data were collected prospectively includes 250 medical centers worldwide and 5495 patients with acute MI and IABCP [37]. Nevertheless, it is a plausible strategy to augment cardiac index but primarily alleviate the left ventricle from added work during an ischemic event. We anticipate in the near future considering levosimendan as an adjunct for cardiogenic shock. There is emerging evidence of its use to include a trial comparing IABCP with levosimendan, in which troponin was lower with levosimendan when compared to IABCP [38]. There is an ongoing trial in the United States to further evaluate the role of levosimendan in perioperative medicine.

## 73.4 Conclusion

Diagnosis of an MI in the postoperative patient requires that the clinician has a high index of suspicion as often this patient population is sedated and intubated or is under the influence of analgesic therapy. Thus reliance on monitors and biomarkers and rapid implementation of a plan to establish reperfusion and anti-ischemic therapy is key. Overall, the oral route of administration for both beta-blocker therapy and ACE-I therapy is more efficacious, even when low-dose therapy is initiated and titrated carefully. Antiplatelet therapy is of utmost importance regardless of whether the patient will receive thrombolytic therapy. Aspirin of 162–325 mg should be initiated and continued indefinitely unless contraindicated. Anticoagulation with unfractionated heparin has been the standard for some time and presently receives the most evidence for its use, but emerging data support superiority of LMWH over unfractionated heparin. Regardless, anticoagulation is an adjuvant to antiplatelet therapy in establishing reperfusion and reducing the risk of restenosis in the acute phase. Finally, implementation of a plan that is easily reproducible and communicated is key to successful delivery of evidence-based care. Development of protocol or algorithm-driven therapy is the key to eliminating deviation from evidence-based practice in a setting of a variety of practitioners from different training backgrounds (Table 73.1).

**TABLE 73.1**

Questions, Levels of Evidence, and References

| | Question | Answer | Grade | References |
|---|---|---|---|---|
| 1 | What beta-blocker is recommended for management of an acute myocardial infarction (MI), and is an intravenous dose superior? | The current ACC/AHA recommendations suggest that an oral dose of beta-blocker therapy (metoprolol) is the optimal treatment. Upon review of IV beta-blocker therapy, mortality is not affected when compared to oral beta-blocker therapy that improved mortality | Class I, Level A | [3,16,17] |
| 2 | What ACE-I is indicated for the management of an acute MI, and is an intravenous dose superior? | The current ACC/AHA recommendations suggest that an oral dose of ACE-I therapy is the optimal treatment. Upon review of IV ACE-I therapy, mortality is not affected when compared to oral ACE-I therapy that improved mortality. For LVEF <40%, it is a class I level A recommendation. For low-risk patients >40% LVEF, it is IIa level B recommendation | Class I, Level A; and Class IIa Level B | [3] |
| 3 | Does the addition of an angiotensin receptor blocker (ARB) improve the benefit of an ACE-I? | Addition of an ARB does not improve the outcome of the patient, and was noted to introduce more adverse effects. ARBs are as effective as ACE-I and can be used when ACE-I are not tolerated by the patient due to adverse reactions | Class I, Level A | [3,29] |
| 4 | Is a baby aspirin 81 mg adequate for management of an acute MI? | A minimum of 162 mg of aspirin should be administered within 10 min of recognizing that the patient is experiencing an acute MI | Class I, Level A | [3] |
| 5 | Is clopidogrel indicated in the management of an acute MI? | Adding clopidogrel to aspirin does improve outcome in non-ST-elevation MI and should be considered. However, caution should be taken we used in postoperative patients | Class I, Level A | [3,31] |
| 6 | What is the optimal time from door to PCI that reduces mortality? | Ninety minutes is the optimal time from door to PCI. Patients that received an intervention within this time frame experienced a reduction in mortality | Class I, Level A | [3,13] |
| 7 | In the absence of a PCI, which agent can be used for anticoagulation with the aim to have lower bleeding? | Fondaparinux is an alternative agent to heparin that has similar outcome with lower bleeding risk profile | Class III, Level B | [23,24] |
| 8 | In the absence of heparin for continuous infusion, what anticoagulant can be used as an anticoagulant? | Bivalirudin can be used at this time pending more evidence | Class I, Level A | [24,25] |

*Note:* These are common questions that need to be addressed while managing a patient with an acute myocardial event. Here, we provide the answers to the specific questions as well as the level of evidence and the respective reference.

## References


1. Go AS, Mozaffarian D, Roger VL, et al. Heart disease and stroke statistics—2014 Update. A report from the American Heart Association. *Circulation*. 2014;128:0–267.
2. Centers for Disease Control and Prevention. Heart disease facts and statistics. Accessed November 5, 2014. http://www.cdc.gov/heartdisease/facts.htm.
3. ACCF/AHA guidelines for the management of ST-elevation myocardial infarction: A report of the American College of Cardiology Foundation/American Heart Association Task Force on Practice Guidelines. *Circulation*. 2013;128(25):e362–e425.
4. Pollack CV, Braunwald E. Update to the ACC/AHA guidelines for the management of patients with unstable angina and non-ST-segment elevation myocardial infarction: Implications for Emergency Department Practice. *Ann Emerg Med*. 2007;51(5):591–606.
5. Shanewise JS, Cheung AT, Aronson S et al. ASE/SCA guidelines for performing a comprehensive intraoperative multiplane transesophageal echocardiography examination: Recommendations of the American Society of Echocardiography Council for Intraoperative Echocardiography and the Society of Cardiovascular Anesthesiologists Task Force for Certification in Perioperative Transesophageal Echocardiography. *Anesth Analg*. 1999;89(4):870–884.
6. Stillman AE, Oudkerk M, Bluemke D et al. Assessment of acute myocardial infarction: Current status and recommendation from the North American society of cardiovascular imaging and the European society of cardiac radiology. *Int J Cardiovasc Imag*. 2011;27:7–24.
7. Heller GV, Stowers SA, Hendel RC et al. Clinical value of acute rest technetium-99 m tetrofosmin tomographic myocardial perfusion imaging in patients with acute chest pain and nondiagnostic electrocardiograms. *J Am Coll Cardiol*. 1998;31:1011–1017.
8. Hilton TC, Thompson RC, Williams HJ, Saylors R, Fulmer H, Stowers SA. Technetium-99 m sestamibi myocardial perfusion imaging in the emergency room evaluation of chest pain. *J Am Coll Cardiol*. 2004; 23:1016–1022.
9. Kontos MC, Jesse RL, Anderson FP, Schmidt KL, Ornato JP, Tatum JL. Comparison of myocardial perfusion imaging and cardiac troponin I in patients admitted to the emergency department with chest pain. *Circulation*. 1999;99:2073–2078.
10. Kontos MC, Jesse RL, Schmidt KL, Ornato JP, Tatum JL. Value of acute rest sestamibi perfusion imaging for evaluation of patients admitted to the emergency department with chest pain. *J Am Coll Cardiol*. 1997;30:976–982.
11. Udelson JE, Beshansky JR, Ballin DS et al. Myocardial perfusion imaging for evaluation and triage of patients with suspected acute cardiac ischemia: A randomized controlled trial. *JAMA*. 2002;288:2693–2700.
12. The Gusto Investigators. An international randomized trial comparing four thrombolytic strategies for acute myocardial infarction. *NEJM*. 1993;329(10):673–682.
13. Khot UN, Johnson ML et al. Emergency Department physician activation of the catheterization laboratory and immediate transfer to an immediately available catheterization laboratory reduce door-to-balloon time in ST-elevation myocardial infarction. *Circulation*. 2007;116(3):67–76.
14. Nallamothu BK, Wang Y, Magid DJ et al. Relation between hospital specialization with primary Percutaneous coronary intervention and clinical outcomes in ST-segment elevation myocardial infarction: National Registry of Myocardial Infarction-4 analysis. *Circulation*. 2006;113:222–229.
15. Pfisterer M, Cox JL, Granger CB et al. Atenolol use and clinical outcomes after thrombolysis for acute myocardial infarction: The (alteplase) for Occluded Coronary Arteries. *JACC*. 1998;32:634–640.
16. Antman EM, Anbe DT, Armstrong PW et al. ACC/AHA guidelines for the management of patients with ST-elevation myocardial infarction: A report of the American College of Cardiology/American Heart Association Task Force on Practice Guidelines (Committee to Revise the 1999 Guidelines for the Management of patients with acute myocardial infarction). *JACC*. 2004;44:e1–e211.
17. Lopez-Sendon J, Swedberg K, McMurray J et al. Expert consensus document on beta-adrenergic receptor blockers. *Eur Heart J*. 2004;25:1341–1362.
18. POISE Study Group. Effects of extended-release metoprolol succinate in patients undergoing non-cardiac surgery (POISE trial): A randomized controlled trial. *Lancet*. 2008;371:1839–1847.
19. ISIS-2 Collaborative Group. Randomized trial of intravenous streptokinase, oral aspirin, both, or neither among 17,187 cases of suspected acute myocardial infarction: ISIS-2. *Lancet*. 1988;2:349–360.
20. Chen ZM, Jiang LX, Chen YP et al. Addition of Clopidogrel t aspirin in 45,852 patients with acute myocardial infarction: Randomized placebo-controlled trial. *Lancet*. 2005;366;1607–1621.
21. Scirica BM, Sabatine MS, Morrow DA et al. The role of Clopidogrel in early and sustained arterial patency after fibrinolysis for ST-segment elevation myocardial infarction: The ECG CLARITY-TIMI 28 study. *JACC*. 2006;48:37–42.
22. The Fifth Organization to Assess Strategies in Acute Ischemic Syndromes Investigators. Comparison of fondaparinux and enoxaparin in acute coronary syndromes. *N Engl J Med*. 2006;354:1464–1476.
23. The OASIS-6 Trial Group. Effects of fondaparinux on mortality and reinfarction in patients with acute ST-segment elevation myocardial infraction. *JAMA*. 2006;295:1519–1530.
24. O'Gara PT, Casey DE, Lemos JA et al. ACCF/AHA guideline for the management of ST-elevation myocardial infarction. *Circulation*. 2013;127:e362–e425.
25. Cavender MA, Sabatine MS. Bivalirudin versus heparin in patients planned for percutaneous coronary intervention: A meta-analysis of randomized controlled trials. *Lancet*. 2014;384:599–606.

26. GISSI-3 Investigators. Causes of death in patients with acute myocardial infarction treated with angiotensin-converting enzyme inhibitors: Findings from the Gruppo Italiano per lo Studio della Sopravvivenza nell'Infarto (GISSI)–3 trial. *Am Heart J.* 2008;155:388–394.
27. Pfeffer MA, Braunwald E, Moye LA et al. Effect of captopril on mortality and morbidity in patients with left ventricular dysfunction after f infarction. Results of the survival and ventricular enlargement trial. The SAVE Investigators. *N Engl J Med.* 1992;327:669–677.
28. Yusuf S, Sleight P, Pogue J et al. Effects of an angiotensin-converting-enzyme inhibitor, ramipril, on cardiovascular events in high-risk patients. The Heart Outcomes Prevention Evaluation Study Investigators. *N Engl J Med.* 2000;342:145–153.
29. Pfeffer MA, McMurray JJ, Velazquez EJ et al. Valsartan, captopril, or both in myocardial infarction complicated by heart failure, left ventricular dysfunction, or both. *N Engl J Med.* 2003;349:1893–1906.
30. Anderson JL, Adams CD, Antman EM et al. ACC/AHA 2007 guidelines for the management of patients with unstable angina/non–ST-elevation myocardial infarction: A report of the American College of Cardiology/American Heart Association Task Force on Practice Guidelines (Writing Committee to Revise the 2002 Guidelines for the Management of Patients With Unstable Angina/Non–ST-Elevation Myocardial Infarction): Developed in collaboration with the American College of Emergency Physicians, American College of Physicians, Society for Academic Emergency Medicine, Society for Cardiovascular Angiography and Interventions, and Society of Thoracic Surgeons. *J Am Coll Cardiol.* 2007;50:e1–e157.
31. Yusuf S, Zhao F, Mehta SR, Chrolavicius S, Tognoni G, Fox KK. Effects of clipidogrel in addition to aspirin in patients with acute coronary syndromes without ST-segment elevation. *N Engl J Med.* 2001;345:494–502.
32. Petersen JL, Califf RM et al. Efficacy and bleeding complications among patients randomized to enoxaparin or unfractionated heparin for antithrombin therapy in non–ST-segment elevation acute coronary syndromes. A systematic overview. *JAMA.* 2004;292:89–96.
33. Antman EM, McCabe CH, Braunwald E. TIMI 11B investigators. Enoxaparin prevents death and cardiac ischemic events in unstable angina/non–Q-wave myocardial infarction results of the thrombolysis in myocardial infarction (TIMI) 11B trial. *Circulation.* 1999;100:1593–1601.
34. Michelakis E, Tymchak W, Archer S et al. Oral sildenafil is an effective and specific pulmonary vasodilator in patients with pulmonary arterial hypertension. comparison with inhaled nitric oxide. *Circulation.* 2002;105:2398–2403.
35. SUPER Study Group. Sildenafil citrate therapy for arterial pulmonary hypertension. *N Engl J Med.* 2005;353:2148–2157.
36. Pepke-Zaba J, Gilbert C, Collings L, Brown, MCJ. Sildenafil improves health-related quality of life in patients with pulmonary arterial hypertension. *Chest.* 2008;133:183–189.
37. Stone GW, Ohman EM, Ferguson JJ, III et al. Contemporary utilization and outcomes of intra-aortic balloon counterpulsation in acute myocardial infarction. *JACC.* 2003;41(11):1940–1945.
38. Lomivorotov VV, Boboshko VA, Efremov SM et al. Levosimendan versus an intra-aortic balloon pump in high-risk cardiac patients. *J Cardiothorac Vasc Anesth.* 2011;25(4):632–636.

## Commentary on Management of Acute Myocardial Infarction and Cardiogenic Shock

*Marvin H. Eng*

Acute myocardial infarctions (AMIs) occur secondary to thrombus formation, platelet activation, and high myocardial oxygen demand, resulting in oxygen deficit for the myocardium. Infarction of myocardium is a life-threatening event, but compounding the complexity with the context of recent surgery presents a particularly challenging clinical dilemma. Patients and providers frequently find themselves without palatable options and usually opt for the best "worst-case scenario." Nevertheless providers must learn to balance multiple clinical variables when managing the infarction and optimizing multiorgan support.

1. Thrombosis and bleeding: The pathophysiology of myocardial infarction, both non-ST elevation myocardial infarction (NSTEMI), or ST-elevation myocardial infarction (STEMI) results from thrombus formation with complete or subtotal vessel occlusion against the background of an unstable plaque. Inactivating both platelets and protein-mediated coagulation pathways with are central to management strategies, but of course, the opportunity to use these agents depends on relative degree of benefit from decreasing thrombosis to the risks associated with bleeding. And these risks must be balanced against the predicted morbidity and mortality of allowing the infarction to complete. As already detailed in Dr. Hernandez's chapter, there is a broad combination of antiplatelet agents (e.g., aspirin, thienopyridines, glycoprotein inhibitors) and anticoagulants (e.g., heparins, direct thrombin inhibitors) at the clinician's disposal.
2. Myocardial oxygen demand: Lowering myocardial oxygen demand remains important in management and can prevent recurrent infarctions in those without the options of revascularization. Decreasing the heart rate is one strategy using beta-blockers as the drug of choice. Minimizing wall-stress is another treatable condition. Recall that wall stress is proportional to the afterload and preload; therefore, lowering blood pressure and filling pressures can relieve stress on the heart. This can be accomplished with any combination of pharmacologic agents and mechanical support devices such as nitroglycerin, nitroprusside, or mechanical support devices, respectively. Mechanical support for myocardial infarction or cardiogenic shock may include intra-aortic balloon counterpulsation (IABCP) or percutaneous left ventricular assist devices.
3. Assessment of myocardial jeopardy and diagnostic angiography: Decisions to revascularize a patient may hinge on the location of the infarction, degree of myocardium affected, and/or ventricular function. Noninvasive means of making the assessment include ECG, echocardiography, nuclear imaging, or MRI. ECG may divulge the general location of the infarction, but it is a crude tool and does not reliably inform providers of the extent of the territory. Location does matter, however, as anterior myocardial infarctions carry a worse inpatient and long-term prognosis than inferior infarctions. Most patients in the perioperative period with an AMI are usually only stable enough to undergo echocardiography, since this is a bedside exam. Instances where the echocardiographer cannot provide detailed images, transesophageal echocardiography, or possible invasive ventriculography may be the best tools for ventricular function measurement.

   At some point, if the patient can tolerate a percutaneous procedure, coronary anatomy should be imaged using angiography. By anatomically defining the lesions and amount of myocardium at stake, we can better understand the type of revascularization needed and thus the risk/benefit ratio of revascularization versus medical management. Many patients presenting with myocardial infarctions may have multivessel coronary disease and risk stratification should occur according to coronary lesion severity, distribution, and left ventricular function. For those patients with a significant risk of bleeding, diagnostic angiography need not require anticoagulation and the catheterization operator may pause and have a multidisciplinary discussion prior to revascularizing the patient.
4. Optimizing perfusion and revascularization: The decision to percutaneously revascularize the patient must be made after duly taking into consideration the risks of bleeding and the ability to continue the patient on dual-antiplatelet therapy. Angioplasty and stenting for AMI involves using some of the most aggressive anticoagulation regiments, either heparin, heparin + glycoprotein inhibitor, or bivalirudin with the combination of aspirin and/or thienopyridines. The most important facet of percutaneous coronary

intervention is restoration of perfusion, whether it is from balloon angioplasty, thrombectomy, or includes implantation of a stent. The liability of stent implantation is the requirement for dual-antiplatelet, because without this, the stent is at high risk for thrombosis, resulting in another myocardial infarction. Therefore, operators may choose to accept balloon angioplasty results with the understanding that stent implantation can be performed at a later time, provided the angioplasty result is stable. If percutaneous intervention is not feasible, increasing perfusion pressure via IABCP may be an option.

5. Hemodynamics and possible mechanical ventricular support: Perfusion assessment clinically (i.e., urine output, warm extremities) or with a pulmonary artery catheter plays a significant role in managing patients. Those patients with cardiogenic shock should undergo revascularization if possible. For those with hypoperfusion, restoration of perfusion is imperative to prevent acidosis and further hemodynamic embarrassment. Therefore, aside from revascularizing the patient, management from interventional cardiology can include IABCP implantation or if needed, a ventricular mechanical assist device such as the Impella (Abiomed, Danvers, Massachusetts) axial flow pump, Tandem Heart (Cardiac Assist, Pittsburg, PA), or extracorporeal membrane oxygenation (ECMO). These devices each have associated bleeding and vascular complications; however, in patients that are not perfusing, they can restore adequate tissue oxygenation and temporarily stabilize patients.
6. Pulmonary status: The first phase of myocardial dysfunction in AMI is stiffening of the ventricle and diastolic dysfunctions. With this, there may be ensuing pulmonary edema and it may be severe depending on the degree of mitral regurgitation in association with the infarction. Certainly, treatment of high-left sided filling pressures (elevated pulmonary capillary wedge pressure) and pulmonary edema will be necessary to optimize oxygenation. In acute situations with unintubated patients call for the use of bi-pap or intubation depending on the mental status and stability. In case of difficulty in oxygenating the patients, use of preload-lowering agents such as nitroglycerin or nitroprusside can be helpful and the patient may require diuresis.
7. Electrical stability: Patients suffering from acute coronary occlusion may manifest arrhythmias anywhere from heart block to ventricular tachycardia storm, a syndrome where the patient has incessant unstable arrhythmias. Certainly, treatment using antiarrhythmic agents is indicated, but unstable electrical arrhythmias may increase the impetus for reperfusion.

#### Postinfarction Care

Whether or not the patient is revascularized, the likelihood of a mechanical complication from the myocardial infarction depends on degree of myocardial damage and adequacy of reperfusion. Patients without revascularization are most susceptible to repeat infarction. Those with completed infarcts may develop complications such as myocardial rupture, ischemic mitral regurgitation, pseudoaneurysm formation, heart block, and aneurysm formation. Postinfarction left ventricular dysfunction can be expected and tailored vasodilator therapy and/or mechanical ventricular support may be required in the convalescent period. Certainly, these are some of the most complex patients and their care should involve the assistance of cardiovascular consultants.

In summary, management of AMI and cardiogenic shock in perioperative patients is one of the most challenging clinical scenarios and requires the careful prioritization and balancing of the aforementioned clinical variables in a thoughtful manner. There is little guidance in managing these patients and a great deal of individualization is required as the breadth and variability of patients is innumerable; however, with careful weighing of these variables, critical care of these patients can be conducted in a more enlightened fashion, hopefully translating into success.

# 74

# *Perioperative Arrhythmias*

**Bipin K. Ravindran and Mohan N. Viswanathan**

**CONTENTS**



## 74.1 Atrial Arrhythmias

Atrial tachyarrhythmias in the early perioperative period are extremely common and encompass atrial fibrillation (AF), atrial flutter, and atrial tachycardia. These rhythm disturbances are similar in terms of their risk factors and management. AF greatly outweighs the incidence of the others and has been the focus of essentially all the existing retrospective, observational, and prospective randomized, controlled trials. Accordingly, AF will be the focus of this discussion.

AF is the most frequently encountered arrhythmia in outpatient clinical practice, and therefore, it is not surprising that AF is also the most commonly encountered perioperative arrhythmia. AF occurs in 4%–20% of patients following noncardiac surgery depending on the complexity of the operation with the highest incidence occurring with cardiac, vascular, and major abdominal surgeries [1–3]. In fact, in coronary artery bypass grafting (CABG), AF occurs in 25%–33% of patients [4–7]. Adding valvular surgery to CABG increases the incidence of AF up to 60% with aortic valve replacement and up to 63% with mitral valve replacement [6].

The exact pathophysiology of AF is still not well defined. The rhythm is characterized by multiple, simultaneously occurring atrial depolarizations that propagate chaotically throughout the atria, the multiple wavelet theory [8–10]. Even less is known about the development of AF in the perioperative setting, but it is thought to be related to (1) catecholamine excess [11], (2) autonomic imbalance [12], (3) inflammation [12,13], and (4) shifts in volume and pressure in the atria that can all affect electrical conduction and stability [14,15].

AF is commonly thought of as a disease of the elderly. Increasing age is the greatest risk factor for incident AF in both the outpatient and perioperative setting. In a study of 570 consecutive patients undergoing CABG, the risk of developing AF in those less than 60 was 18% and in those over 80 was as high as 52% [5]. Additional independent risk factors for AF include prior AF, male gender, reduced left ventricular systolic function, valvular surgery, chronic obstructive pulmonary disease, chronic renal insufficiency, and diabetes mellitus [16].

## 74.2 Prevention

### 74.2.1 What Are Effective and Safe Pharmacologic Strategies for the Prevention of Postoperative AF after Coronary Artery Bypass Surgery?

#### *74.2.1.1 Beta-Adrenergic Receptor Antagonists*

Beta-blockers are the most studied drug class in preventing AF after cardiothoracic surgery and have an established benefit. Although numerous studies have been performed, there exists significant heterogeneity in study designs, specifically with regard to the number of patients enrolled, primary endpoints, specific beta-blocker studied, and even timing of initial therapy. Two meta-analyses looking collectively at these studies demonstrated that beta-blockers reduced the incidence of AF after cardiothoracic surgery by 61%–64% compared with control subjects [17,18].

The largest and probably the best designed beta-blocker study enrolled more than 500 patients in a randomized, double-blinded, placebo-controlled trial, named the beta-Blocker Length of Stay (BLOS) study [19]. The investigators set out to determine whether the expected reduction in postoperative AF with oral metoprolol was associated with a shortened hospital length of stay. The treatment group received either 100 or 150 mg of oral metoprolol daily after arrival to the intensive care unit. Despite a 20% reduction in postoperative AF in the treatment group, the authors were surprised to find that the length of stay was not statistically different between the two groups. This may have been for several reasons. First, all nonstudy beta-blockers were allowed to be continued in both study groups, which accounted for 40% of the control group. This might have decreased the observed effect of beta-blocker therapy. Second, it is also possible that the beta-blockers might have caused adverse complications due to bradycardia or hypotension, which could attenuate any benefits of having reduced the total AF burden. Finally, because the observed reduction in AF from beta-blockers was much lower than expected, this would render this study underpowered to detect a difference in length of stay.

In summary, there is overwhelming evidence that patients on preoperative beta-blockers should be continued on their current therapy and patients who are naïve to beta-blockers should be initiated on beta-blocker therapy and be continued throughout the perioperative period.

#### *74.2.1.2 Amiodarone: Class III Antiarrhythmic*

Amiodarone is a unique antiarrhythmic drug that has been shown to reduce AF after cardiothoracic surgery. The drug works via its multiple actions on potassium, sodium, and calcium channels, as well as possessing anti-adrenergic properties that might aid in attenuating the heightened sympathetic tone seen after surgery. In the Atrial Fibrillation Suppression Trial II (AFIST II) study, an intravenous (IV) amiodarone study, 160 patients undergoing CABG +/− valve surgery received either the treatment drug beginning within the first 6 h postoperatively or received placebo. The treatment group had an encouraging reduction in AF with 22.1% compared to the 38.6% seen in the placebo arm [20]. Instead of IV amiodarone, the PAPABEAR study utilized oral amiodarone, which was initiated 6 days preoperatively, and demonstrated a significant reduction in AF with only 16.1% seen in the treatment group and 29.5% AF seen in the placebo arm [21].

While these results are encouraging, amiodarone is not a completely benign therapy, especially given the numerous reported complications seen in the outpatient setting. Several case reports draw particular attention to the possibility of developing pulmonary toxicity and even fulminant acute respiratory distress syndrome (ARDS). However, two studies looking specifically to identify ARDS as a possible risk failed to demonstrate that amiodarone increases the risk of ARDS in postcardiothoracic surgical patient [22,23].

A recent meta-analysis looked at the safety profile of amiodarone in over 18 different postcardiothoracic surgery trials [24]. This study showed that amiodarone had the benefits of fewer episodes of ventricular arrhythmias and fewer neurologic events (transient ischemic attacks [TIAs] or stroke). However, there were increased episodes of bradycardia and hypotension, but the authors note that more of these episodes were seen using IV amiodarone compared to oral amiodarone.

#### *74.2.1.3 Sotalol: Class III Antiarrhythmic*

Numerous studies have evaluated the potential of sotalol to reduce postcardiothoracic surgery AF due to the effects imparted by both its antiarrhythmic properties and its beta-blocking properties. All of these studies have consistently demonstrated a significant reduction in AF with a recent meta-analysis reporting there to be a 63% risk reduction in AF (odds ratio = 0.37 with 95% confidence interval = 0.29–0.48) [18]. It was found to be more effective than beta-blockers alone by 10%. While these results are certainly promising, there is significant potential for side effects including bradycardia, hypotension, and even proarrhythmia with the development of torsades de pointes (TdP) due to sotalol's QT-prolonging effects. The same meta-analysis noted that sotalol was not tolerated well and that patients discontinued treatment compared to placebo due to side effects of bradycardia, hypotension, and prolongation of the corrected QT (QTc) interval (6.0% vs. 1.9%, $p = 0.004$) [18]. Even though no significant difference was seen with rates of treatment withdrawal between sotalol and beta-blockers, this may have been because the individual studies had small numbers of enrollees and, therefore, may not have adequately represented all the potential for sotalol side effects.

Sotalol does hold promise as an effective prophylactic agent; however, large randomized, placebo-controlled trials need to be performed before it can be recommended as a primary agent.

*Recommendation*: Beta-blockers consistently demonstrate a reduction in AF with an acceptable safety profile (Grade A recommendation). In high-risk patients, amiodarone is also a reasonable strategy; however, there remains some uncertainty regarding its safety profile (Grade B recommendation).

## 74.2.2 Are There Intraoperative Strategies to Consider that may Reduce Incident AF after Cardiothoracic Surgery?

### *74.2.2.1 Intraoperative Techniques*

Varying degrees of hypothermia have demonstrated a significant reduction in postoperative AF, and greater reduction is seen in patients cooled to mild hypothermia (34°C) compared to moderate hypothermia (28°C). Induction of systemic hypothermia is common during CABG surgery for both myocardial and cerebral protection. Although the exact nature of the mechanism of benefit is unclear, it has been proposed that rewarming from only mild hypothermia may reduce autonomic fluctuations that increase the risk of AF [25].

Incision of the posterior pericardium in addition to the typical anterior incision has also been shown to reduce postoperative AF. The typical surgical approach is for the surgeon to make an anterior incision to expose the great vessels and underlying heart. The addition of the posterior incision is thought to facilitate drainage of blood and fluid that collects as a product of peri-myocardial inflammation. This would then theoretically minimize inflammation and irritation to the myocardium [26]. Possibly, with reduced irritation of the pericardium, the incidence of pericarditis should be reduced and, by extension, AF as well.

Cardiac perfusion bypass circuits have long been associated with systemic inflammation and may contribute to AF. Heparin-coated circuits were created in an effort to minimize the inflammation that leads to AF. Results from two randomized, controlled trials looking at the benefits of heparin-coated circuits demonstrated a reduction in AF. The specific brand of heparin-coated circuits used yielded variable results and, thus, should be taken into account [27,28].

### *74.2.2.2 Cardiac Pacing*

The usefulness of atrial pacing to prevent postoperative AF remains inconclusive. The theoretical goals of atrial pacing are to both reduce the premature atrial complexes that are frequently seen in the minutes to hours prior to the onset of AF [29] by overdrive pacing and to minimize dispersion of atrial repolarization [30]. Studies to date have collectively yielded conflicting results. Several studies looking separately at right atrial pacing, left atrial pacing, and biatrial pacing have yielded a reduction in AF in some with no benefit in the others. Of these different modalities, biatrial pacing appears to confer the most benefit with the largest randomized, controlled trial of 130 patients demonstrating a reduction in AF of 13.8% versus 38.5%, $p = 0.001$ [31]. However, these studies all suffer from small sample sizes and variable results, making a clear benefit questionable. At this time, despite the small amount of risk involved in placing epicardial leads at the time of surgery, atrial pacing cannot be strongly recommended for prevention of postoperative AF.

### *74.2.2.3 Treatment*

All hemodynamically *unstable* tachyarrhythmias should receive emergent direct current cardioversion. Otherwise, if hemodynamically *stable*, supraventricular arrhythmias, except for AF, atrial flutter, and most atrial tachycardias, can be terminated using IV adenosine by disrupting conduction at the level of the atrioventricular (AV) node. Typically, this is done using sequential attempts first with 6 mg and then 12 mg and then a repeat attempt with an additional 12 mg of adenosine, each given as a rapid IV bolus.

In hemodynamically stable patients, the management encompasses the control of ventricular rate, mitigating the risk of thromboembolic events and the option of restoring and maintaining normal sinus rhythm (NSR) via direct current cardioversion.

*Recommendation*: Applying mild hypothermia, performing a posterior pericardiotomy, and using heparin-coated bypass circuits have all suggested a benefit in reducing the risk of supraventricular tachycardias (Grade C recommendation).

### 74.2.3 What Drugs Should Be Avoided in Patients with AF with Underlying Wolff–Parkinson–White Syndrome?

It is important to avoid AV nodal blocking agents such as adenosine, beta-blockers, and calcium channel blockers (CCBs) if AF or atrial flutter occurs in a patient known to have ventricular preexcitation, namely, the Wolff–Parkinson–White syndrome [32,33]. If given, AV nodal blocking agents will promote conduction block in the AV node, thereby favoring anterograde over the accessory pathway at dangerously high conduction rates, and the rhythm could then degenerate into ventricular fibrillation (VF).

*Recommendation*: Adenosine, beta-blockers, and CCBs should be avoided in this group of patients (Grade A recommendation).

### 74.2.4 Is Elective Cardioversion, Chemically or by Direct Current Cardioversion, a Reasonable Option in the Postoperative AF Patient?

#### *74.2.4.1 Rate Control and Rhythm Control Strategies*

The first step in managing hemodynamically stable AF is to control the ventricular response, which is often rapid because of the heightened sympathetic tone seen in the immediate postoperative period. Beta-blockers are the first choice with either IV short-acting esmolol or IV metoprolol. Nondihydropyridine CCBs can also be used, but beta-blockers remain first line due to their antiadrenergic properties. Digoxin is considered less useful in the immediate postoperative setting because of its slow onset of action. But it is at times useful in patients with congestive heart failure (CHF) or if added to beta-blockers or CCBs for its synergistic rate-controlling effect. Furthermore, digoxin may be useful in the patient with marginal blood pressures in AF where a beta blocker or CCB would promote undesirable hypotension.

It is important to emphasize that most episodes of AF are self-limited and will frequently spontaneously convert to NSR without antiarrhythmic therapy. In one study, up to 80% of patients spontaneously converted to NSR within 24 h with only an AV nodal blocking agent given for rate control [34]. However, if the patient remains in AF, there are advantages to pursuing elective cardioversion (either chemically or by direct current application) including decreased hospital length of stay and prolonged maintenance of sinus rhythm [35].

Either chemical cardioversion using agents such as amiodarone, ibutilide, sotalol, flecainide, or propafenone or direct current cardioversion is a reasonable option. The advantage of chemical cardioversion is mainly the convenience of its administration; however, all antiarrhythmic medications confer some risk for complications, albeit usually small.

Amiodarone is the agent of choice when looking to chemically convert postoperative AF. When given IV, it will convert AF to NSR ~40%–90% of the time after cardiac surgery in 12–24 h [36–38]. It possesses significant advantages over other Class IC and III agents. Essentially, all antiarrhythmic drugs are associated with an increased risk of proarrhythmia either due to prolongation of the QTc interval resulting in TdP or through their modulation of refractory periods. However, this appears to be a very rare complication of amiodarone. In addition to having less proarrhythmia, its beta-blocking properties help with rate control while the patient is in AF. Finally, it also has the advantage of being easily converted to an oral form if it needs to be taken after discharge to the outpatient setting. Of course, caution should be taken if amiodarone is continued in the outpatient setting, one should be aware of its side effects on the liver, thyroid, and lung.

Ibutilide is a Class III antiarrhythmic that has proven effective in converting AF to NSR after cardiac surgery. In one study, at the 1 mg IV dose, it successfully converted 57% of patients to NSR, which was significantly higher than placebo. There is an increased risk of TdP due to its QT-prolonging effects, which was seen in 1.8% of patients receiving ibutilide. Given this proarrhythmia risk, certain precautions must be taken before administering ibutilide. One must make sure the QTc interval is not prolonged on a 12-lead ECG and that all electrolyte abnormalities have been corrected [39]. Often, pretreatment with magnesium is advocated before administering ibutilide.

*Recommendation*: Yes. Elective cardioversion may reduce length of hospital stay and prolong duration in NSR (Grade B recommendation).

### 74.2.5 Should Warfarin be Given in Postoperative AF that Is Recurrent or Persists for more than 24 h?

#### *74.2.5.1 Anticoagulation*

Anticoagulation for persistent AF (lasting greater than 48 h) must be strongly considered after cardiac surgery to reduce the devastating risk of stroke. The benefits of anticoagulation with heparin or warfarin need to be weighed against the risk of bleeding from the performed surgical procedure. The exact duration of anticoagulation, whether only for the short term or for the long term, needs to be individualized. The major factors that increase the risk of stroke in patients with AF are CHF, diabetes, hypertension, age >75 years, and prior history of TIA, thromboembolism, or stroke [40]; these risk factors comprise the $CHADS_2$ score. In general, patients with two or more $CHADS_2$ risk factors should receive anticoagulation.

#### *74.2.5.2 Bradyarrhythmias*

Conduction system disturbances following noncardiac surgery resulting in permanent pacemaker (PPM) placement are rare. On the other hand, it is relatively common following cardiac surgery, occurring in up to 2%–3% of patients [41,42]. The risk of requiring PPM placement increases with the complexity of the cardiac surgery. Repeat valve surgery results in up to 10% of patients requiring a PPM [43], whereas multivalve surgery results in PPM placement in 10% for aortic + mitral valves, in 16% for mitral + tricuspid valves, and in 25% for aortic + mitral + tricuspid valves [43]. There also has been an increase in the transcatheter aortic valve replacement procedure, and certain replacement valves are associated with an increased rate of postsurgical pacemaker placement.

The conduction disturbances resulting in sinus node dysfunction or varying degrees of heart block are either due to surgical trauma to the areas of the sinoatrial node, AV node, or His–Purkinje specialized conduction system or may be due to ischemic injury associated with cardioplegia.

In sinus node dysfunction or if significant heart block develops, management in the perioperative period is similar to other bradycardic presentations. Electrolyte imbalances need to be corrected and nonessential drugs contributing to bradycardia should be discontinued. Generally, no acute therapy is needed if there is no hemodynamic compromise and, particularly, if the arrhythmia is transient. Most of the bradyarrhythmias that occur immediately postoperatively are self-limited and resolve by postoperative day 7. In fact, it is noteworthy that up to 40% of these patients who receive a PPM, will eventually not require use of their implanted device [44].

In the acute setting, if sinus node dysfunction is persistent and results in end-organ hypoperfusion, then immediate management is needed. The sinus rate can be augmented by giving an anticholinergic agent such as IV atropine or by infusing a beta-agonist such as dopamine or isoproterenol.

If Mobitz type II AV block, high-grade AV block, or complete heart block occurs, then temporary pacing should be sought by either previously placed epicardial pacing wires, percutaneous transvenous pacing, or transcutaneous pacing. Temporary epicardial wires are often routinely implanted at the time of cardiac surgery, especially in patients who are at high risk for developing conduction disturbances.

The long-term management of persistent bradyarrhythmias is essentially the same postoperatively as in the outpatient setting and may require placement of a PPM as detailed by the ACC/AHA/HRS 2008 Guidelines for Device-Based Therapy of Cardiac Rhythm Abnormalities [45].

#### *74.2.5.3 Ventricular Arrhythmias*

Ventricular tachyarrhythmias after noncardiac surgery are uncommon. In two series, the incidence is reported to be up to 3%; however, the vast majority of these included hemodynamically insignificant ectopic ventricular beats [46,47]. Although after cardiothoracic surgery, sustained monomorphic ventricular tachycardia (VT), polymorphic VT, and VF are seen in up to 1%–3% of patients [48,49]. In the same studies, not surprisingly, the presence of ventricular conduction disturbances was associated with a significantly worse outcome compared to similar patients who did not develop these arrhythmias.

The entire spectrum of ventricular arrhythmias that can occur in the perioperative period includes isolated premature ventricular complexes (PVCs), nonsustained ventricular tachycardia (NSVT), sustained monomorphic VT (either with or without hemodynamic compromise), and VF.

PVCs in patients with structurally normal hearts have a benign prognosis and require no further therapy. However, beta-blockers can be used to suppress PVCs in symptomatic patients. In patients with structurally abnormal hearts (including those with either a nonischemic cardiomyopathy or an ischemic cardiomyopathy), like many of those who undergo cardiothoracic surgery, PVCs and nonsustained VT are associated with an increased risk of sudden death. Despite this increased risk, the CAST trials have shown that in patients who have suffered a prior myocardial infarction, suppression of PVCs and episodes of NSVT with Class I antiarrhythmic drugs (encainide, flecainide, and moricizine) increases mortality [50]. Therefore, the use of these drugs for suppression of PVCs and episodes of NSVT should be avoided because of their proarrhythmic nature.

All patients who develop sustained VT and polymorphic VT associated with hemodynamic instability should receive emergent direct current cardioversion. Additionally, an immediate evaluation is required to identify reversible causes such as ischemia, electrolyte imbalances, or the presence of QT-prolonging drugs that may result in a specific type of polymorphic VT, namely, TdP.

Beta-blockers are considered the cornerstone of antiarrhythmic drug therapy and have been shown to safely and effectively reduce the recurrence of the entire spectrum of ventricular arrhythmias in those with and without structural heart disase [51,52]. Patients with structural heart disease should be given beta-blockers as long as patients can hemodynamically tolerate a drug.

Patients with episodes of sustained monomorphic VT at risk of circulatory collapse, but currently

**TABLE 74.1**

Clinical Questions

| Question | Answer | Grade of Recommendation | References |
|---|---|---|---|
| What are effective and safe pharmacologic strategies for prevention of postoperative atrial fibrillation after coronary artery bypass surgery? | Beta-blockers. | A | [19] |
| | Amiodarone. | B | [20–23] |
| Are there intraoperative strategies to consider that may reduce incident atrial fibrillation after cardiothoracic surgery? | Applying mild hypothermia, performing a posterior pericardiotomy, and using heparin-coated bypass circuits. | C | [25–28,31] |
| What drugs should be avoided in patients with atrial fibrillation with underlying Wolff–Parkinson–White syndrome? | Adenosine, beta-blockers, and calcium channel blockers. | A | [32,33] |
| Is elective cardioversion, chemically or by direct current a reasonable option in the postoperative atrial fibrillation patient? | Yes. It may reduce the length of hospital stay and prolong duration in normal sinus rhythm. | B | [34,35] |
| Should warfarin be given in postoperative atrial fibrillation that is recurrent or persists for more than 24 h? | Warfarin anticoagulation should be initiated for at least 4 weeks to mitigate the risk of stroke. | B | [40] |

hemodynamically stable, can be given antiarrhythmic drugs for acute termination and to suppress recurrence. Amiodarone is considered the first-line agent for the acute termination of hemodynamically stable monomorphic VT and to suppress recurrent VT, as outlined in the most recent Advanced Cardiac Life Support (ACLS) guidelines [53,54]. Lidocaine was historically used as a first-line agent [55]; however, it has since fallen out of favor as the first-line agent given that its effectiveness appears to be limited to myocardial tissue subjected to ongoing ischemia [56,57]. Other pharmacologic options include procainamide and sotalol, which is now available in IV formulations.

Polymorphic VT is characterized by a wide complex tachycardia with a continuously shifting QRS morphology, amplitude, and axis. The acute management is similar to monomorphic VT and VF with attention given to immediate direct current cardioversion, antiarrhythmic therapy, and identification of reversible causes. Particular attention needs to given to the patient's 12-lead ECG to accurately measure the QTc interval. If this interval is not prolonged or only mildly prolonged (<440 ms), then this would be highly suggestive of ischemia as a precipitating factor. If this interval is prolonged, then a thorough medication review is warranted to identify and remove any nonessential QT-prolonging drugs.

There are other rare causes for polymorphic VT such as the congenital long-QT syndromes resulting from defects found in ion channels, although the drug-induced causes occur with much more frequency (Table 74.1).

*Recommendation*: Warfarin anticoagulation should be initiated for at least 4 weeks to mitigate the risk of stroke (Grade B recommendation).

## References

1. Goldman L, Caldera DL, Southwick FS et al. Cardiac risk factors and complications in non-cardiac surgery. *Medicine (Baltimore).* 1978;57:357–370.
2. Walsh SR, Thomas C, Manohar S, Coveney EC. Early management of atrial fibrillation in general surgical inpatients. *Int J Surg.* 2006;4:115–117.
3. Polanczyk CA, Goldman L, Marcantonio ER, Orav EJ, Lee TH. Supraventricular arrhythmia in patients having noncardiac surgery: Clinical correlates and effect on length of stay. *Ann Intern Med.* 1998;129:279–285.
4. Almassi GH, Schowalter T, Nicolosi AC et al. Atrial fibrillation after cardiac surgery: A major morbid event? *Ann Surg.* 1997;226:501–511; discussion 11–13.
5. Aranki SF, Shaw DP, Adams DH et al. Predictors of atrial fibrillation after coronary artery surgery. Current trends and impact on hospital resources. *Circulation.* 1996;94:390–397.
6. Creswell LL, Schuessler RB, Rosenbloom M, Cox JL. Hazards of postoperative atrial arrhythmias. *Ann Thorac Surg.* 1993;56:539–549.
7. Fuller JA, Adams GG, Buxton B. Atrial fibrillation after coronary artery bypass grafting. Is it a disorder of the elderly? *J Thorac Cardiovasc Surg.* 1989;97:821–825.
8. Moe GK, Abildskov JA. Atrial fibrillation as a self-sustaining arrhythmia independent of focal discharge. *Am Heart J.* 1959;58:59–70.
9. Moe GK, Rheinboldt WC, Abildskov JA. A computer model of atrial fibrillation. *Am Heart J.* 1964;67:200–220.
10. Waldo AL. Experimental models of atrial fibrillation—What have we learned? *Semin Interv Cardiol.* 1997;2:195–201.
11. Kalman JM, Munawar M, Howes LG et al. Atrial fibrillation after coronary artery bypass grafting is associated with sympathetic activation. *Ann Thorac Surg.* 1995;60:1709–1715.

12. Levy MN. Sympathetic-parasympathetic interactions in the heart. *Circ Res.* 1971;29:437–445.
13. Tselentakis EV, Woodford E, Chandy J, Gaudette GR, Saltman AE. Inflammation effects on the electrical properties of atrial tissue and inducibility of postoperative atrial fibrillation. *J Surg Res.* 2006;135:68–75.
14. Ravelli F, Allessie M. Effects of atrial dilatation on refractory period and vulnerability to atrial fibrillation in the isolated Langendorff-perfused rabbit heart. *Circulation.* 1997;96:1686–1695.
15. Deroubaix E, Folliguet T, Rucker-Martin C et al. Moderate and chronic hemodynamic overload of sheep atria induces reversible cellular electrophysiologic abnormalities and atrial vulnerability. *J Am Coll Cardiol.* 2004;44:1918–1926.
16. Baker WL, White CM. Post-cardiothoracic surgery atrial fibrillation: A review of preventive strategies. *Ann Pharmacother.* 2007;41:587–598.
17. Crystal E, Connolly SJ, Sleik K, Ginger TJ, Yusuf S. Interventions on prevention of postoperative atrial fibrillation in patients undergoing heart surgery: A meta-analysis. *Circulation.* 2002;106:75–80.
18. Burgess DC, Kilborn MJ, Keech AC. Interventions for prevention of post-operative atrial fibrillation and its complications after cardiac surgery: A meta-analysis. *Eur Heart J.* 2006;27:2846–2857.
19. Connolly SJ, Cybulsky I, Lamy A et al. Double-blind, placebo-controlled, randomized trial of prophylactic metoprolol for reduction of hospital length of stay after heart surgery: The beta-Blocker Length Of Stay (BLOS) study. *Am Heart J.* 2003;145:226–232.
20. White CM, Caron MF, Kalus JS et al. Intravenous plus oral amiodarone, atrial septal pacing, or both strategies to prevent post-cardiothoracic surgery atrial fibrillation: The Atrial Fibrillation Suppression Trial II (AFIST II). *Circulation.* 2003;108(Suppl 1):II200–II206.
21. Mitchell LB, Exner DV, Wyse DG et al. Prophylactic oral amiodarone for the prevention of arrhythmias that begin early after revascularization, valve replacement, or repair: PAPABEAR: A randomized controlled trial. *JAMA.* 2005;294:3093–3100.
22. Crystal E, Kahn S, Roberts R et al. Long-term amiodarone therapy and the risk of complications after cardiac surgery: Results from the Canadian Amiodarone Myocardial Infarction Arrhythmia Trial (CAMIAT). *J Thorac Cardiovasc Surg.* 2003;125:633–637.
23. Kaushik S, Hussain A, Clarke P, Lazar HL. Acute pulmonary toxicity after low-dose amiodarone therapy. *Ann Thorac Surg.* 2001;72:1760–1761.
24. Patel AA, White CM, Gillespie EL, Kluger J, Coleman CI. Safety of amiodarone in the prevention of postoperative atrial fibrillation: A meta-analysis. *Am J Health Syst Pharm.* 2006;63:829–837.
25. Adams DC, Heyer EJ, Simon AE et al. Incidence of atrial fibrillation after mild or moderate hypothermic cardiopulmonary bypass. *Crit Care Med.* 2000;28:309–311.
26. Kuralay E, Ozal E, Demirkili U, Tatar H. Effect of posterior pericardiotomy on postoperative supraventricular arrhythmias and late pericardial effusion (posterior pericardiotomy). *J Thorac Cardiovasc Surg.* 1999;118:492–495.
27. Ovrum E, Am Holen E, Tangen G, Ringdal MA. Heparinized cardiopulmonary bypass and full heparin dose marginally improve clinical performance. *Ann Thorac Surg.* 1996;62:1128–1133.
28. Svenmarker S, Sandstrom E, Karlsson T et al. Neurological and general outcome in low-risk coronary artery bypass patients using heparin coated circuits. *Eur J Cardiothorac Surg.* 2001;19:47–53.
29. Maisel WH, Rawn JD, Stevenson WG. Atrial fibrillation after cardiac surgery. *Ann Intern Med.* 2001;135:1061–1073.
30. Satoh T, Zipes DP. Unequal atrial stretch in dogs increases dispersion of refractoriness conducive to developing atrial fibrillation. *J Cardiovasc Electrophysiol.* 1996;7:833–842.
31. Levy T, Fotopoulos G, Walker S et al. Randomized controlled study investigating the effect of biatrial pacing in prevention of atrial fibrillation after coronary artery bypass grafting. *Circulation.* 2000;102:1382–1387.
32. Garratt C, Antoniou A, Ward D, Camm AJ. Misuse of verapamil in pre-excited atrial fibrillation. *Lancet.* 1989;1:367–369.
33. McGovern B, Garan H, Ruskin JN. Precipitation of cardiac arrest by verapamil in patients with Wolff-Parkinson-White syndrome. *Ann Intern Med.* 1986;104:791–794.
34. Soucier RJ, Mirza S, Abordo MG et al. Predictors of conversion of atrial fibrillation after cardiac operation in the absence of class I or III antiarrhythmic medications. *Ann Thorac Surg.* 2001;72:694–697; discussion 7–8.
35. Lee JK, Klein GJ, Krahn AD et al. Rate-control versus conversion strategy in postoperative atrial fibrillation: Trial design and pilot study results. *Card Electrophysiol Rev.* 2003;7:178–184.
36. Cochrane AD, Siddins M, Rosenfeldt FL et al. A comparison of amiodarone and digoxin for treatment of supraventricular arrhythmias after cardiac surgery. *Eur J Cardiothorac Surg.* 1994;8:194–198.
37. McAlister HF, Luke RA, Whitlock RM, Smith WM. Intravenous amiodarone bolus versus oral quinidine for atrial flutter and fibrillation after cardiac operations. *J Thorac Cardiovasc Surg.* 1990;99:911–918.
38. Installe E, Schoevaerdts JC, Gadisseux P, Charles S, Tremouroux J. Intravenous amiodarone in the treatment of various arrhythmias following cardiac operations. *J Thorac Cardiovasc Surg.* 1981;81:302–308.
39. VanderLugt JT, Mattioni T, Denker S et al. Efficacy and safety of ibutilide fumarate for the conversion of atrial arrhythmias after cardiac surgery. *Circulation.* 1999;100:369–375.
40. Fuster V, Ryden LE, Cannom DS et al. ACC/AHA/ESC 2006 guidelines for the management of patients with atrial fibrillation—Executive summary: A report of the American College of Cardiology/American Heart Association Task Force on Practice Guidelines and the European Society of Cardiology Committee for Practice Guidelines (Writing Committee to Revise the 2001 Guidelines for the Management of Patients With Atrial Fibrillation). *J Am Coll Cardiol.* 2006;48:854–906.
41. Goldman BS, Hill TJ, Weisel RD et al. Permanent cardiac pacing after open-heart surgery: Acquired heart disease. *Pacing Clin Electrophysiol.* 1984;7:367–371.

42. Del Rizzo DF, Nishimura S, Lau C, Sever J, Goldman BS. Cardiac pacing following surgery for acquired heart disease. *J Card Surg.* 1996;11:332–340.
43. Lewis JW, Jr., Webb CR, Pickard SD, Lehman J, Jacobsen G. The increased need for a permanent pacemaker after reoperative cardiac surgery. *J Thorac Cardiovasc Surg.* 1998;116:74–81.
44. Glikson M, Dearani JA, Hyberger LK, Schaff HV, Hammill SC, Hayes DL. Indications, effectiveness, and long-term dependency in permanent pacing after cardiac surgery. *Am J Cardiol.* 1997;80:1309–1313.
45. Epstein AE, Dimarco JP, Ellenbogen KA et al. ACC/AHA/HRS 2008 Guidelines for Device-Based Therapy of Cardiac Rhythm Abnormalities: Executive Summary: A Report of the American College of Cardiology/American Heart Association Task Force on Practice Guidelines (Writing Committee to Revise the ACC/AHA/NASPE 2002 Guideline Update for Implantation of Cardiac Pacemakers and Antiarrhythmia Devices): Developed in Collaboration With the American Association for Thoracic Surgery and Society of Thoracic Surgeons. *Circulation.* 2008;117:2820–2840.
46. Walsh SR, Tang T, Wijewardena C, Yarham SI, Boyle JR, Gaunt ME. Postoperative arrhythmias in general surgical patients. *Ann R Coll Surg Engl.* 2007;89:91–95.
47. Batra GS, Molyneux J, Scott NA. Colorectal patients and cardiac arrhythmias detected on the surgical high dependency unit. *Ann R Coll Surg Engl.* 2001;83:174–176.
48. Ascione R, Reeves BC, Santo K, Khan N, Angelini GD. Predictors of new malignant ventricular arrhythmias after coronary surgery: A case-control study. *J Am Coll Cardiol.* 2004;43:1630–1638.
49. Yeung-Lai-Wah JA, Qi A, McNeill E et al. New-onset sustained ventricular tachycardia and fibrillation early after cardiac operations. *Ann Thorac Surg.* 2004;77:2083–2088.
50. Echt DS, Liebson PR, Mitchell LB et al. Mortality and morbidity in patients receiving encainide, flecainide, or placebo. The Cardiac Arrhythmia Suppression Trial. *N Engl J Med.* 1991;324:781–788.
51. Reiter MJ, Reiffel JA. Importance of beta blockade in the therapy of serious ventricular arrhythmias. *Am J Cardiol.* 1998;82:9I–19I.
52. Ellison KE, Hafley GE, Hickey K et al. Effect of beta-blocking therapy on outcome in the Multicenter UnSustained Tachycardia Trial (MUSTT). *Circulation.* 2002;106:2694–2699.
53. Zipes DP, Camm AJ, Borggrefe M et al. ACC/AHA/ESC 2006 guidelines for management of patients with ventricular arrhythmias and the prevention of sudden cardiac death: A report of the American College of Cardiology/American Heart Association Task Force and the European Society of Cardiology Committee for Practice Guidelines (Writing Committee to Develop Guidelines for Management of Patients With Ventricular Arrhythmias and the Prevention of Sudden Cardiac Death). *J Am Coll Cardiol.* 2006;48: e247–e346.
54. Dorian P, Cass D, Schwartz B, Cooper R, Gelaznikas R, Barr A. Amiodarone as compared with lidocaine for shock-resistant ventricular fibrillation. *N Engl J Med.* 2002;346:884–890.
55. Griffith MJ, Linker NJ, Garratt CJ, Ward DE, Camm AJ. Relative efficacy and safety of intravenous drugs for termination of sustained ventricular tachycardia. *Lancet.* 1990;336:670–673.
56. Kowey PR, Marinchak RA, Rials SJ, Bharucha DB. Intravenous antiarrhythmic therapy in the acute control of in-hospital destabilizing ventricular tachycardia and fibrillation. *Am J Cardiol.* 1999;84:46R–51R.
57. Gorgels AP, van den Dool A, Hofs A et al. Comparison of procainamide and lidocaine in terminating sustained monomorphic ventricular tachycardia. *Am J Cardiol.* 1996;78:43–46.

## Commentary on Perioperative Arrhythmias

*Suresh K. Agarwal*

Our understanding of atrial fibrillation has certainly evolved greatly over the past few decades. Not only has our management of these arrhythmias evolved but our consideration of patients at risk and the impact of this irregular heartbeat has advanced.

Drs. Viswanathan and Ravindran have presented a thorough and evidence-based approach to patients who encounter atrial arrhythmias and as cardiologists, they certainly arrive at their conclusions after having had many years of experience in the management of these complex patients. They note that significant numbers of patients who undergo cardiac or vascular procedures may have their postoperative courses complicated by atrial abnormalities.

However, the onset of atrial arrhythmias, particularly fibrillation, is not relegated solely to individuals undergoing vascular operations, although they are far more common in this population. In patients with severe sepsis, the incidence of atrial fibrillation approached 5% and was associated with significantly worsened outcomes.

As the authors mention, an ounce of prevention is worth a pound of cure. Their strategies for preventing atrial fibrillation in cardiac patients are well reasoned; however, data for the prevention of atrial arrhythmias in noncardiac surgery is limited and inconclusive. Expert opinion (Level IV data) warns against overdistending the atria as a method to prevent the onset.

The management of anticoagulation for patients with atrial fibrillation has evolved over the past few years. As the annual risk for stroke for nonanticoagulated individuals with atrial fibrillation remains about 2%, the need for embolic disease prevention remains clear. The formation of clot in the left atrium, and particularly its appendage, remains the source of embolus.

In the past, our only option has been intravenous heparinization followed by oral anticoagulation with Warfarin. This process, although monitored through international normalized ration (INR), requires prolonged hospitalization and is fraught with variability in outpatient INR dependent upon diet, additional medications, and compliance. Reversal of heparin consists of protamine administration or time (half-life of heparin is 2 h). Warfarin reversal consists of fresh frozen plasma (FFP) and prothrombin complex concentrate (PCC) for acute reversal and vitamin K for long-term reversal. Aspirin, by itself, is not an adequate agent for prevention of embolic complications from atrial fibrillation.

Other alternatives for anticoagulation have arisen: Dabigatran (Pradaxa®), Rivaroxaban (Xarelto®), and Apixaban (Eliquis®). Each of these drugs is taken once per day and does not require blood tests to monitor therapeutic levels. That being said, all anticoagulation carries the risks with usage, the most important of which is bleeding. Despite their ease of use, reversal of these anticoagulants remains difficult. In the face of trauma or internal bleeding, rapid reversal may be difficult to achieve as these medications are not responsive to platelet transfusion, fresh frozen plasma, cryoprecipitate, nor vitamin K. PCC and hemodialysis may offer acute reversal of some of these novel agents.

Long-term correction of atrial fibrillation may be necessary, particularly if anticoagulation is contraindicated. This may be a necessity if chemical cardioversion is ineffective or unsustained. In these instances, ablation of cardiac tissue may be recommended via direct cardiac ablation, a Maze procedure (which may or may not be done in conjunction with a separate cardiac procedure), or atrioventricular node ablation.

Overall, the management of atrial arrhythmias has been evolving over time. As Drs. Viswanathan and Ravindran noted, there are many therapeutic options for the management of these patients in the postoperative time period. It is imperative to utilize these guidelines to optimize the delivery of care for our patients.

# 75

## *Feeds and Feeding Surgical Patients*

**Jayson D. Aydelotte, Ben Coopwood, and Oscar Rios**

**CONTENTS**



Nutrition is one of the key components of good wound healing. From the moment a patient is injured or undergoes a significant surgical procedure, he or she is dependent on the building blocks of nutrients. Surgeons have traditionally been faced with answering questions such as when to start someone on enteral feeds? Should patients just get total parenteral nutrition (TPN) instead of tube feeds? Should we feed the stomach or feed past the pylorus? Is immunonutrition beneficial? Is glutamine beneficial as an additive to feedings? And, what is the best way to start someone on an oral diet after abdominal surgery? Nutrition lends itself to quality research. Most of the research is done in controlled hospital settings with a relatively standard patient population. Because of this, there have been many randomized controlled trials looking at many of the questions above.

### 75.1 Do I Have to Use the Gut after a Major Abdominal Operation or Can I Just Give the Patient TPN?

Apprehension in using the bowel after major abdominal surgery or trauma leads many surgeons to deliver nutrition to patients without using the gut. This indicates a certain amount of common sense and several studies have been done to address this very question.

One randomized prospective trial divided two groups of trauma patients at the time of laparotomy into needle jejunostomy enteral feeds versus isocaloric/isonitrogenous TPN starting 12 h after surgery. Eighty-six percent of the patients receiving enteral feeds tolerated a full feeding rate. There were no differences in nitrogen balance in the two groups but the enteral feeding group had significantly less hyperglycemia and septic complications [1] (Level 1b evidence). Another study was done randomizing patients with both blunt and penetrating abdominal trauma to TPN and protein/calorie-matched enteral feeds. The results were very similar. Overall, there were less infections in fewer patients in the enterally fed group. There was no difference in mortality [2] (Level 1b evidence). Another prospective randomized trial looked at standard enteral feeds versus TPN versus immune-enhanced enteral feeds and found that only 94% of the patients receiving enteral feeds tolerated the feeds well [3] (Level 2b evidence). A meta-analysis of 13 prospective random assignment trials concluded enteral nutrition had less infective complications without any decrease in mortality or hospital stay than TPN [4] (Level 1a evidence).

*Recommendation*: Enteral tube feedings started within the first 24 h after abdominal trauma or abdominal surgery is safe and the preferred method of nutrition delivery over parenteral nutrition (Grade A recommendation).

## 75.2 Is TPN Safe?

Traditionally, TPN has been viewed to carry a significant risk of infectious complications. Braunschweig et al. evaluated several prospective randomized trials comparing TPN to EN in a large meta-analysis in 2001. They found that, while there is no mortality differences between the groups, TPN use echoed the historical concern. There were more overall infections and more central line infections in those patients who received TPN [5] (Class 1a evidence). Another Prospective Randomized Trial in 2011 comparing ICU patients started on TPN after 48 h to another group that did not start TPN until after 8 days found the earlier group was less likely to leave the ICU alive, had more ICU infections, had a higher percentage of patients requiring mechanical ventilation over 2 days, and higher healthcare costs [6] (Class 1b evidence). However, a more recent study found that *adding* TPN to EN to reach 100% of goal caloric needs starting 4 days after admission significantly reduced the number of infections for each of the patients in the treatment group [7] (Class 1b evidence). This is a landmark study because it is the first major study to suggest infection rates with TPN use are not *higher* than those patients who did not get TPN. But the jury is still out on TPN and its safety. Historical concerns over infectious risks may be decreasing.

*Recommendation*: It appears TPN is safe and the historical concerns of infectious complications, most notably line infections, have diminished over the past few years (Grade B recommendation).

## 75.3 When Should Enteral Feeds Be Started?

This question was indirectly asked during some of the trials listed in the question regarding TPN versus enteral feeds. Traditionally, surgeons are apprehensive in starting enteral feeds in patients before they demonstrate return of bowel function as manifested by many different clinical signs, such as passing flatus, or return of bowel sounds. In an effort to objectify things, some authors set out to just start tube feeds at a certain time postoperatively or after injury and see how the patients tolerated this, and, more importantly, to see if this made any difference in outcome. In Moore's study, enteral feeding was started in patients who had undergone abdominal surgery 12 h postoperatively. These feeds were tolerated well and the patients fed enterally had less septic complications [1] (Level 1b evidence). Another study looking at non-trauma septic patients with peritonitis from perforation started enteral feeds within 12 h of surgery. Only 18% of the studied subjects needed the feeds temporarily held for abdominal distention. The studied group had a positive nitrogen balance by the third postoperative day and suffered less septic complications than the controls [8] (Level 1b evidence).

*Recommendation*: Enteral feeds can safely be started in trauma patients and patients who undergo major abdominal surgery within the first 24 h in most cases (Grade A recommendation).

## 75.4 Can We Just Feed the Stomach or Do We Need to Feed Past the Pylorus into the Small Bowel?

Much like the notion that not using the gut after major surgery or trauma makes common sense to some surgeons, the idea that feeding beyond the ligament of Treitz or beyond the pylorus makes some sense as well. The idea is that the tube feeds would not be in the stomach and easily aspirated into the lungs. Or, more commonly, the tube feeds would not be in a stomach that may or may not be emptying well because of the overall poor physical condition of the patient. For this reason, many surgeons and non-surgeons advocate the placement of a small bowel feeding catheter instead of feeding the gastric tube. The problem is that placing these tubes is not always as easy as it seems and they often become displaced from the small bowel. Several studies were done to see if feeding the stomach is as safe and effective as feeding the small bowel. Neuman and colleagues randomized 60 patients to receive gastric feeds or have a post-pyloric tube placed. Patients receiving gastric feeds had their feeds started sooner and had an earlier time to goal feeding while having no increased aspiration as compared to the patients randomized to the post-pyloric group [9] (Level 1b evidence). Another study with similar numbers in children came to an opposite conclusion. The post-pyloric group had a higher percentage of daily caloric goal achieved, but had the same complication rate as stomach feeding. However, in this study, the investigators suffered from the same problem that lead to the original question in that nearly 30% of the patients randomized to the post-pyloric group could not have their tube placed properly and were then switched to the gastric feeding group [10] (Level 2b evidence). This study, however, is helpful to answer the question in part. That is to say that there were no significant differences in complications between gastric and post-pyloric tube feeding complications.

*Recommendation*: It is safe to feed a working stomach. Placing a small bowel feeding tube delays time to goal feeds and does not lower complication rates (Grade A recommendation).

## 75.5 Is Immunonutrition Beneficial?

Enteral tube feedings have been adjusted and manipulated for many different reasons to give different desired results. One particular way tube feeds can be adjusted is by adding certain "immune enhancing" agents to the feeding. There are varieties of specific immune enhancing agents that have been studied such as arginine, glutamine, nucleic acids, Eicosapentaenoic acid, and Omege-3 fatty acids. Different manufacturers produce different combinations of these agents to make their own proprietary products. There have been randomized trials looking at specific products and outcomes. One study evaluated preoperative and postoperative immunonutrition with arginine, Omega-3 fats, and RNA nucleotides in patients undergoing upper gastrointestinal surgery for cancer. Treated subjects had a lower incidence of postoperative infective complications with no difference in mortality [11] (Level 1b evidence). Another study evaluated immunonutrition using the same additives in critically ill patients. Subjects receiving immunonutrition had a decrease in ventilator days and hospital stay with no change in mortality [12] (Level 1b evidence). A meta-analysis was done on a total of 15 prospective randomized studies utilizing "immunonutrition" and comprising many different products. Overall conclusions of this study were that immunonutrition as a whole showed a significant decrease in ventilator days, hospital days, and infection complications [13] (Level 1a evidence). However, a recent multi-institutional, prospective random assignment trial in European ICUs showed no difference in hospital infectious complications in those who got immunomodulating feeds and those that did not. In fact, there was a higher age-adjusted 6 month mortality in the treatment group [14] (Level 1b evidence). These new data may dampen the enthusiasm to use immune feeds in critically ill patients.

*Recommendation*: Immunonutrition may be associated with a decrease in hospital days, ventilator days, and postoperative infection in seriously ill patients and may decrease postoperative infections in patients undergoing major abdominal operations for cancer, although more recent data that are emerging may decrease the enthusiasm for recommending its use (Grade B recommendation).

## 75.6 Is Glutamine Helpful as a Feed Additive?

Glutamine is a nonessential amino acid and a preferential nutrient of the enterocyte. Glutamine is relatively cheap and can be easily added to standard tube feed products. Several randomized prospective trials evaluating the addition of glutamine to both tube feeds and parenteral formulas have been done. One randomized study in burn patients found an association of lower mortality and decreased infection [15] (Level 1b evidence). Another study in patients with multitrauma found a lower incidence of pneumonia, bacteremia, and sepsis in the glutamine-treated group [16] (Level 1b evidence). A large, French, multicenter randomized trial found glutamine addition to TPN decreased pneumonia and incidence of hyperglycemia [17] (Level 1b evidence). However, a large, multicentered random assignment trial adding glutamine, antioxidants, or both as supplements to patients with multisystem (two or more) organ failure in Canadian ICUs found no difference in their primary outcome of 28-day mortality in those patients who received glutamine supplementation alone. But those patients in the glutamine group had a higher in-hospital (37.2 vs. 31.0, $p = 0.02$) and 6-month (43.7 vs. 37.2, $p = 0.02$) mortality rates than the other groups who did not get glutamine. In addition, those patients who lived and got glutamine spent a longer time on the ventilator (11 vs. 8.7 days, $p = 0.03$), longer time in the ICU (17.1 vs. 13.1 days, $p = 0.03$), and a longer time in the hospital (51 vs. 41 days, $p = 0.04$) than those that did not [18] (Level 1b evidence). This suggests the original enthusiasm for glutamine's ability to improve infective outcomes should be tempered, so much so that in light of the increased mortality data, glutamine supplementation should be avoided.

*Recommendation*: No. Glutamine supplementation is associated with a decreased infection rate in some studies, but a recent large trial shows it carries an overall in-hospital and 6-month increase in mortality and should be avoided (Grade A Recommendation).

## 75.7 What Is the Best Way to Start and Progress a Diet in a Patient after Abdominal Surgery?

The traditional surgical thinking regarding the starting of oral intake after abdominal surgery is to wait for hard signs of return of bowel function and then slowly progress the diet to a "regular" diet in a stepwise fashion from clear liquids through a range of food qualities to regular diet over the course of several days. Recently, this thought process has been challenged. One trial randomly assigned gynecologic oncology patients into two groups: those who were to be given clear liquids on the first postoperative day and advance as tolerated and those who were to be NPO until passage of flatus. There was no difference in vomiting or other complications, although the treatment group trended toward more nausea. There was a 1 day shorter hospital stay and 2.5 less days to tolerating a regular diet [19] (Level 1b evidence). A similar prospective randomized study by the same authors looked at the same patient population and divided groups into regular diet as first diet of choice versus clear liquids and progression as tolerated. There was no difference in complication or hospital stay but a decrease in time to tolerating regular diet [20] (Level 1b evidence). Another study assigned patients undergoing elective aortic and colorectal surgery randomly to two groups: the treatment group which was provided a patient controlled diet of choice and the control was NPO for 5 days. There was no difference in hospital days, complications, or NGT reinsertion rate. The patients in the treatment group had a shorter time until they were tolerating a diet [21] (Level 1b evidence).

*Recommendation*: Provide a patient-controlled diet as soon as possible postoperatively (Grade A recommendation).

## 75.8 Should Tube Feeds Be Held Prior to Surgery? If So, When?

Historically, there has been consternation about the safety of continuing enteral nutrition (EN) in patients undergoing further operations and, if not, then when would be the safest time to stop the feeds? This concern revolves around two central concepts: The risk of aspiration of tube feeds/enteral contents and the interruption of protein calorie intake. There are no current prospective randomized trials available to address these concerns.

Retrospective data have been collected and published in a variety of studies that help assess the safety and impact of the practice of stopping tube feedings. Passier et al. studied their population of ICU patients in an Australian Trauma ICU and evaluated EN cessations for cause and impact to the patients' protein nutrition. Almost a quarter of patients in that study had unnecessary EN cessation that prevented delivery of planned nutrition. Eighty-nine percent of planned procedures had EN stopped for an average of just over 10 h of stoppage per procedure. The average time tube feeds were held prior to the procedure was 6.5 h. But 27% of the planned procedures ended up being delayed to the next day yielding a cumulative stoppage of just over 30 h per patient, creating a mean protein energy deficit of 7.7% of calculated needs. In this study, EN cessation was associated with a significant decrease in protein nutrition [22] (Level 3 evidence). Likewise, van den Broek et al. studied 55 patients receiving full EN and found 40% of patients had feedings that were significantly lower (13%) than prescribed in patients not in the ICU. The most common reasons for tube feed calorie deficits were interruptions in delivery for diagnostic or therapeutic procedures [23] (Class 3 evidence). Peev et al. prospectively evaluated 94 ICU patients in two groups: those that had an interruption in their EN and those that did not. Those that had interruptions had significantly higher cumulative and daily caloric deficits and higher risk of both prolonged ICU and hospital stays. Twenty-six percent of the interruptions were considered "avoidable" interruptions [24] (Class 3 evidence).

McElroy et al. changed their practice from holding tube feeds for 8 h prior to procedures to NOT holding tube feeds. They evaluated 14 intubated ICU patients receiving nasojejunal tube feedings after their change and studied the EN practice patterns and calorie nutrition in that group of patients during the day of surgery. Still the average interruption of EN in this group was just over 3 h. But the patients overall received a cumulative 11.9 additional hours of EN over their hospital stay and 1065 kcal/day per operation [25] (Class 2 evidence). Pousman et al. changed their practice to continue small bowel tube feedings up to the time of the procedure and interrupted gastric tube feedings 45 min before the procedure in intubated trauma patients. They found no difference in nutritional outcomes but also found no difference in complications to include emesis and pneumonia [26] (Class 2 evidence).

Andel et al. studied two cohorts of burn patients undergoing surgery to evaluate the $CO_2$ gap between the arterial and the gastric mucosa $CO_2$ levels at specific intervals during burn operations. One group of nine patients had duodenal feeds held 1 h prior to the operation and 6 h postoperatively and the treatment group (nine patients) had tube feeds continued through the operation. The $CO_2$ gaps were significantly higher in the fasting group versus those patients who were fed throughout the case, suggesting the splanchnic malperfusion may actually be helped or avoided by continuing tube feeds during the case [27] (Level 2 evidence) (Table 75.1).

*Recommendation*: Tube feedings should not be held 8 or 6 h prior to surgery. There is a knowledge gap in this field and more prospective studies should be done to find the right time, if any, to safely hold tube feeds. Holding small bowel tube feeds at the time of surgery and gastric tube feeds 1 h prior to surgery seems to be a safe practice (Grade B recommendations).

**TABLE 75.1**

Clinical Questions

| Question | Answer | Grade of Recommendation | References |
|---|---|---|---|
| Is TPN or Tube feedings better for the patient? | Enteral feeds have less and less severe infective complications and faster return of bowel function. | A | [1–4,8] |
| What is the safest and most effective, feeding the stomach or the small bowel? | Complication rates are the same for both methods. Gastric feeds have faster onset of goal feeds. | A | [9,10] |
| Does immunonutrition improve outcome? | Yes, immunonutrition is linked to shorter hospital stay and vent days as well as overall infection. Mortality unchanged. | A | [11–13] |
| What is the best way to start and advance postoperative patients on a diet? | Give them a diet of choice as soon as possible. Waiting for flatus and physician dictated diets just drag things out longer with no decrease in complications. | A | [19–21] |
| Is glutamine a beneficial additive to feedings? | No, most recent data suggests glutamine supplementation increases mortality in the severely ill. | A | [15–18,28] |
| How early can tube feeds be safely started? | Enteral feeds can be safely started within 12–24 h. Early tube feeds are linked to lower septic morbidity. | A | [1,2,8] |
| Is TPN safe? | It appears TPN is safe and the historical concerns of infectious complications, most notably line infections, have diminished over the past few years. | B | [5–7] |
| Should tube feeds be held prior to surgery? If so, when? | Tube feedings should not be held 8 or 6 h prior to surgery. There is a huge knowledge gap in this field and more prospective studies should be done to find the right time, if any, to safely hold tube feeds. Holding small bowel tube feeds at the time of surgery and gastric tube feeds 1 h prior to surgery seems to be a safe practice. | B | [22–27] |

## References


1. Moore F, Moore E, Jones T, McCroskey B, Peterson V. TEN versus TPN following major abdominal trauma—Reduced septic morbidity. *J Trauma*. 1989;29(7):916–922.
2. Kudsk K, Croce M, Fabian T, Minard G, Tolley E. Enteral versus parenteral feeding. Effects on septic morbidity after blunt and penetrating abdominal trauma. *Ann Surg*. 215(5):503–511.
3. Braga M, Gianotti L, Vignali A, Cestari A, Bisagni P, Di Carlo V. Artificial nutrition after major abdominal surgery: Impact of route of administration and composition of the diet. *Crit Care Med*. 1998;26(1):24–30.
4. Gramlich L, Krikor K, Pinilla J. Does enteral nutrition compared to parenteral nutrition result in better outcomes in critically ill adult patients? A systematic review of the literature. *Nutrition*. 2004;20:843–848.
5. Braunschweig CL, Levy P, Sheean PM, Wang X. Enteral compared with parenteral nutrition: A meta-analysis. *Am J Clin Nutr*. 2001;74:534–542.
6. Casaer MP, Mesotten D, Hermans G et al. Early versus late parenteral nutrition in critically ill adults. *N Engl J Med*. 2011;365:506–517.
7. Heidegger CP, Berger MM, Graf S et al. Optimisation of energy provision with supplemental parenteral nutrition in critically ill patients: A randomized controlled clinical trial. *Lancet*. 2013;381:9864:385–393.
8. Singh G, Ram RP, Khanna SK. Early postoperative enteral feeding in patients with nontraumatic intestinal perforation and peritonitis. *JACS*. 1989;187(2):142–146.
9. Neumann D, Delegge M. Gastric versus small-bowel tube feeding in the intensive care unit: A prospective comparison of efficacy. *Crit Care Med*. 2002;30(7):1436–1438.
10. Meert K, Daphtary K, Metheny N. Gastric vs small-bowel feeding in critically ill children receiving mechanical ventilation: A randomized controlled trial. *Chest*. 2004;126(3):872–878.
11. Senkal M, Zumtobel V, Bauer K. Outcome and cost-effectiveness of perioperative enteral immunonutrition in patients undergoing elective upper gastrointestinal tract surgery: A prospective randomized study. *Arch Surg*. 1999;134:964–970.
12. Atkinson S, Sieffert E, Bihari D. A prospective, randomized, double-blind, controlled clinical trial of enteral immunonutrition in the critically ill. Guy's Hospital Intensive Care Group. *Crit Care Med*. 1998;26(7):1164–1172.
13. Beale R, Bryg D, Bihari D. Immunonutrition in the critically ill: A systematic review of clinical outcome. *Crit Care Med*. 1999;27(12):2799–2805.
14. van Zanten A, Sztark F, Hofman Z et al. High-protein enteral nutrition enriched with immune-modulating nutrients vs standard high-protein enteral nutrition and nosocomial infections in the ICU. A randomized clinical trial. *JAMA*. 2014;312(5):14–524.

15. Garrel D. Decreased mortality and infectious morbidity in adult burn patients given enteral glutamine supplements: A prospective, controlled, randomized clinical trial. *Crit Care Med.* 2003;31(10):2444–2449.
16. Houdijk A, Alexander PJ, Rijnsburger E, Jansen J. Randomised trial of glutamine-enriched enteral nutrition on infectious morbidity in patients with multiple trauma. *Lancet.* 1998;352(9130):772–776.
17. Saalwachter A, Schulman K, Willcutts J. Does enteral glutamine supplementation decrease infectious morbidity? *Surg Infect.* 2006;7(1):29–35.
18. Heyland D, Muscedere J, Wishmeyer P, Cook D, Jones G, Albert M, Elke G, Berger M, Day A, Canadian Clinical Trials Group. A randomized trial of glutamine and antioxidants in critically ill patients. *N Engl J Med.* 2013;368(16):1489–1497.
19. Pearl M, Valea F, Fischer M. A randomized controlled trial of early postoperative feeding in gynecologic oncology patients undergoing intra-abdominal surgery. *Obstet Gynecol.* 1998;92(1):94–97.
20. Pearl M, Frandina M, Mahler L, Valea F, DiSilvestro P, Chalas E. A randomized controlled trial of a regular diet as the first meal in gynecologic oncology patients undergoing intra-abdominal surgery. *Obstet Gynecol.* 2002;100(2):230–234.
21. Han-Guerts I, Jeekel J, Tilanus H, Brouwer K. Randomized clinical trial of patient-controlled versus fixed regimen feeding after elective abdominal surgery. *Br J Surg.* 2001;88(12):1578–1582.
22. Passier RH, Davies AR, Ridley E, McClure J, Murphy D, Scheinkestel CD. Periprocedural cessation of nutrition in the intensive care unit: Opportunities for improvement. *Intens Care Med.* 2013;39(7):1221–1226.
23. van den Broek PW, Rasmussen-Conrad EL, Naber AH, Wanten GJ. *Br J Nutr.* 2009;101(1):68–71.
24. Peev MP, Yeh DD, Quraishi SA, Osler P, Chany Y, Gillis E, Albano CE, Darak S, Velmahos GC. Causes and consequences of interrupted enteral nutrition: a prospective observational study in critically ill surgical patients. *J Parenter Enteral Nutr.* 2014.
25. McElroy LM, Codner PA, Brasel KJ. A pilot study to explore the safety of perioperative enteral nutrition. *Nutr Clin Pract.* 2012;27(6):777–780.
26. Pousman RM, Pepper C, Pandharipande P, Ayers GD, Mills B, Diaz J, Collier B, Miller R, Jensen G. Feasibility of implementing a reduced fasting protocol for critically ill trauma patients undergoing operative and nonoperative procedures. *J Parenter Enteral Nutr.* 2009;33(2):176–180.
27. Andel D, Kamolz LP, Donner A, Hoerauf K, Schramm W, Meissl G, Andel H. Impact of intraoperative duodenal feeding on the oxygen balance of the splanchnic region in severely burned patients. *Burns.* 2005;31(3):302–305.
28. Dechelotte P, Hasselmann M, Cynober L. L-Alanyl-glutamine dipeptide-supplemented total parenteral nutrition reduces infectious complications and glucose intolerance in critically ill patients: The French controlled, randomized, double-blind, multicenter study. *Crit Care Med.* 2006;34(3):598–604.

## Commentary on Feeds and Feeding Surgical Patients

*Kenneth A. Kudsk*

During my residency years in the 1970s, TPN was a hot topic with its own session at the surgical forum. TPN finally provided a practical way to feed malnourished patients suffering with fistulas, sepsis, bowel obstruction, a "frozen" abdomen, prolonged ileus, and many other problems. With TPN, wounds healed and patients survived. For a decade or more, most work written about TPN stated that it helped patients as long as it was given safely. Articles addressed refeeding syndrome, IV access, and development of organized nutrition support services. But mistakes were made: if 30 kcal/kg was good, perhaps 40 kcal/kg or more would be even better.

Eventually, clinicians recognized that TPN (or hyperalimentation as it was called) was no panacea for critically ill patients with a gradual shift to the concept that feeding the gut was better in the 1980s. About this time the long awaited VA cooperative study demonstrated that only malnourished patients benefited from TPN, with reductions in wound failure and no increase in infections. However, better nourished patients paid a price: infectious complications increased with a modest reduction in healing complications. Studies showed that patients did better when fed enterally. The first studies came from trauma centers where patients could be stratified by risk for infection and other complications. Most patients were young, previously healthy, hypermetabolic, and well-nourished prior to injury—a much different group than the VA cooperative study. These studies showed that enteral feeding improved infectious complications compared to starvation or TPN and it appeared that the more severely injured the patient, the more benefit with enteral nutrition. But to get enteral nutrition, gastric feeding was not feasible; small bowel access with a jejunostomy was the common technique. Subsequent studies suggested additions benefits with "immune-enhancing diets" compared to "standard nutrition" in the trauma patient, which coincided with studies of these diets administered preoperatively, postoperatively, or perioperatively in cancer patients.

Several things transpired. Firstly, clinicians realized that enteral feeding had a dark side with reports of small bowel necrosis occurring in patients not otherwise at risk of gut ischemia. Speculation of a cause included poor gut perfusion but increased metabolic needs during feeding. Gastric feeding under these conditions is probably correct. If the stomach empties feedings whether the patient is hypotensive or on pressor agents, the intestine tolerates the feedings fine—in my experience. This is particularly true of burn patients feed intragastrically while on pressor support but suffer no ill effects. The problem is that clinicians cannot tell this when feeding directly into the small bowel. The clinician must frequently examine a sick patient after initiating small bowel feeding to look for intolerance—reflux of feedings into the stomach, acute tachycardia, increasing abdominal distension, a dramatic fever spike, acutely elevated WBC, and/or acute hemodynamic instability. Without this, opportunities to intervene are missed.

Secondly, studies of "critically ill ICU patients" expanded from trauma patients to both medical and surgical patients with the presumption that one ICU patient is just another looking for similar outcomes as trauma patients. Enteral/TPN studies of trauma patients showed reduced pneumonia, intra-abdominal abscess, and perhaps multiple organ dysfunctions. Most trauma patients are extubated within 1 or 2 days, antibiotics are limited, and few, if any, have pre-existing nutritional deficits or chronic diseases (although drug and alcohol abuse are not uncommon). Compare them to general medical ICU patients: interabdominal abscesses are a rare without a perforated viscus as part of the pathology. Prolonged intubation is common—can pneumonia be prevented when tracheal aspiration of nasopharyngeal secretions occurs in 20%–25% of patients. Multiple organ failure is common (and often unavoidable), since organ failure from pre-existing chronic disease is common at baseline. Gastric feeing might be safe in many patients, but anatomically, the GE junction is the most dependent area of the stomach and gastric contents pool there. Also small bore feeding tubes are notoriously unreliable in monitoring gastric residuals—a perfect condition for aspiration. Is gastric feeding as safe as small bowel feeding? It depends on the patient.

Finally, morality has never been shown to differ between enteral and parenteral feeding. That makes sense—mortality is a poor marker of outcome. Trauma studies of nutrition do not recruit patients likely to die from the most common causes of severe head injury, uncontrollable hemorrhage, or acute early onset of severe organ dysfunction following prolonged hemorrhagic shock, acidosis, and circulatory failure. Death from late-onset organ failure after trauma is very uncommon, so it would require huge numbers to define a difference. This is much different than the medical ICU patient admitted with acute exacerbation of organ dysfunction that was not easy to manage as an outpatient prior to admission. Can any study discern differences in outcome due to the presence or absence of nutrition or the route or type of nutrition in these heterogeneous medical patients? A daunting challenge to be sure.

So does enteral feeding improve outcome compared to TPN? Most likely yes as the authors suggest—particularly in younger, well-nourished patient or patient with pre-existing malnutrition who tolerate preoperative enteral nutrition. Preoperative nutrition will not reverse long-standing protein and energy deficits but can turn a catabolic patient anabolic and benefit wound healing. Severely malnourished patients benefit from both enteral and TPN. A recent study of combining enteral and TPN added TPN on the fourth day only if patients failed to advance on enteral feeding. An extremely important point of this study was that many people will often tolerate tube feeding so that TPN is not necessary. TPN should only be administered to patients who fail after trying enteral if at all feasible. Under these conditions, TPN improves outcome.

But all enteral feeding is not alike. If the stomach empties (sometimes difficult to determine), feed the stomach since it stimulates all systems of digestion and absorption. If, however, the stomach does not empty, attempts may result in aspiration; under these conditions, advance a feeding tube out of the stomach and into the intestine if possible. While blind intestinal placement of small bores tubes is not easy and carries the risks of airway placement, pneumothorax, and death, new technologies can provide immediate feedback to trained tube team members, resulting in a high success rate. The technology does not replace the learned "touch" of a successful advancement, but successful placement is immediately apparent with the technology. An organized tube team using such technology produces immediate results.

But by whatever means small bowel is accessed, feedings must be administered safely. The more unstable the patient, the more important re-examination of the abdomen and vital signs become. Reflux of tube feedings into the stomach, significant complaints of cramping (yes, patients can frequently answer this question), or a fever spike cannot be ignored. In addition, failure to have a bowel movement by 5 days—particularly when using a fiber containing diet mandates an abdominal film, since fecal impaction in the distal small bowel or cecum can precede delayed small bowel necrosis due to feeding an overdistended small bowel. In general, the physician that institutes and advances the tube feeding rate should examine and re-examine the patient. There should never be an order to "advance feedings as tolerated" with small bowel feedings.

Decisions to hold feedings prior to surgery present a fairly complex issue. Stop tube feedings for 6–8 h prior to OR is a not uncommon dogma among anesthesiologists. Communication between surgeons and anesthesiologists can abbreviate this issue particularly if an NG tube is in place. Over time, experience renders stopping small bowel feeding a nonissue if there is a dialogue between surgery and anesthesia. Unfortunately, use of small bore tubes is no assurance that there are no gastric residuals. The question is how to diagnose a large volume of gastric contents pooled at the GE junction and the current literature does not really help.[*†‡]

Over the years, my practice has been influenced by both personal experience and the literature. Don't use TPN immediately in well-nourished patients (who might very well tolerate a diet within a few days) but be more aggressive in patients with severe protein calorie malnutrition unless you feel they may tolerate enteral nutrition via jejunostomy or a nasoenteric tube. Develop a trained team using the current technology to place small bore tubes. Gastroparesis precludes the more desirable intragastric feeding. Finally, it behooves the clinician to closely watch the patients are fed into the small intestine to avoid the infrequent, but very real, complication of intestinal necrosis. Any additional benefits of using glutamine and specialty diets may be related to specific patient populations yet to be defined. A safer bet for using an IED is the trauma patient.

---

* Aguilar-Nascimento JE, Kudsk KA. Clinical costs of feeding tube placement. J Parenter Enteral Nutr. *2007;31(4):269–273.*

† Koopman MC, Kudsk KA, Szotkowski MJ, Rees SM. A team-based protocol and electromagnetic technology eliminate feeding tube placement complications. Ann Surg. *2011 February; 253(2):297–302.*

‡ Aguilar-Nascimento JE, Kudsk KA. Use of small bore feeding tubes: successes and failures. Curr Opin Clin Nutr Metab Care. *2007;10:291–296.*

# 76

# *Acute Lung Injury/Acute Respiratory Distress Syndrome*

**Kristin P. Colling, Juan J. Blondet, and Greg J. Beilman**

**CONTENTS**



## 76.1 Introduction

Acute respiratory distress syndrome (ARDS) is a severe, life-threatening respiratory disease that is characterized by hypoxemia and noncompliant lungs. This condition was first described in a landmark case series of 12 patients in 1967 [1], and since that time, it has been a topic of extensive research. The incidence of ARDS in the United States has been estimated to be 64/100,000 [2], and accounts for a large amount of critical care resources. Recently, in 2012, the European Society of Intensive Care Medicine convened an international panel of experts and created a new consensus definition for ARDS, termed the Berlin definition [3]. In this newest definition, ARDS is characterized by the following criteria: (1) lung injury of acute onset, i.e., within 7 days of a known inciting risk factor or worsening respiratory symptoms; (2) bilateral infiltrates on chest imaging, which are not explained by effusions, lung collapse, or pulmonary nodules; (3) pulmonary edema and respiratory failure that is not *fully* explained by cardiac failure or fluid overload; and (4) hypoxemia defined by $PaO_2/FiO_2$ ratio of less than 300 with a positive end expiratory pressure (PEEP) or continuous positive airway pressure (CPAP) of >5 cm $H_2O$. The $PaO_2/FiO_2$ ratio is used to further characterize ARDS as *mild* ($PaO_2/FiO_2$ 201–300), *moderate* ($PaO_2/FiO_2$ 101–200), or *severe* (<100).

This new definition replaces the 1994 ARDS definition [4], which was often criticized as lacking explicit criteria for the timing of "acute" disease, a lack of inclusion of ventilator settings in the definition, and unclear definitions of radiographic findings. The 1994 definition also stated that the pulmonary artery wedge pressure must be <18 mmHg, however, given the declining use of pulmonary arterial catheters and the fact that ARDS may coexist with elevated pulmonary wedge pressures, this criterion was redefined to state that the primary cause of respiratory failure is not hydrostatic edema. The condition of "acute lung injury," previously defined as $PaO_2:FiO_2$ ratio of 201–300 has been discarded in the Berlin definition. The Berlin definition not only attempts to better define ARDS, but it also has been shown to correlate with mortality and other physiologic factors [2]. The mortality from ARDS increases from 27% for mild disease, to 32% for moderate disease, and 45% for severe disease. Ventilator-free days declined as ARDS severity increased and increased lung weight and pulmonary shunting also correlated with increased ARDS severity.

In this chapter, we will review the latest literature concerning the most relevant questions regarding risk factors, management, and prevention of ARDS and we will seek to provide recommendations as supported by the current level of evidence.

## 76.2 What Are Risk Factors for the Development of ALI/ARDS and Can We Predict Who Is at Risk for ARDS?

Identification of potential risk factors and early identification of patients at risk for ARDS may lead to earlier treatment and decreased severity of the disease. However, this is made somewhat difficult in that ARDS is rarely present at the time of hospital admission and the majority of patients with predisposing conditions never develop ARDS. In their prospective observational study, Ferguson et al. found that in patients with at least one clinical risk factor for ARDS (most commonly sepsis and pneumonia) only 6.5% of patient developed ARDS [5]. This group also found that as the number of risk factors increased, the risk of ARDS increased with each additional associated condition; the presence of one risk factor was associated with only a 2.2% rate of ARDS, but three risk factors were associated with a 21% risk of ARDS.

A two-hit hypothesis has been proposed for the development of ARDS, the first condition leading to a predisposition toward ARDS and a second hit, or a "risk modifier" that increases the likelihood of developing ARDS. Conditions associated with ARDS include pneumonia, sepsis, shock, severe trauma, traumatic brain injury, aspiration, smoke inhalation, pancreatitis, and high-risk surgery [5,6]. The predisposing conditions lead to either direct pulmonary injury via endothelial damage, as in the case of pneumonia, lung contusions, smoke inhalation, and aspiration, or via indirect pulmonary injury via epithelial damage. Sepsis, shock, trauma, and pancreatitis are all examples of conditions that can lead to increased and often unregulated, stimulation of inflammatory cells and cytokine release which then lead to pulmonary injury [7].

A number of risk modifiers have been associated with development of ARDS in these at-risk populations. Patient factors that have been repeated found to be associated with increased risk of ARDS development include alcohol abuse, obesity, active smoking, and hypoalbuminemia [5,6,8]. There are also a number of clinically modifiable factors that have been associated with the development of ARDS. In a prospective study evaluating patients with septic shock, Iscimen et al. found that delays in antibiotic treatment and delays in goal-directed resuscitation were significantly associated with the development of ARDS [8]. Transfusion of packed red blood cells, platelets, and fresh frozen plasma has also been shown to be associated with increased rates of ARDS [9], as well as with mortality from ARDS [10].

There is increasing evidence that mechanical ventilation itself can trigger inflammatory pulmonary edema in both animal models [11] and human patients [12]. Higher tidal volumes have been associated with development of ARDS in patients that did not have evidence of ARDS at the onset of mechanical ventilation [13,14]. A retrospective cohort study that evaluated 1366 ICU patients requiring mechanical ventilation for more than 48 h, who did not have ARDS at admission, found that 19% developed bilateral infiltrates and met ARDS criteria on an average of 3.3 days after initiation of mechanical ventilation [15]. In their univariate and multivariate logistic regression analyses, they found that high airway pressures (high peak inspiratory pressures, plateau pressures, positive end-expiratory pressure [PEEP]) and tidal volumes were the most important ventilator-associated risk factors for the development of new ARDS.

Early identification of patients at greatest risk of ARDS and those patients with early ARDS may allow for prevention of ARDS development and/or the amelioration of the severity of the disease. However, predicting patients that will develop ARDS remains difficult. The group at Mayo Clinic has developed the Lung Injury Prediction Score, which incorporates patient demographics, predisposing conditions, and risk modifiers [16]. The LIPS has been demonstrated to discriminate between patients at high risk for ARDS prior to ICU admission both in an internal prospective validation [16], as well as in a multicenter cohort study [17]. It has high negative predictive value (0.97), and can serve as a good screening tool to rule out those patients at low risk for ARDS; however, its positive predictive value remains low (0.18), therefore its usefulness in clinical practice is low. However, it may help to identify patients at risk for ARDS for enrollment in prospective studies that can help evaluate preventive therapies.

*Recommendation*: Numerous predisposing conditions are associated with ARDS, and should prompt clinicians to be watchful for development of this condition. Early and appropriate management of these predisposing conditions, especially in shock and sepsis, may help decrease the development of ARDS. Appropriate ventilator management and minimizing blood transfusions may also decrease the development of ARDS.

*Level of evidence*: 2c

*Grade of recommendation*: B

## 76.3 What Are the Most Common Causes of Poor Outcome in ALI/ARDS?

In 2004, the ALIVE study (Acute Lung Injury Verification of Epidemiology) published the results of their prospective, multinational, cohort study, conducted in 78 ICUs across 10 European countries [18]. This study evaluated the occurrence, etiologies, outcomes, and risk factors associated with survival in patients with ARDS. In patients with ARDS, mortality rates varied according to the cause of lung injury, and to whether the lung injury was from a direct cause (e.g., pneumonia), an indirect cause (e.g., extrapulmonary sepsis), or a combined insult (pneumonia and septic shock), where the latter had the worst outcome. In univariate analysis, mortality at hospital discharge was the highest in patients with sepsis (43%), lower in patients with pneumonia (36%) or aspiration (37%), and the lowest in patients with trauma (11%). Using multivariable logistic regression analysis, the following variables remained significantly associated with mortality: age, immunocompromise, air leak in the first 2 days, the Simplified Acute Physiology Score (SAPS) II on admission, and a pH of 7.30 or less (OR = 1.88 [1.11–3.18, 95% CI], $p = 0.019$).

*Recommendation*: Factors associated with mortality in patients with ARDS include sepsis, older age, immunosuppression, acidosis, and the presence of nonpulmonary organ failure.

*Level of evidence*: 2b

*Grade of recommendation*: B

## 76.4 What Is the Evidence That Justifies Current Ventilator Management in ALI/ARDS?

Early interest in low tidal volumes ventilation was prompted by animal studies that found that ventilation with large tidal volumes and high inspiratory pressures not only resulted in increased levels of inflammatory mediators (tumor necrosis factor [TNF]-α, interleukin [IL]-6, and IL-10), but also led to the development of ARDS [19–21]. These studies prompted Hickling et al. [22] to use a low tidal volume/low inspiratory pressure strategy of ventilation in patients with severe ARDS. In a retrospective analysis of a series of 50 of these patients, Hickling et al. reported that mortality was significantly lower in patients that were ventilated using protective lung ventilation than the mortality predicted by their APACHE II scores (16% vs. 39.6%, respectively; $p < 0.001$).

Since that study, numerous randomized controlled trials have evaluated low tidal volume ventilation in ARDS patients compared with traditional tidal volume ventilation, however, these have often been criticized, as they did not show concordant differences in mortality and many had small patient populations [23–26]. The largest RCT was conducted by the National Heart, Lung, and Blood Institute (NHLBI) ARDS Network. This was a multicenter RCT that included 861 patients at 10 institutions, known as the Respiratory Management in Acute Lung Injury/ARDS (ARMA) trial [27]. ARMA compared a ventilation protocol using tidal volumes of 6 mL/kg of predicted body weight (calculated from sex and height) and maintaining plateau pressures of ≤30 cm $H_2O$ to a conventional mechanical ventilation using tidal volumes of 12 mL/kg. The hospital mortality rate was significantly reduced in the low tidal volumes group compared with the control group (31% vs. 39.8%, respectively; $p = 0.007$). Additionally, patients treated with low tidal volumes ventilation had a greater mean) number of days free of mechanical ventilation (12 vs. 10 days, respectively; $p = 0.007$) and a greater number of days free of non-pulmonary organ failure (15 vs. 12 days, respectively; $p = 0.006$).

The most recent Cochrane review, which included six studies and 1297 patients, demonstrated that both 28-day mortality and in-hospital mortality were significantly reduced by lung protective ventilation [28]. However, they concluded that there continues to be insufficient evidence regarding long-term outcomes and overall morbidity for lung protective ventilation. This review was limited in that each study had different lengths of follow-up as well as heterogeneous plateau pressure goals in the control arms.

The association between protective ventilation and clinical outcome in patients that did not have ARDS prior to intubation was recently evaluated with a meta-analysis [29]. They found that patients ventilated using lung protective ventilation had a lower risk of developing ARDS (RR, 0.33; 95% CI, 0.23–0.47) and of mortality (RR, 0.64; 95% CI, 0.46–0.89). This study, and others like it, have prompted changes in ventilator management in critically ill patients and surgical patients, and have raised questions whether all patients should be ventilated using lung-protective ventilation.

PEEP is an essential component of mechanical ventilation for patients with ARDS. It can be used to increase the proportion of non-aerated lung, via recruitment of unused alveoli, resulting in improved oxygenation. It has also been hypothesized that PEEP may be protective, in that it may help to decrease the opening and closing of alveoli during ventilation, thereby decreasing "atelectrauma" caused by intermittent alveolar collapse. However, PEEP also may increase the "volutrauma" by increasing end-inspiratory lung volumes. Traditionally, PEEP levels of 5–12 cm $H_2O$ have been used for patients with ARDS; however, the ideal PEEP has yet to be determined. Three large RCTs have evaluated high versus low PEEP in patients ventilated using lung-protective volumes, the ALVEOLI study in the United States [30], LOVS study in Canada [31], and the ExPress study in France [32]. These large, multicenter trials did not find any significant difference in mortality associated with different PEEP levels. The ExPress trial [32] found that the high PEEP group had a greater number of ventilator-free days and nonpulmonary organ failure free days, as well as less refractory hypoxemia. Similarly, in the LOVS trial [31], the high PEEP group had less refractory hypoxemia and needed fewer rescue interventions. Therefore, a meta-analysis of these studies was performed in an attempt to better clarify these findings [33]. This meta-analysis found that if all patients with ARDS were evaluated, there was no difference in mortality for patients treated with high versus low PEEP (adjusted RR, 0.94; 95% CI, 0.86–1.04; $p = 0.25$). However, in their subgroup analysis evaluating only patients with moderate or severe ARDS (P:F ratio <200) there was a survival benefit with high PEEP (adjusted RR, 0.90; 95% CI, 0.81–1.00; $p = 0.049$). A subsequent further analysis of the LOVS and ExPress trials further evaluated how to identify those patients most likely to benefit from increased PEEP [34]. This group found that patients with ARDS that had an improvement in oxygenation (defined as a P:F increase of >25) after an increase in PEEP had significantly lower mortality than patients that did not respond to increased PEEP with improvement in oxygenation (31% vs. 54% mortality; aOR, 0.36; 95% CI, 0.23–0.58) [34]. This mortality effect was even more pronounced in patients with more severe ARDS. Further study needs to be done to better characterize patients that will most benefit from increased PEEP, however, it appears to be beneficial, especially in more severe cases of ARDS.

*Recommendation*: Low tidal volume ventilation (≤6–8 mL/kg of predicted body weight) should be the initial target in all patients with ARDS as it is the only method of mechanical ventilation demonstrating improved survival. After reaching this initial goal, titration of $V_T$ according to indices of pulmonary compliance (such as peak or plateau inspiratory pressures) should be based on clinical judgment:

*Level of evidence*: 1b

*Grade of recommendation*: B

PEEP is an essential component of mechanical ventilation for patients with ARDS. Higher levels of PEEP may improve survival, especially in patients with moderate to severe ARDS and may result in improvement in other respiratory variables (e.g., hypoxemia, ventilator-free days).

*Level of evidence*: 1a

*Grade of recommendation*: B

## 76.5 What Is the Ideal Fluid Management in Patients with ARDS?

Given that ARDS is characterized by pulmonary edema, it stands to reason that conservative fluid management would benefit these patients; however, many of these patients are concomitantly suffering from sepsis or other associated injury that requires fluid resuscitation, therefore achieving a balance between these divergent goals can be challenging. The Surviving Sepsis Campaign has shown that early, goal-directed fluid resuscitation with crystalloids to achieve a normal lactate, CVP of 8–12 mmHg, MAP of >65 mmHg, urine output of >0.5 mL/kg/h and central venous or mixed venous oxygen saturation of 65% or 70% respectively within the first 6 h are associated with improved survival [35]. In contrast, the ProCESS trial, a recent RCT found that early goal-directed resuscitation did not confer a survival benefit compared to patients treated with a protocol-based standard therapy [36]. The protocol-based standard therapy did not mandate placement of central venous catheters (CVC) and did not mandate assessment and treatment based on mixed venous oxygen saturations. Instead, fluid resuscitation was guided by clinical assessment, only 56% of patients in the protocol-based standard therapy group having CVC placed, compared to 93% of the goal-directed group. The main takeaway point would be that treatment and monitoring should be tailored to each patient, but that early resuscitation based on patient's clinical presentation, guided by other monitoring and labs as necessary, improves outcomes. As clinicians, we should continue to be vigilant in order to detect sepsis early, and start appropriate empiric antibiotics early and resuscitate promptly with little delay.

Numerous studies have been conducted to assess the ideal fluid management in ARDS. The Network Fluid and Catheter Treatment Trial was a prospective, RCT comparing conservative fluid management to a liberal fluid management strategy [37]. Patients' fluid status was monitored via CVP, MAP, urine output, and either clinical or physical signs of effective circulation. The conservative fluid management stressed maintaining a relatively low CVP, i.e., diuresis for CVP of 4–8 with adequate urine output, MAPs, and circulation. Conservative fluid management was not associated with any difference in mortality; however, it was associated with significantly more ventilator-free days and decreased the number of days in the ICU. This study evaluated all patients with ARDS, both medical and surgical; recently Stewart et al. conducted a subgroup analysis of only the surgical patients [38]. This group postulated that because surgical patients often have a different pathology behind their ARDS, they may require different fluid managements. However, the results were concordant with the previous study and found that conservative management improved the number of ventilator-free days and the number of ICU-free days. They also found that overall, surgical patients had a lower mortality rate with ARDS than the nonsurgical patients (19% vs. 30%; $p < 0.01$).

*Recommendation*: Currently, initial treatment of ARDS includes early, goal-directed resuscitation to achieve hemodynamic stability and provide adequate treatment of sepsis and shock, however, conservative fluid management should be implemented after hemodynamic stabilization.

*Level of evidence*: 1a

*Grade of recommendation*: B

## 76.6 What Is the Evidence Regarding Use of Pulmonary Arterial Catheters to Monitor Patients with ARDS?

Pulmonary artery catheters (PAC) can provide additional hemodynamic data to clinicians, such as cardiac index, pulmonary artery pressures, and the pulmonary wedge pressure. There has long been a debate whether PACs are needed to guide management for patients with ARDS. These patients require careful fluid status monitoring, and often have increased PEEP, which can lead to decreased cardiac output and venous return via the increased intrathoracic pressures, and many have argued that PAC may help guide or even change management in these patients [38]. A multicenter RCT in 2006 compared the outcomes of ARDS patients monitored using a PAC or a central venous catheter (CVC), as well as numerous other hemodynamic and physical findings, to guide fluid resuscitation and clinical management [40]. This study found that there was no difference in mortality, ventilator-free days or ICU-free days between groups. There was also no difference in rates of kidney dysfunction, hypotension, or vasopressor use in patients monitored with a PAC compared to a CVC. Importantly, they also found that PACs were associated with two times the rate of catheter-related complications, most of which were arrhythmias. As many proponents of the use of PAC in ARDS argue that PAC monitoring may help identify those patients that are subjected to a high PEEP and have a decrease in cardiac output and hemodynamic compromise, Fares and Carson performed a post-hoc analysis of this same study to evaluate the association between PEEP and cardiac output [41]. They found no association between PEEP and cardiac index. Even with PEEP >15 the mean cardiac index was 4.6 + 1.5 which was not different from the cardiac indexes of patients with lower PEEP.

*Recommendation*: Given that PACs are an invasive means of monitoring, which are associated with increased rates of complications and do not provide a benefit in mortality or reduction in organ dysfunction, PACs should not be routinely used to monitor ARDS patients.

*Level of evidence*: 1a

*Grade of recommendation*: B

## 76.7 What Is the Evidence to Support Salvage Therapies for Severe Hypoxemia?

In the most severe, refractory cases of ARDS, there are numerous salvage therapies that have been described. One ventilatory strategy that has been evaluated for severe ARDS is high-frequency oscillatory ventilation (HFOV). Some investigators have proposed that high-frequency oscillatory ventilation is an ideal mode of ventilation for ARDS patients as it is the natural culmination of low tidal volume ventilation. This mode of ventilation rapidly delivers small tidal volumes that are typically 1–5 mL/kg [42], possibly improving gas exchange and reducing ventilator-induced lung injury. However, in both, a large meta-analysis of 8 RCT which included 419 patients [43], and a recent large RCT which included 795 patients [44], HFOV was associated with no difference in mortality when compared to conventional ventilation. The most recent trial, the OSCILLATE trial [45], was a large multicenter study that aimed to evaluate early application of HFOV. However, this trial was stopped prematurely after enrolling only 548 of the planned 1200 patients, due to a significantly increased mortality in the HFOV group compared to the control group (47% vs. 35%). Currently, HFOV is not recommended as an early ventilation strategy for ARDS.

Prone positioning has also been proposed as a potential therapy for ARDS. It is thought to function via improving gas exchange and oxygenation through several hypothesized mechanisms, such as redistribution of perfusion and recruitment of dorsal alveoli, as well as lessening any cardiac or diaphragmatic compression of the lungs. Guerin et al. recently published a randomized controlled trial evaluating prone positioning for at least 16 h a day in patients with severe ARDS [46]. They found that mortality was significantly less with prone positioning, with a mortality rate of 16% in the prone group compared to a 32% mortality rate in the supine group. A recent meta-analysis was conducting including Guerin's study as well as five other evaluating prone-positioning for severe ARDS was performed in 2014 [47]. This large meta-analysis found that compared to supine position, prone positioning was associated with decreased mortality in patients with severe ARDS and in patients requiring ventilation with PEEP >10. They also found that prone positioning for >16 h a day was associated with a decrease in mortality. There was no benefit identified for patients with mild ARDS. They concluded that prone positioning is a noninvasive intervention that provides significant benefit to patients with severe ARDS and those requiring high PEEP, but that it is unlikely to provide significant benefit to patients with mild and moderate ARDS.

ECMO has recently also been increasingly used as a salvage treatment for severe ARDS. After the increase in ARDS due to H1N1 outbreak in 2009, there was a significant rise in the use of this modality to treat ARDS. The Australia and New Zealand ECMO group reported that they had a 21% mortality rate in an observational study on H1N1 patients with ARDS treated with ECMO [47]. The increasing evidence in observational studies that ECMO benefited patients with ARDS led to the CESAR trial, a large RCT conducted in the United Kingdom from 2001 to 2006 [48]. This study included patients with severe ARDS, but potentially reversible ARDS and found that 63% of patients survived to 6 months after ECMO treatment, compared to 47% treated with conventional management. This study has been criticized in that the benefit may have been more from the referral to a high volume center, well versed in the management of ARDS, which led to the mortality benefit. This is highlighted by the fact that 93% of the ECMO group and only 70% of the non-ECMO group received low volume, low pressure lung protective ventilation. Further study needs to be done to confirm or negate these findings.

Many other modalities have been studied on their effectiveness in ARDS, including steroids, neuromuscular blockade, nitric oxide, etc., however, as of yet, none of these have been shown to have any significant effect on outcomes from ARDS.

*Recommendation*: Current evidence supports the use of prone positioning as a viable treatment modality associated with decreased mortality from ARDS. ECMO may also be associated with decreased mortality from severe ARDS. Currently, these modalities have not been shown to be of benefit in less severe cases of ARDS. The use of these therapies is at the discretion of the treating physician.

*Level of evidence*: 1b

*Grade of recommendation*: B

## 76.8 What Is the Current Evidence to Support Use of Weaning Protocols for Mechanical Ventilation?

In 1999, the Agency for Healthcare Policy and Research (AHCPR) and the McMaster University Evidence Based Practice Center published the first evidence-based report on the criteria for discontinuation of mechanical ventilation [49]. At the same time, the American College of Chest Physicians, the Society for Critical Care Medicine, and the American Association for Respiratory Care formed a task force to incorporate the recommendations from the AHCPR–McMaster University and produce evidence-based clinical practice guidelines for managing the weaning process of mechanically ventilated patients [50]. These guidelines were developed from data derived from multiple meta-analyses and individual RCTs. The most important of their recommendations include the

**TABLE 76.1**

Levels of Evidence

| Question | Answer | Level of Evidence | Grade of Recommendation | References |
|---|---|---|---|---|
| What are risk factors for the development of ALI/ARDS? | Risk factors for ARDS/ALI include severe sepsis, multiple system trauma, massive blood transfusion, aspiration, and others | 2c | B | [5–16] |
| What are common causes of poor outcome in ARDS? | Age, immunocompromise, severity of illness, organ failure | 2b | B | [17] |
| What is appropriate ventilator management in ARDS? | Low tidal volume ventilation with PEEP. Higher PEEP benefits those with severe ARDS | 1a | A | [18–41] |
| What is optimum fluid management in ARDS? | Early, goal-directed resuscitation to achieve hemodynamic stability and provide adequate treatment of sepsis and shock, followed by conservative fluid management after hemodynamic stabilization | 1a | A | [35–38] |
| What is the evidence regarding use of pulmonary arterial catheters to monitor patients with ARDS? | PACs do not lead to improved outcomes, and have higher rates of catheter-related complications | 1b | A | [39–41] |
| Salvage therapies for severe hypoxemia? | Prone positioning improves survival in severe ARDS. Other modalities, such as ECMO, HFOV, etc., are still unclear, although they may be used in refractory cases | 1b | A | [42–49] |
| How should I wean my patient from the ventilator? | Daily spontaneous breathing trial (SBT) in appropriate patients | 1a | A | [50–52] |
| | Method of SBT: Pressure support, continuous positive airway pressure, T-piece all equivalent | 1a | | |
| | Daily interruption of sedation decreased time on ventilator, ICU, hospital | 1b | | |

use of spontaneous breathing to assess the potential for formal discontinuation of ventilatory support. The technique as described includes the use of a 30–120 min spontaneous breathing trial (SBT) to identify candidates for permanent ventilator discontinuation, evaluation, and treatment of causes of failed SBT, and daily reevaluation with SBT. Candidates for SBT include those patients with evidence for improvement in their underlying process, adequate oxygenation (PEEP <5–8 cm $H_2O$, and $FiO_2$ <0.4–0.5), hemodynamic stability, and the capability to initiate an inspiratory effort. SBT can be accomplished by utilizing low levels of continuous positive airway pressure (CPAP) (5 cm $H_2O$), low levels of pressure support (5–7 cm $H_2O$), or "T-piece" breathing.

Spontaneous awakening trials (SAT) (daily interruption of sedatives) followed by an SBT [51] has been shown in an RCT to be associated with more ventilator-free days (14.7 vs. 11.6 days; mean difference 3.1 days, 95% CI, 0.7–5.6; $p$ = 0.02), and earlier discharge from the ICU (median time in the ICU 9.1 vs. 12.9 days, $p$ = 0.01) and from the hospital (median time in the hospital 14.9 vs. 19.2 days; $p$ = 0.04) compared to patients with SBT alone [52]. SAT are associated with higher rates of self-extubation than patients with SBT without daily interruption of sedatives; however, the number of patients that required re-intubation were similar. Patients given SAT while intubated were 32% less likely to die than were patients without SAT (hazard ratio, 0.68; 95% CI, 0.5–0.92; $p$ = 0.01). This survival benefit remains to be validated in a larger study.

*Recommendation*: The use of an SBT is the most direct way to assess how a patient will perform without ventilatory support. Use of SBT to evaluate candidates for liberation from the ventilator has been shown to reduce ventilator, ICU, and hospital days.

*Level*: 1a

*Grade of recommendation*: A (Table 76.1).

Daily removal of sedation (spontaneous awakening trial) coupled with SBT has been shown to decrease ICU, hospital, and ventilator days and should be utilized in appropriate ventilated patients. Additional multicenter trials should be conducted to confirm the benefits of this approach.

*Level of evidence*: 1b

*Grade of recommendation*: B

## References


1. Ashbaugh DG, Bigelow DB, Petty TL et al. Acute respiratory distress in adults. *Lancet.* 1967;2:319–323.
2. Goss CH, Brower RG, Hudson LD, Rubenfeld GD. Incidence of acute lung injury in the United States. *Crit Care Med.*2003;31:1607–1611.
3. Ranieri VM, Rubenfeld GD, Thompson BT et al. Acute respiratory distress syndrome. The Berlin Definition. *JAMA.* 2012;307:E1–E8.
4. Bernard GR, Artigas A, Brigham KL et al. The American-European Consensus Conference on ARDS: Definitions, mechanisms, relevant outcomes, and clinical trial coordination. *Am J Respir Crit Care Med.* 1994;149:818–824.
5. Ferguson ND, Frutos-Vivar F, Esteban A et al. Clinical risk conditions for acute lung injury in the intensive care unit and hospital ward: A prospective observation study. *Crit Care.* 2007;11:R96.
6. Gajic O, Dabbagh O, Park P et al. Early identification of patients at risk of acute lung injury: Evaluation of lung injury prediction score in a multicenter cohort study. *Am J Respir Crit Care Med.* February 15, 2011;183(4): 462–470.
7. Perl M, Lomas-Neira J, Venet F, Chung CS, Ayala A. Pathogenesis of indirect (secondary) acute lung injury. *Expert Rev Respir Med.* 2011;5(1):115–126.
8. Iscimen R, Cartin-Ceba R, Yilmaz M et al. Risk factors for the development of acute lung injury in patients with septic shock: An observational cohort study. *Crit Care Med.* 2008:36:1518–1522.
9. Khan H, Belsher J, Yilmaz M et al. Fresh-frozen plasma and platelet transfusions are associated with development of acute lung injury in critically ill medical patients. *Chest.* 2007;131:1308–1314.
10. Gong N, Thompson BT, Williams P et al. Clinical predictors of and mortality n acute respiratory distress syndrome: Potential role of red cell transfusion. *Crit Care Med.* 2005;33:1191–1198.
11. Gurkan OU, O'Donell C, Brower R et al. Differential effects of mechanical ventilatory strategy on lung injury and systemic organ inflammation in mice. *Am J Physiol Lung Cell Mol Physiol.* 2003;285:L710–L718.
12. Slutsky AS. Lung injury caused by mechanical ventilation. *Chest.* 1999;116(1 Suppl):9S–15S.
13. Gajic O, Dara SI, Mendez JL et al. Ventilator-associated lung injury in patients without acute lung injury at the onset of mechanical ventilation. *Crit Care Med.* 2004;32: 1817–1824.
14. Gajic O, Frutos-Vivar F, Esteban A et al. Ventilator settings as a risk factor for acute respiratory distress syndrome in mechanically ventilated patients. *Intensive Care Med.* 2005;31:922–926.
15. Jia X, Malhotra A, Saeed M et al. Risk factors for ARDS in patients receiving mechanical ventilation for >48h. *Chest.* 2008;133(4):853–861.
16. Trillo Alvarez C, Cartin-Ceba R, Kor DJ et al. Acute lung injury prediction score: Derivation and validation in a population-based sample. *Eur Respir J.* 2001;37:604–609.
17. Gajic O, Dabbagh O, Park PK et al. Early identification of patients at risk of acute lung injury: Evaluation of the lung injury prediction score in a multicenter cohort study. *Am J Resp Crit Care Med.* 2010;183:462–470.
18. Brun-Buisson C, Minelli C, Bertolini G et al. for the ALIVE study group. Epidemiology and outcome of acute lung injury in European intensive care units. Results from the ALIVE study. *Intensive Care Med.* 2004;30:51–61.

19. Kolobow T, Moretti MP, Fumagalli R et al. Severe impairment in lung function induced by high peak airway pressure during mechanical ventilation: An experimental study. *Am Rev Respir Dis.* 1987;135:312–315.
20. Dreyfuss D, Basset G, Soler P et al. Intermittent positive-pressure hyperventilation with high inflation pressures produces pulmonary microvascular injury in rats. *Am Rev Respir Dis.* 1985;132:880–884.
21. von Bethmann AN, Brasch F, Nusing R et al. Hyperventilation induces release of cytokines from perfused mouse lung. *Am J Respir Crit Care Med.* 1998;157:263–272.
22. Hickling KG, Henderson SJ, Jackson R. Low mortality associated with low volume pressure limited ventilation with permissive hypercapnia in severe adult respiratory distress syndrome. *Intensive Care Med.* 1990;16:372–377.
23. Amato MB, Barbas CS, Medeiros DM et al. Effect of a protective-ventilation strategy on mortality in the acute respiratory distress syndrome. *N Engl J Med.* 1998;338:347–354.
24. Stewart TE, Meade MO, Cook DJ et al. Evaluation of a ventilation strategy to prevent barotrauma in patients at high risk for acute respiratory distress syndrome: Pressure- and Volume-Limited Ventilation Strategy Group. *N Engl J Med.* 1998;338:355–361.
25. Brochard L, Roudot-Thoraval F, Roupie E et al. Tidal volume reduction for prevention of ventilator-induced lung injury in acute respiratory distress syndrome. Multicenter Trial Group on Tidal Volume Reduction in ARDS. *Am J Respir Crit Care Med.* 1998;158:1831–1838.
26. Brower RG, Shanholtz CB, Fessler HE et al. Prospective, randomized, controlled clinical trial comparing traditional versus reduced tidal volume ventilation in acute respiratory distress syndrome patients. *Crit Care Med.* 1999;27:1492–1498.
27. The Acute Respiratory Distress Syndrome Network. Ventilation with lower tidal volumes as compared with traditional tidal volumes for acute lung injury and the acute respiratory distress syndrome. *N Engl J Med.* 2000;342:1301–1308.
28. Petrucci N, De Feo C. Lung protective ventilation strategy for the acute respiratory distress syndrome. *Cochrane Database Syst Rev.* 2013;2:CD003844.
29. Neto AS, Cardoso SO, Manetta JA et al. Association between use of lung-protective ventilation with lower tidal volumes and clinical outcomes among patients without acute respiratory distress syndrome: A meta-analysis. *JAMA.* 2012;308(16):1651–1659.
30. Brower RG, Lanken PN, MacIntyre N et al. National Heart, Lung, and Blood Institute ARDS Clinical Trials Network. Higher versus lower positive end-expiratory pressures in patients with the acute respiratory distress syndrome. *N Engl J Med.* 2004;351:327–336.
31. Mercat A, Richard JC, Vielle B et al. Expiratory Pressure (Express) Study Group. Positive end-expiratory pressure setting in adults with acute lung injury and acute respiratory distress syndrome: A randomized controlled trial. *JAMA.* 2008;299:646–655.
32. Meade MO, Cook DJ, Guyatt GH et al. Lung Open Ventilation Study Investigators. Ventilation strategy using low tidal volumes, recruitment maneuvers, and high positive end-expiratory pressure for acute lung injury and acute respiratory distress syndrome: A randomized controlled trial. *JAMA.* 2008;299:637–645.
33. Briel M, Meade M, Mercat A et al. Higher vs lower positive end-expiratory pressure in patients with acute lung injury and acute respiratory distress syndrome: Systematic review and meta-analysis. *JAMA.* 2010;303(9):865–873.
34. Goligher EC, Kavanagh BP, Rubenfeld GD et al. Oxygenation response to positive end-expiratory pressure predicts mortality in acute respiratory distress syndrome. A secondary analysis of the LOVS and ExPress trials. *Am J Respir Crit Care Med.* 2014;190(1):70–76.
35. Dellinger RP, Levy MM, Rhodes A et al. Surviving sepsis campaign: International guidelines for management of severe sepsis and septic shock: 2012. *Crit Care Med.* 2013;41(2):580–637.
36. Yealy DM, Kellum JA, Huang DT, Barnato AE, Weissfeld LA, Pike F, The ProCESS Investigators et al. A randomized trial of protocol-based care for early septic shock. *N Engl J Med.* 2014;370(18):1683–1693.
37. Wiedemann HP, Wheeler AP, Bernard GR et al. Comparison of two fluid-management strategies in acute lung injury. *N Engl J Med.* 2006; 354:2564–2575.
38. Stewart RM, Park PK, Hunt JP et al. Less is more: Improved outcomes in surgical patients with conservative fluid administration and central venous catheter monitoring. *J Am Coll Surg.* 2009;208(5):725–735.
39. Fergeson ND, Meade MO, Hallett DC, Stewart TE. High values of the pulmonary artery wedge pressure in patients with acute lung injury and acute respiratory distress syndrome. *Intensive Care Med.* 2002;298:1073–1077.
40. Wheeler AP, Bernard GR, Thompson BT et al. Pulmonary-artery versus central venous catheter to guide treatment of acute lung injury. *N Engl J Med.* 2006;354:2213–2224.
41. Fares WH, Carson SS. The relationship between positive end-expiratory pressure and cardiac index in patients with acute respiratory distress syndrome. *J Crit Care.* 2013;28:6.
42. Ferguson ND, Stewart TE. New therapies for adults with acute lung injury: High-frequency oscillatory ventilation. *Crit Care Clin.* 2002;18:91–106.
43. Young D, Lamb SE, Shah S et al. High-frequency oscillation for acute respiratory distress syndrome. *N Engl J Med.* 2013;368:806–813.
44. Sud S, Sud M, Friedrich JO et al. High frequency oscillation in patients with acute lung injury and acute respiratory distress syndrome (ARDS): Systematic review and meta-analysis. *BMJ.* 2010;340:c2327.
45. Ferguson ND, Cook DJ, Guyatt GH et al. High-frequency oscillation in early acute respiratory distress syndrome. *N Engl J Med.* 2013;368:795–805.
46. Guerin C, Reignier J, Richard JC et al. Prone positioning in severe acute respiratory distress syndrome. *N Engl J Med.* 2013;368:2159–2168

47. Sud S, Friedrich JO, Adhikari NKJ et al. Effect of prone positioning during mechanical ventilation on mortality among patients with acute respiratory distress syndrome: A systematic review and meta-analysis. *CMAJ*. 2014;186:E381–E390.
48. Noah MA, Peek GJ, Finney SJ. Referral to an extracorporeal membrane oxygenation center and mortality among patients with severe 2009 influenza A(H1N1). *JAMA*. 2011;306(15):1659–1668.
49. Peek GJ, Mugford M, Tiruvoipati R et al. Efficacy and economic assessment of conventional ventilatory support versus extracorporeal membrane oxygenation for severe adult respiratory failure (CESAR): A multicentre randomised controlled trial. *Lancet*. 2009;374:1351–1363.
50. Cook D, Meade M, Guyatt G et al. 1999. *Evidence Report on Criteria for Weaning from Mechanical Ventilation*. Agency for Health Care Policy and Research: Rockville, MD.
51. MacIntyre NR, Cook DJ, Ely EW, Jr. et al. Evidence-based guidelines for weaning and discontinuing ventilatory support: A collective task force facilitated by the American College of Chest Physicians; the American Association for Respiratory Care; and the American College of Critical Care Medicine. *Chest*. 2001;120:375S–395S.
52. Girard TD, Kress JP, Fuchs BD et al. Efficacy and safety of a paired sedation and ventilator weaning protocol for mechanically ventilated patients in intensive care (Awakening and Breathing Controlled trial): A randomised controlled trial. *Lancet*. 2008;371:126–134.

## Commentary on Evidence-Based Surgery: Acute Lung Injury/Acute Respiratory Distress Syndrome

*Robert C. MacKersie*

The adult respiratory distress syndrome (ARDS) continues to plague trauma and acute care surgeons as a source of significant morbidity and mortality. The underlying inflammatory response and related clinical management has been the subject of innumerable clinical and basic research studies. Despite these long-standing efforts, no "magic bullet" to prevent or tame the inflammatory response has been discovered and progress in improved clinical management has been slow. Fortunately, likely due to number of improvements in general intensive care, both the mortality associated with and directly attributable to ARDS have been declining steadily over the last 20+ years.

Colling and colleagues have provided a concise and important overview of the current state-of-the-art in the management of ARDS, emphasizing those areas where evidence has resulted in a change in clinical practice. The current "Berlin" consensus definition of ARDS is less confusing than previous definitions and still enables clinicians to classify mild, moderate, and severe forms of the disease—a feature particularly important in comparing randomized clinical trials and for the analysis of comparative outcomes.

The author's evidence-based review highlights three primary areas of essential knowledge for intensivists caring for ARDS patients: (1) What, if anything, can be done to minimize the risk of ARDS or even prevent the disease itself? (2) What current strategies in the management of ARDS have demonstrated efficacy in ameliorating the course of established disease? (3) What strategies are effective in the "rescue" of patients with the most severe ARDS.

### Preventing ARDS

While general risk factors for ARDS are becoming better recognized (shock, sepsis, pneumonia, pancreatitis, etc.), the seemingly capricious nature of ARDS has impaired our ability to more precisely predict or even accurately assess risk on an individual patient basis. The evidence for the effectiveness of risk-reduction strategies, however, is growing and includes such practices as adherence to clinical guidelines for goal-directed resuscitation (including sepsis and traumatic shock), and the avoidance of "unnecessary" transfusion of blood and blood products to reach goals that are not indicated from a clinical standpoint.

Following the landmark ARDS-net study in 2000,* most centers began a transition to protocolized ARDS care involving low tidal volume ventilation. The logical progression of this management philosophy was, of course, to extend "ARDS-net" protocols to high-risk patients *before* they developed ARDS. The effectiveness of this approach has been a source of debate for a number of years. One of the more notable papers cited by the authors was the 2012 meta-analysis by Neto and colleagues,† reporting an aggregate improvement in clinical outcomes, (lower mortality, fewer pulmonary infections, less ARDS) associated with the use of preemptive low tidal volume ventilation in an at-risk population. While not a well-established guideline as yet, it is likely that the detrimental effects of higher tidal volume ventilation have been underestimated in patients without ARDS and that ventilator management will increasingly utilize lung protective strategies in all at-risk patients.

### Current Strategies in the Management of ARDS

Outside of low tidal volume ventilation, there have been relatively few strategies that have been convincingly shown to improve the outcomes from ARDS. The high PEEP trials have been disappointing as have the oscillatory ventilation studies. The fluid and catheter therapy trial (FACTT trial)‡ suggested a benefit to "conservative" fluid management, but the definition used for the study was very complicated and difficult to reproduce in day-to-day clinical management. A number of interventions have been shown to improve oxygenation, but this physiological effect has not yet translated into a survival benefit. Some of these include: (1) nitric oxide (expensive and cumbersome—abandoned by many ICUs), (2) aerosolized prostaglandins (epoprostenol), a relatively effective alternative to nitric oxide, (3) neuromuscular blockade (NMB, chemical paralysis), potentially important in some patients with ventilator dyssychrony and in some TBI patients,

* The Acute Respiratory Distress Syndrome Network. Ventilation with lower tidal volumes as compared with traditional tidal volumes for acute lung injury and the acute respiratory distress syndrome. *N Engl J Med.* 2000;342:1301–1308.

† Neto AS, Cardoso SO, Manetta JA et al. Association between use of lung-protective ventilation with lower tidal volumes and clinical outcomes among patients without acute respiratory distress syndrome: A meta-analysis. *J Am Med Assoc.* 2012;308(16):1651–1659.

‡ Yealy DM, Kellum JA, Huang DT et al. A randomized trial of protocol-based care for early septic shock. *N Engl J Med.* 2014;370(18):1683–1693.

but NMB creates concerns regarding ICU polymyopathies, particularly when coupled with steroids.

#### Strategies for "Rescue" in Patients with Severe ARDS

Rescue therapy for ARDS typically applied to patients with PF ratios consistently well less than 100 who have exhausted most of the interventions designed to improve oxygenation. The two most commonly used interventions now are probably prone ventilation and ECMO. Prone ventilation, pioneered in Europe decades ago, has gradually gradually gained ground in the United States, it is used routinely for the most severe ARDS in many ICUs. For many years, prone ventilation had been associated with improvements in oxygenation (much like several of the interventions noted above), but not survival benefit. The survival benefit to prone ventilation has finally been established in a multicenter, RTC by Guerin et al.,* and a meta-analysis by Sud and colleagues.† As prone ventilation has been increasingly used and experience has accumulated, patients with difficult to manage conditions such as open abdomens and more severe traumatic brain injuries have become candidates for this intervention.

The use of ECMO as a rescue modality has also seen broader use and acceptance in many ICUs, with a gradual increase in overall survival over the past 35 years. As a "rescue" modality for ARDS however, its survival benefit still remains to be demonstrated. In the first two RTCs for ECMO (EC CO2 removal), there was no survival benefit to extracorporeal treatment.‡§ In the 2009 CESAR trial,¶ the primary analysis was by intention to treat. Twenty-four percent (24%) of the intent-to-treat ECMO group did not actually get ECMO and demonstrated a remarkable 70% survival. The overall survival between those patients who received ECMO versus conventional management was not statistically significant. This is an important study that should not be interpreted as showing benefit attributable solely to ECMO—it should be read carefully. The CESAR trial demonstrated that relative risk was reduced by referral to a sophisticated center capable of treating advanced ARDS, and not by ECMO for per se. Study should not be interpreted showing survival benefit attributable solely to ECMO.

In summary, the management of established or incipient ARDS probably should involve the following elements: (1) Adequate and close hemodynamic and ventilatory monitoring in an ICU appropriately staffed to provide 24/7 in-house physician care. (2) Goal-directed resuscitation for various shock states using guideline-driven management with fluids, blood, inotropes, and vasopressors, with a more fluid restrictive approach to preload management. (3) Preemptive low tidal volume ventilation in patients deemed to be at high risk for the development of ARDS. (4) Hemodynamic assessment (more often than not now involving echocardiography) for those patients with severe ARDS to ensure that depressed cardiac output is not contributing to aberrant gas exchange. (5) A trial of aerosolized prostacyclin to determine patient's response in improved oxygenation. (6) The institution of neuromuscular blockade, particularly in patients with ventilator dyssynchrony. (7) Prone ventilation as a rescue strategy. (8) Consider ECMO in patients unresponsive to prone ventilation in centers with appropriate capability and expertise.

* Guerin C, Reignier J, Richard JC et al. Prone positioning in severe acute respiratory distress syndrome. *N Engl J Med.* 2013;368:2159–2168.

† Sud S, Friedrich JO, Adhikari NKJ et al. Effect of prone positioning during mechanical ventilation on mortality among patients with acute respiratory distress syndrome: A systematic review and meta-analysis. *CMAJ.* 2014;186:E381–E390.

‡ Zapol. *J Am Med Assoc.* 1979.

§ Morris. *Am J Respir Crit Care Med.* 1994.

¶ Peek GJ, Mugford M, Tiruvoipati R et al. Efficacy and economic assessment of conventional ventilatory support versus extracorporeal membrane oxygenation for severe adult respiratory failure (CESAR): A multicentre randomised controlled trial. *Lancet.* 2009;374:1351–1363.

# 77

## *Acute Renal Dysfunction*

**David Bennett, Meghan E. Sise, Catherine S. Forster, Matthew O'Rourke, Katherine Xu, and Jonathan Barasch**

**CONTENTS**



Acute renal dysfunction is a common complication of hospitalized patients that is associated with significant morbidity and mortality. Multiple classification systems have been developed, including risk, injury, failure, loss, end-stage renal disease (RIFLE), Acute Kidney Injury Network, and more recently, the Kidney Disease: Improving Global Outcomes (KDIGO). These classification systems are thought to identify acute kidney injury (AKI) and allow for severity grading based on changes in the level of serum creatinine (sCr) and urine output. However, there are significant limitations to the use of sCr. These limitations are highlighted by the recent discovery of serum and urinary biomarkers, as well as kidney-specific genes, expressed soon after kidney injury, which are changing that paradigm in which we view AKI. At present, there are multiple forms of kidney stress and damage that are known to raise sCr in hospitalized patients including prerenal, intrinsic renal, and postrenal causes. Sepsis, hypovolemia, chronic kidney disease, major trauma, and surgery all confer significantly increased risk of the most severe form of azotemia, called intrinsic AKI. Unfortunately, medical therapies to limit or reverse the intrinsic forms of AKI have thus far eluded researchers, and while the judicious use of fluids is appropriate in volume-depleted prerenal patients with renal failure, they may be dangerous in patients with renal failure of the edematous states such as heart failure. Neither the timing of renal replacement therapy nor its modality or intensity has been consistently shown to impact mortality or renal recovery. Intermittent hemodialysis is used for hemodynamically stable patients, whereas continuous renal replacement therapy is typically used for patients who are unstable or in shock. Peritoneal dialysis has fallen out of favor for the treatment of AKI, albeit a useful modality for chronic kidney disease.

### 77.1 Introduction

Acute renal dysfunction is a commonly encountered clinical entity with profound implications. In the United States, one million patients are diagnosed annually with acute renal dysfunction, and the incidence is rising [1,2]. In its most severe form, called intrinsic acute kidney injury (AKI), acute renal dysfunction is a rapidly progressive disease that predicts morbidity and mortality. Patients with AKI often require admission to the intensive care unit (ICU), initiation of dialysis, and prolonged hospitalization. They encounter significant risk of both in-hospital death and the development of chronic kidney disease (CKD) [3]. Even small changes in serum creatinine (sCr) are associated with significant morbidity and mortality, underscoring the significance of this condition [4].

In 2004, the Acute Dialysis Quality Initiative Group published a consensus definition known as the risk, injury, failure, loss, end-stage renal disease (RIFLE) classification system of AKI. This scheme identified three grades of AKI severity (risk, injury, and failure) based on relative changes in sCr and/or glomerular filtration rate (GFR) over a 7-day time period and/or absolute changes in urine output. There were also two AKI outcome classes (loss- and end-stage) determined by the duration of renal replacement therapy (RRT) [5]. From this definition, it is clear that the term "AKI" can encompass a spectrum of renal dysfunction: AKI does not represent only acute tubular necrosis (ATN) or acute hemodynamic stress; it encompasses both less severe alterations in kidney function, including the rapidly reversible physiologic changes typical of prerenal azotemia and slowly reversible tubular cell death. Despite its imprecision, the RIFLE criteria have been validated as an independent predictor of in-hospital mortality, with an increased risk of death found in all RIFLE grades, which increases with each subsequent grade [6]. These criteria have established a degree of uniformity required for research on the prevention and treatment of AKI.

In 2007, the Acute Kidney Injury Network (AKIN) published their own diagnostic criteria based on relative changes in sCr within a 48 h time period and/or absolute changes in urine output. However, the AKIN criteria do not include GFR [7]. In 2012, the Kidney Disease: Improving Global Outcomes (KDIGO) classification was established as a hybrid of the RIFLE and AKIN classifications using both absolute changes of the sCr (≥0.3 mg/dL) within a 48 h time period, and relative changes (≥50% from baseline) within 7 days. It also included urine output in the criteria [8]. In each of these classification systems, hospital mortality has been shown to increase in accordance with staging. However, in a retrospective observational study, Fujii et al. found that the RIFLE and KDIGO classification systems had a superior predictive ability for hospital mortality [9].

Despite the development of multiple new classification schemes for AKI, the reliance on the sCr as a marker of kidney damage has limited their ability to accurately distinguish structural kidney damage from reversible prerenal stress. More sensitive and specific biomarkers are needed to better identify patients with reversible causes of AKI from those with more severe etiologies.

## 77.2 Risk Factors

### 77.2.1 Who Is at Risk for AKI?

A combination of vascular, tubular, and inflammatory factors is known to be responsible for renal injury in most cases of AKI. Several cohort studies have attempted to define risk factors for the development of AKI. Among critically ill patients, sepsis is the most common condition associated with AKI. Bagshaw et al. found that AKI occurred in 42% of septic patients admitted to ICUs [10]. In a prospective cohort study, Uchino et al. studied 30,000 patients admitted to 54 ICUs and found that sepsis contributed to 47% of cases of AKI [11]. Additionally, many of the patients who develop AKI have a history of CKD. This finding is supported by data from Hsu et al., who reported that CKD is a risk factor for AKI that is severe enough to require RRT during hospitalization [12]. CKD limits renal reserve during stress [13], and this may contribute to the elevated rates of AKI seen in patients with baseline renal dysfunction. Diminished renal reserve during stress also appears to place older patients at risk for severe AKI [14]. Retrospective reviews of both public and private health delivery systems data in the United States demonstrate that older patients have an elevated rate of AKI compared to younger patients [2].

Hypovolemia is also a risk factor for renal ischemia and thus AKI. Reduced effective intravascular volume (i.e., from cirrhosis or congestive heart failure), which causes renal vasoconstriction and ischemia, also predisposes to AKI from further insults, such as contrast or nephrotoxins.

Perioperative AKI is associated with distinct set of risk factors. Preexisting conditions such as diabetes, CKD, cardiac disease, and advanced age increase the risk of perioperative AKI [15]. Surgical procedures that produce higher rates of AKI include cardiac surgery requiring cardiopulmonary bypass, major intraabdominal surgery, vascular surgery requiring aortic manipulation, and/or cross-clamping and organ transplantation. Trauma patients are also at risk for AKI, particularly those with rhabdomyolysis. In a review of 436 consecutive admissions to a Level 1 trauma center, Gomes et al. found that 50% patients satisfied the RIFLE criteria, and that patients with higher severity trauma scores were more likely to develop in AKI [16].

*Recommendation*: Acute kidney injury (AKI) occurs in numerous clinical settings and, therefore, has a variety of risk factors. Conditions that confer significant risk of AKI include sepsis, baseline CKD, advanced age, hypovolemia, major surgery, and trauma (Grade B recommendation).

## 77.3 Diagnosis

### 77.3.1 What Is the Optimal Diagnostic Test to Establish AKI?

Despite its prevalence, the timely and early recognition of AKI remains difficult due to the inadequacies of sCr to definitively identify AKI. RIFLE, AKIN, and KDIGO criteria require an increase in sCr from baseline. This creates several problems: (1) baseline sCr may be unknown; (2) sCr is a delayed marker and, therefore, significant time may elapse after an injury until sCr reaches a diagnostic threshold; (3) the level of sCr may not accurately reflect the degree of renal injury since the kinetics of sCr are influenced by age, gender, muscle mass, nutritional status, hemodynamics, fluid status, and medications [17]. These limitations have generated intense interest in the identification of sensitive and specific biomarkers that allow for the early diagnosis of AKI.

In recent years, a number of urinary proteins have been shown to be associated with AKI. These proteins are normally present at low concentration in the urine, but stressors activate their expression in different cells of the kidney, resulting in an increase in their urinary concentrations. The hope is that these proteins may serve as sCr-independent "biomarkers," providing prospective data on the effects of toxic stimulation of the kidney.

These biomarkers include neutrophil gelatinase-associated lipocalin (NGAL), kidney injury molecule 1 (KIM-1), interleukin-18 (IL-18), liver fatty acid-binding protein (L-FABP), and cystatin C [18]. Multiple studies have shown the promise of these biomarkers in identifying patients with AKI, and in predicting postoperative AKI [19,20]. NGAL has been studied in over 16 [500], patients [21] including patients in the emergency room where it has been shown to be predictive of AKI and adverse clinical outcomes [22]. NGAL is significantly elevated in intrinsic AKI, but NGAL is not elevated in rapidly reversible prerenal stress in humans or mice [23].

More recently, Kashani et al. found that urine insulin-like growth factor-binding protein 7 (IGFBP7) and tissue inhibitor of metalloproteinases-2 (TIMP-2) both individually and in combination ([TIMP-2] × [IGFBP7]) were more predictive of moderate to severe AKI within 12 h than other biomarkers, including urine or plasma NGAL, plasma cystatin C, urine KIM-1, urine IL-18, and urine L-FABP [24]. Meersch et al. found that in addition to a rise in urinary [TIMP-2] × [IGFBP7] that is predictive of AKI within 4 h of cardiac surgery, a decline in its levels were predictive of renal recovery from AKI after cardiac surgery [25]. However, these results need to be further validated in larger studies. Additionally, these genes are expressed predominately in glomeruli (http://www.gudmap.org; http://www.proteinatlas.org), and are also found in normal urine.

It is important to note that biomarkers are a relatively new concept in the field of nephrology. Validation of these biomarkers necessitates comparison to sCr, and this comparison has intrinsic difficulties given that sCr is an imperfect marker of AKI. As noted in Figure 77.1,

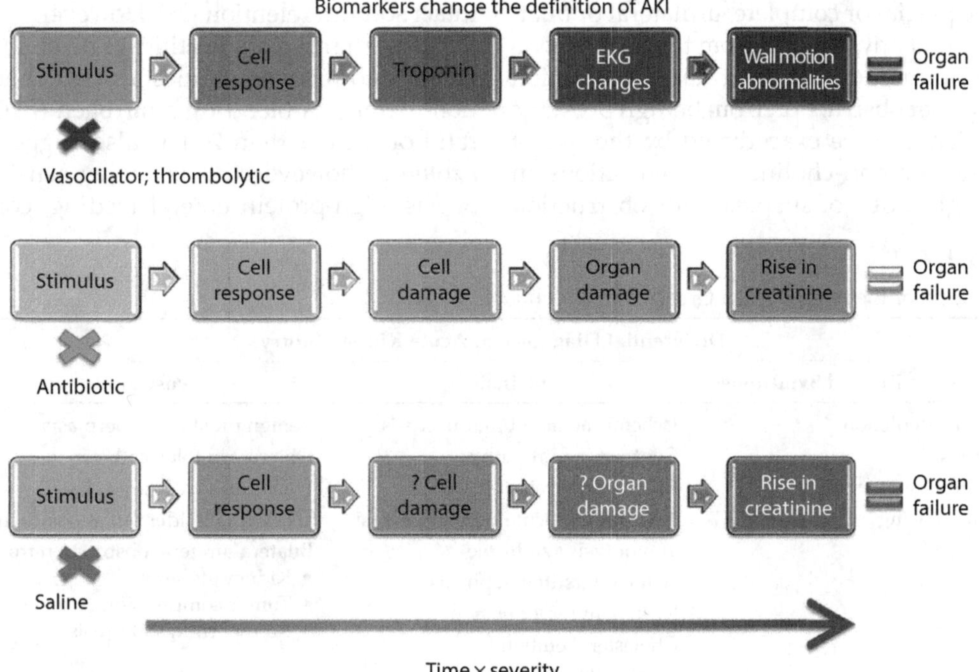


**FIGURE 77.1**
Progressivity and severity of AKI. AKI starts with an injurious stimulus (e.g., sepsis, ischemia, and volume depletion) that activates a biological pathway that includes cellular responses, cellular damage, organ damage, and organ failure. Biomarkers such as troponin and NGAL activate long before and at lower severity of damage than measures of organ failure such as sCr. Many stimuli can activate sCr, but each may activate a distinct biological pathway (e.g., sepsis, shown in the middle panel compared with volume depletion shown in the bottom panel) and deserve a different treatment (antibiotics versus saline).

cellular stress, cellular damage, organ damage, and organ failure form a pathway of increasing severity that has been well studied with cardiology, but is a new paradigm within the field of nephrology. In the former case, the appearance of troponin defines a myocardial infarction, while the presence of troponin in addition to EKG changes and subsequently echocardiographic changes represents an ascending scale of severity of tissue damage. In AKI, only sCr has been recognized as a marker of kidney distress (Figure 77.1). Within this new paradigm of AKI, biomarkers that are upregulated in response to a weak stimulus without elevation of sCr indicate an earlier or less severe level of renal injury. Conversely, a strong stimulus will activate both the biomarkers and sCR, indicating a more severe injury. The utilization of biomarkers will allow for the identification of renal injury in the absence of overt renal failure.

*Answer*: While standardized creatinine-based definitions of AKI now exist, novel biomarkers hold great promise for expedient and accurate diagnosis (Grade B recommendation).

### 77.3.2 What Is the Best Approach to the Differential Diagnosis of AKI?

AKI is classically divided into three large categories: prerenal, intrinsic renal, and postrenal causes (Table 77.1).

Postrenal causes refer to any obstruction of urinary flow. This may be partial or complete, unilateral or bilateral, and may occur at any location from the renal pelvis to the urethra. Common causes of urinary obstruction include bladder outlet obstruction from benign prostatic hypertrophy, which may be exacerbated by the use of narcotic analgesics or anti-cholinergic medications in the hospital; a high index of suspicion for obstruction is necessary in any older man with unexplained AKI. Severe cystitis or obstruction of a Foley catheter may cause bladder outlet obstruction. An obstructing kidney stone may cause AKI in patients with single functioning kidney or baseline CKD. Obstruction can be evaluated by renal ultrasonography demonstrating hydroureter or hydronephrosis; however, it should be noted that in patients with early obstruction, significant volume depletion, or retroperitoneal fibrosis, normal ultrasound findings are expected despite urinary tract obstruction [26]. Moreover, normal urine output does not exclude partial urinary tract obstruction, nor do normal creatinine values (e.g., unilateral kidney obstruction) [27], and, in fact, are likely to delay the diagnosis.

Distinguishing prerenal kidney stress from intrinsic AKI is more difficult, but necessary, given the significant increase in morbidity and mortality in the latter. Prerenal causes include volume depletion from dehydration, blood loss, and diuretics. Prerenal AKI can also result from volume overloaded or edematous states including congestive heart failure or cirrhosis, in which the total body fluid is increased, but the effective circulating volume is decreased due to movement of fluids from the intravascular into the extravascular space, causing decreased renal blood flow. Urinary studies can be helpful in distinguish prerenal from intrinsic renal causes. Prerenal causes are associated with low urine sodium (i.e., <20 mEq/L) and low fractional excretion of sodium <1%, indicating intact sodium retention [28]. However, several factors can decrease the diagnostic utility of urine sodium, including recently administered diuretics, CKD, and acute rehydration therapy. A blood urea nitrogen (BUN) to creatinine ratio of greater than 20:1 is also suggestive of prerenal azotemia; however, this is neither sensitive nor specific. Sepsis, high-protein enteral feeding, corticosteroid use,

**TABLE 77.1**

Etiology of Elevated Serum Creatinine which Defines AKI

| Differential Diagnosis of Acute Kidney Injury | | |
|---|---|---|
| **Prerenal + Related Syndromes** | **Intrinsic** | **Postrenal** |
| Volume depletion | Ischemic acute tubular necrosis | Benign prostatic hyperplasia |
| Cirrhosis | Contrast nephropathy | Obstructed foley catheter |
| Congestive heart failure | Rhabdomyolysis | Hematuria with large clots |
| Third-spacing | Nephrotoxic acute tubular necrosis | UTI with bladder outlet obstruction |
| | Tumor lysis syndrome | Bilateral ureteral obstruction from: |
| | Acute interstitial nephritis | • Kidney stones |
| | Malignant hypertension | • Tumor compression |
| | Cholesterol emboli | • Retroperitoneal fibrosis |
| | Glomerulonephritis | |
| | • Lupus | |
| | • Post-infectious | |
| | • Anti-GBM | |
| | • ANCA vasculitis | |
| | • Cryoglobulinemia | |

and upper gastrointestinal bleeding can all elevate BUN out of proportion to the creatinine and, conversely, liver disease and poor nutritional status will depress the BUN. Therefore, prerenal disease cannot be excluded by a normal BUN/creatinine ratio. It is important to note that fluid management cannot be determined based on serum or urinary findings alone, but must incorporate history and physical examination findings, since both volume depletion and congestive heart failure are "prerenal" causes of AKI, yet are managed very differently: IV fluids in the former group and IV diuresis and possible inotropic support in the latter group.

Urinary biomarkers are currently under investigation to determine if they can distinguish intrinsic renal failure from prerenal causes. Certain biomarkers, such as NGAL, are upregulated in response to tubular damage rather than quickly reversible prerenal azotemia, and, therefore, high urinary levels are expected in intrinsic renal failure but not prerenal azotemia [29,30]. Genetic studies are now ongoing to identify novel biomarkers in the kidney. Ongoing studies have demonstrated that gene expression differs in subjects with different types of AKI, even when sCr levels are equivalent. Many genetic pathways are activated in ischemia, while fewer genes are activated in prerenal azotemia, with only a small degree of overlap between the two conditions. This suggests that there should be distinct molecular identifications to each state.

*Recommendation*: When evaluating AKI, a systematic approach that includes prerenal, intrinsic renal, and postrenal causes is critical as therapy is substantially different between these groups. Urinary studies can help distinguish prerenal AKI from intrinsic AKI. Urinary biomarkers, including NGAL, have been repeatedly shown to separate subsets of AKI (Grade B recommendation).

### 77.3.3 What Are Common Causes of Intrinsic AKI Seen on Surgical Services

Causes of intrinsic renal failure commonly encountered on surgical services include ischemic and nephrotoxic ATN, contrast-induced nephropathy (CIN), and allergic interstitial nephritis. Postoperative AKI may occur to up to 25% of patients undergoing coronary artery bypass grafting [31]. Medications including vancomycin and aminoglycosides are an important cause of nephrotoxic ATN [32]. Beta-lactam and sulfonamide antibiotics, flouroquinolonnes, proton pump inhibitors, and non-steroidal anti-inflammatory drugs (NSAIDs) are associated with acute interstitial nephritis. The clinical scenario is important in diagnosing acute interstitial nephritis as these patients may have other allergic symptoms including rash, fever, and peripheral eosinophila [33]. NSAIDs, such as ketorolac and ibuprofen, can also cause ischemic ATN, and should be used with caution in elderly patients and avoided entirely in patients with CKD or cardiac disease [34].

CIN typically occurs in patients with other underlying risk factors including hypotension, use of an intraaortic balloon pump, congestive heart failure, older age, anemia, diabetes, high contrast volumes, and elevated sCr or low GFR. Using a score model developed for patients undergoing percutaneous coronary intervention, the risk of CIN ranges from 7.5% for low-risk patients to ≥57.3% for the patients at the highest risk [35]; findings have been validated in other studies [36,37]. Strategies for preventing CIN include discontinuing furosemide and angiotensin-converting enzyme inhibitors or angiotensin receptor blocking medications prior to contrast exposure. Patients should be hydrated with either normal saline or sodium bicarbonate at a rate of 1 mL/kg/h for 12 h prior to contrast and 12 h after contrast exposure. If a patient is known to have congestive heart failure, then the rate of IV fluid administration should be decreased to 0.5 mL/kg/h [38]. Once CIN is established and urine output has decreased, it is wise to stop standing IV fluids to prevent worsening volume overload.

Pigment-induced nephropathy, due to either rhabdomyolysis (myoglobin pigment) or massive hemolysis (hemoglobin pigment), results from direct tubular damage from these substances. Prophylaxis with judicious IV fluids are recommended to prevent AKI in patients with rhabdomyolysis or hemolysis [39].

## 77.4 Management

### 77.4.1 Does Time of RRT Initiation, Modality, or Intensity Impact Mortality?

RRT is the definitive treatment for complications of AKI (extracellular fluid volume overload, solute imbalance, and uremia) that are intractable to medical management. Nevertheless, the current literature offers incomplete guidance as to the optimal timing, method, and intensity of such therapy. While case–control and retrospective studies suggested "early" dialysis reduces mortality, two randomized clinical trials produced conflicting results. In 2002, a trial of 106 patients initiated "early" dialysis if urine output was less than 30 mL/h after 6 h but did not find a difference with regard to mortality or recovery of renal function in survivors [40]. A 2004 trial found a large reduction in mortality with early dialysis, defined by postoperative urine output (RR = 0.17; 95% CI = 0.05–0.61), but weak methods and a small sample size ($N$ = 28) temper this conclusion [41]. The lone observational study in this area found that the risk of death in critically ill AKI patients was significantly decreased by initiating RRT before levels of BUN were greater than 76 mg/dL (adjusted hazard ratio = 0.54; 95% CI = 0.34–0.86) [42]. Based on this evidence, a 2008 systematic review of adult patients concluded that the available literature does not permit a definitive statement as to the optimal timing of acute RRT initiation [43]. However, the pediatric literature suggests that there may at least be a mortality benefit to treating patients with RRT before they become significantly volume-overloaded [44–46]. This fits with a model developed by Goldstein for patients with AKI in which there are three phases to fluid management: (1) fluid resuscitation/repletion, (2) fluid balance maintenance, and (3) fluid removal/recovery [47]. This model requires clinicians to diligently monitor patients' volume status.

Debate also persists regarding the preferred mode of dialysis. Available methods include intermittent hemodialysis (IHD) and continuous renal replacement therapy (CRRT), with significant differences between these two techniques. IHD is conventionally performed three times a week in 4 h sessions via venovenous access. Because of more rapid fluid shifts, IHD requires hemodynamic stability. Conversely, CRRT is performed continuously using venovenous or arteriovenous access and reduced blood flow and ultrafiltration rates. In doing so, CRRT offers gradual solute and fluid clearance and, therefore, is the preferred choice in patients who are not hemodynamically stable. Despite the theoretical advantage of more "physiologic" restoration of solute and fluid balance, CRRT has not been found to offer a survival benefit compared with IHD. While methodological concerns, such as patient selection, plague this literature, no recent randomized control trial has demonstrated a mortality advantage to CRRT [48–52]. Similarly, numerous meta-analyses have concluded that CRRT does not appear to confer a survival advantage over IHD [53,54]. On the other hand, it is likely that sicker patients are offered CRRT, rather than IHD.

Six randomized trials have analyzed whether the dose of dialysate administered with CRRT impacts mortality. Two early studies produced preliminary evidence to suggest that increased CRRT intensity decreases mortality. Ronco et al. found that patients who received doses of 45 or 35 mL/kg/h demonstrated reduced mortality compared to patients who received doses of 20 mL/kg/h (RR = 0.72; 95% CI = 0.54–0.94 and RR = 0.73; 95% CI = 0.56–0.96, respectively) [55]. However, the preponderance of subsequent evidence has come to suggest that CRRT dose does not affect mortality. In 2002, Bouman et al. found no decrease in mortality among 106 patients who sustained higher hemofiltration volumes compared to lower volumes (48 versus 20 mL/kg/h) [40]. Similarly, Tolwani et al. found no difference in mortality between 200 patients randomized to receive CRRT dose of 35 or 20 mL/kg/h [56]. In a multicenter 1100 patient randomized trial, Palevsky et al. did not note a mortality difference between patients receiving CRRT dose of 35 versus 20 mL/kg/h [57]. Bellomo et al. conducted a 1500 patient trial and found no mortality difference at 90 days between patients who received a dose of 40 mL/kg/h and those who received 25 mL/kg/h [58]. In addition, none of these studies reported a difference in rates of recovery of renal function following a more intense CRRT treatment. Given this body of evidence, most authors recommend achieving flow rates of 20 mL/kg/h. Higher rates may be used in cases with clinically significant metabolic acidosis or hyperkalemia or severe catabolic disease.

Early studies implied that more frequent IHD might also reduce mortality among critically ill patients with AKI. Schiffl et al. studied 160 patients and found reduced mortality among patients treated with daily IHD as compared to an alternating day schedule [59]. Another group found reduced mortality among 34 patients randomized to receive either IHD to maintain BUN levels less than 60 mg/dL and sCr levels less than 5 mg/dL as compared to conventional IHD schedule [60]. In spite of these early reports, a more recent, large randomized trial with 1100 patients failed to demonstrate a mortality benefit to daily IHD in AKI [57].

*Recommendation*: Neither the exact timing of RRT initiation, modality of dialysis, or intensity of the therapy above a minimum seem to impact mortality or renal recovery (Grade B recommendation).

### 77.4.2 What Are Potential Pharmacologic Treatments of AKI?

Initial therapy for suspected prerenal AKI secondary to volume depletion includes a judicious trial of fluid repletion in the appropriate clinical setting, unless evidence of congestive heart failure or pulmonary edema is present. Conversely, diuretics are useful in right-sided congestion that may cause congestive nephropathy [61], but more commonly diuretics are utilized in an attempt to improve urine output and manage volume overload in a patient with AKI. Nonetheless, numerous studies have found that diuretics do not decrease mortality or improve renal outcomes in established renal failure [62,63], albeit that both higher fluid balance and lower urine volumes were shown to be independently associated with 28-day mortality of AKI patients in one multicenter ICU study [64].

Various vasoactive substances have also been trialed in AKI. Low- or renal-dose dopamine has been proposed to preferentially reduce renal vasoconstriction and thus advocated as a technique to ameliorate renal dysfunction. Several recent meta-analyses have not documented reduced mortality or improved renal function with low-dose dopamine and have explicitly argued against its use [65,66]. Fenoldapam is a pure dopamine A-1 receptor agonist that increases blood flow to the renal cortex and outer medulla. Two meta-analyses, one in critically ill patients

**TABLE 77.2**
Clinical Questions Summary

| Question | Answer | Grade of Recommendation | References |
|---|---|---|---|
| Who is at risk for AKI? | Acute kidney injury (AKI) occurs in numerous clinical settings and therefore has a variety of risk factors. Conditions which confer significant risk of AKI include sepsis, baseline CKD, advanced age, hypovolemia, major surgery, and trauma. | B | [2,10–16] |
| What is the optimal diagnostic test to establish AKI? | While standardized creatinine-based definitions of AKI now exist, novel biomarkers hold great promise for expedient and accurate diagnosis. | B | [17–25] |
| What is the best approach to the differential diagnosis of AKI? | When evaluating AKI, a systematic approach that includes prerenal, intrinsic renal, and post-renal causes is critical as therapy is substantially different between these groups. Urinary studies can help distinguish pre-renal AKI from intrinsic AKI. Urinary biomarkers, including NGAL, have been repeatedly shown to separate subsets of AKI. | B | [26–30] |
| Does time of RRT initiation, modality, or intensity impact mortality? | Neither the exact timing of RRT initiation, nor modality of dialysis, nor intensity of the therapy above a minimum seem to impact mortality or renal recovery. | B | [40–60] |
| What are potential pharmacologic treatments of AKI? | Medical therapies to limit or reverse AKI have thus far eluded researchers. | B | [61–72] |

following cardiac surgery and one in critically ill patients with or at risk for AKI, found that fenoldapam reduced the need for renal replacement therapy, decreased mortality, and reduced length of stay [67,68]. Heterogeneity among the analyzed studies limited this conclusion, and when Bove et al. randomized postcardiac surgery patients to fenoldopam or placebo, there was no difference in the rate of renal replacement therapy or mortality, although those receiving fenoldopam had a higher rate of hypotension [69]. Atrial natriuretic peptide (ANP) is produced by modified cardiac myocytes and increases GFR through afferent arteriolar vasodilation and efferent arteriolar vasoconstriction. ANP has been mainly studied in the setting of postcardiac surgery AKI. While systematic reviews found a reduced need for RRT in AKI patients, other meta-analyses have concluded that the lack of high-quality studies limits this conclusion [70].

Another area of active research concerns the use of growth factors in the treatment of AKI. Noting that expression in animal models of insulin-like growth factor (IGF) decreased during ischemia and increased coincident with renal recovery, Hammerman et al. found that IGF administration ameliorated AKI in animal models [71]. Translation of this concept from animals to humans has, however, proven difficult. Similarly, while large doses of erythropoietin improved AKI in animal models, a randomized, placebo-controlled trial of erythropoietin revealed that prophylactic administration did not decrease rates of AKI in the intensive care setting [72].

*Recommendation*: Medical therapies to limit or reverse AKI have thus far eluded researchers (Grade B recommendation).

Table 77.2 summarizes the clinical questions posed by practicing clinicians regarding AKI and assigns a grade based on the level of evidence.

## References


1. Chertow GM, Burdick E, Honour M, Bonventre JV, Bates DW. Acute kidney injury, mortality, length of stay, and costs in hospitalized patients. *J Am Soc Nephrol.* 2005;16(11):3365–3370.
2. Hsu CY, McCulloch CE, Fan D, Ordonez JD, Chertow GM, Go AS. Community-based incidence of acute renal failure. *Kidney Int.* 2007;72(2):208–212.
3. Venkatachalam MA, Griffin KA, Lan R, Geng H, Saikumar P, Bidani AK. Acute kidney injury: A springboard for progression in chronic kidney disease. *Am J Physiol Renal Physiol.* 2010;298(5):F1078–F1094.
4. Lassnigg A, Schmidlin D, Mouhieddine M et al. Minimal changes of serum creatinine predict prognosis in patients after cardiothoracic surgery: A prospective cohort study. *J Am Soc Nephrol.* 2004;15(6):1597–1605.
5. Hoste EA, Clermont G, Kersten A et al. RIFLE criteria for acute kidney injury are associated with hospital mortality in critically ill patients: A cohort analysis. *Crit Care.* 2006;10(3):R73.
6. Abosaif NY, Tolba YA, Heap M, Russell J, El Nahas AM. The outcome of acute renal failure in the intensive care unit according to RIFLE: Model application, sensitivity, and predictability. *Am J Kidney Dis.* 2005;46(6):1038–1048.
7. Mehta RL, Kellum JA, Shah SV, Molitoris BA, Ronco C, Warnock DG, Levin A. Acute Kidney Injury Network: Report of an initiative to improve outcomes in acute kidney injury. *Crit Care.* 2007;11(2):R31.

8. Kidney Disease: Improving Global Outcomes (KDIGO) Acute Kidney Injury Work Group. KDIGO Clinical Practice Guideline for acute kidney injury. *Kidney Int.* 2012;Suppl. 2:1–138.
9. Fujii T, Uchino S, Takinami M, and Bellomo R. Validation of the kidney disease improving global outcomes criteria for AKI and comparison of three criteria in hospitalized patients. *Clin J Am Soc Nephrol.* 2014;9(5):848–854.
10. Bagshaw SM, George C, Bellomo R, Committee ADM. Early acute kidney injury and sepsis: A multicentre evaluation. *Crit Care.* 2008;12(2):R47.
11. Uchino S, Kellum JA, Bellomo R et al. Acute renal failure in critically ill patients: A multinational, multicenter study. *JAMA.* 2005;294(7):813–818.
12. Hsu CY, Ordonez JD, Chertow GM, Fan D, McCulloch CE, Go AS. The risk of acute renal failure in patients with chronic kidney disease. *Kidney Int.* 2008;74(1):101–107.
13. Sharma A, Mucino MJ, Ronco C. Renal functional reserve and renal recovery after acute kidney injury. *Nephron Clin Pract.* 2014;127:94–100.
14. Rosner MH. The pathogenesis of susceptibility to acute kidney injury in the elderly. *Curr Aging Sci.* 2009;2(2):158–164.
15. Thakar CV, Arrigain S, Worley S, Yared JP, Paganini EP. A clinical score to predict acute renal failure after cardiac surgery. *J Am Soc Nephrol.* 2005;16(1):162–168.
16. Gomes E, Antunes R, Dias C, Araujo R, Costa-Pereira A. Acute kidney injury in severe trauma assessed by RIFLE criteria: A common feature without implications on mortality? *Scand J Trauma Resusc Emerg Med.* 2010;18(1):1–6.
17. Waikar SS, Bonventre JV. Creatinine kinetics and the definition of acute kidney injury. *J Am Soc Nephrol.* 2009;20(3):672–679.
18. Coca SG, Yalavarthy R, Concato J, Parikh CR. Biomarkers for the diagnosis and risk stratification of acute kidney injury: A systematic review. *Kidney Int.* 2008;73(9):1008–1016.
19. Liu S, Che M, Xue S et al. Urinary L-FABP and its combination with urinary NGAL in early diagnosis of acute kidney injury after cardiac surgery in adult patients. *Biomarkers.* 2013;18(1):95–101.
20. Portilla D, Dent C, Sugaya T et al. Liver fatty acid-binding protein as a biomarker of acute kidney injury after cardiac surgery. *Kidney Int.* 2008;73(4):465–472.
21. Haase-Fielitz A, Haase M, Devarajan P. Neutrophil gelatinase-associated lipocalin as a biomarker of acute kidney injury: A critical evaluation of current status. *Ann Clin Biochem.* 2014;51(3);335–351.
22. Nickolas TL, Schmidt-Ott KM, Canetta P et al. Diagnostic and prognostic stratification in the emergency department using urinary biomarkers of nephron damage: A multicenter prospective cohort study. *J Am Coll Cardiol.* 2012;59(3):246–255.
23. Paragas N, Qiu A, Zhang Q et al. The Ngal reporter mouse detects the response of the kidney to injury in real time. *Nat Med.* 2011;17:216–222.
24. Kashani K, Al-Khafaji A, Ardiles T et al. Discovery and validation of cell cycle arrest biomarkers in human acute kidney injury. *Crit Care.* 2013;17:R25.
25. Meersch M, Schmidt C, Van Aken H et al. Urinary TIMP-2 and IGFBP7 as early biomarkers of acute kidney injury and renal recovery following cardiac surgery. *PLoS One.* 2014;9(3):e93460.
26. Webb JA. Ultrasonography in the diagnosis of renal obstruction. *BMJ.* 1990;301(6758):944–946.
27. Sise ME, Forster C, Singer E et al. Urine neutrophil gelatinase-associated lipocalin identifies unilateral and bilateral urinary tract obstruction. *Nephrol Dial Transplant.* 2011;26(12):4132–4135.
28. Lameire N, Van Biesen W, Vanholder R. Acute renal failure. *Lancet.* 2005;365(9457):417–430.
29. Nickolas TL, O'Rourke MJ, Yang J et al. Sensitivity and specificity of a single emergency department measurement of urinary neutrophil gelatinase-associated lipocalin for diagnosing acute kidney injury. *Ann Intern Med.* 2008;148(11):810–819.
30. Bagshaw SM, Bennett M, Devarajan P, Bellomo R. Urine biochemistry in septic and non-septic acute kidney injury: A prospective observational study. *J Crit Care.* 2013;28(4):371–378.
31. Del Duca D, Iqbal S, Rahme E, Goldberg P, de Varennes B. Renal failure after cardiac surgery: Timing of cardiac catheterization and other perioperative risk factors. *Ann Thorac Surg.* 2007;84(4):1264–1271.
32. Rybak MJ, Albrecht LM, Boike SC, Chandrasekar PH. Nephrotoxicity of vancomycin, alone and with an aminoglycoside. *J Antimicrob Chemother.* 1990;25(4):679–687.
33. Farrington K, Levison DA, Greenwood RN, Cattell WR, Baker LR. Renal biopsy in patients with unexplained renal impairment and normal kidney size. *Quart J Med.* 1989;70(263):221–233.
34. Schneider V, Levesque LE, Zhang B, Hutchinson T, Brophy JM. Association of selective and conventional nonsteroidal antiinflammatory drugs with acute renal failure: A population-based, nested case-control analysis. *Am J Epidemiol.* 2006;164(9):881–889.
35. Mehran R, Aymong ED, Nikolsky E et al. A simple risk score for prediction of contrast-induced nephropathy after percutaneous coronary intervention: Development and initial validation. *J Am Coll Cardiol.* 2004;44:1393–1399.
36. Parfrey PS, Griffiths SM, Barrett BJ et al. Contrast material-induced renal failure in patients with diabetes mellitus, renal insufficiency, or both. A prospective controlled study. *N Engl J Med.* 1989;320(3):143–149.
37. Manske CL, Sprafka JM, Strony JT, Wang Y. Contrast nephropathy in azotemic diabetic patients undergoing coronary angiography. *Am J Med.* 1990;89(5):615–620.
38. Asif A, Epstein M. Prevention of radiocontrast-induced nephropathy. *Am J Kidney Dis.* Jul 2004;44(1):12–24.
39. Melli G, Chaudhry V, Cornblath DR. Rhabdomyolysis: An evaluation of 475 hospitalized patients. *Medicine (Baltimore).* 2005;84(6):377–385.
40. Bouman CS, Oudemans-Van Straaten HM, Tijssen JG, Zandstra DF, Kesecioglu J. Effects of early high-volume continuous venovenous hemofiltration on survival and recovery of renal function in intensive care patients with acute renal failure: A prospective, randomized trial. *Crit Care Med.* 2002;30(10):2205–2211.

41. Sugahara S, Suzuki H. Early start on continuous hemodialysis therapy improves survival rate in patients with acute renal failure following coronary bypass surgery. *Hemodial Int.* 2004;8(4):320–325.
42. Liu KD, Himmelfarb J, Paganini E et al. Timing of initiation of dialysis in critically ill patients with acute kidney injury. *Clin J Am Soc Nephrol.* 2006;1(5):915–919.
43. Pannu N, Klarenbach S, Wiebe N, Manns B, Tonelli M, Alberta Kidney Disease N. Renal replacement therapy in patients with acute renal failure: A systematic review. *JAMA.* 2008;299(7):793–805.
44. Goldstein SL, Somers MJ, Baum MA et al. Pediatric patients with multi-organ dysfunction syndrome receiving continuous renal replacement therapy. *Kidney Int.* 2005;67:653–658.
45. Modem V, Thompson M, Gollhofer D, Dhar AV, Quigley R. Timing of continuous renal replacement therapy and mortality in critically ill children. *Crit Care Med.* 2014;42(4):943–953.
46. Sutherland SM, Zappitelli M, Alexander SR et al. Fluid overload and mortality in children receiving continuous renal replacement therapy: The prospective pediatric continuous renal replacement therapy registry. *Am J Kidney Dis.* 2010;55(2):316–325.
47. Goldstein SL. Fluid management in acute kidney injury. *J Intensive Care Med.* 2012;29(4):183–189.
48. Mehta RL, McDonald B, Gabbai FB et al. A randomized clinical trial of continuous versus intermittent dialysis for acute renal failure. *Kidney Int.* 2001;60(3):1154–1163.
49. Uehlinger DE, Jakob SM, Ferrari P et al. Comparison of continuous and intermittent renal replacement therapy for acute renal failure. *Nephrol Dial Transplant.* 2005;20(8):1630–1637.
50. Augustine JJ, Sandy D, Seifert TH, Paganini EP. A randomized controlled trial comparing intermittent with continuous dialysis in patients with ARF. *Am J Kidney Dis.* 2004;44(6):1000–1007.
51. Vinsonneau C, Camus C, Combes A et al. Continuous venovenous haemodiafiltration versus intermittent haemodialysis for acute renal failure in patients with multiple-organ dysfunction syndrome: A multicentre randomised trial. *Lancet.* 2006;368(9533):379–385.
52. Cho KC, Himmelfarb J, Paganini E et al. Survival by dialysis modality in critically ill patients with acute kidney injury. *J Am Soc Nephrol.* 2006;17(11):3132–3138.
53. Bagshaw SM, Berthiaume LR, Delaney A, Bellomo R. Continuous versus intermittent renal replacement therapy for critically ill patients with acute kidney injury: A meta-analysis. *Crit Care Med.* 2008;36(2):610–617.
54. Rabindranath K, Adams J, Macleod AM, Muirhead N. Intermittent versus continuous renal replacement therapy for acute renal failure in adults. *Cochrane Database Syst Rev.* 2007(3):CD003773.
55. Ronco C, Bellomo R, Homel P et al. Effects of different doses in continuous veno-venous haemofiltration on outcomes of acute renal failure: A prospective randomised trial. *Lancet.* 2000;356(9223):26–30.
56. Tolwani AJ, Campbell RC, Stofan BS, Lai KR, Oster RA, Wille KM. Standard versus high-dose CVVHDF for ICU-related acute renal failure. *J Am Soc Nephrol.* 2008;19(6):1233–1238.
57. Network V, Palevsky PM, Zhang JH et al. Intensity of renal support in critically ill patients with acute kidney injury. *N Engl J Med.* 2008;359(1):7–20.
58. Investigators RRTS, Bellomo R, Cass A et al. Intensity of continuous renal-replacement therapy in critically ill patients. *N Engl J Med.* 2009;361(17):1627–1638.
59. Schiffl H, Lang SM, Fischer R. Daily hemodialysis and the outcome of acute renal failure. *N Engl J Med.* 2002;346(5):305–310.
60. Gillum DM, Dixon BS, Yanover MJ et al. The role of intensive dialysis in acute renal failure. *Clin Nephrol.* 1986;25(5):249–255.
61. Li X, Liu M, Bedja D et al. Acute renal venous obstruction is more detrimental to the kidney than arterial occlusion: Implication for murine models of acute kidney injury. *Am J Physiol Renal Physiol.* 2012;302(5):F519–F525.
62. Bagshaw SM, Delaney A, Haase M, Ghali WA, Bellomo R. Loop diuretics in the management of acute renal failure: A systematic review and meta-analysis. *Crit Care Resusc.* 2007;9(1):60–68.
63. Mehta RL, Pascual MT, Soroko S, Chertow GM. Diuretics, mortality, and nonrecovery of renal function in acute renal failure. *JAMA.* 2002;288(20):2547–2553.
64. Teixeira C, Garzotto F, Piccinni P et al. Fluid balance and urine volume are independent predictors of mortality in acute kidney injury. *Crit Care.* 2013;17:R14.
65. Holmes CL, Walley KR. Bad medicine: Low-dose dopamine in the ICU. *Chest.* 2003;123(4):1266–1275.
66. Friedrich JO, Adhikari N, Herridge MS, Beyene J. Meta-analysis: Low-dose dopamine increases urine output but does not prevent renal dysfunction or death. *Ann Intern Med.* 2005;142(7):510–524.
67. Landoni G, Biondi-Zoccai GG, Tumlin JA et al. Beneficial impact of fenoldopam in critically ill patients with or at risk for acute renal failure: A meta-analysis of randomized clinical trials. *Am J Kidney Dis.* 2007;49(1):56–68.
68. Landoni G, Biondi-Zoccai GG, Marino G et al. Fenoldopam reduces the need for renal replacement therapy and in-hospital death in cardiovascular surgery: A meta-analysis. *J Cardiothorac Vasc Anesth.* 2008;22(10):27–33.
69. Bove T, Zangrillo A, Guarracino F et al. Effect of fenoldopam on use of renal replacement therapy among patients with acute kidney injury after cardiac surgery: A randomized clinical trial. *JAMA.* 2014;312(21):2244–2253.
70. Nigwekar SU, Navaneethan SD, Parikh CR, Hix JK. Atrial natriuretic peptide for preventing and treating acute kidney injury. *Cochrane Database Syst Rev.* 2009;(4):CD006028.
71. Hammerman MR. Growth factors and apoptosis in acute renal injury. *Curr Opin Nephrol Hypertens.* 1998;7(4):419–424.
72. Endre ZH, Walker RJ, Pickering JW et al. Early intervention with erythropoietin does not affect the outcome of acute kidney injury (the EARLYARF trial). *Kidney Int.* 2010;77(11):1020–1030.

# 78

## *Evidence-Based Electrolyte Management*

**Brian O'Gara, Balachundhar Subramaniam, and Alan Lisbon**

**CONTENTS**



### 78.1 Introduction

Electrolyte disorders are among the most common and potentially lethal conditions that accompany a variety of surgical diseases. Although the knowledge behind the etiology of certain electrolyte disorders and the strategies to manage them have in certain cases been practiced and commonly accepted for decades, recent investigations have sought to shed scientific light as to what is to be considered best practice. This chapter aims to summarize both historical and novel investigations into the etiology and treatment of commonly encountered electrolyte disorders and to provide evidence-based recommendations to guide the perioperative physician in the ideal management of the acute surgical patient.

### 78.2 Glucose

#### 78.2.1 What Is the Optimal Target for Glycemic Control in Perioperative and Intensive Care Unit Patients?

Hyperglycemia has been shown to have a significant impact on the perioperative outcome of surgical patients and the critically ill. Because of the relationship between hyperglycemia and microvascular injury, physicians have sought to seek the optimal glycemic control strategy in order to prevent patient harm from uncontrolled perioperative and critical illness hyperglycemia. Most of the data surrounding perioperative glycemic control come from the care of cardiac surgical patients. Uncontrolled hyperglycemia in cardiac surgical patients has been shown to result in higher rates of both mortality and wound infection [1–3]. In the early 2000s, there were two landmark prospective trials that investigated the effect of glycemic control in the critically ill. These two trials found a significant reduction in mortality for a wide range of both medical and surgical critically ill patients through achieving glycemic control within the strict control range of 80–110 mg/dL, as opposed to the "conventional" treatment group that strived to maintain glucose levels in between 180 and 200 mg/dL [4,5]. These studies also found that strict glycemic control was associated with reductions in sepsis by 46%, blood transfusion by 50%, critical illness polyneuropathy by 44%, and renal failure requiring dialysis by 41%. The main criticism of these trials was that the strictly controlled group experienced major hypoglycemic events at a rate nearly fivefold that of the conventional group. Logistic regression analysis found that hypoglycemia was found to be an independent predictor of mortality, and thus at the time, it was proposed that the higher risk of hypoglycemia with a strict glucose control regimen could offset the benefits of controlling hyperglycemia.

In 2009, an international multicenter, prospective randomized controlled trial named NICE-SUGAR involving over 6000 patients was published that investigated the potential effect of strict glucose control on mortality in a mix of critically ill surgical and medical patients [6]. Strict glucose control was again defined as 80–110 mg/dL, but the conventional group was designed to have glycemic control in the 140–180 mg/dL range. The investigators found an odds ratio for death in the strict control group of 1.14 compared with the conventional group. This represented a number needed to harm of 38. In addition, they found none of the previously reported benefits of strict glycemic control in terms of the rates of blood-borne infection, renal replacement therapy, or blood transfusion. Subgroup analysis did not reveal any differences in the treatment effect between the two groups for diabetics, operative versus nonoperative patients, septic patients, or those with higher severities of illness, as graded by the APACHE2 scoring system. Severe hypoglycemia, defined as a serum glucose level being below 40 mg/dL, was found in 6.8% of strictly controlled patients as opposed to 0.5% in the conventional group. Although it can be inferred that the markedly higher rates of hypoglycemia in the control group may have led to higher mortality, the investigators properly maintained that their study was not designed to evaluate the mechanism of this association. A subsequent ancillary study using the same data set showed a dose–effect relationship of hypoglycemia on mortality beginning at levels of less than 70 mmol/dL, adding evidence to the argument that hypoglycemia is associated with increased mortality [7].

In an effort to generalize the findings from NICE-SUGAR in critically ill patients to the larger general surgical population, an independent review was performed in 2012 to evaluate the effects of strict perioperative glycemic control in diabetic patients [8]. The analysis of 12 trials involving nearly 1400 patients found that strict perioperative glycemic control in diabetic patients was not associated with any statistically significant reductions in mortality, infectious complications, or renal failure. Post hoc analysis did show a statistically significant higher incidence of hypoglycemia in strictly controlled patients. The authors' recommendations summarized the apparent lack of evidence for strict glucose control in diabetics undergoing surgery.

*Recommendations*: A strategy for avoidance of both hyperglycemia and hypoglycemia, with target serum glucose levels in the 110–180 mg/dL range, should be employed for perioperative and critically ill patients. While the strategy of strict glycemic control (80–110 mg/dL) has been shown to be beneficial as compared with patients allowed to have a higher serum glucose level (above 180 mg/dL), this strategy has been shown to lead to a higher incidence of mortality when compared with a patients treated within a range of 140–180 mg/dL, which may be related by a higher incidence of hypoglycemia in strictly controlled patients.

*Strength of evidence*: 1a

*Grade of recommendation*: A

### 78.2.2 Can Variability in Blood Glucose Levels Affect the Outcome Independent of Set Target Blood Glucose Levels?

Clearly, the selection of an appropriate target range for glycemic control has dramatic effect on patient mortality, but recently, additional data have also arisen that evaluates the impact of fluctuation in blood glucose levels and its relationship to patient outcome. Less variability in blood glucose values was associated with a survival benefit in a retrospective study of 7049 critically ill patients [9]. The standard deviation of the values of blood glucose recorded in each patient was closely related to survival in a multivariate logistic regression analysis. The authors showed that the variability of glucose levels was a stronger predictor of ICU mortality than the absolute blood glucose value. They also found that unlike nondiabetic subjects, patients with diabetes did not display an association between increasing levels of blood glucose or glucose variability and ICU or hospital mortality. This suggests that diabetic patients may have a unique response to the biologic effects of hyperglycemia. Hirsh and Brownlee, in a review of the care of chronically ill diabetic patients, stressed the potential importance of minimizing glucose variability in the prevention of long-term diabetic vascular complications [10]. Glucose fluctuations may increase oxidative stress, as cellular damage has been shown to be most prominent when glucose levels increase rapidly from a normal level [11]. Decreasing variability of blood glucose concentration might be an important factor by which intensive insulin therapy exerts its beneficial effects. Continuous intravenous administration has been suggested to be more effective in minimizing glycemic variability than continuous and subcutaneous administration, which in turn may be better than bolus intravenous administration [12].

*Recommendation*: Reducing variability in perioperative blood glucose levels can lead to improved patient survival.

*Strength of evidence*: 2a

*Grade of recommendation*: C

## 78.3 Sodium

### 78.3.1 What Is the Prevalence of Hypernatremia in Hospitalized Patients and What Is Its Relationship to Mortality?

There are many retrospective studies performed in both hospitalized and ICU patients evaluating the presence of hypernatremia on admission, its development during the course of the admission, and its association with mortality. The most frequently cited study looking at the incidence of hypernatremia in hospitalized patients is by Palevsky et al. [13]. In a retrospective review of 7,836 patients admitted to a single center over the course of 3 months, 18 patients (0.2%) were admitted with a serum sodium concentration exceeding 150 mmol/L. An additional 85 patients (1%) developed hypernatremia over the course of their admission. Investigation into possible explanations for this fivefold increase in the development of hypernatremia revealed that over 75% of patients who developed hypernatremia over the course of their admission were either completely restricted from free water intake or were prescribed to ingest <1 L/day. This finding illustrates not only the potential iatrogenic contribution to hypernatremia from restricted fluid intake and the importance of patient inability to ingest fluid associated with other causes (intubated patients, altered mental status, etc.) but also the highly important regulatory role that thirst plays in the homeostatic mechanisms that limit hypernatremia.

Hypernatremia is more prevalent both on admission and during the course of stay for critically ill patients. Between 2% and 6% of ICU patients will be hypernatremic on admission, and they have between a 4% and 26% chance of developing the condition during admission. A recently published review of the retrospective studies that observed these incidences also noted a consistent and significant association between the development of hypernatremia and mortality, with hypernatremic patients experiencing between an 11% and 38% increased incidence in mortality [14–22]. An additional study involving over 150,000 ICU patients with hypernatremia on admission found that an elevation of serum sodium above 145 mmol/L was found to be independently associated with an adverse effect on mortality after adjusting for patient age, admission type, and severity of disease [23]. Although this evidence of a clear association between hypernatremia and mortality is very strong, a true causal relationship cannot clearly be defined based on these data without prospective studies.

*Recommendation*: Hypernatremia is a commonly encountered electrolyte disorder on admission and is also likely to develop during the course of a patient's stay. Elevations in serum sodium above 145 mmol/L should be avoided and treated appropriately as it has been shown to be independently associated with increased mortality.

*Strength of evidence*: 2a

*Grade of recommendation*: B

### 78.3.2 What Is the Role of Therapeutic Hypernatremia in Brain Injury?

Induced and sustained hypernatremia has been used in various states of brain injury with the rationale of avoiding secondary brain injury through the prevention and treatment of cerebral edema by removing brain water via an osmotic gradient to reduce intracranial pressure. To date, therapeutic hypernatremia has been achieved mainly through the use of two agents, hypertonic (3% or higher) saline (HS) and 20% mannitol solution. Despite the widespread use of these agents to control intracranial pressure in various states of brain injury, to date, there are no Level I data available to support their use. In general, a strategy involving maintenance of serum sodium concentration between 145 and 155 mmol/L is employed, due to evidence that patients with higher degrees of hypernatremia may experience worse neurologic outcomes, as judged by the Glascow Coma Scale [24]. Both agents have been shown to be effective in lowering intracranial pressure in numerous retrospective studies with few rare side effects such as pulmonary edema, acute kidney injury, and worsened or rebound intracranial hypertension secondary to presumed osmolyte accumulation in brain parenchyma in the setting of a disrupted blood–brain barrier [25].

As to whether one solution is more effective than another in treating patients with traumatic brain injury, a meta-analysis in 2011 involving five randomized trials comparing equiosmolar doses of HS and mannitol in the care of 112 patients with traumatic brain injury showed a relative risk of intracranial pressure control favoring HS, but there was a mild degree of heterogeneity between the studies included [26]. The purported mechanism for HS's superiority in lowering intracranial pressure is that it acts more as a volume expander, avoiding the reduction in cerebral perfusion pressure via osmotic diuresis that can accompany mannitol therapy. Therapeutic hypernatremia has also been evaluated by retrospective studies in other brain injury states such as intracranial hemorrhage and cerebrovascular disease. Both Hauer and Wagner found that the use of 3% HS was more effective in limiting intracranial pressure crisis, reducing cerebral edema volume, and reducing mortality when compared with historical controls without additional adverse effects [27,28].

*Recommendation*: Therapeutic hypernatremia is effective in lowering intracranial pressure in various causes of brain injury. Hypertonic saline may be superior to mannitol for lowering intracranial pressure in traumatic brain injury, but more definitive prospective studies need to be performed.

*Strength of evidence*: 2a

*Grade of recommendation*: B

### 78.3.3 When Does Hyponatremia Require Treatment and What Is the Optimal Rate of Correction?

Hyponatremia is the most commonly encountered laboratory abnormality in clinical practice with an incidence of up to 15%–30% in both acutely and chronically hospitalized patients [29]. Despite its pervasiveness in clinical practice, there is much confusion as to its risk to patients and the optimal management strategy. Signs and symptoms of acute surgical patients with hyponatremia range from drowsiness, nausea, and gait disturbances to seizures, coma, and death secondary to cerebral edema and herniation. In general, the most important implications for both the indication for treatment and the rate of correction have been found to involve determination of the chronicity of the hyponatremia and the presence of symptoms.

Acute hyponatremia is often defined as occurring within a period of 48 h and is most commonly associated with toxic water ingestion (marathon runners, users of MDMA, and psychotics), iatrogenic fluid administration, or in postneurosurgical patients. Acute hyponatremia in these situations is classically thought of as a medical emergency, with a 50% mortality rate found in one classic case series in patients with a serum sodium less than 115 mmol/L [30]. This same case series noted a markedly lower mortality rate and incidence of seizure in patients who developed hyponatremia over the course of greater than 72 h. Subsequent investigations into the mechanism behind this finding revealed that the brain employs a homeostatic strategy of extruding intracellular organic osmolytes to maintain its cellular volume under conditions of hyponatremia [31]. This process is thought to occur over the course of 1–2 days; thus, patients who have not had enough time to allow this process to occur are thought to be at higher risk for the most severe complications of the condition. The high mortality reported in the cases mentioned above have led to a consensus that acute hyponatremia should be treated regardless of the presence of symptoms, especially in the case of marathon runners [32]. The incidence of mortality and seizure has been shown to be much lower in chronic hyponatremics [33]. However, treatment of chronic hyponatremia is often advocated in the presence of symptoms, as even mild symptoms such as gait instability can lead to adverse outcomes in certain patient populations such as the elderly, and in cases where even mild cerebral edema can lead to disastrous complications, such as in postneurosurgical patients and intracranial hemorrhage [34].

The same process that allows the brain to accommodate hyponatremia is also thought to be responsible for the most feared complication of the rapid correction of hyponatremia in the form of central pontine myelinolysis (CPM). There appears to be a marked difference in the incidence of this condition depending on the chronicity of the condition, with acutely hyponatremic patients exhibiting a higher tolerance for rapid correction without neurologic sequelae. Although there is prospective evidence that acutely hyponatremic patients can safely tolerate correction at a rate of 25 mmol/L in 48 h, there exist data that neither this rate nor magnitude of correction are necessary even in emergencies [35]. Specifically, a review by Sterns et al. in 2006 found that increases of 7–9 mmol/L were safely tolerated even if conducted over as little as 10 min, but increases in serum sodium in the range of 4–6 mmol/L were sufficient to halt hyponatremic seizures [36].

The pathogenesis of CPM in the rapid correction of chronic hyponatremics is thought to involve the deformation of intracranial endothelial cells surrounding areas of the brain that have adjusted to hyponatremia, leading to gaps in tight junctions that form during rapid correction that allow for inflammatory mediators access to oligodendrocytes, initiating an inflammatory demyelination [37]. To date, there have been five cohort studies and three independent reviews of the literature that have found that rapid rates of correction in chronically hyponatremic patients result in adverse neurologic sequelae [34]. One such study at multiple centers showed that patients who have been corrected at rates of 18–25 mmol/L in 48 h showed a lower incidence of neurologic complications when compared with higher rates, but neurologic complications did still exist in this group at a rate of 50% [38]. Patients treated below this rate did not experience any neurologic complications. Citing several case reports of demyelination occurring at rates exceeding 10 mmol/L in 24 h, the authors have suggested a limit of <10 mmol/L/day and <18 mmol/L in 48 h as an absolute maximum rate of correction [36].

*Recommendations*: Acute hyponatremia from any cause should be treated regardless of presence or absence of patient symptoms due to a high incidence of patient mortality in these cases.

*Strength of evidence*: 1a

*Grade of recommendation*: A

Chronic hyponatremia should be treated in the presence of symptoms or in cases where even mild cerebral edema can be injurious to the patient.

*Strength of evidence*: 2a

*Grade of recommendation*: B

Chronic hyponatremia should be corrected with a maximum rate of correction of 10 mmol/L in 24 h or 18 mmol/L in 48 h to avoid adverse neurologic outcomes.

*Strength of evidence*: 1a

*Grade of recommendation*: A

Acute hyponatremia can be corrected aggressively at rates above those prescribed for chronic hyponatremics but increases in serum sodium above the range of 4–6 mmol/L may not be necessary to halt hyponatremic seizures.

*Strength of evidence*: 2a

*Grade of recommendation*: B

## 78.4 Calcium

### 78.4.1 What Is the Optimal Timing for Calcium Administration in Massive Transfusion?

The rapid transfusion of multiple stored units of packed red blood cells (PRBC) can result in hypocalcemia. The mechanism behind the development of hypocalcemia is via citrate toxicity. Citrate is used in stored blood products as an anticoagulant because it binds and chelates calcium, a necessary part of the coagulation cascade. Each unit of PRBC contains 3 g of citrate, and the normal healthy human liver metabolizes approximately 3 g of citrate in 5 min [39]. Therefore, transfusion rates exceeding 1 U of PRBC every 5 min or multiple transfusions in the surgical patient with impaired liver function can lead to citrate toxicity and hypocalcemia. Of note, in vitro studies suggest that hypocalcemia can result from rapid transfusion of fresh frozen plasma [40].

Hypocalcemia in these settings can lead to QT segment prolongation and myocardial and peripheral vasculature depression. It can be assumed that patients with hypocalcemia would be expected to experience higher mortality rates in the setting of massive hemorrhage. In fact, three large cohort studies found that hypocalcemia was found to be an independent predictor of mortality in patients undergoing massive transfusion [41–43]. In all three of these studies, serum ionized calcium concentration appeared to be negatively associated with mortality, with higher mortality rates seen for any amount of hypocalcemia, but especially at concentrations below 0.07 mmol/L.

*Recommendation*: Citrate toxicity and hypocalcemia can be expected to occur with transfusion rates exceeding 1 U PRBC every 5 min and perhaps even faster in patients with liver disease. Supplemental calcium should be administered to maintain a serum ionized calcium above 0.07 mmol/L.

*Strength of evidence*: 2b

*Grade of recommendation*: B

## 78.5 Potassium

### 78.5.1 What Is an Ideal Strategy for the Preoperative Management of the Hyperkalemic Surgical Patient with Preexisting End-Stage Renal Disease?

Since the introduction of intravenous dialysis in the 1960s, the number of patients with end-stage renal disease (ESRD) on dialysis has grown exponentially. Not surprisingly, both elective and emergent surgical procedures for these patients have also become more commonplace. A review of ESRD patients undergoing general surgical procedures revealed a mortality rate of nearly 4%, with the rate increasing nearly fivefold for emergency cases [44]. ESRD patients often have an extensive list of comorbidities to blame for this increased mortality rate, but there is likely an association with their propensity to develop perioperative hyperkalemia, which in a large case series was found to be the most common postoperative complication [45]. This propensity to develop potentially lethal hyperkalemia often complicates the management of the acute surgical ESRD patient. The general consensus is that emergency surgery should be performed on the hyperkalemic patient with proper ongoing pharmacologic treatment if the benefit from surgery is going to include saving the life of the patient or preventing significant morbidity.

**TABLE 78.1**

Evidence-Based Recommendations for Electrolyte Management

| Question | Answer | Level of Evidence | Grade of Recommendation | References |
|---|---|---|---|---|
| What is the optimal target for glycemic control in perioperative and intensive care unit patients? | A target serum glucose of 110–180 mg/dL may provide the benefits of glycemic control while avoiding severe hypoglycemia. | 1a | A | [1–8] |
| Can variability in blood glucose levels affect the outcome independent of set target blood glucose levels? | Reducing variability in perioperative blood glucose levels can lead to improved patient survival. | 2a | C | [9–12] |
| What is the prevalence of hypernatremia in hospitalized patients and what is its relationship to mortality? | Hypernatremia is commonly present on admission and commonly occurs over the course of a hospital stay. Serum sodium >145 mmol/L is independently associated with increased mortality. | 2a | B | [13–23] |
| What is the role of therapeutic hypernatremia in brain injury? | Therapeutic hypernatremia is effective in lowering intracranial pressure in various states of brain injury. HS may be more effective than mannitol in traumatic brain injury. | 2a | B | [23–28] |
| When does hyponatremia require treatment and what is the optimal rate of correction? | Acute hyponatremia should be corrected regardless of symptoms as it is associated with increased mortality. | 1A | A | [30,32] |
| | Chronic hyponatremia should be treated in the presence of symptoms or when even small amounts of cerebral edema can be disastrous. | 2A | B | [33,34] |
| | Chronic hyponatremia should be corrected with a maximum rate of correction of 10 mmol/L in 24 h or 18 mmol/L in 48 h to avoid adverse neurologic outcomes. | 1A | A | [34,36,38] |
| | Acute hyponatremia can be corrected more rapidly, but corrections greater than 4–6 mmol/L may not be necessary to halt seizures. | 2A | B | [35,36] |
| What is the optimal timing for calcium administration in massive transfusion? | Citrate toxicity can occur quickly with transfusion rates exceeding 1 U PRBC in 5 min, and in cirrhotics. Calcium should be administered to maintain an ionized calcium level of at least 0.07 mmol/L. | 2B | B | [41–43] |
| What is an ideal strategy for the preoperative management of the hyperkalemic surgical patient with preexisting ESRD ? | Patients with ESRD can safely tolerate chronically elevated potassium levels and can be given succinylcholine during induction of anesthesia. Conditions that result in rapid potassium loading should be avoided when possible. | 2B | B | [46–48] |

For the ESRD patient who requires nonemergent surgery and presents to the preoperative area with hyperkalemia, however, there is frequent discussion over the risk:benefit ratio and to which degree the patient may be subjected to potential harm by proceeding with the case.

To date, there are no Level 1 or Level 2 studies that evaluate for the specific level of hyperkalemia that can be recommended as safe for patients undergoing surgical procedures, but retrospective data exist as to the levels of hyperkalemia that they can safely tolerate in the nonoperative setting. ESRD patients often have increased total body stores of potassium and, therefore, do not exhibit a change in their transmembrane gradient even at high serum potassium levels, and have therefore been reported to tolerate chronically elevated serum potassium levels of above 6.5 mEq/L without exhibiting EKG changes [46]. However, experimental data have shown that ESRD patients have impaired ability to handle a potassium load, with patients with higher baseline elevations in potassium having the least reserve [47]. This finding suggests that ESRD patients cannot tolerate a rapid increase in extracellular potassium, with a resultant effect on the transmembrane gradient leading to myocardial instability. There are many perioperative conditions that can result in potassium loading including fasting, tissue and red blood cell lysis, and the administration of the muscle relaxant succinylcholine. The safety of the latter in these patients is often the subject of debate among anesthesiologists. A recent review showed that the administration of a single dose of succinylcholine in the setting of both acute and chronic renal disease results in similar elevations in serum potassium as compared with patients with no renal dysfunction [48]. A standard one-time dose used for the patients in the nine studies evaluated did not result in a markedly elevated rate of hyperkalemic arrest.

*Recommendations*: Surgical patients with ESRD can safely tolerate chronically elevated serum potassium levels and can be given succinylcholine safely without a markedly increased risk of hyperkalemic arrest. Attention should be given to conditions that can result in rapid potassium loading, however, as these conditions can lead to lethal hyperkalemia and should be avoided.

*Strength of evidence*: 2b

*Strength of recommendation*: B

Please refer to Table 78.1 for a list of recommendations with references for evidence-based electrolyte management.

## References


1. Golden SH, Peart-Vigilance C, Kao WH, Brancati FL. Perioperative glycemic control and the risk of infectious complications in a cohort of adults with diabetes. *Diabetes Care.* 1999;22(9):1408–1414.
2. Latham RMD, Lancaster ADRN, Janet F. Covington RN, Pirolo JSMD, Thomas CSJMD. The association of diabetes and glucose control with surgical-site infections among cardiothoracic surgery patients. *Infect Contr Hosp Epidemiol.* 2001;22(10):607–612.
3. Furnary AP, Gao G, Grunkemeier GL et al. Continuous insulin infusion reduces mortality in patients with diabetes undergoing coronary artery bypass grafting. *J Thorac Cardiovasc Surg.* 2003;125(5):1007–1021.
4. Van den Berghe G, Wouters P, Weekers F et al. Intensive insulin therapy in critically ill patients. *N Engl J Med.* 2001;345(19):1359–1367.
5. Van den Berghe G, Wilmer A, Hermans G et al. Intensive insulin therapy in the medical ICU. *N Engl J Med.* 2006;354(5):449–461.
6. NICE SUGAR Investigators. Intensive versus conventional glucose control in critically ill patients. *N Engl J Med.* 2009;360(13):1283–1297.
7. NICE SUGAR Investigators. Hypoglycemia and risk of death in critically ill patients. *N Engl J Med.* 2012;367(12):1108–1118.
8. Buchleitner AM, Martinez-Alonso M, Hernandez M, Sola I, Mauricio D. Perioperative glycaemic control for diabetic patients undergoing surgery. *Cochrane Database Syst Rev.* 2012;Issue 9, Art. No. CD007315.
9. Egi M, Bellomo R, Stachowski E, French CJ, Hart G. Variability of blood glucose concentration and short-term mortality in critically ill patients. *Anesthesiology.* 2006;105(2):244–252.
10. Hirsch IB, Brownlee M. Should minimal blood glucose variability become the gold standard of glycemic control? *J Diabetes Complications.* 2005;19(3):178–181.
11. Brownlee M. Biochemistry and molecular cell biology of diabetic complications. *Nature.* 2001;414(6865):813–820.
12. Ouattara A, Grimaldi A, Riou B. Blood glucose variability: A new paradigm in critical care? *Anesthesiology.* 2006;105(2):233–234.
13. Palevsky PM, Bhagrath R, Greenberg A. Hypernatremia in hospitalized patients. *Ann Intern Med.* 1996;124(2):197–203.
14. Lindner G, Funk G-C, Schwarz C et al. Hypernatremia in the critically ill is an independent risk factor for mortality. *Am J Kidney Dis.* 2007;50(6):952–957.
15. Darmon M, Timsit J-F, Francais A et al. Association between hypernatraemia acquired in the ICU and mortality: A cohort study. *Nephrol Dial Transplant.* 2010;25(8):2510–2515.
16. Lindner G, Funk G-C, Lassnigg A et al. Intensive care-acquired hypernatremia after major cardiothoracic surgery is associated with increased mortality. *Intensive Care Med.* 2010;36(10):1718–1723.
17. Stelfox H, Ahmed S, Khandwala F, Zygun D, Shahpori R, Laupland K. The epidemiology of intensive care unit-acquired hyponatraemia and hypernatraemia in medical-surgical intensive care units. *Crit Care.* 2008;12(6):R162.
18. Stelfox H, Ahmed S, Zygun D, Khandwala F, Laupland K. Characterization of intensive care unit acquired hyponatremia and hypernatremia following cardiac surgery. *Can J Anesth.* 2010;57(7):650–658.
19. O'Donoghue SD, Dulhunty JM, Bandeshe HK, Senthuran S, Gowardman JR. Acquired hypernatraemia is an independent predictor of mortality in critically ill patients. *Anaesthesia.* 2009;64(5):514–520.
20. Hoorn EJ, Betjes MGH, Weigel J, Zietse R. Hypernatraemia in critically ill patients: Too little water and too much salt. *Nephrol Dial Transplant.* 2008;23(5):1562–1568.
21. Polderman KH, Schreuder WO, van Schijndel RJMS, Thijs LG. Hypernatremia in the intensive care unit: An indicator of quality of care? *Crit Care Med.* 1999;27(6): 1105–1108.
22. Lindner G, Funk G-C. Hypernatremia in critically ill patients. *J Crit Care.* 2013;28(2):e211–e216, e220.
23. Funk G-C, Lindner G, Druml W et al. Incidence and prognosis of dysnatremias present on ICU admission. *Intensive Care Med.* 2010;36(2):304–311.
24. Peterson B, Khanna S, Fisher B, Marshall L. Prolonged hypernatremia controls elevated intracranial pressure in head-injured pediatric patients. *Crit Care Med.* 2000;28(4):1136–1143.
25. Ryu J, Walcott B, Kahle K et al. Induced and sustained hypernatremia for the prevention and treatment of cerebral edema following brain injury. *Neurocrit Care.* 2013;19(2):222–231.
26. Kamel H, Navi BB, Nakagawa K, Hemphill JCI, Ko NU. Hypertonic saline versus mannitol for the treatment of elevated intracranial pressure: A meta-analysis of randomized clinical trials. *Crit Care Med.* 2011;39(3):554–559.
27. Hauer E-M, Stark D, Staykov D, Steigleder T, Schwab S, Bardutzky J. Early continuous hypertonic saline infusion in patients with severe cerebrovascular disease. *Crit Care Med.* 2011;39(7):1766–1772.

28. Wagner I, Hauer E-M, Staykov D et al. Effects of continuous hypertonic saline infusion on perihemorrhagic edema evolution. *Stroke.* 2011;42(6):1540–1545.
29. Upadhyay A, Jaber BL, Madias NE. Incidence and prevalence of hyponatremia. *Am J Med.* 2006;119(7, Suppl 1): S30–S35.
30. Arieff A, Llach F, Massry S. Neurological manifestations and morbidity of hyponatremia: Correlation with brain water and electrolytes. *Medicine.* 1976;55: 121–129.
31. Sterns RH, Silver SM. Brain Volume Regulation in Response to Hypo-osmolality and Its Correction. *Am J Med.* 2006;119(7, Suppl 1):S12–S16.
32. Hew-Butler C, Almond C, Ayus J, Panel E-AHEC et al. Consensus statement of the 1st International Exercise-Associated Hyponatremia Consensus Development Conference, Cape Town, South Africa 2005. *Clin J Sports Med.* 2005;15:208–213.
33. Sterns RH. Severe symptomatic hyponatremia: Treatment and outcome. A study of 64 cases. *Ann Intern Med.* 1987;107(5):656–664.
34. Verbalis JG, Goldsmith SR, Greenberg A, Schrier RW, Sterns RH. Hyponatremia treatment guidelines 2007: Expert panel recommendations. *Am J Med.* 2007;120(11, Suppl 1):S1–S21.
35. Ayus JC, Krothapalli RK, Arieff AI. Treatment of symptomatic hyponatremia and its relation to brain damage. *N Engl J Med.* 1987;317(19):1190–1195.
36. Sterns RH, Nigwekar SU, Hix JK. The treatment of hyponatremia. *Semin Nephrol.* 2009;29(3):282–299.
37. DeLuca G, Nagy Z, Esiri M, Davey P. Evidence for a role for apoptosis in central pontine myelinolysis. *Acta Neuropathol.* 2002;103(6):590–598.
38. Sterns RH, Cappuccio JD, Silver SM, Cohen EP. Neurologic sequelae after treatment of severe hyponatremia: A multicenter perspective. *J Am Soc Nephrol.* 1994;4(8):1522–1530.
39. Sihler KC, Napolitano LM. Complications of massive transfusion. *Chest.* 2010;137(1):209–220.
40. Sulemanji DS, Bloom JD, Dzik WH, Jiang Y. New insights into the effect of rapid transfusion of fresh frozen plasma on ionized calcium. *J Clin Anesth.* 2012;24(5):364–369.
41. KM H, AD, L. Concentration-dependent effect of hypocalcaemia on mortality of patients with critical bleeding requiring massive transfusion: A cohort study. *Anaesth Intensive Care.* 2011;39(1):46–54.
42. Gunter OLJ, Au BK, Isbell JM, Mowery NT, Young PP, Cotton BA. Optimizing outcomes in damage control resuscitation: Identifying blood product ratios associated with improved survival. *J Trauma Acute Care Surg.* 2008;65(3):527–534.
43. Wilson RF, Binkley LE, Jr., Sabo FM et al. Electrolyte and acid-base changes with massive blood transfusions. *Am Surg.* 1992;58(9):535–544.
44. Kellerman PS. Perioperative care of the renal patient. *Arch Intern Med.* 1994;154(15):1674–1688.
45. Pinson CW, Schuman ES, Gross GF, Schuman TA, Hayes JF. Surgery in long-term dialysis patients: Experience with more than 300 cases. *Am J Surg.* 1986;151(5):567–571.
46. Ahmed J, Weisberg LS. Hyperkalemia in dialysis patients. *Semin Dial.* 2001;14(5):348–356.
47. RH S, PU F, M P, J G, I S. Disposition of intravenous potassium in anuric man: A kinetic analysis. *Kidney Int.* 1979;15(6):651–660.
48. Thapa S, Brull SJ. Succinylcholine-induced hyperkalemia in patients with renal failure: An old question revisited. *Anesth Analg.* 2000;91(1):237–241.

## Commentary on Evidence-Based Electrolyte Management

*David B. Hoyt*

### Introduction

The management of electrolytes has always been essential to prevent catastrophic complications. Recent evidence in the last 15–20 years has shown that precise management leads to improved surgical outcomes. Assuring preoperative readiness by correcting risk factors associated with chronic disease, managing current patient medications, improving nutritional status, and encouraging smoking cessation all improve outcomes. The precise management of critical electrolyte status before and during the course of surgical care will also contribute to optimal outcomes.

### Glucose

The evidence shows that glucose control enhances outcomes. Controlling too tightly (80–110 mg/dL) is associated with increased hypoglycemia and worse outcomes. This has led to agreement to target glucose levels in the range 110–180 mg/dL (avoiding the lower limit) for perioperative and critically ill surgical patients. Evidence also shows that controlling *variability* within this range also improves outcome. Mechanisms that achieve this higher reliability involve use of computer-based algorithms, which lead to good control and less variability within a target range. Their use is inexpensive and effective.*

### Sodium

Hypernatremia is associated with increased mortality and this may be due to water loss and underresuscitation, chronically inadequate $H_2O$ ingestion, or iatrogenic causes.

Hypernatremia is used as therapy for ICP control in brain injury. Use can be supported as an alternative to other osmotic therapy and some data suggests hypertonic saline is superior to mannitol.

Hyponatremia is common. Corrective therapy is guided by symptom presence and reversal timed to the chronicity of the condition (general rule—correct over the same time taken to acquire it). Rapid-onset hyponatremia should be treated regardless of symptoms and is well tolerated with little risk of central pontine myelinolysis if treated quickly. In chronic conditions, correction should be limited to <10 mmol/L the first day and <18 mmol/L the first 48 h.

The benefits of hypertonic saline treatment as an immune adjuvant strategy have been well supported with much basic and mechanism-based research. Clinical trials evaluating this as a resuscitation strategy for shock or early treatment of head injured patients have not proven to be more effective than traditional resuscitation.

### Calcium

Hypercalcemia and hypocalcemia are frequently seen in surgical patients with malignancies, hyperparathyroidism, and other conditions affecting overall parathyroid hormone homeostasis and bone physiology. One condition where hypocalcemia can occur is following massive transfusion where chelation of $Ca^{++}$ by citrate may lead to a coagulopathy in a patient where excessive bleeding is the reason for the massive transfusion in the first place. Prolonged QT segments and myocardial depression are associated with increased mortality, which may occur with transfusion rates > 1 unit/5 min. Supplemental $Ca^{++}$ should be anticipated with these high transfusion rates and given to maintain a serum ionized $Ca^{++}$ above 0.07 mmol/L.

### Potassium

Patients with renal failure are particularly prone to hyperkalemia and patients undergoing rapid correction of hypokalemia can develop hyperkalemia in the preoperative setting. Lethal hyperkalemia can be treated and the surgery can proceed if the benefit from surgery is lifesaving. Generally, hyperkalemia is tolerated in patients with end-stage renal disease. In elective or less urgent surgery, correction should be attempted and surgery delayed. Any condition, which can lead to rapid extracellular release, can aggravate hyperkalemia that is present. Fasting, blood lysis, tissue injury, and use of succinylcholine are traditional risks of surgery and hyperkalemia. Use of succinylcholine in renal disease does not actually elevate potassium seriously compared to patients with no renal dysfunction. A single dose during induction in these patients can be tolerated.

### Conclusions

Many aspects of electrolytes are managed in the course of caring for surgical patients, particularly when conditions altering acid/base balance contribute to electrolyte distribution or overall supply (hypochloremic, hypokalemic, metabolic alkalosis after vomiting, lactic acidosis, and potassium distribution following hypovolemic shock).

Awareness of the relative importance of these states, in a particular clinical condition, will triage the efforts and urgency to correcting them.

* Lee J, Fortlage D, Box K, Sakarafus L, Bhavsar D, Coimbra R, Potenza B. Computerized insulin infusion programs are safe and effective in the burn intensive care unit. *J Burn Care Res.* 2012 May–June;33(3):e114–e119.

# 79

# *Abdominal Compartment Syndrome*

**J. Kayle Lee, Damaris Ortiz, Shanel B. Bhagwandin, and James C. Doherty**

**CONTENTS**



## 79.1 Introduction

Abdominal compartment syndrome (ACS) has evolved conceptually from a postoperative concern of trauma surgeons to a potential preventable cause of multiple organ dysfunction for all critically ill patients. Since the first description of ACS by Kron et al. in 1984, increasing awareness of research regarding ACS has resulted in a need for consensus definitions and clinical management guidelines [1]. The World Society of the Abdominal Compartment Syndrome (WSACS) met in 2004, established consensus definitions in 2006 to guide clinicians in the diagnosis of ACS, published evidence-based recommendations for the diagnosis, management, and prevention of ACS in 2007, and released research recommendations in 2009 [2,3]. An update of definitions and guidelines using the Grading of Recommendations Assessment, Development, and Evaluation (GRADE) methodology was published by WSACS in 2013 [4].

The WSACS defined intraabdominal hypertension (IAH) as a "sustained or repeated pathological elevation in intraabdominal pressure (IAP) ≥12 mmHg." Furthermore, it defined ACS as "sustained IAP >20 mmHg that is associated with new organ dysfunction/failure." It also subclassified ACS into primary ACS (due to primary abdominal or pelvic pathology), secondary ACS (due to non-abdominopelvic pathology), and recurrent ACS (redevelopment of ACS after treatment). New definitions added in 2013 by the WSACS included polycompartment syndrome (elevated compartment pressures in two or more anatomic regions) and abdominal compliance (change in volume over change in IAP). Also, a classification of open abdomen complexity was created [4].

The remainder of this chapter presents a systematic review of the medical literature to provide timely, evidence-based recommendations for the diagnosis and treatment of ACS. Specific questions will be used to frame the discussions and to develop appropriate recommendations supported by the existing literature. Table 79.1 summarizes the questions and answers discussed in the text.

## 79.2 Questions and Answers

### 79.2.1 Are There Risk Factors for IAH/ACS That Can Be Used to Identify Patients to Be Screened for the Development of IAH/ACS?

Given that there has only been a recent consensus on the definitions of IAH and ACS, no consistent data exist regarding the incidence of these entities in clinical practice. Nevertheless, IAH and ACS do occur with some

**TABLE 79.1**

Clinical Questions

| Question | Answer | Level of Evidence | Grade of Recommendation | References |
|---|---|---|---|---|
| Are there risk factors that can be used to identify patients at risk for IAH/ACS? | Abdominal surgery; ileus; pulmonary, hepatic, or renal dysfunction; >3.5 L/24 h resuscitation, hypothermia, oliguria, anemia, base deficit, high GAP $CO_2$, pelvic fracture in setting of abdominal trauma, severe burns, and severe acute pancreatitis are risk factors for IAH/ACS. | 2B | B | [4–12] |
| How should patients be screened for IAH/ACS? | Screening for IAH/ACS can be done by serial intermittent IAP measurement via a urinary bladder catheter. | 1B | B | [4,14–19] |
| Is there a threshold level of IAP that mandates intervention? | There appears to be benefit in keeping APP ≥50–60 mmHg. | 2B | C | [19–22] |
| Are there any effective nonsurgical strategies for treating IAH/ACS? | There are no systematic reviews or randomized controlled trials that compare decompressive laparotomy to nonsurgical strategies in patients with ACS.<br>Neuromuscular blockade and supine positioning may be used as adjunctive measures.<br>In patients at risk for IAH or ACS, care must be taken to provide sufficient resuscitation to support adequate organ perfusion while avoiding overly zealous volume administration.<br>Percutaneous catheter decompression may be an option in cases of IAH/ACS due to intraperitoneal fluid collections. | 1B, 3, 4 | C, B, C | [23–30] |
| Is there a preferred technique for temporary abdominal closure after decompressive laparotomy? | Constant negative wound therapy affords a preferred approach to temporary abdominal closure.<br>No technique for temporary abdominal closure is favored by the existing medical literature, and thus no recommendation can be made. | 1B, 3, 4 | D | [31–34] |
| Is there a predictable time frame or preferred technique for definitive abdominal closure after decompressive laparotomy? | In general, primary fascial closure is usually possible within 5–7 days if critical illness resolves and if progressive organ failure does not occur.<br>No predictable time frame or preferred technique for definitive abdominal closure is favored by the existing medical literature, and thus no recommendation can be made. | 3, 4 | D | [35] |

frequency in the ICU and are associated with organ dysfunction and mortality. Through varying types of studies, many risk factors for ICH/ACS have been identified. The WSACS classifies 34 risk factors into five categories: diminished abdominal wall compliance, increased intraluminal contents, increased intraabdominal contents, capillary leak/fluid resuscitation, and miscellaneous [4]. Prospective studies have associated the development of IAH with the presence of abdominal surgery, ileus, pulmonary dysfunction, liver dysfunction, renal dysfunction, and large-volume fluid administration (>3.5 L/24 h) [5]. In a prospective study of blunt torso trauma, hypothermia, anemia, oliguria, base deficit, large volume of crystalloid resuscitation, and high arterial-mucosal $CO_2$ gap by gastric tonometry were found to be predictors of ACS development [6]. Additional risk factors identified in prospective studies include pelvic fracture in the setting of abdominal trauma [7], severe acute pancreatitis [8], and major burns [9]. Holodinsky et al. identified several candidate risk factors for ACS in a meta-analysis that, while heterogeneous, gives direction for future studies. Large-volume crystalloid resuscitation, respiratory status of the patient, and hypotension/shock were factors that were broadly relevant, while other factors were specific to certain patient populations. For example, crystalloid resuscitation was the most common associated factor for ACS in trauma and surgical patients, while higher APACHEII/Glasgow–Imrie scores and elevated serum creatinine were more commonly associated with ACS in severe acute pancreatitis [10].

Given the frequent association of fluid resuscitation with IAH and ACS in studies, it warrants further attention. Gonzalez-Fajardo et al. found that a restriction in postoperative fluids (1500 vs. 2500 mL/day) was associated with a significant decrease in hospital stay in patients who had open abdominal vascular surgery [11]. In a prospective study comparing plasma vs. crystalloid fluid resuscitation in severe burn patients, the patients who received more volume had higher intraabdominal pressures. Two patients died from complications due to ACS [9]. A recent evaluation of sepsis in European intensive care units suggests that positive fluid balance is an independent predictor of outcome, associated with increased mortality in septic patients [12].

*Recommendation*: Given the presence of identifiable risk factors for IAH and ACS and the high morbidity and mortality associated with untreated ACS, identification of at-risk individuals using criteria, such as those listed above, may provide an opportunity for screening and early intervention in IAH and ACS. This Grade B recommendation in favor of risk assessment and screening is offered with the recognition that future prospective multicenter studies may identify additional risk factors to be considered in specific patient populations.

### 79.2.2 How Should Patients Be Screened and/or Monitored for the Development of IAH/ACS?

Physical examination has been shown to lack sufficient sensitivity to diagnose IAH [13]. Thus, direct measurement of IAP is the preferred diagnostic test for IAH. The WSACS recommends intermittent IAP measurement via the urinary bladder with an instillation volume of 25 mL of sterile saline, the pressure transducer zeroed at the midaxillary line, the patient in supine position, and at end-expiration [4]. This determination was based on reliability, simplicity, and low cost, especially when performed in a standardized fashion [14,15].

Little data exist regarding the ideal frequency of IAP measurements in at-risk individuals. Zengerink et al. demonstrated that a continuous IAP measurement technique utilizing a standard three-way bladder catheter yields IAP measurements that closely correlate with those obtained using the intermittent technique [16]. Moreover, specialized catheters placed in the esophagus, stomach, and bladder designed for continuous measurement of IAP are commercially available [17]. If such techniques prove to be cost-effective and can be further validated clinically, continuous monitoring may replace traditional intermittent monitoring, and the frequency issue may become irrelevant.

According to surveys of surgeons and anesthesiologists in multiple countries, detection and management of IAH and ACS are inconsistent, and physicians tend to wait until there is an associated organ dysfunction before proceeding to decompressive laparotomy instead of using a critical threshold IAP [18]. Cheatham and Safcsak demonstrated in a prospective observational study that routinely monitoring IAP in ICU patients at risk for IAH/ACS every 4 h in the ICU via the intravesicular technique to guide resuscitation and need for decompression, as per the WSACS guidelines, significantly increases patient survival and the rate of fascial closure following abdominal decompression [19].

*Recommendation*: Intermittent IAP measurement via the urinary bladder should be performed in patients identified to be at risk for IAH/ACS, based on assessment of the risk factors mentioned earlier (Grade B recommendation). At-risk individuals demonstrating IAH (IAP ≥12 mmHg) should have serial measurements performed during their ICU course to monitor for the development of worsening IAH or ACS requiring intervention (Grade B recommendation).

### 79.2.3 Is There an IAP Threshold Level That Mandates Intervention in IAH/ACS?

As mentioned previously, IAP >20 mmHg in the presence of organ dysfunction defines ACS, a condition requiring acute intervention. Nevertheless, no threshold value for IAP exists that can be universally applied to all patients. An alternative parameter, abdominal perfusion pressure (APP), defined as the difference of mean arterial pressure and intraabdominal pressure, has been studied as a resuscitation endpoint. One retrospective trial identified an APP value of ≥50 mmHg as being correlated with lower mortality in surgical and trauma patients [20]. Several other studies in mixed populations of medical and surgical patients identified a critical APP value of ≥60 mmHg as imparting improved survival [21,22]. Unfortunately, there are no studies to date that define one threshold IAP value for intervention, but the aforementioned study by Cheatham demonstrated that surgical decompression as a prophylactic intervention for IAP of 28 ± 8 and APP of 46 ± 15 mmHg improved survival and the subsequent fascial closure [19].

*Recommendation:* In patients being monitored for IAP, there appears to be benefit in keeping APP ≥50–60 mmHg (Grade C recommendation).

### 79.2.4 Are There Any Effective Nonsurgical Strategies for Treating IAH/ACS?

The standard treatment for ACS remains decompressive laparotomy, and the progression of IAH, organ failure, or failed management of nonoperative strategies should not delay its utilization. Nevertheless, the use of screening IAP measurement inevitably leads to the identification of a population of patients with isolated IAH or with evolving ACS. Such patients may be candidates for nonsurgical interventions aimed at reducing IAP. Such interventions may theoretically prevent the development of ACS and its associated organ dysfunction while simultaneously sparing the patient the morbidity associated with a decompressive laparotomy and an open abdomen. These interventions include sedation, analgesia, diuretics, hemofiltration/ultrafiltration, gastric/colonic decompression, prokinetic agents, neuromuscular blockade, supine positioning, limitation of fluid resuscitation, albumin resuscitation, damage control resuscitation, and catheter decompression. These nonsurgical strategies of treating IAH/ACS revolve around the principles of improving abdominal wall compliance, decreasing intraabdominal and intraluminal volume, decreasing capillary leak, and other measures to optimize regional perfusion. Achieving an ideal fluid balance that maintains perfusion yet does not unnecessarily increase third-space volume is also synergistic with decreasing ACS and its associated morbidity.

Although sedation and analgesia might be expected to have favorable effects on IAH by decreasing abdominal muscle tone, no clinical data exist to support such intervention. Similarly, no clinical studies of active fluid withdrawal by either diuretic therapy or renal replacement therapies have been conducted. Similarly, neither gastrointestinal decompression nor prokinetic drug therapy has been studied as treatments for IAH.

A small prospective trial of 10 patients using a single-dose cisatracurium demonstrated the effectiveness of neuromuscular blockade in reducing IAP, but the effectiveness of therapy appeared to be diminished at higher levels of IAP [23]. There is one retrospective cohort study that was able to demonstrate improved time to fascial closure among trauma patients who underwent damage control laparotomy. Patients who were administered a continuous infusion of neuromuscular blockade were more likely to achieve primary fascial closure by postlaparotomy day 7. Although this has not been replicated in patients with IAH, neuromuscular blockade was an independent predictor of time to fascial closure that suggests that brief trials can be utilized as a temporizing measure [24]. The adverse effects of paralytics (myopathy, neuropathy, and prolonged mechanical ventilation) must be carefully weighed into the decision to use these agents to decrease abdominal muscle tone and increase abdominal compliance.

Both prone positioning and elevation of the head of the bed have been shown to increase IAP, and both of these positioning maneuvers are becoming more commonplace in the ICU. Head elevation is used to reduce aspiration risk, and prone positioning is used as an adjunct to mechanical ventilation in the management of patients with adult respiratory distress syndrome (ARDS). A prospective cohort of 37 patients quantified that head of bed increases more than 45° correlated with an increase in IAP being 7.4 mmHg compared with when the patient was supine [25]. Although supine positioning may minimize IAP, no evidence exists as to whether the IAP benefit is of sufficient magnitude to offset the greater risk of aspiration or to preclude prone positioning in the ARDS patient.

Fluid administration is a critical consideration in the management of IAH/ACS. Volume resuscitation is necessary to maintain adequate intravascular volume and support organ perfusion in the critically ill patient. However, excessive or supranormal fluid resuscitation is an independent risk factor for IAH/ACS and is a frequent cause of secondary ACS. In one retrospective study, volume resuscitation to a supranormal level of oxygen delivery was found to be associated with a significantly increased incidence of IAH and ACS, organ failure, and decreased survival [26]. A single prospective, randomized controlled trial of fluid administration in IAH/ACS has also been performed. This study demonstrated higher IAP in burn patients receiving large-volume crystalloid resuscitation, as opposed to those receiving a lower-volume, colloid-based resuscitation strategy [27]. In another study, limitation of fluid administration accomplished by the use of a hypertonic resuscitation has been associated with higher APP, lower IAP, and lower peak inspiratory pressures [28].

The use of catheter decompression to reduce IAP may be an effective alternative to decompressive laparotomy, especially when the elevation in IAP results from intraperitoneal fluid accumulations such as hemoperitoneum, ascites, or abscess. Percutaneous decompression has been reported as a successful treatment for ACS in a number of retrospective case series [29,30]. Furthermore, a small prospective study demonstrated its effectiveness in decreasing IAP in 33 of 35 patients with IAH secondary to malignant ovarian ascites [29]. A second small prospective study demonstrated that percutaneous catheter drainage performed in conjunction with aggressive IAP and APP monitoring resulted in successful reduction of IAP and augmentation of APP in 8 of 12 trauma patients [30].

*Recommendation*: Decompressive laparotomy remains the standard treatment of ACS (Grade B recommendation). There are no systematic reviews or randomized controlled trials that compare decompressive laparotomy to nonsurgical strategies in patients with ACS. Neuromuscular blockade and supine positioning may be used as adjunctive measures in the treatment of IAH after careful consideration of the potential adverse consequences of such therapies (Grade C recommendation). In patients at risk for IAH or ACS, care must be taken to provide sufficient resuscitation to support adequate organ perfusion while avoiding overly zealous volume administration (Grade B recommendation). Colloids and hypertonic crystalloid administration may serve as alternatives to conventional isotonic crystalloid resuscitation to prevent IAH/ACS (Grade C recommendation). Percutaneous catheter decompression may be an option in cases of IAH/ACS due to intraperitoneal fluid collections (Grade C recommendation).

### 79.2.5 Is There a Preferred Technique for Temporary Abdominal Closure after Decompressive Laparotomy?

Once abdominal decompression is completed, the patient's abdomen must be left open to prevent recurrence of IAH/ACS. Maintenance of the open abdomen requires some type of protective dressing to isolate the exposed abdominal contents from the external environment while accommodating further postoperative visceral expansion. Failure to provide for such expansion may lead to recurrence of IAH/ACS, and constant negative wound therapy affords a preferred approach to temporary abdominal closure. This technique also allows for preventing visceral adhesions to the anterolateral abdominal wall with a certain degree of medial fascial approximation [31]. The application of an abdominal negative pressure device removes inflammatory cytokines and fluid from third-space expansion that contribute to the systemic inflammatory response and organ failure [32]. Although some commercial techniques are available that may achieve more effective negative IAP, there are no studies that compare commercial negative pressure wound therapy to noncommercial techniques such as the "vacuum pack" closure, the "Bogota bag," or other negative pressure modalities. However, most contemporary studies describing temporary abdominal closure utilize a vacuum-assisted closure device [33]. One prospective randomized trial compared outcomes related to using either polyglactin mesh or vacuum-assisted closure without any significant difference in time to delayed fascial closure or fistula rate [34]. If ACS recurs following placement of a temporary abdominal closure device, it should be removed immediately to relieve the IAP.

*Recommendation*: No technique for temporary abdominal closure is favored by the existing medical literature, and thus no recommendation can be made.

### 79.2.6 Is There a Predictable Time Frame or Preferred Technique for Definitive Abdominal Closure after Decompressive Laparotomy?

In general, primary fascial closure is possible within 5–7 days if critical illness resolves and if progressive organ failure does not occur. The development of cardiovascular, renal, and/or hepatic failure often leads to worsening of visceral edema. Such edema combined with retraction of the fascia and loss of domain may render primary fascial closure impossible. When fascial closure is no longer possible, alternative long-term wound management strategies must be considered. These include split-thickness skin grafting of the exposed abdominal contents, closure of cutaneous advancement flaps over the viscera, fascial closure via components separation, and fascial replacement with one of the many types of commercially available biological and prosthetic mesh materials [35]. While each of these techniques is well-described in the literature, no comparative studies or relevant evidence exists that would favor the routine use of any one approach over the others. In practice, most surgeons use a variety of techniques depending on the specific situation and financial implications of routine utilization.

*Recommendation*: No predictable time frame or preferred technique for definitive abdominal closure is favored by the existing medical literature, and thus no recommendation can be made.

## 79.3 Discussion

There has been advancement in the understanding of IAH and ACS and the WSACS has developed a standardized method of measuring IAP. Consensus definitions have also been made that facilitate a common discussion regarding diagnosis and management. With an increase in awareness, there will naturally be issues related to extrapolating principles to different patient populations. Nonsurgical approaches have been supported by only anecdotal or retrospective study support. Prospective, randomized controlled studies are eagerly anticipated. The WSACS has made available detailed recommendations for research and information on current trials. The next decade could potentially be invaluable to the management of IAH/ACS, as future research projects play out.

## References


1. Kron IL, Harman PK, Nolan SP. The measurement of intra-abdominal pressure as a criterion for abdominal re-exploration. *Ann Surg.* 1984;199:28–30.
2. Malbrain ML, Cheatham ML, Sugrue M et al. Results from the International Conference of Experts on Intra-abdominal Hypertension and Abdominal Compartment Syndrome. I. Definitions. *Intensive Care Med.* 2006;32:1722–1732.
3. Cheatham MI, Malbrain ML, Kirkpatrick A et al. Results from the International Conference of Experts on Intra-abdominal Hypertension and Abdominal Compartment Syndrome. II. Recommendations. *Intensive Care Med.* 2007;33:951–962.
4. Kirkpatrick AW, Roberts DJ, Waele JD et al. Intra-abdominal hypertension and the abdominal compartment syndrome: Updated consensus definitions and clinical practice guidelines from the World Society of the Abdominal Compartment Syndrome. *Intensive Care Med.* 2013;39:1190–1206.

5. Malbrain ML, Chiumello D, Pelosi P et al. Incidence and prognosis of intra-abdominal hypertension in a mixed population of critically ill patients: A multiple-center epidemiological study. *Crit Care Med.* 2005;33:315–322.
6. Balogh Z, McKinley BA, Holcomb JB et al. Both primary and secondary abdominal compartment syndrome can be predicted early and are harbingers of multiple organ failure. *J Trauma.* 2003;54:848–859.
7. Ali SR, Mohammad H, Sara S. Evaluation of the relationship between pelvic fracture and abdominal compartment syndrome in traumatic patients. *J Emerg Trauma Shock.* 2013;6(3):176–179.
8. Blaser AR, Par P, Kitus R et al. Risk factors for intra-abdominal hypertension in mechanically ventilated patients. *Acta Anaesthesiol Scand.* 2011;55:607–614.
9. O'Mara MS, Slater H, Goldfarb W et al. A prospective, randomized evaluation of intra-abdominal pressures with crystalloid and colloid resuscitation in burn patients. *J Trauma.* 2005;58(5):1011–1018.
10. Holodinsky JK, Roberts DJ, Ball CG et al. Risk factors for intra-abdominal hypertension and abdominal compartment syndrome among adult intensive care unit patients: A systematic review and meta-analysis. *Crit Care.* 2013;17:R249.
11. Gonzalez-Fajardo JA, Mengibar L, Brizuela JA et al. Effect of postoperative restrictive fluid therapy in the recovery of patients with abdominal vascular surgery. *Eur J Vasc Endovasc Surg.* 2009;37:538–543.
12. Vincent J-L, Sakr Y, Sprung CL et al. Sepsis in European intensive care units: Results of the SOAP study. *Crit Care Med.* 2006;34(2):344–353.
13. Sugrue M, Bauman A, Jones F et al. Clinical examination is an inaccurate predictor of intraabdominal pressure. *World J Surg.* 2002;26:1428–1431.
14. Malbrain ML. Different techniques to measure intra-abdominal pressure (IAP): Time for a critical re-appraisal. *Intensive Care Med.* 2004;30:357–371.
15. Malbrain ML, Cheatham ML, Kirkpatrick A et al. Results from the International Conference of Experts on Intra-abdominal Hypertension and Abdominal Compartment Syndrome. I. Definitions. *Intensive Care Med.* 2006;32:1722–1732.
16. Zengerink I, McBeth PB, Zygun DA et al. Validation and experience with a simple continuous intra-abdominal pressure measurement technique in a multidisciplinary medical/surgical critical care unit. *J Trauma.* 2008;64(5):1159–1164.
17. Wauters J, Spincemaille L, albrain ML et al. A Novel method (CiMON) for continuous intra-abdominal pressure monitoring: Pilot test in a pig model. *Crit Care Res Pract.* 2012;2012:181563.
18. Kaussen T, Otto J, Schachtrupp A. Recognition and management of abdominal compartment syndrome among German anesthetists and surgeons: A national survey. *Ann Intensive Care.* 2012;2(Suppl 1):S7.
19. Cheatham ML, Safcsak K. Is the evolving management of intra-abdominal hypertension and abdominal compartment syndrome improving survival? *Crit Care Med.* 2010;38(2):402–407.
20. Cheatham ML, White MW, Sagraves SG et al. Abdominal perfusion pressure: A superior parameter in the assessment of intra-abdominal hypertension. *J Trauma.* 2000;49:621–626.
21. Malbrain ML. 2002. Abdominal perfusion pressure as a prognostic marker in intra-abdominal hypertension. In: Vincent JL, ed. *Yearbook of Intensive Care and Emergency Medicine.* Springer: New York, pp. 792–814.
22. Cheatham ML, Malbrain ML. 2006. Abdominal perfusion pressure. In: Ivatury RR, Cheatham ML, Malbrain ML, Sugrue M, eds. *Abdominal Compartment Syndrome.* Landes Biomedical: Georgetown, Guyana, pp. 69–81.
23. De Waele J, Delaet I, Hoste E et al. The effect of neuromuscular blockers on intraabdominal pressure. *Crit Care Med.* 2006;34:A70.
24. Abouassaly CT, Dutton WD, Zaydfudimv et al. Postoperative neuromuscular blocker use is associated with higher primary fascial closure rates after damage control laparotomy. *J Trauma.* 2010;69: 557–561.
25. McBeth PB, Zygun DA, Widder S et al. Effect of patient positioning on intra-abdominal pressure monitoring. *Am J Surg.* 2007;193:644–647.
26. Balogh Z, McKinley BA, Cocanour CS et al. Supranormal trauma resuscitation causes more cases of abdominal compartment syndrome. *Arch Surg.* 2003;138:637–642.
27. O'Mara MS, Slater H, Goldfarb IW et al. A prospective, randomized evaluation of intra-abdominal pressures with crystalloid and colloid resuscitation in burn patients. *J Trauma.* 2005;58:1011–1018.
28. Oda J, Ueyama M, Yamashita K et al. Hypertonic lactated saline resuscitation reduces the risk of abdominal compartment syndrome in severely burned patients. *J Trauma.* 2006;60:64–71.
29. Reckard JM, Chung MH, Varma MK et al. Management of intraabdominal hypertension by percutaneous catheter drainage. *J Vasc Interv Radiol.* 2005;16:1019–1021.
30. Parra MW, Al-Khayat H, Smith HG et al. Paracentesis for resuscitation-induced abdominal compartment syndrome: An alternative to decompressive laparotomy in the burn patient. *J Trauma.* 2006;60:1119–1121.
31. Batacchi S, Matano S, Nella A et al. Vacuum-assisted closure device enhances recovery of critically ill patients following emergency surgical procedures. *Crit Care.* 2009;13:R194.
32. Kubiak BD, Albert SP, Gatto LA et al. Peritoneal negative pressure therapy prevents multiple organ injury in a chronic porcine sepsis and ischemia/reperfusion model. *Shock.* 2010;34:525–534.
33. Roberts DJ, Zygun DA, Grendar J et al. Negative-pressure wound therapy for critically ill adults with open abdominal wounds: A systematic review. *J Trauma Acute Care Surg.* 2012;73:629–639.
34. Bee TK, Croce MA, Magnotti LJ et al. Temporary abdominal closure techniques: A prospective randomized trial comparing polyglactin 910 mesh and vacuum-assisted closure. *J Trauma.* 2008;65:337–342.
35. Diaz JJ, Jr., Dutton WD, Ott MM et al. Eastern Association for the Surgery of Trauma: A review of the management of the open abdomen—Part 2 "Management of the open abdomen". *J Trauma.* 2011;71:502–512.

## Commentary on Abdominal Compartment Syndrome

*David H. Wisner*

It is with some chagrin that I realize my career is now long enough to have witnessed several major shifts in both my individual thinking and our collective thinking about abdominal compartment syndrome.

In the earliest stages of my career, we were dimly aware that patients who were not doing well and had major organ dysfunction sometimes also had really tight abdomens, but we did not appreciate that there might be at least a partial cause and effect relationship between the tight belly and the stiff lungs or the failing kidneys. We gradually started to understand that high intra-abdominal pressure could itself constitute a pathology and have negative consequences for different organ systems. We aggressively sought to characterize the effects on as many different organ systems as we could imagine: pulmonary (decreased diaphragmatic excursion and lung compliance), cardiac (decreased venous return, reorientation of the heart with elevation of the diaphragm), renal (increased renal venous pressure, redistribution of cortico-medullary blood flow), gastrointestinal (decreased venous outflow, perhaps decreased blood supply), and neurologic (increased intracranial pressure).

We also eventually concluded that we could do something about the pathology of increased intra-abdominal pressure and there was growing enthusiasm for opening the abdomen if the measured intra-abdominal pressure was higher than some predetermined number, even if the associated physiologic derangement was not that bad. We opened a lot of abdomens.

We then developed an increased appreciation that an open abdomen generated both short- and long-term problems of its own, and the pendulum swung back to a slower trigger for decompressive laparotomy and a more measured response to the numbers we generated when measuring intra-abdominal pressure.

Our latest maturation has been a better understanding of when to leave the abdomen open in the first place, thereby leaving fewer patients set up for the need for decompression of an abdomen that should never have been closed in the first place. Sometimes the abdomen is intentionally left open solely to avoid abdominal compartment syndrome. Sometimes the abdomen is left open as part of a damage control strategy and avoiding abdominal compartment syndrome is just a byproduct of that approach. Often, the abdomen is left open for both of those reasons. Regardless of the rationale for leaving the abdomen open, it is happening more now than it used to and we are as a consequence seeing fewer cases of postoperative abdominal compartment syndrome than we used to see.

To comment briefly on the questions addressed in the chapter.

### Are There Risk Factors for Abdominal Compartment Syndrome and Can Patients Be Screened for the Development of Abdominal Compartment Syndrome?

The risk factors listed by the authors are interesting and correct but of limited usefulness. Their greatest utility, as implied earlier, is in the operating room when deciding whether to close a laparotomy incision. In the ICU, perhaps the simplest thing to do is to measure intra-abdominal pressure in sick patients with organ dysfunction, particularly pulmonary or renal dysfunction, regardless of the presence or absence of risk factors, to see if increased intra-abdominal pressure might be contributing to their difficulties. The observation that patients given lots of fluid are more likely to develop abdominal compartment syndrome is just that, an observation. It probably implies a causal relationship but, as the authors point out, it would be incorrect to come to the blanket conclusion that the best way to avoid abdominal compartment syndrome is to be stingy with fluids. Inadequate intravascular volume is bad, also, and shock can exacerbate the factors leading to the elevated abdominal compartment pressure in the first place.

### How Should Patients Be Screened and Monitored for the Development of Abdominal Compartment Syndrome?

Bladder pressure measurements seem to be pretty reliable compared to direct measurements and they have the added advantage of being simple to do. Our group long ago concluded that we did not need fancy measuring devices and that simply raising the urinary catheter tubing and measuring the distance of the column of fluid in the tube above the heart of pubic symphysis correlated quite well with more complicated transducer-based measurements.* The authors' discussion of the appropriate frequency of measurement is somewhat obviated if this simple measurement technique is used, because measurements can be done pretty easily as often as you like.

I do think it is probably worth emphasizing that measurements should be done with the patient

* Lee SL, Anderson JT, Kraut EJ, Wisner DH, Wolfe BM. A simplified approach to the diagnosis of elevated intra-abdominal pressure. *J Trauma*. 2002;52:1169–1172.

pharmacologically relaxed in order to avoid spuriously high values from voluntary muscle contraction.

### Is There an Intra-Abdominal Pressure Threshold Level That Mandates Intervention?

I think a value of >20 mmHg (or cm $H_2O$ if you use a simple measurement technique) is as good as any. I do agree that there should be associated organ dysfunction and that blind obeisance to the number is too aggressive. Markedly decreased pulmonary compliance is the most important thing I look for, along with decreased urine output with no other satisfactory explanation. Both of those observations should be triggers for measuring intra-abdominal pressure.

I have never been able to make the abdominal perfusion pressure work for me and worry that patients with a somewhat high blood pressure can still have pulmonary dysfunction for mechanical reasons even with a reassuring abdominal perfusion pressure.

### Are There Any Effective Nonsurgical Strategies for Treating Abdominal Compartment Syndrome?

The chapter has a very interesting discussion of this question. I agree with the authors' essential conclusion that the answer is largely "No." Sedation may not have a direct effect on the pathophysiology, but it is important to ensure reliable measurement and also to help with the pulmonary compliance issues that come with an elevated intra-abdominal pressure, so I think it should be fairly routine at least while the patient remains at high risk.

The pulmonary benefits of keeping the head of the bed at 30 degrees trump the theoretical benefits on intra-abdominal pressure of lying the patient flat. Finally, I really do not think catheter decompression helps. Serous fluid is the only kind of fluid you could reliably remove in large volumes with a small tube, and in my experience, the relief you get from removing that fluid is short-lived; it reaccumulates pretty rapidly.

### Is There a Preferred Technique for Temporary Abdominal Closure after Decompressive Laparotomy?

Experience with both vacuum-based closures and non-vacuum-based closures has convinced me of the virtues of vacuum-based closure. In the early experience with open abdomens, we tried all sorts of temporary closure techniques and none were very satisfactory. I am not sure that use of a vacuum closure makes much difference with the underlying pathophysiology of abdominal compartment syndrome or the speed with which things get better but the bedside nursing management is cleaner and simpler with a vacuum-based approach and the vacuum approach keeps the wound edges and the underlying viscera mobile for much longer, which enhances our ability to get abdomens closed primarily.

### Is There a Predictable Timeframe or Preferred Technique for Definitive Abdominal Closure after Decompressive Laparotomy?

In general, I think if you cannot get the abdomen closed primarily within about 2 weeks, it is necessary to accept an open abdomen for a number of months and the need for another operation down the road for definitive closure. Placement of a skin graft on a piece of bridging absorbable mesh is the tried and true method for covering the patient until the definitive closure can be done. While this approach does not feel very elegant, trying to force a definitive closure in a relatively fresh abdomen in which the abdominal wall has retracted and become immobile is asking for trouble. Component separation works well when done by someone with the necessary expertise, and we have found that a simple and easy way to decide when the abdomen is ready for that technique is to see if the skin graft that was applied can be easily pinched. If it can be, the implications are that the abdomen is quiescent enough to go back in and also that the skin graft will be relatively easy to remove.

# 80

# *Pain, Agitation, and Delirium in the ICU*

**Abdul Alarhayem and Natasha Keric**

**CONTENTS**



## 80.1 Introduction

There seems to be no chronologic landmarks in intensive care units (ICUs). Activity seems continuous; the stimulation from sound, sight, and touch never stops, nor does it seem predictable, further disrupting a patient's usual daily rhythm. Recovering patients have described experiences of fear, panic, and helplessness in such a surreal environment.

Pain, agitation, and delirium (PAD) are arguably the most common patient issues challenging clinicians on a daily basis. An emergent understanding of the inextricable link of each component of the "ICU triad" forms the basis of the 2012 Society of Critical Care Medicine (SCCM) guidelines for management of PAD through an integrating multiprofessional approach.

## 80.2 How Can Sedation Needs Be Assessed?

*Agitation*, originally described as "violent motion, tumultuous emotion," is a psychomotor disturbance characterized by neuropsychological dysfunction *and* excessive motor activity that is either nonpurposeful, such as flailing in bed, or counterproductive, such as removing medical devices and/or attempted assault of a care provider [1,2]. Fifty to seventy percent of patients in ICUs have some degree of agitation during their stay.

Agitation has been shown to be an independent predictor of morbidity and mortality [3]. It is also associated with an increase in ICU and overall hospital length of stay (LOS), increased cost [4,5], and long-term adverse outcomes such as posttraumatic stress disorder [6].

Clinical evidence continues to suggest that most patients are treated for agitation using informal criteria.

With over 10 different scoring systems for the monitoring of sedation at the clinicians' disposal, objectively determining how well they measure the construct of interest is critical. Psychometric properties most frequently used in comparing ICU scoring systems include the following:

1. *Reliability* is defined as a test's ability to measure the construct of interest consistently. Inter-rater reliability allows health-care providers to agree in the way they score condition severity (e.g., agitation), with obvious diagnostic and therapeutic implications.
2. *Validity* refers to how well a test accurately correlates with the measure of interest. Discriminant validity is demonstrated when scores on the test being examined do not correlate with a test meant to measure a different construct (i.e., an agitation scale should measure agitation, not pain).
3. *Responsiveness* is defined as the ability of an instrument to accurately detect change when it has occurred.
4. *Feasibility* refers to the ease with which clinicians can apply a particular scale in the clinical setting [7].

The Richmond Agitation–Sedation Scale (RASS) and Sedation–Agitation Scale (SAS) (see Table 80.1) have yielded the highest psychometric scores and were found to be the most *valid, reliable, and discriminatory* sedation assessment tools for measuring quality and depth of sedation in adult ICU patients [8–10]. Moderate to high correlations were found between these scales and electroencephalogram (EEG) or bispectral index (BIS) values [11,12]. In head-to-head comparison, neither is demonstrably superior to the other.

The BIS provides a discrete value from 100 (completely awake state) to <60 (deep sedation) and ≤40 (deep hypnotic state or barbiturate coma) by incorporating several EEG components. Although the technique has been shown to be a valid and reliable measure in the operating room, no recommendation can be made supporting the use of BIS, EEG, or any other objective measure of brain function in the noncomatose, nonparalyzed critically ill adult. Their use should be limited to patients receiving neuromuscular blocking agents, when subjective sedation assessments may be unobtainable, and in monitoring nonconvulsive seizure activity in adult ICU patients with either known or suspected seizures. They may also be used to titrate electrosuppressive medication to achieve burst suppression in adult ICU patients with elevated intracranial pressure.

Lack of validation and lower psychometric scores associated with scales such as Sheffield and Ramsay, make them less appealing for clinical use.

**TABLE 80.1**

Riker Sedation Agitation Scale and the Richmond Agitation–Sedation Scale

| Score | Term | Description |
|---|---|---|
| *Riker sedation agitation scale* | | |
| 7 | Dangerous agitation | Pulling at ET tube, trying to remove catheters, climbing over bedrail, striking at staff, thrashing side-to-side |
| 6 | Very agitated | Requiring restraint and frequent verbal reminding of limits, biting ETT |
| 5 | Agitated | Anxious or mildly agitated, attempts to sit up. Calms down with verbal instructions |
| 4 | Calm and cooperative | Calm, awakens easily, follows commands |
| 3 | Sedated | Difficult to arouse, awakens to verbal stimuli or gentle shaking but drifts off again, follows simple commands |
| 2 | Very sedated | Arouses to physical stimuli but does not communicate or follow commands, may mow spontaneously |
| 1 | Unarousable | Minimal or no response to noxious stimuli, does not communicate or follow commands |
| *Richmond agitation sedation scale* | | |
| +4 | Combative | Overtly combative or violent and an immediate danger to staff |
| +3 | Very agitated | Pulls on or removes tube(s) or catheter(s) or has aggressive behavior toward staff |
| +2 | Agitated | Frequent nonpurposeful movement or patient ventilator dyssynchrony |
| +1 | Restless | Anxious or apprehensive but movements not aggressive or vigorous |
| 0 | Alert and calm | |
| −1 | Drowsy | Not fully alert but has sustained (>10 s) awakenings, with eye contact, to voice |
| −2 | Light sedation | Briefly (<10 s) awakens with eye contact to voice |
| −3 | Moderate sedation | Any movement (but no eye contact) to voice |
| −4 | Deep sedation | No response to voice, but any movement to physical stimuli |
| −5 | Unarousable | No response to voice or physical stimulation |

*Sources:* Riker, RR et al., *Crit Care Med*, 27, 1325, 1999; Brandl, KM et al., *Pharmacother J Human Pharmacol Drug Ther*, 21, 431, 2001; Ryder-Lewis, MC and Nelson, KM, *Intensive Crit Care Nurs*, 24, 211, 2008; Riker, RR et al., *Intens Care Med*, 27(5), 853, 2001; Ely, EW et al., *JAMA*, 289, 2983, 2003.

*Recommendation*: RASS and SAS are valid and reliable sedation assessment tools for measuring quality and depth of sedation in adult ICU patients (Grade B).

Routine use of objective measures of brain function (BIS and EEG) to monitor sedation in noncomatose, nonparalyzed patients is not recommended (Grade B).

## 80.3 How Should Sedation in the ICU Be Managed?

Traditionally, our attempts at addressing anxiety and agitation associated with the inherently distressing nature of critical illness were directed toward suppressing patients' awareness of and responses to their environment, primarily through the use of sedatives [13]. It was also thought deep sedation mitigated patients' traumatic perceptions of their ICU experience.

We now know that administering sedatives in response to agitation serves only to mask the symptoms rather than treat the underlying etiology.

The recent SCCM guidelines highlight the need to promptly address the underlying causes of agitation and minimize the use of sedatives, except in very select circumstances.

## 80.4 Addressing the Underlying Causes of Agitation

Providing directed therapy in treating ICU agitation can prove difficult given its multifactorial and enigmatic nature. Unrelieved pain and delirium are among the most commonly cited causes of agitation. A newer analgesia-first approach, in which opiates are administered and only supplemented with sedatives if patients are not at the goal sedation level, has been found to shorten time on mechanical ventilation and minimize sedative use [14]. One should also evaluate for the presence of hypoxemia, hypotension, temperature and metabolic derangements, infections, and an underlying history of substance abuse or psychiatric disorders. Of interest, in 33% of patients, no definite cause can be found [6].

## 80.5 Nonpharmacological Strategies and Light Sedation

In nearly all ICU patients, the goal should be to establish a state where the patient is calm, lucid, pain-free, and cooperative with his/her care.

Current expert opinion favors nonpharmacological methods prior to administrating sedatives. Maintenance of patient comfort, provision of adequate analgesia, frequent reorientation, and optimization of the environment to maintain normal sleep patterns have been shown to minimize the need for pharmacotherapy.

Even when they are to be used, sedative medications should be titrated to maintain a light rather than a deep level of sedation, unless contraindicated.

Deep sedation is associated with an increased duration of mechanical ventilation, ICU LOS, morbidity, mortality, and expenditure.

Although lighter sedation has been shown to increase physiologic stress in terms of increased catecholamine concentrations and/or oxygen consumption, this has not translated into worsened clinical outcomes.

Only in a minority of ICU patients is there truly an indication for continuous deep sedation, namely, treatment of intracranial hypertension, severe respiratory failure, refractory status epilepticus, and prevention of awareness in patients treated with neuromuscular blocking agents [15].

## 80.6 Protocolized Sedation Is Preferred Over Daily Sedation Interruption

The following two strategies may be used to minimize sedation:

1. A nursing-implemented sedation titration protocol that specifies clear targets for level of awareness, such as a target RASS level.
2. Daily interruption of sedation (i.e., drug holiday) with infusions resumed only when necessary and at half the previous dose.

A systematic review of five trials concluded that daily interruption of sedation was not associated with a significant reduction in the duration of mechanical ventilation, ICU and hospital LOS, or mortality [16].

Data from a randomized controlled trial published after the issuance of the 2012 SCCM guidelines found that daily sedation interruption offered no advantage in patients managed with protocolized sedation [17].

*Recommendation*: Analgesia-first sedation should be used in mechanically ventilated adult ICU patients (Grade B). Sedative medications should be titrated to maintain a light rather than a deep level of sedation in adult ICU patients, unless clinically contraindicated (Grade B). Either daily sedation interruption or a light target level of sedation should be routinely used in adult ICU patients using mechanical ventilation (Grade B).

## 80.7 Should Non-Benzodiazepine-Based Sedation, Instead of Sedation with Benzodiazepines, Be Used in Mechanically Ventilated Adult ICU Patients?

As discussed earlier, minimizing sedation such that patients are calm, lucid, pain-free, and cooperative with their care is encouraged. Factors taken into consideration while selecting a sedative agent include sedation goals for the individual patient, the drugs' pharmacokinetic properties, and overall cost. Regardless of the particular agent used to provide sedation, it is important to appreciate that the central nervous system (CNS)-depressant effects of these drugs proceed in a dose–response manner.

Outcome studies in ICU patients typically compare benzodiazepines with either propofol or dexmedetomidine for sedation.

### 80.7.1 Benzodiazepines (Midazolam and Lorazepam)

The therapeutic effects of benzodiazepines are attributed to their ability to potentiate the inhibitory influences of gamma-aminobutyric acid (GABA). At supratherapeutic levels, all benzodiazepines can reduce ventilation and lower blood pressure in a dose-dependent manner. Midazolam is the benzodiazepine of choice for intravenous (IV) sedation. Compared with lorazepam, it is more lipid soluble (thus a more rapid onset) and has a shorter distribution and elimination half-life. Both undergo hepatic metabolism prior to renal elimination [18].

### 80.7.2 Propofol

Propofol is short-acting, IV nonbarbiturate hypnotic. At room temperature, it is very lipid-soluble, allowing for rapid onset and offset of drug effect and fast elimination from the body. Its CNS-depressant properties are facilitated through activating GABA A receptors, directly inhibiting the *N*-methyl-D-aspartate receptor and modulating calcium influx through slow calcium-ion channels. Although propofol has no analgesic effects, its antiemetic properties and ability to produce anterograde amnesia make it one of the most widely used sedatives in the ICU. Propofol has also been reported to have neuroprotective effects, mainly mediated through reducing cerebral blood flow and intracranial pressure, and antioxidant and anti-inflammatory effects [19,20]. Propofol has a remarkable safety profile; its most common side effects, however, are dose-dependent hypotension and cardiorespiratory depression. Other side effects include hypertriglyceridemia, acute pancreatitis, myoclonus, and rarely (<1%), propofol infusion syndrome.

### 80.7.3 Dexmedetomidine

Dexmedetomidine is a potent α2-receptor agonist with sedative, anxiolytic, analgesic/opioid sparing, and sympatholytic properties [21]. Patients sedated with dexmedetomidine are more easily arousable and interactive, with reduced analgesic requirements [22]. It does not significantly affect respiratory drive, and is thus the only sedative approved for administration in nonintubated ICU patients [23]. Dexmedetomidine is rapidly redistributed into peripheral tissues and is metabolized by the liver. It has only been approved in the United States for short-term sedation of ICU patients (<24 h) at a maximal dose of 0.7 μg/kg/h. The most common side effects of dexmedetomidine are hypotension and bradycardia (see Table 80.2).

Two systemic reviews of trials ranked as moderate to high quality suggest that using a dexmedetomidine- or propofol-based sedation regimen rather than a benzodiazepine-based sedation regimen may reduce ICU LOS and duration of mechanical ventilation [24,25]. Similar results were noted in two large randomized controlled trials [26].

*Recommendation*: Sedation strategies using nonbenzodiazepine sedatives (either propofol or dexmedetomidine) may improve clinical outcomes in mechanically ventilated adult ICU patient compared with benzodiazepines (either midazolam or lorazepam) (Grade B).

**TABLE 80.2**
Sedatives and Analgesics in Common Use in the ICU

| Agent | Onset after IV Loading Dose | Elimination Half-Life | Active Metabolites | Loading Dose (IV) | Maintenance Dosing (IV) |
|---|---|---|---|---|---|
| Midazolam | 2–5 min | 3–11 h | Yes | 0.01–0.05 mg/kg over several minutes | 0.02–0.1 mg/kg/h |
| Lorazepam | 15–20 min | 8–15 h | None | 0.02–0.04 mg/kg (≤2 mg) | 0.01–0.1 mg/kg/h (≤10 mg/h) |
| Propofol | 1–2 min | Short-term use = 3–12 h<br>Long-term use = 50 ± 18.6 h | None | 5 μg/kg/min over 5 min | 5–50 μg/kg/min |
| Dexmedetomidine | 5–10 min | 1.8–3.1 h | None | 1 μg/kg over 10 min | 0.2–0.7 μg/kg/h |

*Source:* Barr, J et al., *Crit Care Med*, 41, 263, 2013.

## 80.8 How Is Delirium Identified?

The most common feature of delirium, thought by many to be its cardinal sign, is inattention [15]. Delirium is a clinical- and criterion-based diagnosis; the four domains of the *Diagnostic and Statistical Manual of Mental Disorders*, 5th edition (DSM-V), are as follows:

1. Disturbance of awareness
2. Change in cognition not secondary to dementia
3. Development over a short period and fluctuation
4. Instigated by an underlying medical condition, toxin, or medication

Patients with delirium may be agitated (hyperactive delirium), lethargic (hypoactive delirium), or may fluctuate between the two subtypes (mixed).

In the absence of formal monitoring criteria, one report found ICU staff members unable to diagnose delirium in almost three quarters of patients with the condition [27]. This may be due to hypoactive delirium, which is more difficult to recognize, being more frequent than hyperactive delirium.

The SCCM thus issued strong recommendations that ICU patients at moderate to high risk for delirium be routinely monitored, at least once per nursing shift, using valid and reliable delirium assessment tools.

A meta-analysis of five ICU delirium screening tools found the Confusion Assessment Method for the ICU (CAM-ICU) and the ICU Delirium Screening Checklist (ICDSC) to be the most sensitive and specific tools for detecting delirium [28]. They are valid, reliable, and feasible in patients both on and off mechanical ventilation [29,30].

The CAM-ICU reports a dichotomous assessment at a single time point, whereas the ICDSC lists signs that can be observed over a period of time [15].

Scoring is positive or negative according to the presence or absence of criteria listed (see Table 80.3).

*Recommendation*: Routine monitoring of delirium in adult ICU patients is feasible and recommended (Grade B). The CAM-ICU and the ICDSC are the most valid and reliable delirium monitoring tools in ICU patients (Grade A).

**TABLE 80.3**

Confusion Assessment Method for the ICU

| | |
|---|---|
| *Feature 1*—Acute Onset or Fluctuating Course. | Is patient at their baseline mental status and have they been there for the last 24 hours? If not, then patient scores positive. |
| *Feature 2*—Inattention SAVEAHAART or pictures. | >2 *Errors* scores positive |
| *Feature 3*—Altered LOC. | Anything other than *RASS = 0* score is positive |
| *Feature 4*—Disorganized Thinking. | 4 yes/no questions and 1 command. >*1 error* is positive. |

*Sources:* Ely, EW et al., *JAMA*, 286, 2703, 2001; Ely, EW et al., *Crit Care Med*, 29, 1370, 2001.
CAM-ICU positive if the patient is positive for *both* features 1 and 2 and *either* feature 3 or 4.

## 80.9 What Is the Impact of Delirium in the ICU?

Numerous studies with high-quality evidence have shown delirium to be an independent predictor of mortality [31,32]. Two cohort studies found the duration of delirium consistently portended a 10% increased risk of death per day [32]. Delirium was also found to be an independent predictor of duration of mechanical ventilation and of ICU LOS [33] (see Table 80.4).

Patients have also been found to have a higher incidence of cognitive dysfunction postdischarge [34].

Although these associations are well established, it is difficult to determine causality given the presence of numerous confounders (severe illness and multiple organ dysfunction, prolonged exposure medications, etc.) [35].

*Recommendation*: Delirium is associated with increased mortality (Grade A), prolonged ICU and hospital LOS (Grade A), and the development of post-ICU cognitive impairment in adult ICU patients (Grade B).

## 80.10 How Should Delirium Be Treated?

The SCCM recommends identifying underlying etiologies as the first step in delirium management. Infectious processes, metabolic and electrolyte derangements, strokes, seizures, and overdose/withdrawal syndromes should all be investigated.

The use of pharmacotherapy to treat delirium is modestly successful at best and has clear potential to harm. Nevertheless, expert guidelines still recommend antipsychotic agents as the treatment of choice for delirium, especially when it persistent, interferes with patient care, or is associated with significant agitation.

Haloperidol remains the drug of choice for delirium, despite the lack of evidence that it actually reduces the duration of delirium in adult ICU patients. Haloperidol is also associated with corrected QT interval (QTc) interval prolongation, and this can precipitate fatal arrhythmias.

In contrast, the use of atypical antipsychotics (e.g., quetiapine) was found to reduce the duration of

**TABLE 80.4**

Intensive Care Delirium Screening Checklist

| Patient Evaluation | Score |
|---|---|
| Altered level of consciousness[a] | No, 0; Yes, 1 |
| Inattention | No, 0; Yes, 1 |
| Disorientation | No, 0; Yes, 1 |
| Hallucination—delusion—psychosis | No, 0; Yes, 1 |
| Psychomotor agitation or retardation | No, 0; Yes, 1 |
| Inappropriate speech or mood | No, 0; Yes, 1 |
| Sleep/wake cycle disturbance | No, 0; Yes, 1 |
| Symptom fluctuation | No, 0; Yes, 1 |
| Total score (0–8) | |

*Sources:* Bergeron, N et al., *Intensive Care Med*, 27, 859, 2001; Ouimets S et al., *Intensive Care Med*, 33, 1007, 2007.
*Note:* Score 1 point for each of the following features, as assessed in the manner thought appropriate by the clinician. A score of ≥4 is positive for delirium (with scores of 1–3 termed "subsyndromal delirium").
[a] Patient must show at least a response to mild or moderate stimulation.

delirium and improve discharge rates in a small randomized controlled trial [36].

A high-quality randomized trial also noted a more rapid resolution of delirium in patients randomized to dexmedetomidine compared to those receiving midazolam [37]. Due to the deliriogenic properties of benzodiazepines, they should be avoided.

Despite the neuropathogensis of delirium implicating a central cholinergic deficiency, a multicenter trial found rivastigmine, a cholinesterase inhibitor, to be associated with more severe and longer durations of delirium, with a trend toward higher mortality [38].

*Recommendation*: Atypical antipsychotics may reduce the duration of delirium in adult ICU patients (Grade C). In mechanically ventilated ICU patients at risk for delirium, dexmedetomidine infusions are associated with a lower prevalence of delirium compared to benzodiazepine infusions (Grade B).

## 80.11 What Are Some Preventative Strategies That Can Reduce the Incidence of Delirium?

Identifying patients at risk of delirium allows for early institution of preventative measures and can help minimize the detrimental effects associated with delirium. Four baseline risk factors have been associated with the development of delirium in the ICU: preexisting dementia, history of hypertension or alcoholism, a high severity of illness at admission, and coma.

The relationship between the use of opiates and the development of delirium in adult ICU patients is less clear. The anxiolytic, amnesic, and anticonvulsant properties of benzodiazepines make them attractive to the ICU clinician.

Routine use of simple preventative measures in patients at risk of delirium has been shown to significantly reduce the incidence of delirium, depth of sedation, and hospital and ICU LOS.

In a landmark trial, there was a significant decrease in the incidence of delirium (15.0% vs. 9.9%) in patients managed with nonpharmacologic delirium prevention protocols [39].

A large randomized control trial found similar results when early mobilization strategies were used [40].

## 80.12 Pharmacological Prevention

Evidence supporting the routine use of haloperidol or atypical antipsychotics to prevent delirium in adult ICU patients is lacking.

A recent multicenter, randomized controlled trial of delirium prophylaxis with either haloperidol or ziprasidone versus placebo found no benefit with either treatment compared to placebo [41].

*Recommendation*: Early mobilization of adult ICU patients has been found to reduce the incidence and duration of delirium (Grade B). The use of haloperidol or atypical antipsychotics be administered to prevent delirium in adult ICU patients is not recommended (Grade C).

## 80.13 What Is the Impact of Alcohol on the Critically Ill Patient?

More than 50% of Americans adults are considered to be regular drinkers and 10% are excessive alcohol consumers. Alcohol misuse is the leading risk factor for serious injury and the third leading cause of preventable death in the United States. Studies have shown that 40%–50% of trauma patients are injured while under the influence of alcohol, and over 40% of trauma deaths have a positive screen for alcohol, drugs, or both [42,43]. The annual economic cost of alcohol misuse is estimated to be $185 million [44].

Due to its CNS-depressant effects, alcohol adversely impacts fine motor tasks and judgment, leading to increasing aggression and risk-taking behavior, thus predisposing to motor vehicle collisions and interpersonal violence-related injuries [45]. Alcohol intoxication is estimated to double the severity of traumatic brain injury. A study of assault victims found intoxication was associated with a higher incidence of depressed mental status (Glasgow Coma Score <8) [46].

Acute alcohol ingestion is associated with a significantly lower systolic blood pressure on admission that responds poorly to volume resuscitation, especially in the presence of hemorrhage [47,48]. This blunted physiologic response is secondary to inhibition of the release of epinephrine, norepinephrine, and vasopressin, as well as a direct depressive effect upon the myocardium. The net result is inadequate oxygen delivery to tissue. Alcohol also reduces the electrical threshold for ventricular arrhythmias.

Acute alcohol exposure is also directly immunosuppressive, increasing the risk for postinjury infections, acute respiratory distress syndrome, and multiple organ failure [49,50].

Up to 25% of patients with an alcohol use disorder will have a metabolic acidosis on presentation and up to two-thirds may have raised lactate concentrations. This can limit the use of lactic acid and base deficit as markers of organ perfusion. However, even in the presence of ethanol, a base deficit <–6 remains a powerful indicator of major injury [51].

Pain control can prove challenging in sober alcoholics due to cross-tolerance to opioids. The acutely intoxicated patient, however, may require less opioids due to the additive effect with narcotics.

In 2007, the American College of Surgeons Committee on Trauma implemented a requirement that Level I trauma centers must have a mechanism to identify patients who are problem drinkers and the capacity to provide an intervention for patients who screen positive.

There is evidence that these interventions are cost-effective and reduce alcohol use through follow-up surveys and trauma recidivism [52,53].

*Recommendation*: Given the high prevalence of alcohol use among trauma admission; routine screening for alcoholism is warranted. If identified, a brief intervention is warranted (Grade A).

## 80.14 How Is Alcohol Withdrawal Identified and How Should It Be Treated?

Approximately 500,000 episodes of withdrawal severe enough to require pharmacologic treatment occur each year. Symptoms of alcohol withdrawal occur because alcohol is a CNS-depressant; abrupt cessation unmasks the adaptive responses to chronic ethanol use resulting in overactivity of the CNS. Symptoms of alcohol withdrawal syndrome (AWS) develop 6–24 h after a patient's last drink, with the majority of patients experiencing minor withdrawal symptoms. Less than 5% of patients with AWS suffer from delirium tremens (DTs), a clinical syndrome characterized by hallucinations, psychomotor agitation, profound autonomic hyperactivity, and tonic–clonic seizures in the setting of abrupt alcohol cessation. DT is associated with a mortality rate of up to 5% [54].

No prospective data support the use of a formal tool to identify ICU patients at risk for AWS; however, a prior history of AWS or seizures constitutes the greatest risk for withdrawal symptoms [55]. There is no evidence for the prophylactic treatment of alcohol withdrawal, even in high-risk patients. However, once withdrawal occurs, early and frequent assessment of withdrawal symptoms is essential. The most commonly studied tool for the diagnosis and monitoring of withdrawal is the revised Clinical Institute Withdrawal Assessment for Alcohol scale. It is a multidimensional scale that rates 10 objective and subjective symptoms of withdrawal. With a total possible score of 67, a score >20 reflects full-blown AWS in most studies.

Administering benzodiazepines in a symptom-driven approach is the standard of care for AWS treatment [56,57]. Prospective randomized control trials have demonstrated that symptom-triggered administration leads to a shorter duration of treatment, as compared with fixed-dose regimens and less medication [58,59]. Current evidence does not suggest that one benzodiazepine is more efficacious than another. DTs unresponsive to high-dose benzodiazepines may be treated with propofol or even phenobarbital [60].

The use of ethanol in the treatment of acute alcohol withdrawal is not recommended due to difficult titration, its narrow therapeutic index, and the presence of superior alternatives. Drugs like haloperidol may lower the seizure threshold in AWS and should be avoided [61]. There is insufficient evidence to support the use of clonidine or dexmedetomidine, alone or in combination with benzodiazepines, for the treatment of AWS [62] (Table 80.5).

*Recommendation*: High-quality evidence supporting the prophylactic treatment of alcohol withdrawal is lacking. Alcohol withdrawal should be treated using benzodiazepines in a symptom-driven approach, employing a validated assessment tool (Grade A).

**TABLE 80.5**

Pain, Agitation, and Delirium in the ICU: Evidence and Grades of Recommendation

| Question | Answer | Level of Evidence | Grade of Recommendation | References |
|---|---|---|---|---|
| How can sedation needs be assessed? | RASS and SAS are valid and reliable sedation assessment tools for measuring quality and depth of sedation in adult ICU patients. | 2 | B | [8–12] |
| | Routine use of objective measures of brain function (BIS, EEG, etc.) to monitor sedation in noncomatose, nonparalyzed patients is not recommended. | 2 | B | |
| How should sedation in the ICU be managed? | Analgesia-first sedation be used in mechanically ventilated adult ICU patients. | 2 | B | [14] |
| | Sedative medications be titrated to maintain a light rather than a deep level of sedation in adult ICU patients, unless clinically contraindicated. | 1 | B | [1,13–17] |
| | Either daily sedation interruption or a light target level of sedation be routinely used in adult ICU patients using mechanical ventilation. | 1 | B | |
| Should nonbenzodiazepine-based sedation, instead of sedation with benzodiazepines, be used in mechanically ventilated adult ICU patients? | Sedation strategies using nonbenzodiazepine sedatives (either propofol or dexmedetomidine) may improve clinical outcomes in mechanically ventilated adult ICU patient compared to benzodiazepines (either midazolam or lorazepam). | 2 | B | [24–26] |
| How is delirium identified? | Routine monitoring of delirium in adult ICU patients is feasible and recommended. | | B | [28–30] |
| | The CAM-ICU and the ICDSC are the most valid and reliable delirium monitoring tools in ICU patients. | | A | |
| What is the impact of delirium in the ICU? | Delirium is associated with increased morbidity, mortality, prolonged ICU, and hospital LOS. | | A | [31–35] |
| | It has also been linked to the development of post-ICU cognitive impairment in adult patients. | | B | |
| How should delirium be treated? | Atypical antipsychotics may reduce the duration of delirium in adult ICU patients. | | C | [36–38] |
| | In mechanically ventilated adult ICU patients at risk for delirium, dexmedetomidine infusions may be associated with a lower prevalence of delirium compared with benzodiazepine infusions. | | B | |
| What are some preventative strategies that can reduce the incidence of delirium? | Early mobilization of adult ICU patients has been found to reduce the incidence and duration of delirium. | | B | [39–41] |
| | The use of haloperidol or atypical antipsychotics be administered to prevent delirium in adult ICU patients is not recommended. | | C | |
| What is the impact of alcohol on the critically ill patient? | Given the high prevalence of alcohol use among trauma admission, routine screening for alcoholism is warranted. If identified, a brief intervention is warranted. | 1 | A | [42–51] |
| How is alcohol withdrawal identified, and how should it be treated? | High-quality evidence supporting the prophylactic treatment of alcohol withdrawal is lacking. Alcohol withdrawal should be treated using benzodiazepines in a symptom-driven approach, employing a validated assessment tool. | 1 | A | [54–62] |

*Sources:* Dailey, RW et al., *Am J Respir Crit Care Med*, 183, A3164, 2011; Muzyk, AJ et al., *J Neuropsychiatry Clin Neurosci*, 24, 3, 2012; Tolonen, J et al., *Eur J Emerg Med*, 20, 425, 2013; U.S. National Institutes of Health, Dexmedetomidine (Precedex®) for severe alcohol withdrawal syndrome (AWS) and alcohol withdrawal delirium (AWD). http://clinicaltrials.gov/show/NCT01362205%5D, accessed November 20, 2013.

## References


1. Cohen IL, Gallagher TJ, Pohlman AS, Dasta JF, Abraham E, Papadokos PJ. Management of the agitated intensive care unit patient. *Crit Care Med.* 2002;30(1):S97–S123.
2. Burk RS, Grap MJ, Munro CL, Schubert CM, Sessler CN. Agitation onset, frequency, and associated temporal factors in critically ill adults. *Am J Crit Care.* 2014;23(4):296–304.
3. Ely EW, Shintani A, Truman B et al. Delirium as a predictor of mortality in mechanically ventilated patients in the intensive care unit. *JAMA.* 2004;291(14): 1753–1762.
4. Woods JC, Mion LC, Connor JT et al. Severe agitation among ventilated medical intensive care unit patients: Frequency, characteristics and outcomes. *Intensive Care Med.* 2004;30(6):1066–1072.
5. Jaber S, Chanques Gr, Altairac C et al. A prospective study of agitation in a medical-surgical ICU incidence, risk factors, and outcomes. *Chest J.* 2005;128(4): 2749–2957.
6. Parker A, Raparla S, Schneck K, Bienvenu O, Needham D. A meta-analysis of post-traumatic stress disorder (ptsd) symptoms in intensive care unit survivors. *Am J Respir Crit Care Med.* 2014;189:A2534.
7. Streiner DL, Norman GR. 2008. *Health Measurement Scales: A Practical Guide to Their Development and Use.* Oxford University Press: Oxford, U.K.
8. Brandl KM, Langley KA, Riker R, Dork LA, Qualls CR, Levy H. Confirming the reliability of the sedation-agitation scale administered by ICU nurses without experience in its use. pharmacotherapy. *J Human Pharmacol Drug Ther.* 2001;21(4):431–436.
9. Sessler CN, Gosnell MS, Grap MJ et al. The Richmond Agitation–Sedation Scale: Validity and reliability in adult intensive care unit patients. *Am J Respir Crit Care Med.* 2002;166(10):1338–1344.
10. Ryder-Lewis MC, Nelson KM. Reliability of the Sedation-Agitation scale between nurses and doctors. *Intensive Crit Care Nurs.* 2008;24(4):211–217.
11. Deogaonkar A, Gupta R, DeGeorgia M et al. Bispectral index monitoring correlates with sedation scales in brain-injured patients. *Crit Care Med.* 2004;32(12):2403–2406.
12. Riker RR, Fraser GL, Simmons LE, Wilkins ML. Validating the Sedation-Agitation Scale with the Bispectral Index and Visual Analog Scale in adult ICU patients after cardiac surgery. *Intensive Care Med.* 2001;27(5):853–858.
13. Rowe K, Fletcher S. Sedation in the intensive care unit. Continuing education in anaesthesia. *Crit Care Pain.* 2008;8(2):50–55.
14. Strøm T, Martinussen T, Toft P. A protocol of no sedation for critically ill patients receiving mechanical ventilation: A randomised trial. *Lancet.* 2010;375(9713):475.
15. Reade MC, Finfer S. Sedation and delirium in the intensive care unit. *N Engl J Med.* 2014;370(5):444–454.
16. Augustes R, Ho KM. Meta-analysis of randomised controlled trials on daily sedation interruption for critically ill adult patients. *Anaesth Intensive Care.* 2011;39(3):401–409.
17. ILL C. Daily sedation interruption in mechanically ventilated critically ill patients cared for with a sedation protocol. *JAMA.* 2012;308(19):1985–1992.
18. Becker DE. Pharmacodynamic considerations for moderate and deep sedation. *AnesthProg.* 2012;59(1):28–42.
19. Kotani Y, Shimazawa M, Yoshimura S, Iwama T, Hara H. The experimental and clinical pharmacology of propofol, an anesthetic agent with neuroprotective properties. *CNS Neurosci Ther.* 2008;14(2):95–106.
20. Vanlersberghe C, Camu F. Propofol. *Handb Exp Pharmacol.* 2008(182):227–252.
21. Bhana N, Goa KL, McClellan KJ. Dexmedetomidine. *Drugs.* 2000;59(2):263–268; discussion 9–70.
22. Triltsch AE, Welte M, von Homeyer P et al. Bispectral index-guided sedation with dexmedetomidine in intensive care: A prospective, randomized, double blind, placebo-controlled phase II study. *Crit Care Med.* 2002;30(5):1007–1014.
23. Venn RM, Hell J, Michael Grounds R. Respiratory effects of dexmedetomidine in the surgical patient requiring intensive care. *Crit Care.* 2000;4(5):302–308.
24. Barr J, Fraser GL, Puntillo K et al. Clinical practice guidelines for the management of pain, agitation, and delirium in adult patients in the intensive care unit. *Crit Care Med.* 2013;41(1):263–306.
25. Fraser GL, Devlin JW, Worby CP et al. Benzodiazepine versus nonbenzodiazepine-based sedation for mechanically ventilated, critically ill adults: A systematic review and meta-analysis of randomized trials. *Crit Care Med.* 2013;41(9):S30–S38.
26. Jakob SM, Ruokonen E, Grounds RM et al. Dexmedetomidine vs midazolam or propofol for sedation during prolonged mechanical ventilation: Two randomized controlled trials. *JAMA.* 2012;307(11):1151–1160.
27. van Eijk MM, van Marum RJ, Klijn IA, de Wit N, Kesecioglu J, Slooter AJ. Comparison of delirium assessment tools in a mixed intensive care unit. *Crit Care Med.* 2009;37(6):1881–1885.
28. Neto AS, Júnior AN, Cardoso SO et al. Delirium screening in critically ill patients: A systematic review and meta-analysis. *Crit Care.* 2012;16(Suppl 1):P337.
29. Ely EW, Margolin R, Francis J et al. Evaluation of delirium in critically ill patients: Validation of the Confusion Assessment Method for the Intensive Care Unit (CAM-ICU). *Crit Care Med.* 2001;29(7):1370–1379.
30. Bergeron N, Dubois M-J, Dumont M, Dial S, Skrobik Y. Intensive Care Delirium Screening Checklist: Evaluation of a new screening tool. *Intensive Care Med.* 2001;27(5):859–864.
31. Shehabi Y, Riker R, Bokesch P, Wisemandle W, Shintani A, Ely E. SEDCOM (Safety and Efficacy of Dexmedetomidine Compared With Midazolam) Study Group: Delirium duration and mortality in lightly sedated, mechanically ventilated intensive care patients. *Crit Care Med.* 2010;38(12):2311–2318.

32. Pisani MA, Kong SYJ, Kasl SV, Murphy TE, Araujo KL, Van Ness PH. Days of delirium are associated with 1-year mortality in an older intensive care unit population. *Am J Respir Crit Care Med.* 2009;180(11):1092–1097.
33. Ouimet S, Kavanagh BP, Gottfried SB, Skrobik Y. Incidence, risk factors and consequences of ICU delirium. *Intensive Care Med.* 2007;33(1):66–73.
34. Girard TD, Jackson JC, Pandharipande PP et al. Delirium as a predictor of long-term cognitive impairment in survivors of critical illness. *Crit Care Med.* 2010; 38(7):1513.
35. MacLullich AM, Beaglehole A, Hall RJ, Meagher DJ. Delirium and long-term cognitive impairment. *Int Rev Psychiatry.* 2009;21(1):30–42.
36. Devlin JW, Roberts RJ, Fong JJ et al. Efficacy and safety of quetiapine in critically ill patients with delirium: A prospective, multicenter, randomized, double-blind, placebo-controlled pilot study. *Crit Care Med.* 2010;38(2): 419–427.
37. Riker RR, Shehabi Y, Bokesch PM et al. Dexmedetomidine vs midazolam for sedation of critically ill patients: a randomized trial. *JAMA.* 2009;301(5):489–499.
38. Gamberini M, Bolliger D, LuratiBuse GA et al. Rivastigmine for the prevention of postoperative delirium in elderly patients undergoing elective cardiac surgery—A randomized controlled trial. *Crit Care Med.* 2009;37(5):1762–1768.
39. Inouye SK, Bogardus ST, Jr., Charpentier PA et al. A multicomponent intervention to prevent delirium in hospitalized older patients. *N Engl J Med.* 1999;340(9): 669–676.
40. Schweickert WD, Pohlman MC, Pohlman AS et al. Early physical and occupational therapy in mechanically ventilated, critically ill patients: a randomised controlled trial. *Lancet.* 2009;373(9678):1874–1882.
41. Girard TD, Pandharipande PP, Carson SS et al. Feasibility, efficacy, and safety of antipsychotics for ICU delirium: The mind randomized, placebo-controlled trial. *Crit Care Med.* 2010;38(2):428–437.
42. Mukamal KJ, Kuller LH, Fitzpatrick AL, Longstreth W, Jr., Mittleman MA, Siscovick DS. Prospective study of alcohol consumption and risk of dementia in older adults. *JAMA.* 2003;289(11):1405–1413.
43. Plurad D, Demetriades D, Gruzinski G et al. Pedestrian injuries: The association of alcohol consumption with the type and severity of injuries and outcomes. *J Am Coll Surg.* 2006;202(6):919–927.
44. Abuse NIoA, Alcoholism. 2000. *10th Special Report to the US Congress on Alcohol and Health.* U.S. Department of Health and Human Services: Washington, DC.
45. Taylor B, Irving H, Kanteres F et al. The more you drink, the harder you fall: A systematic review and meta-analysis of how acute alcohol consumption and injury or collision risk increase together. *Drug Alcohol Depend.* 2010;110(1):108–116.
46. Cherpitel CJ, Ye Y, Bond J. Alcohol and injury: Multilevel analysis from the emergency room Collaborative alcohol analysis project (ercaap). *Alcohol Alcoholism.* 2004;39(6):552–558.
47. Blomqvist S, Thörne J, Elmér O, Jönsson B-A, Strand S-E, Lindahl SG. Early post-traumatic changes in hemodynamics and pulmonary ventilation in alcohol-pretreated pigs. *J Trauma Acute Care Surg.* 1987;27(1): 40–44.
48. Bilello J, McCray V, Davis J, Jackson L, Danos LA. Acute ethanol intoxication and the trauma patient: Hemodynamic pitfalls. *World J Surg.* 2011;35(9):2149–2153.
49. Messingham KAN, Faunce DE, Kovacs EJ. Review article: Alcohol, injury, and cellular immunity. *Alcohol.* 2002;28(3):137–149.
50. Moore EE. Alcohol and trauma: The perfect storm. *J Trauma.* 2005;59(3):S53–S56.
51. Davis JW, Kaups KL, Parks SN. Effect of alcohol on the utility of base deficit in trauma. *J Trauma Acute Care Surg.* 1997;43(3):507–510.
52. Gentilello LM, Ebel BE, Wickizer TM, Salkever DS, Rivara FP. Alcohol interventions for trauma patients treated in emergency departments and hospitals: A cost benefit analysis. *Ann Surg.* 2005;241(4):541.
53. Soderstrom CA, DiClemente CC, Dischinger PC et al. A controlled trial of brief intervention versus brief advice for at-risk drinking trauma center patients. *J Trauma.* 2007;62(5):1102–1112.
54. DeBellis R, Smith BS, Choi S, Malloy M. Management of delirium tremens. *J Intensive Care Med.* 2005;20(3): 164–173.
55. Dissanaike S, Halldorsson A, Frezza EE, Griswold J. An ethanol protocol to prevent alcohol withdrawal syndrome. *J Am Coll Surg.* 2006;203(2):186–191.
56. Mayo-Smith MF, Beecher LH, Fischer TL et al. Management of alcohol withdrawal delirium: An evidence-based practice guideline. *Arch Intern Med.* 2004;164(13):1405–1412.
57. Holbrook AM, Crowther R, Lotter A, Cheng C, King D. Meta-analysis of benzodiazepine use in the treatment of acute alcohol withdrawal. *Can Med Assoc J.* 1999;160(5):649–655.
58. Saitz R, Mayo-Smith MF, Roberts MS, Redmond HA, Bernard DR, Calkins DR. Individualized treatment for alcohol withdrawal: A randomized double-blind controlled trial. *JAMA.* 1994;272(7):519–523.
59. Daeppen J-B, Gache P, Landry U et al. Symptom-triggered vs fixed-schedule doses of benzodiazepine for alcohol withdrawal: A randomized treatment trial. *Arch Intern Med.* 2002;162(10):1117–1121.
60. McCowan C, Marik P. Refractory delirium tremens treated with propofol: A case series. *Crit Care Med.* 2000;28(6):1781–1784.
61. Blum K, Eubanks JD, Wallace JE, Hamilton H. Enhancement of alcohol withdrawal convulsions in mice by haloperidol. *Clin Toxicol.* 1976;9(3):427–434.
62. Lansford CD, Guerriero CH, Kocan MJ et al. Improved outcomes in patients with head and neck cancer using a standardized care protocol for postoperative alcohol withdrawal. *Arch Otolaryngol Head Neck Surg.* 2008;134(8):865–872.

## Commentary on Pain, Agitation, and Delirium in the ICU

*Kelly Vogt and Heidi L. Frankel*

It is perhaps fitting that we have been selected to comment on this excellent review of pain, agitation, and delirium in critically ill patients by Drs. Alarhayem and Keric. As one of us is somewhat long in the tooth (HF) and one of us just starting a career (KV), we truly appreciate and represent the before and after of the sea change in ICU management addressing the provision of comfort and maintenance of mobility and cognitive integrity in our patients. The senior member of our pair recalls past instances of signing out to her colleagues (we did that even then!) when, upon hearing about a brain dead patient, the partners would look out over the ICU of motionless and (iatrogenically) comatose patients and query: "Which one?" The junior author (and now the senior one as well) finds it routine to engage in conversation with most of her ICU patients, including those intubated and receiving mechanical ventilation.

In some institutions, surgeons have been late to adopt this management strategy, even positing that it is cruel to allow ICU patients to be mobile and interactive in the face of critical illness and injury and the interventions (including ventilators) required for recovery. But, as Alarhayem and Keric note, nothing could be further from the truth. In fact, the traditional approach yielded patients with longer ventilator and overall ICU stays and long-term cognitive and musculoskeletal deficits, the extent of which we are now just appreciating. This paradigm shift has been the result of significant work on the part of many intensivists, surgeons, nurses, therapists, and other health professionals, much of which is summarized in this chapter. To be clear, the contemporary approach to the care of pain, agitation, and delirium is labor-intensive for frontline providers. Much of our current understanding is addressed in the recent SCCM guidelines for the general ICU population* and in a review of the Surgical ICU population specifically.†

So what does the surgeon really need to know about pain, agitation, and delirium in the ICU?

* Barr J, Fraser GL, Puntillo K et al. Clinical practice guidelines for the management of pain, agitation and delirium in adult patients in the intensive care unit. *Crit Care Med.* 2013;41(1):263–306.

† Vogt KN, Frankel HL. Maintaining comfort, cognitive function and mobility in surgical ICU patients. *J Trauma Acute Care Surg.* 2014;77(2):364–375.

### The Need to Look for the Problem

You cannot identify a problem if you do not search for it, and you cannot manage a problem that you have not identified. The fact that we are routinely assessing the need for sedation and pain management is a major advancement in the care of our SICU patients. While any reproducible method is good, there are reliable, valid, and reproducible scales for both sedation and pain that should be used consistently in the SICU. While some of these scales can be complex, it is important to remember that it may be as simple as asking the awake and interactive patient if he or she is having pain—believe us, he or she will tell you! Finally, daily assessments for the presence of delirium, and recognition that patients are more likely to present with the hypoactive form of this disease, will help to identify patients early in their course, so that corrective measures may be instituted to reduce the negative consequences associated with this iatrogenic complication. Most ICUs screen adequately for pain and agitation, particularly with the regulatory demands for the former, but are less successful in the realm of delirium. It is difficult to appreciate that the withdrawn, but docile, ICU patient could be delirious and at a greater risk for long-term harm than the hallucinatory, "difficult" patient with hyperactive delirium.

### What Is the Best Management Strategy for Pain and Sedation in the SICU?

The management of sedation and pain in the SICU has undergone a revolution. From the historical strategy of maximum sedation, up to and including paralysis, and pain management largely as an afterthought, we have evolved to the recommended strategy of analgesia-based sedation. This so-called analgesiosedation is achieved by first adequately controlling that patient's pain and agitation using a combination of pharmacologic (opioid- and nonopioid-based regimens) and nonpharmacologic (reorientation, noise reduction, music, pet therapy) strategies. Once pain and agitation are adequately controlled, many patients will not require further sedation. In patients who do require additional agents, a nonbenzodiazepine-based sedation regimen, using agents such as dexmedetomidine or propofol, should be chosen to achieve light to moderate sedation. The use of these agents can be expected to minimize the duration of mechanical ventilation and ICU length of stay, and to reduce the incidence of delirium that is nearly universal with the use of benzodiazepines. No matter what agent is used, patients should be maintained on as little sedation as possible for as short a time as possible, as heavier and longer-term use results in worse cognitive and overall outcome. Paradoxically, in patients undergoing alcohol withdrawal who display delirium, benzodiazepines remain the therapeutic agent of choice, although practitioners are now using other medications as well.

### How Should We Prevent the Development of Problems?

In addition to the use of frequent assessments for pain, agitation, and delirium, and management of these conditions if they are present, additional preventative strategies have been used successfully to improve patient outcomes in the SICU. One of the most important is early mobilization of SICU patients. Of course, ambulation of mechanically ventilated patients poses many logistic challenges and the need for dedicated personnel. Other strategies, including noise regulation and patient-directed music through noise cancelling headphones, have also shown benefit in the prevention of delirium. Maintaining a sense of normalcy in the decidedly abnormal environment of the SICU is the key to preventing the development of delirium—in fact, no pharmacologic agent has proved successful instead.

### How Should We Manage Delirium Once We Identify It?

If appropriately managing pain and agitation and instituting prophylactic measures are not sufficient to prevent the development of delirium, treatment should be aimed at minimizing additional risks and shortening the course of the delirium episode. Any previously neglected prophylactic strategies should be added, and attempts made to restore the patient's orientation and sleep–wake cycle. The use of atypical antipsychotics may help to shorten the duration of the delirium episode; however, more work is needed to identify novel strategies to manage delirium once it develops. Reliance on old-school sedation strategies yields nearly universal delirium. This results in increased ICU and hospital length of stay, short- and long-term cognitive deficits that may persist as long as 5 years, posttraumatic stress disorder, and even increased mortality.

# 81

# Malignant Hypertension: An Evidence-Based Surgery Review

**Marshall A. Corson and David S. Owens**

CONTENTS



## 81.1 Introduction

Hypertension is a common but incompletely understood disorder that may result in injury, either acute or chronic, to the end organs exposed to elevated blood pressure (BP). It is a particularly menacing problem in the perioperative period due to increased catecholamine states related to anxiety or pain, the frequent inability to take oral medications, and the potential effects of anesthetic agents. Preexisting hypertension is the largest risk factor for postoperative hypertension [1,2], and longstanding preexisting hypertension can complicate perioperative clinical management due to coexistent left ventricular hypertrophy, heart failure, chronic kidney disease, and cerebrovascular or coronary vascular stenoses. In this chapter, we will provide an evidence-based review of the management of hypertension in the perioperative period, with particular attention to the management of accelerated malignant hypertension, in which an acute elevation in BP raises the risk of life-threatening end-organ injury. The management of intraoperative hypertension will not be addressed.

## 81.2 What Is the Optimal Target BP for Chronic Therapy?

There is a vast body of literature informing the management of chronic hypertension, which has been summarized in detail in the Seventh Report of the Joint National Committee (JNC 7) on the Prevention, Evaluation and Treatment of High Blood Pressure [3]. Although epidemiologic studies have suggested that the risk of clinical events increases at BP levels above 115/75 mmHg [4], recent well-powered clinical trials have not demonstrated further reduction of death, myocardial infarction, and stroke in most patients with more aggressive therapeutic lowering of systolic BP (SBP) to <140 mmHg and diastolic BP (DBP) to <90 mmHg [5]. Consistent with observational data that BP increases as the population ages, several trials enrolling older individuals with predominant systolic hypertension have shown that SBP lowering to the mid-140s mmHg is sufficient to reduce cardiovascular complications. The most recent JNC 8 guidelines endorse targets of SBP <150 mmHg and DBP <90 mmHg for individuals ≥60 years of age, and these guidelines maintained targets of SBP <140 mmHg and DBP <90 mmHg for most others [5]. Preferred classes of therapy for patients with hypertension, including those with diabetes, are thiazide-like diuretics, calcium channel blockers (CCB) and either angiotensin-converting enzyme inhibitors (ACE-I) or angiotensin receptor blockers (ARB). Upward titration using combinations of diuretic, CCB, and ACE-I or ARB is encouraged prior to the addition of other classes, such as beta-blockers [5].

*Recommendations*: Optimal management of chronic hypertension includes adherence to lifestyle measures, self-monitoring, and pharmacotherapy to maintain SBP <140 mmHg and DBP <90 mmHg in the general population, with goals of SBP <150 mmHg and DBP <90 mmHg for individuals over 60 years of age.

## 81.3 How Should Preexisting Hypertension Be Managed in the Perioperative Setting?

Preexisting hypertension raises the risk for intraoperative hemodynamic instability [4–7] and perioperative events [6–8], and preoperative BP elevation may prompt consideration of postponing surgery to allow for intensification of therapy [2,4,8,9]. In a meta-analysis of 30 trials, Howell et al. found that the odds ratio for the association between established hypertension and adverse perioperative cardiac outcomes was 1.35 (95% confidence interval: 1.17–1.56), but there was little evidence for an association between preoperative SBP <180 mmHg or DBP <110 mmHg and perioperative complications [7]. Asymptomatic patients with higher presenting BPs may be more prone to ischemia, arrhythmias, and cardiovascular instability, but there is no clear evidence indicating that deferring surgery reduces the risk of such complications [9].

The 2007 American Heart Association guidelines on preoperative risk stratification for noncardiac surgeries [10] recommended that for patients with advanced elevation of BP (SBP >180 mmHg and/or DBP >110 mmHg), the risks of perioperative clinical events should be weighed against the risks in delaying surgery, and the surgery should potentially postponed to allow more optimal BP control [10,11]. However, the updated 2014 version of these guidelines no longer addresses the triage of such patients, potentially reflecting less focus on absolute level of BP elevation in clinical decision-making and more on co-morbidities and functional status [11].

In patients with preexisting hypertension, antihypertensive therapy should be continued throughout the perioperative period as tolerated. This is especially important for beta-blockers and alpha-blockers (e.g., clonidine), in which abrupt discontinuation can cause rebound tachycardia and hypertension. Although the benefits of routine preoperative use of beta-blockers for high-risk patients has recently been called into question [11], discontinuation of beta-blockers has been shown to significantly increase perioperative cardiovascular events and 1-year mortality [12]. If the patient is unable to take oral medications, similar-acting parental or transcutaneous alternatives are available [13]. Data from observational studies and a single randomized trial suggest ACE-inhibitor or angiotensin-blocking agents may be associated with intraoperative hypotension, leading some authors to recommend they be held prior to surgery and restarted postoperatively [14]. However, holding these medications has not been convincingly shown to improve clinical outcomes, in cardiothoracic [15] or general [16] surgery patients.

*Recommendations*: Antihypertensive therapy should be continued preoperatively, and throughout the perioperative period, using parenteral or transcutaneous alternatives if needed. This recommendation is strongest for patients on alpha- and beta-blockers. It is generally not necessary to postpone surgery for patients with asymptomatic elevation of SBP to <180 mmHg and/or DBP to <110 mmHg.

## 81.4 What Is the Threshold for Pharmacologic Treatment of Elevated BP Preoperatively?

*Hypertensive urgency* or accelerated hypertension is defined as a resting SBP >180 mmHg and/or DBP >110 mmHg in the absence of signs or symptoms of end-organ dysfunction [3]. After verification that the BP is elevated, the next step is the identification of potentially reversible causes of hypertension. Pain, anxiety, agitation (e.g., emergence from anesthesia), hypercarbia, hypoxia, hypovolemia or hypervolemia, and other irritants (e.g., bladder distention) can all increase sympathetic tone and are frequent causes of perioperative hypertension [9]. These causes should be considered and addressed prior to the initiation of antihypertensive therapy. While perioperative patients with hypertensive urgency merit consideration for pharmacologic intervention, it must be kept in mind that chronic hypertension can perturb normal cerebral or coronary arterial autoregulation, which normally protects vital organs by maintaining perfusion at constant levels within a BP range of 20–30 mmHg. In patients with preexisting hypertension and altered autoregulation, overly rapid reduction in BP may precipitate ischemic events. Thus, when preoperative SBP is elevated to >180 mmHg or DBP to >110, in the absence of signs or symptoms of end-organ compromise, pharmacologic therapy should be given with the goal to reduce ~BP 20%, or to below 160/100 mmHg, over several hours to days, with a time frame appropriate to the clinical context [13,17].

Severely elevated SBP or DBP may also cause acute dysfunction of multiple organs, including the brain (encephalopathy, hemorrhage, or stroke), heart (myocardial infarction or heart failure), kidneys (acute renal failure), or vasculature (aortic dissection). Severe hypertension with the presence of any of these signs or symptoms is referred to as *hypertensive emergency*, or accelerated malignant hypertension [3] and requires prompt therapy. If patients have signs or symptoms of end-organ compromise, more immediate therapy is justified, as outlined later in the text.

*Recommendations*: Elevation of SBP to >180 mmHg and/or DBP to >110 mmHg, or an acute increase by >15%–20% over prior baseline in the absence of organ dysfunction, merits pharmacologic intervention. BP should be lowered ~20% or to a target of <160 and <100 mmHg with a time frame appropriate for the clinical context, typically over hours.

## 81.5 What Are the Clinical Implications of Acute Postoperative Hypertension (APH)?

APH is broadly defined as a significant elevation in BP in the immediate postoperative period, and can be associated with severe clinical sequelae including strokes, intracranial hemorrhage, myocardial ischemia, heart failure, acute renal failure, and surgical anastomotic or site complications [18]. BP typically becomes elevated less than 2 h postoperatively, remaining elevated for several hours, although persistent BP elevation for up to 48 h has been reported. APH is believed to be caused by adrenergic stimulation, with significant elevations in plasma catecholamine levels, resulting in vasoconstriction and elevation in systemic vascular resistance. Anesthetic and procedural factors may influence the incidence of APH, which may complicate as many as 50% of surgical procedures [19] and is most common following cardiovascular, neurosurgical, abdominal aortic, and head and neck surgeries [18].

The link between APH and postoperative complications has been most clearly defined for cardiovascular surgeries [8,20], wherein a threshold BP of 140/90 mmHg or a mean arterial BP of 105 mmHg have often been used for initiation of parenteral therapy. A recent prospective analysis of the relationship between BP and mortality risk in the ECLIPSE Trials (a comparison of four first-line parenteral agents in the control of perioperative BP in cardiac surgery patients) demonstrated a linear relationship between time with SBP outside the range of 75–135 mmHg intraoperatively, or time with SBP outside the range of 85–145 mmHg pre- or postoperatively, and attendant mortality risk [20].

For noncardiovascular postoperative patients with APH, an SBP >160 and/or DBP >90 mmHg, mean arterial pressure (MAP) >110 mmHg, or a relative 20% increase in SBP or DBP compared to preoperative levels have all been used in clinical trials as thresholds for intervention. In a population of 254 noncardiac surgery patients with elevated risk due to a high prevalence of diabetes and/or hypertension, two patterns of intraoperative BP predicted postoperative complications, namely, >1 h of ≥20 mmHg decrease in MAP, or <1 h of ≥20 mmHg decrease in MAP with >15 min of ≥20 mmHg increase in MAP. Interestingly, the overall mean intraoperative MAP was not a significant predictor of complications [21]. Together, these findings should reorient the treating clinician to consider not only the patient's absolute BP level but also the prior ambient BP levels in the decision to initiate therapy. Given that the risk increases with such short-term BP deviations, the value of rapidly acting, titratable, and parenteral agents is intrinsically increased.

*Recommendations*: APH may be associated with adverse clinical outcomes, and in postcardiac surgery patients, it should be treated to maintain SBP <140 and DBP <90 mmHg; for other postoperative patients, the goal should be to maintain BP at or near the prior baseline levels. For perioperative patients with severe BP elevation and impending or evident organ dysfunction, parenteral therapy is indicated to achieve a 10%–15% reduction over the first hour with continued reduction toward SBP <160 and DBP <100 mmHg over the next 2–6 h as tolerated by the patient [22]. In all cases, it is critical for outcome to avoid wide swings in BP.

## 81.6 What Are the Best Therapies for APH?

Choice of agent should be made with consideration of the patient's current and preoperative BPs, the presence and severity of comorbidities, the type of surgery performed, and an evaluation of the risk of surgical complications. Because APH is a short-lived process with often rapidly fluctuating BPs, the ideal pharmacologic treatments are fast-acting and possess short half-lives to allow rapid titration to effect. Adverse outcomes are not only linked to the absolute levels of BP deviation but also to rapid BP fluctuations and the presence of an elevated pulse pressure [20]. Evidence supports the use of the following classes of parenteral antihypertensive agents: nitrovasodilators (nitroglycerin and nitroprusside), adrenergic antagonists (esmolol and labetalol), CCBs (clevidipine and nicardipine), and the dopamine-type 1 receptor blocker fenoldopam. There are no placebo-controlled trials demonstrating improvement in clinical outcomes, and only limited data comparing the effectiveness of different agents in lowering BP are available.

1. *Sodium nitroprusside*: Sodium nitroprusside is a very potent and rapidly acting, direct arterial vasodilator. It has been used for decades in postoperative patients requiring rapid BP lowering, before the availability of alternative short-acting potent agents. Nitroprusside has a number of major adverse effects including hypotension,

reflex tachycardia, myocardial ischemia, intrapulmonary shunting (from reversal of physiologic hypoxemic vasoconstriction), decreased cerebral blood flow with increased intracerebral pressures, and the potential for cyanide toxicity. It is contraindicated in patients with myocardial ischemia, encephalopathy, acute cerebrovascular accident (CVA), and liver or renal failure. When sodium nitroprusside is used, intra-arterial BP monitoring and thiocyanate surveillance are recommended.

Sodium nitroprusside has been shown to be effective in treating APH following both cardiovascular and noncardiac surgeries, with the vast majority of patients achieving target BPs. It has been shown to achieve equal BP lowering as nitroglycerin, labetalol, esmolol, fenoldopam, and nicardipine [23]. However, because of its potential for serious adverse end-organ effects, the use of sodium nitroprusside should be limited to situations where these risks are justified, such as the treatment of accelerated malignant hypertension following cardiac surgery.

2. *Nitroglycerin*: Intravenous nitroglycerin is predominantly a venodilator, which results in a reduction in myocardial preload; it produces limited direct arterial or coronary vasodilation. Advantages of using nitroglycerin include a quick onset of action, a short half-life, a reduction in pulmonary vascular resistance, and a reduction in myocardial oxygen demand. Potential disadvantages include tachyphylaxis (occurs after 48–72 h, not usually limiting in APH treatment), reflex tachycardia, headaches (which often limit dosing), and a reduction in cardiac output in patients that are preload-dependent.

   Intravenous nitroglycerin has been shown to be effective in treating APH following cardiac surgery [24–26], but has not been as extensively investigated after neurosurgical, head and neck, or other noncardiac procedures. Several trials have compared its efficacy against sodium nitroprusside [23] and suggest equivalent BP control, although nitroglycerin treatment has been associated with lower cardiac filling pressures and better arterial oxygenation.

3. *Labetalol*: Labetalol is a nonselective beta-adrenergic receptor antagonist which also offers partial antagonism of alpha adrenergic receptors. It thus acts as a myocardial depressant, with both negative inotropic and chronotropic effects, and as a direct vasodilator. When given parenterally, it has a short onset of action, but a 3–6 h duration of effect. Advantages of labetalol include reducing myocardial oxygen demand and lack of effect on cerebral perfusion and intracerebral pressures. It is, therefore, a good treatment option for patients with myocardial ischemia or following neurosurgical procedures. It is contraindicated in patients with heart failure, low cardiac output, severe bronchospasm, bradycardia, or impaired atrioventricular nodal conduction.

   Labetalol is a widely studied treatment for APH, and has proven efficacy following cardiovascular [27], neurologic [28], carotid endarterectomies [29], and other general surgeries [30]. It has been tested against sodium nitroprusside and esmolol, and found to be equally efficacious in lowering BP.

4. *Esmolol*: Esmolol is a specific beta-1 adrenergic antagonist, which lowers BP by decreasing heart rate and myocardial contractility, with little effect on systemic vascular resistance. In addition to its more focused effects, it has a very rapid onset of action and a very short half-life, as it is metabolized intravascularly by red blood cell esterase. Advantages and contraindications for esmolol are similar to labetalol, although with less potential for pulmonary bronchospasm and with more rapid clearance.

   Esmolol would appear to be an ideal agent for the management of APH, and it has been studied following cardiac [31] and neurologic [32,33], surgeries and following repair of aortic coarctations [34]. Two recent meta-analyses compared the use of esmolol versus placebo or comparator agents following cardiac surgery (20 trials with $N = 778$ patients) [35] and noncardiac surgery (32 trials with $N = 1765$ patients) [36]; esmolol was associated with significant reductions in myocardial ischemia in all patients and arrhythmias in cardiac surgery patients, with a trend toward reduction in myocardial infarction. This evidence base supports the first-line use of esmolol, especially in patients after cardiovascular surgery.

5. *Nicardipine*: Nicardipine is a parenteral dihydropyridine CCB whose primary mechanism of action is arterial vasodilation, with limited direct effects on cardiac function. Importantly, it has direct coronary and cerebral vasodilating effects, and results in an improvement in myocardial perfusion and metabolism. Potential adverse effects include reflex tachycardia, hypotension, nausea and vomiting [37], and a 2–6 h duration of action, depending on dose administered [9].

   Nicardipine has been well-studied for the treatment of APH, including randomized, placebo-controlled trials [37], with proven efficacy following cardiovascular [38] and other procedures [37,39]. Most of these studies show that less dose titration is needed with nicardipine compared with nitroprusside, esmolol, and labetalol, with variable effects on heart rate [23].

6. *Clevidipine*: Clevidipine is an ultra-short-acting third-generation dihydropyridine CCB, recently approved for the parenteral treatment of hypertension. Its advantages include reduction of BP via a direct effect on arterioles without affecting venous preload, achieving ~15% reduction in SBP with intravenous infusion (no bolus) in 5–6 min, with low frequency of "overshoot" hypotension. No tolerance to clevidipine has been reported, reversal of its BP lowering effect within 5–15 min after discontinuation should be expected, and there are no interactions with hepatic CYP-450 enzyme systems at therapeutic concentrations. At medium to higher doses of clevidipine (>1.5 mcg/kg/min), stroke volume is increased, in conjunction with a modest increase in heart rate [40].

   Three prospective random open-label multicenter trials compared clevidipine with nitroglycerin or nitroprusside perioperatively in 1125 patients, or with nicardipine in 381 postoperative patients, undergoing cardiac surgery [41]. There were no differences in the incidence of myocardial infarction, stroke, or renal dysfunction among any of the treatment groups and no difference in mortality rates between clevidipine- and nitroglycerin- or nicardipine-treated subjects. Although the trial was not powered to detect a mortality difference, mortality was significantly higher in nitroprusside-treated subjects compared with clevidipine-treated subjects. Clevidipine was more effective than nitroglycerin or nitroprusside in keeping BP within a prespecified range during the treatment period and equivalent to nicardipine in this regard. However, when the target BP range was narrowed, clevidipine was associated with fewer BP deviations beyond these limits when compared with nicardipine. The ECLIPSE trials provide the most highly powered and methodologically sound comparison of the nitrovasodilators and parenteral CCBs in cardiac surgery patients.

7. *Fenoldopam*: Fenoldopam is a potent agonist of peripheral dopamine type-1 receptors that is Food and Drug Administration-approved for the treatment of acute hypertension. Its quick onset of action, short half-life, and potential for increasing renal perfusion, glomerular filtration rate, and natriuresis make it an attractive choice in the treatment of APH [42]. Potential adverse effects of fenoldopam include hypotension, reflex tachycardia, headache, dizziness, and increased intraocular pressure. Its use should be avoided in patients with or at risk for glaucoma, intracranial hypertension, and sulfite sensitivity (due to sodium metabisulfate in its solution) [22].

   Fenoldopam has been shown to be an effective treatment of severe hypertension, with improved renal perfusion compared to nitroprusside [43]. A systematic review of randomized placebo-controlled trials of postoperative or intensive care patients ($N$ = 1290 patients in 16 studies) demonstrated that fenoldopam consistently and significantly reduced the risk of acute kidney injury and the need for renal replacement therapy [44]. Trials with active comparator agent(s) in postoperative patients are lacking.

8. *Nonrecommended agents*: Although nifedipine has been administered transmucosally for rapid effect in advanced stage hypertension, these delivery methods have been shown to result in unpredictable BP responses, including severe hypotension [45]. Hydralazine is another agent that has been utilized for parenteral BP lowering, but it may have prolonged and unpredictable effects, limiting the ability to effectively titrate its hypotensive effect [22]. Consequently, nifedipine and hydralazine are no longer recommended as the treatment for acute hypertension.

*Recommendations*: Sodium nitroprusside, nitroglycerin, labetalol, esmolol, nicardipine, clevidipine, and fenoldopam have been shown to be effective in the treatment of postoperative hypertension (Table 81.1). The choice of pharmacologic agent(s) should be primarily guided by consideration of patient physiologic conditions and co-morbidities.

## 81.7 What Signs and Symptoms Suggest End-Organ Compromise Due to Acute Hypertension?

Severe hypertension can result in rapid end-organ deterioration, especially when the hypertension develops acutely. APH has been associated with adverse clinical events including encephalopathy, hemorrhagic and ischemic CVAs, myocardial ischemia and infarction, congestive heart failure, aortic dissection, acute renal failure, and surgical site or anastomotic complications.

**TABLE 81.1**

Levels of Evidence for the Use of Specific Pharmacologic Agents in the Treatment of APH

| | Type of Surgery | | | |
|---|---|---|---|---|
| | Cardiovascular | Neurologic | Head and Neck | General |
| Esmolol | 1b | 1b | 5 | 2b |
| Labetalol | 2a | 2a | 2b | 2b |
| Clevidipine | 1b | 2b | 5 | 5 |
| Nicardipine | 2a | 1b | 1b | 1b |
| Nitroprusside | 2b | 5[a] | 2b | 2b |
| Nitroglycerin | 2a | 2b | 2b | 2b |
| Fenoldopam | 2b | 5 | 5 | 1b |

[a] May cause potential harm.

Symptoms of end-organ damage are often masked in the postoperative period due to sedation, analgesia, and impaired levels of consciousness, and severe hypertension may cause a physiologic response to myocardial ischemia, stroke, or increased intracranial pressure. Thus, it is imperative that all patients with significant postoperative hypertension undergo a complete physical examination aimed at determining whether there is impairment in end-organ function.

The rate of change in BP is an important factor in the development of end-organ dysfunction due to limits of autoregulation. Thus, hypertensive urgencies may be more common perioperatively, when hypertensive stimuli are frequently present and BP is more labile. In conscious patients, the most common symptoms of end-organ dysfunction include chest pain, dyspnea, impaired cognition, and headache. Focal stroke-like symptoms cannot be singly attributed to hypertension, and a complete neurologic evaluation is warranted. Signs of end-organ compromise may include pulmonary rales, cardiac murmurs or gallops, ischemic ECG changes, impaired cognition, decreased urine output with hematuria or proteinuria, or papillary edema on fundoscopic examination.

*Recommendation*: Patients with APH merit full evaluation, with attention to signs and symptoms of end-organ (i.e., brain, heart, lung, kidney, and vasculature) involvement. Patients with end-organ involvement should receive prompt therapy targeted at relieving and preventing further end-organ injury.

## 81.8 What Are the Best Pharmacologic Therapies for Management of Acute Hypertension in the Setting of Complicating Conditions?

When signs or symptoms of end-organ involvement are present, prompt treatment of severe hypertension is necessary, and dictated by the clinical syndrome. There is limited clinical trial evidence for the utility of particular pharmacologic agents in given clinical circumstances, especially in the postoperative setting. Thus, the following recommendations are based primarily on knowledge regarding the physiologic effects of the medications and, when available, studies of hypertensive emergency in the nonperioperative setting.

1. *Encephalopathy*: Hypertensive encephalopathy is generally due to the development of cerebral edema [46], and generally manifests as symptoms of nausea, vomiting, headache, or impairment in cognition, although more severe symptoms such as seizure and coma can occur if untreated. If encephalopathy is suspected, computed tomography should be performed to exclude hemorrhage or stroke, as the appropriate level of BP lowering is specific in these more complicated situations. The goal of therapy should be to reduce BP by 20%–25% within the first 2–6 h, aiming for a DBP of 100–105 mmHg [46]. There is no particular agent of choice for the treatment of hypertensive encephalopathy, although sodium nitroprusside should be avoided due to the possibility of increased cerebral pressure and decreased cerebral perfusion.
2. *Stroke*: CVAs often cause a severe reflex elevation in BP, making it difficult to determine whether the CVA or the hypertension is the primary inciting event. This hypertension generally declines within 24 h of the inciting event, and aggressive lowering of BP may result in worse clinical outcomes. The current American Stroke Association and American Heart Association guidelines recommend therapy if BP is severely elevated (SBP >220 or DBP >120 mmHg), if thrombolysis is planned and SBP is >185 or DBP >110 mmHg, or if the hypertension is causing impairment of other organs [47]. In these situations, BP should be lowered incrementally, aiming for an initial

15% reduction in BP followed by clinical reassessment. The guideline-recommended pharmacologic treatment options include labetalol or nicardipine, which have been shown to be effective following both ischemia and hemorrhagic CVAs. Guideline-recommended treatment of hypertension following hemorrhagic CVA is slightly more complex and dependent on whether intracerebral pressure is elevated [48]. It is recommended that neurologic or neurosurgical consultation be obtained for all suspected CVAs.

3. *Myocardial ischemia*: Severe hypertension results in an increase in myocardial wall stress, the principle determinant of myocardial oxygen consumption. In the presence of obstructive lesions in the coronary arteries, this increase in oxygen demand may outstretch the supply of oxygen, resulting in endocardial ischemia, which manifests as ST segment depression on ECG. If untreated, this may result in a non-ST segment elevation myocardial infarction. Beta-blockers and nitroglycerin (sublingual or intravenous) are the cornerstones of therapy in this situation, which will reduce myocardial oxygen demands by reducing heart rate, contractility, and preload (thus reducing wall stress).

   It is crucially important that all patients with perioperative chest pain have an ECG to exclude the presence of ST segment elevation, which indicates a distinct, more severe pathologic mechanism of coronary plaque rupture and *in situ* thrombosis that requires treatment with percutaneous coronary intervention. The increased catecholamines and inflammation seen postoperatively predispose to plaque rupture, which, in turn, may cause reflex hypertension. Importantly, a high percentage of plaques causing ST-segment elevation myocardial infarctions are initially nonobstructive and would not be identified on preoperative stress testing.

4. *Heart failure*: Severe hypertension can cause an increase in intracardiac pressures, which are then transmitted back into the pulmonary

**TABLE 81.2**

Key Points in Management of Peri-Operative Hypertension

| Question | Summary Recommendation | LOE | Grade | References |
|---|---|---|---|---|
| What is the optimal target BP for chronic therapy? | Current care guidelines recommend SBP <140 and DBP <90 mmHg in the general population aged <60 years and SBP <150 and DBP <90 mmHg if ≥60 years old. | 1a | A | [3,5] |
| How should preexisting hypertension be managed in the perioperative setting? | Antihypertensive therapies should be continued throughout the perioperative period; it is generally not necessary to delay or postpone surgery in asymptomatic patients with SBP <180 and DBP <110 mmHg. | 1b | B | [3,10–12,14–16] |
| What is the threshold for pharmacologic treatment of elevated BP preoperatively? | Further elevation beyond SBP >180 or DBP >110 or increase to >15%–20% of prior baseline merits pharmacologic treatment. BP should be lowered with a time frame appropriate to the clinical context, ideally over the course of hours, to targets SBP <160 and DBP <100 mmHg, or to near prior baseline. | 1b | B | [9,17,20,21] |
| What are the clinical and treatment implications of APH? | APH increases the risk for adverse outcomes, and therapy with a rapidly acting titratable agent is indicated to maintain SBP <140 and DBP <90 mmHg following cardiac surgeries, and at or near prior baseline BP after noncardiac surgeries; in the presence of evolving/evident end-organ dysfunction, therapy should be more rapid. In all cases, strive to avoid prolonged BP swings. | 1a | B | [1,2,6,8,19] |
| What are the best therapies for APH? | Agents shown to be equally efficacious at lowering BP acutely include adrenergic antagonists (esmolol/labetalol), CCBs (clevidipine/nicardipine), nitrovasodilators (sodium nitroprusside/nitroglycerin), and a dopamine antagonist (fenoldopam). | 1b | A | [18,22–34,38–40,42,43,45] |
| What signs and symptoms suggest end-organ compromise due to malignant hypertension? | Encephalopathy, CVAs, myocardial ischemia and infarction, acute pulmonary edema, aortic dissection, acute renal failure, or anastomotic complications; these signs may be masked in the perioperative period and should be aggressively sought and treated promptly. | — | — | [11,47,48] |
| What are the best therapies for management of acute hypertension in the presence of complicating conditions? | Society guidelines for treatment of acute stroke and coronary syndromes should guide therapy for these conditions when co-existent (LOE 1a); esmolol or labetalol are first-line therapy for aortic dissection, these agents or CCB for encephalopathy (LOE 1b). Choice of therapy should be tailored to clinical context and patient condition. | | B | [35,36,44,46,49,50] |

vasculature, resulting in pulmonary edema. This may be due to myocardial ischemia, resulting in impaired cardiac systolic function, but may also be seen in the absence of ischemia in patients with impaired baseline systolic function, diastolic dysfunction, or valvular regurgitation. Transthoracic echocardiography can identify contributing factors and guide therapy. The treatment of systolic heart failure primarily involves a reduction of systemic vascular resistance using vasodilators [49], while beta-blockers and nondihyropyridine CCB should be withheld in the absence of myocardial ischemia or arrhythmias owing to their suppressive effects on cardiac contractility. Nitroprusside is a good initial treatment option that can interrupt the cycle of hypertension causing heart failure, which increases catecholamines and BP. Nitroglycerin may also be beneficial, as it can also increase venous capacitance and reduce preload. If the primary mechanism of heart failure is diastolic dysfunction, treatment should be directed at reducing BP and slowing heart rate to allow increased diastolic filling. Together with diuretics, beta-blockers and/or CCB are the preferred agents of choice in this setting.

5. *Aortic dissection*: Aortic dissection should be considered in all patients with chest discomfort, especially if they have a prior history of hypertension, aortic valve pathology, or Marfan syndrome. Given the high early mortality associated with aortic dissection, prompt diagnosis and treatment can be lifesaving [50]. Medical therapy, primarily involving heart rate lowering in conjunction with BP control, is the recommended treatment for Type B (descending aorta) and in the acute, preoperative management of Type A (ascending aorta) dissections. The aim of medical therapy is to reduce aortic wall stress and thus minimize further dissection. Esmolol is recommended as the initial pharmacologic therapy, due to its rapid pharmacokinetics, although treatment with other parenteral or oral beta-blockers may be substituted as clinical condition stabilizes. Vasodilators such as sodium nitroprusside are not the preferred agents, as they may cause reflex tachycardia and a compensatory increase in cardiac contractility and aortic wall stress (Table 81.2).

*Recommendations*: Society guidelines for treatment of acute stroke and coronary syndromes should guide therapy for these conditions when co-existent; esmolol or labetalol are first-line therapy for aortic dissection and adrenergic antagonists or CCB for encephalopathy. Choice of therapy should be tailored to clinical context and patient condition.

## References

1. Gal TJ, Cooperman LH. Hypertension in the immediate postoperative period. *Br J Anaesth*. 1975;47:70–74.
2. Towne JB, Bernhard VM. The relationship of postoperative hypertension to complications following carotid endarterectomy. *Surgery*. 1980;88:575–580.
3. Chobanian AV, Bakris GL, Black HR et al. The Seventh Report of the Joint National Committee on prevention, detection, evaluation, and treatment of high blood pressure: The JNC 7 report. *JAMA*. 2003;289:2560–2572.
4. Lewington S, Clarke R, Qizilbash N et al. Age-specific relevance of usual blood pressure to vascular mortality: A meta-analysis of individual data for one million adults in 61 prospective studies. *Lancet*. 2002;360:1903–1913.
5. James PA, Oparil S, Carter BL et al. 2014 evidence-based guideline for the management of high blood pressure in adults: Report from the panel members appointed to the Eighth Joint National Committee (JNC 8). *JAMA*. 2014;311:507–520.
6. Prys-Roberts C, Meloche R, Foex P. Studies of anaesthesia in relation to hypertension. I. Cardiovascular responses of treated and untreated patients. *Br J Anaesth*. 1971;43:122–137.
7. Howell SJ, Sear JW, Foex P. Hypertension, hypertensive heart disease and perioperative cardiac risk. *Br J Anaesth*. 2004;92:570–583.
8. Aronson S, Boisvert D, Lapp W. Isolated systolic hypertension is associated with adverse outcomes from coronary artery bypass grafting surgery. *Anesth Analg*. 2002;94:1079–1084, Table of Contents.
9. Lonjaret L, Lairez O, Minville V, Geeraerts T. Optimal perioperative management of arterial blood pressure. *Integr Blood Press Control*. 2014;7:49–59.
10. Fleisher LA, Beckman JA, Brown KA et al. ACC/AHA 2007 guidelines on perioperative cardiovascular evaluation and care for noncardiac surgery: Executive summary: A report of the American College of Cardiology/American Heart Association Task Force on Practice Guidelines. *Circulation*. 2007;116:1971–1996.
11. Fleisher LA, Fleischmann KE, Auerbach AD et al. 2014 ACC/AHA guideline on perioperative cardiovascular evaluation and management of patients undergoing noncardiac surgery: A report of the American College of Cardiology/American Heart Association Task Force on Practice Guidelines. *Circulation*. 2014;130:2215–2245.
12. Hoeks SE, Scholte Op Reimer WJ, van Urk H et al. Increase of 1-year mortality after perioperative beta-blocker withdrawal in endovascular and vascular surgery patients. *Eur J Vasc Endovasc Surg*. 2007;33:13–19.
13. Ahuja K, Charap MH. Management of perioperative hypertensive urgencies with parenteral medications. *J Hosp Med*. 2010;5:E11–E16.

14. Comfere T, Sprung J, Kumar MM et al. Angiotensin system inhibitors in a general surgical population. *Anesth Analg.* 2005;100:636–644, Table of Contents.
15. Drenger B, Fontes ML, Miao Y et al. Patterns of use of perioperative angiotensin-converting enzyme inhibitors in coronary artery bypass graft surgery with cardiopulmonary bypass: Effects on in-hospital morbidity and mortality. *Circulation.* 2012;126:261–269.
16. Turan A, You J, Shiba A et al. Angiotensin converting enzyme inhibitors are not associated with respiratory complications or mortality after noncardiac surgery. *Anesth Analg.* 2012;114:552–560.
17. Marik PE, Varon J. Hypertensive crises: Challenges and management. *Chest.* 2007;131:1949–1962.
18. Haas CE, LeBlanc JM. Acute postoperative hypertension: A review of therapeutic options. *Am J Health Syst Pharm.* 2004;61:1661–1673; quiz 1674–1675.
19. Aronson S, Varon J. Hemodynamic control and clinical outcomes in the perioperative setting. *J Cardiothorac Vasc Anesth.* 2011;25:509–525.
20. Aronson S, Dyke CM, Levy JH et al. Does perioperative systolic blood pressure variability predict mortality after cardiac surgery? An exploratory analysis of the ECLIPSE trials. *Anesth Analg.* 2011;113:19–30.
21. Charlson ME, MacKenzie CR, Gold JP et al. Intraoperative blood pressure. What patterns identify patients at risk for postoperative complications? *Ann Surg.* 1990;212:567–580.
22. Varon J, Marik PE. Perioperative hypertension management. *Vasc Health Risk Manage.* 2008;4:615–627.
23. Owens DS, Corson MA. 2010. Malignant hypertension. In: Cohn SM, ed. *Evidenced-Based Surgery.* Informa: London, U.K., pp. 499–507.
24. Flaherty JT, Magee PA, Gardner TL et al. Comparison of intravenous nitroglycerin and sodium nitroprusside for treatment of acute hypertension developing after coronary artery bypass surgery. *Circulation.* 1982;65:1072–1077.
25. Fremes SE, Weisel RD, Mickle DA et al. A comparison of nitroglycerin and nitroprusside: I. Treatment of postoperative hypertension. *Ann Thorac Surg.* 1985;39:53–60.
26. Kaplan JA, Finlayson DC, Woodward S. Vasodilator therapy after cardiac surgery: A review of the efficacy and toxicity of nitroglycerin and nitroprusside. *Can Anaesth Soc J.* 1980;27:254–259.
27. Cruise CJ, Skrobik Y, Webster RE et al. Intravenous labetalol versus sodium nitroprusside for treatment of hypertension postcoronary bypass surgery. *Anesthesiology.* 1989;71:835–839.
28. Orlowski JP, Shiesley D, Vidt DG et al. Labetalol to control blood pressure after cerebrovascular surgery. *Crit Care Med.* 1988;16:765–768.
29. Geniton DJ. A comparison of the hemodynamic effects of labetalol and sodium nitroprusside in patients undergoing carotid endarterectomy. *AANA J* 1990;58:281–287.
30. Malsch E, Katonah J, Gratz I, Scott A. The effectiveness of labetalol in treating postoperative hypertension. *Nurse Anesth.* 1991;2:65–71.
31. Gray RJ, Bateman TM, Czer LS et al. Comparison of esmolol and nitroprusside for acute post-cardiac surgical hypertension. *Am J Cardiol.* 1987;59:887–891.
32. Gibson BE, Black S, Maass L, Cucchiara RF. Esmolol for the control of hypertension after neurologic surgery. *Clin Pharmacol Ther.* 1988;44:650–653.
33. Muzzi DA, Black S, Losasso TJ, Cucchiara RF. Labetalol and esmolol in the control of hypertension after intracranial surgery. *Anesth Analg.* 1990;70:68–71.
34. Smerling A, Gersony WM. Esmolol for severe hypertension following repair of aortic coarctation. *Crit Care Med.* 1990;18:1288–1290.
35. Zangrillo A, Turi S, Crescenzi G et al. Esmolol reduces perioperative ischemia in cardiac surgery: A meta-analysis of randomized controlled studies. *J Cardiothorac Vasc Anesth.* 2009;23:625–632.
36. Landoni G, Turi S, Biondi-Zoccai G et al. Esmolol reduces perioperative ischemia in noncardiac surgery: A meta-analysis of randomized controlled studies. *J Cardiothorac Vasc Anesth.* 2010;24:219–229.
37. Goldberg ME, IV Nicardipine Study Group. Efficacy and safety of intravenous nicardipine in the control of postoperative hypertension. *Chest.* 1991;99:393–398.
38. David D, Dubois C, Loria Y. Comparison of nicardipine and sodium nitroprusside in the treatment of paroxysmal hypertension following aortocoronary bypass surgery. *J Cardiothorac Vasc Anesth.* 1991;5:357–361.
39. Halpern NA, Goldberg M, Neely C et al. Postoperative hypertension: A multicenter, prospective, randomized comparison between intravenous nicardipine and sodium nitroprusside. *Crit Care Med.* 1992;20:1637–1643.
40. Keating GM. Clevidipine: A review of its use for managing blood pressure in perioperative and intensive care settings. *Drugs.* 2014;74:1947–1960.
41. Aronson S, Dyke CM, Stierer KA et al. The ECLIPSE trials: Comparative studies of clevidipine to nitroglycerin, sodium nitroprusside, and nicardipine for acute hypertension treatment in cardiac surgery patients. *Anesth Analg.* 2008;107:1110–1121.
42. Murphy MB, Murray C, Shorten GD. Fenoldopam: A selective peripheral dopamine-receptor agonist for the treatment of severe hypertension. *N Engl J Med.* 2001;345:1548–1557.
43. Gombotz H, Plaza J, Mahla E et al. DA1-receptor stimulation by fenoldopam in the treatment of postcardiac surgical hypertension. *Acta Anaesthesiol Scand.* 1998;42:834–840.
44. Landoni G, Biondi-Zoccai GG, Tumlin JA et al. Beneficial impact of fenoldopam in critically ill patients with or at risk for acute renal failure: A meta-analysis of randomized clinical trials. *Am J Kid Dis.* 2007;49:56–68.
45. Grossman E, Messerli FH, Grodzicki T, Kowey P. Should a moratorium be placed on sublingual nifedipine capsules given for hypertensive emergencies and pseudoemergencies? *JAMA.* 1996;276:1328–1331.
46. Vaughan CJ, Delanty N. Hypertensive emergencies. *Lancet.* 2000;356:411–417.
47. Jauch EC, Saver JL, Adams HP, Jr. et al. Guidelines for the early management of patients with acute ischemic stroke: A guideline for healthcare professionals from the American Heart Association/American Stroke Association. *Stroke.* 2013;44:870–947.

48. Morgenstern LB, Hemphill JC, 3rd, Anderson C et al. Guidelines for the management of spontaneous intracerebral hemorrhage: A guideline for healthcare professionals from the American Heart Association/American Stroke Association. *Stroke*. 2010;41:2108–2129.
49. Elkayam U, Janmohamed M, Habib M, Hatamizadeh P. Vasodilators in the management of acute heart failure. *Crit Care Med*. 2008;36:S95–S105.
50. Ince H, Nienaber CA. Diagnosis and management of patients with aortic dissection. *Heart*. 2007;93:266–270.

# Index

## D

## P

## Q



## R

## S



## T

U